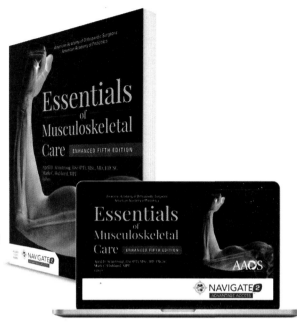
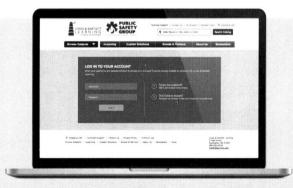
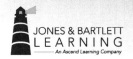
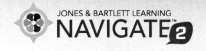

American Academy of Orthopaedic Surgeons
American Academy of Pediatrics

Essentials

of

Musculoskeletal
Care 5

April D. Armstrong, BSc(PT), MSc, MD, FRCSC

Mark C. Hubbard, MPT

Editors

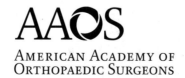

AAOS
AMERICAN ACADEMY OF
ORTHOPAEDIC SURGEONS

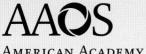

AMERICAN ACADEMY OF ORTHOPAEDIC SURGEONS

Published 2016 by the
American Academy of Orthopaedic Surgeons
9400 West Higgins Road
Rosemont, IL 60018

Fifth Edition
Copyright 2016
by the American Academy of Orthopaedic Surgeons

The material presented in *Essentials of Musculoskeletal Care,* 5th Edition has been made available by the American Academy of Orthopaedic Surgeons for educational purposes only. This material is not intended to present the only, or necessarily best, methods or procedures for the medical situations discussed, but rather is intended to represent an approach, view, statement, or opinion of the author(s) or producer(s), which may be helpful to others who face similar situations.

Some drugs or medical devices demonstrated in Academy courses or described in Academy print or electronic publications have not been cleared by the Food and Drug Administration (FDA) or have been cleared for specific uses only. The FDA has stated that it is the responsibility of the physician to determine the FDA clearance status of each drug or device he or she wishes to use in clinical practice.

Furthermore, any statements about commercial products are solely the opinion(s) of the author(s) and do not represent an Academy endorsement or evaluation of these products. These statements may not be used in advertising or for any commercial purpose.

Library of Congress Control Number: 2015945905

ISBN 978-1-62552-415-7

Printed in the USA

Cover art
Robert Liberace

Anatomic Illustrations
Scott Thorn Barrows, MA, CMI, FAMI

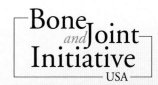

Editorial Board Disclosures

Contributors

Albert J. Aboulafia, MD, FACS, MBA
Medical Director, Weinberg
    Cancer Institute
Director, Sarcoma Services
Associate Professor of Orthopaedics
    and Oncology, Georgetown University
    School of Medicine
Franklin Square Hospital and
    Sinai Hospital
Baltimore, Maryland

Lindsay M. Andras, MD
Assistant Professor of Orthopaedics
Children's Orthopaedic Center
Children's Hospital Los Angeles
Keck School of Medicine of the
    University of Southern California
Los Angeles, California

Laura L. Bellaire, MD
Resident
Orthopaedic Surgery
Emory University
Atlanta, Georgia

John A. Bergfeld, MD
Senior Surgeon
Department of Orthopaedic Surgery
Cleveland Clinic
Cleveland, Ohio

Julie A. Dodds, MD
Associate Clinical Professor
Division of Sports Medicine
Michigan State University
East Lansing, Michigan

Gregory K. Faucher, MD
Resident Physician
Orthopaedic Surgery
Emory University
Atlanta, Georgia

Eli C. Garrard, MD
Resident
Department of Orthopaedic Surgery
Emory University
Atlanta, Georgia

Marcel Gilli, MD
Anesthesiologist
American Anesthesiology of Georgia
Piedmont Hospital
Atlanta, Georgia

Jordyn R. Griffin, MD
Resident Physician
    Internal Medicine, Pediatrics
    University of Kentucky
    Lexington, Kentucky

George N. Guild III, MD
Orthopaedic Surgeon
Peachtree Orthopaedic Clinic
Northside Hospital
Atlanta, Georgia

Stephen C. Hamilton, MD
Orthopaedic Surgeon
Beacon Orthopaedics
Cincinnati, Ohio

Douglas Hollern, MD
Medical Student
College of Medicine
University of Cincinnati
Cincinnati, Ohio

James S. Kercher, MD
Orthopaedic Surgeon
Peachtree Orthopaedic Clinic
Atlanta, Georgia

Lindsey S. Knowles, DPT, STC
Owner, Physical Therapist
Department of Outpatient Orthopaedics
    and Sports Physical Therapy
Atlanta Sport & Spine Physical Therapy
Atlanta, Georgia

L. Andrew Koman, MD
Professor and Chair
Orthopaedic Surgery
Wake Forest Baptist Health
Winston-Salem, North Carolina

Joseph M. Lane, MD
Professor of Orthopaedic Surgery
Department of Orthopaedics
Weill Cornell Medical College
New York, New York

Laurel R. Lemasters, MD
Musculoskeletal Radiologist
Northwest Radiology Consultants
Atlanta, Georgia

Tanya Maxwell, MS, L/ATC
Clinical Coordinator for Dr. Letha Griffin
Peachtree Orthopaedic Clinic
Atlanta, Georgia

Thomas J. Moore, MD
Associate Professor
Department of Orthopaedics
Emory School of Medicine
Atlanta, Georgia

Robert A. Murphy, MS, ATC
Associate Athletic Director for Sports
    Medicine and Nutrition
Athletic Department
Georgia State University
Atlanta, Georgia`

Michael S. Pinzur, MD
Professor of Orthopaedic Surgery
Department of Orthopaedic Surgery
    and Rehabilitation
Loyola University Health System
Maywood, Illinois

David A. Schiff, MD
Orthopaedic Surgeon
Peachtree Orthopaedic Clinic
Atlanta, Georgia

Ted Sousa, MD
Clinical Fellow
Children's Hospital Los Angeles
University of Southern California
Los Angeles, California

Harlan McMillan Starr, Jr, MD
Orthopaedic Surgeon
Georgia Hand, Shoulder, & Elbow
Atlanta, Georgia

Contributors from the American Academy of Pediatrics

American Academy of Pediatrics
DEDICATED TO THE HEALTH OF ALL CHILDREN®

Pooya Hosseinzadeh, MD
Assistant Professor
Department of Pediatric Orthopedics
Baptist Children's Hospital
Miami, Florida

Thomas G. McPartland, MD
Assistant Clinical Professor Orthopedic Surgery
Department of Orthopedic Surgery
Rutgers-Robert Wood Johnson Medical School
New Brunswick, New Jersey

Brien Rabenhorst, MD
Assistant Professor of Orthopaedic Surgery
University of Arkansas for Medical Sciences
Little Rock, Arkansas

Brian A. Shaw, MD
Associate Professor of Orthopaedic Surgery
Children's Hospital Colorado
University of Colorado School of Medicine
Colorado Springs, Colorado

Contributors' Disclosures

Dr. Aboulafia or an immediate family member has received royalties from and has stock or stock options held in Amgen and serves as a board member, owner, officer, or committee member of the Musculoskeletal Tumor Society.

Dr. Andras or an immediate family member serves as a board member, owner, officer, or committee member of the Pediatric Orthopaedic Society of North America and has stock or stock options held in Eli Lilly.

Neither Dr. Bellaire nor any immediate family member has received anything of value from or has stock or stock options held in a commercial company or institution related directly or indirectly to the content of this publication.

Neither Dr. Bergfeld nor any immediate family member has received anything of value from or has stock or stock options held in a commercial company or institution related directly or indirectly to the content of this publication.

Dr. Dodds or an immediate family member serves as a board member, owner, officer, or committee member of the Arthroscopy Association of North America.

Neither Dr. Faucher nor any immediate family member has received anything of value from or has stock or stock options held in a commercial company or institution related directly or indirectly to the content of this publication.

Dr. Garrard or an immediate family member is an employee of Sanofi-Aventis.

Neither Dr. Gilli nor any immediate family member has received anything of value from or has stock or stock options held in a commercial company or institution related directly or indirectly to the content of this publication.

Dr. Griffin or an immediate family member serves as a board member, owner, officer, or committee member of the American Orthopaedic Society for Sports Medicine and the Orthopaedic Research and Education Foundation.

Neither Dr. Guild nor any immediate family member has received anything of value from or has stock or stock options held in a commercial company or institution related directly or indirectly to the content of this publication.

Neither Dr. Hamilton nor any immediate family member has received anything of value from or has stock or stock options held in a commercial company or institution related directly or indirectly to the content of this publication.

Neither Dr. Hollern nor any immediate family member has received anything of value from or has stock or stock options held in a commercial company or institution related directly or indirectly to the content of this publication.

Neither Dr. Hosseinzadeh nor any immediate family member has received anything of value from or has stock or stock options held in a commercial company or institution related directly or indirectly to the content of this publication.

Dr. Kercher or an immediate family member serves as a board member, owner, officer, or committee member of the American Academy of Orthopaedic Surgeons and the American Orthopaedic Society for Sports Medicine.

Neither Dr. Knowles nor any immediate family member has received anything of value from or has stock or stock options held in a commercial company or institution related directly or indirectly to the content of this publication.

Dr. Koman or an immediate family member has stock or stock options held in DT Scimed, KeraNetics, Orthovatum, and Zellko; has received nonincome support (such as equipment or services), commercially derived honoraria, or other non-research–related funding (such as paid travel) from

KeraNetics, Orthovatum, and Zellko; and serves as a board member, owner, officer, or committee member of the Southern Orthopaedic Association and the American Orthopaedic Association.

Dr. Lane or an immediate family member serves as a board member, owner, officer, or committee member of the American Academy of Orthopaedic Surgeons, the Association of Bone and Joint Surgeons, the American Osteopathic Association, the American Society for Bone and Mineral Research, the Musculoskeletal Tumor Society, and the Orthopaedic Research Society; serves as a paid consultant to or is an employee of Bone Therapeutics, Inc., CollPlant, Harvest, Inc., ISTO, BiologicsMD, and Graftys; has stock or stock options held in Dfine and CollPlant; and has received research or institutional support from Merck.

Neither Dr. Lemasters nor any immediate family member has received anything of value from or has stock or stock options held in a commercial company or institution related directly or indirectly to the content of this publication.

Neither Ms. Maxwell nor any immediate family member has received anything of value from or has stock or stock options held in a commercial company or institution related directly or indirectly to the content of this publication.

Dr. McPartland or an immediate family member has stock or stock options held in Johnson & Johnson and serves as a board member, owner, officer, or committee member of the Pediatric Orthopaedic Society of North America.

Neither Dr. Moore nor any immediate family member has received anything of value from or has stock or stock options held in a commercial company or institution related directly or indirectly to the content of this publication.

Mr. Murphy or an immediate family member serves as a board member, owner, officer, or committee member of the College Athletic Trainers' Society.

Dr. Pinzur or an immediate family member serves as a board member, owner, officer, or committee member of the American Academy of Orthopaedic Surgeons; is a member of a speakers' bureau or has made paid presentations on behalf of Smith & Nephew, Stryker, and Wright Medical Technology; and serves as a paid consultant to or is an employee of Wright Medical Technology.

Neither Dr. Rabenhorst nor any immediate family member has received anything of value from or has stock or stock options held in a commercial company or institution related directly or indirectly to the content of this publication.

Neither Dr. Schiff nor any immediate family member has received anything of value from or has stock or stock options held in a commercial company or institution related directly or indirectly to the content of this publication.

Dr. Shaw or an immediate family member serves as a board member, owner, officer, or committee member of the American Academy of Pediatrics and the Pediatric Orthopaedic Society of North America and has stock or stock options held in Biomet, Johnson & Johnson, Medtronic, Merck, Pfizer, Stryker, and Zimmer.

Neither Dr. Sousa nor any immediate family member has received anything of value from or has stock or stock options held in a commercial company or institution related directly or indirectly to the content of this publication.

Neither Dr. Starr nor any immediate family member has received anything of value from or has stock or stock options held in a commercial company or institution related directly or indirectly to the content of this publication.

Dedication

To healthcare providers everywhere—who devote their careers to the health and well-being of individual patients and families, both young and old.

Preface

Essentials of Musculoskeletal Care bridges the gap between what primary care physicians were taught in medical school and what they need to know to evaluate and manage common musculoskeletal conditions. This text is used for immediate, point-of-care guidance in decision making and intervention. Physicians and allied healthcare providers also often use the images in this text to educate their patients regarding conditions and treatments, as well as suggested at-home exercises. Essentials also helps physicians decide which cases to treat themselves and which to refer. Since the first edition of *Essentials of Musculoskeletal Care* was published in 1997, more than 150,000 copies have been sold.

Essentials of Musculoskeletal Care is used by physicians in family practice, internists, specialists in physical medicine and rehabilitation, pediatricians, physicians in the armed forces, physicians in occupational medicine, physicians in sports medicine, athletic trainers, physical therapists, emergency medicine physicians, nurse practitioners, physician assistants, residents in family practice and orthopaedic surgery, orthopaedic surgeons, osteopathic physicians, and many others. In addition, although not designed as a textbook, *Essentials* has been adopted as a required or recommended text by numerous teaching programs, both for clinical rotations and for courses such as Concepts in Primary Care, Orthopaedic Injuries, Primary Care of Adults, and Musculoskeletal Clinical Medicine. Students indicate that *Essentials* is the only text that follows them from the classroom into clinical practice.

This fifth edition of *Essentials of Musculoskeletal Care* has been improved and enhanced with additional illustrations, tables, and injection/aspiration videos. Sections and chapters have been reviewed and updated, and new topics have been added, including a chapter on sports-related concussions in the General Orthopaedics section and another chapter on concussion in the Pediatric Orthopaedics section. In addition, rehabilitation prescriptions with home exercise programs and general musculoskeletal conditioning programs are available in the text and as patient handouts that can be printed from the website that accompanies this publication. This title is also available as an eBook.

I am indebted to the Board of Directors of the American Academy of Orthopaedic Surgeons (AAOS) and to the executive staff of AAOS for their commitment to excellence in education. My thanks also go to the Editorial Board for this fifth edition for their commitment to this project: section editors Letha Yurko Griffin (General Orthopaedics); Robert Z. Tashjian (Shoulder); Joseph A. Abboud (Elbow and Forearm); Julie E. Adams (Hand and Wrist); Kathleen Weber (Hip and Thigh); Robert A. Gallo (Knee and Lower Leg); Umur Aydogan (Foot and Ankle); Daniel T. Altman (Spine); Kelly L. VanderHave and Joseph A. Janicki (Pediatric Orthopaedics); and Mark C. Hubbard, who oversaw the rehabilitation content and served as coeditor. I also would like to thank the following AAOS staff for their work on this publication: Hans Koelsch, Director, Publications; Maureen Geoghegan, Director of Marketing; Monica Baum; Lisa Claxton Moore; Laura Goetz; Genevieve Charet; Courtney Dunker; Abram Fassler; Susan Baim; Charlie Baldwin; Emily Nickel; Hollie Muir; Karen Danca; Suzanne O'Reilly; Michelle Wild; Steven Kellert; Brian Moore; Katie Hovany; Laszlo Dianovsky; Susan Reindl; Mike Johnson; Derrick Philips; and Abel Jimenez.

Once again, the AAOS is grateful for the support of the American Academy of Pediatrics (AAP) and thank them for serving as a valuable professional Academy partner in the *Essentials* project. The comments from the AAP as well as from the internists, physiatrists, family practitioners, orthopaedic residents, medical students, and others who use this book have helped us continuously improve this publication, leading to improvements in musculoskeletal education and patient care.

April D. Armstrong, BSc(PT), MSc, MD, FRCSC

Editor

How to Use
Essentials of Musculoskeletal Care 5th Edition

Essentials of Musculoskeletal Care provides concise content in a practical and easy-to-use format. To access the associated videos (physical examinations, maneuvers, injections, aspirations) and printable PDFs of home exercise programs, follow the instructions provided on the inside cover of this book.

Pain diagram opens each section. Shows areas of pain and identifies conditions typically associated with each pain location. Names chapter in which condition is discussed.

Table of contents lists conditions in alphabetic order as well as procedures and home exercise programs.

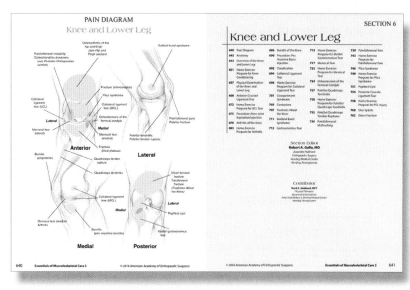

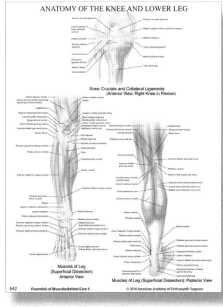

Anatomic art at beginning of section for handy reference.

Physical examination shows photographs and step-by-step descriptions of physical examination maneuvers: inspection and palpation, range of motion, muscle testing, and special tests. Symbol indicates that video is available on the website: www.aaos.org/essentials5.

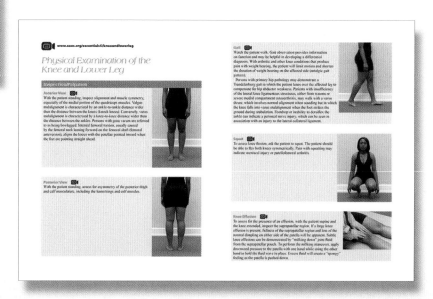

Conditions chapters include:

a. Synonyms
b. Clinical symptoms
c. Physical examination pearls
d. Diagnostic tests
e. Differential diagnosis
f. Adverse outcomes of the disease
g. Treatment
h. Rehabilitation prescription
i. Adverse outcomes of treatment
j. Referral decisions/Red flags

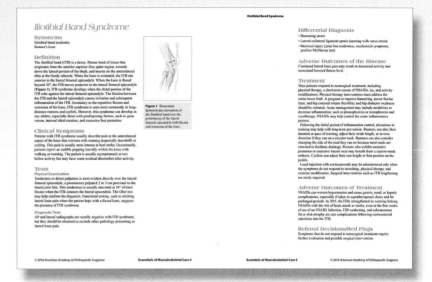

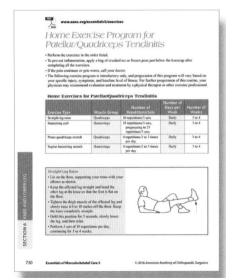

Home exercise program includes:

a. Symbol indicating the availability of a customizable, printable PDF of the home exercise program
b. Concise table of exercises
c. Step-by-step instructions and illustrations

Procedures include:

a. Symbol indicating video is available on the website: www.aaos.org/essentials5.
b. List of materials
c. Step-by-step instructions

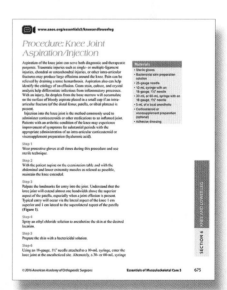

Table of Contents

SECTION ONE
General Orthopaedics

SECTION TWO
Shoulder

SECTION THREE
Elbow and Forearm

SECTION FIVE

Hip and Thigh

SECTION SEVEN
Foot and Ankle

SECTION EIGHT
Spine

PAIN DIAGRAM
General Orthopaedics

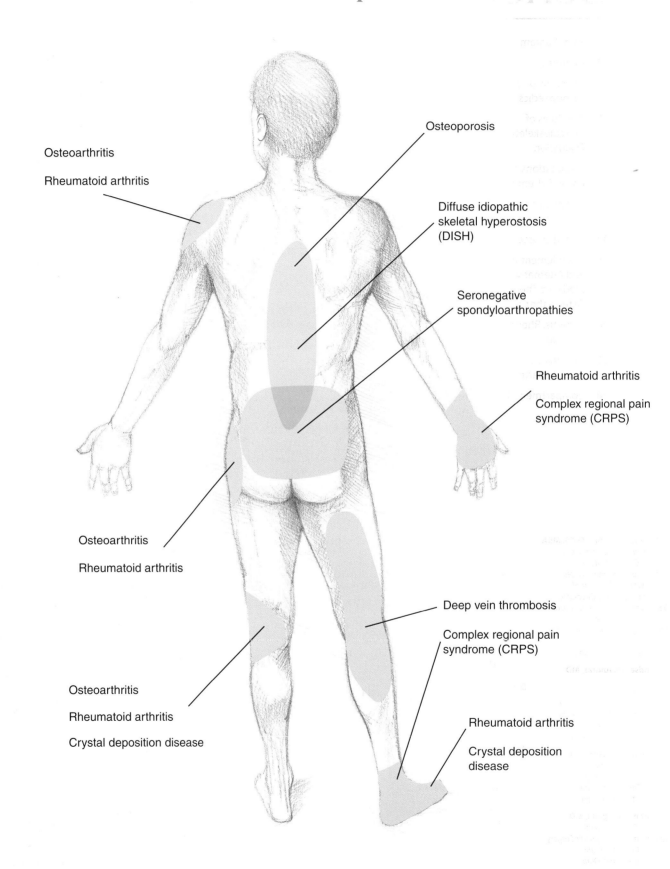

Osteoporosis

Osteoarthritis

Rheumatoid arthritis

Diffuse idiopathic
skeletal hyperostosis
(DISH)

Seronegative
spondyloarthropathies

Rheumatoid arthritis

Complex regional pain
syndrome (CRPS)

Osteoarthritis

Rheumatoid arthritis

Deep vein thrombosis

Complex regional pain
syndrome (CRPS)

Osteoarthritis

Rheumatoid arthritis

Crystal deposition disease

Rheumatoid arthritis

Crystal deposition
disease

General Orthopaedics

Section Editor

Letha Y. Griffin, MD, PhD
Peachtree Orthopaedic Clinic
Team Physician
Georgia State University
Atlanta, Georgia

Contributors

...ert J. Aboulafia, MD, FACS, MBA
Medical Director, Weinberg
Cancer Institute
Director, Sarcoma Services
Associate Professor of
Orthopaedics and Oncology,
Georgetown University School of
Medicine
Franklin Square Hospital and Sinai
Hospital
Baltimore, Maryland

Lindsay M. Andras, MD
Assistant Professor of Orthopaedics
Children's Orthopaedic Center
Children's Hospital Los Angeles
Keck School of Medicine of the
University of Southern California
Los Angeles, California

Laura L. Bellaire, MD
Resident
Orthopaedic Surgery
Emory University
Atlanta, Georgia

John A. Bergfeld, MD
Senior Surgeon
Department of Orthopaedic Surgery
Cleveland Clinic
Cleveland, Ohio

Julie A. Dodds, MD
Associate Clinical Professor
Division of Sports Medicine
Michigan State University
East Lansing, Michigan

Gregory K. Faucher, MD
Resident Physician
Orthopaedic Surgery
Emory University
Atlanta, Georgia

Eli C. Garrard, MD
Resident
Department of Orthopaedic Surgery
Emory University
Atlanta, Georgia

Marcel Gilli, MD
Anesthesiologist
American Anesthesiology of Georgia
Piedmont Hospital
Atlanta, Georgia

Jordyn R. Griffin, MD
Resident Physician
Internal Medicine, Pediatrics
University of Kentucky
Lexington, Kentucky

George N. Guild III, MD
Orthopaedic Surgeon
Peachtree Orthopaedic Clinic
Northside Hospital
Atlanta, Georgia

Stephen C. Hamilton, MD
Orthopaedic Surgeon
Beacon Orthopaedics
Cincinnati, Ohio

Douglas Hollern, MD
Medical Student
College of Medicine
University of Cincinnati
Cincinnati, Ohio

Mark C. Hubbard, MPT
Physical Therapist
Bone and Joint Institute
Penn State Milton S. Hershey
Medical Center
Hershey, Pennsylvania

James S. Kercher, MD
Orthopaedic Surgeon
Peachtree Orthopaedic Clinic
Atlanta, Georgia

Lindsey S. Knowles, DPT, STC
Owner, Physical Therapist
Department of Outpatient
Orthopaedics and Sports
Physical Therapy
Atlanta Sport & Spine Physical Therapy
Atlanta, Georgia

L. Andrew Koman, MD
Professor and Chair
Orthopaedic Surgery
Wake Forest Baptist Health
Winston-Salem, North Carolina

Joseph M. Lane, MD
Professor of Orthopaedic Surgery
Department of Orthopaedics
Weill Cornell Medical College
New York, New York

Laurel R. Lemasters, MD
Musculoskeletal Radiologist
Northwest Radiology Consultants
Atlanta, Georgia

Tanya Maxwell, MS, L/ATC
Clinical Coordinator for Dr. Letha Griffin
Peachtree Orthopaedic Clinic
Atlanta, Georgia

Thomas J. Moore, MD
Associate Professor
Department of Orthopaedics
Emory School of Medicine
Atlanta, Georgia

Robert A. Murphy, MS, ATC
Associate Athletic Director for Sports
Medicine and Nutrition
Athletic Department
Georgia State University
Atlanta, Georgia

Michael S. Pinzur, MD
Professor of Orthopaedic Surgery
Department of Orthopaedic Surgery
and Rehabilitation
Loyola University Health System
Maywood, Illinois

David A. Schiff, MD
Orthopaedic Surgeon
Peachtree Orthopaedic Clinic
Atlanta, Georgia

Ted Sousa, MD
Clinical Fellow
Children's Hospital Los Angeles
University of Southern California
Los Angeles, California

Harlan McMillan Starr, Jr, MD
Orthopaedic Surgeon
Georgia Hand, Shoulder, & Elbow
Atlanta, Georgia

ANATOMY—MAJOR BONES OF THE BODY

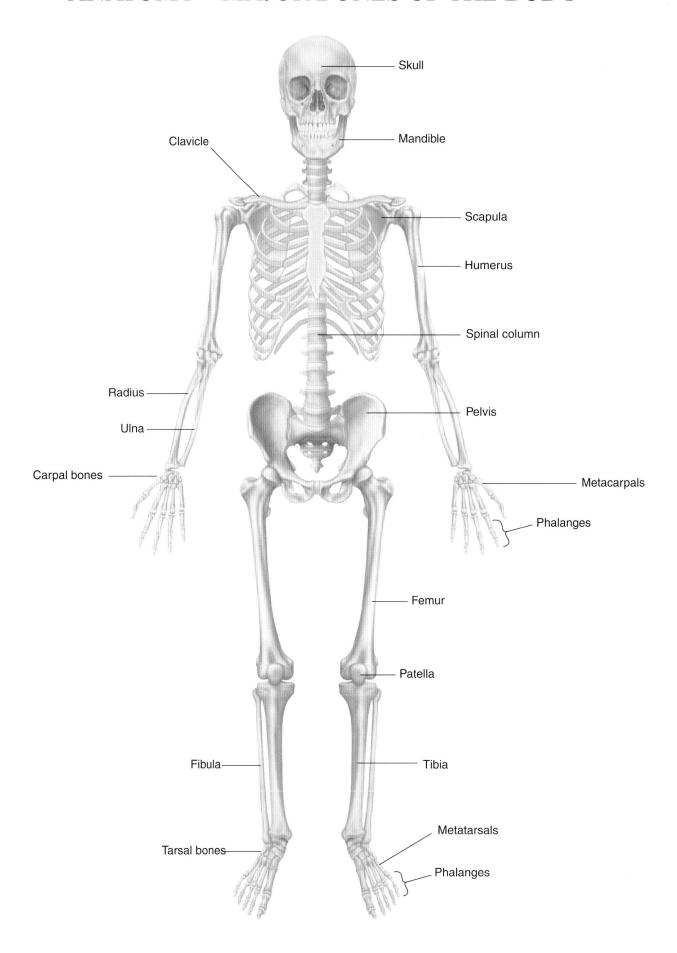

Skull

Mandible

Clavicle

Scapula

Humerus

Spinal column

Radius

Pelvis

Ulna

Carpal bones

Metacarpals

Phalanges

Femur

Patella

Fibula

Tibia

Metatarsals

Tarsal bones

Phalanges

Overview of General Orthopaedics

Bone, cartilage, muscle, tendon, ligament, and their supporting nerve and vascular supplies are the specialized structures that make up the musculoskeletal system. In combination, these structures provide remarkable strength, movement, durability, and efficiency. Disease or injury to any of these tissues may adversely affect function and the ability to perform daily activities. This General Orthopaedics section of *Essentials of Musculoskeletal Care* describes conditions that affect multiple joints, bones, or regions; conditions that have systemic effects; and therapeutic modalities commonly used in the nonsurgical treatment of musculoskeletal conditions. An anatomic drawing showing the major bones of the human body is on page 2; a detailed anatomic drawing showing the bones and muscles of the various anatomic areas appears at the beginning of each anatomic section. A glossary of commonly used orthopaedic terms is provided immediately after section 9.

Arthritis

The etiologies of arthritis range from degenerative processes associated with aging (osteoarthritis) to acute infectious processes (septic arthritis). Likewise, disability from arthritis ranges from stiffness to severe pain and crippling dysfunction. Two of the most common forms of adult arthritis encountered in clinical practice are osteoarthritis and rheumatoid arthritis (**Figure 1**). Distinguishing characteristics are listed in **Table 1**.

Other types of inflammatory arthritis include the seronegative spondyloarthropathies, crystal deposition diseases, and septic arthritis. Of these conditions, septic arthritis is the most urgent because immediate diagnosis and efficacious treatment are required to prevent joint destruction. Diagnosis typically involves joint fluid analysis, in which a leukocyte count greater than 50,000 or a differential count of 90% polymorphonucleocytes is concerning for bacterial arthritis. Joint aspiration and culture, followed by appropriately tailored antibiotics, and in most cases, surgical drainage and lavage, are imperative. The crystal arthropathies present as acute monoarticular arthritis with an abrupt onset of intense pain and swelling. The seronegative spondyloarthropathies are a group of disorders characterized by oligoarticular peripheral joint arthritis, enthesitis, inflammatory changes in axial skeletal joints (sacroiliitis and spondylitis), extra-articular sites of inflammation, association with HLA-B27, and negative rheumatoid factor.

Bursitis and Tenosynovitis

Sterile inflammation of bursae (bursitis) and tendon sheaths (tendinitis) occurs frequently in adults, particularly following an injury or repetitive motion. Characteristic symptoms include

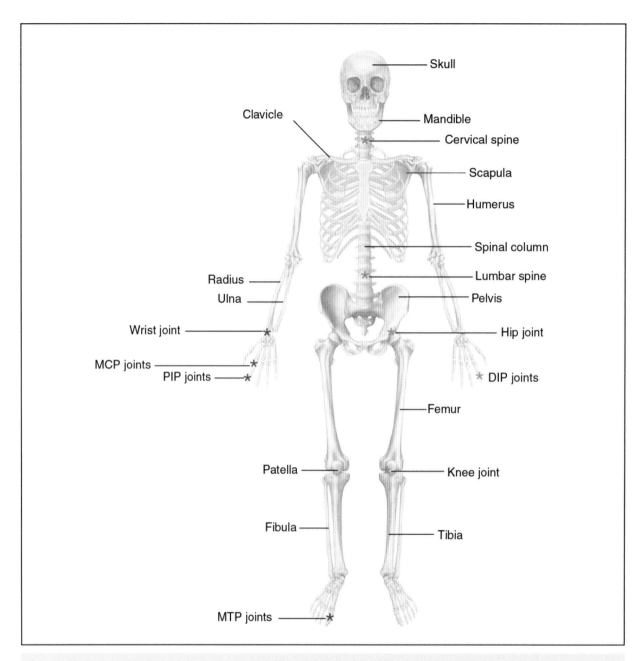

Figure 1 Illustration shows joints commonly affected by arthritis. Blue asterisks indicate joints predominantly affected by osteoarthritis; red asterisks indicate joints predominantly affected by rheumatoid arthritis. DIP = distal interphalangeal, MCP = metacarpophalangeal, MTP = metatarsophalangeal, PIP = proximal interphalangeal.

localized pain that is exacerbated by specific movements and is frequently relieved with rest. Classic locations of bursitis include the olecranon, greater trochanter, and prepatellar bursa, whereas tenosynovitis frequently affects tendon sheaths of the wrist and hand flexor tendons and tendons about the ankle (peroneal, posterior tibial, and Achilles). Common treatments for bursitis and tenosynovitis include activity modification, NSAIDs, splinting, and the judicious use of corticosteroid injections. Infectious tenosynovitis or infectious bursitis can follow minor trauma, especially if the skin is violated.

Table 1		
Characteristics of Osteoarthritis Versus Rheumatoid Arthritis		
Characteristic	**Osteoarthritis**	**Rheumatoid Arthritis**
Pathophysiology	Noninflammatory, asymmetric, articular cartilage deterioration "Wear and tear"	Autoimmune, inflammatory cytokines target synovial membranes
Demographics	Most common arthritis Incidence increases with age Obesity History of joint trauma or other joint disease (secondary to OA)	Affects 1% of population 3:1 female-to-male Peak onset in the fourth and fifth decades
Clinical	Increased pain with use, fast-resolving stiffness Classically affects knees, hips, spine, DIP joints, thumb CMC joint Crepitus, decreased joint ROM	Morning stiffness Classically affects MCP, PIP, wrists, MTP joints Symmetric and deforming joint erosion Synovial thickening and joint tenderness to palpation
Workup	Radiographs: asymmetric joint space narrowing, subchondral sclerosis, osteophytes	Laboratory tests: RF (high sensitivity), anti-CCP (high specificity) Radiographs: bony erosions, symmetric joint space narrowing
Treatment	Exercise and weight loss, NSAIDs, corticosteroid injections, glucosamine and chondroitin sulfate, hyaluronic acid, total joint arthroplasty	NSAIDs, DMARDs, TNF-α antagonists, glucocorticoids Goal of treatment is to prevent irreversible joint erosion and deformity

CCP = cyclic citrullinated peptide, CMC = carpometacarpal, DIP = distal interphalangeal, DMARDs = disease-modifying antirheumatic drugs, MCP = metacarpophalangeal, MTP = metatarsophalangeal, OA = osteoarthritis, PIP = proximal interphalangeal, RF = rheumatoid factor, ROM = range of motion, TNF-α = tumor necrosis factor-α.

The cardinal signs of Kanavel (**Table 2**) signal infection in pyogenic flexor tenosynovitis of the finger; this condition should be addressed urgently with surgery to prevent permanent finger dysfunction. All infectious bursitis or tenosynovitis requires prompt recognition with culture (if feasible) of the area and initial treatment with broad-spectrum antibiotics until culture results are known. Prompt referral for consideration of surgical drainage is essential.

Osteoporosis
Osteoporosis is a common skeletal disorder with significant health cost. Associated fragility (low-energy) fractures seen primarily in the hip, distal radius, proximal humerus, and vertebrae are estimated to total 9 million per year worldwide and are a significant source of morbidity and mortality in an increasingly aging population. Patients who sustain fragility fracture should be evaluated for osteoporosis and treated when appropriate to reduce the risk for future fracture. Dual-energy x-ray absorptiometry (DEXA) is used to screen for

Table 2
Cardinal Signs of Kanavel for Hand Flexor Tendon Sheath Infection
Fusiform swelling of digit
Tenderness along tendon sheath
Digit held in flexed position
Severe pain with passive digit extension

Table 3

Major Risk Factors for Osteoporotic Fractures

Not Modifiable

Advanced age

Female sex

History of fracture as an adult

History of fracture in first-degree relative

Dementia

Poor health/frailty

Caucasian or Asian race

Possibly Modifiable

Low bone mineral density

Oral glucocorticoid use

Recurrent falls

Current tobacco use

Alcoholism

Estrogen deficiency, including menopause onset before age 45 years

Lifelong low calcium intake

Vitamin D deficiency

Low body weight

Little or no physical activity

---

osteoporosis, defined as a bone density 2.5 SDs below the healthy young adult mean. Treatment of osteoporosis includes modifying risk factors (**Table 3**), vitamin D and calcium supplementation, and pharmacologic therapy. All physicians should encourage patients to include calcium-rich foods in their diet, obtain appropriate "sunshine" vitamin D, and exercise regularly to avoid the development of osteoporosis. The high prevalence of vitamin D deficiency in the United States justifies the regular screening of adolescents, adults, and elderly patients for deficiency as part of the health maintenance examination.

Trauma

Trauma to the musculoskeletal system may involve bones, ligaments, or tendons. Initial management should include a thorough history; physical examination, including assessment of neurovascular status; imaging; and appropriate immobilization via splinting or bracing. The skin should be inspected for wounds that extend into fractures or joints. Open injuries necessitate urgent irrigation and débridement to minimize the chance of infection. Injured patients should be monitored for traumatic compartment syndrome, especially in leg and forearm fractures; immediate surgical fasciotomy is required to prevent catastrophic sequelae. Following trauma, immobilization of the injured body part provides pain relief, limits further bone and soft-tissue damage, and may aid in the definitive treatment. Injury type and severity, along with patient-specific considerations, factor into the decision of nonsurgical versus surgical management in musculoskeletal trauma.

Musculoskeletal Oncology

Primary bone malignancy is uncommon. Evaluation involves clinical, laboratory, radiographic, and pathologic correlation. Metastatic bone disease in adults is substantially more prevalent than primary bone cancer. Malignancies frequently associated with bone metastasis include breast, prostate, lung, kidney, and thyroid tumors.

Abuse

Abuse involving children, spouses, or the elderly is a complex social and medical problem. Recognizing abuse can prevent catastrophic consequences; therefore, it is essential that the appropriate social service agencies be notified when a patient's injuries are recognized as potentially resulting from abuse. Child abuse is discussed in the Pediatric Orthopaedics section. Spouse or elder abuse may be identified by recognizing the signs listed in **Table 4**. The complexity of these problems and the seriousness of the consequences demand familiarity with them and with available community resources.

Table 4

Signs of Elder Abuse

Signs of Physical Abuse
Abrasions
Bruises
Fractures
Signs of Emotional Abuse
Overbearing caregiver
New-onset depression
Dementia-like behavior
Signs of Sexual Abuse
Signs of minor trauma to anogenital area
Sexually transmitted disease (STD)
Signs of Neglect
Malnutrition
Failure to take medications
Poor grooming
Bedsores
Signs of Financial Exploitation
Abrupt changes in finances
Failure to pay bills
Suspicious changes in legal documents

SECTION 1 GENERAL ORTHOPAEDICS

Principles of Musculoskeletal Evaluation

Patients presenting with musculoskeletal problems may report pain, stiffness, deformity, or weakness. General principles for evaluating these patients are described here.

History

The history of the presenting condition should include onset, location, duration, aggravators/relievers, character, and temporal factors tailored to the specific symptom or symptoms (**Table 1**). Additional questions about the patient's medical history, social history, and family history, and a review of systems may reveal clues that suggest the correct diagnosis. For example, substantial weight loss in a person who smokes may suggest that low back pain is secondary to metastatic disease, whereas back pain in a postmenopausal woman with a history of a fragility fracture may suggest a vertebral compression fracture. In persons with musculoskeletal disorders, it is important to understand the patient's level of function before the injury or illness.

Physical Examination

The general principles of examining the musculoskeletal system, including inspection, palpation, range of motion, muscle testing, motor and sensory evaluation, and special tests, are described later in this section. The specific techniques are detailed in subsequent anatomic sections. When examining the extremities, comparison with

Table 1

History Questions Pertinent to Musculoskeletal Conditions

Pain	Joints	Back
Nature: sharp, dull, achy, radiating, associated with fatigue or weakness?	Decreased range of motion?	Radiation to buttocks or legs?
	Swelling?	Midline versus paravertebral?
	Warmth/erythema?	Sharp or aching?
Timing: increasing, decreasing, intermittent, related to time of day, related to activity, related to injury?	Morning or activity-related pain/stiffness?	Postural or height change?
	Catching or giving way?	Paresthesias?
	Instability?	Night pain?
	Loss of function?	Bowel or bladder incontinence?
	Unilateral or bilateral?	
	Crepitus?	
	Related to deformity?	

the opposite, asymptomatic extremity often is helpful in defining the specific abnormalities in the symptomatic extremity.

Inspection/Palpation

Inspect the patient's standing posture. Compare the affected extremity with the opposite extremity for any difference in symmetry or length. Note if the patient has any abnormal spine curvature or axial asymmetry. Watch the patient walk. Analyze the stance and swing phases of gait. Look for an antalgic gait, which is characterized by limited stance phase on the affected extremity. Watch for weakness of the swing-phase muscles—for example, weakness of the ankle dorsiflexors (peroneal nerve dysfunction)—which is manifested by a footdrop gait.

Ask the patient to place one finger on the one spot that hurts the most to localize the problem and narrow the differential diagnosis (**Figure 1**). After exposing the area, look for swelling, erythema, ecchymosis, and muscular atrophy.

Palpate the affected area for tenderness, abnormal masses, fluctuance, crepitus, or temperature changes.

Range of Motion

Measure the motion of the joints in the affected extremity or spine and compare with normal range of motion measurements on the unaffected side. Restricted joint motion may herald trauma, infection, arthritis, or another inflammatory process. Measure both passive and active range of motion. A discrepancy between active and passive range of motion may indicate joint injury or may represent an underlying muscle weakness.

Basic Principles

Joint range of motion is an objective measurement. The parameters for rating musculoskeletal disability, whether for government or other agencies, are based on the degree to which joint motion is impaired. Joint motion can be estimated visually, but a goniometer enhances accuracy and is preferred for evaluating motion of the elbow, wrist, digits, knee, ankle, and great toe. A goniometer is less useful in measuring hip and shoulder motion because the overlying soft tissues do not allow the same degree of precision.

Zero Starting Position

Describing joint motion with reference to the accepted Zero Starting Position for each joint is necessary to provide consistent communication between observers. The Zero Starting Position for each joint is described in the examination chapter of each section and in **Figures 2** and **3**. For most joints, the Zero Starting Position is the anatomic position of the extremity in extension.

To measure joint motion, start by placing the joint in the Zero Starting Position. Place the center of the goniometer at the center of the joint. Align one arm of the goniometer with the bony axis of the proximal segment and the other end of the goniometer with the bony axis of the distal segment (**Figure 4**). Hold the upper end of the goniometer in place while the joint is moved through its arc of

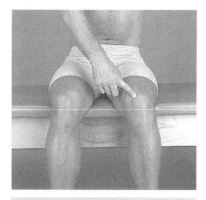

Figure 1 Photograph shows a patient pointing to the one spot that hurts the most, that is, localizing the point of maximal tenderness.

SECTION 1   GENERAL ORTHOPAEDICS

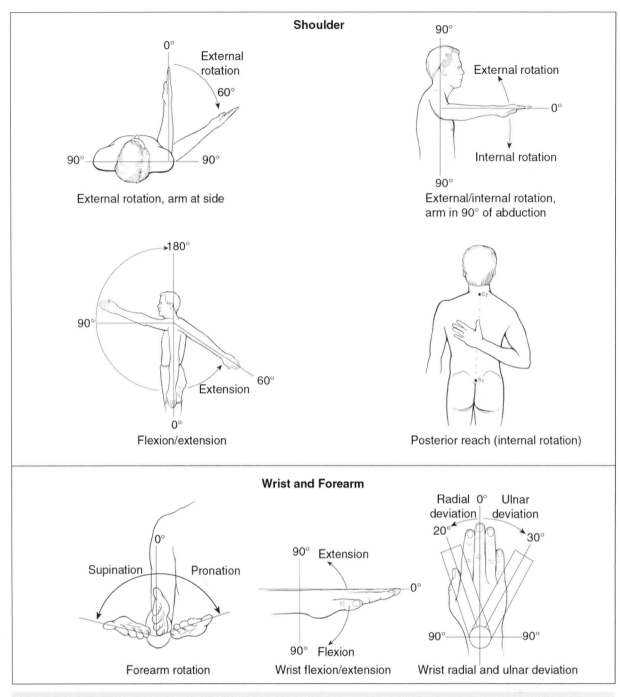

Figure 2 Illustrations show means of measuring joint motion in the upper extremity. (Reproduced from Greene WB, Heckman JD, eds: *The Clinical Measurement of Joint Motion*. Rosemont, IL, American Academy of Orthopaedic Surgeons, 1994.)

motion. When the joint is at the farthest extent of the arc of motion, realign the distal arm of the goniometer with the axis of the distal segment and read the degree of joint motion from the goniometer.

Definitions of Limited Motion

The terminology for describing limited motion is illustrated in **Figure 5**. The knee joint depicted in this photograph can be neither

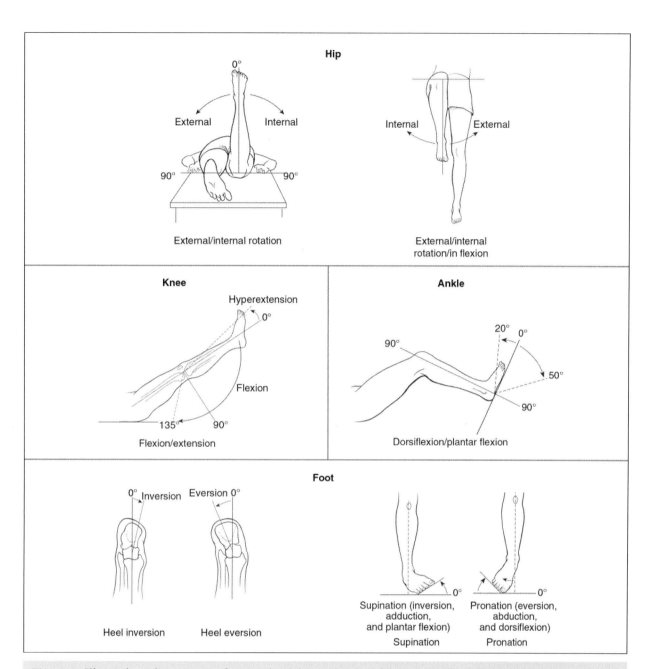

Figure 3 Illustrations show means of measuring joint motion in the lower extremity. (Reproduced from Greene WB, Heckman JD, eds: *The Clinical Measurement of Joint Motion.* Rosemont, IL, American Academy of Orthopaedic Surgeons, 1994.)

fully extended nor fully flexed. The restricted motion is recorded as either "The knee flexes from 30° to 90° (30° → 90°)," or "The knee has a 30° flexion contracture with further flexion to 90° (30° FC → 90° or 30° FC W/FF 90°)."

Range of motion is slightly greater in children, particularly those younger than 10 years. Decreased motion occurs as adults age, but the loss of motion is relatively minimal in most joints. Except for motion at the distal finger joints, it is safe to say that any substantial loss of mobility should be viewed as abnormal and not attributable to aging.

Motion of an injured or diseased joint may be painful. In such a situation, it is better to observe active motion first. The examiner will then know how much support to provide the limb when the passive arc of motion is analyzed.

Muscle Testing

Examination techniques used in muscle testing include placing the muscle in a shortened position and asking the patient to perform an activity that lengthens the muscle while the examiner resists the movement. For example, when testing the biceps muscle, the patient should position the elbow in flexion and supination; the examiner then tests the strength of the biceps by attempting to pull the elbow into extension as the patient resists (**Figure 6**).

Manual muscle testing provides a semiquantitative measurement of muscle strength (**Table 2**). For example, if the patient can actively extend or lift the knee to only 20° of flexion, then, by definition, the quadriceps strength is less than grade 3. A muscle of this strength cannot function against gravity and thus creates a disability for the patient.

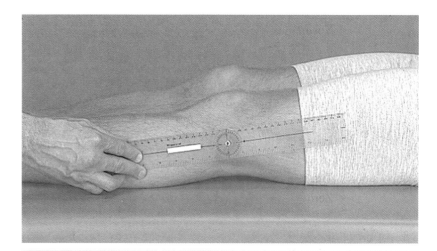

Figure 4   Photograph shows use of a goniometer to measure joint motion.

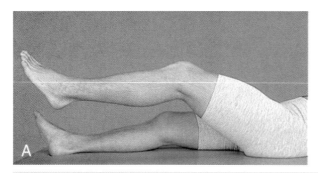
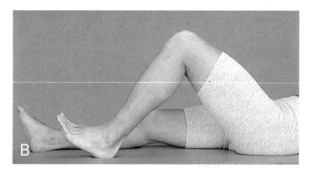

Figure 5   Photographs illustrate the terminology for describing restricted range of motion in a joint. This patient has both restricted extension (**A**) and flexion (**B**) of the knee.

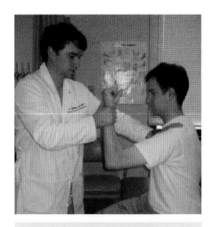

Figure 6 Photograph shows examiner and patient positioning for testing biceps strength.

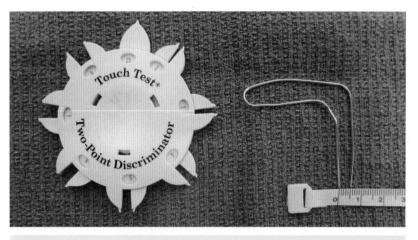

Figure 7 Photograph of a two-point discriminator wheel (left) and a paperclip fashioned to test two-point discrimination at 5 mm (right).

Table 2		
Grading of Manual Muscle Testing		
Numeric Grade	**Descriptive Grade**	**Description**
5	Normal	Complete range of motion against gravity with full or normal resistance
4	Good	Complete range of motion against gravity with some resistance
3	Fair	Complete range of motion against gravity but no motion with resistance
2	Poor	Complete range of motion only with gravity eliminated
1	Trace	Muscle contraction but no joint motion
0	Zero	No evidence of muscle function

Motor and Sensory Evaluation

Nerve root function should be tested if the patient's presenting symptoms suggest a neck or back problem. Peripheral nerve function should be tested if the disorder is localized to the extremities. This is most efficiently accomplished by evaluating one muscle and one area of sensation for each nerve root or peripheral nerve in question. In the case of hand injuries, two-point discrimination is used to evaluate for digital nerve injury. This measurement should be less than or equal to 5 mm at the fingertips. If the examiner does not have access to a formal discriminator wheel, then a paperclip can be fashioned to perform the test (**Figure 7**). The guidelines for assessing nerve root function are presented in the Spine section under Physical Examination of the Spine. A guide to the evaluation of the peripheral nerves is outlined in **Table 3**.

Table 3		
Evaluation of Peripheral Nerves		
Nerve	**Muscle**	**Sensory**
Upper extremity		
Axillary	Deltoid—shoulder abduction	Lateral aspect, arm
Musculocutaneous	Biceps—elbow flexion	Lateral proximal forearm
Median	Flexor pollicis longus—thumb flexion	Tip of thumb, volar aspect
Ulnar	First dorsal interosseous—abduction	Tip of little finger, volar aspect
Radial	Extensor pollicis longus—thumb extension	Dorsum thumb web space
Lower extremity		
Obturator	Adductors—hip adduction	Medial aspect, midthigh
Femoral	Quadriceps—knee extension	Proximal to medial malleolus
Peroneal		
Deep branch	Extensor hallucis longus—great toe extension	Dorsum first web space
Superficial branch	Peroneus brevis—foot eversion	Dorsum lateral foot
Tibial	Flexor hallucis longus—great toe flexion	Plantar aspect, foot

Other Considerations

Stretch exacerbates pain or contracture of an injured or deformed structure. If a muscle/tendon crosses two joints, then both joints must be positioned to stretch the injured part. For example, if the hamstrings are injured, their involvement is elucidated by placing these structures on stretch (such as flexing the hip to 90° and then extending the knee). Pain and/or limited knee extension typically occurs with this maneuver when a patient has an injury or contracture of the hamstring muscles.

Tests specific to individual anatomic injuries are described in the appropriate sections.

Amputations of the Lower Extremity

Definition

Limb amputation is the removal of all or part of an extremity through the level of a bone. Disarticulation is the removal of all or part of an extremity through the level of a joint.

Indications

Certain disease states, particularly diabetes mellitus, severe infections, and peripheral vascular disease, are the cause of approximately 70% of all lower extremity amputations. In fact, these conditions account for more than 100,000 lower extremity amputations performed annually in the United States. Each year, trauma accounts for approximately 20% of lower extremity amputations and tumors for another 5%; another approximately 5% of amputations are related to congenital limb deficiency. Prevalence data, obtained through surveys of all persons living with limb loss, show that approximately 55% of persons who underwent lower limb amputation and 85% of persons who underwent upper limb amputation experienced limb loss as a result of trauma. The differences between the incidence and prevalence data can be explained by understanding that traumatic amputations more often occur in younger individuals, who typically live with the amputation for many more years than do individuals who undergo amputation because of chronic disease.

Amputations frequently are performed after the patient has undergone extensive medical or surgical intervention to salvage the limb. In these situations, the patient and even the medical team may have a negative attitude concerning the amputation and subsequent rehabilitation, regarding it as a sign of failure. This attitude is inappropriate, however, because most persons who undergo lower extremity amputation regain functional ambulation. Almost 90% of patients treated with transtibial (that is, below-knee) amputation achieve a functional ambulatory capacity that approaches their preamputation level. Therefore, the physician should maintain a positive attitude and aggressively pursue early rehabilitation, including prosthesis fitting, to allow patients to resume their normal daily activities.

The energy requirements of walking generally increase with more proximal levels of amputation. Therefore, amputations usually should be performed at the most distal level possible; residual limb (also referred to as stump) length is sometimes sacrificed, however, to create a soft-tissue envelope that will optimize prosthetic limb fitting and comfortable ambulation for the patient. For example, an amputation performed at the hindfoot often compromises prosthetic function. In this case, an amputation at the next higher level (ankle disarticulation) may provide better function.

Levels of Amputation and Prosthetic Considerations

Toe Amputation

Patients with dysvascularity note no substantial loss of function after toe amputation because of their low baseline activity level. Young, active adults with traumatic hallux (great toe) amputations lose some propulsive power and walking stability but are able to walk reasonably well. Little disability is associated with the loss of the lesser toes. Isolated amputation of the second toe should retain the base of the proximal phalanx whenever possible to prevent hallux valgus. In elderly patients, toe amputations often indicate a foot at high risk for ulceration or pressure problems from standard shoes because of poor vascular perfusion and difficulty healing minor injuries and wounds. Therefore, shoes for these individuals should include extra depth and extra width and, often, custom-molded insoles to accommodate and protect a high-risk foot. Following trauma, patients typically are most comfortable in shoes with a more rigid sole and wide toe box to minimize pressure on the amputation site.

Ray Resection

A ray resection includes a toe and all or part of the corresponding metatarsal. A foot with a single-ray resection of ray 2, 3, 4, or 5 will function well in either standard shoes or footwear for individuals with diabetes mellitus, depending on the shape and size of the remaining foot. Amputation of the first ray or resection of more than one ray leads to a residual foot that is more difficult to manage. A custom-molded, multidurometer orthosis is required to load the remaining metatarsal shafts and to unload the amputation site and the remaining metatarsal heads; use of this type of orthosis can improve comfort and lessen the chance of reulceration. Use of a custom-molded, multidurometer orthosis almost always requires footwear with extra depth and extra width.

Midfoot Amputation

Midfoot amputation is performed at either the transmetatarsal or tarsometatarsal level. Muscle rebalancing at the time of surgery and postoperative rehabilitation can help prevent the two most common postoperative contractures of the foot—equinus and varus. Prosthetic requirements vary tremendously at this level. A widened foot at the amputation site is almost universal, and tenderness at the end of the amputation site is common. Because of the increased width of the foot, accommodative footwear and prosthetic or orthotic management usually are needed. A low-profile prosthetic device that cups the heel and provides a long footplate will prevent the shoe from folding and putting pressure on the amputation site. If the foot is hypersensitive, or if balance and weakness are major symptoms, a prosthetic device that encloses the calf may improve function.

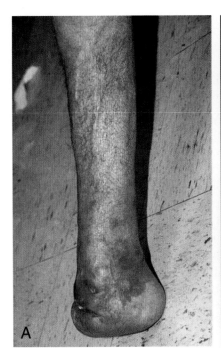 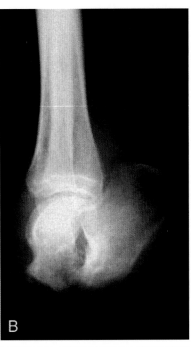

Figure 1 Images show the outcome of hindfoot amputation. **A,** Postoperative photograph obtained following hindfoot amputation performed at the level of the talonavicular joint. Even a successful hindfoot amputation, as shown here, provides a very small surface area for weight bearing and requires custom footwear to prevent the shoe from falling off. The patient also will have an apropulsive gait because of the loss of the forefoot lever arm, which, in the normal foot, is used during the terminal stance phase of gait. **B,** AP radiograph obtained following a hindfoot amputation demonstrates a too-common result, hindfoot equinus. Bearing weight on the plantar surface of the residual foot is painful and is likely to be associated with skin breakdown.

Hindfoot Amputation

Poor function and difficult prosthetic management are common after amputations in the hindfoot (**Figure 1**). The retained talus and calcaneus frequently are pulled into equinus, and attempts at weight bearing put excessive pressure directly on the amputation site. Surgical muscle rebalancing consists of reattachment of the anterior tendons and a complete release of the Achilles tendon. Advances in prostheses have improved function, especially for elderly individuals, and household ambulation and transfer skills can be very successful. Even with state-of-the-art prostheses, however, aggressive walking and impact activities are still very compromised with a hindfoot amputation.

Ankle Disarticulation

Syme ankle disarticulation consists of disarticulation of the entire foot at the ankle and use of the heel pad to cover the amputation site. Surgical revision of the bony malleoli flush with the articular cartilage creates a very smooth weight-bearing surface. When combined with durable heel pad coverage, the resulting residual limb usually can tolerate direct pressure and end weight bearing. A

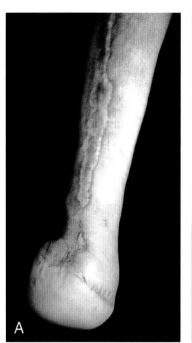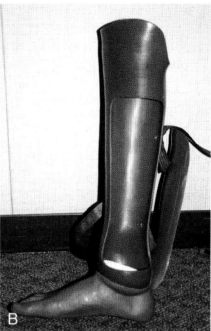

Figure 2 The Syme ankle disarticulation creates an excellent weight-bearing platform. By removing the talus and calcaneus, room is created to place a dynamic elastic-response (that is, energy-storing) prosthetic foot. **A,** Photograph shows the appearance of a lower limb after a Syme ankle disarticulation. **B,** Photograph of the Canadian Syme prosthesis.

prosthesis is required for routine walking, but the amputation site usually can tolerate transfer pressure and the pressure required for a limited number of steps for bathroom activities without a prosthesis, which is a benefit to many patients. The prosthesis socket extends up to the proximal tibia region, very similar to a below-knee prosthesis. The foot component must be very low profile because the amputated limb is almost as long as the nonamputated limb. The gait pattern is stable and requires minimal training (**Figure 2**).

Below-Knee Amputation
As noted previously, transtibial amputation also is referred to as a below-knee, or BK, amputation. Various surgical methods are used, but a long posterior flap usually results in more durable padding over the distal end of the tibia and a cylindrical shape, which tolerates prosthetic fitting better than does a dramatically tapered residual limb. This durable padding can be very important for minimizing residual limb ulcerations, particularly in patients with diabetes mellitus or peripheral vascular disease. The optimal functional length of the remaining tibia is 12 to 15 cm below the knee joint. Some experts recommend longer below-knee amputations in patients with adequate vascular status and skin condition. Amputation in the lower third of the tibia is not recommended because the padding is not adequate below the level of the calf muscle.

Even if walking is expected to be minimal, outfitting the patient with a simple prosthesis and a wheelchair can enhance functional independence following below-knee amputation provided that safe transfer skills can be achieved. New developments in flexible sockets are providing a more comfortable fit and better proprioception through improved suspension. The spring-like design of dynamic elastic-response feet both absorbs the shock and rotation of impact and returns energy at the end of each stride.

Knee Disarticulation

A knee disarticulation extends through the knee joint itself. Like the Syme ankle disarticulation, the goal of knee disarticulation is to create a smooth surface that can tolerate direct end weight bearing, improving function. Early knee disarticulation prostheses had two major drawbacks: they were bulky around the knee area, and the prosthetic knee joint attached below the socket at a level lower than that of the contralateral, unaffected knee. Newer prosthetic knee joints minimize these disadvantages and have greatly improved the walking function of patients with knee disarticulations. For individuals who are nonambulatory because of paraplegia, neurologic conditions, or other chronic diseases, knee disarticulation is preferable to a more proximal amputation because the disarticulation maintains a full-length thigh to maximize sitting support and can improve function. It also minimizes the risk of skin problems associated with more distal amputations.

Above-Knee Amputation

A transfemoral (through the thigh) amputation is commonly referred to as an above-knee, or AK, amputation. Contractures are common following this surgery because the muscle attachments at the hip pull the residual thigh into flexion and abduction. Rebalancing the muscles surgically by attaching the adductor muscle and hamstrings can minimize postoperative problems associated with severe hip joint contractures. Aggressive rehabilitation also is helpful. The energy requirements of walking are substantially higher with this level of amputation than with more distal amputations, and after above-knee amputation, many patients with dysvascularity do not have adequate cardiac function for functional ambulation using a prosthesis. In addition, the power of the knee joint is lost with above-knee amputation, and the prosthesis cannot replace it. Therefore, many patients who undergo above-knee amputation never become very proficient with a prosthesis, and they may find wheelchair ambulation to be more efficient.

The weight of an above-knee prosthesis acts as an anchor and makes transfer more difficult. Therefore, to be a candidate for a prosthetic limb, patients who undergo high-level amputation should have three skills: (1) the ability to independently transfer from bed to chair; (2) the ability to independently rise from sitting to standing; and (3) the ability to ambulate up and down parallel bars with a one-legged gait. Many such patients master these skills within days or weeks of surgery, but others cannot. The ability to go a short distance on the parallel bars without a prosthesis or with a walker is

GENERAL ORTHOPAEDICS

SECTION 1

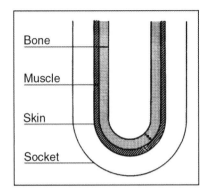

Figure 3 Illustration shows an ideal soft-tissue envelope over the end of the amputation site in a lower limb. This envelope consists of a mobile, nonadherent muscle mass and full-thickness skin that will tolerate the direct pressures and pistoning within the prosthetic socket.

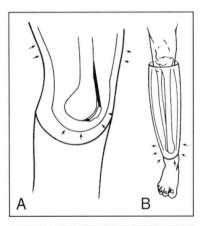

Figure 4 Illustrations of load transfer (arrows) in knee disarticulation and Syme ankle disarticulation. Weight bearing is accomplished directly through the end of the residual limb in knee disarticulations (**A**) and Syme ankle disarticulations (**B**).

an excellent indication that the patient who undergoes above-knee amputation will have the energy to use a prosthesis safely.

Hip Disarticulation

Amputations and disarticulations at the level of the hip and pelvis lead to substantial loss of function. For many individuals, sitting balance and sitting support to prevent decubitus ulcers are the first priority, followed by learning independent transfer and safe toileting skills. The patient should be educated about the importance of mastering the three vital independence skills listed previously under above-knee amputation before the decision is made to proceed with a prosthesis. Even young adults with this level of amputation find the use of a prosthesis very challenging because of the high energy requirements and the need to control three joints (hip, knee, and ankle). Many individuals with amputations at this level prefer walking with crutches rather than using a prosthesis.

Principles of Prosthetic Fitting

The soft-tissue envelope over the end of the amputation site is the interface, or cushion, between the bone of the residual limb and the prosthetic socket (**Figure 3**). Disarticulations at the level of the ankle and the knee can allow weight bearing directly through the end of the residual limb because the bone surface is broad and smooth (**Figure 4**). The soft-tissue envelope acts as a cushion, and the sole function of the prosthetic socket is to prevent the prosthesis from falling off.

In below-knee and above-knee amputations, the bone is transected through the diaphysis and cannot accept much direct force at the end. With these amputations, the socket distributes the load over the entire surface of the residual limb. With below-knee amputations, much more load is directly proximal to the amputation site over the sides of the residual limb and the contours of the knee; with above-knee amputation, the load is placed on the hip area (**Figure 5**). Intimate fit of the prosthetic socket is crucial. If the patient loses weight or the residual limb atrophies, the limb will "bottom out," or drop down in the socket, resulting in the development of a pressure ulcer caused by increased end-bearing pressure. In many cases, a prosthetist can add pads inside the socket to improve the fit of a socket that is too big. Conversely, if the patient gains weight, the residual limb will not fit down into the socket and the end of the limb will swell into the void and create tender, weeping skin lesions from lack of any distal contact. A socket that is too small cannot be modified easily and needs to be replaced.

Perfect, intimate prosthetic fit is impossible; therefore, every patient who uses a prosthesis after amputation experiences pistoning within the prosthetic socket, which produces shear forces. Good surgical technique produces a residual limb composed of mobile muscle and durable skin; however, if the soft-tissue envelope is thin (composed of split-thickness skin graft, or adherent to bone), blisters and shearing ulcers will develop. In this situation, the prosthetist attempts to

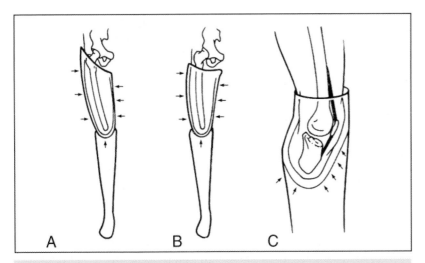

Figure 5 Illustrations of load transfer (arrows) in above-knee and below-knee amputations. The indirect load transfer that is required in above-knee amputations is accomplished with either a standard quadrilateral socket (**A**) or an adducted, narrow, medial-lateral socket (**B**). **C,** The below-knee amputation socket transfers weight indirectly with the knee flexed approximately 10°.

compensate by using pressure- and shear-dissipating materials and by maximizing the suspension of the prosthesis to the residual limb.

A prosthetic socket can be expected to last 18 months to 3 years, but it should be modified or replaced sooner if the fit is poor. Socket liners do not last as long as the socket itself, and they should be replaced when torn or worn out. Liners made of foam may last 6 to 24 months, but the new elastomeric and silicone liners often tear within 3 to 4 months of normal use. Prosthetic components such as feet, ankle units, and knee units should be replaced when they are broken or show signs of fatigue failure. Typically, the components should last 3 to 5 years, and many have warranties for this time span.

Adverse Outcomes

If pressure problems or pain develops, referral to a clinic that specializes in treating patients who have undergone amputation, a certified prosthetist, or a rehabilitation physician should be considered. The initial approach for most pain- and pressure-related problems is to adjust the residual limb/prosthesis interface by modifying the socket. If problems persist, the cause may be heterotopic bone, bone spurs, increased pressure or bruising of the residual nerve ending, or the formation of symptomatic neuromas.

Residual Limb Ulcers or Infection

Most blisters, ulcers, and infections are caused by an inadequate soft-tissue envelope on the residual limb or poor prosthetic fit. If these problems develop, the patient should stop wearing the prosthesis until it can be adjusted. Often, simply modifying the socket will relieve pressure points, and this modification, combined with the use of simple, nonbulky dressings, will allow the wounds to heal.

Antibiotics are necessary only if the patient has signs of local or systemic infection. Surgical revision of the amputation is indicated when superficial wounds fail to heal within 4 to 8 weeks following prosthetic modification; infection fails to resolve with appropriate antibiotics; or wounds become deep, exposing muscle, tendon, or bone.

Skin Conditions

The prosthetic socket is a closed environment, so excessive sweating or poor hygiene will lead to dermatologic eruption on the residual limb. To prevent this, the prosthetic socket and residual limb should be kept clean and dry. Absorbent powders (other than talcum powder) or creams should be used for this purpose.

Folliculitis, which typically develops in the groin following above-knee amputation or in the popliteal area following below-knee amputation, may be just a nuisance or it may be painful, and it can compromise prosthetic fit. Good hygiene, including keeping the prosthesis clean, can help minimize folliculitis. Treatment with warm soaks and topical agents resolves many mild cases. If cellulitis is present, oral antibiotics may be required. When folliculitis becomes chronic or when cystic lesions develop, surgical excision of the involved skin may be required.

Extreme swelling of the residual limb, which is similar in appearance to severe venous insufficiency disease, may develop if the socket fit is not intimate. The hyperemic, weeping skin may become very painful and superficial infection may develop. Treatment includes topical agents and antibiotics as well as improving the fit of the socket.

Amputation-Related Sensation

Various types of sensation are experienced by persons with limb loss, including nonpainful phantom limb sensations, phantom limb pain, residual limb pain, and back and neck pain.

Nonpainful phantom limb sensations may include a feeling that the missing foot is wrapped in cotton or that the missing limb is present. These sensations can take a variety of forms such as touch, pressure, temperature, itch, posture, or location in space. They also can involve feelings of movement in the phantom limb. "Telescoping," the sensation that the distal part of the phantom limb is moving progressively closer to the residual limb, sometimes occurs. Initially, phantom limb sensations may be frightening or annoying, but most patients adjust to these sensations, and they rarely require treatment.

Phantom limb pain refers to painful sensations in the phantom, or missing, portion of the amputated limb. Early reports in the literature suggested that the incidence of chronic phantom limb pain was low, but it is now thought that as many as 55% to 85% of persons who have undergone limb amputation continue to experience phantom limb pain from time to time. Severe, persistent phantom limb pain is unusual. Phantom limb pain tends to be more episodic and more intense than nonpainful phantom limb sensations. Persistent symptoms are best controlled with antiseizure membrane-stabilizing drugs, such as pregabalin and gabapentin. Modalities such as transcutaneous electrical nerve stimulation have been reported as helpful for some individuals, especially for short-term flare-ups, but surgery has not been successful. As in many chronic pain syndromes, treatment often requires multiple modalities. Unrelenting phantom limb pain is best managed as a major causalgia with guidance from a specialist in pain management.

Residual limb pain is pain in the portion of the amputated limb that is still physically present. Existing studies disagree regarding the prevalence of chronic residual limb pain after wound healing. Localized residual limb pain may be caused by poor prosthetic socket fit or alignment, and evaluation and adjustment by a prosthetist often resolves the problem. When persistent residual limb pain is caused by bone spurs, which can be visualized on radiographs, surgical excision is indicated. Painful nodules or masses that cause an electrical sensation when palpated or tapped may indicate symptomatic nerve endings or neuromas. Prosthetic modification to relieve local pressure should be tried initially, but if it is not successful, surgical excision with repositioning of the end of the nerve can help.

Back and neck pain are common following amputation of an extremity. Likely contributing factors are asymmetric pelvic motion, weight shifts, and shoulder motion during gait; asymmetric standing posture; and overuse of the remaining extremities. Such back and neck pain is often more functionally limiting than is phantom limb pain or residual limb pain. A careful examination for spine-related causes of pain is necessary. Treatment typically consists of rehabilitation, stretching, and other physical modalities.

Referral Decisions/Red Flags

Referral for amputation may be required for vascular disease, trauma, diabetes-related ulceration or infection, or complications at the amputation site. Orthopaedic surgeons, vascular surgeons, general surgeons, and plastic surgeons all may have training in amputation-related care. Orthopaedic surgeons and rehabilitation medicine specialists typically have the most experience with prosthetic rehabilitation and complications. The choice between these two specialists will depend on the individual specialist's particular interests in the care and management of limb loss.

Anesthesia for Orthopaedic Surgery

Anesthesia Techniques

General Anesthesia

The safety of general anesthesia has increased over time because of improvements in patient preparation and monitoring and the introduction of modern, short-acting anesthetic agents such as propofol, sevoflurane, and desflurane. Laryngeal mask airways, widely adopted in the 1990s, allow for rapid induction and speedy recovery, especially in the outpatient setting. Expanded use of peripheral nerve blocks and infiltration of local anesthetic agents into the surgical incision reduce the need for potent opioids, decreasing the incidence of respiratory depression, postoperative nausea and vomiting, and prolonged sedation and recovery.

Epidural and Spinal Anesthesia

Epidural and spinal anesthesia techniques for procedures involving the lower extremities decrease postoperative sedation in elderly patients and provide excellent perioperative pain control. Despite the advantages of spinal and epidural anesthesia, no prospective studies have shown improved outcomes compared with general anesthesia. Reports of epidural hematoma following neuraxial anesthesia have become more common because of the use of low-molecular-weight heparins such as enoxaparin for thromboembolic prophylaxis, even when practitioners have followed appropriate safety guidelines. Often, patients presenting for orthopaedic surgery are on antiplatelet medication after cardiovascular interventions. The anesthesiologist and surgeon should discuss the plan for management of anticoagulation during the perioperative period. Given the potential for devastating complications, the use of epidural anesthesia has decreased in many practices in the past several years.

Peripheral Nerve Blocks

Peripheral nerve blocks of the upper and lower extremity are effective and may be used alone or in combination with general anesthesia or monitored anesthesia care (MAC). Potential complications of peripheral blockade are less severe than those seen with epidural or spinal techniques. The use of a peripheral nerve stimulator or ultrasound targeting of the nerves minimizes patient discomfort and allows for successful nerve blocks under minimal sedation. Nerve blocks of the brachial plexus at the level of the interscalene groove, the infraclavicular area, or in the axilla are commonly used for surgery of the upper extremity. Postoperative pain from lower extremity surgery may be managed with femoral and/or sciatic nerve blocks in the groin or popliteal fossa or at the ankle. More recently, the adductor canal block has been advocated as a good alternative to femoral nerve block because the adductor canal block produces only minimal motor blockade of the quadriceps muscle, thereby allowing earlier ambulation without increased risk of falling.

Intravenous Regional Anesthesia

Intravenous regional anesthesia is safe, easy to administer, and effective for short procedures on the forearm, wrist, and hand.

Preoperative Evaluation

Medical centers and outpatient facilities have developed their own preoperative testing and screening protocols based on the characteristics of their particular patient populations. Information from the patient's history, physical examination, and other diagnostic tests can identify the patient's risk factors and guide the anesthesiologist to either a routine or high-risk care plan, taking into account the following:

- The patient's preference and understanding of the proposed procedures
- Procedure-appropriate anesthesia techniques: regional versus general anesthesia, peripheral nerve block
- Need for enhanced intravenous access or invasive monitoring
- Strategies for postoperative pain management
- Perioperative pharmacologic interventions: antacids/H_2 antagonists, β-blockers, inhalers, anticoagulants

The American Society of Anesthesiologists (ASA) Physical Status Classification System (**Table 1**) is widely used to stratify risk before surgical procedures. In general, healthy patients (ASA class I or II) undergoing routine inpatient or outpatient surgery are unlikely to benefit from extensive preoperative testing. Routine laboratory tests are obtained much less frequently in this group. A hematocrit level may be indicated for women beyond menarche and for men older than 65 years. If extensive blood loss is expected, a baseline complete blood count may be helpful. Electrolyte levels may be obtained in elderly patients and in those taking diuretics if renal dysfunction is present. Perioperative glucose testing should be performed on all patients with diabetes. A growing number of studies have shown improved postoperative outcome "in patients in whom blood sugar was strictly controlled perioperatively."

Patients in ASA class III or IV may benefit from preoperative screening for a severe underlying medical condition such as coronary artery disease, particularly if their musculoskeletal condition limits their exercise tolerance. A listing of these tests is included in **Table 2**. Screening tests have limitations, with occasional false-negative results and frequent false-positive results, which may lead to more invasive and costly diagnostic procedures.

Outpatient Surgery Centers

A growing number of orthopaedic procedures are routinely performed in specialty surgery centers outside of the hospital setting. Many orthopaedic procedures, short of total joint arthroplasty,

Table 1

American Society of Aneshesiologists Physical Classification System[a]

Classification	Definition	Examples, Including, but Not Limited To:
ASA I	A normal healthy patient	Healthy, nonsmoking, no or minimal alcohol use
ASA II	A patient with mild systemic disease	Mild diseases only without substantive functional limitations. Examples include (but not limited to): current smoker, social alcohol drinker, pregnancy, obesity (30<BMI<40), well-controlled DM/HTN, mild lung disease
ASA III	A patient with severe systemic disease	Substantive functional limitations; One or more moderate to severe diseases. Examples include (but not limited to): poorly controlled DM or HTN, COPD, morbid obesity (BMI ≥40), active hepatitis, alcohol dependence or abuse, implanted pacemaker, moderate reduction of ejection fraction, ESRD undergoing regularly scheduled dialysis, premature infant PCA < 60 weeks, history (>3 months) of MI, CVA, TIA, or CAD/stents.
ASA IV	A patient with severe systemic disease that is a constant threat to life	Examples include (but not limited to): recent (<3 months) MI, CVA, TIA, or CAD/stents, ongoing cardiac ischemia or severe valve dysfunction, severe reduction of ejection fraction, sepsis, DIC, ARD or ESRD not undergoing regularly scheduled dialysis
ASA V	A moribund patient who is not expected to survive without the operation	Examples include (but not limited to): ruptured abdominal/thoracic aneurysm, massive trauma, intracranial bleed with mass effect, ischemic bowel in the face of significant cardiac pathology or multiple organ/system dysfunction
ASA VI	A declared brain-dead patient whose organs are being removed for donor purposes	

ARD = acute respiratory distress, BMI = body mass index, CAD = coronary artery disease, COPD = chronic obstructive pulmonary disease, CVA = cerebrovascular accident, DIC = disseminated intravascular coagulation, DM = diabetes mellitus, ESRD = end-stage renal disease, HTN = hypertension, MI = myocardial infarction, PCA = postconceptional age, TIA = transient ischemic attack.

[a] Current definitions (NO CHANGE) and Examples (NEW)

[b] The addition of "E" denotes Emergency surgery (An emergency is defined as existing when delay in treatment of the patient would lead to a significant increase in the threat to life or body part).

(Adapted from the ASA website: http://www.asahq.org/~/media/sites/asahq/files/public/resources/standards-guidelines/asa-physical-status-classification-system.pdf. Accessed April 23, 2015.)

Table 2

Preoperative Screening Tests for Orthopaedic Patients

Procedure	Indication	Advantages/Disadvantages
Electrocardiogram	Indicated for men >50 years and women >60 years (younger if diabetes, hypertension, or history of coronary disease is present) If normal, valid for 1 year	Inexpensive Many false-positive and false-negative results Most useful if prior tracing is available
Exercise (treadmill) stress testing	Patient exercises to PMHR; evaluate for ST segment changes, ectopy	Least expensive of "advanced" screening procedures Orthopaedic patients often unable to attain PMHR due to pain or limited mobility
Nuclear stress testing	Imaging obtained with radioactive tracer at rest and under pharmacologic stress; may show areas at risk for ischemia	Expensive Not always predictive of adverse outcome Requires several hours to complete
Dobutamine stress echo	Beta-agonist dobutamine infused during echocardiography; evaluate for appropriate increase in contractility Wall motion abnormalities suggest ischemia	Relatively expensive Risk of dysrhythmia during infusion Echo gives information about valve and ventricular function Requires experienced physician to interpret study

PMHR = predicted maximal heart rate.

complex spine surgery, and surgery for severe fractures, may be performed in an outpatient setting. Patients and families often prefer the convenience of these centers to a hospital experience. A single specialty focus allows for operational efficiencies. Appropriate patient selection, however, is critical to patient safety in these centers, where backup personnel and services for high-risk patients are unavailable. In general, patients who have significant cardiac or pulmonary disease may be better served in a hospital setting. A list of selection criteria is found in **Table 3**.

Surgical Procedures

The various anesthesia considerations for selected orthopaedic surgical procedures are summarized in **Table 4**. Specific procedures are discussed in the following paragraphs.

Hip Fracture

The patient who undergoes surgery for hip fracture is typically an elderly individual, often from a chronic care facility, who sustained the fracture as a result of a fall. The patient's mental and nutritional status must be taken into consideration before induction of general anesthesia, and anesthesia may need to be given before the patient can be moved onto the operating table. The choice of

Table 3

Patient Selection Criteria for Outpatient Orthopaedic Surgery Centers

Condition	Criteria
Cardiac disease	Patients with stable angina should have recent (within 6 months) evaluation by a cardiologist
	Patients with unstable angina, MI, or CHF within the previous 6 months should be cared for in hospital
	Patients with an AICD should be treated in the hospital setting
	Patients with a pacemaker may be treated in an outpatient center depending on the nature of the surgical procedure being considered and the overall health of the patient
Pulmonary disease	If the patient is unable to walk up one flight of steps or is on home O_2, consider hospital setting
	Severe COPD may lead to need for postoperative ventilation in the hospital setting
Morbid obesity	BMI criteria vary among centers; BMI > 40 may lead to difficult airway, which can be difficult for one anesthesiologist to manage
	High risk of postoperative respiratory complications
Sleep apnea/airway	A patient with a history of a difficult airway is best treated in a hospital setting
	A patient with rheumatoid arthritis on gold, methotrexate, or other immunosuppressants may require cervical spine clearance
	Outpatient surgery for a patient with sleep apnea may be safe if body habitus is normal, but a longer postoperative observation period is required
	A patient with sleep apnea with morbid obesity should be operated on in the hospital
Diabetes mellitus	An outpatient setting is most often acceptable, unless the patient also has other diseases
	In young patients or those with the "brittle" type, treatment in the hospital setting may be best
Pregnancy	Fetal monitoring is difficult in a freestanding outpatient setting
Chronic pain	An implanted device or chronic narcotic therapy may make postoperative pain control in the outpatient setting impossible
Latex allergy	A patient with true latex allergy is best treated in the hospital
	A patient with latex sensitivity can usually be treated in the outpatient setting
Malignant hyperthermia	If the patient has a history of disease or is susceptible to it, the procedure should be done in the hospital

AICD = automated implantable cardiovascular defibrillator, BMI = body mass index, CHF = congestive heart failure, COPD = chronic obstructive pulmonary disease, MI = myocardial infarction.

airway management, anesthetic drugs, and extent of intraoperative monitoring is determined by the preoperative assessment. Some practitioners prefer spinal anesthesia; however, this can present challenges with patient positioning.

Hip or Knee Replacement Surgery

In the past, patients undergoing hip or knee replacement surgery received regional anesthesia. The rare but devastating risk of epidural hematoma with common current anticoagulation regimens now outweighs the potential benefits of regional anesthesia (improved

Table 4		

Anesthesia Considerations for Selected Orthopaedic Surgical Procedures

Procedure	Typical Patient/Procedure Characteristics	Common Anesthesia Technique
Repair of hip fracture	Older patient, often >80 years Impaired mental, nutritional status Analgesia required for positioning At risk for thromboembolism, hypothermia, postoperative cognitive dysfunction	General (spinal in some circumstances)
Hip or knee arthroplasty	Predominantly older patients Congenital, rheumatic, or traumatic joint changes, reduced mobility Obesity, often morbid Concurrent health issues, including coronary disease and diabetes At risk for thromboembolism, intraoperative reaction to acrylic bone cement Disabling pain, history of chronic pain therapy	Knee arthroplasty: general with femoral nerve block Hip arthroplasty: general, spinal in some circumstances Postoperative pain therapy directed by consultant
Knee arthroscopy/anterior cruciate ligament reconstruction	Younger patients Outpatient setting Short procedure Minimal blood loss Substantial postoperative pain	General plus local anesthesia and/or nerve block
Shoulder procedures	Arthroscopic or open procedures Beach-chair or lateral position Severe postoperative pain	General plus brachial plexus block
Spine surgery	Chronic pain Potential for difficult airway (cervical) Potential for blood loss Need for specialized monitoring	General
General trauma surgery	Nonorthopaedic injuries, such as cardiac contusion, lung trauma, head injury, blood loss Unstable cervical spine Intoxication	General

postoperative analgesia and cognitive function in the elderly). Postoperative spinal opioids, given using a "single shot" technique without placement of an epidural catheter, may be appropriate, although effective monitoring by a dedicated pain management team and properly trained nursing staff is mandatory. Patient preference and certain conditions, such as an abnormal coagulation profile, previous spine surgery, or morbid obesity (leading to technical difficulty with block placement), may support the use of general

SECTION 1   GENERAL ORTHOPAEDICS

anesthesia in many patients. Intravenous patient-controlled analgesia (PCA) in combination with peripheral nerve block usually provides satisfactory postoperative pain management for these patients. An injectable and long-acting bupivacaine liposome suspension that was recently approved by the FDA has been used in combination with peripheral nerve blocks in the management of postoperative pain after total knee replacement surgery.

Knee Arthroscopy/Anterior Cruciate Ligament Reconstruction

General anesthesia is ideal for the typically young, healthy patient undergoing a knee arthroscopy or anterior cruciate ligament (ACL) reconstruction. This type of anesthesia allows for fast recovery and discharge from the outpatient center. Intra-articular injection of local anesthetics by the surgeon or the administration of a suitable nerve block often provides excellent postoperative analgesia. Preoperative administration of the popular "three-in-one" block (femoral, lateral femoral cutaneous, and obturator nerves) or the ultrasound-guided adductor canal block substantially reduce the amount of general anesthesia needed and provide excellent analgesia during and after ACL reconstruction. The reduced need for postoperative narcotics may contribute to less nausea and vomiting and allow for faster discharge from an outpatient center.

Shoulder Procedures

General anesthesia is the technique of choice for most procedures involving the shoulder. The addition of an interscalene brachial plexus block provides excellent, long-lasting perioperative pain relief and should be considered for procedures on the shoulder. The beach-chair and lateral decubitus positions require careful positioning of the head and neck, as well as meticulous protection of the face and the eyes. Extreme head-up positions may warrant maintenance of higher blood pressure as measured on the arm to maintain adequate cerebral perfusion, especially in older patients. Intraoperative surges in heart rate or blood pressure may be the result of systemic absorption of epinephrine-containing irrigation fluid.

Shoulder replacement surgery is a complex surgical procedure that often is performed in elderly patients. Because of the length of the surgery and the potential for substantial blood loss, close monitoring and adequate intravenous access are required. Postoperative pain control is best achieved with an interscalene brachial plexus block.

Surgical Procedures Involving the Extremities

Patients requiring surgical procedures involving the extremities cannot be characterized by a consistent set of features because their age and health status vary widely. Depending on the particular surgical procedure and the particular patient, any of a wide variety of anesthesia techniques and agents may be appropriate.

Most patients presenting for surgery of the upper extremity, the foot, or the ankle respond well to modern agents used for general anesthesia. In addition, short and minimally invasive procedures can be accomplished by using a peripheral/field block and MAC. Intravenous regional anesthesia (Bier block) may be an excellent choice for short procedures for the hand, wrist, or forearm. Brachial plexus blocks (interscalene, supraclavicular, infraclavicular, axillary) provide excellent, long-lasting anesthesia of the upper extremity. A popliteal or ankle block alone or in combination with general anesthesia or MAC creates excellent surgical conditions for most treatments of the ankle or foot, at the same time reducing postoperative pain, nausea, and vomiting.

Spine Surgery

The most common spine surgery procedures are related to instability and herniation of intervertebral disks. Patients may have a long-standing history of back or neck pain that requires chronic administration of opioid analgesics, which will most likely need to be continued in the immediate postoperative period. After induction of general anesthesia, control of the airway may require fiberoptic intubation if cervical instability or malformation is present. In addition, the competing needs for surgical exposure and controlling and maintaining ventilation and circulation make positioning the patient challenging. Somatosensory-evoked potentials (SSEPs) are useful in assessing spinal cord function during major corrective surgeries of the spine. Potential problems for the anesthesiologist include major blood loss, air embolism, pneumothorax, ventilation perfusion mismatch, and injury to the face and the eyes when the patient is in the prone position. Postoperative bleeding with formation of a hematoma in the neck requires immediate decompression, as would any bleeding in or around the spinal canal that compromises cord function. Postoperative pain can be substantial and is best managed with PCA; help from a pain consultant is often required.

Arthritis: Osteoarthritis

Synonyms

Degenerative joint disease
Osteoarthrosis
Wear-and-tear arthritis

Definition

Osteoarthritis (OA), or osteoarthrosis, is a progressive, irreversible condition involving loss of articular cartilage that leads to pain and sometimes deformity, principally in the weight-bearing joints of the lower extremities and spine. It is the most common type of arthritis and is associated with genetics, age, obesity, and previous trauma or other disorders that change the mechanics of the joint. OA is a leading cause of impaired mobility in the elderly. By the year 2020, 25% of the adult population in the United States, or more than 50 million people, will be affected by OA.

Clinical Symptoms

The common symptoms of OA are stiffness, joint pain, and deformity. Typically, patients report stiffness rather than swelling during an arthritis flare. The joint effusion that is commonly present inhibits pain-free range of motion. Swelling in the back of the knee (a Baker cyst) is a common cause of posterior knee pain. OA occurs frequently in the fingers, knees, hips, and spine and is relatively rare in the elbow, wrist, and ankle. The most common reason patients seek medical attention for OA is joint pain. The pain is deep, poorly localized, and aching and is exacerbated by activity and relieved by rest. Initial signs include decrease in range of motion that may be caused by muscle spasm, a loss of cartilage, and joint capsule contraction. Osteophytes (bone spurs) and articular cartilage fragments also may decrease motion, and the patient may report grating, catching, and grinding (crepitus). With disease progression, pain is noted with less activity and may eventually occur at rest and at night. Joints may enlarge as the disease progresses secondary to adaptive changes in the bone such as sclerosis (increased density of bone) or osteophyte formation. Adaptive changes occur as the articular cartilage pad becomes thinned and the stress to the bone beneath increases. Osteophytes may block motion in advanced disease. The patient may report that changes in symptoms correlate with changes in weather, but the results of studies on the effects of barometric pressure, temperature, and precipitation on OA have been conflicting.

Tests

Physical Examination

On physical examination, a joint with OA may be tender to palpation and have bone spurs and limited range of motion. An effusion may

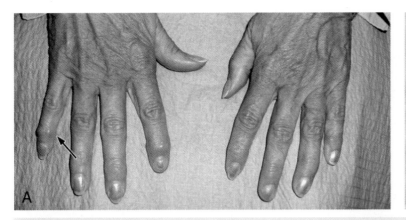
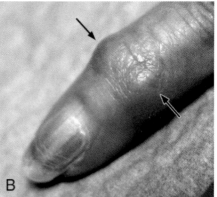

Figure 1 A, Photograph of the hands of a patient with osteoarthritis (OA). Note the prominences at the distal interphalangeal joint caused by osteophytes (arrow). These are called Heberden nodes and are characteristic of OA of the hands. **B,** Photograph shows close-up view of little finger with Heberden nodes (arrows).

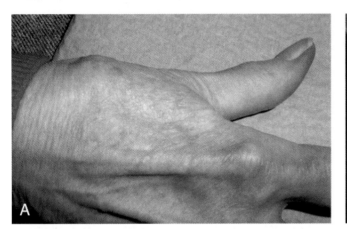
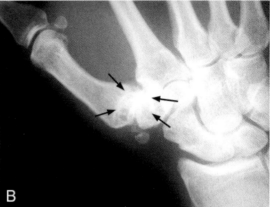

Figure 2 Images of carpometacarpal arthritis of the thumb. **A,** Clinical photograph. Note the typical deformity of adduction of the metacarpal and compensatory hyperextension of the metacarpophalangeal joint. **B,** Radiograph of the hand demonstrates sclerosis (dense bone, arrows), joint space narrowing, osteophytic spur, and cystic changes of the carpometacarpal joint of the thumb.

be present that, on analysis, demonstrates mild pleocytosis, normal viscosity, and slightly elevated protein. Range of motion of the joint may be decreased. The loss of motion typically is mild unless the disease is severe. Joint crepitus (grinding) is a common finding; it results from softening of the articular cartilage.

In the hand, limited range of motion with distal interphalangeal (DIP) and proximal interphalangeal (PIP) joint enlargement is common (Heberden and Bouchard nodes, respectively) (**Figure 1**). OA of the first carpometacarpal joint is common and presents with swelling, bony enlargement of the joint, and restricted motion; the typical deformity is illustrated in **Figure 2**.

Common sites of OA in the foot are the first metatarsophalangeal joint (hallux valgus and rigidus; **Figure 3**), the subtalar joints, and the articulations between the talus, calcaneus, and navicular bones.

In the knee, genu varum (bowleg) or genu valgum (knock-knee) can result from loss of articular cartilage in the medial (genu varum) or lateral (genu valgum) knee compartment. The varus knee is much

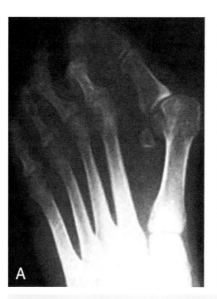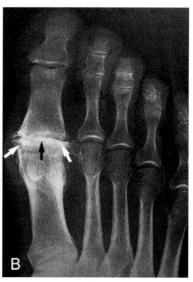

Figure 3 A, AP radiograph of a left foot with hallux valgus and osteoarthritis (OA). **B,** Weight-bearing AP view of a right forefoot shows hallux rigidus (or OA) of the metatarsophalangeal joint of the great toe. Note the joint space narrowing (black arrow), subchondral sclerosis, and medial and lateral osteophytes (white arrows).

more common than the valgus knee. Patellofemoral disease also is common, and joint crepitus often can be felt when palpating the patella while taking the knee through range of motion. A Baker cyst can occur with a knee effusion. This fluid-filled cavity communicates with the joint between the interval of the gastrocnemius and semimembranosus muscles.

With OA of the hip, the patient often walks "toes out," with the limb externally rotated, and tilts or lurches to the affected side with each step. Patients often have pain that radiates to the groin or to the anterior knee as well as pain on internal rotation. Internal rotation also may be limited.

Diagnostic Tests

Radiographs of the affected joint demonstrate loss of joint space, sclerosis, subchondral cysts, and/or osteophytes (bone spurs) at the joint margin (**Figure 4**). The severity of OA based on radiographic criteria has been well described in the Kellgren-Lawrence scale (**Table 1**). Radiographs confirm the disease; however, the correlation between the patient's symptoms and radiographic findings varies. Radiographs are not sensitive in detecting early OA, but they are quite specific when osteoarthritic changes are present. Advanced imaging (for example, MRI, CT) is usually not required if classic signs of OA are present on radiographs. MRI obtained from a patient with moderate to severe OA typically reveals decreased articular cartilage space, subchondral cysts, osteochondral defects, and marrow edema (**Figure 5**).

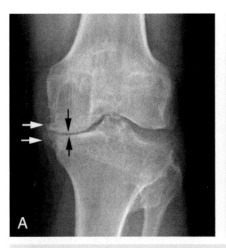 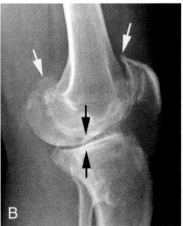

Figure 4 Radiographs of a knee with osteoarthritis (OA). **A,** AP view demonstrates joint space narrowing in the medial compartment (black arrows) and osteophyte formation (white arrows), which are characteristic of OA. **B,** Lateral view demonstrates joint space narrowing (black arrows) and osteophyte formation (white arrows) in the posterior femur and off the superior aspect of the patella. (Reproduced from Johnson TR, Steinbach LS, eds: *Essentials of Musculoskeletal Imaging.* Rosemont, IL, American Academy of Orthopaedic Surgeons, 2004, p 531.)

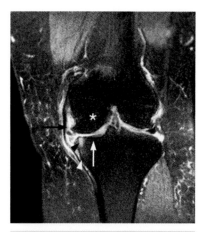

Figure 5 Coronal MRI of a knee with osteoarthritis. Note the decreased joint space (white arrow), flattening of the joint surface (asterisk), osteophyte formation at the joint margin (black arrow), subchondral cyst (black arrowhead), and marrow edema (white arrowhead).

Table 1	

Kellgren-Lawrence Grading Scale for Osteoarthritis

Grade	Radiographic Features
0	No features of osteoarthritis
1	Doubtful: questionable osteophytes or questionable joint space narrowing
2	Minimal: definitive small osteophytes, little or mild joint space narrowing
3	Moderate: definitive moderate osteophytes, joint space narrowing $\geq 50\%$
4	Severe: joint space impaired severely; cysts and sclerosis of subchondral bone

Differential Diagnosis

- Charcot joint (primarily foot and ankle, diabetic neuropathy)
- Chondrocalcinosis (crystals in joint aspirate)
- Degenerative changes secondary to inflammatory arthritis (positive rheumatoid factor)
- Epiphyseal dysplasia (short stature)
- Hemochromatosis (abnormal liver function studies)
- Hemophilia (bleeding tendency)
- Ochronosis (dark urine and pigmentation of cartilage, skin, and/or sclera)
- Osteonecrosis (areas of bone infarcts seen on routine radiographs and/or MRIs)

GENERAL ORTHOPAEDICS

SECTION 1

SECTION 1 GENERAL ORTHOPAEDICS

Adverse Outcomes of the Disease

Pain, deformity, loss of joint motion, loss of limb function, and joint instability are possible. The natural history of OA is classically described as relentless with progressive degeneration of articular cartilage; however, longitudinal studies in patients with OA of the hip and knee report that over a 10-year period, one third to two thirds of patients do not have radiographic progression. Radiographic findings and patient presentation do not always correlate. Over time, OA may remain stable, have periods of symptomatic improvement, or have periods of rapid progression of symptoms and radiographic appearance.

Treatment

Nonpharmacologic treatment includes continued reassurance, patient education, and avoiding activities that cause intense torsional and impact loading of joints. Weight reduction is an essential part of the treatment of lower extremity arthritis in persons with obesity. Weight reduction is critical in arthritis prevention programs. A 10-pound weight loss over 10 years may decrease the risk for OA by 50%. Weight loss for symptomatic OA of the knee in patients with a body mass index greater than 25 received a moderate recommendation from the American Academy of Orthopaedic Surgeons (AAOS) Clinical Practice Guideline *Treatment of Osteoarthritis of the Knee*, 2nd edition. Joint protection is an important concept that includes exercises that do not cyclically load the joint. Gentle, regular joint exercises help maintain function as strong muscle can protect the joint. Water exercise, bicycling, tai chi, and use of an elliptical machine provide nonimpact exercise that can help to reduce symptoms and preserve muscle support in the affected joints without causing increased stress to the joint. Isometric exercises improve strength if patients are unable to tolerate exercises involving joint motion. Data on outcomes regarding rehabilitation show that a standardized knee exercise program can improve pain, function, and stiffness.

Resting the joint is reasonable for acute pain but should not exceed 12 to 24 hours to prevent muscle atrophy and loss of range of motion. Shock-absorbing heel inserts can help decrease weight-bearing stress to the joints of the lower extremities. Braces also may help decrease forces to the joint in some patients; however, the brace should not be too tight, because this will decrease circulation and can increase the risk of deep vein thrombosis (DVT).

Pharmacologic treatment is indicated for patients who do not respond to nonpharmacologic treatment (**Table 2**). NSAIDs are indicated for inflammatory OA and should be given before narcotic medications if the patient has no contraindications. Acetaminophen is an over-the-counter analgesic agent that is superior to placebo but less efficacious than NSAIDs in relieving hip and knee OA pain.

Opioid analgesics such as codeine, hydrocodone, or oxycodone are beneficial for short-term relief of symptoms and are synergistic with NSAIDs. These analgesic agents should be avoided in the

Table 2

Pharmacologic Treatment of Osteoarthritis

Drug	Administration	Indications	Comments
NSAIDs (aspirin, ibuprofen, naproxen)	Oral	Inflammatory OA	Contraindications include stomach ulcers, reflux, liver or kidney disease. Mechanism: NSAIDs block prostaglandin production.
Acetaminophen	Oral; up to 4 g/d	Hip and knee OA	Hepatotoxicity can occur, especially with alcohol use.
COX-2 selective NSAIDs (celecoxib)	Oral	Pain not controlled with acetaminophen	Contraindications include cardiac risk factors
Tramadol	Oral or intramuscular injection	Pain not controlled by NSAIDs or pain not controlled by acetaminophen in a person with GI sensitivity to NSAIDs	Nonaddictive
Corticosteroids	Intra-articular injection	OA or inflammatory arthritis with symptoms not controlled by acetaminophen or NSAIDs	Relief duration variable, may be as little as 1 to 2 weeks
Viscosupplementation	Intra-articular injection	Knee OA	Strong recommendation against use by the AAOS[a]
Glucosamine-chondroitin sulfate	Oral	OA	Benefit not scientifically documented
Opioids (codeine, oxycodone)	Oral	Short-term relief	Addictive Synergistic with NSAIDs Contraindicated in the elderly Not for chronic pain

COX-2 = cyclooxygenase-2, GI = gastrointestinal, OA = osteoarthritis.

[a]American Academy of Orthopaedic Surgeons: *Treatment of Osteoarthritis of the Knee: Evidence-Based Guideline, 2nd Edition.* Available at: http://www.aaos.org/Research/guidelines/TreatmentofOsteoarthritisoftheKneeGuideline.pdf. Accessed April 29, 2015.

elderly because they may cause increased confusion, sedation, and delirium. Moreover, for chronic arthritis pain, opioids should be avoided because of their addictive potential. Tramadol, a nonaddictive pain reliever, is useful especially when used in combination with acetaminophen or NSAIDs and has been shown in meta-analysis to be more efficacious than placebo in improving pain scores.

Cyclooxygenase-2 (COX-2)–selective NSAIDs such as celecoxib have gastrointestinal side effects similar to acetaminophen. Celecoxib is acceptable for patients with no cardiac risk factors and pain not controlled by acetaminophen. Adverse side effects of NSAIDs include hypersensitivity reaction, platelet inhibition, nephrotoxicity, hypersensitivity, and central nervous system disturbances in the elderly. Glucosamine and chondroitin sulfate are other popular options for pain management.

Intra-articular corticosteroids often relieve symptoms, but the duration of relief is variable and can be as short as 1 to 2 weeks. Viscosupplementation injections are no longer recommended by the AAOS for nonsurgical management of knee OA; the Clinical Practice Guideline on the topic indicates that administration of viscosupplementation has similar outcomes to placebo. (See the chapter on Complementary and Alternative Medicine Therapies for Osteoarthritis in this section for further details.)

The use of stem cells has been well described for the treatment of cartilage defects in vitro and in animal models. More recently, interest in using mesenchymal stem cells (MSCs) as an injectable agent for OA has increased. Injection of MSCs is known to have a potential for articular cartilage regeneration. Although MSC injections are commercially available, there is a paucity of prospective randomized evidence to support their routine use in clinical practice.

Joint arthroplasty or arthrodesis (joint fusion) is appropriate for patients with unacceptable loss of joint function or those who have pain at rest or at night that is unresponsive to nonsurgical management. Hip, knee, ankle, and shoulder replacement surgery is especially effective in reducing pain and increasing function. Arthrodesis may relieve the joint pain, but the fusion will result in increased stress above and below the fused level.

Adverse Outcomes of Treatment

Salicylates and NSAIDs often help but can be associated with renal, hepatic, or gastric problems. In 2015, the FDA strengthened its warning linking NSAIDs with the risk of heart attack or stroke, even in the first weeks of use of an NSAID.

Removal of prosthetic implants because of infection or loosening may be required in rare circumstances. Patients who have undergone an earlier, preemptive procedure, such as an arthroscopic joint débridement or osteotomy, may ultimately require a second operation (that is, joint arthroplasty).

Referral Decisions/Red Flags

Referral should be considered for patients who have pain at rest, pain at night, a rapid onset of disabling pain, pain unrelieved by nonsurgical methods, or unacceptable loss of joint function.

Complementary and Alternative Medicine Therapies for Osteoarthritis

Osteoarthritis (OA) is the most common form of arthritis and is a leading cause of disability. NSAIDs are commonly used to alleviate the symptoms of OA, but these medications have significant side effects. In 2015, the FDA strengthened its warning linking NSAIDs with the risk of heart attack or stroke, even in the first weeks of use of an NSAID. For this and other reasons, the field of complementary and alternative medicine (CAM) has grown, especially as it relates to OA. In 2012, more than 34% of adults in the United States used some type of CAM therapy. In fact, a 2007 study from the National Institutes of Health, which included a comprehensive survey on the use of complementary health approaches in the United States, indicated that 5.2% of adults used a CAM therapy specifically for joint pain or stiffness and that 3.5% used a CAM therapy to manage arthritis. This chapter reviews just a few of the complementary and alternative practices sought out by patients for the treatment of OA.

CAM Providers

Certification and/or licensing are available in specific CAM specialties (**Table 1**). The amount of training required for licensing or certification varies from hundreds of hours to several years.

Chiropractic Care

Chiropractic care is currently the most widely used CAM modality in the United States, used by more than 50 million Americans per year. The most common applications of chiropractic care are for back pain and arthritis, but chiropractors often also treat extremity pain, including pain from OA. The main focus of chiropractic treatment is manipulation, or "adjustment," aimed at realigning spinal segments. Chiropractic treatment may be beneficial in shortening the duration of acute back pain, but caution must be exercised in applying manipulative therapy to patients with OA and osteoporosis because of the risk of fracture. Although no evidence exists that chiropractic care can reverse the joint degeneration associated with OA, some clinical studies suggest that spinal manipulation may increase range of motion, relax the muscles, improve joint coordination, and reduce pain.

Acupuncture

Acupuncture is an ancient Chinese practice consisting of the placement of needles in specific acupuncture points on the body to

Table 1

Complementary and Alternative Medicine Providers

Type of Provider	Complementary or Alternative Medicine Therapeutic Principles/Techniques
Acupuncturist	The acupuncturist inserts fine needles at points along the body's meridians to correct the flow of life energy, or "chi," to restore health and relieve pain.
Ayurvedic practitioner	Ayurveda, the traditional system of medicine in India, focuses on wellness and healthy living through diet, exercise, moderation, and meditation; practitioners advise patients on practices to restore mental, physical, and spiritual well-being.
Chinese herbalist	Herbalists prepare various formulations of herbs in an attempt to restore balance to the body.
Chiropractor	Chiropractic is based on the theory that misalignment of vertebrae is the cause of most neuromuscular and related functional diseases and disorders. Chiropractors use spinal manipulation to restore proper vertebral alignment.
Homeopath	Homeopathy is based on the theory that "like cures like." Homeopaths administer minuscule amounts of natural substances such as herbs, minerals, and animal products in serially diluted preparations in an attempt to induce the patient's body to heal itself.
Massage therapist	Massage uses manual touch to improve health and well-being.
Naturopath	Naturopathy encourages healthy living habits, especially proper nutrition, and allowing the body to heal itself. Naturopaths often work closely with physicians and other healthcare providers.

promote the flow of "chi," or body energy, throughout the body in pathways called meridians. Acupuncture has been used for a variety of purposes, including weight loss and smoking cessation, as well as for decreasing pain and swelling such as that associated with OA. Several studies have shown that acupuncture can ease the pain of arthritis, back pain, and fibromyalgia. Several controlled clinical trials suggest that acupuncture is an effective treatment of pain associated with OA, as well as for other aspects of the condition, including diminished joint function and reduced walking ability. In fact, a few clinical studies have shown that people with OA experience better pain relief and improvement in function from acupuncture than from certain NSAIDs.

Qi Xiong and Tai Chi

Qi xiong and tai chi have recently gained popularity for increasing the activity level and enhancing the feeling of well-being of elderly individuals. These ancient Chinese practices, which are based on meditation and gentle movements based on the movements of animals in nature, have been credited with decreasing the rate of falls and hip fractures, increasing circulation, and improving mobility in the elderly.

Magnet Therapy and Copper Garments

Relatively inexpensive and easy to use, magnets have become a $1.5 billion-per-year business. Both magnets and copper bracelets or garments have been used to reduce pain and swelling associated with OA. It is said that Cleopatra slept with a magnet to prevent aging. Magnets often come with wraps or bandages to hold them in place. Little scientific evidence supports the claims that magnets or copper garments alleviate arthritis symptoms, although anecdotal evidence abounds.

Nutritional Supplements

In the United States, more than one third of the population uses nutritional supplements for health purposes, spending more than $3.5 billion annually. The content of these supplements is poorly regulated, and potential interactions of these supplements with prescribed medications are not well publicized. In addition, many supplements are contraindicated in the presence of certain medical conditions. Some studies have shown nutritional supplements to be beneficial, but the physician should exercise caution when recommending any supplement. Commonly used herbal supplements and the potential hazards they pose are listed in **Table 2**. Unlike conventional medications, herbal medications are not regulated by governmental agencies such as the FDA. Patients should be reminded that "natural" is not synonymous with "safe."

Glucosamine and Chondroitin

Glucosamine and chondroitin are the most commonly used herbal supplements marketed for the treatment of OA. Articular cartilage is composed of chondrocytes, water, collagen, and proteoglycans. OA is associated with a breakdown of the proteoglycans, resulting in increased water permeability and deterioration of cartilage. Glycosaminoglycans are an important component of proteoglycans.

Glucosamine is hexosamine sugar and a building block for glycosaminoglycans, including chondroitin sulfate and hyaluronic acid. The nutritional supplement is extracted from cow tracheas and is sold in either a sulfate or hydrochloride form. Chondroitin sulfate is a glycosaminoglycan that is found in proteoglycans. Proteoglycans are important for maintaining the extracellular matrix of articular cartilage. Chondroitin is usually derived from shellfish. Glucosamine and chondroitin are often sold in combination as over-the-counter supplements, with recommended dosages of 1,500 mg/d and 1,200 mg/d, respectively. Only mild side effects such as dyspepsia have been reported in humans, but glucosamine has been shown to increase blood glucose levels in laboratory animals, and some concern exists that chondroitin may increase clotting times in patients who are taking anticoagulants. A large study published by the National Institutes of Health in 2008 showed that in patients with moderate to severe pain, relief was noted with the combination of glucosamine and chondroitin; no difference was shown in patients

Table 2

Herbal Supplement/Drug Interactions

Herbal Supplement	Common Uses	Potential Problems	Potential Interactions
Dong quai (*Angelica*)	To treat menopausal symptoms, PMS, dysmenorrhea	Enhances bleeding	Anticoagulants
Echinacea	To treat colds, influenza, and mild infections, especially upper respiratory infections	Hepatotoxicity; intestinal upset	Other hepatotoxic drugs; anabolic steroids; methotrexate
Garlic	To decrease cholesterol and blood clot formation	Enhances bleeding	Anticoagulants
Ginger	To relieve nausea, decrease inflammation	Enhances bleeding; CNS depression; hypotension; cardiac arrhythmia; hypoglycemia	Anticoagulants; enhances the effects of barbiturates; antihypertensives; cardiac drugs; hypoglycemic drugs
Ginkgo biloba	To improve circulation, especially to the brain; for memory loss, dizziness, and headache	Enhances bleeding; cramps, muscle spasms	Anticoagulants
Ginseng	To increase energy and reduce stress, decrease inflammation	Enhances bleeding; tachycardia and hypertension; mania	Anticoagulants; stimulants; antihypertensives; antidepressants/phenelzine; digoxin; potentiates the effects of corticosteroids and estrogens
Goldenseal	To treat sore throats and upper respiratory infections (as a mild antibiotic)	Increases fluid retention; hypertension; nausea; nervousness	Diuretics; antihypertensives
Kava kava	To treat anxiety, nervousness, and insomnia	Upset stomach; allergic skin reaction, yellow discoloration of skin; CNS depression, liver toxicity	Potentiates the effects of antidepressants, barbiturates, and benzodiazepines; skeletal muscle relaxants; anesthetics
Licorice	To treat hepatitis and peptic ulcers	Hypertension; hypokalemia; edema	Antihypertensives; potentiates the effects of corticosteroids
SAMe (S-adenosyl-methionine)	To treat depression or osteoarthritis	Mimics serotonin; nausea, upset stomach	Drugs that can increase or mimic serotonin, such as antidepressants
St. John's wort	To treat mild depression, anxiety, seasonal affective disorder	Enhances bleeding; hastens metabolic breakdown of drugs; contraindicated for organ transplant recipients	Anticoagulants; antidepressants; decreases the effectiveness of cyclosporine, antiviral drugs; digoxin; dextromethorphan; prolongs the effects of general anesthetics; MAO inhibitors
Valerian	To treat insomnia, anxiety	Sedation; digestion problems	Potentiates the effects of barbiturates

CNS = central nervous system, MAO = monoamine oxidase, PMS = premenstrual syndrome.

This table was compiled by the AAOS Committee on Complementary and Alternative Medicine. The information contained here is based on literature searches conducted in July and August of 2001 and was updated in 2003, and it may not be exhaustive. User physicians should rely on their own judgment concerning the care of specific patients and should use this table for general guidance only. Common medical practice is that patients cease using most of these preparations at least 2 weeks before surgical interventions.

with mild pain. In this study, the supplements showed no slowing of the progression of OA as compared with control patients, although other studies have suggested this benefit.

S-Adenosylmethionine

S-adenosylmethionine (SAMe) is available as an over-the-counter dietary supplement used to manage OA and depression. The usual dosage is 200 to 400 mg three times a day. SAMe is synthesized in the body from the essential amino acid methionine. In theory, SAMe augments cartilage formation by forming sulfur compounds. Some clinical studies have shown SAMe to be as effective as NSAIDs in relieving pain and to have fewer side effects; however, more evidence is needed to prove whether SAMe promotes cartilage repair. Caution is required when combining SAMe with some antidepressants because of the possibility of serotonin syndrome.

Methylsulfonylmethane

Methylsulfonylmethane (MSM) is a sulfur compound formed in the breakdown of dimethyl sulfoxide (DMSO). It is sold as an over-the-counter nutritional supplement and lotion that has been touted as a cure for arthritis. DMSO has been widely used in veterinary medicine for musculoskeletal problems, including arthritis. Both DMSO and MSM are proposed to act as potent anti-inflammatory agents. Results of a few clinical studies have shown that MSM modestly reduced pain and swelling associated with OA.

Omega-3 Fatty Acids

Omega-3 fatty acids are essential for human health but cannot be manufactured by the human body; therefore, they must be obtained through food or supplements. Certain fish, such as salmon and tuna, are especially high in this nutrient. Extensive research indicates that omega-3 fatty acids reduce inflammation and help prevent risk factors associated with chronic diseases such as heart disease, some cancers, and arthritis. Omega-3 fatty acids have been more extensively studied for the control of symptoms associated with rheumatoid arthritis than for OA, but it has been suggested that they have similar beneficial effects on decreasing stiffness and pain associated with OA. Omega-3 fatty acids should be used with caution because they may increase the effect of prescription blood thinners (warfarin [Coumadin] or clopidogrel bisulfate [Plavix]), and taking more than 3 g/d of this supplement has been associated with increased risk of bleeding and severe disorders such as hemorrhagic stroke.

Viscosupplementation

A relatively common treatment of OA is viscosupplementation. This involves injecting hyaluronic acid (HA) into a joint to improve joint function and decrease pain. HA is a large glycosaminoglycan that is usually produced by chondrocytes and type B synoviocytes. HA is essential for synovial viscoelasticity, joint lubrication, and joint motion. Patients with OA have a diminished concentration of HA within the affected joint or joints. Because it is poorly absorbed in the

Table 3

Comparative Prescribing Information for Viscosupplements

Viscosupplement[a]	Description	HA Dose per Injection	Volume per Injection	Injections per Course	Source
Gel-One hyaluronate (Zimmer)	Cross-linked hyaluronate	30 mg	3 mL	1	Avian (rooster combs)
Supartz (Bioventus)	Sodium hyaluronate	25 mg	2.5 mL	3 or 5	Avian (rooster combs
Hyalgan (Fidia Pharma USA)	Sodium hyaluronate	20 mg	2 mL	3 or 5	Avian (rooster combs)
Euflexxa (Ferring Pharmaceuticals)	Sodium hyaluronate	20 mg	2 mL	3	Bacterial fermentation
Orthovisc (DePuy Mitek)	High-molecular-weight hyaluronan	30 mg	2 mL	3 or 4	Bacterial fermentation
Monovisc (DePuy Synthes)	High-molecular-weight hyaluronan	88 mg	4 mL	1	Bacterial fermentation
Synvisc (Sanofi-Aventis)	Hylan G-F 20 Hylan A and hylan B (cross-linked polymers of hyaluronan)	16 mg	2 mL	3	Avian (rooster combs)
Synvisc-One (Sanofi-Aventis)	Hylan G-F 20 Hylan A and hylan B (cross-linked polymers of hyaluronan)	48 mg	6 mL	1	Avian (rooster combs)
Gel-Synm (Institut Biochimique)	Low- to medium-weight hyaluronic acid chains	16 mg	2 mL	3	Bacterial fermentation

HA = hyaluronic acid.

[a] Refer to prescribing information for each product. The information given here is not intended to imply a comparison of efficacy or safety.

gastrointestinal tract, HA must be injected into the joint rather than taken orally. Possible mechanisms by which HA may be therapeutic include (1) providing additional lubrication of the synovial membrane; (2) controlling permeability of the synovial membrane, thus diminishing joint effusions; and (3) directly blocking inflammation by scavenging free radicals. Several clinical trials have shown decreased pain and improved function, especially at 5 to 12 weeks after injection.

Currently, the FDA approves viscosupplementation for OA of the knee only. Viscosupplements are considered investigational for other joints (hip, ankle, and shoulder). Several preparations produced either from rooster combs or from bacterial cultures are available, with varying molecular weights (**Table 3**). Intra-articular injections are administered weekly for 3 or 5 weeks, or as a one-time injection of a larger volume of HA. Local reactions of increased joint pain, swelling, erythema, and itching have been reported. Viscosupplementation has been most effective in less severe OA (that is, OA without bone-on-bone changes).

Arthritis: Rheumatoid Arthritis

Definition

Rheumatoid arthritis (RA) is a systemic autoimmune disorder characterized by acute and chronic inflammation in the synovium, causing proliferative and erosive joint changes. The etiology is unknown, but it is theorized that an unknown agent activates an immune response in synovial tissue. Genetic predisposition, hormonal changes, infectious agents, and immunologic cytokines all have been postulated to trigger the abnormal immune response seen in RA.

RA affects women more often than men (ratio, 3:1). The prevalence increases with age, with peak onset in the late 40s and early 50s. The arthritis typically is symmetric and most often involves the joints of the hands, wrist, knees, feet, and ankles (**Figure 1**).

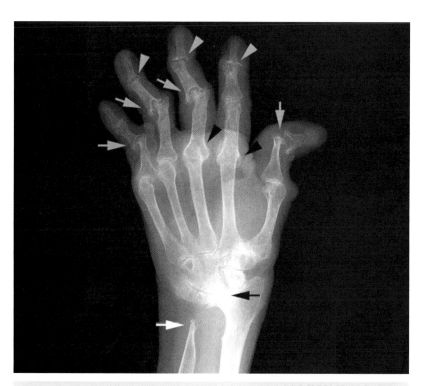

Figure 1 PA radiograph of the left hand of a 42-year-old woman with advanced rheumatoid arthritis (RA). Note the ulnar translocation of the carpus (black arrow); the pencil shape of the ulna (white arrow); the dislocation of the metacarpophalangeal joints of the index and middle fingers (black arrowheads); the destruction of the interphalangeal joint of the thumb and the proximal interphalangeal joints of the long, ring, and little fingers (gray arrows); and the arthritic changes in the distal interphalangeal joints (gray arrowheads). (Reproduced from Johnson TR, Steinbach LS, eds: *Essentials of Musculoskeletal Imaging.* Rosemont, IL, American Academy of Orthopaedic Surgeons, 2004, p 394.)

Table 1	
2010 American College of Rheumatology/European League Against Rheumatism Classification Criteria for Rheumatoid Arthritis	
Criteria	**Points**
Joint Distribution (0-5)	
1 large joint	0
2-10 large joints	1
1-3 small joints[a] (large joints not counted)	2
4-10 small joints (large joints not counted)	3
>10 joints (at least one small joint)	5
Serology (0-3)	
Negative RF and negative ACPA	0
Low positive RF or low positive ACPA	2
High positive RF or high positive ACPA	3
Symptom Duration (0-1)	
<6 wk	0
≥6 wk	1
Acute-Phase Reactants (0-1)	
Normal CRP and normal ESR	0
Abnormal CRP or abnormal ESR	1

ACPA = anticitrullinated protein antibody, CRP = C-reactive protein level, ESR = erythrocyte sedimentation rate, RF = rheumatoid factor.

[a] For example, the metacarpophalangeal, proximal interphalangeal, second to fifth metatarsophalangeal, and wrist.

(Adapted with permission from American College of Rheumatology: *2010 ACR-EULAR Classification Criteria for Rheumatoid Arthritis*. American College of Rheumatology, Atlanta, GA. Available at: https://www.rheumatology.org/ practice/clinical/classification/ra/ra_2010.asp. Accessed April 29, 2015.)

Clinical Symptoms

Pain, morning stiffness, swelling, and systemic symptoms are common. Symptoms of two or more swollen joints, morning stiffness lasting more than 1 hour at a time for at least 6 weeks, or the detection of rheumatoid factors (RFs) or anticyclic citrullinated peptides (anti-CCPs) should raise suspicion for RA.

The 2010 American College of Rheumatology/European League Against Rheumatism (ACR/EULAR) classification criteria for RA are designed to identify patients with unexplained inflammatory arthritis in at least one peripheral joint and a short duration of symptoms who would benefit from early therapeutic intervention (**Table 1**). The four criteria included in the diagnosis are joint involvement, serology test results, acute-phase reactant test results, and patient self-reporting. A diagnosis of definitive RA requires a score of at least 6 out of 10. Patients who present with erosive changes characteristic of RA meet the definition of RA.

The onset of RA is typically insidious. The patient reports pain, stiffness, and swelling in many joints. Joints of the hands and feet are usually affected first; proximal joint involvement occurs later in

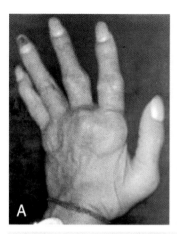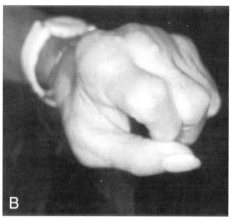

Figure 2 Clinical photographs of the left hand of a patient with rheumatoid arthritis. Note the characteristic volar subluxation (**A**) and ulnar drift of the digits at the metacarpophalangeal joints (**B**). (Reproduced from Abboud JA, Beredjiklian PK, Bozentka DJ: Metacarpophalangeal joint arthroplasty in rheumatoid arthritis. *J Am Acad Orthop Surg* 2003;11[3]:184-191.)

the disease course. The distal interphalangeal joints of the hands are spared from rheumatic changes.

The hypertrophic synovium stretches the ligaments and joint capsules. As a result, these supporting structures become less effective. Erosion of the articular cartilage in combination with the ligamentous changes results in deformity and contractures such as ulnar drifting and subluxation of the metacarpophalangeal joints in the hand (**Figure 2**) and hallux valgus and claw toe deformities in the foot. Although involvement of the joints is symmetric in RA, the severity of joint disease and deformity is commonly asymmetric. This asymmetry is attributed to increased use of a dominant extremity or protection of a painful extremity. Peripheral joint involvement is almost universal in RA, and 20% to 50% of patients have involvement of central and axial joints. Neck pain and stiffness occur, and with atlantoaxial subluxation, cervical myelopathy develops rarely.

Extra-articular symptoms are more common in patients who are seropositive for RF and rarely occur in the absence of clinical arthritis. In patients with extra-articular symptoms, anemia, generalized malaise, fatigue, vasculitis, scleritis, rheumatoid nodules, pleuropericarditis, and renal disease may develop (**Table 2**). Tenosynovitis causes carpal tunnel syndrome in 1% to 5% of patients with RA. Nodules along the tendon sheath may cause trigger finger or tendon ruptures, most commonly in the extensor pollicis longus, resulting in lack of thumb extension.

Both the course of disease activity and the speed of joint destruction vary markedly in patients with RA. In most patients, disease activity fluctuates over periods lasting from weeks to months throughout the disease course. In 10% to 20% of patients, however, disease activity does not subside. Remission is rare without disease-modifying antirheumatic drugs (DMARDs). Studies have demonstrated

SECTION 1   GENERAL ORTHOPAEDICS

Table 2		
Extra-articular Manifestations of Rheumatoid Arthritis		
System	**Manifestation**	**Symptoms**
Pulmonary	Nodules, fibrosis	Pleurisy, effusion
Cardiovascular	Vasculitis, pericarditis	Digital infarcts, ischemic mononeuropathy
Musculoskeletal	Nodules, tenosynovitis	Carpal/tarsal tunnel syndrome, trigger finger
Ocular	Keratoconjunctivitis, scleritis	Dry eyes, corneal ulcer, scleritis

remission rates up to 25% after 3 years of DMARD therapy and 20% after 5 years of DMARD therapy. Even though disease activity is variable, joint structural damage is cumulative and irreversible.

Tests
Physical Examination
Pain and swelling of the affected joints, along with diminished range of motion and pain elicited by pressure, are the predominant physical findings in early RA. Erythema and marked warmth are not predominant physical examination findings. Synovial hypertrophy causes a boggy feeling in swollen joints. Joint aspirations often produce less fluid than expected because much of the enlargement comes from synovial hypertrophy, not effusions. The characteristic joint deformities seen in RA are late manifestations of the disease.

Swelling of the proximal interphalangeal joints and stiffness in the hands usually occur early. Distal interphalangeal joints are typically spared. Reduced grip strength is common, as is carpal tunnel syndrome as noted by symptoms of numbness and tingling in the median nerve distribution of the hand and as tested by the Phalen test. The elbow is the most common site of subcutaneous rheumatoid nodules. Lateral drift of the toes and plantar subluxation of the metatarsal heads are common foot deformities in patients with RA (**Figure 3**).

Heel pain can be caused by retrocalcaneal bursitis or tarsal tunnel syndrome, which is caused by impingement of the posterior tibial nerve. In the knee, ligamentous laxity, effusion, and genu valgum deformity (knock-knee) are common.

Diagnostic Tests
Laboratory tests are used for diagnostic purposes and to assess disease activity in persons with RA. RF, an immunoglobulin M (IgM) antibody against the Fc portion of immunoglobulin G (IgG), is elevated in 75% to 90% of patients. Higher titers are seen in patients with more severe disease, but this test is not specific for RA. Anti-CCP antibodies are as sensitive as RF and are more specific. When both RF and anti-CCPs are tested in patients with early-stage

GENERAL ORTHOPAEDICS   SECTION 1

GENERAL ORTHOPAEDICS

SECTION 1

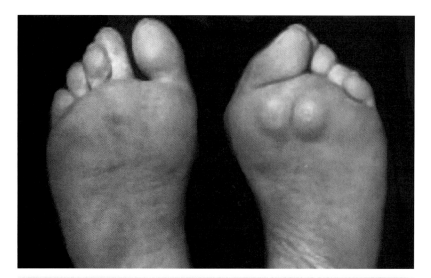

Figure 3 Clinical photograph of the plantar aspect of the feet of a patient with rheumatoid arthritis (RA). The left foot demonstrates forefoot deformities typical of RA, including hallux valgus, claw toes, and plantar keratoses beneath the second and third metatarsal heads. The right forefoot has been surgically reconstructed. (Reproduced from Abdo RV, Iorio LJ: Rheumatoid arthritis of the foot and ankle. *J Am Acad Orthop Surg* 1994;2[6]:326-333.)

arthritis, the tests are 55% sensitive and 97% specific in identifying patients in whom clinical RA would develop. The C-reactive protein level and erythrocyte sedimentation rate are acute-phase reactants that correlate with the degree of joint inflammation. Platelet counts are typically elevated in patients with an acute flare. Serum albumin has been shown to be decreased in active disease and to correlate with disease activity.

Radiographic changes vary according to disease activity. Common signs are periarticular osteopenia and bony erosion at the joint margin, which correlates with the insertion site of the synovium. Lateral flexion and extension views of the neck may demonstrate C1-C2 instability secondary to erosion of the ligaments that hold the odontoid in place. These findings are important if the patient is anticipating any surgery that involves intubation or manipulation of the neck, because it could lead to quadriparesis or death (**Figure 4**). Regional anesthesia should be considered in all patients with RA. If general anesthesia is necessary, an awake patient and fiber-optic intubation may be warranted if substantial instability exists at C1-C2.

Differential Diagnosis

• Hepatitis (abnormal liver function tests)
• Lyme disease (serology, rash, anemia)

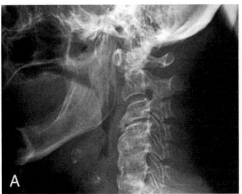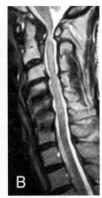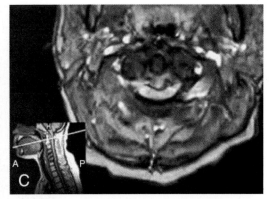

Figure 4 Images from a patient with rheumatoid arthritis. **A,** Lateral cervical spine radiograph demonstrates atlantoaxial subluxation. Sagittal (**B**) and axial (**C**) T2-weighted MRIs of the cervical spine show decreased space available for the spinal cord and a soft-tissue pannus posterior to the odontoid. The line on the inset indicates the level at which the image was obtained. (Reproduced from Kim DH, Hilibrand AS: Rheumatoid arthritis in the cervical spine. *J Am Acad Orthop Surg* 2005;13[7]:463-474.)

- Seronegative arthropathies (HLA tests, abnormal radiographs, urethritis)
- Systemic lupus erythematosus (antinuclear antibodies, peripheral blood smear)

Adverse Outcomes of the Disease

Joint contractures, pain, loss of function, loss of ambulation, and multisystem disorders resulting in death are possible. Osteoporosis is common, in part related to the disease, inactivity, and steroids that are commonly used in managing the disease. Patients can have impaired immune function when using DMARDs.

Treatment

Drug therapy is the main treatment of patients with RA to prevent complications and reduce morbidity. DMARDs alter the inflammatory cascade on a molecular level. Two classes of DMARDs have been developed: nonbiologic and biologic. These drugs reduce or prevent articular damage and the development of joint deformities. The nonbiologic agents include hydroxychloroquine, sulfasalazine, and methotrexate. These nonbiologic DMARDs are the first-line treatment in RA. The biologic agents are produced with recombinant DNA technology and target cytokines or their receptors in the inflammatory cascade. Biologic agents include tumor necrosis factor–α (TNF-α) inhibitors (etanercept, infliximab, adalimumab), interleukin-1 (IL-1) antagonists (anakinra), and anti-CD20 B-cell depleting monoclonal antibodies (rituximab).

Analgesics are available in both topical (capsaicin) and oral forms. Oral agents such as acetaminophen, tramadol, and opioids are used in RA, but opioids should be used with great discretion in managing chronic pain caused by RA. NSAIDs, which provide both analgesic and anti-inflammatory benefits, can be used as adjunctive treatment. Glucocorticoids have anti-inflammatory properties and are administered by various routes in the treatment of RA, including orally, intravenously, and intra-articularly. Corticosteroid injections into selected joints and the carpal tunnel may relieve acute synovitis and thereby decrease pain and improve function.

Splints and orthoses may help manage acute episodes of pain associated with synovitis as well as position joints to minimize progressive deformity and improve function. Custom shoes are helpful for patients with severe foot deformities. Physical and occupational therapy for modalities to decrease swelling and pain as well as for information on range-of-motion and strengthening exercises should be part of a multidisciplinary treatment program. Selective surgical intervention by synovectomy or tenosynovectomy may prevent tendon rupture and progression of joint deformity. End-stage arthritis requires total joint arthroplasty or arthrodesis.

Adverse Outcomes of Treatment

Infection secondary to injections or surgery; gastric, hepatic, or renal complications associated with NSAID use; and osteonecrosis of bone or osteoporosis associated with steroid use are possible. In 2015, the FDA strengthened its warning linking NSAIDs with the risk of heart attack or stroke, even in the first weeks of use of an NSAID. Skin rash and other side effects of various medications also can develop. DMARDs weaken the immune system, so patients should be monitored for serious infections.

Referral Decisions/Red Flags

Patients whose symptoms persist for more than 3 months or who have uncontrollable joint pain at rest despite nonsurgical care, as well as those who have substantial deformity or extra-articular manifestations of the disease, are appropriate for referral for consideration of surgical options.

Arthritis: Seronegative Spondyloarthropathies

Synonyms
Ankylosing spondylitis
Psoriatic arthritis
Psoriatic arthropathy
Reactive arthritis
Reiter syndrome

Definition
The seronegative spondyloarthropathies—including ankylosing spondylitis, reactive arthritis (Reiter syndrome), psoriatic arthritis, and arthritis associated with inflammatory bowel disease—are a group of arthritides that have common clinical and genetic features (**Table 1**). They are called seronegative because laboratory results are negative for rheumatoid factor and antinuclear antibodies. The axial skeleton is commonly involved, and patients report back pain. Ocular, dermatologic, and gastrointestinal manifestations are frequent. Enthesitis, an inflammation at the site of ligament and tendon insertions onto bone, can develop in some patients. These arthropathies share a common genetic factor, HLA-B27, so a strong familial association exists. However, not all patients with seronegative spondyloarthropathies are positive for the HLA-B27 antigen. The strongest association is found in ankylosing spondylitis, with an 88% positive rate for HLA-B27.

Table 1				
Seronegative Spondyloarthropathies				
Condition	**Arthritis Characteristics**	**Commonly Affected Joints**	**Associated Conditions**	**Treatment**
Ankylosing spondylitis	Sacroiliitis	Sacroiliac joint; rarely peripheral joints	Uveitis, carditis, enthesitis	NSAIDs, exercise
Arthritis associated with inflammatory bowel disease	Asymmetric, oligoarticular	Sacroiliac joint, knee, ankle	Crohn disease, ulcerative colitis, enthesitis	NSAIDs
Psoriatic arthritis	5 clinical patterns, erosive	Hands, wrist, ankle, sacroiliac joint	Skin lesions, nail involvement, dactylitis, iritis, enthesitis	NSAIDs, methotrexate, biologics
Reiter syndrome	Asymmetric, oligoarticular	Knee, ankle, sacroiliac joint	Iritis, urethritis, dactylitis, enthesitis	Treatment of precipitating infection, NSAIDs

GENERAL ORTHOPAEDICS

SECTION 1

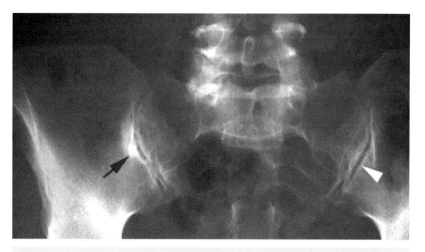

Figure 1 AP radiograph of the pelvis demonstrates iliac sclerosis at the middle aspect of the right sacroiliac joint (arrow). The left sacroiliac joint appears normal (arrowhead). Lack of involvement of the inferior sacroiliac joint excludes sacroiliitis.

Ankylosing Spondylitis

Ankylosing spondylitis is a systemic inflammatory disorder that primarily affects the axial skeleton. Sacroiliitis (**Figure 1**) and kyphosis are seen on radiographic imaging. Ankylosing spondylitis typically begins in the second or third decade of life and is three times more common in men than in women. Peripheral joint involvement correlates with the severity of the disease but is typically less severe than that observed in the other seronegative spondyloarthropathies. The ankle, hip, and shoulder are the peripheral joints most commonly affected by arthritic changes. Association with the HLA-B27 antigen is high, particularly in white patients, who have an HLA-B27–positive rate of approximately 92%. Systemic manifestations, including uveitis, iritis, aortitis, and cardiac conduction abnormalities, occur in 33% of patients.

Reactive Arthritis

Reactive arthritis is an acute spondyloarthropathy precipitated by gastrointestinal or genitourinary infection. The HLA-B27 antigen has been documented in 63% to 96% of patients with reactive arthritis. Reiter syndrome is a type of reactive arthritis that causes arthritis, urethritis, conjunctivitis, and mucocutaneous lesions. Sexually transmitted and dysenteric diseases are common 2 to 6 weeks before the onset of joint pain. *Chlamydia trachomatis, Shigella, Salmonella, Yersinia, Clostridium difficile*, and *Campylobacter* are common inciting pathogens.

Psoriatic Arthritis

Psoriatic arthritis affects approximately 5% to 14% of patients with psoriasis. The sex ratio is approximately equal, and age of onset is typically in the late 30s. Five patterns of psoriatic arthritis have been described: distal interphalangeal (DIP) joint arthritis, asymmetric

Table 2

Patterns of Psoriatic Arthritis

Type	Diagnostic Pattern	Commonly Affected Joints
DIP joint	Nail involvement common (5% to 10% of patients)	DIP
Asymmetric oligoarthritis	Fewer than 5 joints affected, dactylitis	Hands, feet
Symmetric polyarthritis	Similar to rheumatoid arthritis, but DIP joint involvement and negative rheumatoid factor	Hands, wrist, ankles, feet
Arthritic mutilans	Osteolysis at joint	DIP
Sacroiliitis	Asymmetric vertebral involvement	Sacroiliac

DIP = distal interphalangeal.

oligoarthritis, symmetric polyarthritis, arthritic mutilans, and sacroiliitis (**Table 2**). DIP joint involvement and the absence of rheumatoid nodules differentiates symmetric polyarthritis from rheumatoid arthritis.

Arthritis Associated With Inflammatory Bowel Disease

Arthritis associated with inflammatory bowel disease occurs in patients with ulcerative colitis or Crohn disease. The incidence is 10% to 20% and is more common in patients with Crohn disease. The HLA-B27 antigen is present in 50% to 70% of these patients.

Clinical Symptoms

Back pain may be the presenting symptom in all seronegative spondyloarthropathies, particularly in young men with ankylosing spondylitis. With ankylosing spondylitis, patients report nocturnal back pain and morning stiffness that is relieved by activity and leaning forward.

Patients with reactive arthritis report pain in the large joints of the lower extremity. Joint involvement is typically an asymmetric oligoarthritis involving the large joints of the lower extremity. Other musculoskeletal manifestations include enthesitis of the Achilles tendon or plantar fascia, dactylitis (also known as sausage digit, that is, swelling of an entire toe or finger), and sacroiliitis. Conjunctivitis and nongonococcal urethritis commonly develop. Other associated lesions include iritis and cutaneous ulcerations. Reactive arthritis commonly resolves in 3 to 4 months, but up to 50% of patients experience recurrent symptoms lasting years.

DIP joint pain associated with scaly, cutaneous lesions is the usual clinical presentation of psoriatic arthritis. Skin disease usually, but not always, precedes joint symptoms. Patients with joint problems

SECTION 1 GENERAL ORTHOPAEDICS

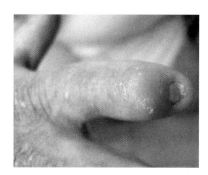

Figure 2 Photograph of the finger of a patient with psoriatic arthritis. Note the pitting, ridging, and oncolysis of the nail.

commonly have nail disorders, including pitting, ridging, and oncolysis (**Figure 2**).

Sacroiliitis, spondylitis, and arthritis of the knee and ankle are common in patients with arthritis that is associated with inflammatory bowel disease. Peripheral arthritis symptoms usually worsen during gastrointestinal flares, but the spondylitis symptoms typically do not.

Enthesitis, particularly at the Achilles tendon insertion, and extraskeletal manifestations, such as iritis, conjunctivitis, and urethritis, are common manifestations in patients with seronegative spondyloarthropathies.

Tests
Physical Examination
With ankylosing spondylitis, limited spinal motion is common. A 15-cm span should be measured in the midline distally from the posterior iliac spine (dimples of Venus) to the upper lumbar region. Then the patient should flex (lean forward) as much as possible. The distance between the two points should increase by 5 to 7 cm. With ankylosing spondylitis, spinal motion is limited, and the skin distraction on forward flexion is decreased. The FABER maneuver (flexion, abduction, and external rotation of the hip) places stress across the sacroiliac joint; patients with sacroiliitis have increased pain with this maneuver. The patient's hands must be examined carefully for swelling, inflammation, and nail abnormalities. The patient should be examined as well for enthesitis, particularly of the lower extremity.

Diagnostic Tests
Laboratory Tests
Although many of these patients are positive for the HLA-B27 antigen, the test for this antigen is relatively expensive and usually is not needed to make the diagnosis. The erythrocyte sedimentation rate and C-reactive protein level are inconsistently elevated during acute episodes. Rheumatoid factor and antinuclear antibody tests are negative. A detailed history and physical examination are more important than laboratory testing.

Radiographs
Resorption of terminal phalanges and proliferative bone reaction are common radiographic findings in the DIP joints of patients with psoriatic arthritis. In diagnosing sacroiliitis, radiographs demonstrating narrowing of the sacroiliac joints can be helpful. With ankylosing spondylitis, early radiographic findings in the spine include squaring of the superior and anterior margins of the vertebral bodies, which is thought to be caused by enthesitis at the attachment of the anulus fibrosus onto the vertebral body. Later findings include ossification of the anterior longitudinal ligament of the spine and autofusion of the facet joints leading to the classic "poker spine." The spine may be fused along the entire length.

Differential Diagnosis

- Achilles tendinitis or plantar fasciitis (no associated symptoms)
- Degenerative disk disease (no associated symptoms, normal skin distraction on flexion of the spine)
- Rheumatoid arthritis (positive rheumatoid factor, peripheral joint involvement)

Adverse Outcomes of the Disease

Severe spinal deformity may occur in ankylosing spondylitis. End-stage arthritis may affect the peripheral joints. Uveitis with visual impairment may occur. Occasionally, carditis may cause aortic insufficiency in patients with ankylosing spondylitis.

Treatment

NSAIDs, particularly indomethacin, are effective in controlling symptoms in many patients with seronegative spondyloarthropathies. Tumor necrosis factor-α (TNF-α) inhibitors, such as etanercept, infliximab, and adalimumab, are administered to patients with ankylosing spondylitis when symptoms are not controlled by NSAIDs. Regular exercise is important, particularly for patients with ankylosing spondylitis. An occasional patient may require a spinal osteotomy for correction of deformity associated with ankylosing spondylitis. Treatment of the inciting genitourologic or gastrointestinal infection is imperative in the management of reactive arthritis. Sulfasalazine may be useful for chronic reactive arthritis. Both nonbiologic and biologic disease-modifying antirheumatic drugs (DMARDs) are effective in treating psoriatic arthritis. The dermatologic manifestations of psoriatic arthritis are often treated with phototherapy. Surgery (total joint arthroplasty) can provide relief for end-stage arthritic pain.

Adverse Outcomes of Treatment

NSAIDs can cause gastric, renal, or hepatic complications. In 2015, the FDA strengthened its warning linking NSAIDs with the risk of heart attack or stroke, even in the first weeks of use of an NSAID. Postoperative infection and/or loosening of total joint implants is possible, and heterotopic ossification can complicate total hip arthroplasty.

Referral Decisions/Red Flags

Patients with kyphosis, pain at rest, or pain at night in a weight-bearing joint may benefit from orthopaedic evaluation. Accompanying problems with the eyes, skin, or pulmonary system may require referral to an ophthalmologist, dermatologist, or pulmonologist.

Compartment Syndrome

Definition

A muscle compartment is defined as a group of one or more muscles and their associated nerves and vessels surrounded by fascia that is relatively unyielding. Compartment syndrome occurs when intracompartmental pressure exceeds vascular perfusion pressure, leading to ischemia of the muscles, nerves, and vessels in the closed fibro-osseous space. Historically, an absolute compartment pressure of 35 mm Hg was thought to be diagnostic of acute compartment syndrome. Currently, perfusion pressure (calculated by subtracting the compartment pressure from the diastolic pressure to determine the ΔP value) of 20 mm Hg is diagnostic of acute compartment syndrome. Multiple etiologies of acute compartment syndrome exist. Trauma is the most common cause of acute compartment syndrome; other etiologies are burns, coagulopathies, snake bites, reperfusion syndrome, and unrelieved pressure necrosis. Extremity gunshot wounds are particularly susceptible to acute compartment syndrome, especially gunshot wounds at the level of the proximal fibula, where several arteries lie in close proximity.

There are multiple muscle compartments in the body, including the brachium, forearm, hand, gluteal compartment, thigh, tibia, and foot. The most common anatomic locations of acute compartment syndrome are the leg and the forearm. The leg has four compartments (**Figure 1**): anterior, lateral, superficial posterior, and deep posterior.

The forearm comprises three compartments (**Figure 2**): volar (flexors, pronators, supinators), dorsal (extensors), and mobile wad (brachioradialis, extensor carpi radialis longus, extensor carpi radialis brevis). The thigh has three compartments (**Figure 3**): medial, anterior, and posterior.

Chronic exertional compartment syndrome (CECS) occurs when muscle compartments are subjected to strenuous activity over a prolonged period, with resultant muscle edema and elevated compartment pressure. Diagnosis is made by measuring compartment pressures before and after exertion. CECS may develop in long-distance runners, new military recruits, or others involved in a major change in activity level. The pain associated with CECS usually diminishes with cessation of activity. So-called shin splints are a common complaint in adolescent athletes, and stress fractures and CECS should be ruled out. The differences in presentation, diagnosis, and management between acute compartment syndrome and CECS are outlined in **Table 1**.

As an acute compartment syndrome develops, the increased pressure in the compartments precipitates a cascade of physiologic events. As the pressure within the compartment approaches critical value (diastolic pressure), an increasing amount of muscle damage occurs, causing more swelling and increased compartment pressure and, subsequently, additional muscle necrosis. Animal studies and clinical observation indicate that muscles within a compartment

SECTION 1 GENERAL ORTHOPAEDICS

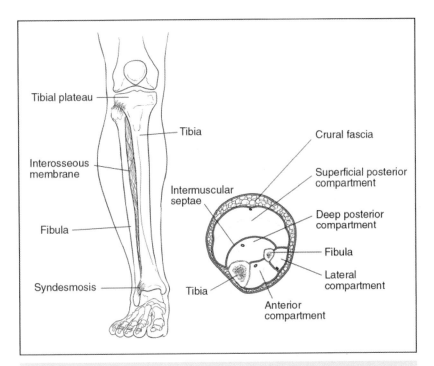

Figure 1 Illustration of the muscle compartments of the leg. These compartments are enveloped by strong septae. Swelling within a compartment increases the pressure on the nerves and compromises the perfusion of the muscles.

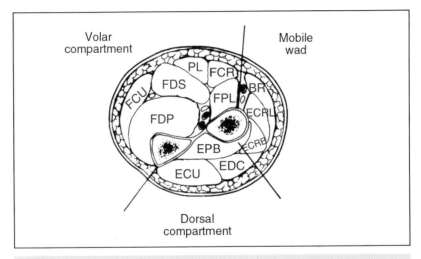

Figure 2 Illustration of the cross section of the midportion of the forearm shows the location of the various compartments. BR = brachioradialis, ECRB = extensor carpi radialis brevis, ECRL = extensor carpi radialis longus, ECU = extensor carpi ulnaris, EDC = extensor digitorum communis, EPB = extensor pollicis brevis, FCR = flexor carpi ulnaris, FCU = flexor carpi ulnaris, FDP = flexor digitorum profundus, FDS = flexor digitorum superficialis, FPL = flexor pollicis longus, PL = palmaris longus.

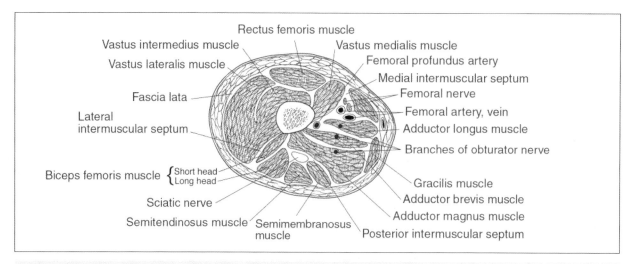

Figure 3 Illustration of a cross section of the left thigh, 10 to 15 cm distal to the inguinal ligament. Note the intermuscular fascial septae. (Reproduced from Fraipont MJ, Adamson GJ: Chronic exertional compartment syndrome. *J Am Acad Orthop Surg* 2003;11[4]:268-276.)

Table 1

Acute Compartment Syndrome Versus Chronic Exertional Compartment Syndrome

Parameter	Acute Compartment Syndrome	Chronic Exertional Compartment Syndrome
Mechanism	Usually traumatic	Overuse
Population	Any	Athlete
Area of body most commonly affected	Leg, forearm, thigh	Leg, forearm, thigh
Symptoms	7 Ps: pain, pallor, paresthesias, paresis, poikilothermia, pressure, pulselessness	Cramping, weakness, paresthesias
Diagnosis	Compartment pressures	Rest/exertional compartment pressures
Rest provides relief?	No	Yes
Treatment	Emergent fasciotomies	Elective fasciotomies
Permanent damage	Yes, if untreated	No
Notification	Immediate referral to surgeon	Nonurgent referral to surgeon's clinic

can withstand 4 hours of critical pressure without the occurrence of muscle necrosis. At 6 hours of critical pressure within a compartment, intermediate muscle damage occurs; however, this damage may be reversed by release of the compartment (fasciotomy). At 8 hours of critical pressure within a compartment, irreversible muscle necrosis occurs.

Acute compartment syndrome must be diagnosed and managed before irreversible muscle damage occurs. Failure to recognize an acute compartment syndrome can lead to serious sequelae, including muscle necrosis and joint contractures. Unrecognized and untreated acute compartment syndrome is a major source of medical malpractice claims.

Clinical Symptoms and Diagnostic Tests

The clinical diagnosis of acute compartment syndrome has traditionally utilized the "6 Ps": pain, pallor, paresthesias, paresis, poikilothermia (cool extremity distally), and pulselessness. Recently, some physicians have begun to consider pressure as the seventh "P." As with any clinical examination or test, reliability is dependent on the sensitivity (true positive rate) and specificity (true negative rate) of the test. The specificity of the 6 Ps is high (that is, most patients with acute compartment syndrome have the symptoms of the 6 Ps). The most specific test is pain out of proportion to what would normally be expected, especially pain with passive stretch of the muscles of the suspected compartment. Pulselessness and paresis are extremely late clinical findings. The sensitivity of the 6 Ps is low; multiple other clinical syndromes have similar physical findings. In general, the clinical assessment for acute compartment syndrome involves evaluation of the history, physical examination findings, and diagnostic tests. A history of known etiologies of acute compartment syndrome, such as trauma, coagulopathy, or rapid reperfusion for hypovolemia, should raise the index of suspicion for acute compartment syndrome. Restrictive dressings and splints should be removed. Palpation for so-called tight compartments is not completely accurate for acute compartment syndrome. Instead, the patient should be evaluated for the 6 Ps. The patient's medication record should be assessed for escalating analgesic usage. Nerve blocks for substantial pain should never be administered in clinical situations in which acute compartment syndrome is suspected.

In certain clinical situations, especially in obtunded patients from whom the history and physical findings cannot be obtained, compartment pressures can be measured directly. Historically, the Whitesides infusion technique was used to measure compartment pressure (**Figure 4**). However, the Whitesides technique has largely been replaced by other, more user-friendly techniques. One such technique uses an arterial line in which saline is used to return the measurement to zero before each subsequent compartment is measured. Other advances include handheld devices such as the one shown in **Figure 5**. Pressures should be measured in each suspected compartment within 5 cm of the level of injury, because studies have shown that the compartment pressure is highest at the level of injury. Ischemic damage begins when tissue pressure is within 10 to 20 mm Hg of the diastolic pressure. Compartment pressures should be measured to confirm the patient history and physical examination findings. Some general guidelines regarding when to measure compartment pressures are listed in **Table 2**. Emergent fasciotomy should be performed in cases of clinically significant pressures. Each compartment measurement indicates one moment in time, and sequential measurements may be necessary. Studies have been done

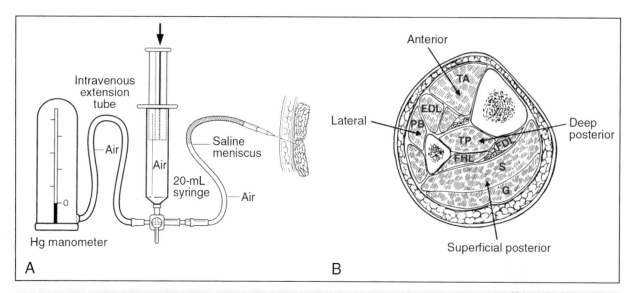

Figure 4 Illustration shows one manner of testing compartment pressure. **A,** The Whitesides infusion technique. **B,** Cross section of the proximal half of the leg shows the direction of needle insertion for testing each compartment. EDL = extensor digitorum longus, FDL = flexor digitorum longus, FHL = flexor hallucis longus, G = gastrocnemius, PB = peroneus brevis, S = soleus, TA = tibialis anterior, TP = tibialis posterior.

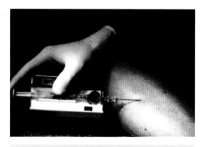

Figure 5 Photograph of an intracompartmental pressure monitoring system that is used to measure the pressure in the deep posterior compartment of the leg.

Table 2

Indications for Compartment Pressure Measurement

One or more symptoms of compartment syndrome with confounding factors (eg, neurologic injury, regional anesthesia, undermedication)

No symptoms other than increased firmness or swelling in the limb in an awake, alert patient receiving postoperative pain control

Unreliable or unobtainable examination with firmness or swelling in the injured extremity

Prolonged hypotension and a swollen extremity with equivocal firmness

Spontaneous increase in pain in the limb after receiving adequate pain control

(Reproduced from Olson SA, Glasgow RR: Acute compartment syndrome in lower extremity musculoskeletal trauma. *J Am Acad Orthop Surg* 2005;13[7]:436-444.)

on continuous monitoring of at-risk compartments by measuring the percentage of oxyhemoglobin in the compartment, thus monitoring perfusion rather than pressure.

In CECS, pressures are measured a variety of ways. The commonly accepted criteria for diagnosis are (1) a resting pressure measurement of 15 mm Hg or higher; a measurement of 30 mm Hg or higher obtained after 1 minute of exercise; or (3) a measurement of 20 mm Hg or higher obtained after 5 minutes of exercise. The differential diagnoses for CECS are listed in **Table 3**.

Table 3

Differential Diagnosis for Chronic Exertional Compartment Syndrome

Diagnosis	Findings	Confirmatory Studies
Stress fracture	Localized tenderness directly over the tibia; pain with torsional or bending stress	Plain radiograph, bone scan, MRI
Medial tibial stress syndrome (periostitis at the muscular attachment site along the posteromedial tibia)	Manual resistance to active plantar flexion and inversion leading to pain along the distal posteromedial aspect of the tibia; localized to diffuse tibial tenderness	Bone scan, MRI
Complex regional pain syndrome (reflex sympathetic dystrophy)	Allodynia and trophic skin changes	Three-phase bone scan, thermography, sympathetic block
Tenosynovitis of the ankle dorsiflexors or the posterior tibialis tendon	Tenderness along the extent of the tendon aggravated by flexion and extension maneuvers	MRI
Peripheral nerve entrapment syndromes	Tingling or numbness associated with a specific location (Tinel sign)	EMG, nerve conduction velocity study
Venous stasis disease	Trophic skin changes	Duplex ultrasonography
Deep vein thrombosis	Palpable cords or pain with plantar flexion; calf swelling	Duplex ultrasonography, venogram
Radiculopathy	Sensory losses, weakness	EMG, central nervous system evaluation
Arterial vascular disease	Pain, paresthesias, and coolness with activity; claudication	Ankle-brachial index
Popliteal artery entrapment syndrome	Pain and coolness; paradoxical claudication	Arteriogram

EMG = electromyogram.

(Reproduced from Fraipont MJ, Adamson GJ: Chronic exertional compartment syndrome. *J Am Acad Orthop Surg* 2003;11[4]:268-276.)

Differential Diagnosis

• Arterial injury (pulse deficit)
• Muscle contusion (local soft-tissue bleeding)

Adverse Outcomes of the Disease

Without immediate treatment, acute compartment syndrome may result in permanent loss of function. The muscles undergo necrosis, fibrosis, and shortening; fingers and toes are often clawed and have little motion. The wrist is held in flexion, and sensation is impaired. Late reconstructive surgery, usually involving tendon transfers, has little chance of restoring normal function.

Treatment

After a clinical diagnosis of acute compartment syndrome is made, emergent fasciotomies should be done. Fasciotomies of the leg can be done through either medial and lateral incisions or a single-incision perifibular approach. In the forearm, decompression is achieved either with a volar approach or with combined volar and dorsal approaches. The wounds are left open, supported by vessel loops or a wound vacuum, and delayed closure or skin grafting is performed after swelling subsides. Postfasciotomy pressures should be measured intraoperatively. So-called mini-incision fasciotomies should be avoided, because the skin has a small but clinically important contribution to compartment pressures.

Adverse Outcomes of Treatment

Treating an acute compartment syndrome with fasciotomy carries very little risk, except that the scar may be unsightly. Failure to perform a fasciotomy can be catastrophic for the patient.

Referral Decisions/Red Flags

Even a tentative diagnosis of compartment syndrome requires urgent evaluation so that surgical decompression by emergency fasciotomy can be considered. Surgery is indicated for the patient with CECS who is unwilling to modify or restrict provocative activities.

Complex Regional Pain Syndrome

Synonyms
Algodystrophy
Causalgia
Pain dysfunction syndrome
Reflex sympathetic dystrophy (RSD)
Shoulder-hand syndrome
Sudeck atrophy
Sympathetically maintained pain (SMP)

Definition
Complex regional pain syndrome (CRPS), also known as reflex sympathetic dystrophy (RSD), algodystrophy, and causalgia, is a clinical diagnosis composed of pain, autonomic dysfunction, trophic changes, and functional impairment. CRPS is classified as type 1 (RSD, algodystrophy) if there is no identifiable nerve injury or type 2 (causalgia) if an identifiable nerve lesion exists. CRPS, which is part of the spectrum of pain dysfunction syndromes, is characterized by pain that is generally out of proportion to what would be expected after the original injury or initiating event and that persists despite the absence of ongoing cellular damage or death. CRPS is the abnormal prolongation of normal postinjury physiologic responses and, in part, involves receptor dysfunction. It is a dynamic process that is initiated and manifested in the extremity but is affected by spinal cord and cortical events. The precise etiology of CRPS has not been defined, and no pathognomonic marker has been identified.

The worldwide incidence of CRPS is unknown; however, one report from Minnesota showed an incidence of 5.5 per 100,000 person years and a period prevalence of 20.7 per 100,000 residents. In the Netherlands, the incidence was 26.2 per 100,000 residents. Women are affected at a rate three to four times that of men, and smokers are at higher risk than nonsmokers. Individuals between ages 30 and 50 years are most likely to be affected; however, CRPS does occur at any age in children. No identifiable psychological profile or psychiatric disorder is linked causally to CRPS.

Although CRPS is classically associated with the upper extremity, the lower extremity is affected almost as often. Injuries that commonly precipitate CRPS include fracture of the distal radius and injury of the infrapatellar branch of the saphenous nerve; injury of the infrapatellar branch of the saphenous nerve occurs after contusion or arthroscopy. Up to 30% of patients have no apparent injury, indicating the seemingly innocuous nature of the events that may precipitate CRPS. A persistent and associated nociceptive focus—either neural or mechanical—is identifiable in less than 50% of patients. Early, appropriate treatment is important for the best prognosis. However, CRPS after fracture of the distal radius (in which poor finger function

3 months after the fracture correlates significantly with sequelae of CRPS [algodystrophy] after 10 years) is an exception. Anecdotal experience suggests that approximately 80% of patients who are diagnosed and treated within 1 year of injury experience substantial improvement. Similarly, 50% of patients for whom treatment is initiated later than 1 year after injury have substantial long-term morbidity. Some patients experience deterioration and manifest long-term disability despite early diagnosis and appropriate intervention.

Clinical Symptoms and Signs

The clinical presentation of CRPS varies from classic dystrophy to indolent forms. A delay in the onset of dystrophic pain is common. Classic symptoms of CRPS may not be present for 3 to 14 or more days after the initiating event, with progression of the affected area from localized to diffuse pain that involves the entire extremity. Patients with classic symptoms have difficulty sleeping, and narcotics provide incomplete pain relief. The injured body part and surrounding area are hot and/or swollen and allodynic and manifest autonomic dysfunction. In addition, temperature changes and abnormal sweat gland function compared with the contralateral extremity is common. Variant presentations are common, and classic staging with time intervals is often unreliable. The hallmark pain of CRPS is described as "burning," "tearing," "searing," and "throbbing;" this pain is associated with allodynia (pain caused by a normally nonpainful stimulus), hyperpathia (perception of pain that is delayed and extends beyond the normal nerve distribution), and hyperesthesia.

Signs associated with CRPS include abnormal vasomotor function, abnormal pseudomotor function, abnormal motor function or coordination, and trophic changes. Commonly noted findings of the skin are color changes, temperature asymmetry, and color asymmetry. Edema, abnormal (increased or decreased) sweating, and sweating asymmetry may occur. Stiffness, decreased range of motion, trophic changes, contracture weakness, tremor, dystonia, and functional impairment may occur. The Budapest criteria provide a standardized approach to diagnosis (**Tables 1** and **2**). In later or chronic presentations, pain, autonomic dysfunction, and functional impairment persist, and trophic changes are often obvious. Contractures are common, and the involved part of the extremity is often cool.

Tests/Instruments

The use of functional and health-related quality-of-life instruments such as the Disabilities of the Arm, Shoulder and Hand (DASH) questionnaire; the Rand 36-Item Health Survey; and the McGill Pain Questionnaire may be helpful for documenting symptoms in patients with CRPS.

Diagnostic Tests

Plain radiographs may show spotty areas of osteopenia or demineralization in the bones of the affected extremity. Three-phase

Table 1

International Association for the Study of Pain Diagnostic Criteria for Complex Regional Pain Syndrome (CRPS)[a]: Budapest Criteria

1. The presence of an initiating noxious event, or a cause if immobilization[b]
2. Continuing pain, allodynia, or hyperalgesia in which the pain is disproportionate to any known inciting event
3. Evidence at some time of edema, changes in skin blood flow, or abnormal sudomotor activity in the region of pain (can be a sign or a symptom)
4. This diagnosis is excluded by the existence of other conditions that would otherwise account for the degree of pain and dysfunction

[a] If seen without major nerve damage, diagnose CRPS I; if seen in the presence of "major nerve damage," diagnose CRPS II.

[b] Not required for diagnosis; 5% to 10% of patients will not have a known inciting event.

(Reproduced with permission from Harden RN, Bruehl S, Stanton-Hicks M, Wilson PR: Proposed new diagnostic criteria for complex regional pain syndrome. *Pain Med* 2007;8[4]:326-331.)

bone scans may show increased uptake in the extremity, especially in the third phase of the scan. Autonomic function may be evaluated with temperature and laser Doppler fluxometry measurements obtained after cold stress testing, quantitative sudomotor axon reflex testing (QSART), and sweat testing. Functional impairment may be quantified with endurance testing. Nutritional blood flow may be analyzed with vital capillaroscopy. Response to sympatholytic oral or injectable drugs should be evaluated to assess whether the patient has sympathetically maintained pain (SMP) or sympathetically independent pain (SIP). Pain relief after sympatholysis from intravenous phentolamine defines SMP, which has a more favorable prognosis than SIP. Similarly, a positive response to stellate block, other autonomic blocks, and/or oral agents supports the diagnosis and suggests SMP. It should be remembered, however, that CRPS is a dynamic process, and the pain of CRPS can change from SMP to SIP.

Differential Diagnosis
- Factitious syndromes (such as SHAFT—sad, hostile, anxious, factitious, tenacious syndrome; Munchausen syndrome); malingering (skin breakdown, unexplainable and massive edema, recurrent and mixed flora infections, abnormal posturing, spread to other areas beyond the affected extremity)
- Other neuropathic pain disorders (localized to the site of nerve damage)

Table 2

Budapest Clinical Diagnostic Criteria for Complex Regional Pain Syndrome

1. Continuing pain, which is disproportionate to any inciting event

2. Must report at least one symptom *in three of the four* following categories:
   - *Sensory:* reports of hyperesthesia and/or allodynia
   - *Vasomotor:* reports of temperature asymmetry and/or skin color changes and/or skin color asymmetry
   - *Sudomotor/edema:* reports of edema and/or sweating changes and/or sweating asymmetry
   - *Motor/trophic:* reports of decreased range of motion and/or motor dysfunction (weaknesses, tremor, dystonia) and/or trophic changes (hair, nails, skin)

3. Must display at least one sign at time of evaluation in *two or more* of the following categories:
   - *Sensory:* evidence of hyperalgesia (to pinprick) and/or allodynia (to light touch and/or deep somatic pressure and/or joint movement)
   - *Vasomotor:* evidence of temperature asymmetry and/or skin color changes and/or asymmetry
   - *Sudomotor/edema:* evidence of edema and/or sweating changes and/or sweating asymmetry
   - *Motor/trophic:* evidence of decreased range of motion and/or motor dysfunction (weakness, tremor, dystonia) and/or trophic changes (hair, nails, skin)

4. There is no other diagnosis that better explains the signs and symptoms

(Reproduced with permission from Harden RN, Bruehl S, Perez RS, et al: Validation of proposed diagnostic criteria [the "Budapest Criteria"] for complex regional pain syndrome. *Pain* 2010;150[2]:268-274.)

Adverse Outcomes of the Disease

Chronic, possibly debilitating, pain; joint contractures and stiffness; and skin and muscle atrophy may develop. Loss of function in the affected extremity, osteopenia, and delayed healing also may occur.

Treatment

Early recognition and prompt treatment of CRPS are crucial. Treatment includes rehabilitation, oral medications (**Table 3**), biofeedback, therapeutic modalities, parenteral medications, and surgery. Generally, several modalities are used simultaneously, starting with less invasive treatments and progressing to more invasive treatments if the response to the initial interventions is unsatisfactory. A prophylactic use of vitamin C (500 IU/d orally) has been demonstrated in randomized clinical trials to decrease the incidence of CRPS after fractures of the distal radius.

Table 3

Oral Medications Used to Treat Complex Regional Pain Syndrome

Drug	Usual Dosage	Mechanism	Major Short-term Disadvantage or Side Effects
Vitamin C	500 IU/d	Unknown	None
Amitriptyline hydrochloride	25 mg tid or 50 mg qhs	Inhibits amine pump–decreased norepinephrine reuptake	Drowsiness; should not be taken with guanethidine sulfate
Pregabalin (Lyrica [Pfizer])	50-200 mg tid	Antinociceptive-binding α-2 delta subunit, blocks calcium channels	Dizziness, somnolence, peripheral edema
Gabapentin (Neurontin [Pfizer])	300-600 mg tid	Blocks calcium channels	Dizziness, peripheral edema, asthenia
Fluoxetine (Prozac [Eli Lilly])	20 mg/d in the morning	Serotonin inhibitor	Minimal drowsiness
Phenytoin (Dilantin [Pfizer])	100 mg tid	Decreases resting membrane potential, inhibits amine pump, stabilizes synaptic membrane	Minimal drowsiness
Phenoxybenzamine hydrochloride (Dibenzyline [Wellspring Pharmaceuticals])	40-120 mg/d	α-1 receptor blocking agent	Orthostatic hypotension
Nifedipine (Procardia [Pfizer])	10 mg tid, may increase slowly to 30 mg tid	$Ca^{2}+$ channel blocking agent, prevents arteriovenous shunting, increases nutritional flow	Headache, postural hypotension
Amlodipine besylate (Norvasc [Pfizer])	5-10 mg qd	$Ca^{2}+$ channel blocking agent; prevents arteriovenous shunting; increases nutritional flow	Headache, postural hypotension
Corticosteroids	20-80 mg/d, prednisone equivalents × 5-40 days	Stabilizes membranes, increases nutritional flow, decreases inflammatory pain	Adrenal suppression, osteonecrosis (dose-related)

qd = once a day, qhs = before bed, tid = three times a day.

First-line treatment includes a combination of oral sympatholytic medications, rehabilitation with physical therapy or occupational therapy, counseling, and parenteral interventions. Although analgesics (nonnarcotic and narcotic) and NSAIDs treat pain resulting from underlying nociceptive insults and trauma, pharmacologic management of CRPS is designed to block sympatholytic events and/or improve nutritional blood flow. Pharmacologic management is accomplished with the use of multiple drug classes, most of which are not FDA-labeled for managing CRPS. Commonly used drug classes include antidepressants (tricyclic type preferred), antihypertensive agents, anticonvulsants, membrane stabilizers (steroid), and calcium channel blockers (α-2 agonists). Effective oral medications include prednisone, amitriptyline, gabapentin, pregabalin, phenytoin, amlodipine besylate, clonidine, and calcitonin. Two or more of these oral agents are commonly prescribed together.

Although therapy programs to manage CRPS include passive range of motion, they emphasize active range of motion, including stress loading. Frequently, adaptive modalities such as contrast baths, transcutaneous electrical nerve stimulation (TENS), or iontophoresis are used.

Psychological counseling may be helpful and often incorporates coping techniques and biofeedback to control the autonomic functions of the body that regulate sweating, skin temperature, and blood flow. Injections of corticosteroid and local anesthetic into trigger points also can provide transient pain relief; acupuncture has been reported to be helpful.

Bupivacaine may be used for stellate blocks. Continuous brachial plexus autonomic blocks may be used for diagnosis and/ or management of symptoms; they may also be curative in rare instances.

Continuous intrathecal administration of drugs such as clonidine (an α-2 agonist) and ziconotide (a snail venom that produces an N-type voltage-gated calcium channel blocker) are used as salvage treatments for refractory symptoms, as are dorsal column stimulators, brainstem stimulators, and other implanted central nervous system devices. Phenol or partial radiofrequency stellate ganglion interruption can provide palliative relief, but sympathetic nerve transection should be avoided to prevent receptor upregulation and potential late exacerbation of symptoms. Dorsal column stimulators may be beneficial in patients with chronic refractory symptoms.

In acute CRPS, identification and surgical management of associated nerve injury (compression or mechanical injury) is desirable. Perioperative continuous or intermittent autonomic blockade may be used to prevent dystrophic exacerbation if less invasive modalities are ineffective (**Figure 1**). The sequelae of CRPS, including compression neuropathy, neuroma in continuity, neuroma, mechanical pain as a result of initial injury, joint contractures, and deformity, can be managed surgically, using appropriate monitoring and pharmacologic management (such as postoperative medications or continuous block) as needed. Patients with CRPS can undergo surgical intervention throughout the dystrophic process to decrease pain caused by neurologic or mechanical mechanisms. Amputation usually is not effective and is best reserved to manage refractory infection.

Adverse Outcomes of Treatment

Side effects of treatment are minimal when the therapeutic modalities are used judiciously. Undertreatment is common. Serious side effects of stellate ganglion blocks, which include hoarseness, weakness,

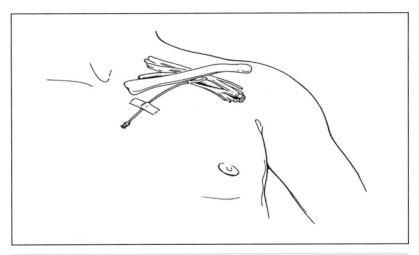

Figure 1 Illustration of the technique for administering continuous axillary or subclavian block. (Reproduced with permission from Koman LA, Poehling GG: Reflex sympathetic dystrophy, in Gelberman RH, ed: *Operative Nerve Repair and Reconstruction*. Philadelphia, PA, JB Lippincott, 1991, pp 1497-1523.)

numbness in the arm, pneumothorax, and possible seizures from vertebral artery injection, are infrequent and usually resolve uneventfully within a few hours. The use of narcotics may lead to addiction, and the excessive use of NSAIDs may result in gastric, hepatic, and renal symptoms. In 2015, the FDA strengthened its warning linking NSAIDs with the risk of heart attack or stroke, even in the first weeks of use of an NSAID. Fractures also may occur from too-vigorous manipulations during therapy sessions. Generally, amputation is contraindicated.

Referral Decisions/Red Flags
If symptoms fail to respond to initial sympatholytic pharmacologic and therapeutic treatments, consultation with a pain specialist should be considered. Additional evaluations performed at a center at which a multidisciplinary team is available to manage this difficult problem may be beneficial.

Concussion: Sports-Related

Definition

A concussion is a traumatic brain injury caused by a sudden blow to the head or to the body that causes the brain to come in contact with the inside of the skull. A concussion is typically characterized by the rapid onset of short-lived impairment of neurologic function. Neuropathologic changes may occur, but the acute symptoms reflect a functional disturbance rather than a structural injury.

Clinical Symptoms

Clinical symptoms associated with concussion include physical signs, behavioral changes, cognitive impairment, balance problems, and sleep disturbances. Several common symptoms and signs of concussion are listed in **Table 1**. Loss of consciousness may or may not occur with concussion. Symptoms should progressively decrease in the days after injury. In 80% to 90% of cases, symptoms completely resolve within 10 days after injury. Anyone who sustains a concussion should be closely monitored for the first few hours after injury. Signs and symptoms that may indicate a more serious head injury and warrant referral either to a physician who is trained in concussion management or to an emergency care facility are listed in **Table 2**.

Table 1

Signs and Symptoms of Concussion

Balance problems
Blurred vision
Confusion
Difficulty concentrating
Disorientation
Dizziness
Fatigue or low energy
Feeling as if one is "in a fog"
Feeling sluggish
Headache
Irritability
Lack of coordination/delayed response
Memory abnormalities
Nausea/vomiting
Neck pain
Nervousness or anxiety
Not "feeling right"
Personality change
Pressure in head
Ringing in ears
Seeing stars
Sensitivity to light
Sensitivity to noise
Sleep disturbances
Slurred speech

Table 2

Signs and Symptoms That Warrant Immediate Referral to a Physician Trained in Concussion Management or to an Emergency Care Facility

Loss of consciousness
Amnesia lasting longer than 15 minutes
Deterioration of neurologic function
Decreasing level of consciousness
Decrease or irregularity in pulse and/or respirations
Increase in blood pressure
Unequal, dilated, or unreactive pupils
Seizure
Symptoms that worsen over time
Vomiting

Essentials of Musculoskeletal Care 5   *© 2016 American Academy of Orthopaedic Surgeons*

Tests

Physical Examination

Steps in concussion management include evaluation on the field (in the case of sports-related injury), clinical examination, and cognitive evaluation. In the sports setting, an athlete with suspected concussion should be removed from activity and evaluated immediately. Standardized tests are readily available for assessment of concussion at the time of injury. These brief sideline tests assess attention, memory function, and balance. The tests can be administered by a physician or other licensed healthcare professional who is trained in concussion assessment. The Standardized Concussion Assessment Tool 3 (SCAT 3™) is one example of a sideline test for use in persons age 13 years and older. A child SCAT3 has been developed for persons younger than 13 years. An athlete who sustains a concussion should not be allowed to return to play until a comprehensive concussion evaluation has been conducted.

In the office setting, evaluation of a patient with suspected concussion should begin with a review of current symptoms—the symptoms the patient is experiencing, the severity of each symptom, and how the symptoms have changed since the initial injury. Concussion history and history of other relevant conditions (such as migraine or other headaches, mental dysfunctions, and learning disabilities) should be discussed. The evaluation should also include a thorough medical assessment and detailed neurologic examination.

Neuropsychologic testing can be done while the patient is recovering from concussion. Several computerized neuropsychologic screening tools exist. In some cases, an athlete may be administered baseline neuropsychologic testing for comparison to postinjury test results. Formal neuropsychologic testing is not required for all cases of concussion; however, it can be considered for persons with prolonged concussion symptoms or those with concurrent mental dysfunctions.

Diagnostic Tests

Typically, neuroimaging findings are normal in persons with concussion; thus, it is recommended that it be reserved for patients in whom severe skull or brain injury is suspected.

Differential Diagnosis

• Depression
• General trauma or injury to the body not involving the head
• Headache disorder
• Seizure disorder
• Severe/moderate traumatic brain injury

Adverse Outcomes of the Disease

Postconcussion syndrome, in which symptoms related to the concussion are present for weeks or months after the initial injury, may occur. Persons who sustain a concussion may have a lower

SECTION 1 | GENERAL ORTHOPAEDICS

Table 3

Gradual Progression of Return to Activity

Step	Description
1	No activity
2	Light aerobic exercise (walking, swimming, stationary cycling)
3	Sport-specific exercise (without head contact)
4	Noncontact training drills and weight lifting
5	Full-contact practice
6	Return to competition

threshold for subsequent concussions and may experience symptoms for a longer period of time after injury.

Treatment

If symptoms stabilize and do not worsen after a concussion occurs, daily monitoring of symptoms is recommended. Certain signs and symptoms warrant immediate referral to a physician who is experienced in concussion management or to an emergency care facility (**Table 2**). Regardless of concussion severity, an athlete who sustains a concussion should be evaluated by a physician who is experienced in concussion management before returning to play.

Treatment for concussion consists of physical and mental rest. Patients who sustain a concussion should not participate in any activity that exacerbates symptoms until all symptoms subside for at least 24 hours and medical clearance is granted. Patients should then proceed through a gradual, stepwise return to activity (**Table 3**). If concussion symptoms return during the return-to-activity process, exertional activity should cease until symptoms are absent for at least 24 hours, after which the process should resume at the stage at which symptoms developed. A slower, more conservative plan for return to activity should be considered for the child or adolescent athlete, as noted in the Concussion chapter in Pediatric Orthopaedics section.

Patients who sustain concussion also should be advised to take mental rest. Mental rest includes avoiding any activities that stimulate the visual or auditory senses, such as using a computer or smartphone or watching television, or being in environments that are bright or loud. For students, an excuse from class for multiple days after a concussion may be appropriate.

Pharmacologic treatment for a concussion can be used to manage symptoms. Drug treatment for headache should be avoided the first few hours after injury to prevent masking of worsening symptoms and of a possibly more severe injury.

Adverse Outcomes of Treatment

Patients who return to activity too soon after a concussion may risk prolonged concussion symptoms.

Referral Decisions/Red Flags

Patients who experience prolonged loss of consciousness, focal neurologic deficit, or worsening symptoms after concussion should be referred to an emergency care facility for further evaluation (**Table 2**). Patients who experience postconcussion symptoms that do not improve over time or who wish to return to high-risk or contact sports or activities after concussion should be referred to a physician who is experienced in concussion management.

Crystal Deposition Diseases

Synonyms
Calcium pyrophosphate crystal deposition disease
Calcium pyrophosphate deposition disease (CPDD)
Calcium pyrophosphate dihydrate crystal deposition disease
Gout
Podagra
Pseudogout

Definition
Crystal deposition disease is an arthritis characterized by abrupt episodes of severe joint pain and swelling, typically involving a single joint. The pain and swelling result from the lysis of polymorphonuclear cells triggered when these cells engulf crystals deposited in synovium, cartilage, and other tissues.

Gout
All patients with gout have hyperuricemia (elevated serum levels of uric acid), but not all patients with hyperuricemia have gout. Uric acid is a by-product of purine metabolism. Urine excretion levels are used to categorize patients as overproducers or underexcretors of uric acid. In certain patients with hyperuricemia, the excess monosodium urate crystals deposit in tissue, causing the inflammatory process of gout. Gout is relatively common, and its prevalence increases with age. The most frequent manifestation of gout is recurrent attacks of acute inflammatory arthritis, but the uric acid crystals may also be deposited in other tissues. Accumulation of urate crystals causes the formation of tophaceous deposits, or tophi (soft-tissue masses from urate crystal deposition noted several years after the onset of gout [**Figure 1**]), and renal manifestations, such as uric acid nephrolithiasis and chronic nephropathy.

Calcium Pyrophosphate Deposition Disease
Calcium pyrophosphate deposition disease (CPDD), which is caused by the precipitation of calcium pyrophosphate dihydrate (CPPD) crystals in connective tissues, has a wide spectrum of clinical manifestations. The clinical spectrum includes asymptomatic disease, pseudogout (**Table 1**), pseudorheumatoid arthritis, pseudo-osteoarthritis, and pseudoneuropathic joint disease. Most patients with radiographic evidence of crystal deposition resulting from CPDD are asymptomatic.

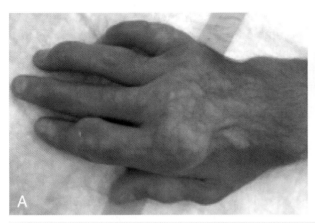 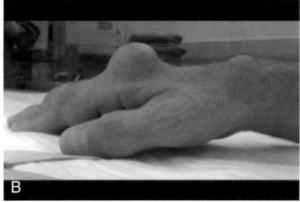

Figure 1 Dorsal (**A**) and lateral (**B**) photographs of tophi affecting the hand, primarily the metacarpophalangeal joints. (Reproduced from Fitzgerald BT, Setty A, Mudgal CS: Gout affecting the hand and wrist. *J Am Acad Orthop Surg* 2007;15[10]:625-635.)

Table 1

Characteristics of Crystal Deposition Diseases

Disease	Crystals	Arthritis	Commonly Affected Joints	Treatment
Gout	Monosodium urate monohydrate, negative birefringence	Acute monoarticular	First MTP joint, ankle, knee	Colchicine, indomethacin, NSAIDs, allopurinol
Pseudogout	Calcium pyrophosphate, positive birefringence	Acute monoarticular or oligoarticular	Knee, wrist	Joint aspiration, intra-articular steroids, NSAIDs

MTP = metatarsophalangeal.

Clinical Symptoms

Gout

Acute gouty arthritis, interval gout, and chronic tophaceous gout represent three stages of progressive urate crystal deposition. Acute gouty arthritis occurs after years of asymptomatic hyperuricemia. At least 80% of initial attacks involve a single joint. The metatarsophalangeal joint of the great toe is most commonly affected (podagra), accounting for approximately 50% of the initial episodes of gouty arthritis. Other frequent sites of involvement include the ankle, the tarsal joints, and the knee. Gout can occur in the spine and sacroiliac joints, as well, although those presentations are much less common than is peripheral involvement. Most proven cases of gouty back pain have been associated with the tophaceous type.

Patients with acute gouty arthritis report severe pain, redness, and swelling in the affected joint, with maximal severity of symptoms reached over several hours. The overlying erythema may be confused with cellulitis or a septic joint. During the acute event, serum uric acid concentrations are often normal or low. After resolution of the acute attack, patients are often asymptomatic for a variable period of time, with most patients experiencing another attack within

2 years. Tophi develop in only approximately 5% of patients who are compliant with antihyperuricemic therapy. Tophi can develop in many locations, including the olecranon bursa, the extensor surface of the forearm, the Achilles tendon, or the tendon sheaths in the hand. Tophi may be confused with rheumatoid nodules.

Calcium Pyrophosphate Deposition Disease
CPDD commonly affects patients older than 65 years. It is characterized by acute or subacute attacks of arthritis and radiographic evidence of CPPD crystal deposition. Chondrocalcinosis is the calcification of articular cartilage or menisci caused by deposition of CPPD crystals. Most patients with chondrocalcinosis are asymptomatic or have only mild arthritic symptoms. This disorder is more common in women and increases with age, affecting approximately one half of the population older than 80 years.

Patients with pseudogout experience acute or subacute attacks of arthritis, usually in one joint. The knee joint is affected in more than 50% of patients, and CPPD crystals are found on examination of synovial fluid aspirate.

Progressive joint degeneration in a pattern similar to osteoarthritis affects 50% of patients with symptomatic CPDD. The knees are the most commonly affected joints, followed by the wrist, metacarpophalangeal joints, hips, shoulders, elbows, and spine. Evidence of CPPD crystals in synovial fluid and radiographic evidence of CPPD crystal deposition help distinguish this clinical entity from osteoarthritis. Approximately half of the patients experience intermittent acute inflammatory attacks similar to pseudogout.

CPPD arthropathy may be confused with rheumatoid arthritis (RA), but patients with CPPD do not have bony erosions or other features of RA, such as tenosynovitis. CPDD crystal deposition has been associated with severe neuropathic joint degeneration, but patients with severe neuropathic joint degeneration typically present with underlying conditions such as diabetes mellitus or tabes dorsalis.

Tests
Physical Examination
In both gout and pseudogout, examination of the affected joint reveals marked tenderness to palpation, swelling, erythema, and limited motion.

Diagnostic Tests
Laboratory serum analysis for calcium, phosphorous, magnesium, alkaline phosphatase, ferritin, iron, transferrin, and thyroid-stimulating hormone are performed to screen for gout and pseudogout.

Gout
The clinical picture of acute gouty arthritis is similar to that of acute septic arthritis. Common findings include fever with accompanying leukocytosis and an elevated erythrocyte sedimentation rate. Serum

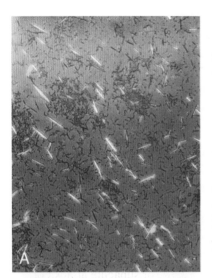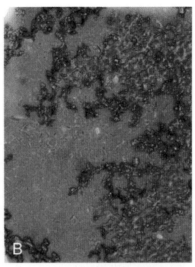

Figure 2 **A,** Microscopic image of monosodium urate crystals as seen under polarized light. These crystals are characteristic of gout and are found in the fluid of the inflamed joint and in other affected tissues. **B,** Microscopic image of birefringent rhomboid-shaped calcium pyrophosphate crystals, which are characteristic of pseudogout. (Courtesy of Ann Faber, photographer.)

uric acid levels should be checked; however, these levels may be normal during an acute episode. Joint aspiration and analysis of synovial fluid with white blood cell count, Gram stain, and culture are critical in distinguishing gout from septic arthritis. Ultrasonography of joints and adjacent soft tissues is useful for guiding fluid aspiration and can aid in identifying urate crystal deposition. Examination of joint fluid under polarized microscopy reveals the characteristic negatively birefringent urate crystals (**Figure 2**). Early in the disease, radiographs are normal except for soft-tissue swelling. Radiographs of established gout are characterized by subchondral bony erosions and peripheral articular spurs (**Figure 3**).

Calcium Pyrophosphate Deposition Disease
Patients with acute CPDD inflammatory arthritis present with a clinical picture similar to that of an acute gout attack, hence the name pseudogout. Common findings include fever with accompanying leukocytosis and an elevated erythrocyte sedimentation rate. Joint aspiration and synovial fluid analysis with cell count, Gram stain, culture, and polarized microscopy help distinguish this clinical entity from gout or a septic joint. CPPD crystals in synovial fluid appear as weakly positive, birefringent rhomboid-shaped crystals (**Figure 2, B**). The deposition of CPPD crystals in soft tissues can cause chondrocalcinosis, which is visualized on radiographs as punctate or linear calcification of articular cartilage and internal joint structures, such as menisci in the knee or the triangular fibrocartilage in the wrist (**Figure 4**). Some metabolic disorders, such as hyperparathyroidism, hemochromatosis, hypophosphatasia, and hypothyroidism, are associated with CPPD.

SECTION 1 GENERAL ORTHOPAEDICS

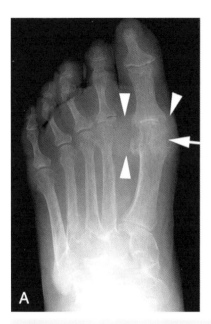
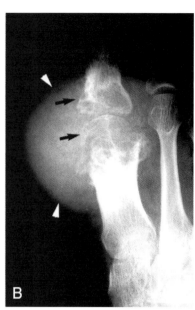

Figure 3 **A,** AP radiograph of the foot of a patient with gout. Note the erosions with sharp margins, the overhanging edge in the metatarsophalangeal joint of the great toe (arrow), and a soft-tissue mass around the first metatarsal consistent with a deposit of sodium urate (arrowheads). **B,** AP radiograph of the great toe of a patient with advanced gout. The black arrows indicate large, well-marginated erosions on both sides of the metatarsophalangeal joint, and the white arrowheads indicate a large soft-tissue mass. These findings are consistent with advanced gout. (Reproduced from Johnson TR, Steinbach LS, eds: *Essentials of Musculoskeletal Imaging.* Rosemont, IL, American Academy of Orthopaedic Surgeons, 2004, p 627.)

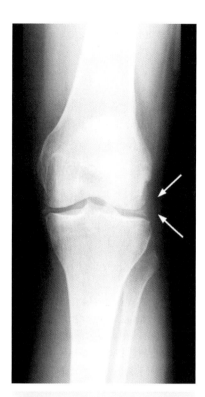

Figure 4 AP radiograph of the knee of a 48-year-old patient with pseudogout. The crystals in the meniscal cartilage demonstrate the linear calcifications characteristic of chondrocalcinosis (arrows).

Differential Diagnosis

- Cellulitis (joint not involved and motion only mildly affected by overlying skin infection)
- Lyme disease (chronic fatigue, memory loss, history of rash, immunoglobulin M [IgM] or immunoglobulin G [IgG] antibody titer)
- Neuropathic arthropathy (underlying neurologic disorder such as diabetes, insignificant pain)
- Osteoarthritis (less acute, pain proportionate to activity)
- RA (younger age, multiple joints involved, associated tenosynovitis)
- Septic arthritis (severe pain, systemic signs, positive Gram stain and culture)
- Trauma (history, hemarthrosis, or fracture)

Adverse Outcomes of the Disease

Before effective control of hyperuricemia was common, the development of tophi and chronic gouty arthritis was the expected course. Chronic hyperuricemia also leads to nephropathy and renal stones. End-stage arthritis may occur with CPPD, but this is infrequent.

Treatment

Gout

Treatment of acute episodes of gout should focus on relieving pain and inflammation. NSAIDs are first-line agents. Indomethacin is a commonly used NSAID; it is dosed at 50 mg every 8 hours until symptoms subside. Naproxen 500 mg twice daily has yielded similar relief. The use of oral NSAIDs is limited in patients with gastrointestinal complications. NSAIDs are most effective when treatment is initiated within 48 hours of the onset of symptoms.

Colchicine is a second-line agent in treating acute gouty arthritis because side effects such as nausea, diarrhea, and bone marrow suppression often limit administration of therapeutic doses. Oral glucocorticoids are also second-line agents and should be used cautiously in patients with diabetes mellitus. Intra-articular corticosteroid injections can be used to manage acute gout in a single joint. The goal of long-term management of gout is to limit hyperuricemia using drugs such as probenecid and allopurinol. Probenecid increases the urinary excretion of uric acid and should not be administered to patients with renal insufficiency. Allopurinol is a xanthine oxidase inhibitor that decreases production of uric acid in purine metabolism. Allopurinol should not be used in the acute setting because it can exacerbate symptoms.

Calcium Pyrophosphate Deposition Disease

Joint aspiration serves both a diagnostic and therapeutic role in pseudogout. Joint aspiration is commonly followed by intra-articular corticosteroid injections if one or two joints are involved. Oral NSAIDs or colchicine are administered during acute attacks if multiple joints are affected. Short-term joint immobilization plays a role in reducing pain and inflammation. In patients who have experienced three or more attacks of pseudogout, prophylaxis with colchicine has yielded decreased frequency of subsequent attacks.

Adverse Outcomes of Treatment

NSAIDs can interfere with drugs used concomitantly to control hypertension and often produce gastrointestinal side effects. In 2015, the FDA strengthened its warning linking NSAIDs with the risk of heart attack or stroke, even in the first weeks of use of an NSAID. Complications of corticosteroid use include osteonecrosis, osteoporosis, glaucoma, and elevated blood glucose levels.

Referral Decisions/Red Flags

Joint deformity or destruction, large tophaceous masses, or drainage of tophaceous material may require surgical attention.

Deep Vein Thrombosis

Table 1

Risk Factors for Deep Vein Thrombosis

Major musculoskeletal injuries (especially pelvic fractures) or surgery

Polytrauma

Immobilization

Malignancy

Obesity

Smoking

Estrogen replacement or use of oral contraceptives

Spinal cord injury

History of deep vein thrombosis

Inherited thrombophilia

Myeloproliferative disease

Inflammatory bowel disease

Diabetes

Congestive heart disease

Stroke

Synonym

Venous thromboembolism (VTE)

Definition

Deep vein thrombosis (DVT) is a cause of substantial morbidity and mortality, and pulmonary embolism (PE), a direct result of venous thrombosis, is responsible for between 60,000 and 100,000 deaths per year in the United States. Pulmonary emboli, which have been estimated to be the cause of 5% to 10% of all hospital deaths, are the most preventable cause of in-hospital deaths and are the third overall cause of death in polytrauma patients. The etiologies of DVT are venous stasis, intimal damage to the vein, and a hypercoagulable state (Virchow triad). Certain intraoperative and postoperative factors and conditions predispose patients to DVT. Intraoperatively, the supine position as well as various surgical positions (such as abduction, internal rotation and flexion of the hip during hip arthroplasty) cause venous stasis and intimal damage of the veins. General anesthesia causes vasodilatation and stasis, and the release of bioactive substances such as histamines and leukotrienes during surgery may cause venous stasis and endothelial damage to the veins. A hypercoagulable state, which is a risk factor for DVT, can be caused by a genetic abnormality. In addition, decreased levels of antithrombin III have been noted after total joint arthroplasty, with resultant impaired modulation of the clotting cascade, which leads to venous stasis and DVT.

Clinical Symptoms

It has been estimated that two thirds of clinically significant cases of DVT go unrecognized. The most important factor in recognizing DVT is an understanding of who is at risk for it (**Table 1**).

The American College of Chest Physicians stratified the risk of DVT based on type of surgical procedure. High-risk surgeries such as total joint arthroplasties or internal fixation of hip fracture and those involving polytrauma or spinal cord injuries carry a 40% to 80% risk of DVT in the absence of adequate prophylaxis. Clinically, an edematous, painful limb is indicative of DVT. DVT is much more common in the lower extremity than the upper extremity. Pain on stretch of the limb, such as Homan sign in the lower extremity, is suggestive of DVT. Postoperatively, an unexplained fever or leukocytosis can be indicative of DVT. A PE resulting from DVT clinically presents with tachycardia, tachypnea, chest pain, and occasional hemoptysis.

Diagnostic Tests

The use of screening tests for DVT in asymptomatic patients in high-risk groups (that is, polytrauma, postoperative) has not been recommended. In patients in whom DVT is suspected (such as an edematous limb), venography has been the standard diagnostic test. Ultrasound is increasingly being used to rule out DVT. In patients with suspected PE, initial evaluation findings of right-sided stress or tachycardia on electromyography, low oxygen saturation levels, and infiltrate on a chest radiograph are all suggestive of PE. CT scan of the chest has supplanted CT scan of the lungs as the definitive test for diagnosing PE. In general, screening tests for inherited thrombophilia (**Table 2**) are not indicated unless the patient has a personal history of recurrent idiopathic DVTs or substantial family history of DVT.

Treatment
Prophylaxis
Most DVTs and PEs are clinically silent, and it is difficult to know in which patients they will be symptomatic. Trying to identify at-risk individuals with a physical examination and screening modalities has been largely ineffective. The cost of treating the sequelae of venous thromboembolism (VTE) is substantial, and each event carries with it an increased risk of recurrent disease and its sequelae (chronic postthrombotic syndrome). The ultimate goal of prophylaxis is to prevent a symptomatic PE, which is the end point of research in the orthopaedic literature.

Most patients who die as a result of a PE do so within 30 minutes of the acute event, which is too soon for therapeutic anticoagulation to be effective or interventional radiologic catheter-based measures to begin. Consequently, prevention of PE depends on prevention of lower extremity thromboses. General agreement exists that patients undergoing total hip or knee arthroplasty and polytrauma patients (including those with spinal injuries) require DVT prophylaxis. Despite extensive research, however, controversy remains regarding the best regimen. The ideal prophylactic regimen would be practical, easy to use, and cost effective, would have no side effects, and would require no monitoring. Unfortunately, this regimen does not exist. Anticoagulants require constant balancing of the risk of clots against the risk of bleeding. Most orthopaedic surgeons' practices are based on the literature concerning arthroplasty procedures. American Academy of Orthopaedic Surgeons' guidelines for the prevention of symptomatic PE, published in *Preventing Venous Thromboembolic Disease in Patients Undergoing Elective Hip and Knee Arthroplasty*, are available at http://www.aaos.org/research/guidelines/VTE/VTE_full_guideline.pdf. Current guidelines for venous prophylaxis in orthopaedics are listed in **Table 3**.

The current mainstays of prophylaxis include parenteral heparin (including low-molecular-weight heparin [LMWH] formulations), fondaparinux, oral warfarin, and aspirin. Desirudin, a hirudin derivative, is approved by the FDA for VTE prevention. Many more medications are in various stages of development, including oral heparin and direct and indirect inhibitors of factors IIa, IXa, and Xa. Zontivity (Merck) has recently been approved by the FDA, and other medications for VTE prevention are in development. The

Table 2

Increased Risk of Thromboembolism Associated With Factors of Inherited Thrombophilia

Disorder	Risk
Factor V Leiden mutation	
Heterozygous	7×
Homozygous	80×
Protein C deficiency	2-10×
Protein S deficiency	2-10×
Hyperhomocystein-emia	2.5×
Elevated factor VIII	5×
Elevated factor XI	2.2×

Table 3

Current Guidelines for Venous Prophylaxis in Orthopaedics

Source	Guidelines
Orthopaedic Trauma Association[a]	Major orthopaedic surgery LMWH is considered the agent of choice and should be initiated within 24 hr provided there are no contraindications (Strong) Combined LMWH and calf pneumatic compressive devices over either regimen alone (Strong) Continuation of VTE prophylaxis for at least 1 mo after discharge (Limited) Recommend against routine screening protocols for DVT in asymptomatic trauma patients (Strong) Isolated lower extremity injury Do not recommend routine chemical prophylaxis in patients who do not have additional risk factors and are independently mobile (Moderate) Recommend against routine screening protocols for DVT in asymptomatic trauma patients (Strong)
American College of Chest Physicians[b]	Major orthopaedic surgery Extend outpatient prophylaxis for up to 35 d postop (2B) Dual prophylaxis with pharmacologic agent and IPCD while inpatient (2C) Recommend against screening Doppler ultrasonography before discharge (1B) Hip fracture surgery Prophylaxis for a minimum of 10-14 d (1B) Start LMWH either 12 h or more preop or 12 h or more postop (1B) Recommend use of LMWH, fondaparinux, LDUH, adjusted-dose aspirin (1B) or IPCD (1C) LMWH is preferred to other agents (2B/2C) Isolated lower extremity injury No prophylaxis in patients who require leg immobilization (2C)
American Academy of Orthopaedic Surgeons[c]	Elective total joint arthroplasty Pharmacologic agents and/or mechanical compressive devices for VTE prevention for those who are not at elevated risk (Moderate) No specific agent recommended (Inconclusive) Patients and physicians discuss duration of treatment (Consensus)

characteristics of some of the most commonly used medications in DVT prevention are listed in **Table 4**.

Enoxaparin is the most commonly used LMWH for hip and knee arthroplasty. Enoxaparin and heparin are both frequently used in the setting of polytrauma or long-bone fractures. Enoxaparin is renally cleared, so heparin may be a better choice in patients with underlying renal insufficiency.

Oral warfarin is the agent most commonly used for anticoagulation. Studies indicate that an international normalized ratio (INR) of

Table3 (Continued)

Current Guidelines for Venous Prophylaxis in Orthopaedics

Source	Guidelines
Eastern Association for the Surgery of Trauma[d]	LDH has little proven efficacy in prevention of VTE as sole agent in high-risk trauma patients (Level II)
	IPCD may have some benefit in isolated studies (Level III)
	LMWH can be used in trauma patients with pelvic fractures, complex lower extremity fractures, and spinal cord injury when bleeding risk is acceptable (Level II)
	IVCF should be considered in very high-risk trauma patients who cannot receive pharmacologic prophylaxis or have an injury pattern that would leave them immobilized for long periods of time (Level III)
	Duplex ultrasonography may be used to diagnose symptomatic patients with suspected DVT without venography (Level I)
Cochrane Review	No evidence that prophylaxis reduces mortality or secondary outcome of pulmonary embolus
	Pharmacologic prophylaxis is more effective than mechanical prophylaxis
	LMWH is more effective than UH
	Insufficient studies for comparison between pharmacologic agents vs placebo or pharmacologic prophylaxis vs mechanical prophylaxis

DVT = deep vein thrombosis, IPCD = intermittent pneumatic compression devices, IVCF = inferior vena cava filter, LDH = low-dose heparin, LDUH = low-dose unfractionated heparin, LMWH = low-molecular-weight heparin, UH = unfractionated heparin, VTE = venous thromboembolism.

[a]OTA recommendation strengths: Strong = greater than two high-quality (level I) studies to support the recommendation; Moderate: one high-quality (level I) or two moderate-quality (level II or III) studies to support the recommendation; Limited = one moderate-quality (level II or III) or two low-quality (level IV) studies to support the recommendation; Inconclusive = one low-quality (level IV) study or lack of evidence to support the recommendation; Consensus = expert work-group opinion (no studies)

[b]American College of Chest Physicians recommendation strengths: 1B = strong recommendation, moderate-quality evidence, benefits clearly outweigh risk and burdens or vice versa; 1C = strong recommendation, low-quality or very low–quality evidence, benefits clearly outweigh risks and burdens or vice versa; 2B = weak recommendation, moderate-quality evidence, benefits closely balanced with risks and burdens; 2C = weak recommendation, low-quality or very low–quality evidence, uncertainty in the estimates of benefits, risks, and burdens; benefits, risk, and burden may be closely balanced

[c]American Academy of Orthopaedic Surgeons recommendation strengths: Consensus = expert opinion supports the guideline even though there is no available empirical evidence that meets the inclusion criteria of the guideline's systematic review; Strong = benefits of the recommended approach clearly exceed the potential harm and the quality of supporting evidence is high; Moderate = the benefits exceed the potential harm but the quality/applicability of the supporting evidence is not strong; Inconclusive = lack of compelling evidence that has resulted in an unclear balance between benefits and potential harm

[d]Eastern Association for the Surgery of Trauma recommendation strengths: Level I recommendation = convincingly justifiable on the basis of scientific information alone through class I data; Level II recommendation = reasonably justifiable on the basis of a preponderance of class II data; Level III recommendation = supported only by class III data; Class I data = prospective randomized controlled trial; Class II data = clinical study with prospectively collected data or large retrospective analyses with reliable data; Class III data = retrospective data, expert opinion, or a case report

(Reproduced from Scolaro JA, Taylor RM, Wigner NA: Venous thromboembolism in orthopaedic trauma. *J Am Acad Orthop Surg* 2015;23[1]:1-6.)

Table 4

Characteristics of Some Common Pharmacologic Prophylactic Agents

Medication	Mechanism of Action	Advantages	Disadvantages
Heparin (including LMWH)	Activation of antithrombin III	Can be used in patients with renal insufficiency	Risk of bleeding; can lead to HIT; can cause hyperkalemia; can cause elevation in serum aminotransferase levels
Dabigatran (Pradaxa)	Direct thrombin inhibitor	Can be used in patients with a history of or at risk for HIT; monitoring usually not required	Risk of bleeding; requires renal monitoring
Enoxaparin (Lovenox [Sanofi], Clexane [Sanofi])	Activation of antithrombin III	Rapid onset; linear pharmacokinetics; little variability among patients; monitoring not required; practical for outpatient use; can be dosed every 12 or 24 h	High cost; risk of bleeding (intraoperative and postoperative); use prohibited with epidural catheters; renally cleared
Warfarin (Coumadin [Bristol-Myers Squibb])	Inhibits vitamin K–dependent carboxylation of factors II, VII, IX, X, protein C, and protein S	Proved efficacy; oral administration; effects reversed using vitamin K	Requires outpatient monitoring; low but real risk of bleeding; possibly inferior to LMWH for primary thrombosis prevention; Warfarin alone not sufficient for clot prevention; multiple drug and dietary interactions
Aspirin (ASA)	Inhibits platelet aggregation via inhibition of COX-1 and thus production of thromboxane A_2	Inexpensive; easy to take; monitoring not required; safe; combats heterotopic ossification	Efficacy inferior to LMWH, warfarin; no rapid reversal, as this is a permanent inhibition of COX-1
Fondaparinux (Arixtra [GlaxoSmithKline])	Factor Xa inhibitor	Effectively prevents VTE; lower risk of HIT	Risk of major bleeding; risk of thrombocytopenia

ASA = acetylsalicylic acid, COX = cyclooxygenase, HIT = heparin-induced thrombocytopenia, LMWH = low-molecular-weight heparin, VTE = venous thromboembolism.

2.0 to 2.5 is associated with the lowest bleeding risk while maintaining efficacy. Warfarin alone is not sufficient for clot prevention, and it has been shown to be more effective in preventing proximal clots than distal ones in patients undergoing total hip arthroplasty.

Aspirin, although inferior in effectiveness to LMWH and warfarin, may be effective if combined with mechanical prophylaxis.

Mechanical prophylaxis reduces VTE disease secondary to increased fibrinolysis and decreasing stasis with accelerated venous emptying. Foot, calf, and calf/thigh pumps are the three basic devices. They work using pneumatic compression, sequential inflation, or rapid inflation. Elastic stockings are useful as well. The stockings or other mechanical devices should be applied preoperatively, intraoperatively, and postoperatively. Mechanical devices have very low complication rates. Patient compliance can be a problem, however, so the modality that the patient will be most compliant with should be used. Mechanical devices should be used as an adjunct to pharmacologic prophylaxis.

Procoagulant medication should be discontinued before admission. Autologous blood donation is encouraged because it has been proven to substantially reduce the prevalence of DVT in total hip and knee arthroplasty. Regional anesthesia decreases blood loss and the rate of DVT. A surgical time of less than 70 minutes decreases the rate of DVT in patients undergoing total knee arthroplasty, and a single, intraoperative dose of unfractionated heparin may do so in patients undergoing total hip arthroplasty. The effect of early hospital discharge on the duration of prophylaxis and the prevalence of symptomatic thromboembolism following discharge is unclear.

The standard inpatient regimen for patients treated with arthroplasty is intermittent pneumatic compression and pharmacologic prophylaxis (warfarin or aspirin if warfarin is contraindicated). Some authors have even advocated and achieved excellent results with low-dose oral chemoprophylaxis before surgery. Prophylaxis should continue after discharge, and patients should be educated on signs and symptoms of VTE. Studies have shown that even if screening tests are negative, discharging patients after total knee and hip arthroplasty without continuing prophylaxis is not cost effective. Other regimens exist and are usually used according to the surgeon's preference. LMWH has a short half-life and therefore should not be administered immediately after surgery. Depending on the drug used, the first dose is started 6 to 24 hours postoperatively and may be started later at the discretion of the surgeon if intraoperative blood loss was high or a concern exists for compartment syndrome. LMWH has been found to be more effective than warfarin in reducing the overall rates of asymptomatic DVT, but no difference has been noted in reducing the prevalence of death from PEs. **Table 5** details inpatient and outpatient care to optimize DVT prevention.

The duration of prophylaxis remains controversial. After total hip arthroplasty, total knee arthroplasty, and hip fracture surgery, 7 to 10 days of prophylaxis has been recommended, although some authors recommend up to 30 days of prophylaxis. Recent large studies of patients who underwent total hip arthroplasty have shown that if a diligent multimodal approach in the form of preoperative

SECTION 1 GENERAL ORTHOPAEDICS

Table 5

Perioperative Modalities for Optimization of Deep Vein Thrombosis Prophylaxis

Timing	Modality
Preoperative	Cessation of procoagulant medication
	Physical therapy
	Weight loss
	Smoking cessation
	Low-dose chemoprophylaxis in select cases
Intraoperative	Pneumatic compression of uninvolved extremity
	Autologous blood for transfusion if required
	Regional anesthesia
	Short surgical time
	Intraoperative dose of heparin in select cases
Postoperative	Pharmacologic prophylaxis (eg, warfarin, enoxaparin)
	Pneumatic compression bilaterally
	Physical therapy
	Adherence to outpatient pharmacologic regimen for instructed duration
	Patient education with regard to signs/symptoms of DVT/PE

DVT = deep vein thrombosis, PE = pulmonary embolism.

and intraoperative measures combined with pneumatic compression, compression stockings, early mobilization, and 4 to 6 weeks of oral warfarin or aspirin is administered, then chemoprophylactic agents that carry an increased risk of bleeding (such as LMWH) may be unnecessary. Chemical anticoagulation is usually withheld for 7 to 10 days to reduce the risk of an epidural hematoma after surgery. Patients with spinal trauma may require an inferior vena cava filter when (1) a history of VTE exists despite appropriate prophylaxis, (2) prolonged immobilization is expected, or (3) chemical anticoagulation is contraindicated. Filter placement is not without risk, is invasive, and exposes the patient to contrast dye loads. Current models are retrievable, but some may be left in place permanently.

In the near future, the number of total knee arthroplasties performed is expected to increase, especially in younger, healthier individuals whose risk for VTE is decreased. The judicious use of more aggressive chemoprophylactic regimens is warranted, both for cost reasons and to avoid placing patients who are at low risk for DVT at risk for complications such as bleeding and wound infection.

Treatment of Distal Clots
The risk of PE and subsequent death is substantially lower for a distal clot than for a proximal one; therefore, many physicians do not treat

distal thromboses. Instead, they monitor them with serial duplex ultrasonographic imaging, and, if the clot migrates proximally (as occurs in 20% of patients), they treat the DVT. No consensus exists as to how long to follow patients, although one accepted regimen recommends following patients every 7 to 10 days for 3 weeks, discontinuing follow-up if the clot does not progress.

Treatment of Proximal Clots

Anticoagulation is recommended in patients in whom a proximal venous thrombosis has been diagnosed. This can be done by hospitalization for an intravenous, therapeutic heparin drip or as an outpatient with LMWH. The patient is usually bridged to warfarin with a goal INR of 2 to 3. This bridging with parenteral therapy is necessary because it takes a few days to achieve a therapeutic INR and warfarin initially reduces circulating protein C and S levels, placing the patient in a temporarily hypercoagulable state. Popliteal clots are considered proximal clots. Warfarin therapy is usually continued for 3 months. Therapeutic heparin can be monitored with serial activated partial thromboplastin time measurements. Therapeutic enoxaparin monitoring, if warranted and available, is best done with anti–factor Xa levels.

  Contraindications to long-term warfarin therapy include pregnancy, liver insufficiency, severe liver disease, noncompliance, severe alcoholism, uncontrolled hypertension, active major hemorrhage or recent hemorrhagic stroke, and an inability to return for monitoring.

Treatment of Acute PE

Admission to the hospital for intravenous therapeutic heparin, supplemental oxygen, and close monitoring is advised. Warfarin therapy is then initiated, and when INR levels reach the therapeutic range, the intravenous heparin may be discontinued. Oral anticoagulation is typically continued for 6 months for a first episode of PE, including idiopathic cases. With any PE or DVT, it is important to evaluate for causative factors before declaring the event idiopathic.

Adverse Outcomes of Treatment

Bleeding has been associated with anticoagulants. Reports documenting death from postoperative bleeding with aggressive chemoprophylaxis have been rare. Immune-mediated heparin–induced thrombocytopenia (HIT) type II, which is also known as white clot syndrome, is a prothrombotic adverse effect of unfractionated heparin and, less frequently, LMWH. Venous limb gangrene may complicate the transition from heparin to warfarin in HIT type II. Skin necrosis can develop with warfarin but is uncommon.

Referral Decisions/Red Flags

None

Diffuse Idiopathic Skeletal Hyperostosis

Synonyms

Ankylosing hyperostosis
Vertebral osteophytosis

Definition

Diffuse idiopathic skeletal hyperostosis (DISH) is an idiopathic disease characterized by striking osteophyte formation in the spine. Patients with DISH have confluent ossification spanning three or more intervertebral disks, most commonly in the thoracic and thoracolumbar spine. The bridging osteophytes follow the course of the anterior longitudinal ligaments and the peripheral disk margins. The disease primarily affects white men (the male-to-female ratio is 2:1) who are age 60 years or older.

Clinical Symptoms

The principal symptom is stiffness in the spine, especially in the morning and evening. Patients often report that symptoms have been present for several months or even years. Nonradicular back pain, especially in the lumbar and thoracolumbar junction area, is mild (**Figure 1**). Patients with cervical spine involvement may notice dysphagia related to a large anterior cervical osteophyte located behind the esophagus. Other weight-bearing joints can be painful, but spinal pain is the most common.

Tests

Physical Examination

Examination reveals stiffness in the spine on forward flexion and on extension. Reduced hip motion or associated knee arthritis also is possible.

Diagnostic Tests

Radiographs of the thoracic and lumbar spine, especially the lateral view, show confluent ossification spanning the intervertebral disks of at least four contiguous vertebral bodies (three disks) (**Figure 2**). The intervertebral disk height is preserved in the fused segments. The posterior apophyseal joints and sacroiliac joints are normal in contrast to the findings characteristic of ankylosing spondylitis.

In the cervical spine, ossification of the posterior longitudinal ligament occurs and is the second most common cause of cervical myelopathy, after cervical spondylosis.

The pelvis often shows "whiskering," or shaggy hyperostotic bone at the pelvic rim. Hyperostotic changes may be seen in the ribs as well.

No HLA association exists.

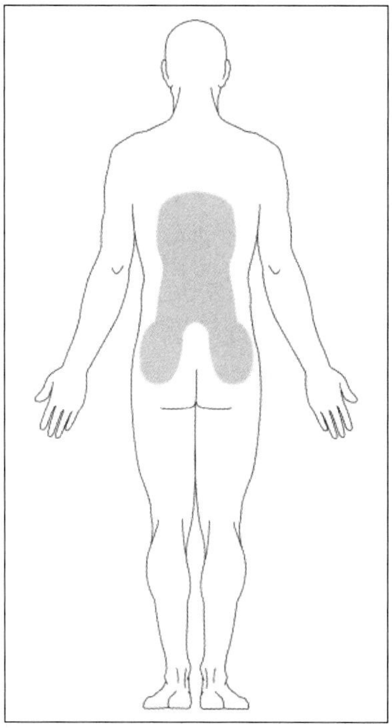

Figure 1 Illustration shows distribution of pain in diffuse idiopathic skeletal hyperostosis.

Differential Diagnosis

- Acromegaly (facial and phalangeal changes)
- Ankylosing spondylitis (sacroiliac and apophyseal joint involvement, positive HLA-B27)
- Degenerative disk disease (reduced disk height)
- Paget disease (bowing of legs, enlarging head, hearing loss; 32% of patients also have DISH)
- Polymyalgia rheumatica (muscle and joint pain and stiffness associated with systemic symptoms)

Adverse Outcomes of the Disease

Spinal stiffness is common. With widespread involvement, a single mobile segment can remain, but it may become unstable and painful.

Treatment

Walking and exercise programs are recommended as initial treatment. Intermittent NSAIDs may be useful, but pain usually is mild and tolerable.

Adverse Outcomes of Treatment

Heterotopic ossification following hip replacement surgery occurs five times more often in patients with DISH. Preventive intervention may be indicated. NSAIDs can cause gastric, renal, or hepatic complications. In 2015, the FDA strengthened its warning linking NSAIDs with the risk of heart attack or stroke, even in the first weeks of use of an NSAID.

Referral Decisions/Red Flags

Symptoms of neurogenic claudication, myelopathy, or dysphagia indicate the need for further evaluation.

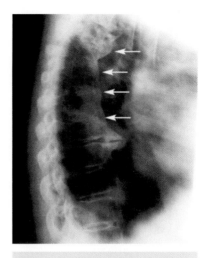

Figure 2 Lateral radiograph of the thoracic spine demonstrates confluent ossification anteriorly spanning multiple disk levels (arrows).

GENERAL ORTHOPAEDICS

SECTION 1

Drugs: Corticosteroid Injections

Introduction

Corticosteroid injections (**Table 1**) are a mainstay of treatment of several common musculoskeletal conditions, particularly osteoarthritis and inflammatory arthritis. Steroid injections provide substantial pain relief for many patients while avoiding the side effects of systemic steroids. Steroid injections function primarily by suppressing synovial inflammation. Although the effects are largely limited to the single joint injected, several studies have demonstrated improvement in inflammatory markers (erythrocyte sedimentation rate and C-reactive protein level) and clinical improvement of other joints, which suggests that a broader systemic effect is possible. Depot formulations remain at the injected site for an extended time and have limited systemic effects. The most common depot corticosteroids used are methylprednisolone acetate, triamcinolone hexacetonide, and triamcinolone acetonide. Injection principles are provided in **Table 2**. The use of a particular depot corticosteroid is based on cost, availability, and pharmacokinetics of the agent.

Intra-articular Injections

Corticosteroids have long been used in the management of a variety of intra-articular conditions, including rheumatoid arthritis, degenerative arthritis, crystal deposition diseases (such as gout), systemic lupus erythematosus arthrosis, and posttraumatic arthritis. Although few high-level studies (randomized clinical trials) have investigated the long-term efficacy of intra-articular corticosteroid injections, clinical experience has demonstrated that this therapy provides substantial pain relief for many patients, allowing them to delay surgical intervention while maintaining function. The duration of pain relief with intra-articular injections of corticosteroids is widely variable, ranging from 1 to 13 weeks.

Table 1

Characteristics of Common Injectable Corticosteroids

Corticosteroid	Relative Potency	Onset	Duration
Hydrocortisone	1	Fast	Short
Prednisolone tebutate	4	Fast	Intermediate
Methylprednisolone acetate	4	Slow	Intermediate
Triamcinolone acetonide	5	Moderate	Intermediate
Triamcinolone hexacetonide	5	Moderate	Intermediate
Betamethasone	25	Fast	Long

Table 2

Corticosteroid Injection Principles

1. Scrub the intended injection site with a bactericidal solution. Wear sterile gloves and handle the syringes and needles with strict aseptic technique. Observe universal precautions.
2. Cleanse the top of the solution vial with an antiseptic solution.
3. Use an 18- or 20-gauge needle for easy withdrawal of solution. Discard this needle.
4. Consider anesthetizing the injection site with a small amount of local anesthetic administered with a 25- or 27-gauge needle.
5. Do not use local anesthetics that contain epinephrine when injecting the hand or foot; these can cause arterial constriction and infarction of a digit.
6. Corticosteroid and local anesthetic solutions can be mixed in the same syringe, usually in a 1:2 ratio. Injection of the site with 2 to 3 mL of a rapid-acting local anesthetic solution, advancing the same needle into the joint or tendon sheath, and injecting additional local anesthetic followed by the steroid through the same needle is less traumatic to the patient. Large joints (knee and shoulder) may need an additional 4 mL of local anesthetic. Alternatively, a mixture of the local anesthetic and steroid can be injected simultaneously into the affected joint.
7. Inject anesthetic or corticosteroid preparation with a sterile 22- to 25-gauge needle.
8. Do not inject anesthetic or corticosteroid into a nerve, tendon, ligament, or subcutaneous fat.
9. Use multiple injections only if clear improvement has occurred. Limit the number of injections to three.
10. Following the injection, have the patient rest the extremity for 24 h and avoid the precipitating cause of the problem.

Table 3

Usual Doses of Methylprednisolone or Equivalent by Site

Dose Range (mg)	Anatomic Site
5-10	Phalangeal joints
20-30	Wrist
20-30	Elbow and ankle
40-80	Shoulder, hip, or knee

Little evidence exists on which to base the time sequence of serial intra-articular injections. Animal studies have shown hyaline cartilage damage with serial corticosteroid injections, but in patients with osteoarthritis who underwent intra-articular knee injections every 3 months for up to 2 years, no significant joint space narrowing was seen on weight-bearing radiographs. In patients with rheumatoid arthritis, serial corticosteroid joint injections did not increase the frequency of joint arthroplasty surgery in comparison to patients who did not receive injections. It is generally accepted that the same joint should not be injected with corticosteroids more often than every 3 months. The suggested dose of methylprednisolone or equivalent by site are noted in **Table 3**.

The use of glucosamine and chondroitin sulfate as alternatives to intra-articular corticosteroids is somewhat controversial. These agents, which are considered to be chondroprotective, are purported

SECTION 1 GENERAL ORTHOPAEDICS

to increase the activity of chondrocytes while suppressing the destruction caused by inflammatory mediators such as cytokines. These promising effects, however, have yet to be borne out in long-term, randomized studies. Thus, the most recent guideline published by the American Academy of Orthopaedic Surgeons on the treatment of osteoarthritis in the knee recommends against the use of these agents for symptomatic osteoarthritis of the knee. This second-edition clinical practice guideline, which was published in 2013, is available at http://www.aaos.org/Research/guidelines/TreatmentofOsteoarthritisoftheKneeGuideline.pdf. Some patients still use glucosamine and chondroitin sulfate because they believe that these agents improve their symptoms.

Extra-articular Injections

Corticosteroid injections also are used for several nonarticular conditions, including overuse syndromes, athletic injuries, selected neuropathies, bursitis, and tendinitis. The most common nonarticular injection sites are the subacromial shoulder for rotator cuff tendinitis, the lateral elbow for lateral epicondylitis (tennis elbow), the lateral wrist for de Quervain tenosynovitis and trigger finger, the lateral knee for iliotibial band tendinitis, the lateral hip for trochanteric bursitis, and the lateral heel for plantar fasciitis. A corticosteroid injection into the carpal canal is frequently helpful in alleviating the pain and numbness associated with carpal tunnel syndrome. In the spine, epidural injections can be used for discogenic pain, and facet injections can be used for axial spine pain. These spinal injections may require radiographic guidance.

Contraindications to Injections and Adverse Outcomes

Although corticosteroid injections can provide substantial pain relief and allow patients to delay or avoid surgical intervention, they also entail certain risks. Intra-articular injection of corticosteroids is contraindicated in the presence of a pyarthrosis. The clinical presentation of a pyarthrosis and nonseptic inflammation of a joint is often similar. If clinical signs of infection are present (fever, leukocytosis, elevated inflammatory markers, or cellulitis), a preliminary aspiration of the joint should be done to obtain a joint fluid leukocyte count and culture. Intra-articular fractures and the presence of prosthetic joint components (such as total knee replacement) are contraindications to intra-articular corticosteroid injections.

The complication rate for corticosteroid injections is very low, with transient injection pain the most common complication. Postinjection joint pain occurs in 1% to 10% of patients and may be related to crystal inflammation caused by the injected steroid. Facial flushing, focal skin discoloration, or subcutaneous lipodystrophy (fat atrophy) rarely occurs. Tendon rupture has been associated with corticosteroid injection into the tendon itself or from masking of pain by the corticosteroid. A serious complication of intra-articular injection of corticosteroids is iatrogenic joint infection, which is reported to occur in 1 in 3,000 to 5,000 injections. Meticulous care must be taken while performing these injections to maintain sterile technique and avoid this devastating complication.

Recent debate also has centered on the possible chondrotoxic effects of both corticosteroids and the local anesthetics that are almost always co-administered during these injections. Steroids have been linked with decreased protein synthesis and increased chondrocyte cell death in animal studies. Local anesthetics, including bupivacaine and lidocaine, which are commonly mixed with steroids in varying ratios (**Table 2**), have been hypothesized to be involved in disrupting cell membranes and contributing to decreased chondrocyte density. Local anesthetics have been linked with an increase in the rate of chondrocyte death in in-vitro studies. These effects are both dose- and time-dependent, and the long-term clinical effects of a single injection have not yet been determined.

Drugs: Nonsteroidal Anti-Inflammatory Drugs

Definition

NSAIDs are a group of drugs used to treat inflammatory conditions such as arthritis, bursitis, and tendinitis (**Table 1**). Aspirin is an NSAID, but the term usually is reserved for the newer aspirin-like agents that were developed to decrease the severity of gastritis associated with long-term use of aspirin. The American Academy of Orthopaedic Surgeons (AAOS) gives a strong recommendation for the use of NSAIDs in the treatment of osteoarthritis of the knee.

Inflammation is an essential, normal protective mechanism associated with injury to the musculoskeletal system. Inflammation can be caused by trauma or triggered by infection, allergy, or an autoimmune response, as in rheumatoid arthritis. The inflammatory response is mediated by chemicals, such as prostaglandins, that are released from mast cells, granulocytes, and basophils. NSAIDs block prostaglandin by interfering with the action of the cyclooxygenase (COX) enzyme. Corticosteroids also block the formation of prostaglandins but at a different step in the production chain.

In addition to their anti-inflammatory properties, NSAIDs exhibit analgesic and antipyretic activity. These drugs also decrease platelet adhesiveness and may inhibit the production of prothrombin. Aspirin is often used for thromboembolic prophylaxis following hip and knee arthroplasty and is administered to patients with lower extremity trauma who consequently require long-term immobilization. However, NSAID use can result in a bleeding diathesis intraoperatively. As a result, many physicians recommend cessation of NSAID use 5 to 10 days before elective surgery.

NSAIDs vary in chemical structure, cost, frequency of side effects, and duration of action. The effective use of these drugs often requires some trialing because a patient may respond to one NSAID but not another, and an initial good response may wane with time. Switching to another class of NSAID as opposed to switching within the class is likely to be more effective. **Table 1** lists NSAIDs by class.

Two forms of COX have been identified. COX-1 is expressed in many tissues, but COX-2 primarily mediates the inflammatory response. Most NSAIDs inhibit COX-1 and COX-2 production, thereby affecting gastric mucosa, renal blood flow, and platelet aggregation as well as inflammation. COX-2 inhibitors selectively affect COX-2 enzymes and are therefore less likely to cause gastric ulcers and bleeding. Renal and hepatic complications have been reported in patients taking COX-2 inhibitors. COX-2 inhibitors also have been associated with an increased risk of stroke and myocardial infarction and should be used with great caution in a susceptible patient population.

Table 1

Types of NSAIDs

Drug	Strength (mg)	Trade Name	Typical Dosage
Salicylates			
Aspirin	300, 325, 600, 650	Several	325 mg qid
Choline magnesium trisalicylate	500, 750, 1,000	—	1,500 mg bid
Salsalate	500, 700	—	1,000 mg tid, 1,500 mg bid
Diflunisal	500	Dolobid (Merck)	250 mg bid or tid, 500 mg bid
Propionic Acids			
Naproxen sodium	220	Aleve (Bayer)	220 mg bid
	375, 500	Naprelan 375, 500 (Almatica Pharma)	750-1,000 mg/d
	275, DS 550	Anaprox (Roche Laboratories)	275 mg bid or tid, 500 mg bid
Naproxen	250, 375, 500	Naprosyn (Roche Laboratories)	250, 375, or 500 mg bid
Naproxen EC	375, 500	EC Naprosyn (Roche Laboratories)	375 or 500 mg/d
Flurbiprofen	50, 100	Ansaid (Pfizer)	100 mg bid
Oxaprozin	600	Daypro (Pfizer)	600-1,200 mg/d
Ibuprofen	400, 600, 800	Motrin (McNeil Consumer Healthcare)	400-800 mg bid or tid
Ibuprofen (over the counter)	200	Motrin IB, Advil (Pfizer), Nuprin (McNeil)	200-400 mg bid or tid
Ketoprofen	25, 50, 75	—	50 mg qid, 75 mg tid
Ketoprofen extended release	100, 150, 200	Oruvail (Sanofi-Aventis)	200 mg/d
Ketorolac tromethamine	10	—	10 mg qid; 5 d maximum of oral and IM combined
Indoleacetic Acids and Related Compounds			
Sulindac	150, 200	Clinoril (Merck)	150-200 mg bid
Indomethacin	25, 50	Indocin (Iroko Pharmaceuticals)	25-50 mg tid
Indomethacin sustained release	75	Indocin SR (Iroko Pharmaceuticals)	75 mg/d
Etodolac	200-500	—	200-400 mg tid, 500 mg bid

bid = twice a day, DS = double strength, IM = intramuscular, qid = four times a day, tid = three times a day.

Side Effects

NSAIDs cause similar side effects, but in varying degrees. Minor dyspepsia is common, even with COX-2 drugs. Gastric ulcers and bleeding are less common but are more serious side effects. In patients older than 65 years, approximately 30% of hospitalizations and deaths from gastrointestinal hemorrhage are secondary to NSAID treatment.

In 2015, the FDA strengthened its warning linking NSAIDs with the risk of heart attack or stroke, even in the first weeks of use of an NSAID. Reversible hepatotoxicity is observed with long-term use of some NSAIDs in 10% to 15% of patients. Nephrotoxicity is less common but can develop early in treatment; it results from the loss of vasodilatory effects of renal prostaglandins. Fluid retention can increase blood pressure in susceptible patients. The inhibition of prostaglandin synthesis also can be responsible for hives and acute episodes of asthma in some patients.

Use of NSAIDs for pain management in patients with fracture warrants special mention. The initial stimulus for fracture healing involves an inflammatory response that is regulated primarily by prostaglandin E_2. Animal studies dating back to the 1970s have shown that NSAIDs can dampen this process and thus impede fracture healing. This finding has been validated by more recent clinical studies showing higher rates of delayed healing and nonunion in patients who are taking NSAIDs.

Choice of Therapeutic Agents

When choosing an NSAID, cost, side effects, dosage schedule, and physician familiarity should be considered. Once- or twice-daily dosage schedules are optimal for patients with poor compliance. Although long-term use is standard practice in patients with rheumatoid arthritis or osteoarthritis, short-term use is encouraged for most other conditions. For osteoarthritis that has a minimal inflammatory component, acetaminophen can be taken for primary management and supplemented with the intermittent use of NSAIDs for breakthrough pain. This dual therapy helps reduce gastric complications caused by NSAIDs. In patients who cannot tolerate oral NSAIDs because of the associated gastrointestinal side effects, topical NSAIDs may be a viable alternative. Clinical studies have shown that topical NSAIDs provide local analgesia equivalent to that of oral agents with fewer gastrointestinal complications.

In general, NSAIDs should be taken with food to decrease gastric irritation. Oral hypoglycemic agents or warfarin sodium may be unfavorably potentiated by some NSAIDs in some patients. Full-dose aspirin or other NSAIDs should not be taken at the same time as another NSAID; however, low-dose aspirin often is used with other NSAIDs in patients with cardiac disease. NSAIDs should be used with caution in patients with hypertension; indomethacin is particularly hazardous in elderly patients.

Patients who are at risk for gastric complications can choose from the following alternatives, in addition to those described previously:

• Nonacetylated NSAIDs such as salsalate (These drugs appear to cause less mucosal injury.)

• NSAIDs that are nonacidic, such as nabumetone

• Prodrugs (drugs that must undergo biotransformation to an active metabolite). These drugs are reported to cause less gastric injury.

• NSAIDs of the pyranocarboxylic acid class, such as etodolac. These drugs are appropriate in high-risk patients.

• COX-2 inhibitors. These drugs cause the lowest incidence of gastritis; however, they are more expensive than generic NSAIDs that inhibit both COX-1 and COX-2. Given findings of increased risk of cardiovascular events and stroke associated with COX-2 inhibitors, caution must be exercised when prescribing these anti-inflammatory agents.

Falls and Traumatic Injuries in the Elderly Patient

Definition

Epidemiology

The elderly are the fastest growing segment of the US population, due in part to the aging of the baby boomers. The population of persons age 65 years and older is expected to double between 2012 and 2050, and this cohort will comprise nearly 20% of the US population by 2030. Although older adults currently benefit from healthier lifestyles, better nutrition, and advancements in medical care, many still require acute care for traumatic injuries, including falls.

For adults 65 years and older, falls are the leading cause of both fatal and nonfatal injuries. Nearly one third of elderly people fall each year, and of these patients, approximately 50% will fall repeatedly. In fact, in the United States in 2012, nearly 2.4 million people age 65 years and older were seen in emergency departments for nonfatal falls. This accounts for 62% of all visits to the emergency department for this segment of the population. The most common serious injuries are head injuries, wrist fractures, spine fractures, and hip fractures. The total cost to treat the elderly after falls in year 2012 alone was a staggering $30 billion, and this number is expected to more than double by 2020, to almost $68 billion (2012 dollars). Only 78% of these costs are estimated to be covered by Medicare. Thus, the prevention of falls and treatment of elderly patients after fall-induced injuries is an important health economics issue, and it will only increase in importance as the population of adults older than 65 years continues to grow. (See **Sidebar: Quick Facts About Falls in the Elderly**.)

Risk Factors

Several factors increase the elderly person's risk of falling. These may be categorized as medical risk factors, personal risk factors, and environmental risk factors (**Table 1**).

Medical risk factors are known medical conditions that increase the risk of falling. Several medical conditions lead to an increased risk of falling, but gait and balance disturbance from any cause are the most recognized and well-studied risk factors. Medications, especially concerns of polypharmacy and the use of psychotropic medications, is the most easily modifiable medical risk factor. Cognitive impairment and generalized age-related muscle weakness are two common medical risk factors seen in the elderly population.

Personal risk factors are unique to the individual patient. Age contributes significantly, with the rate of hip fracture increasing in patients older than 50 years and nearly doubling at 5-year increments thereafter. A lack of weight-bearing activity contributes to decreased bone strength and thus, increased risk of falling. Decreased bone

Table 1
Risk Factors for Falls in the Elderly

Medical Risk Factors

Cardiac arrhythmias

Fluctuant blood pressure

Cancer

Arthritis, joint weakness

Preexisting orthopaedic conditions

Gait/balance disturbance

Cognitive impairment (Alzheimer/Parkinson disease)

Stroke/vascular disease

Multiple sclerosis

Urinary/bladder dysfunction

Vision loss

Hearing loss

Medications (polypharmacy, psychotropic drugs)

Personal Risk Factors

Age

Activity (lack of weight-bearing activity)

Sex (women at greater risk than men)

Habits (eg, smoking, heavy alcohol use)

Heredity

Nutrition

Environmental Risk Factors

Wet/slippery surfaces

Poor lighting

Cluttered pathways

Poor home layout/design

Inadequate footwear/clothing

Poor supervision

strength resulting from decreasing estrogen levels puts women at a greater risk than men, as demonstrated by the fact that women have two to three times as many hip fractures and falls as men. Habits that increase risk include smoking and heavy alcohol use. Poor nutrition, low calcium intake or absorption, and inadequate vitamin D intake can all lead to osteoporosis, which is known to drastically increase a patient's risk for fall and traumatic injury.

Environmental risk factors may be considered extrinsic factors. Approximately 60% of falls occur at home, 30% occur in the community, and 10% occur in nursing homes/institutions. The risk of falls in hospitals and nursing homes is rising, and falls or injuries occurring in these institutions are associated with increased morbidity. One quarter of all falls are the result of hazards such

Table 2

Tests Administered and Imaging Modalities Used to Identify Increased Risk of Fall

Clinical Competency Tests

Tinetti Performance Oriented Mobility Assessment (POMA)

Get Up and Go

Short Physical Performance Battery (SPPB)

Simultaneous manual and cognitive testing

Functional reach test

Laboratory Tests

Complete blood count

Basic metabolic panel

Vitamin D level

Imaging Studies

Radiography

CT/MRI

Dual-energy x-ray absorptiometry (DEXA) scan

as slippery or wet surfaces, poor lighting, and cluttered pathways. Although nearly 4.5 million elderly adults need assistance with activities of daily living, most do not receive the supervision or support that they require. Therefore, they are often forced to engage in activities that put them at risk for a fall and serious injury, including climbing to reach objects high in closets or cabinets, bathing alone, or ambulating through difficult terrain without assistance.

Clinical Symptoms

Symptoms depend on the specific injury sustained as a result of the fall or trauma.

Wrist fractures most often follow a fall on an outstretched hand. Presenting symptoms include pain, swelling, and usually an obvious deformity.

Spine fractures in the elderly are often compression fractures, which are the result of osteoporosis and usually occur in the low thoracic and upper lumbar region. The patient reports pain and occasionally deformity; neurologic complaints are rare.

An elderly patient presenting with a hip fracture is usually nonambulatory. The patient may report pain in the groin, and the leg is shortened and externally rotated.

Tests

Clinical testing, laboratory testing, and routine imaging may suggest an increased risk of falling (**Table 2**).

There are five well-studied clinical tests that can aid in determining whether a patient is at increased risk of falling or traumatic injury. The Tinetti Performance Oriented Mobility Assessment (POMA) is a scored tool that is used to assess balance and gait (**Figure 1**). The Get Up and Go test is used to observe a patient rising from a chair, walking, and returning to the seated position (**Table 3**). A longer than average time to complete this action is associated with an increased risk of falling and injury; however, no clear cutoff score at which an individual patient is at risk of falling/injury has been established for either of these tests. Therefore, the POMA and the Get Up and Go test should be used as part of a more global assessment of gait and balance disturbance. Similarly, the Short Physical Performance Battery (SPPB) allows a physician to better characterize a patient's lower extremity function; impaired lower extremity function may contribute to overall instability and an increased risk of falling and serious injury. Patients age 60 years and older who have difficulty performing a manual and a cognitive task simultaneously, such as walking and singing the alphabet, are at increased risk of falling. The fifth test, the functional reach test, is the only clinical tool with an objective cutoff score to indicate an increased risk of falling. The patient who is unable to reach past 6 inches (15 cm) is at increased risk of falling (**Figure 2**).

Laboratory testing may include a complete blood count, basic metabolic panel, and vitamin D level. Anemia, uremia, electrolyte

NYC Health — Tinetti Performance Oriented Mobility Assessment

POMA is a task-oriented test that measures an older adult's gait and balance abilities by an ordinal scale of 0 (most impairment) to 2 (independence). The assessments takes **10 - 15 minutes to complete.**

(See: Tinetti ME. Performance-oriented assessment of mobility problems in elderly patients. JAGS 1986; 34: 119-126. Scoring description: PT Bulletin Feb. 10, 1993)

Name: **Date:**

Location: **Administrator:**

Balance Assessment

Instructions: Subject is seated in a hard, armless chair. The following maneuvers are tested.

Task	Description of Balance	Possible	Score
1 Sitting Balance	Leans or slides in chair	0	
	Steady, safe	1	
2 Arises	Unable without help	0	
	Able, uses arms to help	1	
	Able without using arms	2	
3 Attempts to arise	Unable without help	0	
	Able, requires > 1 attempt	1	
	Able to rise, 1 attempt	2	
4 Immediate standing balance (first 5 seconds)	Unsteady (swaggers, moves feet, trunk sway)	0	
	Steady but uses walker or other support	1	
	Steady without walker or other support	2	
5 Standing Balance	Unsteady	0	
	Steady but wide stance (medial heels > 4 inches apart) and uses cane or other support	1	
	Narrow stance without support	2	
6 Nudged (subject at max position with feet as close together as possible, examiner pushes lightly on subject's sternum with palm of hand 3 times)	Begins to fall	0	
	Staggers, grabs, catches self	1	
	Steady	2	
7 Eyes closed (at maximum position #6)	Unsteady	0	
	Steady	1	
8 Turning 360 degrees	Discontinuous steps	0	
	Continuous steps	1	
	Unsteady (grabs, swaggers)	0	
	Steady	1	
9 Sitting Down	Unsafe (misjudged distance, falls into chair)	0	
	Uses arms or not a smooth motion	1	
	Safe, smooth motion	2	

0 = highest level of impairment
2 = independent

Total Balance Score (out of 16) =

Figure 1   Tinetti Performance Oriented Mobility Assessment. (Available at http://www.nyc.gov/html/doh/downloads/pdf/win/tinetti-test.pdf. Accessed July 21, 2015.)

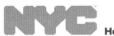

Tinetti Performance Oriented Mobility Assessment

Patient Name: Date:

Location: Administrator:

Gait Assessment

Instructions: Subject stands with examiner, walks down hallway or across the room, first at "usual" pace, then back at "rapid, but safe" pace (using usual walking aids).

	Task	Description of Gait	Possible	Score
10	Initiation of gait (immediately or after told to "go")	Any hesitancy or multiple attempts to start	0	
		No hesitancy	1	
11	Step length and height	a. Right swing foot does not pass left stance foot with step	0	
		b. Right foot passes left stance foot	1	
		c. Right foot does not clear floor completely with step	0	
		d. Right foot completely clears floor	1	
		e. Left swing foot does not pass right stance foot with step	0	
		f. Left foot passes right stance foot	1	
		g. Left foot does not clear floor completely with step	0	
		h. Left foot completely clears floor	1	
12	Step Symmetry	Right and left step length not equal (estimate)	0	
		Right and left step appear equal	1	
13	Step Continuity	Stopping or discontinuity between steps	0	
		Steps appear continuous	1	
14	Path (estimated in relation to floor tiles, 12-inch diameter; observe excursion of 1 foot over about 10 feet of the course).	Marked deviation	0	
		Mild/moderate deviation or uses walking aid	1	
		Straight without walking aid	2	
15	Trunk	Marked sway or uses walking aid	0	
		No sway but flexion of knees or back, or spreads arms out while walking	1	
		No sway, no flexion, no use of arms, and no use of walking aid	2	
16	Walking Stance	Heels apart	0	
		Heels almost touching while walking	1	

0 = highest level of impairment
2 = independent

Total Gait Score (out of 12) =

Balance + Gait Score=

< 19 = HIGH FALL RISK   19-24 = MEDIUM FALL RISK   25-28 = LOW FALL RISK

Figure 1 (continued) Tinetti Performance Oriented Mobility Assessment. Available at: http://www.nyc.gov/html/doh/downloads/pdf/win/tinetti-test.pdf. Accessed July 21, 2015.)

Table 3

Get Up and Go Test

Have the patient sit in a straight-backed high-seat chair

Instructions for the patient:

Get up (without the use of arm rests if possible)

Stand still momentarily

Walk forward 10 ft (3 m)

Turn around and walk back to the chair

Turn and be seated

Factors to note:

Sitting balance

Transfers from sitting to standing

Pace and stability of walking

Ability to turn without staggering

Modified qualitative scoring

1) No fall risk	1) Well coordinated movements, no walking aid
2) Low fall risk	2) Controlled but adjusted movements
3) Some fall risk	3) Uncoordinated movements
4) High fall risk	4) Supervision necessary
5) Very high fall risk	5) Physical support necessary

Timed test (from initial rising to re-seating)

Age (years)	Mean Time (seconds)
60-69	8.1 (7.1-9.0)
70-79	9.2 (8.2-10.2)
80-89	11.3 (10.0-12.7)

(Reproduced with permission from Mathias S, Nayak US, Isaacs B: Balance in elderly patients: The "get-up and go" test. *Arch Phys Med Rehabil* 1986;67[6]:387-389.)

disturbance, and vitamin D deficiency can all lead to an increased risk of falling and traumatic injury in the elderly.

Radiographs are used to evaluate bone integrity. CT and MRI may be necessary to evaluate soft-tissue injury and may reveal bony injury when radiographs are inconclusive. A dual-energy x-ray absorptiometry (DEXA) scan may be appropriate to diagnose osteoporosis.

Adverse Outcomes of the Disease

Falls and the serious injuries that result can be catastrophic for the older adult. Serious injury occurs in 5% of falls sustained by community dwellers and in 10% of falls sustained by persons living in an institution such as a nursing home or staying in a hospital. Prolonged immobility can result in a permanent decrease in mobility

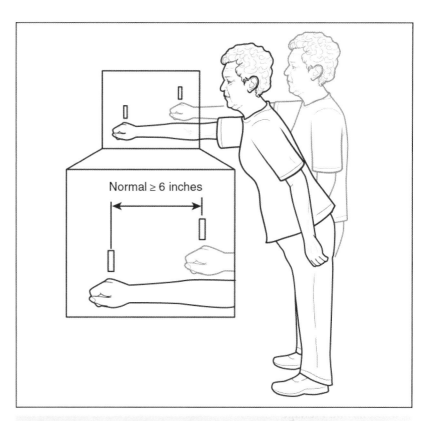

Normal ≥ 6 inches

Figure 2 Illustration of the functional reach test. The patient stands with the arm and fist extended alongside a wall. The patient then leans forward as far as possible, moving the fist along the wall without taking a step or losing stability. The length of the first movement is measured. A distance of less than 6 in (15 cm) indicates an increased risk of falling.

and a loss of independence. Many elderly patients with fractures as a result of a fall do not return to their functional baseline, with hip fractures being responsible for the greatest morbidity and mortality in the older adult population. Although approximately 25% of hip fracture patients make a full recovery, 40% require nursing home admission, 50% are dependent on a cane or walker, and 20% die within 1 year. Additionally, many patients develop a subsequent fear of falling or postfall anxiety syndrome. This is believed to affect nearly one half of patients following a hip fracture and is associated with increased mortality and risk for institutionalization.

Prevention and Treatment
Prevention
Given the high morbidity, mortality, and financial burden associated with falls and traumatic injury in the elderly, it is imperative to consider how to prevent falls from occurring. This can best be accomplished by examining each risk factor category and devising an individualized, multifactorial plan to diminish or eliminate the known risks.

It may be impossible to eliminate a preexisting medical condition or risk factor. However, seeing a physician regularly to monitor known

Table 4					
Modifying the Home Environment to Prevent Falls					
Stairs	**Bathroom**	**Kitchen**	**Living Room**	**Bedroom**	**Footwear**
Keep adequately lighted	Use a night-light	Avoid climbing to reach high shelves	Leave open pathways	Use a night-light	Wear low-heeled shoes
Remove clutter	Use rugs with nonskid backing	Arrange cabinets so frequently used items are easily accessible	Remove low tables and footrests	Remove throw rugs and extension cords	Ensure shoes have nonskid soles
Cover with carpet or nonslip tread	Install handrails in the shower	Clean up spills immediately	Keep cords out of walkways	Avoid beds that are too high or too low	Avoid shoes with heavy soles
Install steady handrails	Use a rubber mat on shower floor				
	Leave door unlocked				

conditions and manage any new risk factors that may develop can help to decrease the number of falls and injuries in patients older than 65 years. Physicians should ask about falls and assess a patient's risks at least once per year. A thorough history should be obtained at each visit to ensure that known chronic medical conditions are adequately controlled and that no new conditions have developed that may lead to an increased risk of falling and serious injury. Additionally, the medication list should be reviewed at each visit. A comprehensive physical examination should be done, including both visual and hearing assessments. Neurologic and musculoskeletal examinations are critically important. Many studies show that lower extremity weakness has a higher correlation with risk of falling than does a prior history of falls. If a new condition is diagnosed, appropriate treatment plans can be instituted to help mitigate the risk of falling and traumatic injury.

Personal risk factors, such as age, sex, and heredity, are nonmodifiable, but activity level, habits, and diet can be modified. Weight-bearing exercise helps to strengthen bone and improve coordination, resulting in a decreased risk of falling and a decreased risk of fracture after a fall. Consuming adequate calcium and vitamin D also strengthens bone. Avoiding smoking and alcohol also lowers the risk of falling and subsequent injury.

With 60% of falls occurring in the home, this is the most obvious place to make environmental modifications. For example, stairwells and hallways should be clutter free and well lit, handrails and nonskid rubber mats should be placed in the shower, and throw rugs and loose cords should be removed (**Table 4**).

Treatment

The goal of treatment is to restore the patient to his or her preinjury level of function. The intervention must be tailored to the specific injury and to the patient, including the patient's ability to participate in and comply with rehabilitation. The presence of comorbid, complex medical conditions in the elderly patient complicates injury management. For example, cardiopulmonary disease increases risks associated with general anesthesia and surgery. These risks must be taken into account when weighing treatment options.

Wrist fractures are most often treated with closed reduction followed by splinting or casting for 6 weeks. Some wrist fractures require surgical intervention.

Compression fractures of the spine without neurologic compromise often can be treated with rest and pain medication followed by short-term bracing and early mobilization. Follow-up with a spine specialist is encouraged because although neurologic damage is rare, it can occur. Severe collapse (compression) of the vertebral body may require surgical stabilization even in the absence of neurologic symptoms.

Most hip fractures require surgical intervention. Morbidity and mortality have been shown to increase substantially with a surgical delay of more than 3 days following injury. After surgery, early mobilization and appropriate rehabilitation are essential.

It is crucial to involve not only the patient and the patient's family in the management of these traumatic injuries, but also the patient's primary care physician (if the primary care physician is not the treating physician). This will ensure a coordinated approach that includes early mobility, adequate control of any preexisting medical conditions, continued supervision, and continued follow-up care. These simple measures may prevent a loss of independence, which can lead to devastating psychiatric, social, and physical consequences for the elderly patient.

Referral Decisions/Red Flags

Referral decisions depend on the specific injury; however, referral is indicated if the patient has a loss of distal pulses, evidence of nerve damage (failure to use certain muscle groups or changes in sensation), evidence of bleeding in the brain, displaced or open fractures, deformity, or increasing pain despite appropriate care. It also is important to note that the incidence of elder abuse is increasing. Therefore, if the circumstances surrounding the fall are suspect or the injuries do not fit the proposed mechanism of injury, it is appropriate to seek intervention by a social worker to investigate the possibility of abuse or neglect.

Fibromyalgia Syndrome

Definition

Fibromyalgia syndrome (FMS) is a chronic, non–life-threatening condition characterized by generalized pain, fatigue, and tender areas in the soft tissues. The joints, however, are spared. This syndrome is the second most common disorder encountered by rheumatologists, with rheumatoid arthritis being the first. Women between ages 20 and 60 years are primarily affected. The exact cause of FMS is unknown. Historically, many physicians questioned the validity of a diagnosis of FMS, resulting in a delay in care. Increasing evidence suggests, however, that genetic and environmental factors (**Table 1**) are responsible for FMS, and the diagnosis is becoming more widely accepted. Unfortunately, no cure is available for this often debilitating disease.

Clinical Symptoms

Prejudices should always be set aside in the evaluation of patients with symptoms of FMS. A careful history and thorough examination is much more valuable than advanced imaging and laboratory tests in arriving at the correct diagnosis. Patients typically report "hurting all over all the time." In 1992, the American College of Rheumatology established the following criteria for the diagnosis of FMS:

- Widespread pain in all four quadrants of the body, usually waxing and waning, that has been present continuously for 3 months. Pain is considered widespread when all of the following are present: pain in the left side of the body, pain in the right side of the body, pain above the waist, and pain below the waist. In addition, axial skeletal pain must be present (neck, anterior chest, or thoracic or low back). Low back pain is considered pain below the waist.

- Pain and tenderness at 11 or more of 18 tender point sites (9 pairs) on digital palpation with an approximate force of 4 kg (enough force to cause the examiner's nail bed to blanch). A dolorimeter is an examination tool that applies exactly 4 kg of pressure. For a tender point to be considered positive, the patient must state that the palpation was "painful" in contrast to "tender" (**Table 2**).

A wide variety of symptoms and conditions can accompany FMS (**Table 3**). The history should always include questions about a patient's diet, exercise regimen, medication list, allergies, and perpetuating factors.

Table 1
Current Theories of Causation for Fibromyalgia Syndrome
Hyperexcitability of central nervous system pain receptors, termed "central sensitization"
Abnormal central processing of nociceptive input
Dysfunction of hypothalamic-pituitary-adrenal axis, specifically dopaminergic neurotransmission

Table 2

Tender Point Sites

Location	Characteristics
Posterior	
Occiput	Bilateral, at the occipital muscle insertions
Supraspinatus	Bilateral, at origins, above the scapular spine near the medial border
Trapezius	Bilateral, at the midpoint of the upper border
Gluteal	Bilateral, in upper outer quadrants of buttocks in anterior fold of muscle
Greater trochanter	Bilateral, posterior to the trochanteric prominence
Anterior	
Low cervical	Bilateral, at the anterior aspects of the intertransverse spaces at C5-7
Second rib	Bilateral, at the second costochondral junctions, just lateral to the junctions on upper surfaces
Lateral epicondyle	Bilateral, 2 cm distal to the epicondyles
Knee	Bilateral, at the medial fat pad proximal to the joint line

(Reproduced with permission from the Arthritis Foundation, Atlanta, GA.)

An important distinction should be made between FMS and myofascial pain syndrome (MPS). MPS involves trigger points, which, like FMS tender points, have reproducible tenderness with pressure at the muscular and fascial sites; unlike FMS, however, with MPS, pain also is experienced distally, at a zone of referred pain. Trigger points are found in firm, elongated bands in muscle fibers and are associated with a local twitch response. This response is an involuntary, transient contraction of the bands and can be elicited by snapping or pinching. **Table 4** contains a comprehensive list of differences between the two syndromes.

Tests

Physical Examination

Examination reveals tenderness to palpation over 11 or more of the 18 tender point sites (**Figure 1**). These tender points are limited to the soft tissues (muscle, tendon, ligament, or bursa); examination of the joints is normal. Additionally, a patient's gait and posture should be evaluated. Patients often report a sensation of swelling, tingling, or numbness, but objective and other neurologic findings are usually absent. Chest pain, shortness of breath, and palpitations are common, and studies to rule out serious cardiac problems should be pursued. Upon auscultation, a midsystolic click followed by a late systolic murmur heard best at the apex, consistent with mitral valve prolapse, may be appreciated.

Table 3

Symptoms and Conditions Associated With Fibromyalgia Syndrome

Associated Symptoms

Sleep disturbances

Stiffness

Bursitis and tendinitis

Short-term memory loss

Fatigue

Mood changes: depression, anxiety

Headaches: migraines, tension

Substernal chest pain

Urinary frequency and urgency

Paresthesias in hands/feet

Associated Conditions

Restless legs syndrome (RLS)

Temporomandibular joint syndrome

Silicone breast implant syndrome

Irritable bowel syndrome

Premenstrual syndrome

Dysmenorrhea

Cystitis

Mitral valve prolapse

Myofascial pain syndrome

Systemic lupus erythematosus

Table 4

Differences Between Fibromyalgia Syndrome and Myofascial Pain Syndrome

Characteristic	FMS	MPS
Point type	Tender	Trigger
Twitch response	None	Local
Sex predilection	Females	None
Pain	Diffuse	Localized or regional
Associated symptoms	Associated with fatigue	None
Associated entities	Associated conditions	None
Response	None	Responds to manual muscle therapies

FMS = fibromyalgia syndrome, MPS = myofascial pain syndrome.

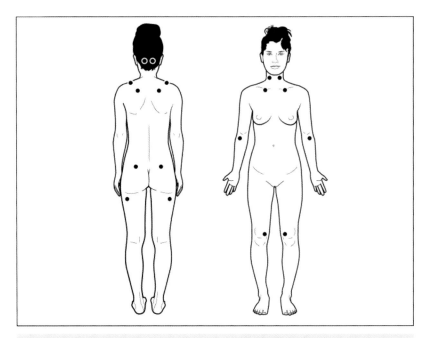

Figure 1   Illustration shows the posterior and anterior trigger points for fibromyalgia syndrome.

Diagnostic Tests

Imaging and laboratory studies should be ordered to evaluate coexisting conditions and rule out other disease processes. Although no laboratory test can definitively diagnose FMS, research suggests that several laboratory findings are associated with FMS (**Table 5**).

Differential Diagnosis

- AIDS (blood test)
- Bursitis or tendinitis (usually single joint or extremity)
- Complex regional pain syndrome (usually a single extremity)
- Hypothyroidism (abnormal thyroid function tests)
- Lyme disease (serology test)
- Multiple sclerosis (abnormal MRI of the brain)
- Polymyalgia rheumatica (elevated erythrocyte sedimentation rate)
- Polymyositis (skin rash)
- Rheumatoid arthritis (positive rheumatoid factor)
- Systemic lupus erythematosus (antinuclear antibodies, elevated erythrocyte sedimentation rate)
- Tenosynovitis (single focus, associated with tendon motion)

Adverse Outcomes of the Disease

The chronic pain associated with FMS can result in depression, anxiety, and inactivity. The multiple tests ordered and the multiple clinicians consulted to make the correct diagnosis can be expensive.

Table 5

Laboratory Findings Associated With Fibromyalgia Syndrome

Reduced central serotonin

Elevated nerve growth factor

Elevated substance P

Reduced insulinlike growth factor-1, implicated in reduced stage 4 (delta) sleep

Table 6	
Treatments of Fibromyalgia Syndrome	
Type	**Treatment Modalities**
Medicinal	Antidepressants (duloxetine, milnacipran)
	Anticonvulsants (pregabalin)
	Nonbenzodiazepine hypnotics
	Benzodiazepines
	Muscle relaxants
	Dopamine agonists
	NSAIDs
	Topical agents
	Alternative therapies
Mechanical	Injections
	Massage
	Physical therapy
	Stretching
	Exercise
Psychologic	Cognitive or behavioral therapy
	Support groups
Other	Electrical stimulation
	Cryotherapy
	Heat therapy

Treatment

Patients should be advised that FMS is not a life-threatening or progressive disease. No cure is available, but symptomatic relief is possible. The optimal treatment program is multifaceted and should include a team consisting of the patient, a physician, a psychologist, physical and massage therapists, and an exercise physiologist.

The FDA has approved three drugs specifically for the treatment of FMS: pregabalin (Lyrica [Pfizer]), duloxetine (Cymbalta [Eli Lilly]), and milnacipran (Savella [Forest Pharmaceuticals]). Available treatment modalities are listed in **Table 6**. Patients with FMS are usually very sensitive to medication, and adverse effects are common, so pharmacologic therapy should begin with low doses. Narcotics should be used only rarely, and steroids should be avoided. Antidepressants, anticonvulsants, nonbenzodiazepine hypnotics, muscle relaxants, dopamine agonists, and NSAIDs can be effective. NSAIDs accompanied by a tricyclic antidepressant may offer some analgesia. Amitriptyline in doses of 10 to 50 mg or cyclobenzaprine in doses of 10 to 40 mg taken at bedtime can be useful. Fluoxetine taken in the morning is useful to reduce severe depression. The nonnarcotic analgesic tramadol taken in divided doses of 50 to 400 mg per day has been shown to help the pain in FMS. Topical agents such as capsaicin cream applied to the tender point areas and even guaifenesin may be beneficial. For sleep initiation, trazodone at a starting dose of 25 mg is helpful, and for sleep maintenance, selective serotonin reuptake inhibitors are effective. Tricyclic antidepressants are the most efficacious for sleep maintenance, but some patients cannot tolerate them. Tiagabine (titrated from 2 to 12 mg) and gabapentin also can be useful for sleep maintenance. If the patient has concomitant restless legs syndrome (RLS) or mitral valve prolapse, low-dose clonazepam (0.125 or 0.25 mg) may be taken in the evening. Pramipexole also may be used to treat RLS. Alternative therapies, including vitamins, minerals, herbs, and supplements, have a limited role.

Injections, when combined with massage, rehabilitation, and stretching, are effective for providing mechanical disruption (myolysis) of tender points. Needling and infiltration with a local anesthetic (usually lidocaine; saline if the patient is allergic) is most effective. Steroids are generally not indicated or recommended. When properly administered, injections lead to pain reduction, improvement in range of motion and exercise tolerance, and enhanced circulation. These injections are contraindicated in the setting of a local or systemic infection, a bleeding disorder, or the use of anticoagulation medication.

Patients with FMS should be enrolled in a rehabilitation program, sometimes combined with cognitive and behavioral therapy. Stretching programs increase flexibility, and massage may be helpful. Electrical stimulation, cryotherapy, and heat may also be helpful. Initiation of an aerobic exercise program to increase cardiac fitness is recommended. The patient should begin slowly and increase gradually to build endurance while minimizing pain. The patient's target regimen should be 20 to 30 minutes of aerobic exercise four to five times per week. Aquatic exercise is well tolerated and helpful for some patients. Referral to a dietitian for weight-loss supervision often is indicated. Many patients will benefit from participation in FMS support groups, which are a useful source of information and encouragement. Many larger medical centers have established FMS clinics, which use a multidisciplinary approach in the treatment of patients with FMS.

Adverse Outcomes of Treatment

Patients can become dependent on narcotics and tranquilizers. Medications also have side effects, including drowsiness, dry mouth, change in appetite, and constipation. Tachyphylaxis (decreased response) can develop with long-term use of amitriptyline and/or cyclobenzaprine. In 2015, the FDA strengthened its warning linking NSAIDs with the risk of heart attack or stroke, even in the first weeks of use of an NSAID.

Referral Decisions/Red Flags

Severe symptoms that interfere with the patient's ability to work or the presence of serious psychiatric problems indicate the need for evaluation at an FMS treatment center.

Fracture Evaluation and Management Principles

Definition

Bones form the framework of the human body and provide many functions, including stability, mobility, hematopoiesis, and protection of vital organs. Bone has a hard outer layer known as the cortex and a softer inner layer known as cancellous bone. The periosteum is a thick layer that covers the cortex and contains vessels, nerve endings, and cells capable of repairing fractures. The endosteum is the inner lining of the cancellous bone (**Figure 1**).

In persons who are skeletally immature, long bones grow through specialized regions known as the physis. The physis is highly vascular and is prone to infections and fractures in children. The metaphysis consists largely of spongy, trabecular, cancellous bone and is the region most susceptible to compression fractures. The diaphysis has thick cortical bone and provides most of the structural support.

A fracture is defined as a disruption in the continuity or structural integrity of bone. A fracture occurs when the stress applied to the bone is greater than the bone's intrinsic strength. Bone can withstand very high compressive forces, but it is susceptible to breaks from tension and torsional forces (**Figure 2**).

Fractures involve not only injury to bone but also injury to the surrounding soft tissues, including the periosteum, muscles, and

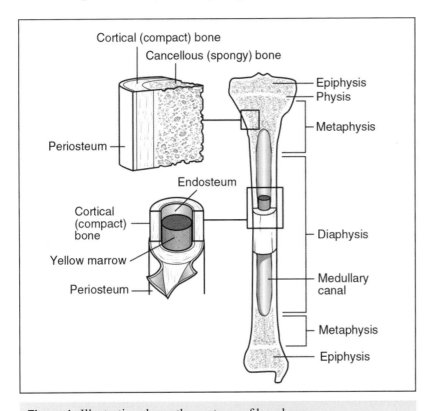

Figure 1 Illustration shows the anatomy of long bones.

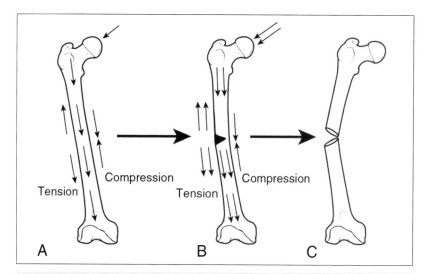

Figure 2 Illustration shows tension versus compression loads and fracture propagation. During loading (**A**), the convex side of the bone is under tension, and the concave side is under compression. Ultimately, the bone will fail in tension (**B**) and the crack will propagate across the bone (**C**), creating a fracture.

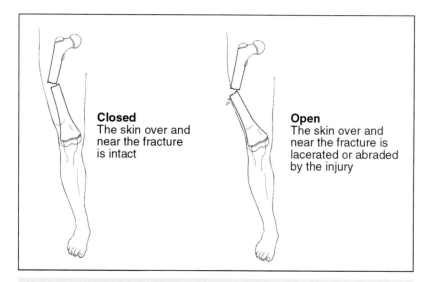

Figure 3 Illustration shows closed and open fractures, showing the integrity of the skin and soft-tissue envelope around the fracture. (Reproduced from Johnson TR, Steinbach LS, eds: *Essentials of Musculoskeletal Imaging*. Rosemont, IL, American Academy of Orthopaedic Surgeons, 2004, p 40.)

surrounding vessels. A fracture that compromises the skin and overlying soft tissue resulting in bone exposure is called an open fracture (**Figure 3**).

Fractures are classified by location, orientation and extent of fracture lines, amount of displacement, and soft-tissue integrity (**Figures 4** and **5**).

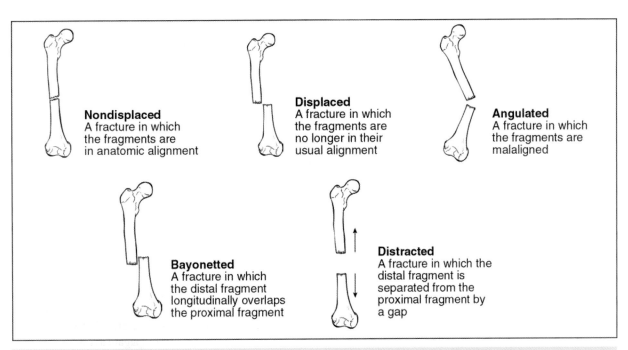

Figure 4 Illustration of types of fracture displacement. Bayonetted fractures are also called "shortened" fractures. For angulated fractures, valgus angulation is when the distal fragment is displaced away from the midline; varus angulation is when the distal fragment is displaced toward the midline. (Reproduced from Johnson TR, Steinbach LS, eds: *Essentials of Musculoskeletal Imaging.* Rosemont, IL, American Academy of Orthopaedic Surgeons, 2004, p 40.)

Clinical Symptoms

Patients with acute fractures present with pain, swelling, and decreased function. Pain is worsened by movement and may limit weight-bearing capacity. Displaced fractures commonly produce visible deformity in the injured extremity. Stress fractures present more insidiously, with pain during weight bearing. Numbness and tingling in an extremity may suggest neurologic or vascular injury.

Tests

Physical Examination

Fracture evaluation begins with a comprehensive history and physical examination that is focused on mechanism of injury, location, radiating symptoms, and timing of onset. The entire injured extremity, including the bones and joints above and below the injury, should be inspected for pain, swelling, ecchymosis, deformity, and skin integrity. Lacerations and abrasions in the vicinity of the fracture should be inspected closely because their presence may indicate an open fracture. Periarticular lacerations should be inspected closely because lacerations into a joint require surgical irrigation and débridement. Open fractures require expedient care and evaluation by a specialist.

On physical examination, the extremity should be palpated for tenderness, crepitus, and compartment tightness. Extreme swelling in a fractured extremity may suggest impending compartment syndrome. When feasible, the surrounding joints should be evaluated

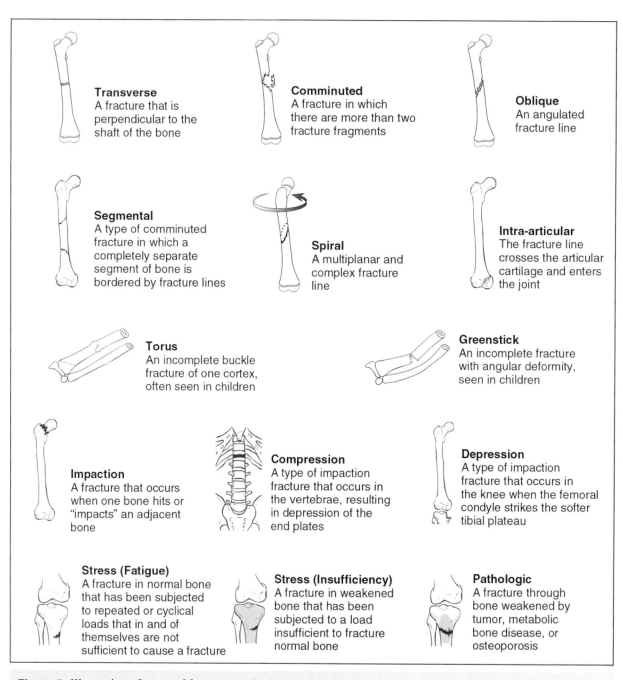

Figure 5   Illustration of types of fractures and orientation of the fracture lines. (Reproduced from Johnson TR, Steinbach LS, eds: *Essentials of Musculoskeletal Imaging.* Rosemont, IL, American Academy of Orthopaedic Surgeons, 2004, p 41.)

and taken through passive motion to assess stability. Neurologic and vascular status should be evaluated and documented in detail. In the patient with suspected vascular injury who exhibits symptoms such as increased capillary refill time or weak pulses, an ankle-brachial index, which compares systolic blood pressure in the arm and the leg, can be done to detect arterial injury.

Diagnostic Tests

Radiographs are an important initial diagnostic test for the evaluation of suspected fractures. At a minimum, AP and lateral views are required to properly assess a fracture. For complete evaluation of the wrist, ankle, and foot, an oblique view may be required. Imaging should always include the joints above and below the injury.

A CT scan is indicated to evaluate bony anatomy in detail, especially if concern exists for joint involvement or bone loss or if the bones are difficult to visualize on plain radiographs, such as the spine, scapula, knee, foot, and hand. In general, the cost and amount of radiation involved with CT scans are substantial, and this test should be ordered by an orthopaedic consultant. MRI is indicated to evaluate soft-tissue injuries such as ligamentous injuries, soft-tissue involvement of tumors, and osteomyelitis.

Differential Diagnosis

- Infection (fever; tenderness; gross purulence or draining sinus; elevated erythrocyte sedimentation rate, C-reactive protein level, or white blood cell count; may have no history of trauma)
- Joint dislocation (deformity, tenderness, abnormal joint alignment on radiographs, inability to range the joint in comparison with the contralateral extremity)
- Sprain/strain (tenderness, normal radiographs, possible ecchymosis or swelling)
- Tumor (insidious pain; possible constitutional symptoms, swelling, mass, or radiographic findings)

Adverse Outcomes of the Disease

A fracture that does not heal properly may result in a delayed union, a nonunion, or a malunion. Delayed unions are fractures that heal at a slower rate than anticipated by the treating physician. Nonunions are fractures that do not unite because of lack of biologic environment, inadequate stability, or both. Malunions are fractures that heal in an unacceptable alignment that may compromise the function of that extremity.

Fractures that extend into the articular surface may result in joint stiffness, chronic pain, or contractures. Osteonecrosis (bone death) occurs when the blood supply to a bone is compromised during an injury. Osteonecrosis is more likely to develop in bones that have a tenuous blood supply, such as the talus, scaphoid, and femoral head. In addition, osteonecrosis can occur with systemic disease, such as the altered fatty metabolism associated with alcoholism or corticosteroid use.

Severe injury can result in damage to surrounding nerves and blood vessels such that limb viability and function may be threatened, leading to long-lasting disability. Substantial soft-tissue loss, infection, and osteomyelitis all can result after significant open fractures. Compartment syndrome is a serious complication that should be considered in any injured extremity with pain with passive

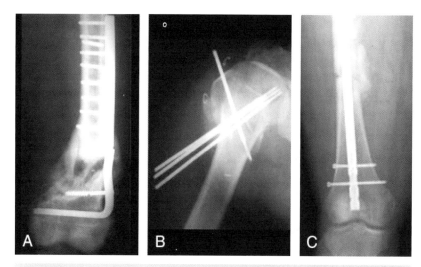

Figure 6 Radiographs demonstrate fractures stabilized with a plate-and-screw construct (**A**), percutaneous pins (**B**), and an intramedullary implant (**C**).

stretching of intracompartmental muscles, substantial swelling, or pain out of proportion to the injury. Compartment syndrome is a clinical diagnosis. Measuring intracompartmental pressures may aid in this diagnosis in the setting of an equivocal clinical examination.

Treatment

After a fracture is identified, a specialist should be notified to determine the need for manipulation and reduction and to determine the urgency of fracture stabilization. Management is guided by the bone involved, the fracture location and type, and the degree of displacement. In general, fractures require immobilization for proper healing. Fractures of the extremities are commonly immobilized with a cast, splint, or sling as determined by the fracture-specific variables mentioned previously. Axial fractures, such as those in the hip, pelvis, and spine, require bed rest and non–weight-bearing precautions before evaluation and treatment by a specialist.

Nondisplaced or minimally displaced fractures do not require acute fracture reduction. However, displaced and angulated fractures typically require early reduction to avoid subsequent swelling and vascular compromise. In some fractures, acceptable alignment and stability may be achieved definitively following reduction and proper immobilization consisting of a properly molded splint or cast. Immobilization is continued until the fracture unites.

Displaced, angulated, or unstable fractures often require surgical intervention to achieve acceptable alignment and stability with either closed or open reduction and placement of an external fixation device. Open reduction entails the anatomic restoration of the fracture site using direct visualization of the fragments. Following fracture reduction, implants such as plates, screws, pins, or intramedullary devices may be needed to maintain alignment and stability (**Figure 6**).

Table 1
Factors That Influence Fracture Healing

Factors That Improve Stability or Prognosis

Skeletal immaturity: increased remodeling potential, thick periosteum, decreased time to union

Nondisplaced fractures

Single bone fracture of the forearm (radius/ulna) or lower leg (tibia/fibula)

Thoracic spine fractures (support of the rib cage provides added stability)

Factors That Worsen Stability or Prognosis

Skeletal maturity: less remodeling capability, thin periosteum, increased time to union

Marked displacement or segmental fractures indicating possible soft-tissue disruption

Intra-articular fractures

Nerve or vascular injury

Compartment syndrome

Osteonecrosis

Oblique fracture patterns

Open fractures require urgent treatment that includes broad-spectrum intravenous antibiotic coverage and copious irrigation of soft tissue and exposed bone with application of sterile dressings. The fractured extremity is initially splinted for stability on presentation. Prompt administration of parenteral antibiotics has been shown to decrease the incidence of long-term infection. Rehabilitation may be necessary given muscle atrophy and joint stiffness that naturally occur during immobilization. Different fractures and stabilization methods require specific rehabilitation protocols that should be directed by the treating specialist.

Adverse Outcomes of Treatment

Most fractures unite uneventfully, but certain factors can influence healing (**Table 1**). Inadequate reduction may lead to fracture malunion. Fracture immobilization may lead to stiffness or contractures of the affected joint and the surrounding joints. Posttraumatic arthritis may develop following fractures involving articular surfaces. Other possible complications following fracture treatment include vascular and nerve injury, amputation, compartment syndrome, osteonecrosis, and infection.

Referral Decisions/Red Flags

Patients with open, displaced, unstable, or irreducible fractures, suspected compartment syndrome, nerve injury, or vascular injury require further evaluation and treatment by a specialist.

Fracture Healing

Definition

Following a fracture, bone has the inherent capacity for complete structural regeneration (healing), provided an appropriate environment is present. Fracture healing involves two pathways: surgical (primary or intramembranous healing) and nonsurgical (secondary or endochondral healing). Each pathway is mediated by bioactive cells and proteins, and fracture healing usually occurs, barring certain intrinsic factors (patient factors) or extrinsic factors (errors in surgical technique). Fracture healing is difficult to define, but it must be evident both clinically (functional use of the fractured extremity and absence of pain) and radiographically (progression of increasing callus in secondary fracture healing or decreasing fracture line in primary fracture healing).

Principles of Fracture Healing

Fracture healing involves three overlapping phases (**Figure 1**). The first phase (inflammation) begins with bleeding from the fracture site and surrounding soft tissues. This peaks after several days, during which time numerous bioactive cells migrate to the fracture site hematoma under the direction of cell mediators. Granulation tissue is formed during this phase.

During the second phase (repair), new blood vessels are formed and deliver cells essential to the healing process. Necrotic tissue and debris is removed by phagocytes, and fibroblasts begin to produce collagen. Soft cartilaginous callus is produced first and is then mineralized. Mineralized callus is then slowly converted to woven bone (immature bone).

The final phase (remodeling) overlaps with the repair phase and can continue for several months. During this phase, woven bone is replaced by more mature lamellar bone. Typically, union occurs at approximately 6 to 10 weeks; however, the remodeling process can last for months.

Primary Fracture Healing Pattern

Primary or intramembranous fracture healing involves a direct reestablishment of the bony cortex following fracture. Primary

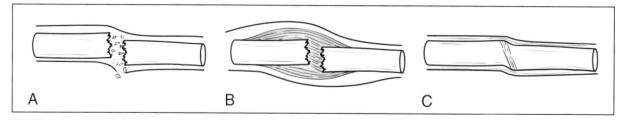

Figure 1 Illustration shows the stages of secondary fracture healing. **A,** Inflammatory phase: migration of bioactive cells. **B,** Repair phase: formation of bridging callus. **C,** Remodeling phase: remodeling of the fracture.

fracture healing requires anatomic reduction of the fracture with no or minimal fracture gaps. In addition, rigid stabilization of the fracture is necessary for primary fracture healing to occur. Typically, primary fracture healing requires plate-and-screw stabilization. With primary fracture healing, no callus is formed. Radiographic evidence of callus is suspicious for inadequate fixation and motion at the fracture site. Primary fracture healing is desirable in fractures in which callus could impede motion, as in fractures of the radius and ulna (pronation and supination could be limited). Intra-articular and periarticular fractures are often treated with rigid plate fixation because the rigid stabilization of the fracture allows early motion of the joints, which prevents adhesions and enhances cartilage nutrition (**Figure 2**).

Secondary Fracture Healing Pattern

Secondary or endochondral fracture healing requires controlled stress or motion at the fracture site; such healing usually occurs in nonsurgical management of fractures (that is, casting). Healing of endochondral fracture involves three phases. The first is the inflammatory phase, which usually lasts for approximately 2 weeks. In this phase, there is a marked inflammatory response that is mediated by prostaglandins and cytokines and by migration of pluripotent cells to the fracture site. If possible, the use of anti-inflammatory medications should be avoided during this phase because they may inhibit fracture healing. In certain polytrauma patients, this inflammatory response, along with the additional inflammation caused by surgical procedures, may trigger excessive inflammation, resulting in multiple organ failure. In polytrauma patients, damage control treatment often takes precedence, and fracture stabilization is delayed until after the initial inflammatory phase has abated. The second phase of fracture healing is the repair or callus-forming phase. The initial callus is cartilaginous and is not apparent on routine radiographs. Different signaling proteins, of which bone morphogenetic protein (BMP) is the most important, mediate the differentiation of the callus into bone. BMP has been isolated from bone and can be used either to accelerate fracture healing or, in the case of nonunions, cause fractures to heal. The last phase of endochondral fracture healing is the remodeling phase, which is particularly important in children. Radiographs of a tibial fracture with endochondral fracture healing are shown in **Figure 3**. For endochondral fracture healing to occur, stress or motion must be present at the fracture site; weight bearing in a cast is required to achieve endochondral healing of lower extremity fractures.

Hybrid Fracture Healing

Recently, a hybrid fracture healing model was developed that involves the achievement of relative stability of the fracture. Percutaneous plate stabilization preserves the biologic environment for fracture healing by minimally disturbing the blood supply. A less rigid construct is deliberately created by using fewer screws

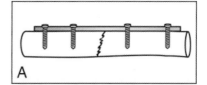
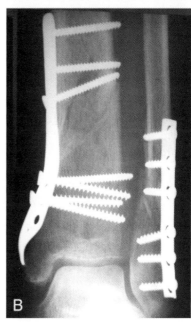

Figure 2 Primary fracture healing. **A,** Illustration shows primary fracture healing. **B,** Radiograph demonstrates healing without fracture callus following rigid fixation. This is indicative of intramembranous healing.

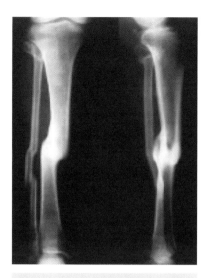

Figure 3 Radiographs of a tibia fracture treated nonsurgically. Note the exuberant callus present at the healed fracture site. (Reproduced from Sarmiento A, Latta LL: Functional fracture bracing. *J Am Acad Orthop Surg* 1999;7[1]:66-75.)

Risk Factors for Impaired Fracture Healing

Smoking

Indolent infection

Inadequate immobilization

Malnutrition

NSAID use

Significant soft-tissue injury

than in rigid fixation, thereby placing stress on the fracture site and promoting callus formation. In addition, intramedullary nails are inserted percutaneously. These nails often are made of titanium; of the available materials for nails, titanium has a modulus of elasticity that is closest to bone, which allows stress to the bone and callus formation. Typically, external fixators are used for temporary fracture stabilization, such as in damage-control orthopaedics, but external fixators can be used in special clinical cases to lengthen bone (such as the Ilizarov technique).

Impaired Fracture Healing
Malunion
Malunion is defined as an inadequately aligned union of a fracture and is commonly a result of inadequate fracture reduction, immobilization, or possible surgical error in alignment during fixation. Each bone has defined ranges for acceptable alignment. For example, more malalignment is tolerated in humeral fractures than in tibial fractures. Tibial malalignment can result in altered biomechanical stresses on the knee and the ankle.

Delayed Union and Nonunion
Delayed union is a prolonged time to union. Healing beyond 16 to 20 weeks typically is considered delayed. Nonunion is failure of normal fracture healing and is defined as (1) a fracture that has not healed following 6 months of treatment, or (2) a fracture that demonstrates no healing progress on radiographs for 3 consecutive months. It has been demonstrated that in patients allowed unrestricted weight bearing, delayed weight bearing usually results in delayed fracture healing. Nonunions usually are the result of an impaired biologic environment (poor blood supply, indolent infection, diabetes), inadequate immobilization, or poor surgical technique. Smoking has been shown to be a causative factor for nonunion (**Sidebar: Risk Factors for Impaired Fracture Healing**).

   Treatment of nonunions varies based on the etiology of the nonunion (**Table 1**). Evaluation of patients with nonunions should include testing of inflammatory markers (white blood cell count, erythrocyte sedimentation rate, C-reactive protein level) to rule out indolent infection. Although malnutrition has not been definitively proved to cause nonunion, it should be ruled out. Recently, low serum levels of vitamin D has been implicated in nonunions. Cessation of smoking is a requirement for treatment of nonunions. After performing this basic work-up, the physician should classify the radiographic fracture pattern. Hypertrophic nonunions demonstrate abundant callus but exhibit a persistent fracture line. Hypertrophic nonunion can be managed either by stabilizing the fracture with internal fixation or by stimulating fracture healing with either electrical or ultrasonic stimulation. Atrophic nonunions result from a poor biologic environment or inadequate blood supply. Treatment of atrophic nonunions involves enhancing the fracture healing environment by either inserting cells (autogenous bone graft) or inserting

Table 1

Classification of Nonunions

Type	Cause	Treatment
Hypertrophic	Inadequate stability	Revision to more stable fixation
Atrophic	Inadequate biologic conditions	Bone grafting
Fibrous	Inadequate reduction	Débridement, bone grafting
	Inadequate biologic conditions	Débridement, bone grafting
	Inadequate stability	Débridement, bone grafting
Oligotrophic	Inadequate reduction	Revision of reduction
Septic	Infection	Débridement, antibiotics

osteoinductive substances (BMP) that recruit pluripotential cells to the fracture. Ideally, both methods are used to enhance healing of atrophic nonunion.

Treatment

Nonsurgical

Nonsurgical management is appropriate for stable fracture patterns that can be immobilized with a splint or cast. For fractures managed in this manner, follow-up radiographs should be obtained to assess healing and maintenance of acceptable alignment. Loss of reduction or a lack of healing may require surgical intervention. Electrical and ultrasound stimulation may be used as an adjunct to enhance the healing of fractures prone to nonunion as well as delayed unions and established nonunions.

Surgical

Surgical treatment of fractures is indicated for unstable fractures and fractures that do not respond to nonsurgical treatment. Surgery may range from closed reduction with percutaneous pinning to allograft reconstructions for massive bone defects.

Open fractures require urgent irrigation and débridement to minimize the development of infection. Intra-articular fractures often require open treatment to reduce the articular cartilage as a way of minimizing future posttraumatic arthritis.

Malunions may require an osteotomy, or bone cuts, to restore the anatomic alignment of the bone. Nonunions from infection are treated with extensive débridement of infected bone and tissue followed by intravenous antibiotics and delayed reconstruction.

Bone grafting is often necessary in the treatment of nonunions as well as for fractures with bone loss. Available graft properties and graft options are shown in **Tables 2** and **3**. Autograft and allograft tissue have osteoinductive and osteoconductive properties. Autograft

Table 2

Properties of Bone Grafts

Graft Type	Description
Osteogenic	Contains cells capable of bone formation
Osteoinductive	Induces mesenchymal cells to differentiate into osteoblasts
Osteoconductive	Provides structural stability and forms a scaffold on which bone-forming cells can build

Table 3

Descriptions of and Indications for Bone Grafts

Type	Properties	Advantages	Disadvantages
Autogenous bone	Osteogenic Osteoconductive Osteoinductive	Reference standard	Donor site morbidity, limited supply
Allograft bone	Osteoconductive	Structural grafts	Disease transmission, infection
Synthetic bone substitutes	Osteoconductive	Large supply for filling voids, high compressive strength	Nonstructural graft
Demineralized bone matrix	Osteoconductive Osteoinductive	Bioactive, fills voids	Disease transmission, expensive
Recombinant bone proteins	Osteoinductive	Improves fracture and wound healing	Expensive

is considered the reference standard and may be harvested from the patient's iliac crest, proximal tibia, or, less commonly, local bone near the surgical site. Allograft tissue is taken from cadavers and has a very small risk of bacterial or viral disease transmission. Newer processing procedures have decreased this risk dramatically. Demineralized bone matrix is an allograft product processed to remove calcium hydroxyapatite without disrupting the osteoinductive proteins or osteoconductive substrate. Recombinant human BMP is a potent osteoinductive agent useful for treating difficult nonunions and open fractures. Osteoconductive synthetic bone substitutes, including calcium phosphate, also are available for situations involving bone loss or poor bone production.

Fracture Splinting Principles

Splinting of fractures, dislocations, or tendon ruptures often is required as part of initial emergent management. A well-applied splint reduces pain, bleeding, and swelling by immobilizing the injured soft and hard tissue. Splinting also helps prevent several problems:

- Further damage of muscles, nerves (including the spinal cord), and blood vessels by the sharp bony cortices
- Laceration of the skin by the sharp fracture ends
- Compression of vascular structures by malaligned bone ends
- Further contamination of an open wound

General Principles of Splinting

1. Remove clothing from the area of any suspected fracture or dislocation to inspect the extremity for open wounds, deformity, swelling, ecchymosis, and additional injuries.

2. Note and record the pulse, capillary refill, and neurologic status, including motor and sensory examinations, distal to the site of injury.

3. Cover all wounds with a dry, sterile dressing before applying a splint. If it is necessary to transfer the patient, notify the receiving physician of all open wounds, including location and extent of the soft-tissue injury as well as the neurovascular status of the extremity.

4. Ensure that the splint immobilizes the joint above and below the suspected fracture.

5. With intra-articular injuries, ensure that the splint immobilizes the bones above and below the injured joint.

6. Sufficiently pad all bony prominences prior to application of rigid splints to prevent local pressure sores and soft-tissue compromise.

7. During application of the splint, use your hands to minimize movement of the limb and to support the injury site until the splinting material has hardened and the limb is completely immobilized. Some splints require the help of an assistant to ensure proper application.

8. Align a severely deformed and shortened limb with constant, gentle traction to ensure appropriate reduction and immobilization in the splint.

9. If you encounter resistance to limb alignment when you apply traction, splint the limb in the position of deformity.

10. When in doubt, temporarily immobilize the suspected area of injury with a splint.

Table 1

Splinting Materials

Thumb/Finger	Wrist and Forearm	Arm	Long Leg Splint	Short Leg Splint
1 to 2 rolls 4″ cast padding (adults) or 3″ cast padding (children)	2 rolls 4″ cast padding (adults) or 3″ cast padding (children)	2 or 3 rolls 4″ cast padding (adults) or 3″ cast padding (children)	3 to 4 rolls 6″ cast padding	2 rolls 4″ to 5″ cast padding
4″ × 15″ splints, six thicknesses (adults), or 3″ roll folded into splint of appropriate length (children)	5″ × 30″ splints, six thicknesses (adults), for sugar tong; or 4″ × 15″ splints, six thicknesses (children), for simple dorsal or volar splint	5″ × 30″ splints, six thicknesses (adults), or 4″ plaster rolls folded to necessary length (children)	3 to 4 rolls 5″ or 6″ wide plaster or 5″ × 45″ plaster splints	12 to 14 thicknesses of 5″ × 30″ or 5″ × 45″ plaster strips; one 3″ to 4″ wide roll of plaster
2″ or 3″ elastic bandage	2″ or 3″ elastic bandage	3″ or 4″ elastic bandage	One roll each of 4″ and 6″ elastic bandages	One roll 4″ elastic bandage
Tepid water (≈24°C)	Tepid water (≈24°C)	Tepid water (≈24°C)	One bucket of tepid water (≈24°C)	One bucket of tepid water (≈24°C)
Nonsterile gloves	Nonsterile gloves	Nonsterile gloves	Nonsterile gloves	Nonsterile gloves

Materials

Although prefabricated plastic, fabric, and metal splints are available, the immobilization provided by these devices is generally unsatisfactory except when used in the emergent setting and for short periods of time. If a splint must remain in place for more than several hours, custom application of a well-padded plaster or fiberglass splint is preferred. Although plaster splints are cheaper than fiberglass and may better hold fractures reduced, fiberglass splints are lighter, stay cleaner, and often are more durable. During the curing process, multilayered "homemade" splints or thick commercial plaster splints can generate heat sufficient to burn the patient; thus, such splints should be used with caution. See **Table 1** for the materials needed for splinting. Store these materials in a dry cabinet or closet. With the advent of three-dimensional printing, it may one day be possible and cost-effective to print custom splints tailored to particular fractures and patients.

Splinting the Upper Extremity
Fractures or Injuries of the Hand or Wrist

1. Position the patient supine or sitting and have an assistant hold the patient's thumb and/or index fingers.

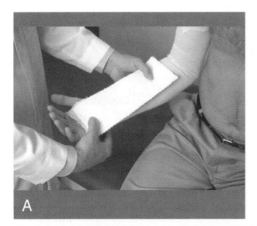
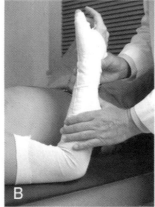

Figure 1 Photographs show splinting of an injury of the hand or wrist. **A,** Begin in the palm and extend up the volar surface of the forearm to below the elbow. **B,** Apply the splint along the volar aspect of the thumb, extending across the wrist to the proximal forearm.

2. Loosely wrap cast padding from the palm to the elbow, ensuring that there are three layers of padding at all bony prominences.

3. Place a 4″ × 15″ preassembled splint in the palm and carry it up the volar aspect of the forearm to just below the elbow (**Figure 1, A**). If the injury involves the thumb, wrap it separately with 2″ or 3″ of cast padding.

4. Place the splint on the volar or radial aspect and fold the plaster around the thumb, extending across the wrist to the proximal forearm. Leave the dorsal or ulnar side open for swelling (**Figure 1, B**).

5. Wrap the cast padding loosely over the plaster. Wrap an elastic bandage loosely over the cast padding as you mold the splint.

6. Trim the palmar portion of the splint back to the distal palmar flexion crease, proximal to the metacarpophalangeal (MCP) joint.

7. Ensure complete hardening of the splint material with proper alignment before leaving the patient. Constantly mold the splint as it dries for an anatomic fit.

Fractures or Injuries of the Forearm and Elbow

1. With the patient sitting or supine, have an assistant support the patient's hand with the elbow flexed to 90°. If sitting, the patient should lean slightly to the affected side so that the elbow falls away from the body.

2. Loosely wrap cast padding from the palm to above the elbow, taking care to avoid creating a constriction in the elbow crease, or antecubital fossa. Make sure that there are three layers of padding at all bony prominences, such as the wrist and the elbow.

3. For a sugar tong splint, begin the splint in the palm at the level of the distal palmar flexion crease, proximal to the MCP joint as described previously. Carry the splint up the volar forearm to the elbow, and around the posterior elbow, and then continue back

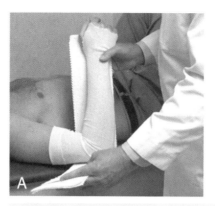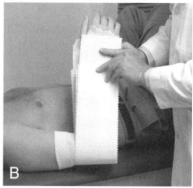

Figure 2 Photographs show splinting of an injury of the elbow and forearm. **A,** Begin in the palm and extend proximally around the posterior elbow. **B,** Complete the splint distally on the extensor aspect of the forearm to the dorsum of the hand.

toward the hand over the dorsal forearm distally on the extensor aspect of the forearm to the dorsum of the hand (**Figure 2**). Use multiple 4″ × 15″ preassembled splints or a 5″ × 30″ preassembled splint if that size is appropriate.

4. Wrap cast padding loosely over the plaster, then wrap an elastic bandage loosely over the cast padding as you mold the splint.

5. Trim the palmar portion of the splint back to the distal palmar flexion crease, proximal to the MCP joint.

6. Ensure complete hardening of the splint material with proper alignment before leaving the patient. Constantly mold the splint as it dries for an anatomic fit.

Fractures or Injuries of the Humerus

1. With the patient sitting, have an assistant support the patient's hand with the elbow flexed to 90°. The patient should lean slightly to the affected side so that the elbow falls away from the body.

2. Loosely wrap cast padding from the palm to the upper arm. Begin the splint below the axilla, carry it under the elbow, and then proceed distally along the lateral aspect of the forearm.

3. For unstable humeral fractures, use an elephant ear splint: continue the splint over the top of the shoulder, cover the plaster with a layer of cast padding, and then loosely wrap the entire arm with an elastic bandage (**Figure 3**).

4. For lower humeral fractures or elbow injuries, use a coaptation splint: end the splint below the lateral shoulder, cover the plaster with a layer of cast padding, and then loosely wrap the entire arm with an elastic bandage. Provide the patient with a strap sling that loops around the wrist, then around the neck, and back to the wrist (**Figure 4**). The sling should be long enough to allow the elbow to be maintained at 90°.

5. Make sure that the sling has padding at the neck and wrist; these straps do not slide at night and can be adjusted for different arm lengths.

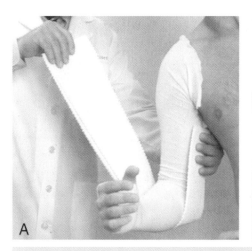

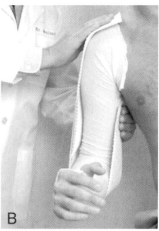

Figure 3 Photographs show proper splinting of an injury of the humerus. **A,** Begin the splint below the axilla, extending it under the elbow, and then proceed up the lateral aspect of the arm. **B,** For unstable humeral fractures, continue the splint over the top of the shoulder.

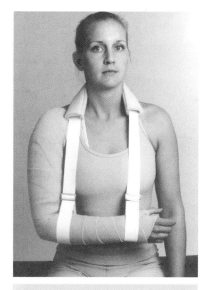

Figure 4 Photograph shows proper positioning of a sling to maintain the elbow at 90°.

6. Ensure complete hardening of the splint material with proper alignment before leaving the patient. Constantly mold the splint as it dries for an anatomic fit.

Patient Instructions

Patients should be advised to protect the splint for 24 hours, until the plaster cures and hardens completely. Fiberglass splints harden faster than plaster splints. A splinted arm should not be placed on any plastic-covered surfaces (including pillows) until the plaster has cooled. Patients also should be reminded to watch for changes in skin color (circulation), sensation, and motion in the hand.

Splinting the Lower Extremity
Long Leg Splint for Fractures and Injuries of the Lower Leg

1. For unstable fractures of the leg or ankle, a long leg splint is appropriate with the knee flexed slightly at 25° to 30° of flexion and the ankle flexed to neutral or 90°.

2. The patient should be supine, with the buttock on the affected side at the edge of the table, allowing the entire leg to hang suspended as an assistant holds the patient's forefoot and toes. Ask the patient to relax the calf muscles to allow the ankle to be maintained at 90° during splinting.

3. Use either a stirrup-type splint or a long posterior splint. For a stirrup splint, have an assistant hold the patient's forefoot as you wrap the leg with three layers of 6″ cast padding. Place extra padding over the bony prominences, such as the kneecap and lateral knee (fibular head).

4. Begin the plaster on the lateral aspect of the mid thigh, extending it distally along the lateral aspect of the leg, around the heel, and then proximally back up the medial side to the level of the mid thigh (**Figure 5, A**).

SECTION 1 GENERAL ORTHOPAEDICS

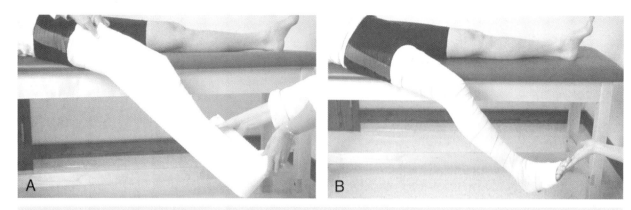

Figure 5 Photographs of a long leg splint. **A,** Begin the splint on the lateral aspect of the thigh, extending it down the lateral aspect of the leg, under the heel, and then back up the medial side. **B,** Maintain the knee in 25° to 30° of flexion and the ankle at 90° as the splint hardens.

5. Start a second splint on the plantar surface of the foot and extend it proximally to the level of the mid thigh.

6. Apply a layer of cast padding over the plaster, and wrap a 5″ or 6″ elastic bandage over the padding as you mold the splint.

7. Ensure that the knee is positioned in slight flexion (approximately 25° to 30°) and the foot is positioned at 90° to the tibia (**Figure 5, B**).

Avoid folds in the plaster over the area of the peroneal nerve below the lateral knee (fibular head) or around the ankle. Preassembled foam-padded splints are convenient, but use them with caution because they may develop folds or ridges in critical areas.

Use tepid or cool—never hot—water when applying the splint. The heat generated by the reaction of the plaster, when coupled with the use of hot water, can seriously burn the patient's skin. For the same reason, place the leg on a cloth (not plastic) pillow and leave it uncovered for approximately 10 minutes following application to allow better heat convection away from the soft tissue.

Hold the splint in place with a loosely applied elastic bandage or bias-cut stockinet, rolled on with almost no tension. As the splint hardens, maintain the ankle at 90°. Mold or support the splint with the flat of the hand—only while it hardens—to avoid causing dents. Dents not only make the splint uncomfortable but can cause cast sores or peroneal nerve palsy and footdrop.

Short Leg Splint for Fractures and Injuries of the Ankle and Foot

1. With the patient sitting, have an assistant hold the forefoot and toes to maintain the ankle at a 90° angle. Wrap the foot, ankle, and leg loosely with three layers of cast padding.

2. Fashion a splint using either 4″ or 5″ plaster splinting rolls folded to length.

3. Begin the splint laterally, three fingerbreadths below the knee flexion crease, and extend it distally around the heel and then proximally up the medial side of the leg to the level of the splint on the lateral aspect of the leg (**Figure 6, A**).

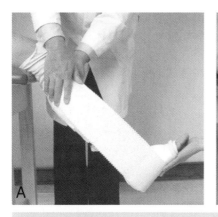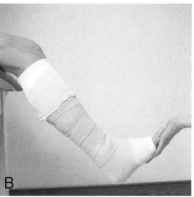

Figure 6 Photographs of application of a short leg splint. **A,** Begin the splint laterally, three fingerbreadths below the knee flexion crease, and extend it down and wrap it under the heel and then up the medial side of the leg. **B,** Maintain the angle of the ankle at 90° as the splint hardens.

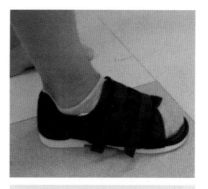

Figure 7 Photograph of a postoperative shoe used in the management of fractures of the midfoot or forefoot.

4. Apply the splint like a stirrup, extending material under the foot, covering the heel and arch.

5. Place a single layer of cast padding over the splint, and loosely wrap a 4″ elastic bandage to secure the splint as you mold it to the extremity.

6. Maintain the ankle at 90° as the splint hardens (**Figure 6, B**).

Leave the plaster open in front and/or back so that the patient can unwrap the elastic bandage and spread the splint if needed to accommodate swelling.

Postoperative Shoe for Fracture or Injuries of the Midfoot and Forefoot

A commercially available hard-soled, wide shoe with Velcro straps can be used to support fractures of the midfoot and forefoot (**Figure 7**). An elastic bandage is frequently wrapped around the foot before applying the shoe. A bulky sock can be substituted for the elastic bandage.

Patient Instructions

Patients should be advised to keep the injured leg elevated to the level of the heart as much as possible to decrease soft-tissue swelling. Sitting in a reclining chair with a pillow beneath the leg is a useful position for this. In addition, cold therapy such as application of ice should be incorporated for 2 to 3 days after the injury to reduce pain and minimize swelling.

If the pain increases substantially, the foot or toes feel numb or tingly, or the patient notes a change in his or her ability to move the toes up and down, the splint should be loosened by unwrapping the elastic bandage and tearing the padding down the front of the leg. If the leg does not feel better within 20 to 30 minutes, the patient should be advised to call the treating physician or seek immediate medical attention because the vascular circulation to the leg may be compromised. Vascular compromise has serious consequences and must be managed promptly.

The splint must be kept clean and dry. To bathe, the patient should place a plastic bag or commercially available cast cover over the leg, prop the leg on the side of the tub, and then fill the tub, keeping the splinted leg out of the water. The patient should not shower. Sponge bathing is another option to maintain hygiene while wearing an extremity splint.

The patient should be advised to contact the physician if the splint feels as though it is chafing or digging into the skin. The patient also should be reminded to watch for changes in skin color (circulation), sensation, and motion in the foot (including the toes).

Adverse Outcomes of Treatment

Compartment syndrome, soft-tissue burns, nerve compression injuries, and pressure sores can occur in splinted upper or lower extremities. Plantar flexion or equinus contractures of the ankle can develop if the ankle is splinted for prolonged periods with the ankle plantarflexed beyond the neutral position.

Imaging: Principles and Techniques

Imaging studies are essential in the evaluation and management of musculoskeletal pathology. Each imaging modality provides unique and valuable information (**Table 1**). Before ordering imaging studies, a thorough history and physical examination should be performed to formulate a working diagnosis. This will help guide imaging selection. In general, the most basic imaging should be ordered first, and if further information is needed, more invasive and advanced imaging studies may be necessary. *Essentials of Musculoskeletal Imaging*, another volume in this series, describes appropriate imaging studies for more than 300 musculoskeletal conditions.

Radiography

Radiographic images are obtained by projecting x-ray beams through a subject onto an image detector. As the beam traverses the tissues, radiation is absorbed, which decreases the amount of radiation projected onto the detector. Decreased-intensity radiation produces a bright (or white) image on the x-ray film (**Figure 1**).

Table 1

Imaging Modalities

Modality	Advantages	Disadvantages
Radiography	Simple, inexpensive, readily available, easily interpreted	Radiation, poor tissue contrast, relies on technician for adequate images, two-dimensional
CT	Three-dimensional capability, axial imaging, high bony detail, rapid	Highest radiation, motion and metal artifact, poor soft-tissue contrast
MRI	Superior contrast resolution	Expensive, motion and metal artifact, contraindicated with certain indwelling devices
Arthrography	Combined with other modalities to improve contrast	Radiation, invasive, allergic reactions
Bone scan	Images metabolic activity, especially in bones	Nonspecific, poor detail, radiation exposure
Ultrasonography	Very safe, inexpensive	Small field of view, technician- and radiologist-dependent, artifacts

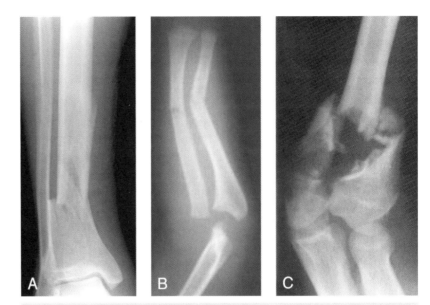

Figure 1 Radiographs of distal tibia fracture (**A**), radius and ulna fracture (**B**), and distal humerus fracture (**C**). (Panel A reproduced from Bedi A, Le TT, Karunakar MA: Surgical treatment of nonarticular distal tibia fractures. *J Am Acad Orthop Surg* 2006;14[7]:406-416. Panel B reproduced from Ring D, Jupiter JB, Waters PM: Monteggia fractures in children and adults. *J Am Acad Orthop Surg* 1998;6[4]:215-224. Panel C reproduced with permission from Mayo Foundation for Medical Education and Research.)

Radiographs are effective for the initial evaluation of musculoskeletal pathology. Radiographic evaluation should include a minimum of two views of the bone in perpendicular planes (AP and lateral). In fracture evaluation, the joints above and below the area of interest are imaged to assess for joint dislocations or associated fractures. In specific scenarios, such as wrist, elbow, pelvic, and ankle fractures, specialized views should be obtained (**Table 2**).

Views of the contralateral asymptomatic limb may be beneficial in children with suspected physeal injuries and for comparison of irregularities, which may be benign variants.

Lead shields should be used whenever possible to protect patients from radiation exposure, especially in areas of radiation-sensitive tissue and in children.

Indications

The most common indications for radiographic imaging include the following:

• Deformity of a bone or joint
• Pain or decreased motion of a bone or joint
• Unexplained or disproportionate localized tenderness
• Abnormal asymmetry or mass
• Evaluation for foreign bodies

Table 2

Radiographic Views Commonly Ordered to Evaluate Various Anatomic Regions

Anatomic Region	Radiographic Views
Upper Extremity	
Fingers	PA, lateral, and oblique with fingers separated
Hand	PA, lateral (oblique)
Wrist	PA, lateral with wrist in neutral position (consider scaphoid views for anatomic snuffbox tenderness)
Forearm	AP, lateral
Elbow	AP in supination, lateral in 90° flexion (consider radial head views for direct tenderness over radial head)
Humerus	AP, lateral
Shoulder	AP in internal and external rotation, scapular-Y lateral, axillary lateral view (for all trauma/suspected dislocations), consider Zanca view for AC joint pathology
Lower Extremity	
Hip	AP in internal rotation, frog-lateral or cross-table lateral if necessary
Femur	AP, lateral
Knee	AP, lateral, and tunnel views; oblique view to see fibular head; add AP weight-bearing for arthritis evaluation
Tibia/fibula	AP, lateral
Ankle	AP, lateral, mortise
Foot	AP, lateral, internal oblique (weight-bearing views for Lisfranc injury, alignment abnormalities)
Calcaneus	AP, lateral, Harris axial view
Toes	AP, lateral, oblique
Axial Skeleton	
Cervical spine	AP, lateral (trauma series also should include odontoid view and C7 swimmer's view; consider lateral flexion/extension views for patients with rheumatoid arthritis and suspected instability)
Thoracic spine	AP, lateral
Lumbar spine	AP, lateral
Pelvis	AP (consider Judet views for acetabular fractures, inlet/outlet views for pelvic ring injuries)

AC = acromioclavicular.

Computed Tomography

CT offers detailed axial and three-dimensional imaging by detecting variable tissue absorption of x-rays, much like plain radiographs (**Figure 2**). A computer manipulates and reconstructs the data into contiguous axial images as well as multiplanar reconstructions. CT is useful for detailed examination of bone, and it is the best modality for evaluating intra-articular and complex fractures such as those in the scapula, spine, and pelvis. Three-dimensional CT reconstructions provide spatial information, which is useful in surgical planning. Soft-tissue evaluation is limited; however, the addition of intravenous

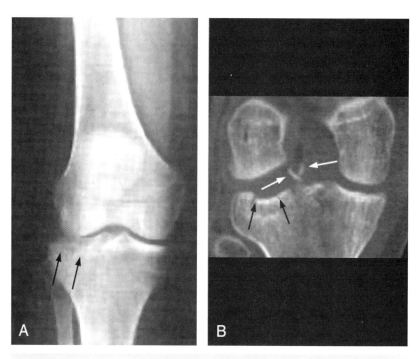

Figure 2 Images of depressed tibial plateau fracture. **A,** AP radiograph of the knee demonstrates an irregularity of the lateral tibial plateau (arrows) consistent with a fracture. **B,** Coronal reformatted CT scan of the knee demonstrates depression of the posterior lateral articular surface (black arrows) consistent with a fracture. Note the two intra-articular fracture fragments about the tibia (white arrows), as well as the bony detail of fracture pattern seen on CT. (Reproduced from Johnson TR, Steinbach LS, eds: *Essentials of Musculoskeletal Imaging.* Rosemont, IL, American Academy of Orthopaedic Surgeons, 2004, p 501.)

contrast dye can be used to evaluate tumors and other soft-tissue masses. CT myelography is typically used for evaluation of spinal cord and nerve root pathology in patients following surgical instrumentation. Intravenous contrast is contraindicated in certain patients with kidney disease, and a small percentage of patients may have an allergy to the dye. CT also can be used to guide difficult joint aspirations. The major drawback of CT imaging is that it subjects patients to considerable radiation exposure. Claustrophobic patients and those with a larger body habitus may be unsuitable for this imaging modality because of the enclosed space of the CT scanner.

Indications
The most common indications for CT imaging include the following:
• Complex or intra-articular fracture evaluation
• Preoperative planning to evaluate bone fragment size and location
• Evaluation of bone tumors

Magnetic Resonance Imaging
MRI uses a powerful magnet to align the hydrogen atoms of water, which are present in varying concentrations in tissues. Radiofrequency (RF) fields are used to alter the alignment of these

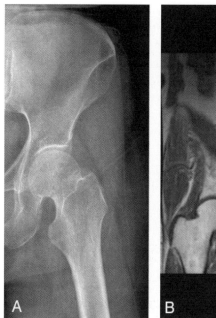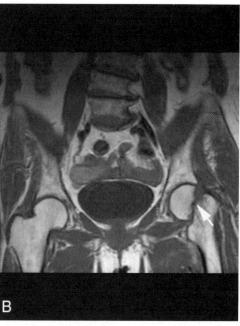

Figure 3   Fracture of the femoral neck seen on MRI but not on radiograph. **A,** AP radiograph of the left femur does not reveal a fracture line. **B,** A T1-weighted MRI of the same patient shows the low–signal intensity fracture line across the left femoral neck (arrow). (Reproduced from Johnson TR, Steinbach LS, eds: *Essentials of Musculoskeletal Imaging.* Rosemont, IL, American Academy of Orthopaedic Surgeons, 2004, p 435.)

atoms, producing a magnetic field detectable by the scanner. MRI provides the most detail for evaluation of soft tissues and the spine. MRI also is useful to evaluate tumors and certain bone conditions such as osteonecrosis, osteomyelitis, and stress fractures (**Figure 3**). MRI should not be used as an initial screening study because of its high cost. MRI may be used to further clarify a particular problem. Radiologists have several different techniques available to further enhance the information provided by MRI, including T1-weighted, T2-weighted, proton density, fat suppression or saturation, gradient echo, and short tau inversion recovery (STIR) sequences (**Table 3**). Gadolinium-based contrast agents can be injected into a joint or delivered intravenously to provide further contrast detail.

Caution should be used when MRI is ordered in patients who have implanted ferromagnetic metal in their body that may heat up, malfunction (cardiac pacemakers), or dislodge (aneurysm clips in the brain) when placed in a strong magnetic field. Common metals used for orthopaedic stabilization such as titanium are nonferromagnetic and are typically safe for MRI; however, images lose value in the presence of these materials because they are blurred by artifact. Care should be taken to avoid delivering contrast in patients with kidney disease or contrast material allergy. Open MRI scanners are available for patients who are claustrophobic and for patients who have a larger body habitus.

Table 3

Signal Intensities for Selected Structures on Different MRI Sequences

Structure	Sequence		
	T1-weighted; short TR/short TE	Proton-density; long TR/short TE	T2-weighted; long TR/long TE
Fat[a]	Bright	Bright	Intermediate
Fluid[b]	Dark	Intermediate	Bright
Fibrocartilage[c]	Dark	Dark	Dark
Ligament, tendon[d]	Dark	Dark	Dark
Muscle	Intermediate	Intermediate	Dark
Bone marrow	Bright	Intermediate	Dark
Nerve	Intermediate	Intermediate	Intermediate

TE = echo time (short, < 20 to 30 msec; long ≥ 90 msec), TR = repetition time (short, < 600 to 700 msec; long, > 2,000 msec).

[a] Includes yellow marrow. Signal will be dark if fat-suppressed techniques (eg, fat-saturation, short tau inversion recovery [STIR]) are used

[b] Includes edema, most tears, and most cysts

[c] Includes labrum, menisci, triangular fibrocartilage complex

[d] Signal may be increased because of artifacts (eg, magic angle artifact seen in the rotator cuff or the ankle tendons)

(Reproduced from Johnson TR, Steinbach LS, eds: *Essentials of Musculoskeletal Imaging.* Rosemont, IL, American Academy of Orthopaedic Surgeons, 2004, p 12.)

Indications

The most common indications for MRI include the following:

• Disk disease and spinal cord abnormalities

• Tendon and ligamentous injuries

• Meniscal and cartilaginous injuries

• Stress and occult fractures

• Evaluation of soft tissue and bone tumor

• Osteonecrosis or osteomyelitis

Arthrography

Arthrography is the imaging of a joint following the injection of contrast medium. This modality provides further information about joint congruity and the capsule, cartilage, and surrounding soft tissues (**Figure 4**). Contrast also enhances the differentiation of tissues in and around the joint. Arthrography is usually combined with CT or MRI, using different contrast agents in the joint to provide detailed imaging. Delivering contrast is minimally invasive and subjects the patient to a small risk of joint infection or allergic reaction. Delivering contrast adds complexity and cost, however.

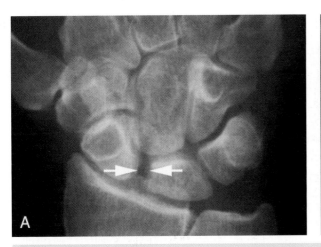 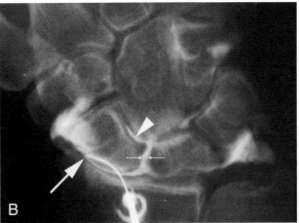

Figure 4 Examples of arthrography of the radiocarpal joint. **A,** Preinjection PA view demonstrates a wide scapholunate interval (arrows), which is suspicious for scapholunate dissociation and tear. **B,** PA view obtained after injection of iodinated contrast medium into the radiocarpal joint (long arrow) of the same wrist demonstrates the flow of the contrast medium through the defect in the scapholunate ligament (short arrows) into the midcarpal joint (arrowhead). (Reproduced from Johnson TR, Steinbach LS, eds: *Essentials of Musculoskeletal Imaging.* Rosemont, IL, American Academy of Orthopaedic Surgeons, 2004, p 20.)

Indications

Common indications for arthrography include the following:

- Wrist cartilage injury (triangular fibrocartilage complex) or ligament tears
- Knee postoperative menisci or joint bodies
- Shoulder labral tears or recurrent rotator cuff tears after repair
- Hip labral tears (femoroacetabular impingement [FAI])
- Elbow ulnar collateral ligament tears
- Ankle talar dome osteochondritis dissecans or joint bodies

Scintigraphy (Bone Scan)

A bone scan, like other scintigraphic studies, detects the distribution of a radioactive agent throughout the body after the agent is injected intravenously. The agent (typically technetium Tc 99m–methylene diphosphonate for bone studies) emits gamma radiation, which is then detected by a scintillation camera to form two-dimensional images. In bone scans, the radioactive agent localizes to areas of metabolic bone activity. Bone scans are sensitive but not specific for bone lesions.

During a three-phase bone scan, the camera detects emission at different times following administration of the contrast agent. This technique is helpful in evaluating fractures and infections (**Figure 5**). Special tracers can be ordered specifically for evaluation of infection (indium and indium-tagged white blood cells).

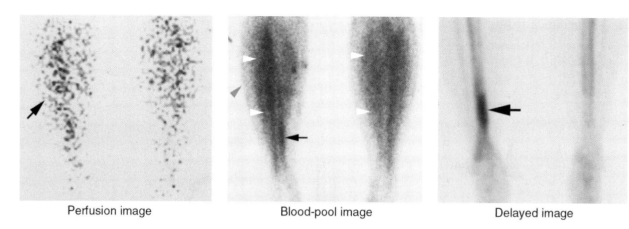

Perfusion image   Blood-pool image   Delayed image

Figure 5   Images from a three-phase bone scan of a tibial stress fracture. Perfusion image demonstrates relatively increased radiotracer flow (arrow) to the symptomatic right leg. Blood-pool image shows relatively increased tracer delivery (gray arrowhead) to the right leg. Note extensive soft-tissue activity (white arrowheads) during this phase and early accumulation of radiotracer in the right tibial stress fracture (black arrow). Delayed image shows clearance of the soft-tissue uptake compared with the blood-pool image. The stress fracture is clearly visible as a linear band of increased uptake in the tibia (arrow). (Reproduced from Johnson TR, Steinbach LS, eds: *Essentials of Musculoskeletal Imaging.* Rosemont, IL, American Academy of Orthopaedic Surgeons, 2004, p 17.)

Indications

The most common indications for a bone scan include the following:

• Infections and inflammatory disorders

• Whole-body imaging for metastatic disease

• Tumors

• Metabolic bone diseases

Ultrasonography

The use of ultrasonography (also called ultrasound) in the evaluation of the musculoskeletal system has increased because of its safety and low cost. Ultrasound relies on the interaction of pulsed sound waves with tissue interfaces. When sound waves bounce off certain structures, echoes are produced. Different tissue characteristics produce specific echo patterns. Echoes are then picked up by a transducer and converted into images and viewed. Ultrasound is noninvasive and the equipment is easy to transport. The major downside is that it is highly technician-dependent and technically difficult to perform and interpret.

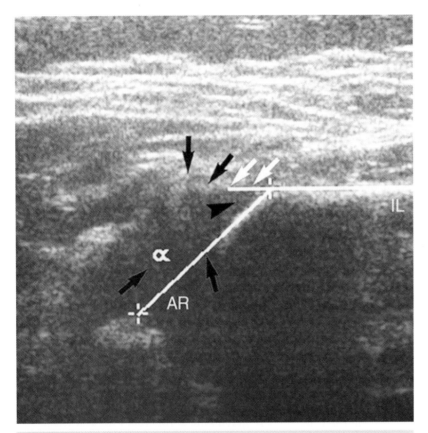

Figure 6 Coronal ultrasonogram of pediatric hip dysplasia demonstrates the cartilaginous femoral head (black arrows), labrum (white arrows), and α angle (arrowhead). AR = bony acetabular roof, IL = iliac wing. (Reproduced from Johnson TR, Steinbach LS, eds: *Essentials of Musculoskeletal Imaging*. Rosemont, IL, American Academy of Orthopaedic Surgeons, 2004, p 801.)

Indications

The most common indications for musculoskeletal ultrasonography include the following:

- Joint effusions or fluid collections
- Tendinopathy—rotator cuff, ankle, elbow, wrist
- Ligament pathology
- Soft-tissue masses
- Infantile hip dysplasia (**Figure 6**)

Infection: Osteomyelitis

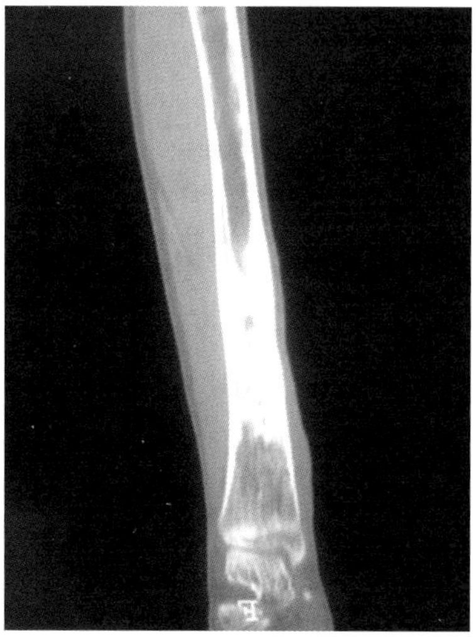

Synonym
Bone infection

Definition
Osteomyelitis is defined as an infection in bone. Osteomyelitis can occur in both pediatric and adult patients. In pediatric patients, the usual etiology of infection is hematogenous, with the highly vascular metaphysis of long bones the most common anatomic area of presentation. Almost one half of pediatric osteomyelitis occurs in patients younger than 5 years. In adult patients, osteomyelitis usually occurs from inoculation of organisms through either open fractures or following surgical fixation of fractures.

Clinical Symptoms
In pediatric patients, osteomyelitis is often difficult to diagnose. Neonates can present with vague symptoms of malaise, including pseudoparalysis, excessive crying, local swelling, and pain with palpation at the affected site. In older children and adults, acute osteomyelitis clinically presents with fever as well as pain and swelling at the infected site. In patients with either previous open fractures or following surgical stabilization of fractures, osteomyelitis presents with drainage or substantial delay in fracture healing.

Tests
The leukocyte count is usually elevated in acute osteomyelitis, but it may be normal in chronic osteomyelitis or in patients with immune suppression. Two markers of inflammation, the erythrocyte sedimentation rate and the C-reactive protein level, are typically elevated in acute and chronic osteomyelitis and therefore can be used as markers of the disease process. Radiographic diagnosis of osteomyelitis is difficult. Plain radiographs show focal osteopenia, soft-tissue swelling, periosteal elevation, and focal lucency around surgical implants. Plain radiographs have a sensitivity of only 14% and a specificity of 76% for osteomyelitis. CT better demonstrates cortical bony details and can detect the presence of early cortical erosions associated with osteomyelitis. MRI reliably detects marrow changes associated with osteomyelitis (**Figure 1**). Nuclear medicine imaging has high sensitivity but low specificity for diagnosing osteomyelitis, so it is not always productive in differentiating osteomyelitis from other clinical entities (**Figure 2**). The best method for diagnosing osteomyelitis is either open biopsy or aspiration, preferably performed before the initiation of antibiotics. In pediatric patients, the most common organism is *Staphylococcus aureus*, followed by group A β-hemolytic streptococci. *Haemophilus influenzae*, a previously prevalent organism in pediatric osteomyelitis, has a diminishing prevalence secondary to immunization. In

Figure 1 MRI demonstrates features consistent with chronic intramedullary osteomyelitis.

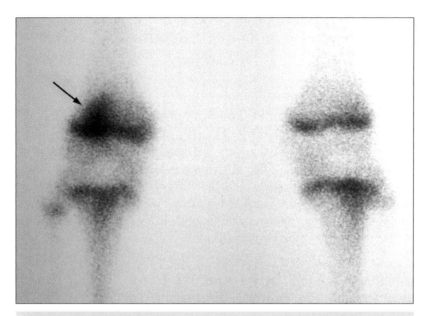

Figure 2 Bone scan from a patient with osteomyelitis demonstrates increased uptake at the metaphysis of the right distal femur (arrow). (Reproduced from Johnson TR, Steinbach LS, eds: *Essentials of Musculoskeletal Imaging.* Rosemont, IL, American Academy of Orthopaedic Surgeons, 2004, p 829.)

adult osteomyelitis, the most common infecting organism is *S aureus*, followed by *Pseudomonas aeruginosa*. In significantly immunocompromised patients, atypical organisms may be the infecting agent. In patients with AIDS, a low CD4 count (< 200 cells/mm^3) or malnutrition (serum albumin level < 2.5 g/dL) is predictive of surgical site infection.

Differential Diagnosis

Several clinical conditions can be confused with osteomyelitis. Neuropathic arthropathy (Charcot arthropathy), a progressive destructive condition associated with denervated limbs, can be confused radiographically with osteomyelitis. Certain tumors, especially tumors that produce lytic lesions in bones, also can mimic osteomyelitis radiographically. Biopsy or aspiration confirms the diagnosis. Tuberculosis may initially manifest in the form of musculoskeletal lesions. Tuberculosis of the musculoskeletal system presents in patients with immunosuppression.

Adverse Outcomes of the Disease

Much advancement has been made in the diagnosis and treatment of osteomyelitis; nonetheless, 5% to 33% of cases remain refractory to treatment. Refractory osteomyelitis is often related to the patient's overall medical status. Diabetes mellitus, peripheral vascular disease, smoking, malnutrition, and immunosuppression are related to failure of treatment. Occasionally, refractory osteomyelitis can be treated with long-term suppressive antibiotic therapy. Amputation may be required in some cases. Rarely, a chronic osteomyelitic sinus will undergo metaplasia and develop squamous cell carcinoma, called a Marjolin ulcer.

Treatment

Treatment of osteomyelitis is different from the treatment of other infections. Bacteria adhere to avascular bone by a glycocalyx that makes antibiotic treatment largely ineffective without débridement of the osteomyelitic bone. Therefore, surgical excision of osteomyelitic bone is absolutely necessary. Antibiotic therapy, either parenterally or locally by antibiotic-impregnated methyl methacrylate beads, is effective following adequate débridement. Bony reconstruction can proceed after the infection is eradicated.

Referral Decisions/Red Flags

In pediatric patients, focal extremity tenderness or fever warrants referral. In adult patients, drainage following surgery for fracture indicates the need for further evaluation.

Infection: Septic Arthritis

Synonyms
Pyogenic arthritis
Suppurative arthritis

Definition
Septic arthritis, also called pyogenic or suppurative arthritis, describes an infection of the joint space. Septic arthritis can affect a variety of joints throughout the body and may occur from direct inoculation, hematogenous spread from concomitant infectious processes, or extension from a contiguous bone infection. Several infectious agents (including bacteria, viruses, mycobacteria, and fungi) can cause septic arthritis; however, *Staphylococcus aureus* is the most common source of acute bacterial arthritis in adults and children older than 2 years and may result in rapid joint destruction. Common sites for septic arthritis include the knee, hip, shoulder, elbow, and wrists. Certain host conditions, such as intravenous (IV) drug abuse, predispose uncommon locations such as the sternoclavicular and sacroiliac joints to infection with *Pseudomonas aeruginosa*.

Septic arthritis in children most commonly results from hematogenous spread. Seeding of the joint may occur, however, from metaphyseal osteomyelitis, particularly if the metaphysis is intra-articular, as it is in the shoulder, elbow, hip, and ankle. In adults, immunocompromised or immunosuppressed patients as well as those with joint-damaging conditions such as rheumatoid arthritis and systemic lupus erythematosus are at increased risk for septic arthritis.

Periprosthetic joint infection may result from intraoperative contamination, local infection, or hematogenous spread. Periprosthetic joint infection is separated into three main categories: acute postoperative, hematogenous, and chronic infection (**Table 1**).

Clinical Symptoms
A thorough history is necessary when evaluating a patient with a suspected septic joint. Key points to elucidate from the patient's history are listed in **Table 2**.

Table 1

Classification of Periprosthetic Joint Infection

Type	Duration
Acute postoperative	Within 3 weeks of joint arthroplasty surgery
Hematogenous	Within 3 weeks of hematogenous seeding
Chronic infection	More than 3 weeks after joint arthroplasty or hematogenous seeding

Key Patient History Points for Septic Arthritis

Number of joints involved

Underlying joint disease or trauma

Prior illnesses or infections

Previous intra-articular injections or joint surgery

Intravenous drug abuse

Time of onset

A high index of suspicion for septic arthritis is required when examining young patients presenting with joint pain. Symptoms may be mild in the early stages, and children will commonly report a vague history of trauma that can confuse the picture. A common scenario is a previously ambulatory child who now refuses to bear weight or move the symptomatic extremity. Other children with septic arthritis will have symptoms of systemic infection such as fever, tachycardia, irritability, and decreased appetite. In addition, it is important to note that knee pain may reflect hip joint pathology.

Joint pain, swelling, and limited range of motion are the most common symptoms and are accompanied by redness and warmth of the joint in question. However, these signs may be muted in elderly or immunocompromised patients who are unable to mount the appropriate inflammatory response to infection. Patients with periprosthetic joints should be carefully evaluated for new-onset pain and swelling, which should always raise the suspicion of infection.

Tuberculous and fungal infections are typically indolent in their presentation. Gonococcal joint infections from *Neisseria gonorrhoeae* are more common in young, sexually active patients, who present with multiple joint arthralgias and skin lesions.

Tests

Physical Examination

The evaluation of a patient with a suspected septic joint begins with a history and physical examination to identify any possible sources of infection such as breaks in the skin and penetrating injuries, as well as skin and tooth abscesses. All joints should be inspected, palpated, and examined for range of motion. Joint tenderness, effusion, and erythema with marked limitation in passive range of motion are the hallmark clinical signs of septic arthritis. Patients with septic arthritis guard the affected joint and report severe pain with joint motion. The affected joint may be held in flexion secondary to the painful joint effusion. The hip will generally be flexed and abducted.

Diagnostic Tests

Laboratory tests for septic arthritis include a white blood cell (WBC) count with differential, erythrocyte sedimentation rate (ESR), and C-reactive protein (CRP) level. These tests are very sensitive but are nonspecific and may not distinguish between infection and other inflammatory processes. The WBC count and ESR may be normal initially, and normal levels do not preclude the diagnosis of septic arthritis. The CRP level increases in response to infection, rising earlier than ESR (within 6 to 8 hours) and normalizing more rapidly. Therefore, monitoring CRP is of value in assessing response to therapy.

Joint fluid aspirate should be evaluated for crystal analysis, Gram stain, cell count, and cultures with sensitivities. Most joints are easy to aspirate; however, ultrasonographic guidance may facilitate aspiration in difficult joints. In a native joint, analysis of the synovial fluid with a WBC count greater than 50,000/mm³ is indicative of infectious arthritis. In the prosthetic joint, synovial fluid with a WBC count greater than 1,100/mm³ with neutrophils greater than 64% is useful to diagnose infection. The glucose level is typically low, and the protein level may be elevated.

Blood cultures should be performed and may help identify the causative organism. If gonococcus is suspected, throat cultures, cervical cultures in females, or urethral cultures in males should be obtained. In addition, the laboratory should be notified if *Haemophilus influenzae*, *N gonorrhoeae*, or *Kingella kingae* are suspected, because these cultures require special considerations. In the setting of chronic infections, cultures should include studies for acid-fast and fungal organisms. Lyme disease titers should be added in regions in which the disease is endemic.

AP and lateral radiographs should be obtained. Radiographs usually are normal but may show soft-tissue swelling around the joint and widening of the joint space. In patients with prosthetic joints, radiographs may reveal radiolucent lines around the prosthesis; the presence of these lines is suggestive of loosening. Ultrasonography is particularly helpful in detecting joint effusion and fluid collection in the surrounding soft tissues. MRI may be useful in excluding adjacent osteomyelitis. A technetium Tc-99m bone scan may be obtained and is useful in identifying the site of infection. Equal uptake on both sides of the joint is suggestive of septic arthritis, but it is difficult to differentiate osteomyelitis from septic arthritis.

Differential Diagnosis

- Acute rheumatic fever (migratory arthralgia, carditis, increased antistreptolysin titer, group A streptococcal infection)
- Bursitis (effusion of the bursa overlying the joint, usually does not limit range of motion, typically afebrile unless infected)
- Crystal-induced arthritis (gout, calcium pyrophosphate dihydrate deposition disease, painful joint, history of flare-ups and normal WBC count)
- Hemarthrosis (hemophilia or traumatic effusions)
- Juvenile rheumatoid arthritis (morning stiffness, usually mild joint swelling, multiple joints involved)
- Lyme disease (indolent onset, erythema migrans, cardiac and neurologic manifestations)
- Osteoarthritis (evident on radiographs)
- Rheumatoid arthritis (morning stiffness, symmetric involvement, positive rheumatoid factor, elevated ESR, elevated leukocyte count in synovial fluid analysis)
- Transient synovitis of the hip (painful joint with prior respiratory infection, afebrile)

Adverse Outcomes of the Disease

Irreversible damage to the joint can occur without or, in some cases, despite proper treatment. Major complications of septic arthritis

SECTION 1 GENERAL ORTHOPAEDICS

Table 3

Causative Organisms and Empiric Antibiotic Regimens for Septic Arthritis

Age/Category	Likely Organism	Initial Antibiotic Regimen
Neonate	*Staphylococcus aureus*, group B streptococcus	Oxacillin + gentamicin
Child < 5 years	*S aureus*, group A streptococcus	Second-generation cephalosporin
	Streptococcus pneumoniae	
	Kingella kingae	
	Haemophilus influenzae	
Child 5 years to adolescence	*S aureus*	Oxacillin
Adolescence to adult	*Neisseria gonorrhoeae, S aureus*	Ceftriaxone (third-generation cephalosporin)
Older adult	*S aureus*	Oxacillin or cefazolin, aminoglycoside
Intravenous drug abuse	*Pseudomonas aeruginosa, Serratia marcescens*	Intravenous aminoglycoside + antipseudomonal cephalosporin (ceftazidime, cefepime, cefoperazone)
Prosthetic joint	*S epidermidis, S aureus*	Vancomycin

include degenerative joint disease, soft-tissue injury and contractures, osteomyelitis, and fibrous or bony ankylosis. The most serious associated outcomes are sepsis and death.

Treatment

After septic arthritis has been diagnosed, empiric IV antibiotic therapy should be initiated following the collection of synovial fluid and blood cultures. Administering antibiotics before obtaining cultures may decrease the likelihood of identifying the infecting organism. Empiric antibiotic coverage is based on patient-specific factors (**Table 3**).

Emergent surgical decompression and lavage of a septic joint is the cornerstone of successful treatment. In special situations in which the patient may not be medically fit for surgery, it may be necessary to perform serial needle aspiration and lavage. The affected extremity should be splinted to rest the soft tissues following surgical intervention. Clinical improvement (afebrile, increased range of motion, and decreased swelling and pain) as well as CRP levels should be monitored postoperatively for resolution. The antimicrobial regimen is adjusted according to culture and sensitivity results, and an infectious disease consultation should be obtained. In uncomplicated infections, IV antibiotics are typically transitioned to oral antibiotics with a total therapy duration of 4 to 6 weeks.

In patients with a periprosthetic joint infection, surgical decisions are based on how long the infection has been present. In the acute setting, an attempt at surgical débridement and prosthesis retention should be made. A chronic periprosthetic infection may require staged revision surgery or possibly prosthetic joint removal and fusion. Antibiotics are then generally administered for 4 to 6 weeks.

Adverse Outcomes of Treatment

Patients may have allergic reactions or adverse drug interactions related to certain antibiotic regimens. Strict adherence to aseptic technique must be followed during joint aspiration to avoid inoculating a joint that is not infected.

Referral Decisions/Red Flags

Patients with a swollen, painful joint with markedly decreased range of motion should be strongly suspected of having septic arthritis and require emergent evaluation by a specialist. An erythematous or swollen joint without limited range of motion may represent overlying cellulitis or septic bursitis. This scenario would preclude arthrocentesis because such action could spread infection from overlying tissues to the joint.

Lyme Disease

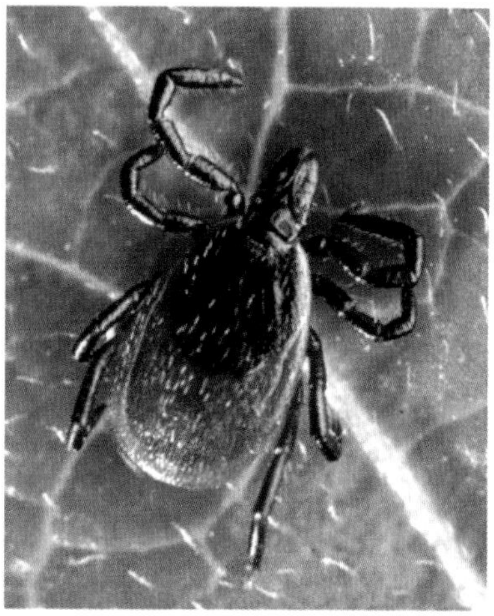

Synonym

Lyme arthritis

Definition

Lyme disease is a multisystem illness caused by the spirochete *Borrelia burgdorferi* that is borne by the deer tick *Ixodes dammini* (**Figure 1**). Lyme disease was first described in 1977 as Lyme arthritis when a group of children in Connecticut had symptoms similar to juvenile rheumatoid arthritis. Lyme disease is the most prevalent vector-borne illness in the United States, with an infection rate of 7.9 cases per 100,000 persons according to the Centers for Disease Control and Prevention (CDC). The incidence is highest in the Northeast (Maryland to northern Massachusetts), the upper Midwest (Wisconsin and Minnesota), and the far West (northern California and Oregon) (**Figure 2**). Lyme disease has been reported in all 50 states, as well as in Asia and Europe. Two additional pathogenic species, *B afzelii* and *B garinii*, are endemic in both Europe and Asia.

Figure 1 Photograph of *Ixodes dammini*, the deer tick that transmits Lyme disease. (Reproduced with permission from the US Department of Agriculture, Washington, DC. http://www.ars.usda.gov/is/graphics/photos/mar98/k8002-3.htm. Accessed June 29, 2015. Photo by Scott Bauer.)

Clinical Symptoms

The clinical symptoms associated with Lyme disease have been divided into three distinct phases: early localized, early disseminated, and late. The characteristic feature of early localized disease is the characteristic skin lesion, erythema migrans (**Figure 3**). Erythema migrans lesions typically occur within 1 month of a tick bite and occur in 80% of patients infected with Lyme disease. The lesions expand over the course of days or weeks, reaching a diameter of up to 20 cm. Erythema migrans lesions are classically described as displaying central clearing, but this has been reported in only 9% of lesions. In the early localized phase, patients may report symptoms similar to a viral syndrome including fatigue, anorexia, headache, neck stiffness, myalgias, arthralgias, and fever. The early disseminated phase typically occurs weeks to several months after the tick bite and can include cardiac or neurologic involvement. The three most common neurologic abnormalities are meningitis, cranial neuropathy, and radiculopathy. Bell palsy (paralysis of the facial nerve) is the most common neurologic manifestation. Pericarditis and atrioventricular heart block are the common cardiac manifestations of early disseminated Lyme disease. Ocular manifestations have been described in the early disseminated phase. Conjunctivitis is the most common manifestation and has been reported in 10% of patients. Arthritis and neurologic symptoms are manifestations of late Lyme disease and occur several months to years after the tick bite; joint pain and swelling develop within several months of infection in 60% of patients who go untreated. Intermittent or persistent arthritis in large joints is commonly seen several months after infection in

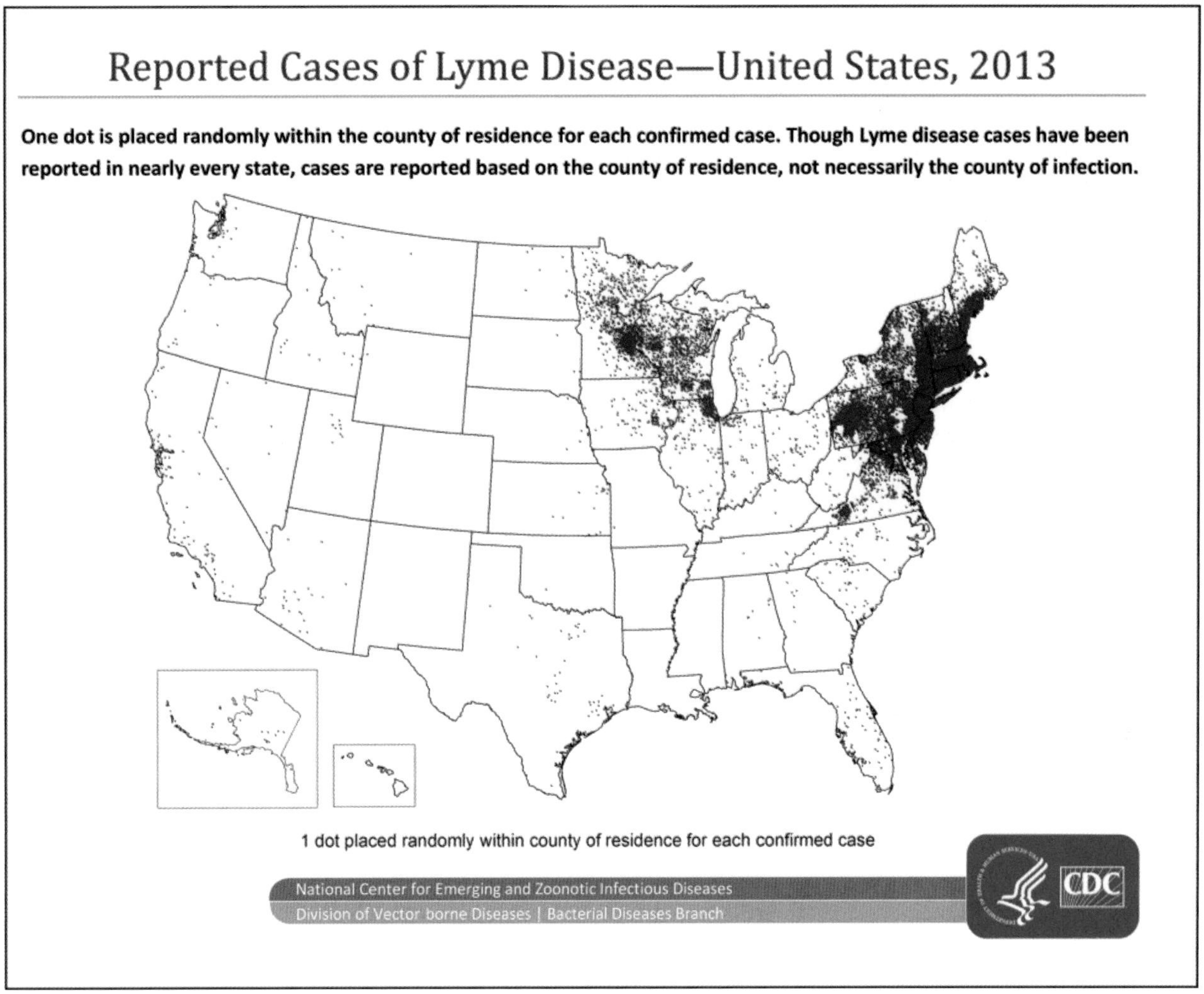

Reported Cases of Lyme Disease—United States, 2013

One dot is placed randomly within the county of residence for each confirmed case. Though Lyme disease cases have been reported in nearly every state, cases are reported based on the county of residence, not necessarily the county of infection.

1 dot placed randomly within county of residence for each confirmed case

National Center for Emerging and Zoonotic Infectious Diseases
Division of Vector borne Diseases | Bacterial Diseases Branch

CDC

Figure 2 Image depicts the approximate risk of Lyme disease in the United States by county. The true relative risk in any given county compared with other counties might differ from that shown here and might change from year to year. Risk categories are defined at www.cdc.gov. Information on risk distribution within states and counties is best obtained from state and local public health authorities. (Reproduced with permission from the Centers for Disease Control and Prevention, Atlanta, GA. http://www.cdc.gov/lyme/resources/ reportedcasesoflymedisease_2013.pdf. Accessed June 16, 2015.)

untreated patients. Lyme arthritis remains the second most frequent manifestation of Lyme disease. Nearly one third of patients with Lyme disease are affected by arthritis that is characterized by brief attacks of joint swelling. The knee is the most commonly affected joint, followed by the shoulder, ankle, and elbow. Lyme encephalopathy, which is characterized by mild cognitive difficulties, occurs in the late phase. Radicular pain and distal paresthesias also have been associated with late Lyme disease. In Europe, cutaneous manifestations have been associated with Lyme disease, but these symptoms have not been reported in the United States.

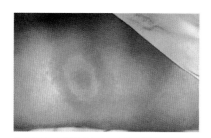

Figure 3 Photograph depicts the appearance of a lesion that developed after a bite by a tick harboring *Borrelia burgdorferi*. (Reproduced from Browner BD, Pollak AN, Gupton CL, eds: *Emergency Care and Transportation of the Sick and Injured*, ed 8. Boston, MA, Jones and Bartlett, 2002, p 427.)

Tests

Physical Examination

Patients with the characteristic erythema migrans skin lesion and constitutional symptoms should be examined for synovitis and restricted joint motion. The axilla, inguinal region, and popliteal fossa are common locations for tick bites. Twenty-five percent of patients with early Lyme disease recall sustaining a tick bite.

Diagnostic Tests

Early Lyme disease can be diagnosed based on clinical examination and the presence of an erythema migrans lesion. In patients with no erythema migrans lesion but clinical features consistent with Lyme disease, serologic studies can be used to confirm the diagnosis. Patients should not be treated for Lyme disease based on serologic test results alone. When a patient begins to manifest symptoms of the early disseminated phase of Lyme disease, serologic tests are positive for both immunoglobulin M (IgM) and immunoglobulin (IgG) *Borrelia* antibodies. Enzyme-linked immunosorbent assay (ELISA) is the initial serologic test, but it has a high false-positive rate: 5% of the normal population has a positive ELISA. If the ELISA is positive or equivocal, Western blot for IgM and IgG *Borrelia* antibodies can be ordered to confirm the diagnosis. A newer serologic test, the VlsE C6 ELISA, is FDA approved for use as the first test in the two-tier approach. The VlsE C6 ELISA is more sensitive than the standard ELISA. Polymerase chain reaction can be run on synovial or cerebrospinal fluid for *Borrelia* DNA, but this is not recommended because of a high false-positive rate and low sensitivity.

Differential Diagnosis

- Acute rheumatic fever (serologic tests, distinctive rashes)
- Idiopathic Bell palsy (physical examination)
- Meningitis (lumbar puncture)
- Multiple sclerosis (abnormal MRI of the brain)
- Peripheral neuritis (specific nerve involvement)
- Reiter syndrome (iritis, urethritis)

Adverse Outcomes of the Disease

Lyme disease can be complicated by arthritis in major weight-bearing joints, facial paralysis, chronic fatigue, concentration defects, cardiac conduction block, and peripheral neuritis.

Prevention and Treatment

People in high-risk areas should wear long-sleeved shirts tucked into trousers with the trouser legs tucked into socks when in heavily wooded areas. Most important, the skin and clothing should be checked for ticks. Insect repellants can be used to minimize the risk of tick bites. If the tick is removed within 24 to 36 hours, the risk of Lyme disease is minimal. Ticks should be removed by grasping the tick close to the skin with tweezers and applying steady, straight traction. Heat and chemicals should not be used to remove ticks from the skin.

When diagnosed early, Lyme disease can be treated effectively with antibiotics. Doxycycline 100 mg twice a day for 28 days, or amoxicillin 500 mg three times a day for 28 days has been shown to be effective. For children younger than 8 years, amoxicillin 20 mg/kg in divided doses is indicated.

Adverse Outcomes of Treatment

Allergic reactions or adverse drug interactions to antibiotics can occur.

Referral Decisions/Red Flags

Patients with suspected Lyme disease may require evaluation by an infectious disease specialist.

Osteoporosis

Synonyms

Porous bone disease

Weak bone disease

Definition

Osteoporosis is a disease of low bone strength, characterized by inadequate bone mass and quality leading to microarchitectural deterioration. As a result, increased fragility of the bone and an increased risk of fracture exist. Other adverse outcomes of osteoporosis include deformity, pain, loss of independence, and premature death, particularly following hip fracture. According to a report released by the National Osteoporosis Foundation in 2013, approximately 54 million adults in the United States older than 50 years have osteoporosis or low bone mass (10.2 million and 43.4 million, respectively). The disease is associated with 2 million fractures per year, resulting in $17 billion in healthcare costs. Although osteoporosis has long been considered an inevitable consequence of aging, the natural history can be altered by diet and treatment strategies.

Osteoporosis is defined as primary (type I or II) or secondary. Type I osteoporosis, frequently called postmenopausal osteoporosis, is six times more common in women than in men. Estrogen deficiency in women and testosterone deficiency in men lead to trabecular bone loss. Patients with type I osteoporosis commonly present with vertebral compression fractures or fractures of the distal radius (**Figure 1**). Type II osteoporosis, previously called senile osteoporosis, occurs twice as frequently in women as in men and occurs more commonly in persons older than 70 years. Altered calcium metabolism and intrinsic problems in bone formation lead to a decrease in the formation of new bone. Hip and pelvic fractures are common in patients with type II osteoporosis. In secondary osteoporosis (male-to-female ratio, 65:45), an identifiable agent or disease process causes bone loss. Among men with a low-energy fracture, most have an underlying disorder.

Clinical Symptoms

Osteoporosis frequently is not recognized until a patient seeks medical attention for back pain, fracture, loss of height, or spinal deformity (**Figure 2**). With the greater availability of dual-energy x-ray absorptiometry (DEXA) and quantitative ultrasonography, screening examinations for osteoporosis, especially in women with risk factors, is becoming more common. **Table 1** summarizes risk factors for osteoporotic fractures. In 2008, the World Health Organization (WHO) developed the fracture risk assessment tool (FRAX), which merges bone density and other factors to establish the 10-year fracture risk assessment. The factors of old age and

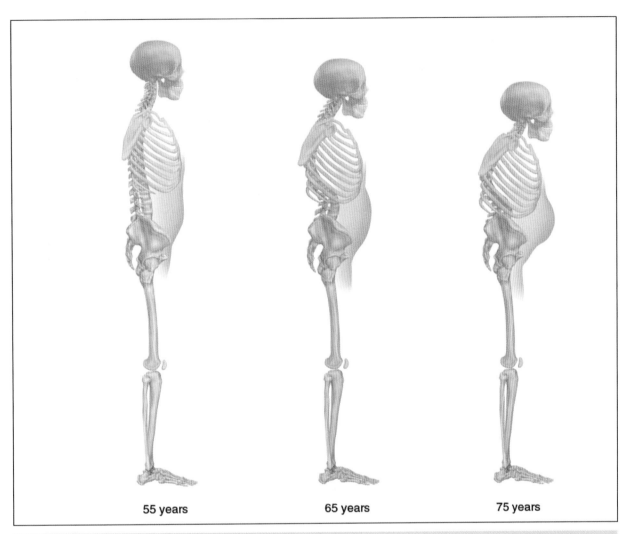

55 years   65 years   75 years

Figure 1 Illustration depicts progressive spinal deformity in osteoporosis. Compression fractures of thoracic vertebrae lead to loss of height and progressive thoracic kyphosis (dowager's hump). The lower ribs eventually rest on the iliac crests, and downward pressure on the viscera causes abdominal distention.

prior low-energy fracture are as important as low bone mass in determining fracture risk.

Secondary osteoporosis is seen commonly in patients undergoing long-term steroid therapy. It also is seen in a wide range of disorders such as hormone abnormalities (hyperthyroidism, hyperparathyroidism), neoplastic disorders (multiple myeloma), metabolic abnormalities (osteomalacia), and connective tissue diseases (osteogenesis imperfecta). Most men who have osteoporotic fractures have secondary osteoporosis.

Osteoporosis is a serious problem for patients who require prolonged immobilization.

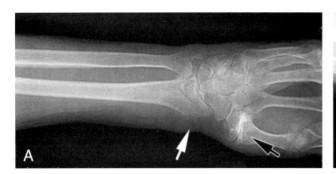
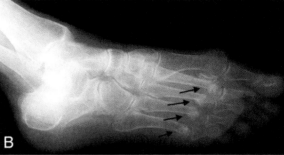

Figure 2 A, AP radiograph of the forearm and wrist of a 74-year-old woman who fell on her outstretched hand, sustaining a fracture of the distal radius and ulna (white arrow). Carpometacarpal arthritis of the thumb (black arrow) is an incidental finding. **B,** Oblique radiograph of the right foot and ankle of an 82-year-old woman who sustained fractures of the necks of metatarsals 2 through 5 (arrows). In both patients, the generalized lack of bone mineral density (BMD) is suggestive of osteopenia or frank osteoporosis, and further studies to evaluate BMD are indicated.

Table 1

Conditions, Diseases and Medications That Cause or Contribute to Osteoporosis and Fractures

Factor	Description
Lifestyle factors	Low calcium intake, high caffeine intake, alcohol (3 or more drinks/d), smoking (active or passive), vitamin D insufficiency, high salt intake, inadequate physical activity, falling, excess vitamin A, aluminum (in antacids), immobilization, thinness
Genetic factors	Cystic fibrosis, Ehlers-Danlos syndrome, Gaucher disease, glycogen storage diseases, hemochromatosis, homocystinuria, hypophosphatasia, idiopathic hypercalciuria, Marfan syndrome, Menkes steely hair syndrome, osteogenesis imperfecta, parental history of hip fracture, porphyria, Riley-Day syndrome
Hypogonadal states	Androgen insensitivity, anorexia nervosa and bulimia, athletic amenorrhea, hyperprolactinemia, panhypopituitarism, premature ovarian failure, Turner and Klinefelter syndromes
Endocrine disorders	Adrenal insufficiency, Cushing syndrome, diabetes mellitus, hyperparathyroidism, thyrotoxicosis
Gastrointestinal disorders	Celiac disease, gastric bypass, gastrointestinal surgery, inflammatory bowel disease, malabsorption, pancreatic disease, primary biliary cirrhosis
Hematologic disorders	Hemophilia, leukemia and lymphomas, multiple myeloma, sickle cell disease, systemic mastocytosis, thalassemia
Rheumatic and autoimmune disease	Ankylosing spondylitis, lupus, rheumatoid arthritis
Miscellaneous conditions and diseases	Alcoholism, amyloidosis, chronic metabolic acidosis, congestive heart failure, depression, emphysema, end-stage renal disease, epilepsy, idiopathic scoliosis, multiple sclerosis, muscular dystrophy, parenteral nutrition, post-transplant bone disease, prior fracture as an adult, sarcoidosis
Medications	Anticoagulants (heparin), anticonvulsants, aromatase inhibitors, barbiturates, cancer chemotherapeutic drugs, cyclosporine A and tacrolimus, depo-medroxyprogesterone, glucocorticoids ($\geq$5 mg/d of prednisone or equivalent for $\geq$3 mo)

(Adapted from *National Osteoporosis Foundation: Clinician's Guide to Prevention and Treatment of Osteoporosis.* Washington, DC, National Osteoporosis Foundation, 2010.)

Tests

Physical Examination

The physical examination is normal in the early stages. In advanced disease, findings may include tenderness to palpation over an area of fracture, spinal deformity, loss of height (often more than 2 inches), lax abdominal musculature with a protuberant abdomen, hypermobility, and exaggerated thoracic kyphosis (dowager's hump).

Low bone density and subsequent stress or overt fractures may develop in female athletes, particularly those participating in endurance activities, gymnastics, skating, and dance, because of overtraining, inadequate diet, and menstrual cessation. It is imperative to thoroughly question female athletes about their menstrual history and to question all athletes about their diet and exercise habits.

Diagnostic Tests

Diagnostic tests are performed to identify the presence and severity of osteoporosis, measure response to therapeutic interventions, and rule out secondary causes of the disease.

Because no specific measurement exists for bone strength, bone mineral density (BMD) is used as a surrogate. DEXA is currently the reference standard for BMD measurement (**Figure 3**). This quick, painless test helps estimate bone strength and predicts future fracture risk. It is fast, reproducible, and involves very low radiation exposure. Bone mass is reported as a real density and compared with both peers (Z score) and young healthy individuals (T score). Z and T scores represent standard deviations (SDs) lower than the comparison group. Bone density is characterized by the lowest value at the spine, femoral neck, trochanter, or total femur. Values of 0 to −1 are normal; −1 to −2.5 indicates osteopenia; lower than −2.5 indicates osteoporosis. DEXA currently is the best test for monitoring the results of osteoporosis treatment. For reasons of cost, speed, and availability, however, quantitative ultrasonography may be used as a screening tool in younger patients.

Because osteoporosis typically is a "silent" disease, the decision to test should be based on a patient's risk profile. The National Osteoporosis Foundation (NOF) recommends BMD testing for the following individuals:

- All women age 65 years or older, regardless of risk factors

- Postmenopausal women younger than 65 years who have one or more of the following risk factors: family history of osteoporosis, personal history of low-trauma fracture at older than 45 years, current cigarette smoker, or low body weight (< 127 lb)

- Men with a history of a low-trauma fracture or of treatment with a gonadotropin-releasing hormone (GnRH) agonist for prostate cancer

- Individuals with primary hyperparathyroidism who are undergoing long-term glucocorticoid treatment, with diseases or conditions known to cause bone loss, or using medications known to cause bone loss.

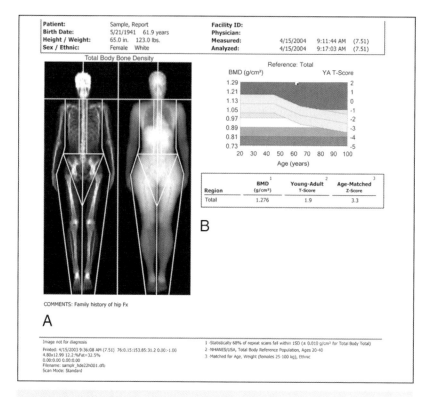

Figure 3 A dual-energy x-ray absorptiometric scan (**A**) and report (**B**) for a white woman who was age 61 years at the time her findings were analyzed. The report provides a reference database of bone mineral density (BMD) as a function of age. The middle line is the mean BMD, and the lines above and below the line represent 1 standard deviation (SD) above and below the mean, respectively. Findings are compared with young adults (T scores) and with age-matched adults (Z scores). The World Health Organization (WHO) bases management guidelines on T scores. According to the WHO, a T score of −1.0 SD or higher is normal; a T score between −1.0 and −2.5 indicates osteopenia; and a T score of −2.5 SD or lower indicates osteoporosis.

Osteoporosis may be either high-turnover osteoporosis (increased rate of absorption) or low-turnover osteoporosis (decreased rate of bone formation). The cross-linked N-telopeptide (NTx) test measures bone collagen breakdown products, with a high NTx level indicating high turnover and a low NTx level indicating low turnover. Tests to rule out secondary causes of osteoporosis include a complete blood cell count, erythrocyte sedimentation rate, C-reactive protein level, serum protein level, and immunoelectrophoresis (serum/urine) to rule out a bone marrow disorder. Thyroid function tests and parathyroid hormone (PTH) level tests are performed to rule out hyperthyroidism or hyperparathyroidism. Cushing disease and diabetes are ruled out by patient history. Tests performed for serum levels of calcium, phosphorus, alkaline phosphatase, and 25-hydroxyvitamin D (along with PTH levels) rule out osteomalacia. Other studies include renal and liver function tests and a 24-hour urine calcium test.

Differential Diagnosis

- Disuse osteopenia (history of prolonged immobilization or bed rest)
- Multiple myeloma (anemia, elevated erythrocyte sedimentation rate, bone pain, immunoelectrophoresis results)
- Osteomalacia (deformity, renal osteodystrophy) (bone pain, low hydroxyvitamin D level, high intact PTH level, elevated alkaline phosphatase, low calcium, low urinary calcium)
- Poor imaging technique on radiographs (overpenetration may be suspected when soft tissues are not visible on radiographs; all radiographic diagnoses are optimally confirmed by DEXA)
- Primary osteoporosis (type I or type II) (by exclusion, all low-energy fracture patients, a loss of > 2 inches in height)
- Secondary osteoporosis (history, occurs in men)

Adverse Outcomes of the Disease

Adverse outcomes of osteoporosis include fracture, deformity, chronic pain, social withdrawal, loss of independence, and death, particularly following hip fracture.

Treatment

Prevention

Because peak bone mass is achieved in patients younger than 25 to 28 years, women should be encouraged to maximize bone formation during youth with proper diet and exercise and minimize bone loss during adulthood. Recommendations for the general population include an adequate intake of calcium and vitamin D, regular weight-bearing exercise, and avoidance of tobacco use and alcohol abuse.

Older patients should be educated about the importance of maintaining their body weight and reducing their risk factors for falls by walking for exercise, avoiding long-acting benzodiazepines, minimizing caffeine intake, and treating impaired visual function (**Table 1**).

Standards for the optimal type and duration of exercise have not been established. The ideal exercise program includes impact-loading exercise (such as walking), strength training, and balance training (such as tai chi).

Recommendations for calcium intake are listed in **Table 2**. The combined recommended dose is 750 to 1,000 mg per day. Most Americans consume far less calcium than is recommended, particularly in their elder years. Calcium supplements are frequently required. The two main forms of calcium are carbonate and citrate. Carbonate requires an acid environment to dissolve; H_2 blockers and indigestion impair its availability. Citrate forms dissolve at all pH levels and decrease the risk of kidney stones. As a consequence, citrate is preferred to carbonate unless chewed. Because calcium levels vary by individual, the proper calcium level is consistent with an intact PTH of 25 through 45.

Table 2

Dietary Reference Intake Values for Calcium by Life-stage Group

Life-stage Group	Adequate Calcium Intake (mg/d)
Males and Females	
0 to 6 mo	210
6 to 12 mo	270
1 through 3 y	500
4 through 8 y	800
9 through 13 y	1,300
14 through 18 y	1,300
19 through 30 y	1,000
31 through 50 y	1,000
51 through 70 y	1,200
>70 y	1,200
Women only	
Pregnancy	
≤18 y	1,300
19 through 50 y	1,000
Lactation	
≤18 y	1,300
19 through 50 y	1,000

(Adapted from *National Osteoporosis Foundation: Physician's Guide to the Prevention and Treatment of Osteoporosis.* Washington, DC, National Osteoporosis Foundation, 1998.)

Vitamin D is essential for intestinal absorption of calcium, and requirements increase with age. Vitamin D is also important because it enhances muscle function and balance. Because skin production of this vitamin decreases even with adequate sun exposure, 25(OH) vitamin D levels should be higher than 15 ng/mL to avoid insufficiency, and levels higher than 30 ng/mL have been recommended. Current recommendations for vitamin D intake are under review; 800 to 1,200 IU/d appear to be appropriate. Higher replacement (2,000 to 4,000 IU/d) is required in patients with vitamin D insufficiency. Fractures resulting from falls can be decreased by 20% with a minimum vitamin D intake of 800 IU/d. A combination of vitamin D and calcium can decrease the risk of hip fracture in the elderly by approximately 25%. The third most common cause for delayed fracture healing is low vitamin D levels.

Intervention

In the best circumstances, treatment of osteoporosis is initiated before a fracture occurs. Physicians should encourage all patients to follow the prevention strategies listed earlier. The NOF recommends pharmacologic intervention for osteoporosis in white women whose

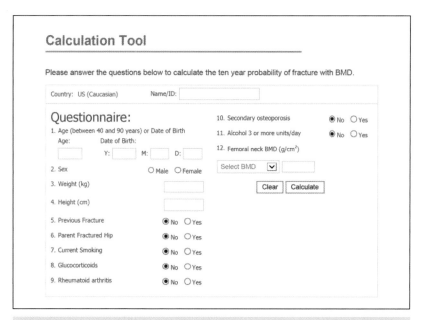

Figure 4 US version of the World Health Organization Fracture Risk Assessment (FRAX) tool. The tool and information on using it is available at http://www.shef.ac.uk/FRAX/tool.jsp?country=9. (© World Health Organization Collaborating Centre for Metabolic Bone Diseases, University of Sheffield, United Kingdom.)

BMD scores are 2 SDs lower than those of a "young healthy" adult in the absence of risk factors and in women whose BMD scores are 1.5 SDs lower than those of a "young healthy" adult if other risk factors are present. The NOF also notes that white women older than 70 years with multiple risk factors (especially those with previous fractures not occurring in the hip or spine) are at a high enough risk of fracture to initiate treatment without BMD testing. Currently, the FRAX provides an estimated fracture risk for an individual (**Table 2**; **Figure 4**). All patients who sustain a low-energy fracture of the hip, spine, pelvis, or proximal humerus should be started on osteoporosis treatment.

All interventions include appropriate calcium and vitamin D intake. Treatment classes include antiresorptive agents (diphosphonates [alendronate, risedronate, ibandronate, zoledronic acid], selective estrogen receptor modulators [SERMs], denosumab), which are prescribed for patients with high NTx levels; and anabolic agents (intermittent PTH), prescribed for patients with low NTx levels or patients who sustained a low-energy fracture subsequent to prior use of diphosphonate (**Table 3**). Diphosphonates decrease the fracture risk in all bones at least 50%. For individuals who cannot tolerate oral diphosphonates, intravenous forms are efficacious in protecting bone mass. Diphosphonates are indicated for all forms of osteoporosis, glucosteroid use, and acute fractures. Although estrogen prevents fractures, it is no longer recommended by the FDA for the treatment of osteoporosis because of its increased risk for myocardial infarction, stroke, breast cancer, and possibly dementia. Raloxifene is a SERM that enhances spinal bone mass and decreases vertebral fractures, but

Table 3

Drugs Used to Treat Osteoporosis

Classification	Drug	Dosage/Administration	Side Effects	Contraindications
A: Antiresorptive agents (indication: high NTx)				
Diphosphonates	Alendronate	70 mg po weekly	GI disturbance	Cannot sit upright or stand for 30 min, premenopausal women, esophageal dysfunction, hypocalcemia
	Risedronate	35 mg po weekly	Same as above	Same as above
	Ibandronate	150 mg po monthly	Same as above	Same as above
	Ibandronate	3 mg IV every 3 mo	Bladder pain, cloudy urine	Hypocalcemia
	Zoledronic acid	5 mg IV every 12 mo	Osteonecrosis of the jaw	Low renal clearance
Nondiphosphonates	Denosumab	60 mg subcutaneous injection every 6 mo	Affects ability to fight infections	Pregnancy, hypocalcemia
	SERMs (raloxifene)	60 mg daily po	DVT/PE, stroke	History of DVT
	Calcitonin	1 spray (200 units)/d	Nosebleed	Hypersensitivity to calcitonin-salmon
B: Anabolic agents (indication: low NTx)				
	PTH	20 µg daily, subcutaneously	Cramps, orthostatic hypotension in very elderly	Children; patients with prior radiation therapy; patients with Paget disease

DVT = deep vein thrombosis, GI = gastrointestinal, IV = intravenous, NTx = crosslinked N-telopeptide, PE = pulmonary embolism, po = per os (by mouth), PTH = parathyroid hormone, SERMs = selective estrogen receptor modulators.

it does not prevent hip fractures. Denosumab is an effective inhibitor of osteoclast formation, has a short half-life, and can be given to patients with compromised renal function. Calcitonin provides minor spinal fracture protection and possibly some pain relief, but it affords no protection against nonvertebral fracture and is associated with an increased rate of cancer.

Anabolic agents are recommended for low-turnover states, failures of diphosphonates, premenopausal women, and in the setting of impaired fracture healing. Intermittent PTH (1 to 34 amino acids) is given only subcutaneously and results in marked enhancement of bone mass, fracture protection comparable to diphosphonates, and enhancement of fracture healing. It is contraindicated in children, patients who have undergone prior radiation, and patients with Paget disease. In randomized studies, use of intermittent PTH resulted in faster and more complete fracture healing (radius, pelvis) and spinal fusion.

Adverse Outcomes of Treatment

Estrogen hormone replacement therapy is associated with an increased risk of breast cancer, heart disease, and deep vein thrombosis. Side effects can include vaginal bleeding, breast tenderness, mood disturbances, and gallbladder disease. Consequently, estrogen is not recommended for osteoporosis. Diphosphonates must be administered on an empty stomach, and some patients report upper gastrointestinal disturbance. Also, some animal studies suggest a delay of maturation during fracture healing. Intravenous diphosphonates do not interfere with fracture healing, and they decrease the rate of myocardial infarctions. Prolonged diphosphonate use is associated with atypical femoral fractures and osteonecrosis of the jaw. After 5 years, diphosphonates should be halted until bone markers rise or until a 5% increase in DEXA exists. Although calcitonin has fewer side effects, it should be avoided because of its low efficacy and association with an increased rate of cancer. Raloxifene has been shown to increase the risk of deep vein thrombosis at the same rate as estrogen, and it provides no hip fracture protection. Raloxifene also causes hot flashes and does not treat menopausal symptoms. PTH may cause cramps and orthostatic hypotension in the very elderly (**Table 3**). The concern for osteosarcoma from a rat study has not been noted with the lower dose used in humans.

Referral Decisions/Red Flags

Osteoporosis and fragility fractures are not inevitable in any age group. All appropriate patients should be referred for BMD testing and offered treatment.

Many physicians may feel uncomfortable evaluating BMD studies, ruling out secondary causes of osteoporosis, or initiating pharmacologic treatment. Referral to an osteoporosis specialist may be appropriate. Many trauma units have established fracture liaison teams to transition the patient into an osteoporosis drug program.

Overuse Syndromes

Synonyms

Cumulative trauma disorder
Repetitive strain injury
Repetitive stress injury
Occupational overuse

Definition

Overuse syndromes encompass many diagnoses that involve inflammatory responses as well as compression and pain syndromes. These conditions typically involve overuse resulting from repetitive motions, stresses, or sustained exertion of a particular body part. Overuse conditions can affect muscles, tendons, nerves, bones, or the physeal plate in skeletally immature patients. In adults, overuse conditions most commonly involve the musculotendinous unit and the surrounding soft tissues. In the pediatric population, growth plates are commonly affected because of repetitive stress across the physis. Overuse syndromes can occur in the upper or lower extremities. Some of the most common forms of tendinopathies associated with overuse injuries and their anatomic locations are listed in **Table 1**.

A wide population is at risk; however, overuse conditions commonly affect athletes, laborers, or persons who perform repetitive, stressful movements at work. At least 25% of adult athletes have experienced overuse injuries. Sporting activities typically associated with overuse injuries include baseball, dancing, tennis, golf, rowing, and long-distance running. In the workplace, contributing factors may include repetitive tasks, forceful exertions, and exposure to vibration or cold

Table 1

Most Common Diagnoses and Locations of Chronic Tendinitis

Diagnosis	Location
Rotator cuff tendinitis	Supraspinatus tendon insertion
Lateral epicondylitis (tennis elbow)	Common wrist extensor tendon origin
de Quervain disease and trigger finger	Sheath/pulley of abductor pollicis longus and long finger flexors
Hamstring tendinitis	Hamstring tendon origin
Quadriceps tendinitis	Quadriceps tendon insertion
Patellar tendinitis (jumper's knee)	Patellar tendon origin
Achilles tendinitis	Sheath, midsubstance, or calcaneal insertion
Posterior tibial tendinitis	Midsubstance

(Reproduced from Almekinders LC: Tendinitis and other chronic tendinopathies. *J Am Acad Orthop Surg* 1998;6[3]:157-164.)

Sport	Overuse Injury
Baseball	Little Leaguer's shoulder
	Little Leaguer's elbow
	Ulnar collateral ligament strain
Gymnastics	Wrist sprain
	Distal radial stress fracture
Dancing	Ankle sprain
	Tendinitis
Swimming	Shoulder instability
Basketball	Patellar tendinitis

Table 2

Common Overuse Injuries in Pediatric Athletes by Sport

Table 3

Extrinsic and Intrinsic Factors in Chronic Tendon Problems

Extrinsic Factors

Repetitive mechanical load
Increased duration
Increased frequency
Increased intensity
Technique errors

Equipment problems
Footwear
Racquet size
Running surface
Protective gear

Intrinsic Factors

Anatomic factors
Malalignment
Inflexibility
Muscle weakness
Muscle imbalance
Decreased vascularity

Age-related factors
Tendon degeneration
Decreased healing response
Increased tendon stiffness
Decreased vascularity

Systemic factors
Inflammatory enthesopathy
Quinolone-induced tendinopathy

(Reproduced from Almekinders LC: Tendinitis and other chronic tendinopathies. *J Am Acad Orthop Surg* 1998;6[3]:157-164.)

SECTION 1 GENERAL ORTHOPAEDICS

temperatures, awkward postures, or poor ergonomic environment. Injury also can occur as the result of or can be exacerbated by incorrect mechanics or kinematics during activities. In the pediatric population, overuse injuries usually are the result of either year-round participation in one sport or improper training. Common overuse injuries incurred by pediatric athletes are listed in **Table 2**.

Overuse tendon injuries can be related to several extrinsic and intrinsic factors (**Table 3**).

Overuse syndromes are typically secondary to repetitive microtrauma, which can produce either acute inflammation or a chronic degenerative state. Reactive or acute inflammatory overuse syndromes are a result of repetitive microtrauma that produces fatigue and inflammation. This is termed tendinitis and represents infiltration of the tendon or fibrous sheath (epitenon) with inflammatory cells and mediators. In the acute setting, the injury typically is not associated with degeneration to the musculotendinous unit. A persistent inflammatory state, however, can eventually lead to tissue breakdown over time. Chronic tendon injuries are a degenerative process rather than an inflammatory process. The term tendinosis defines chronic degeneration without inflammation of the tendon, epitenon, or tendon-bone interface secondary to prolonged microtrauma. Inflammation can be involved in the initial stages; however, later stages demonstrate failed healing and disruption of the tendon structure. Degeneration often occurs in areas of diminished blood flow, and age appears to be an important factor associated with tendon injuries. In skeletally immature athletes, high stress loading and repetitive trauma can lead to inflammation at the growth plate. Inflammation at the growth plate is termed apophysitis, and traumatic widening of the physis is termed epiphysiolysis.

Clinical Symptoms

Overuse syndromes develop over time and patients may not report their problems early, in anticipation that the condition will improve. Symptoms include pain, fatigue, numbness, swelling, or any combination thereof. With repetitive microtrauma–induced overuse syndromes, pain is usually localized to the tendinous insertion and exacerbated with muscle stretch or contraction. With chronic, degenerative overuse syndromes, rupture can cause substantial pain and dysfunction. In syndromes affecting nerve tissue, there will be numbness and/or tingling in the distribution of that particular nerve. Over time, muscle weakness or muscle atrophy may develop secondary to nerve compression.

In exertional compartment syndrome, the patient may report worsening pain with activity or exercise. The only relieving factor may be extended rest from the activity. The patient also may report numbness in the foot, swelling in the lower leg, and pain that is aggravated by passive stretch of the ankle joint. Stress fractures demonstrate exquisite bony tenderness and localized pain at the site of the fracture. Pain typically is worsened with activity.

History and Physical Examination

Patients should be questioned specifically about sporting activities, job-related tasks, exposures, and recent changes in activity level. With regard to occupational overuse syndromes, job satisfaction, working conditions, exposure to repetitive and forceful exertions, vibration, or cold temperature should be investigated. In addition, it is important to identify the type of industry and job specificity because the incidence of overuse syndromes is higher for certain industries and occupations, such as meat packers, assembly line workers, grocery store cashiers, and clerical workers.

Physical examination should be thorough, and comparison should be made with the contralateral extremity. The injured extremity should be inspected for signs of swelling, erythema, pallor, or muscle atrophy. After inspection, the area of complaint should be palpated to determine the area of maximal tenderness. This will help shorten the differential diagnosis. Next, range of motion should be tested both passively and actively and compared with the contralateral extremity. Strength is assessed, paying particular attention to pain with resistance. A thorough neurovascular examination should also be conducted. For example, in de Quervain tenosynovitis, the patient will report pain when moving the thumb and will have tenderness to palpation over the radial-dorsal aspect at the base of the first metacarpal when moving the thumb because this is the location of the inflamed tendons (**Figure 1**). Flexion of the thumb with ulnar deviation of the wrist typically reproduces the pain (a positive Phalen test).

Diagnostic Tests

Diagnostic evaluation begins with radiographic evaluation of the affected extremity, although plain radiographs are typically normal. Radiographs can help rule out fractures, joint pathology, masses, or lesions. Radiographs also may demonstrate calcifications within the tendon, or bone spurs at the tendon insertion sites in cases of chronic tendinosis (**Figure 2**).

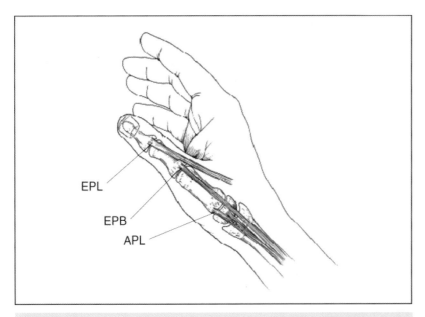

Figure 1 Anatomic drawing of the first dorsal compartment shows tendon insertion points involved in de Quervain tenosynovitis. APL = abductor pollicis longus, EPB = extensor pollicis brevis, EPL = extensor pollicis longus. (Reproduced from Ilyas AM, Ast M, Schaffer AA, Thoder J: De Quervain tenosynovitis of the wrist. *J Am Acad Orthop Surg* 2007;15[12]:757-764.)

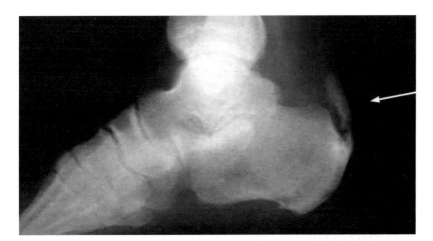

Figure 2 Lateral radiograph demonstrates calcification (arrow) in a patient with chronic Achilles tendinosis.

Bone scans or MRIs may be necessary to identify a stress fracture. Bone scans can detect occult, osseous pathology; MRIs are important for both osseous and soft-tissue pathologies that are not adequately visualized on plain radiographs. **Figure 3** shows a tibial stress fracture seen on MRI that was not seen on initial radiographs of the tibia. MRI also is useful to diagnose certain tendon tears or areas of chronic tendon injury, but it should be ordered with discretion. **Figure 4** demonstrates an Achilles tendon injury seen on MRI.

Nerve compression syndromes can be evaluated with nerve conduction velocity (NCV) studies or electromyelographic (EMG)

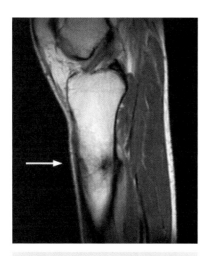

Figure 3 Sagittal MRI demonstrates a tibial stress fracture (arrow).

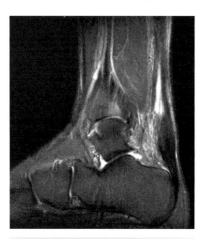

Figure 4 Sagittal MRI demonstrates an Achilles tendon injury. Note the fluid (white area) within the tendons.

studies. NCV or EMG studies are ordered to rule out carpal tunnel syndrome or ulnar nerve entrapment at the elbow. An NCV study will show latency in conduction of nervous impulses, and an EMG study will show decreased electric potential produced by particular muscle cells, which may present as muscle atrophy or weakness in chronic nerve compression syndromes.

Exertional compartment syndrome can be confirmed by measuring compartment pressures before and after exercise. Intracompartmental pressure measurements that confirm the diagnosis of chronic exertional compartment syndrome are as follows: at rest, greater than 15 mm Hg; 1 minute after exercise, greater than 30 mm Hg; 5 minutes after exercise, greater than 20 mm Hg.

Differential Diagnosis

- Deep vein thrombosis (abnormal venogram, Doppler ultrasonogram)
- Fibromyalgia (11 of 18 tender points in four body quadrants)
- Fracture
- Herniated cervical or lumbar disk (abnormal spine radiographs, myelogram, and MRI)
- Ligament or tendon rupture
- Tumor

Adverse Outcomes of the Disease

With overuse conditions, patients often lose time from work or sport and may experience psychologic changes. In chronic conditions, especially those arising from work injuries, patients may become dependent on pain medication. Persistent activity in patients with tendinosis can result in tendon ruptures. Continued activity in athletes with stress fractures can result in a truly displaced fracture. Persistent pressure on nerves in carpal tunnel syndrome, cubital tunnel syndrome, or compartment syndrome can result in irreversible damage. Physeal injuries in the skeletally immature patient can result in growth disturbances and alignment discrepancies.

Treatment

Most overuse syndromes are mild and resolve spontaneously with time and rest. With overuse injuries in the workplace, satisfactory outcomes for many patients depend on the cooperative efforts of the employer, the insurance carrier, and a physician-directed healthcare team including rehabilitation specialists. A case manager, such as an occupational health nurse, can be invaluable in coordinating the efforts of these groups to return the patient to work.

Initial treatment should include protection, ice, and rest of the affected extremity. A progressive exercise program that includes eccentric strengthening has been shown to be helpful in tendinitis. At the workplace, modification of tasks or work schedules and even vocational changes should be considered if the symptoms persist.

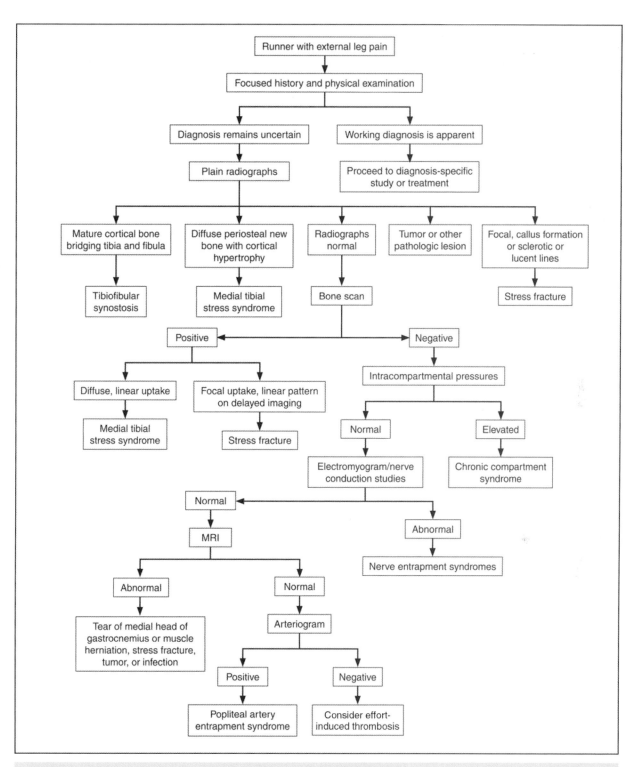

Figure 5 Algorithm used in the work-up for the runner with leg pain. (Reproduced from Pell RF VI, Khanuja HS, Cooley GR: Leg pain in the running athlete. *J Am Acad Orthop Surg* 2004;12[6]:396-404.)

NSAIDs and analgesic creams are beneficial in reducing pain associated with these conditions. Corticosteroid injections can be helpful in carpal tunnel syndrome, plantar fasciitis, lateral epicondylitis, and chronic tendinosis of the shoulder. Narcotics should be avoided because of the possibility of addiction. Antidepressants can be a useful adjunct if depression is a significant part of the clinical picture.

Although surgery may be indicated, it is seldom urgent and the results of surgery have been found to be less predictable in patients with workplace-associated overuse injuries. In workplace overuse injuries, lack of job satisfaction, depression, and litigation also are important predictors of recovery.

Overuse syndromes associated with running are very common in both the young and old. **Figure 5** is an algorithm that can be used for the work-up of a runner who presents with leg pain.

Adverse Outcomes of Treatment

Drug dependence on narcotics or antidepressants is possible. If the patient has undergone multiple ill-advised surgeries, persistently tender scars may remain. Patients may become depressed and lose conditioning if they are unable to perform their sport. It is important to keep patients physically active in alternative activities, such as swimming, which do not aggravate the injured area.

Referral Decisions/Red Flags

Persistent pain despite appropriate care merits referral to a specialist for further evaluation. In the workplace, after the diagnosis of overuse syndrome is suspected, treatment by a team of healthcare professionals may be helpful in managing these difficult problems.

Pain Management in the Orthopaedic Patient

Treatment of orthopaedic pain should be a collaborative effort among the orthopaedic surgeon, pain specialist, anesthesiologist, and nursing staff to ensure the best possible outcome. Providing adequate pain relief can result in increased patient satisfaction and faster rehabilitation while preventing atrophy of the affected tissues and decreasing the risk of deep vein thrombosis. Knowledge of and willingness to adopt the most appropriate available methods and drugs to bring about full functional and emotional recovery are essential.

Definition

Skeletal pain is a deep somatic pain resulting from injuries to the periosteum, matrix, ligaments, or joints. Nociceptors activated by release of potent prostaglandins relay nervous impulses through myelinated or unmyelinated fibers via the spinal cord to the somatosensory cortex. Understanding the mechanism by which the nervous system produces and transmits pain impulses from the periphery to the brain can aid in better understanding how to manage pain in the orthopaedic patient.

Agents used to manage pain include opioids, NSAIDs, centrally acting nonopioids, and local anesthetics. Opioids block pain in the central nervous system, NSAIDs decrease pain by reducing the inflammatory response, centrally acting nonopioid analgesics interact with certain neurotransmitters and *N*-methyl-D-aspartate (NMDA) receptors (acetaminophen, tramadol), and local anesthetics prevent pain impulses from reaching the spinal cord.

Agents Used to Manage Pain

Opioids

Opioids are the most effective and widely used medicines for the treatment of moderate to severe pain. They bind to specific receptors in the brain, spinal cord, and gastrointestinal (GI) tract, causing dose-dependent analgesia, drowsiness, respiratory depression, urinary retention, nausea, vomiting, and constipation. Opioids can be administered via intravenous, oral, rectal, or transcutaneous means. Delivery method has an effect on the onset and duration of the drug. In addition, the effect of opioids can be affected by the concomitant use of other centrally acting drugs and by alcohol in particular. Individualized dosing is strongly advised in the elderly population and in patients with long-standing opioid use. Intravenous administration causes a rapid rise in plasma levels and fast onset, whereas oral administration results in a more gradual onset of analgesia. Transdermal fentanyl consists of a patch that releases a predetermined dose of the active substance over a period of up to 3 days; this patch should only be used for a select group of patients, such as those with metastatic disease or certain chronic pain conditions.

Short-acting opioids such as oxycodone and hydrocodone are now available as extended release tablets, which allows for more stable plasma levels over a longer period of time. However, prescription of these opioids is carefully monitored because of the potential for abuse. Adherence to strict guidelines and thorough follow-up with patients taking opioids is necessary to ensure a safe and successful therapy.

NSAIDs

NSAIDs are readily available and have been widely used over the past 50 years. They affect transmission of pain by primarily reducing the production of prostaglandins at the site of injury. All NSAIDs exhibit similar characteristics and tolerability when used at a comparable dosing regimen. They are classified based on their chemical structure or mechanism of action. Cyclooxygenase (COX)-1 inhibitors are known for producing adverse effects in the GI tract and the kidney and for interfering with platelet adhesion. The use of COX-2 inhibitors has been shown to increase the risk of cardiovascular events. Among the many COX-1 inhibitors currently available, ibuprofen and naproxen seem to be reasonably safe. Celecoxib (Celebrex [Pfizer]) is an extensively used COX-2 inhibitor. It is most commonly prescribed to patients with a history of GI problems or certain allergic reactions.

Cross-sensitivity between NSAIDs and other commonly used drugs such as warfarin, blood pressure medicines (angiotensin-converting enzyme [ACE] inhibitors), and antidepressants (selective serotonin reuptake inhibitors [SSRIs]) are well documented, and the physician must take a careful medication history before prescribing NSAIDs. In 2015, the FDA strengthened its warning linking NSAIDs with the risk of heart attack or stroke, even in the first weeks of use of an NSAID. However, the opioid-sparing effect of NSAIDs makes them an excellent adjunct to the more potent centrally acting opioids and may reduce side effects.

Centrally Acting Nonopioid Analgesics

Acetaminophen and tramadol are the most widely prescribed centrally acting nonopioid analgesics. Although tramadol has a weak affinity to opioid receptors, its analgesic properties are mostly a result of inhibiting the release of serotonin and blocking the reuptake of norepinephrine. In addition, tramadol has the ability to block NMDA receptors in the spinal cord, which prevents or modulates the transmission of afferent nervous impulses from the periphery to the brain. Although tramadol has approximately one-tenth the potency of morphine, it shows similar effectiveness for mild to moderate pain. The most common interaction occurs with antidepressants (SSRIs), meperidine, and the antinausea medication ondansetron, which may antagonize the effect of tramadol. Acetaminophen is widely used as an analgesic in patients with osteoarthritis. It has analgesic properties similar to aspirin but is not considered an anti-inflammatory

GENERAL ORTHOPAEDICS

SECTION 1

Table 1

Critical Factors in Prescribing Pain Medication

Know all of your patient's medications

Check for drug interactions

Ask your patient about his or her previous experience with pain medication

Find out whether the patient can afford pain medication (eg, expensive designer drugs)

Check for allergies

Consider special situations (elderly, pregnant status, malnutrition)

Evaluate for drug or alcohol abuse

Adjust prescription to severity and/or length of expected pain

Write prescriptions for drugs with which you are familiar

Combine drugs with different mechanisms of action

Consult a pain specialist for patients with refractory or severe pain

Ensure regular follow-up by your office staff

medication. Acetaminophen is more effective when used in combination with weak opioids and has few side effects when taken in recommended doses (maximum dose < 4,000 mg/day). Unlike NSAIDs, acetaminophen can be prescribed to pregnant patients in their third trimester for management of pain without running the risk of premature closure of the ductus arteriosus in the fetus. Factors to consider when prescribing pain medication are listed in **Table 1**.

Local Anesthetics

It has become routine to administer peripheral nerve blocks with long-acting local anesthetics to eliminate pain after orthopaedic procedures in the upper or lower extremities. Increased interest and technical advances such as the use of ultrasound with or without nerve stimulation have made it possible to selectively produce profound anesthesia and analgesia at the surgical site. Duration of analgesia with a single injection lasts up to 24 hours, whereas techniques using an indwelling catheter can provide excellent pain relief for several days. Peripheral nerve injury or local anesthetic toxicity is of concern, but these complications can be avoided with meticulous adherence to guidelines published by the American Society of Anesthesiologists.

Both spinal and epidural anesthesia provide excellent pain relief intraoperatively, and their postoperative effect can be augmented by the addition of opioids into the epidural space or the spinal fluid. Spinal and epidural anesthesia are more appropriate for inpatient surgical procedures, which require continuous monitoring of respiratory and cardiovascular functions. However, the use of potent blood thinners in the early postoperative phase is considered a contraindication for neuraxial anesthetic techniques because it markedly increases the risk of epidural hematomas.

Addition of the long-acting local anesthetic bupivacaine in a liposomal suspension enables several-day extension of postoperative analgesia when the drug is appropriately infiltrated at the surgical site. The FDA has not yet approved the use of bupivacaine in peripheral nerve blocks.

Alternative Treatments

In addition to rest, elevation, and ice, the use of transcutaneous electrical nerve stimulation and acupuncture has been shown to be beneficial in reducing pain without adverse effects. Psychological methods such as relaxation techniques and hypnosis may require the participation of a physician trained in psychologic care.

Pain: Nonorganic Symptoms and Signs

Synonyms

Functional overlay
Psychosomatic illness

Definition

Patient responses or symptoms that do not fit known patterns of illness or injury are considered nonorganic. These physical signs were described early in the 20th century following the development of the Compensation Acts and the development of the medicolegal arena. These findings are not considered malingering; rather, they often are the way in which some patients communicate their perception of the seriousness of their problem or that they are not receiving the care they think they need. True malingering is rare and typically is a manifestation of bizarre social behavior.

Nonorganic findings should not be construed as indicating a lack of concomitant disease because significant underlying pathology can be present. Nonorganic findings occur three to four times more often in situations in which workers' compensation and litigation are issues. Such findings are often a clue that further psychologic assessment should be pursued. A standard examination is valuable preoperatively to determine and arrange postoperative pain expectations and treatment requirements. Additionally, with a thorough history and physical examination that includes a few of the standardized tests detailed later in this chapter, addressing unrealistic expectations before treatment initiation may save the clinician and patient a few ill emotions at the end of the day.

Clinical Symptoms

It should be assumed that all patients with pain have a physical source and it is only human nature to have an emotional and behavioral reaction to that pain. The clinician should always be cognizant of external factors that may influence the patient's presentation, including compensation, family, or employment issues. Nonorganic physical signs are most recognizable in relation to low back pain, most notably the five signs of Waddell, originally described in 1979 (see **Sidebar: Waddell Signs**).

Waddell considered three or more signs as clinically significant. Pain or symptoms that appear to "travel" from one side or area of the body to another in a nonanatomic fashion and global pain are characteristic. Nonsegmental numbness (numbness that does not fit a nerve root or peripheral nerve pattern) also occurs.

Waddell Signs

Overreaction to examination

Simulation testing (axial loading, rotation)

Distraction with straight leg raising and other tests

Regional symptoms of weakness and sensation

Tenderness (superficial and nonanatomic)

Tests

Physical Examination

Exaggerated responses: Light touch causes a jerk or withdrawal. Other findings include grimacing, groaning, and grabbing the affected extremity during examination when no obvious trauma or medical problem exists.

Axial loading (low back pain): With the patient standing, place both hands on the patient's head and push down, asking if it causes pain. Low back pain elicited in this position is a nonorganic finding; however, neck pain may be a legitimate finding.

Axial rotation (spine): With the patient's hands on the iliac crests, grasp and rotate the pelvis, asking the patient if this causes pain. This maneuver should not elicit back pain, because the motion occurs at the hips, not in the back. Because this test may be positive in 20% of patients, it is not as sensitive in identifying nonorganic behavior as are exaggerated responses and axial loading.

Flip sign: This sign is elicited with the patient seated and leaning slightly forward, with his or her hands on the edge of the examination table. While asking if the patient has knee problems, lift the foot and extend the knee. This maneuver increases tension on the sciatic nerve, and patients with lower lumbar herniated disks or other similar conditions will involuntarily "flip" back against the wall, reporting back and leg pain. A negative flip sign in the presence of a supine straight leg raise test that produces leg and back pain at less than 45° of leg elevation is a significant nonorganic finding because these maneuvers are the same test.

Distraction: A provocative test (such as palpation) may be negative when the patient is distracted with conversation, but positive when attention is drawn to the test or body part.

Giving way: During muscle testing, a nonorganic finding is a lack of sustained effort. Typically, the patient "gives way" or "lets go" in a ratchety, uneven pattern. Another variant is the patient who gives a poor effort on muscle testing and then, with coaxing, may intermittently contract the muscle, then let go.

Stocking or nonanatomic numbness: Some patients report hypoesthesia that affects the extremity in a circumferential (stocking-glove) distribution or covers nonanatomic patterns. Sensory abnormalities in a stocking-glove or nonsegmental pattern may develop in patients with diabetes mellitus or multiple sclerosis.

Pain diagram: On a diagram of the body, ask the patient to draw representations of symptoms, using marks such as dashes, slashes, or Xs. Bizarre drawings do not indicate malingering or mental disease. Many people have perceptual disorders that blunt the scientific validity of these drawings, but they often yield insight into how pain is perceived by patients and what areas of the body they believe are related in their current problem (**Figure 1**).

The kneeling bench test of Burns: This is another test of exaggerated response. Ask a patient who reports back pain to kneel on a stool. Hold the patient's ankles to ensure confidence and ask the patient to bend forward and touch the floor. Patients who are

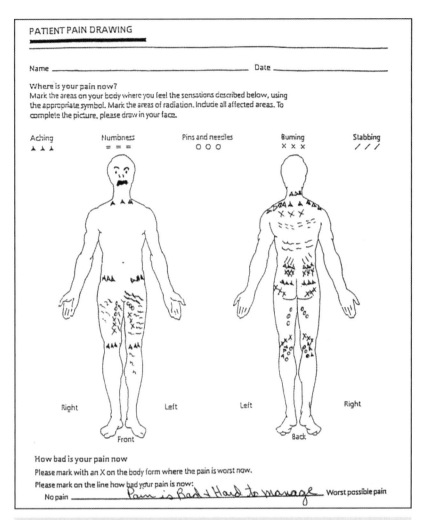

Figure 1 Pain diagram for self-assessment of the patient with nonorganic physical findings.

exaggerating symptoms will bend forward a few degrees and then grab their back, saying they cannot bend. Note that these patients are already bending forward significantly.

A thorough neurologic examination is always required to give the aforementioned tests perspective and to rule out concomitant disease.

Diagnostic Tests
None

Differential Diagnosis

- Acute injury (withdrawal from a painful examination maneuver may be an appropriate response)
- Diabetes mellitus (stocking-type peripheral neuropathy)
- Multiple sclerosis (bizarre sensory patterns that are not segmental)
- Stroke or other central lesions with altered sensory appreciation

Treatment

Serious disorders that may be masked by the aforementioned symptoms should be ruled out and the absence of specific disorders discussed with the patient. Because patients with this condition often are indirectly indicating that they are not getting the support or help they need, psychologic and social support interventions should be discussed and contributing factors such as occupational stress and marital difficulties inquired about.

Adverse Outcomes of Treatment

Failure to identify an associated serious condition is possible. Patients should always be screened for constitutional symptoms including fevers, chills, night sweats, unexpected weight loss, and incontinence. These alert the physician to other entities including infection, malignancy, and neural compression.

Referral Decisions/Red Flags

True diminished pinprick or light touch sensation with or without areflexia, brisk reflexes, clonus, spasticity, or a positive Babinski reflex usually indicates neurologic involvement.

Preoperative Evaluation of Medical Comorbidities

Definition

Surgical risk is the likelihood of an adverse outcome or death for a given surgery and associated anesthesia. A thorough preoperative evaluation allows both the medical team and patient to make a more informed decision regarding the timing and tactics for surgical management of musculoskeletal problems.

Both the patient and the procedure must be evaluated to determine the appropriate preoperative workup. The presence and severity of the patient's medical comorbidities need to be assessed. Additionally, consideration should be given as to whether these factors are modifiable. The procedure must be evaluated for both complexity and timing (that is, whether the surgery is elective, necessary, or emergent; **Table 1**).

Table 1			
Classification of Orthopaedic Procedures			
Parameter	**Elective**	**Necessary**	**Emergent**
Time frame for intervention	At the patient's request and convenience, depending on surgeon availability	Poorly defined, case independent	Within hours or even minutes, depending on the situation
Success of nonsurgical options	Variable depending on the procedure	Usually poor	Usually poor or even fatal to the patient or limb
Importance relative to other surgical cases	Equal to other elective cases; secondary to necessary or emergent cases	Secondary only to emergent cases	Highest importance; warrants "bumping" of nonemergent cases
Timing and extent of medical evaluation	May schedule in conjunction with the patient's primary care physician	Should be performed expeditiously, but also as thoroughly as possible	If condition permits, should be performed emergently and only include life- or limb-saving tests or procedures
Examples	Total joint arthroplasty, anterior cruciate ligament reconstruction, ganglion cyst excision, carpal tunnel release, bunionectomy	Fixation of hemiarthroplasty for hip fracture, treatment of unstable fractures or dislocations in which closed reduction fails	Fasciotomy for compartment syndrome, stabilization of open book pelvis, treatment of open fracture

(Adapted from Bushnell BD, Horton JK, McDonald MF, Robertson PG: Perioperative medical comorbidities in the orthopaedic patient. *J Am Acad Orthop Surg* 2008;16[4]:216-227.)

Table 2

Clinical Predictors of Increased Perioperative Cardiovascular Risk

Coronary artery disease

Heart failure (especially with left ventricular ejection fraction < 30%)

Cardiomyopathy (nonischemic)

Valvular heart disease

Arrhythmias

Cardiovascular implantable electronic device (pacemaker)

Pulmonary hypertension

Adult congenital heart disease

(Adapted from Fleisher LA, Fleischmann KE, Auerbach AD, et al: 2014 ACC/AHA Guideline on Perioperative Cardiovascular Evaluation and Management of Patients Undergoing Noncardiac Surgery: A Report of the American College of Cardiology/American Heart Association Task Force on Practice Guidelines. *J Am Coll Cardiol* 2014;64[22]:e77-e137.)

General Principles

Preoperative testing should be tailored to the group of patients that is more likely to have an abnormal result and only should be ordered if the result will affect management. This helps to avoid both unnecessary cost and delay in surgical treatment.

Cardiac

In 2014, the American College of Cardiology and the American Heart Association issued revised guidelines for the cardiac evaluation of patients undergoing noncardiac surgery. The guidelines are based on the risk factors listed in **Table 2**. Most orthopaedic procedures are deemed to be intermediate risk, and patients with major cardiac clinical predictors require a cardiac workup before undergoing elective orthopaedic surgery. Heart rate control is indicated preoperatively for surgical candidates with the other clinical risk factors listed in **Table 2**.

Anticoagulation

Many patients with coronary artery disease have been treated with percutaneous coronary angioplasty and stent placement. Antiplatelet therapy is used to prevent thrombosis of these stents and subsequent acute myocardial infarction. The increased risk of major bleeding postoperatively in these patients must be weighed against the risk of cessation of antiplatelet therapy. It is recommended that elective procedures be delayed at least 12 months after an acute coronary event and at least 6 weeks after stent placement. Patients should be counseled regarding the risks of possible myocardial infarction with the temporary discontinuation of therapy for surgical procedures.

Similarly, patients with atrial fibrillation are commonly treated with warfarin, and the risks of discontinuing that therapy must be weighed against the need for surgery. A preoperative international normalized ratio (INR) of less than 1.4 has been associated with reduced

Table 3

Recommendations for Preoperative Testing

Preoperative Test	Characteristics
Hemoglobin	Anticipated blood loss or symptoms of anemia
White blood cell count	Symptoms of infection, myeloproliferative disorder, or myelotoxic medications
Platelet count	History of bleeding, diathesis, myeloproliferative disorder, or myelotoxic medications
Partial thromboplastin time	History of bleeding
Electrolytes	Renal insufficiency, congestive heart failure, medications that affect electrolytes
Renal function	Hypertension, older than 50 years, cardiac disease, major surgery, anticipated use of medications that may affect renal function
Glucose	Obesity or known diabetes
Electrocardiogram	Men older than 40 years, women older than 50 years, known coronary artery disease, diabetes mellitus, or hypertension
Chest radiograph	Older than 50 years, known cardiac or pulmonary disease, symptoms or examination suggestive of cardiac or pulmonary disease

(Adapted from Argyros G: Perioperative medical management, in Vaccaro AR, ed: *Orthopaedic Knowledge Update*, ed 8. Rosemont, IL, American Academy of Orthopaedic Surgeons, 2005, p 138.)

intraoperative and postoperative bleeding. An INR greater than 1.7 is an independent risk factor for major postoperative hemorrhage. In elective surgery, warfarin typically can be discontinued 5 days before surgery to achieve an INR of less than 1.4.

Pulmonary

Routine chest radiographs are not recommended for all patients but should be obtained for a clinically significant subset (**Table 3**). Elective surgery should be delayed for active respiratory infections and acute exacerbations of obstructive lung disease. Patients with chronic pulmonary disease should be maintained on their regular medications. With patients who require frequent doses from rescue inhalers preoperatively, the pulmonary team should be involved early in the perioperative period.

Smoking Cessation

Large prospective studies are not available, but other studies have shown that smokers have higher rates of postoperative complications than nonsmokers. These complications are not limited to an increased risk of pulmonary complications but include wound complications, infections, and nonunions as well. Conflicting evidence exists regarding the timing of smoking cessation and lowering risk of complications, but an 8-week period of abstinence prior to surgery is probably ideal.

Renal

In patients who have chronic kidney disease, the leading cause of death is cardiac, and a full cardiac assessment is indicated. Particular attention needs to be paid to volume status, electrolytes, acid/base status, anemia, bleeding diatheses, and blood pressure. In the setting of acute or chronic renal failure, the use of nephrotoxins, such as NSAIDs, some antibiotics, angiotensin-converting enzyme inhibitors, and contrast agents, should be minimized. In 2015, the FDA strengthened its warning linking NSAIDs with the risk of heart attack or stroke, even in the first weeks of use of an NSAID.

Diabetes Mellitus

Patients with diabetes mellitus have more comorbid health conditions than the general population, including obesity, sleep apnea, and renal disease, and diabetes mellitus is considered to be a cardiac risk equivalent. These patients are at an increased risk of postoperative complications including infection, metabolic/electrolyte abnormalities, renal issues, and cardiac issues. Hyperglycemia substantially impairs wound healing and the ability to fight infection. Preoperative evaluation should include evaluating recent blood glucose and hemoglobin A1C measurements. The American Diabetes Association recommends a hemoglobin A1C target value of less than 7%, average preprandial plasma glucose between 90 and 130 mg/dL, and average postprandial plasma glucose < 180 mg/dL before proceeding with elective surgery.

For patients taking oral hypoglycemics, their medications should be withheld in the 24 hours before surgery. The long-acting sulfonylureas (such as chlorpropamide, glyburide) can cause prolonged hypoglycemia and should be withheld for at least 48 to 72 hours before surgery. Persons with diabetes mellitus who are on insulin should take one half to two thirds of their normal dose at their last regularly scheduled dose the day before surgery. The American Association of Clinical Endocrinologists and the American Diabetes Association recommend a target glucose level of less than or equal to 180 mg/dL in critically ill patients, with a maintenance goal between 140 and 180 mg/dL. In noncritically ill patients, target glucose levels should generally be less than 140 mg/dL as long as this can be safely achieved. In general, the target glucose level for an orthopaedic patient is between 110 and 180 mg/dL; however, the level should be individualized to the particular patient.

Rheumatologic Disease

Several additional perioperative concerns exist for patients with rheumatologic disease. For example, these patients carry an increased risk of cardiac events. Additionally, bleeding times may be prolonged by the use of salicylates or NSAIDs. Furthermore, both rheumatologic disease and many of the medications used to treat them are associated with an increased risk for infection. Patients who discontinued methotrexate were found to have the highest infection rate and therefore should be continued on this medication throughout the perioperative period. Infection risk is higher in patients managed with corticosteroid than with methotrexate; the risk of infection is directly proportional to the dose of corticosteroids. Additionally, patients who have taken systemic steroids for more than 1 week in the 6 months

Table 4

Biologic Medications Commonly Used in the Management of Inflammatory Arthritis

Medication (Pharmacologic Half-life)	Stop Date Prior to Elective Surgery
Etanercept (102 h)	1 wk
Infliximab (8-9.5 d)	2-3 wk
Adalimumab (14 d)	2 wk
Golimumab (14 d)	3 wk
Certolizumab pegol (14 d)	4 wk
Tocilizumab (11-13 d)	3-4 wk
Abatacept (13.1-14.3 d)	4 wk
Rituximab (effect lasts > 6 mo)	Prolonged activity. Check gamma globulin levels if infection risk is high. Wait 4 mo if possible.

(Adapted from Goodman SM, Figgie M: Lower extremity arthroplasty in patients with inflammatory arthritis: Preoperative and perioperative management. *J Am Acad Orthop Surg* 2013;21[6]:355-363.)

preceding surgery require a stress dose of steroids to decrease the risk of adrenal suppression. A typical regimen begins with 100 mg of intravenous (IV) hydrocortisone every 8 hours on the day of surgery, followed by 50 mg IV every 8 hours on postoperative day 1, 25 mg IV every 8 hours on postoperative day 2, 25 mg IV every 12 hours on postoperative day 3, and ends by resuming the patient's maintenance dose on postoperative day 4. Biologic medications commonly used in the management of inflammatory arthritis should be stopped preoperatively (**Table 4**). Time from surgery varies by medication. The mechanism for hydroxychloroquine is poorly understood but is believed to be immune modulating. In general, hydroxychloroquine can be safely continued throughout the perioperative period.

Anesthesia in patients with rheumatoid arthritis can be challenging because of either cervical instability or cricoarytenoid arthritis (seen in up to 50% of patients). Evaluation performed with lateral, flexion, and extension radiographs of the cervical spine is needed preoperatively to assess for atlantoaxial instability. Although an anterior atlantodental interval of more than 3 mm or subaxial subluxation of more than 3 mm have been classically used as markers of instability, studies suggest that a posterior atlantodental interval of less than 14 mm or a subaxial space available for the cord measuring less than 14 mm may be more accurate predictors of paralysis.

Nutrition
Nutrition plays an important role in wound healing and the ability to fight infection. Risk factors for malnutrition are listed in **Table 5**. A serum total lymphocyte count of less than 1,500 cells/mm^3, a body mass index less than 20, total cholesterol less than 160 mg/dL, and

SECTION 1 | GENERAL ORTHOPAEDICS

Table 5

Risk Factors for Malnutrition

Prior surgery

Gastrointestinal disease

Advanced age

Depression

Poverty

Recent weight loss

Systemic disease

Alcohol abuse

Medications that interfere with eating/appetite

(Adapted from Bushnell BD, Horton JK, McDonald MF, Robertson PG: Perioperative medical comorbidities in the orthopaedic patient. *J Am Acad Orthop Surg* 2008;16[4]:216-227.)

an albumin level less than 3.5 mg/dL are all markers of malnutrition that are correlated with impaired wound healing. In these patients, nutrition consultation should be obtained and malnourishment addressed preoperatively to reduce complications. Maintenance fluids should contain carbohydrates; nothing-by-mouth (nil per os [NPO]) periods should be minimized; and protein supplements and vitamins should be given to optimize nutritional status in the perioperative period.

Obesity

Obesity affects nearly every organ system, and increasing body mass index (BMI) is correlated with a greater number of comorbidities. All patients with obesity should undergo a preoperative evaluation that includes electrolyte and glucose levels, complete blood count, electrocardiogram, assessment of renal function, and screening for obstructive sleep apnea. An echocardiogram is indicated if there are any signs of congestive heart failure.

Obesity increases the perioperative risk of complications, including higher rates of prosthetic failure, infection, hardware failure, fracture malunion, venous thromboembolism, and pulmonary embolism. Additionally, obesity is associated with longer intensive care unit and hospital stays. One study found a relative risk of deep vein thrombosis (DVT) of 2.5 in patients with obesity compared with patients without obesity. The Workgroup of the American Association of Hip and Knee Surgeons recommends preoperative patient counseling in cases of morbid obesity (BMI > 40) and that consideration be given to delaying total joint arthroplasty, especially in the presence of comorbid conditions. However, although orthopaedic surgical interventions performed on patients with obesity have higher complication rates, these procedures may offer notable improvement in pain and function. Care should be taken to optimize these patients during the perioperative period.

DVT Prophylaxis

An important part of perioperative management of the orthopaedic patient is appropriate DVT prophylaxis. Venographic studies have shown an absolute risk of DVT of 40% to 60% in patients who have undergone hip or knee arthroplasty. Although most of these DVTs are asymptomatic, they have the potential to result in a pulmonary embolism, a potentially fatal complication. Patients who are hypercoagulable, have endothelial damage, or experience decreased activity are at increased risk of DVT (**Table 6**).

The use of prophylaxis after orthopaedic procedures is controversial. No studies compare different agents and the rate of symptomatic DVT or pulmonary embolism. The American Academy of Orthopaedic Surgeons advises using pharmacologic and/or mechanical prophylaxis but does not recommend the use of one specific prophylactic agent or length of therapy. Many hospitals use as quality measures the guidelines established by the Surgical Care Improvement Project (SCIP), which are in turn based on guidelines

Table 6
Risk Factors for Venous Thromboembolism

Surgery

Trauma (major or lower extremity)

Immobility, paresis

Malignancy

Cancer therapy (hormonal, chemotherapy, or radiation therapy)

Previous venous thromboembolic disease

Increasing age

Pregnancy and the postpartum period

Estrogen-containing oral contraception or hormone replacement therapy

Selective estrogen receptor modulators

Acute medical illness

Heart or respiratory failure

Inflammatory bowel disease

Nephrotic syndrome

Myeloproliferative disorders

Paroxysmal nocturnal hemoglobinuria

Obesity

Smoking

Varicose veins

Central venous catheterization

Inherited or acquired thrombophilia

(Adapted from Bushnell BD, Horton JK, McDonald MF, Robertson PG: Perioperative medical comorbidities in the orthopaedic patient. *J Am Acad Orthop Surg* 2008;16[4]:216-227.)

of the American College of Chest Physicians. The SCIP recommends the use of low-molecular-weight heparins, warfarin, or fondaparinux for lower extremity arthroplasty.

Rehabilitation and Therapeutic Modalities

Table 1

Common Impairments Found During Physical Therapy Evaluation

Acute swelling

Chronic inflammation

Restricted joint mobility with or without inflammation

Joint instability

Muscle atrophy

Decreased strength

Muscle imbalances

Loss of flexibility with or without injury

Proprioceptive deficits

Gait deviations

Decreased aerobic capacity and endurance

Postural deviations

Balance deficits

Inability to perform activities of daily living

Rehabilitation is a critical component of maximizing function after musculoskeletal injuries and surgery, and physical therapists (PTs) and athletic trainers (ATs) play a critical role in this process. PTs and ATs are highly educated, licensed healthcare professionals trained to help patients reduce pain, improve function, and restore mobility—in many cases without expensive surgery. Rehabilitation often reduces the need for long-term use of prescription medications, thus sparing patients the resulting side effects. PTs and ATs not only evaluate each patient and develop individualized treatment plans incorporating techniques that promote mobility, reduce pain, restore function, and prevent disability, they also teach patients how to prevent or manage their condition to achieve long-term health benefits. Developing a home exercise program and helping the patient become independent with his or her program is a priority.

Rehabilitation has evolved into an evidence-based multidisciplinary profession with advancements in kinesiology, physiology, and soft-tissue management. The main objective of rehabilitation is to return the patient to maximum function as quickly and safely as possible following injury or surgery. A collaborative effort and communication among the physician, PT, and AT is essential to ensure optimum recovery for an athlete following a musculoskeletal injury or surgery.

In addition to expediting healing times, proper rehabilitation also plays a critical role in allowing patients to maximize their function following surgery and prevent future injuries or surgeries resulting from muscle imbalances and compensatory movement patterns. PTs and ATs can teach patients how to prevent or manage their condition so that they will achieve long-term health benefits. In addition, PTs and ATs work with individuals to prevent the loss of mobility by developing fitness- and wellness-oriented programs for healthier and more active lifestyles. The rehabilitation specialist can design conditioning programs for healthy and injured individuals to facilitate improved strength, speed, balance, and overall cardiovascular fitness, thereby reducing future musculoskeletal injuries. Patients may also benefit from so-called prehab to help reduce swelling and improve range of motion (ROM) and strength before surgery.

Rehabilitation

Evaluation by the physician, PT, and/or AT is essential to identify a patient's specific impairments or weaknesses. Following the evaluation, a problem list (or list of impairments or weaknesses) is created and serves to generate treatment goals for the patient (**Table 1**). The goals of rehabilitation are specific for each patient and often include the following: decreasing inflammation; increasing joint ROM and flexibility; and increasing muscle strength, neuromuscular

Table 2			
Guidelines for Athletic Injury Rehabilitation			
Phase	**Pathologic Process**	**Functional Goals**	**Rehabilitation**
I—Acute injury	Tissue injury (hematoma, edema, inflammation, necrosis)	Protection; limit injury, swelling, and pain	PRICE (protection, rest, ice, compression, elevation)
II—Initial rehabilitation	Fibroblastic stage, decreasing inflammation, edema waning, minimal tensile strength (0%-15%)	Progressive pain-free ROM	Active/assisted ROM, limited short-arc resistance, cold, gentle isometrics, early aerobics
III—Progressive rehabilitation	Early tissue repair, primitive collagen and early tissue maturation, moderate tensile strength (15%-50%)	Improve ROM, increase strength, limited activity skills, ongoing protection	Passive and active ROM and stretching, progressive resistive exercises with isotonic and/or isokinetic exercise, increased aerobic activities
IV—Integrated functions	Mature collagen, tissue characteristics evident, tensile strength improved (50%-90%)	Increase skills and strength, enhance flexibility	Advanced progressive resistive exercises, flexibility exercises, coordination training, proprioceptive training
V—Return to sport	Tissue remodeling, tissue characteristics maturing, tensile strength increased (90%-99%)	Maximize skills, simulated participation, prevent reinjury	Maintain strength and flexibility, advanced coordination activities, protect previously injured area from reinjury

ROM = range of motion.

(Adapted with permission from Skerker RS, Schulz LA: Principles of rehabilitation of the injured athlete, in Pappas AM, Walzer J, eds: *Upper Extremity Injuries in the Athlete.* New York, NY, Churchill Livingstone, 1995, p 31; and Morgan WJ, Slowman LS: Acute hand and wrist injuries in athletes: Evaluation and management. *J Am Acad Orthop Surg* 2001;9[6]:389-400.)

function, proprioception, and balance. The end goals of rehabilitation may range from the ability to successfully perform activities of daily living to returning to a high level of athletic participation. It is important to set realistic and achievable goals specific to each patient. Goals should be reviewed regularly and adjusted accordingly. To maximize patient compliance, it is ideal to prescribe a rehabilitation program that complements the exercise preferences of the patient and involves the participation of family and friends.

Rehabilitation for musculoskeletal injuries generally progresses in stepwise fashion through five main phases, and the rehabilitation specialist must take into account the pathologic processes for the involved tissue (**Table 2**).

GENERAL ORTHOPAEDICS

SECTION 1

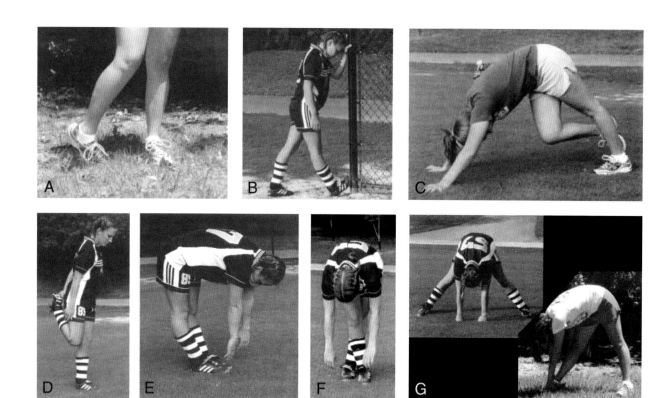

Figure 1 Photographs of commonly used stretching exercises for the muscles of the upper and lower extremities. **A,** Ankle roll. Loosen the tibiotalar and subtalar joints by placing the toes on the ground and gently rolling the ankle. **B,** Plantar fascia and calf. Stand back several feet from a fence or wall, place the toes of one foot against the object, and lean forward. Hold for 30 seconds. Repeat with the opposite extremity. **C,** Alternate calf stretch. Lean forward on the hands, gently arching the back while keeping the foot flat on the ground, and slowly lift the other leg. Hold for 30 seconds and switch legs. **D,** Standing quadriceps stretch. Stand on one leg (may brace yourself against a stationary object), bend the knee toward your buttock, and grasp the ankle. Hold for 30 seconds. Repeat with the opposite leg. **E,** Lower body and hip stretch. Slowly bend forward at the hips. Keep the knees slightly bent during the stretch so that the lower back is not stressed. Let the neck and shoulders relax. Bend to the point where you feel a stretch in the back of the legs. Hold for 30 seconds. **F,** Calf, hamstring, and spine stretch. Stand with your legs crossed. Keep your feet together and your legs straight. Slowly bend forward toward your toes. Hold for 30 seconds. Repeat with the opposite leg crossed in front. **G,** Low back, hips, and hamstring stretch. Stand with the feet at a comfortable distance apart. To stretch the inside of your upper legs and hips, slowly lean forward from the hips, trying to touch the ground in front of you (upper). Hold for 30 seconds. Then slowly reach both hands toward the right ankle (lower). Hold for 30 seconds. Repeat, reaching for the left ankle.

Restoring full ROM is a primary goal of rehabilitation. Flexibility exercises, passive low-load prolonged stretching, and manual therapy are the most successful approaches to restoring full ROM. Flexibility exercises should be performed daily by those recovering from an injury. Stretching techniques include static (slow, gentle stretching), ballistic (quick, repetitive stretching), and proprioceptive neuromuscular function (PNF; a slow stretch followed by isometric contraction against a partner's resistance for 5 to 10 seconds, followed by relaxation and slow stretch). Caution should be taken during ballistic stretching because injury can result. Hence, many rehabilitation specialists prefer static and PNF stretching techniques (**Figure 1**).

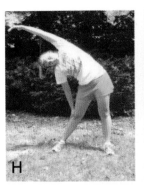
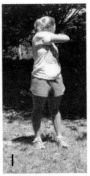
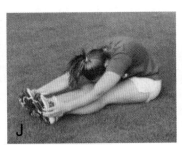
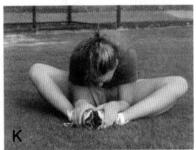

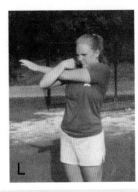
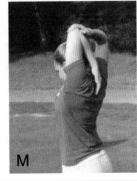
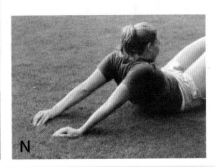

Figure 1 (continued) **H,** Side stretch. Stand with your weight evenly distributed and your feet shoulder width apart. Place one hand at your side and the other above your head, leaning to the opposite side. Hold for 30 seconds. Repeat three times on each side. **I,** Trunk rotation. Stand with your weight evenly distributed and your feet shoulder width apart. Slowly rotate your upper body to one side while keeping your hips still. Hold for 30 seconds. Alternate sides. Repeat 10 times. This stretch may also be performed in a seated position with good posture. **J,** Low back and hamstring stretch. Sit with both legs straight out in front of you. Reach forward with both hands toward your feet. Hold for 30 seconds. Feel the stretch at the back of the thighs. Try not to bend at the knees. This stretch also can be done with one knee bent out to the side (figure-of-4 position). **K,** Groin and low back stretch. Sit on the floor, place the soles of your feet together, and drop your knees toward the floor. Place your forearms on the insides of your knees and gently push your knees toward the floor. Lean forward, bringing your chin to your feet. Hold for 30 seconds. **L,** Crossover arm. Grasp the elbow of one arm with your opposite hand and pull the arm across the front of your chest. **M,** Overhead arm. Raise your injured arm above your head, as high toward the ear as possible, and bend the elbow with the palm up. Use your opposite hand to help pull the arm toward the ear. Hold for 30 seconds and then relax. Perform 25 times, 3 times per day. **N,** Front of shoulder. Put your arms behind your back, shoulder width apart. Move your hands slowly toward each other and hold for 30 seconds.

As ROM improves, it is important to strengthen the muscles surrounding the joint and to improve muscle endurance. Three general types of strengthening exercises can be used: isometric, isotonic, and isokinetic, so named based on the type of muscle contraction elicited (**Table 3**). Isometric exercises produce a muscle contraction without measurable change in joint angle and position. These exercises are often indicated early in a rehabilitation program when muscle contraction is desired without excessive stress on the joint. They can be performed by the therapist or the patient. The therapist can easily match the force that the patient is able to produce without pain and can work to safely achieve strengthening in multiple angles. An example of isometric exercise is a patient or rehabilitation specialist applying a force to the forearm with the elbow at 90° of

Table 3

Muscle Contraction Terminology

Type of Muscle Contraction	Definition	Indications	Example
Isometric	A muscle contraction that produces force without a measurable change in the joint angle	Increasing strength at a specific point in the ROM	The patient or therapist applies a force to the patient's forearm at 90° of elbow flexion. This produces a contraction of the biceps without moving the joint.
Isotonic	A manual or mechanical resistance remains constant while the joint moves through some ROM (may be concentric or eccentric)	—	—
Concentric	An isotonic contraction that occurs as the muscle shortens	Important for producing acceleration of a body segment	Patient performs a bicep curl with resistance from full extension to full elbow flexion
Eccentric	An isotonic contraction that occurs as the muscle lengthens	Important for deceleration of a body segment and shock absorption	Patient lowers a heavier weight from full elbow flexion to extension
Isokinetic	A muscle contraction that occurs at a constant rate of speed	Strengthening throughout the ROM	Therapist applies manual accommodating resistance throughout elbow ROM. This can be performed concentrically or eccentrically.

ROM = range of motion.

flexion while the patient resists or pushes against the applied force. Isotonic exercises consist of a fixed resistance applied to a joint while it moves through ROM. These exercises can be further classified as concentric (contraction occurs as the muscle shortens) or eccentric (contraction occurs as the muscle lengthens). Eccentric exercises are a great choice to improve tensile strength of tendons. Isotonic exercises are used as the rehabilitation program advances to increase muscle strength and endurance. An example is a biceps curl performed with a dumbbell. Isokinetic exercises consist of a varied resistance applied to a joint moving at a constant rate of speed. These exercises can be performed manually by the rehabilitation specialist or with specialized equipment. Isokinetic exercises can be used to decrease the stress on a muscle or joint at points of the ROM at which the joint may be less capable of producing a strong counterforce (that is, at the beginning or end of the ROM versus the midrange). Isokinetic exercise can be used following an injury or surgery to test muscular

Table 4

Open- Versus Closed-Chain Exercises

Exercise	Characteristics	Examples
Open chain	Distal segment is free; non–weight bearing; muscle contraction is primarily concentric; proprioceptive carryover to functional activities is questionable	Knee extension machine; hamstring curl machine; non–weight-bearing isometrics; straight leg raises; stationary bike; terminal knee extension
Closed chain	Distal segment is not free; partial weight bearing; muscle contraction includes concentric, eccentric, isometric and isotonic; movements are functional; significant proprioceptive carryover to functional activities	Partial weight bearing: mini wall squats, proprioceptive exercises with BAPS board Full weight bearing: elliptical machine, agility drills, step ups, mini wall squats

BAPS = biomechanical ankle platform system.

strength, although use of isokinetic evaluations is decreasing in favor of functional movement screenings.

As progress in rehabilitation advances, strength training with heavier weights and lower repetitions may be initiated as long as no pain is present during the exercise. Strengthening exercises for rehabilitation should be performed 3 or 4 days per week. Both closed-chain and open-chain exercises are used to improve strength and function during the rehabilitation program (**Table 4**). Closed-chain exercises are generally safer and more functional, and they are used at the beginning of a rehabilitation program. Typically, the patient begins closed-chain exercises with use of both limbs and smaller joint ROM, progresses to a larger ROM, and then performs the exercises using a single (involved) limb. Open-chain exercises are used to strengthen a particular muscle or muscle group, such as a muscle that has atrophied from disuse or immobilization. Open-chain exercises can place greater stress on a joint, so these exercises should begin with low weight and a higher number of repetitions and advance accordingly.

Proprioception (awareness of the body's position in space) exercises must be included in any rehabilitation program, especially those for lower extremity injuries, so the patient can regain and enhance neuromuscular control. Initially, the patient simply stands on one leg, then progresses to maintaining balance with eyes closed or while standing on an unstable or soft surface. After a patient can safely perform single leg balance activities on an unstable surface, the PT can progress the rehabilitation to include various degrees of unstable surfaces and perturbations (ball toss, manual perturbations) to achieve maximum function. It is critical for all patients to be able to control their own body weight throughout daily activities, and athletes must also be able to maintain control of their body while running, cutting, and jumping, often on uneven terrain.

After normal ROM, strength, and neuromuscular control/balance are achieved, the patient can progress to activity-specific exercises

Table 5

Postoperative Rehabilitation Protocols

Phase	Goals
I—Immediate postoperative	Protect surgical repair
	Promote healing of involved tissues
	Decrease swelling and inflammation
	Gradually improve passive and active ROM (per protocol)
	Educate patient in precautions and HEP
II—Maximum protection	Control of external forces on the surgical site
	Decrease swelling and inflammation
	Gradually increase ROM (per protocol)
	Prevent muscular atrophy
	Stimulate collagen healing
III—Moderate protection	Progress ROM
	Improve muscular strength and endurance while protecting surgical site and healing tissues
	Gradually increase joint stresses and tissue loading
	Improve confidence and function for the patient
IV—Light activity	Increase tensile strength of tendons
	Develop strength, power, and endurance
	Begin to prepare for return to functional activities
V—Return-to-sport/activity	Achieve maximal strength and endurance
	Begin return-to-sport activities

HEP = home exercise program, ROM = range of motion.

designed to achieve the end goals of rehabilitation. A common principle used in rehabilitation includes the specific adaptation to imposed demands principle (SAID), which states that the human body will specifically adapt to the stressors put on the body. Therefore for athletes, as noted previously, rehabilitation would include sport-specific exercises, such as change-of-direction ("cutting") activities, jumping, and throwing. Sport-specific exercises should begin in a controlled setting under the watchful eye of a licensed rehabilitation professional to ensure proper form and technique followed by progression onto the field or court. Athletes must meet return-to-play criteria with agreement among the physician, PT, and AT before returning to his or her sport. At this point, general physical conditioning also may be included in the rehabilitation plan.

Postoperative rehabilitation protocols (**Table 5**) are specific to the surgical procedure and specific ligaments, tendons, and tissues involved. Time frames and exercises are patient-specific and adapted to the individual's specific return-to-sport requirements. Patients must meet the goals and criteria of each phase before progressing to the next one.

Table 6

Therapeutic Modalities, Exercises, and Equipment

Impairments, Symptoms, and Physical Findings	Goals of Treatment	Rehabilitation Principles, Exercises, and Treatment	Equipment	Comments
Acute swelling	Reduce swelling	PRICE, vasopneumatic cold compression, manual therapy, HVPGS, exercises in uninjured areas only	Vasopneumatic compression unit, braces and splints for immobilization as needed	—
Chronic inflammation	Decrease inflammation	Ice, phonophoresis, iontophoresis, NSAIDs, stretching, joint mobilization, isometric and short-arc strengthening	Tape, soft braces, neoprene sleeves	—
Restricted joint motion with inflammation	Restore joint mobility, decrease inflammation	Ice, manual therapy (grade I/II joint mobilizations,[a] gentle soft-tissue massage), isometric strengthening, therapeutic exercises (passive and active ROM in the pain-free range only)	Compression wraps, functional braces	Assess for intra-articular pathology
Restricted joint motion without inflammation	Restore joint mobility	Heat, ultrasound, manual therapy (grade III/IV joint mobilizations and soft-tissue massage), therapeutic exercises (active, passive, and active-assisted ROM)	Progressive splints to maintain motion, night splints	Rule out systemic disease, CRPS
Joint instability	Regain joint stability and improve proprioception for joint protection	Strengthening in ROM without pain, closed-chain kinetic exercises, proprioception exercises	Immobilize acute injury, functional braces later	Distinguish between static and functional instability
Muscle atrophy	Restore muscle tone and strength	PREs, NMES	Weights and tubing for home exercise program	Distinguish between disuse and neurologic injuries
Muscle imbalances	Identify imbalances and restore symmetry bilaterally	Objective measurement to identify deficits, selective strengthening exercises	None	Distinguish between disuse and neurologic injuries
Loss of flexibility with injury	Promote healing of injured site and safely restore flexibility	Ice, HVPGS, ultrasound, manual therapy (myofascial work, manual stretching), static stretching, massage, PREs, dry needling as indicated	Compression with and without immobilization	—

SECTION 1 GENERAL ORTHOPAEDICS

Table 6 (continued)

Therapeutic Modalities, Exercises, and Equipment

Impairments, Symptoms, and Physical Findings	Goals of Treatment	Rehabilitation Principles, Exercises, and Treatment	Equipment	Comments
Loss of flexibility without injury	Restore flexibility	Active stretching with and without assistance; contract-relax, low-load prolonged stretches; dynamic active warm-up; manual therapy (myofascial release); dry needling as indicated	None	Address underlying cause of muscle tightness
Proprioceptive/ balance deficits	Improve proprioception and neuromuscular control	Balance and proprioceptive exercises, progressing from stable to unstable surfaces and more advanced activities; functional activity training	Neoprene sleeve for warmth, neoprene sleeve or wrap for tactile input, balance board, balance pads, unstable discs, balance ball, rebounder	Modified Romberg test
Postural deviations	Improve posture for ADLs	Identify postural deviation, improve flexibility in shortened muscles, improve postural strength to maintain correct posture	Taping for postural corrections, postural bracing as necessary	—
Gait deviations	Restore normal and safe gait	Identify gait deviations and strengthen specific muscle weakness, improve balance, gait training (may use antigravity treadmill or aquatic programs to reduce weight bearing and enable for proper form), video gait analysis with visual feedback for patient education	Anti-gravity treadmill, slow motion video analysis	Slow motion video gait analysis can be beneficial for runners and high-level athletes to identify deficits and compensations that lead to injuries
Decreased aerobic capacity and endurance	Improve endurance for functional activities	Therapeutic exercises and therapeutic activities to safely improve endurance	Stationary bike, elliptical machine, other cardiovascular equipment	Monitor heart rate and perceived rate of exertion
Inability to perform ADLs	Maximize function with ADLs	Identify safety issues and functional deficits; therapeutic exercises specific to deficits	None	—

ADLs = activities of daily living; CRPS = complex regional pain syndrome; HVPGS = high voltage pulsed galvanic stimulation; NMES = neuromuscular electrical stimulation; PREs = passive resistance exercises; PRICE = protection, rest, ice, compression, elevation; ROM = range of motion.

[a] Grades of manual therapy: I = small amplitude rhythmic oscillating mobilization in early ROM, II = large amplitude rhythmic oscillating mobilization in mid ROM, III = large amplitude rhythmic oscillating mobilization to point of limitation in ROM, IV = small amplitude rhythmic oscillating mobilization at end ROM.

Therapeutic Modalities

Rehabilitation specialists use therapeutic modalities to decrease pain and inflammation following an acute injury or surgery. Certain modalities also can be used to assist in reestablishing neuromuscular control in atrophied muscles and are a useful adjunct to strengthening exercises. For example, good evidence exists that neuromuscular electrical stimulation (NMES) used in conjunction with a closed kinetic chain anterior cruciate ligament rehabilitation program enhances quadriceps strength. Transcutaneous electrical nerve stimulation is designed to help control pain through a proposed spinal cord gating mechanism and can be useful to prepare the soft tissue before manual therapy or passive and active stretching exercises. Therapeutic ultrasound can be used to increase tissue elasticity, increase blood flow to tissues, and promote good alignment of scar tissue. Low-level or cold laser therapy has become more popular as a technique to promote tissue healing by increasing cell metabolism. Dry needling is a treatment approach used by some PTs to manage impairments ranging from scarring and myofascial pain to problems with motor recruitment. Preliminary research supports the use of these techniques, which employ thin filament needles, without medication, to stimulate various muscular and connective tissues. The indications for various therapeutic modalities, exercises, and equipment are listed in **Table 6**.

Adverse Outcomes of Treatment

Untimely or overaggressive therapy may disrupt the healing process, as can therapy that does not respect weight-bearing limitations. Good communication between the physician and rehabilitation professional is of the utmost importance for optimal patient care. Additional contraindications to rehabilitation exercises are listed in **Table 7**.

Preparation for activity-related emergencies, preparticipation physical examinations, and proper hydration and nutrition must also be instituted for competitive athletes to prevent possible adverse outcomes from conditioning and rehabilitation programs.

Referral Decisions/Red Flags

Referral to physical therapy is a critical adjunct to many surgical procedures. Proper rehabilitation can expedite healing times, and it plays a critical role in allowing patients to maximize their function following surgery and prevent future injuries or surgeries resulting from muscle imbalances and compensatory movement patterns. When ordering rehabilitation, the physician should specify the diagnosis and the limitations of the patient.

Table 7
Contraindications to Exercise

Absolute

Recent myocardial infarction

Ischemic electrocardiographic changes

Unstable angina

Uncontrolled arrhythmia

Third-degree heart block

Acute congestive heart failure

Relative

Uncontrolled hypertension

Valvular heart disease

Cardiomyopathies

Complex ventricular ectopy

Uncontrolled metabolic disease

(Reproduced from Galloway MT, Jokl P: Aging successfully: The importance of physical activity in maintaining health and function. *J Am Acad Orthop Surg* 2000;8[1]:37-44.)

GENERAL ORTHOPAEDICS

SECTION 1

Musculoskeletal Conditioning: Helping Patients Prevent Injury and Stay Fit

Over the past 50 to 75 years, the United States has experienced a shift in lifestyle. Once a society in which most individuals worked in physically stressful jobs (such as farming, steelmaking, road and railroad building); walked to work, to visit friends, and to shop; and climbed stairs rather than riding elevators, ours is now a society in which individuals may sit in offices during most of their workday and drive to their activities. The mental stresses may be great, but the physical stresses of most jobs are small. Yard and household chores have also become physically less demanding, thanks to technologic advances: lawn mowers are motorized, and sweepers, floor waxers, dishwashers, and clothes washers have replaced manual activities for these tasks.

As physical inactivity has become more common, health issues associated with this inactivity have become all too prominent. Obesity and associated diseases such as heart disease, diabetes mellitus, and hypertension have been reported to be "epidemic" in the United States.

One responsibility of a physician is to educate patients on the importance of physical activity as a part of a healthy lifestyle. Such an exercise prescription typically includes not only instruction in a general aerobic exercise program for cardiovascular fitness (such as swimming, cycling, or walking) but also exercise to strengthen areas weakened by injury or inactivity or areas that would be particularly challenged by a new activity. For example, a 50-year-old man who wishes to play tennis or a 45-year-old woman who recently secured a job as a painter would benefit from both cardiovascular exercise to increase endurance and specific exercises for conditioning the shoulders and trunk. A body made fit by musculoskeletal stretching, strengthening, and proprioceptive exercises is less likely to sustain injury during sport- or work-related activities or daily activities such as gardening or housekeeping. This chapter provides examples of these exercises.

A conditioning program for either the body as a whole or a specific targeted anatomic area of the body consists of three basic phases: stretching exercises to restore range of motion, strengthening exercises to improve muscle power, and proprioceptive exercises to enhance balance and agility. Stretching and strengthening exercises are generally begun first, followed by proprioceptive exercises. Patient handouts for the stretching and strengthening exercises are provided on the website that is associated with this publication, and additional proprioceptive exercises for beginners are described in the text. Plyometric exercises may also be added for power after basic strength and flexibility have been achieved. Advanced proprioceptive exercises and plyometric exercises should be done under the supervision of a rehabilitation specialist (such as a physical therapist, athletic trainer, or occupational therapist) or other exercise professional (such as a strength and conditioning personal trainer).

The goal of a conditioning program is to enable people to live a fit and healthier lifestyle by being more active. A well-structured conditioning program will also prepare the individual for participation in sports and recreational activities. The greater the intensity of the activity in which the individual engages or wishes to engage, the greater the intensity of the conditioning that will be required. If the individual attends supervised rehabilitation (including all specialists listed previously) for instruction in a conditioning routine rather than using only an exercise handout such as provided in this publication, the focus should be on developing and committing to a home exercise fitness program.

The following are conditioning exercises, arranged by anatomic area. Musculoskeletal conditioning of the shoulder is discussed first, followed by the hip, knee, foot and ankle, and lumbar spine. Each section describes a home exercise program and includes patient exercise handouts that may be printed out from the website that accompanies this publication.

Shoulder Conditioning

The shoulder is a complex structure that allows movement in many different planes. The glenohumeral and scapular rotators are important muscle groups for overhead sports activities such as tennis, baseball, and swimming. Strengthening the scapular stabilizers, as well as the rotator cuff and deltoid muscles, is important to assist with the stability of the glenohumeral joint and help prevent injury when engaging in activities that involve repetitive upper extremity motion such as gardening, housekeeping, or sports. Increased strength in these muscles can also translate to a higher velocity tennis serve or baseball pitch.

Proprioceptive and balance exercises enhance the individual's perception of the position of the body and arm in space. Scapular retraction performed while prone on a large exercise ball, push-ups performed on an air mattress, and ball rolling on a wall are examples of proprioceptive exercises for the shoulder. These exercises should be done only after adequate flexibility and strength have been achieved. Instruction and supervision in such exercises is recommended to ensure that they are performed safely.

For individuals beginning a new sport activity, a period of sport-specific training should begin only after the prescribed goals of strengthening, stretching, and proprioceptive conditioning have been met. During this period, the individual would perform the actions normally required by the sport with gradually increasing intensity and duration.

Forcing stretching or strengthening to the point of pain is always deleterious and should be avoided. Progress is achieved by performing these exercises frequently (2 to 3 times per day, 4 to 5 days per week) and making gradual improvement toward goals. The patient should be instructed to call the physician if any exercises cause pain.

Stretching Exercises

The capsule and muscles of the posterior shoulder may be tight, especially in individuals who participate in repetitive overhead activities, including overhead throwing sports and swimming. Horizontal adduction stretching and the sleeper stretch are helpful to relax these posterior shoulder tissues. Static stretching is performed at the end of the range of painless motion of the shoulder.

Strengthening Exercises

Exercises to strengthen the deltoid and rotator cuff muscles are often performed using commercially available elastic therapy bands. These bands are available in different thicknesses, which provide predictable levels of resistance. Similar exercises can also be performed with pulleys or free weights. It usually takes 2 to 3 weeks to progress to the next band or weight. For strength training, the patient should perform 3 sets of 8 repetitions, progressing to 3 sets of 12 repetitions. After 12 repetitions are reached, the resistance should be increased and the repetitions started over at 8. The patient should be advised not to progress to the next level of resistance if he or she still has difficulty at the current level or if pain develops. The patient should also be instructed to continue stretching exercises during this stage to maintain shoulder range of motion.

Proprioceptive Exercises

In addition to adequate strength, athletes benefit from improved control and coordination. Neuromuscular training, which improves the communication between the muscles and nervous system, includes balance and proprioceptive exercises. Balance involves the visual, vestibular, and proprioceptive systems. With balance training, the athlete may be instructed to hold a posture for 30 to 60 seconds at the limits of his or her stability.

Proprioceptive exercises for the shoulder often involve weight bearing through the arms. For example, push-ups performed with the hands on an exercise ball are an excellent advanced exercise for improving dynamic glenohumeral and scapular stability. For the novice athlete, standing push-ups done against a wall provide good proprioceptive training. This exercise can be performed with the hands directly on the wall or, to provide an additional challenge, the hands can be placed on one large or two smaller exercise balls during the push-up motion.

www.aaos.org/essentials5/exercises

Home Exercise Program for Shoulder Conditioning

- Perform 10 minutes of general warm-up activity such as using an arm bike or elliptical before doing these exercises.
- When performing the stretching exercises, stretch slowly to the limit of motion, taking care to avoid pain. If you experience pain with the exercises, call your doctor.
- For the exercises that use a stick, you may use a yardstick or stick of similar size.
- The following exercise program is introductory only, and progression of this program will vary based on your specific injury, symptoms, and baseline level of fitness. For further progression of this routine, your physician may recommend evaluation and treatment by a physical therapist or other exercise professional.

Strengthening and Stretching Exercises for the Shoulder

Exercise	Muscle Group	Number of Repetitions/Sets	Number of Days per Week
Strengthening			
External rotation	Infraspinatus Teres minor	8 repetitions/3 sets, progressing to 12 repetitions/3 sets	3
Standing row	Middle trapezius Rhomboid	8 repetitions/3 sets, progressing to 12 repetitions/3 sets	3
Internal rotation	Pectoralis major and minor Subscapularis	8 repetitions/3 sets, progressing to 12 repetitions/3 sets	3
Bent-over horizontal abduction	Middle and lower trapezius	8 repetitions/3 sets, progressing to 12 repetitions/3 sets	3
Elbow flexion	Biceps	8 repetitions/3 sets, progressing to 12 repetitions/3 sets	3
Elbow extension	Triceps	8 repetitions/3 sets, progressing to 12 repetitions/3 sets	3
External rotation with arm abducted 90°	Infraspinatus Teres minor	8 repetitions/3 sets, progressing to 12 repetitions/3 sets	3
Stretching			
Pendulum	General	10 repetitions/2 sets, progressing to 15 repetitions/3 sets	5 to 6
Passive external rotation	Infraspinatus Teres minor	4 sets	5 to 6
Passive internal rotation	Subscapularis Pectoralis major and minor	4 sets	5 to 6
Horizontal adduction stretch	Posterior deltoid	4 sets	5 to 6
Sleeper stretch	Posterior deltoid	5 repetitions, 2 to 3 times per day, continuing for 3 to 4 weeks	5 to 6

SECTION 1   GENERAL ORTHOPAEDICS

Strengthening Exercises

External Rotation

- Make a 3-foot–long loop with the elastic band and tie the ends together. Attach the loop to a doorknob or other stable object.
- Standing with your side to the wall, hold the loop, as shown in the start position.
- Keeping your elbow close to your side, rotate the arm outward slowly and then slowly return to the start position.
- Perform 3 sets of 8 repetitions, progressing to 3 sets of 12 repetitions, 3 days per week.
- Repeat on the other side.

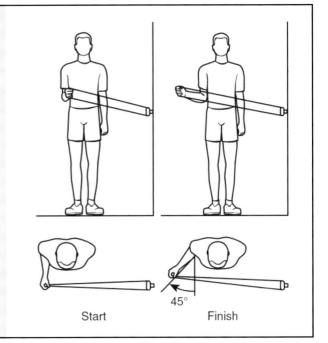

Start   Finish   45°

Standing Row

- Make a 3-foot–long loop with the elastic band and tie the ends together.
- Attach the loop to a doorknob or other stable object.
- Standing while facing the wall, hold the loop with both hands as shown in the start position.
- Keeping your arms close to your sides, slowly pull straight back and squeeze your shoulder blades together.
- Slowly return to the start position.
- Perform 3 sets of 8 repetitions, progressing to 3 sets of 12 repetitions, 3 days per week.
- Repeat on the other side.

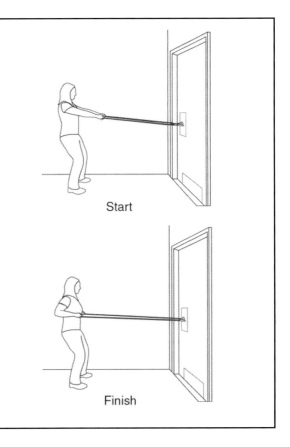

Start

Finish

Internal Rotation

- Make a 3-foot–long loop with the elastic band and tie the ends together. Attach the loop to a doorknob or other stable object.
- Standing with your side to the wall, hold the loop as shown in the start position.
- Keeping your elbow close to your side, rotate the arm across your body slowly, and slowly return to the start position.
- Perform 3 sets of 8 repetitions, progressing to 3 sets of 12 repetitions, 3 days per week.
- Repeat on the other side.

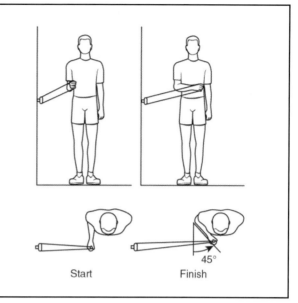

Start   Finish   45°

Bent-Over Horizontal Abduction

- Stand next to a table.
- Bend at the waist with your side supported on the table and the other arm hanging straight down and holding a light weight (up to 5 pounds).
- Keeping the arm straight, slowly raise the hand up to eye level and then slowly lower it back to the start position.
- Perform 3 sets of 8 repetitions, progressing to 3 sets of 12 repetitions, 3 days per week.
- Repeat on the other side.

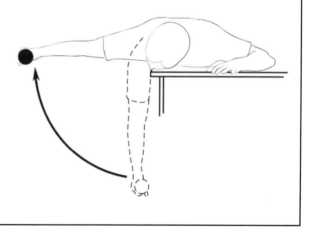

GENERAL ORTHOPAEDICS

SECTION 1

Elbow Flexion

- Stand with your body weight evenly distributed over both feet.
- Holding a light weight (up to 5 pounds) and keeping the arm close to the side, slowly bend the elbow up toward the shoulder as shown; hold for 2 seconds, slowly return to the starting position, and then relax.
- Perform 3 sets of 8 repetitions, progressing to 3 sets of 12 repetitions, 3 days per week.
- Repeat on the other side.

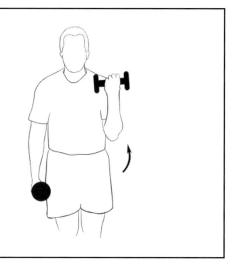

Elbow Extension

- Stand with your body weight evenly distributed over both feet.
- Holding a light weight (up to 5 pounds), raise your arm with the elbow bent and with your opposite hand supporting your elbow. Slowly straighten the elbow overhead, hold for 2 seconds, and then slowly lower the arm to the starting position.
- Perform 3 sets of 8 repetitions, progressing to 3 sets of 12 repetitions, 3 days per week.
- Repeat on the other side.

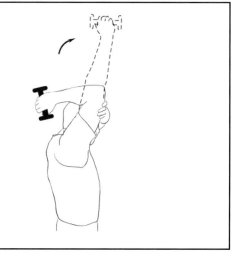

External Rotation With the Arm Abducted 90°

- Make a 3-foot–long loop with the elastic band and tie the ends together. Attach the loop to a doorknob or other stable object.
- Standing facing the wall, hold the loop as shown in the start position, with the arm held straight out from the shoulder and the elbow bent 90°.
- Keeping the shoulder and elbow level, slowly rotate the hand up from the elbow, and then slowly return to the start position.
- Perform 3 sets of 8 repetitions, progressing to 3 sets of 12 repetitions, 3 days per week.

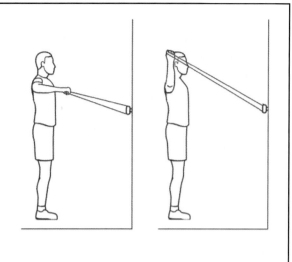

Stretching Exercises

Pendulum

- Lean forward, supporting the body with one arm and relaxing the muscles of the other arm so that it hangs freely.
- Gently move the arm in forward-and-back, side-to-side, and circular motions.
- Perform 2 sets of 10 repetitions, progressing to 3 sets of 15 repetitions, 5 to 6 days per week.
- Repeat on the other side.

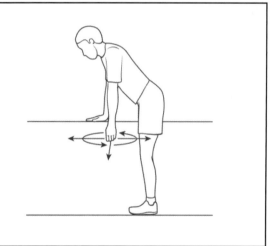

Passive External Rotation

- Grasp the stick with one hand and cup the other end of the stick with the other hand.
- Push the stick horizontally as shown, keeping the elbow against the side of the body so that the arm is passively stretched to the point of feeling a pull without pain.
- Hold for 30 seconds and then relax for 30 seconds.
- Perform 4 sets, 5 to 6 days per week.
- Repeat on the other side.

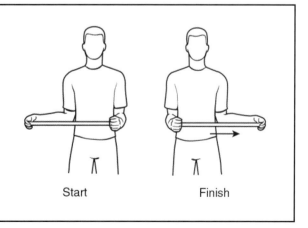

Start   Finish

SECTION 1   GENERAL ORTHOPAEDICS

Passive Internal Rotation

- Behind your back, grasp the stick with one hand and lightly grasp the other end of the stick with the other hand.
- Pull the stick horizontally as shown so that the arm is passively stretched to the point of feeling a pull without pain.
- Hold for 30 seconds and then relax for 30 seconds.
- Perform 4 sets, 5 to 6 days per week.
- Repeat on the other side.

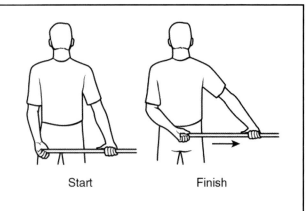

Start   Finish

Horizontal Adduction Stretch

- Gently pull the elbow of one arm across the chest as far as possible without feeling pain.
- Hold the stretch for 30 seconds and then relax for 30 seconds.
- Perform 4 sets, 5 to 6 days per week.
- Repeat on the other side.

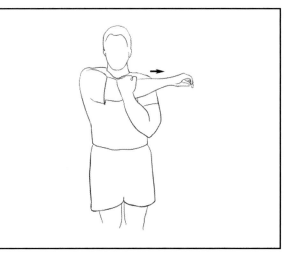

Sleeper Stretch

- Lie on your side on a firm, flat surface with the affected shoulder under you and the arm positioned as shown, keeping your back perpendicular to the surface.
- With the unaffected arm, push the other wrist down, toward the surface. Stop when you feel a stretching sensation in the back of the affected shoulder.
- Hold this position for 30 seconds, then relax the arm for 30 seconds.
- Perform 5 repetitions, 2 to 3 times per day, 5 to 6 days per week, continuing for 3 to 4 weeks.

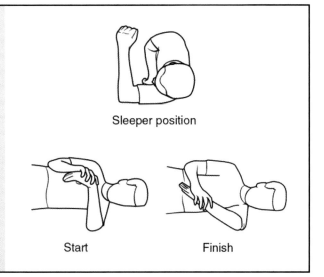

Sleeper position

Start   Finish

Conditioning of the Hip

The muscles of the hip and pelvis are important in walking and running activities. An exercise program for conditioning of the hip should include an active warm-up; stretching, strengthening, and proprioceptive exercises; and, after basic stretching and strengthening have been achieved, plyometrics for power.

Active Warm-Up

The hip muscle groups are large and require an adequate warm-up, such as riding on a stationary bicycle or jogging for 10 minutes to raise the core body temperature. In addition, dynamic stretching exercises such as leg swings can be used to warm up the synovial fluid in the hip joint and actively stretch the muscles before activity.

Strengthening Exercises

Exercises that isolate muscle contraction and do not stimulate co-contractions are important for strengthening the hip muscles. In general, weight-bearing exercises produce co-contractions, and non–weight-bearing exercises do not. Co-contractions are important for stabilizing the joint that is being strengthened. Strengthening of the large hip muscle groups requires heavier weights and few (6 to 12) repetitions. After beginning with a weight that allows the patient to perform 6 to 8 repetitions initially, working up to 12 repetitions should be the goal of the strengthening phase. The exercises described below isolate the gluteus medius (posterior fibers), the gluteus maximus, and the internal and external rotators, which often are weak and can contribute to hip pathology.

Static Stretching Exercises

Static stretching should be done to increase the flexibility of the muscles surrounding the hip. A static stretch is performed at the end of the available range of painless motion of the muscle and joint.

Neuromuscular and Proprioceptive Conditioning

Conditioning programs should enhance neuromuscular control, balance, and functional performance. The program should consist of balance exercises, dynamic joint stability exercises, jump and landing training/plyometric exercises, agility drills, and sport-specific exercises. Neuromuscular training improves the ability to generate fast and optimal muscle firing patterns to improve dynamic joint stability and relearn or improve movement patterns necessary for sports and activities of daily living. Proprioception training improves the awareness of the limb/joint position and joint movement. Training includes balance and perturbation exercises. Balance involves the visual, vestibular, and proprioceptive systems. With balance training, the athlete consciously attempts to hold a posture for 30 to 60 seconds. These exercises might include balancing on one leg or balancing on one leg while touching the other foot to different points within reach on the ground. With perturbation training, the athlete stands on an unstable surface such as a balance board while it is being perturbed by an outside force. Jumping exercises, such as jumping forward and backward over a barrier, are a basic form of plyometrics.

These should be attempted only by individuals with full range of motion and adequate strength in the hip, pelvic and abdominal, and back muscles. These types of plyometric and proprioceptive exercises should be supervised by a rehabilitation specialist or other exercise professional.

www.aaos.org/essentials5/exercises

Home Exercise Program for Hip Conditioning

- Before beginning the conditioning program, warm up the muscles and the hip joint by riding a stationary bicycle or jogging for 10 minutes and performing leg swings as follows: While standing, swing one leg forward and backward 10 times and then side-to-side 10 times. Repeat with the opposite leg. Place one hand against a wall for balance if needed.

- When performing the stretching exercises, stretch slowly to the limit of motion, taking care to avoid pain. If you experience pain with the exercises, call your doctor.

- After performing the active warm-up and strengthening exercises, perform static stretching exercises to maintain or increase flexibility.

- The following exercise program is introductory only, and progression of this program will vary based on your specific injury, symptoms, and baseline level of fitness. For further progression of this routine, your physician may recommend evaluation and treatment by a physical therapist or other exercise professional.

Home Exercises for Hip Conditioning

Exercise	Muscle Group	Number of Repetitions/Sets	Number of Days per Week
Strengthening			
Hip extension (prone)	Gluteus maximus	6 to 8 repetitions, progressing to 12 repetitions	3 to 4
Side-lying hip abduction	Gluteus medius	6 to 8 repetitions, progressing to 12 repetitions	3 to 4
Internal hip rotation	Medial hamstrings	6 to 8 repetitions, progressing to 12 repetitions	3 to 4
External hip rotation	Piriformis	6 to 8 repetitions, progressing to 12 repetitions	3 to 4
Stretching			
Seat side straddle	Adductor muscles Medial hamstrings Semitendinosus Semimembranosus	4 repetitions/2 to 3 sets	Daily
Modified seat side straddle	Hamstrings Adductor muscles	4 repetitions/2 to 3 sets	Daily
Hamstring stretch	Hamstrings	4 repetitions/2 to 3 sets	Daily
Sitting rotation stretch	Piriformis External rotators Internal rotators	4 repetitions/2 to 3 sets	Daily
Knee to chest	Posterior hip muscles	4 repetitions/2 to 3 sets	Daily
Leg crossover	Hamstrings	4 repetitions/2 to 3 sets	Daily
Crossover stand	Hamstrings	4 repetitions/2 to 3 sets	Daily
Iliotibial band stretch	Tensor fascia	4 repetitions/2 to 3 sets	Daily
Foam roller for iliotibial band	Iliotibial band	Once per side, for 2 to 3 minutes each	Daily
Quadriceps stretch (prone)	Quadriceps	4 repetitions/2 to 3 sets	Daily

Strengthening Exercises

Hip Extension (Prone)

- Lie face down with a pillow under your hips and one knee bent 90°. Elevate the leg off the floor, lifting the leg straight up with the knee bent.
- Lower the leg to the floor slowly, to a count of 5. Ankle weights should be used, starting with a weight light enough to allow 6 to 8 repetitions and working up to 12 repetitions.
- Repeat on the other side.
- Perform the exercise 3 to 4 days per week.
- After you have worked up to 12 repetitions, add as much weight as can be lifted only 8 times and work up to 12 repetitions again. Continue this cycle of adding weight and increasing repetitions.

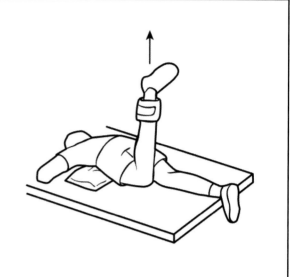

Side-Lying Hip Abduction

- Lie on your side while cradling your head in your arm. Bend the bottom leg for support.
- Slowly move the top leg up and back to 45°, keeping the knee straight. Lower the leg slowly, to a count of 5, and relax it for 2 seconds. Ankle weights should be used, starting with a weight light enough to allow 6 to 8 repetitions and working up to 12 repetitions.
- Repeat on the other side.
- Perform the exercise 3 to 4 days per week.
- After you have worked up to 12 repetitions, add as much weight as can be lifted only 8 times and progress to 12 repetitions again. Continue this cycle of adding weight and increasing repetitions.

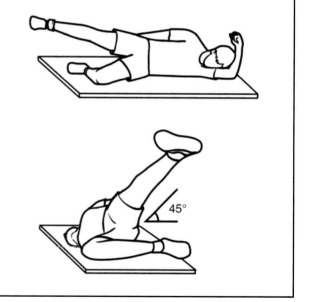

Internal Hip Rotation

- Lie on your side on a table with a pillow between your thighs. Bend the top leg 90° at the hip and 90° at the knee.
- Start with the foot of the top leg below the level of the top of the table; lift to the finish position, which is rotated as high as possible.
- Lower the leg slowly, to a count of 5. Ankle weights should be used, starting with a weight light enough to allow 6 to 8 repetitions, working up to 12 repetitions.
- Repeat on the other side.
- Perform the exercise 3 to 4 days per week.
- After you have worked up to 12 repetitions, add as much weight as can be lifted only 8 times and progress to 12 repetitions again. Continue this cycle of adding weight and increasing repetitions.

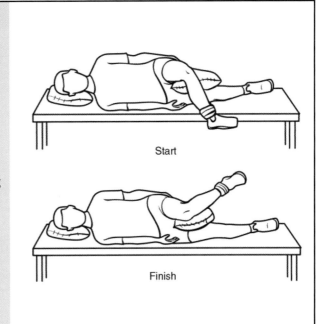

Start

Finish

External Hip Rotation

- Lie on your side on a table with the bottom leg bent 90° at the hip and 90° at the knee.
- Start with the foot below the level of the top of the table; lift to the finish position, which is rotated as high as possible.
- Lower the leg slowly, to a count of 5. Ankle weights should be used, starting with a weight light enough to allow 6 to 8 repetitions and working up to 12 repetitions.
- Repeat on the other side.
- Perform the exercise 3 to 4 days per week.
- After you have worked up to 12 repetitions, add as much weight as can be lifted only 8 times and progress to 12 repetitions again. Continue this cycle of adding weight and increasing repetitions.

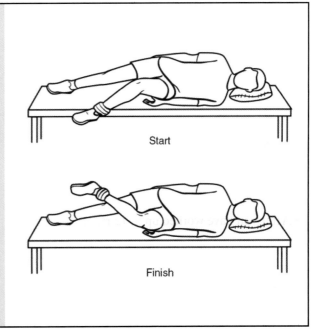

Start

Finish

Stretching Exercises

Seat Side Straddle

- Sit on the floor with your legs spread apart.
- Place both hands on the same knee and slide your hands down the shin toward the ankle until a stretch is felt in the back of the leg. Hold the stretch for 30 seconds and then relax for 30 seconds.
- Attempt to keep your back straight and bend from the hips.
- Repeat on the other side.
- Repeat the sequence 4 times, performing 2 to 3 sets per day.

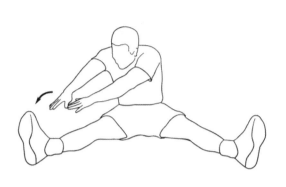

Modified Seat Side Straddle

- Sit on the floor with one leg extended to the side and the other leg bent as shown.
- Place both hands on the knee of your straight leg and slide the hands down the shin toward the ankle until a stretch is felt in the back of the leg. Hold the stretch for 30 seconds and then relax for 30 seconds.
- Attempt to keep your back straight and bend from the hips.
- Reverse leg positions and repeat on the other side.
- Repeat the sequence 4 times, performing 2 to 3 sets per day.

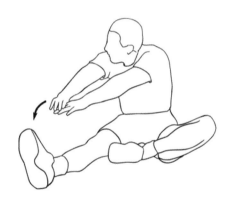

Hamstring Stretch

- Lie on your back with one leg straight and with a strap around your other foot.
- Keeping your knee straight, pull the strap until a gentle stretch is felt in the back of the leg. Hold the stretch for 30 seconds and then return the leg to the resting position on the table or floor and relax for 30 seconds.
- Repeat with the other leg.
- Repeat the sequence 4 times per leg.
- Perform 2 to 3 sets per day.

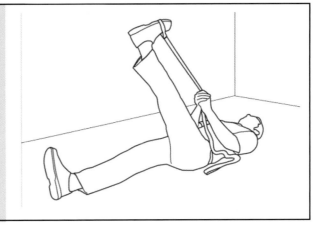

Sitting Rotation Stretch

- Sit on the floor with both legs straight out in front of you.
- Cross one leg over the other, place the elbow of the opposite arm on the outside of the thigh, and support yourself with your other arm behind you.
- Rotate your head and body in the direction of the supporting arm. A gentle stretch will be felt in the outside of the buttock or thigh. Hold the stretch for 30 seconds and then relax for 30 seconds.
- Reverse positions and repeat the stretch on the other side.
- Repeat the sequence 4 times.
- Perform 2 to 3 sets per day.

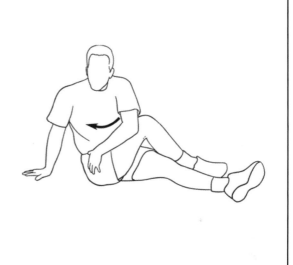

Knee to Chest

- Lie on your back on the floor with your legs straight.
- Grasp one knee and slowly bring it toward your chest as far as it will go. You will feel a stretch in the buttock or back of the leg. Hold the stretch for 30 seconds and then relax for 30 seconds.
- Repeat with the other leg; then do both legs together.
- Repeat the sequence 4 times.
- Perform 2 to 3 sets per day.

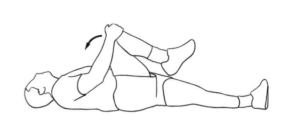

Leg Crossover

- Lie on the floor with your legs spread and your arms at your sides.
- Keeping the leg straight, bring your right toe to your left hand.
- Try to keep the other leg flat on the floor, although you may bend it slightly if needed for comfort. Hold the stretch for 30 seconds and then relax for 30 seconds.
- Repeat with the left leg and the right hand.
- Repeat the sequence 4 times.
- Perform 2 to 3 sets per day.

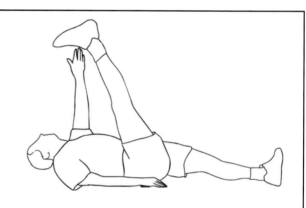

Crossover Stand

- Stand with your legs crossed, with your feet close together and your legs straight.
- Slowly bend forward and try to touch your toes. You will feel the stretch in the back of the leg that is positioned behind. Hold the stretch for 30 seconds and then relax for 30 seconds.
- Repeat with the position of the legs reversed.
- Repeat the sequence 4 times.
- Perform 2 to 3 sets per day.

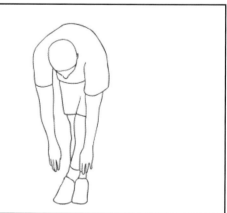

Iliotibial Band Stretch

- Stand next to a wall for support.
- Begin with your weight distributed evenly over both feet, and then cross one leg behind the other.
- Lean the hip of the crossed-over leg toward the wall until you feel a stretch on the outside of the leg. Hold the stretch for 30 seconds and then relax for 30 seconds.
- Repeat on the opposite side.
- Repeat the sequence 4 times.
- Perform 2 to 3 sets per day.

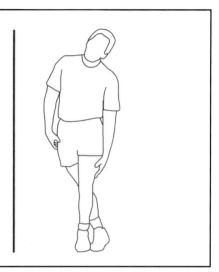

Foam Roller for Iliotibial Band

- Position the foam roller under the outside of your thigh.
- Use your arms to slowly move the lateral or outside portion of your thigh over the foam roller.
- The foam roller should move slowly. Stop and hold the position for 5 to 10 seconds at areas of tightness or discomfort, then proceed up and down the outer thigh.
- Avoid rolling over the bony prominence of the outer hip (arrow) or the knee (double arrow).
- Mild to severe discomfort may be present but should improve with consistent daily use of the foam roller. If the discomfort does not improve within 1 to 2 weeks, seek the advice of your sports medicine physician.
- Perform every day, for 2 to 3 minutes on each leg.

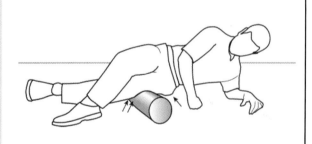

Quadriceps Stretch (Prone)

- Lie on your stomach with your arms at your sides and your legs straight.
- Bend one knee to bring your foot up toward your buttocks and grasp the ankle with the hand on the same side.
- Pull on the ankle. The stretch will be felt on the front of the thigh. Hold the stretch for 30 seconds and then relax for 30 seconds.
- Repeat on the opposite side.
- Repeat the sequence 4 times.
- Perform 2 to 3 sets per day.

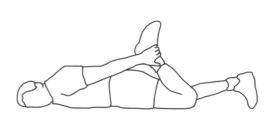

Conditioning of the Knee

The knee has both dynamic and static stabilizers. Muscles provide dynamic stability to the knee joint and the patellofemoral articulation. Strengthening the quadriceps and hamstrings muscle groups provides dynamic stability to the knee. In addition, the hip muscles such as the gluteus maximus, the gluteus medius, and the internal and external rotators help to control the movements of the femur and the position of the patellofemoral articulation. Conditioning of the knee should focus on three phases: strengthening, stretching, and neuromuscular (proprioceptive) training. Plyometric exercises (power training) would be added for the competitive athlete after basic strength and flexibility have been achieved. Advanced proprioception exercises and plyometric exercises should be performed under the supervision of a rehabilitation specialist or other exercise professional.

Strengthening Exercises

Exercises to strengthen the quadriceps and hamstrings can be performed conveniently with progressively heavier ankle weights. The resistance training must be progressive so that the muscle is constantly stimulated to grow. Forward lunges (for the quadriceps), hamstring curls, side-lying hip abductions, and hip extensions are good strengthening exercises. The patient should begin with a weight that allows 6 to 8 repetitions and should work up to 12 repetitions. After reaching 12 repetitions with a given weight, the patient should add weight and drop back to 6 to 8 repetitions.

Stretching Exercises

The effectiveness of strengthening exercises for the quadriceps muscle group can be compromised if the range of motion of the knee is limited. Stretching the soft tissues, especially after trauma or periods of immobilization, can be very effective in increasing range of motion. Hamstring stretching exercises such as leg crossovers and crossover standing increase the range of motion at the knee and hip during functional activities such as walking and running.

After the patient has achieved normal range of motion and strength, sport-specific or work-specific training should begin. The knee musculature needs to be strong and powerful, and protective reflexes need to be optimized to reduce the risk of injury during athletic maneuvers such as sudden changes in direction while running.

Proprioceptive Training

Proprioceptive training is important for balance. Balance, or postural control, is the result of the integration of visual, vestibular, and proprioceptive afferent inputs. The goal of proprioceptive training is to enhance the activity of the proprioceptors, thereby improving their ability to protect the ligaments of the knee. Several commercial devices, such as tiltboards and proprioceptive disks, are available for proprioceptive training. Advanced balance training should be performed under the supervision of a physical therapist, athletic trainer, or other exercise specialist.

SECTION 1 GENERAL ORTHOPAEDICS

Plyometric Exercises

Explosive power of the lower leg is necessary for a high level of athletic performance. Plyometrics and explosive weight training facilitate the development of power in the quadriceps, hamstrings, and gluteal muscles. Examples of plyometric exercises are jumping rope and jumping from side to side over a 6-inch–high barrier. More advanced exercises should be performed under the supervision of a physical therapist, athletic trainer, or other trained professional.

www.aaos.org/essentials5/exercises

Home Exercise Program for Knee Conditioning

- Before beginning the conditioning program, warm up the muscles by riding a stationary bicycle or jogging for 10 minutes.
- After the active warm-up and the strengthening exercises, stretching exercises should be performed to maintain or increase flexibility. When performing the stretching exercises, you should stretch slowly to the limit of motion, taking care to avoid pain.
- If you experience pain with exercising, call your doctor.
- The following exercise program is introductory only, and progression of this program will vary based on your specific injury, symptoms, and baseline level of fitness. For further progression of this routine, your physician may recommend evaluation and treatment by a physical therapist or other exercise professional.

Strengthening and Stretching Exercises for the Knee

Exercise	Muscle Group	Number of Repetitions/Sets	Number of Days per Week	Number of Weeks
Strengthening				
Forward lunge	Quadriceps	Work up to 3 sets of 10 repetitions	3	6 to 8
Hamstring curl	Hamstrings	10 repetitions/3 sets	3	6 to 8
Side-lying hip abduction	Gluteus medius	6 to 8 repetitions, progressing to 12 repetitions	3	6 to 8
Hip extension (prone)	Gluteus maximus	6 to 8 repetitions, progressing to 12 repetitions	3	6 to 8
Straight leg raise	Quadriceps	6 to 8 repetitions, working up to 12 repetitions	3	6 to 8
Straight leg raise (prone)	Gluteus maximus	6 to 8 repetitions, working up to 12 repetitions	3	6 to 8
Wall slide	Quadriceps Hamstrings	Work up to 3 sets of 10 repetitions	3	6 to 8
Stretching				
Hamstring stretch	Hamstrings	3 to 6 repetitions/3 sets	Daily	6 to 8
Leg crossover	Hamstrings	3 to 6 repetitions/3 sets	Daily	6 to 8
Standing crossover	Hamstrings	3 to 6 repetitions/3 sets	Daily	6 to 8

Strengthening Exercises

Forward Lunge

- Stand up with the feet approximately 3 to 4 feet apart and with the forward foot pointing forward and the back foot angled to provide support.
- Lunge forward, bending the forward knee and keeping the back and the back leg straight. You should feel a slight stretch in the left groin area. Do not let the forward-lunging knee pass beyond the toes.
- Hold the stretch for 5 seconds.
- Repeat with the opposite leg.
- Work up to 3 sets of 10 repetitions, 3 days per week. Continue for 6 to 8 weeks.

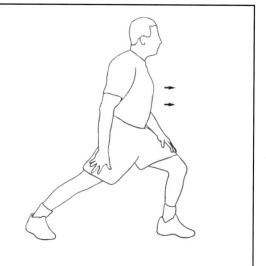

Hamstring Curl

- Stand on a flat surface with your weight evenly distributed over both feet. Hold on to the back of a chair or the wall for balance.
- Raise the heel of one leg toward the ceiling. Hold this position for 5 seconds and then relax.
- Perform 3 sets of 10 repetitions, 3 days per week. Continue for 6 to 8 weeks.

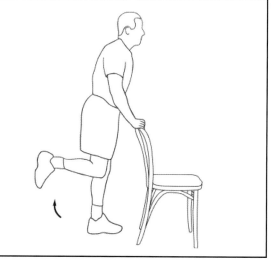

Side-Lying Hip Abduction

- Lie on your side, cradling your head in your arm. Bend the bottom leg for support.
- Slowly move the top leg up and back to 45°, keeping the knee straight. Hold this position for 5 seconds.
- Slowly lower the leg and relax it for 2 seconds.
- Ankle weights should be used, starting with a weight light enough to allow 6 to 8 repetitions, progressing to 12 repetitions. Then add weight and return to 6 to 8 repetitions.
- Repeat on the opposite leg.
- Perform the exercise 3 days per week. Continue for 6 to 8 weeks.

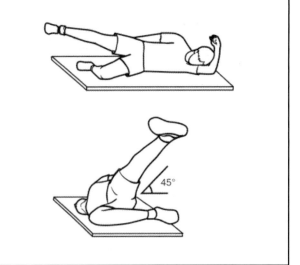

Hip Extension (Prone)

- Lie face down with a pillow under your hips and one knee bent 90°.
- Elevate the leg off the floor approximately 4 inches for a count of 5, lifting the leg straight up with the knee bent.
- Ankle weights should be used, starting with a weight light enough to allow 6 to 8 repetitions, working up to 12 repetitions. Then add weight and return to 6 to 8 repetitions.
- Repeat on the opposite leg.
- Perform the exercise 3 days per week. Continue for 6 to 8 weeks.

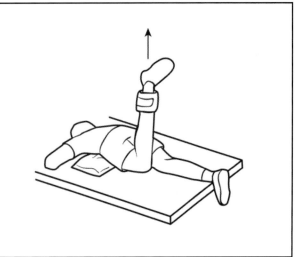

Straight Leg Raise

- Lie on the floor supporting your torso with your elbows as shown, with one leg straight and the other leg bent.
- Tighten the thigh muscle of the straight leg and slowly raise it 6 to 10 inches off the floor. Hold this position for 5 seconds. Repeat with the opposite leg.
- Ankle weights may be used, starting with a weight light enough to allow 6 to 8 repetitions, working up to 12 repetitions. Then add weight and return to 6 to 8 repetitions.
- Perform the exercise 3 days per week, for 6 to 8 weeks.

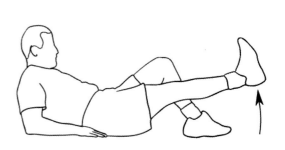

Straight Leg Raise (Prone)

- Lie on the floor on your stomach with your legs straight.
- Keeping the leg straight, tighten the hamstrings of one leg and raise the leg approximately 6 inches. Keep your stomach muscles tight and avoid arching the back.
- Repeat with the opposite leg.
- Ankle weights may be used, starting with a weight light enough to allow 6 to 8 repetitions, working up to 12 repetitions. Then add weight and return to 6 to 8 repetitions.
- Perform the exercise 3 days per week. Continue for 6 to 8 weeks.

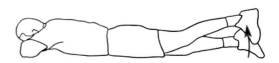

Wall Slide

- Stand with your back against a wall and your feet approximately 1 foot from the wall.
- Tighten your stomach muscles so that your lower back is flat against the wall.
- Stop when your knees are bent 90°. The knees should not pass beyond the toes.
- Hold for 5 seconds and then return to the starting position. Work up to 3 sets of 10 repetitions.
- Perform the exercise 3 days per week, for 6 to 8 weeks.

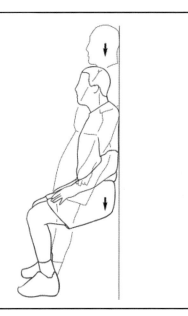

Stretching Exercises

Hamstring Stretch

- Sit on the floor with your legs straight in front of you, and place your hands on the backs of your calves. For comfort, you may slightly bend the leg not being stretched.
- Slowly lift and pull one leg toward your ear, keeping your back straight. Hold the stretch for 5 seconds.
- Alternate from side to side.
- Repeat the exercise with each leg 3 to 6 times. Perform 3 sets per day for 6 to 8 weeks.

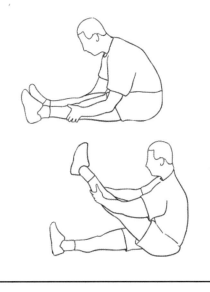

Leg Crossover

- Lie on the floor with your legs spread and your arms out to the sides.
- Bring your right toe to your left hand, keeping the leg straight.
- Hold the stretch for 5 seconds.
- Alternate from side to side.
- Repeat the exercise with each leg 3 to 6 times. For comfort, you may slightly bend the leg not being stretched. Perform 3 sets per day for 6 to 8 weeks.

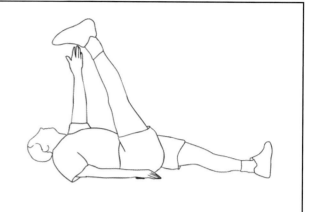

Standing Crossover

- Stand with your legs crossed.
- Keeping your feet close together and your legs straight, slowly bend forward toward your toes.
- Hold the stretch for 5 seconds.
- Repeat with the opposite leg crossed in front for 3 to 6 repetitions. Perform 3 sets per day for 6 to 8 weeks.

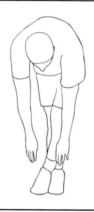

Conditioning of the Foot and Ankle

The foot is the first part of the lower kinetic chain to hit the ground during weight-bearing activities and is therefore the first input to the neuromuscular system of the lower kinetic chain. Dynamic joint stability is critical for injury prevention and improved performance during typical daily activities and sports activities. Whether an individual experiences a single-episode lateral ankle sprain or whether chronic ankle instability develops most likely depends on rehabilitation of the individual's proprioception.

Strengthening Exercises
Strengthening exercises for the foot and ankle include calf raises, ankle dorsiflexion/plantar flexion, and ankle inversion/eversion exercises.

Stretching Exercises
Perform stretching to maintain or increase flexibility. Heel cord stretches performed with the knee both straight and bent are good stretching exercises for the gastrocnemius-soleus muscle complex.

Toe Strengthening Exercises
The toe strengthening program can be helpful for patients with the particular conditions listed, including bunions, hammer toes, plantar fasciitis, and toe cramps.

Proprioceptive Exercises
Optimizing the proprioceptive system is important in preventing injuries such as ankle sprains in both athletes and nonathletes. Balance, or postural control, is the result of the integration of visual, vestibular, and proprioceptive afferent inputs. The goal of proprioceptive training is to enhance the activity of the proprioceptors, thereby improving their ability to protect the ligaments of the foot and ankle. Several commercial devices, such as tiltboards and proprioceptive disks, are available for proprioceptive training. Perturbation training is another way to optimize the proprioceptive system, especially in athletes. Perturbation exercises are performed on an unstable surface with perturbing forces applied in all directions. Perturbation training and advanced balance training should be performed under the supervision of a rehabilitation specialist or other exercise professional.

Plyometrics
Explosive power is necessary for a high level of athletic performance. Plyometrics facilitate the development of power. Examples of plyometric exercises are jumping rope and jumping from side to side over a 6-inch–high barrier. More advanced exercises should be performed under the supervision of a rehabilitation specialist or other trained exercise professional.

SECTION 1 GENERAL ORTHOPAEDICS

www.aaos.org/essentials5/exercises

Home Exercise Program for Foot and Ankle Conditioning

- Performing active warm-up exercises before athletic activities is important for optimal neuromuscular control and for maintaining normal range of motion.
- Before beginning the conditioning program, warm up the muscles of the lower extremities by riding a stationary bicycle or jogging for 10 minutes and performing leg swings as follows: While standing, swing one leg forward/backward 10 times and then side-to-side 10 times. Repeat with the opposite leg. Place one hand against a wall for balance if needed.
- Perform the exercises indefinitely or as directed by your physician. Contact your physician if the exercises cause pain.
- The following exercise program is introductory only, and progression of this program will vary based on your specific injury, symptoms, and baseline level of fitness. For further progression of this routine, your physician may recommend evaluation and treatment by a physical therapist or other exercise professional.

Strengthening and Stretching Exercises for the Foot and Ankle

Exercise	Muscle Group	Number of Repetitions/Sets	Number of Days per Week
Strengthening			
Calf raise	Gastrocnemius-soleus complex	10 repetitions/3 sets	3 to 4
Ankle dorsiflexion/plantar flexion	Anterior tibialis Gastrocnemius-soleus complex	10 repetitions/3 sets	3 to 4
Ankle eversion/inversion	Posterior tibialis Peroneus longus and peroneus brevis	10 repetitions/3 sets	3 to 4
Stretching			
Heel cord stretch	Knee straight: Gastrocnemius Knee bent: Soleus	4 to 5 repetitions/2 to 3 sets	Daily

SECTION 1   GENERAL ORTHOPAEDICS

Toe Strengthening Exercises

Exercise	Condition Recommended For	Repetitions or Duration	Number of Days per Week
Toe squeeze	Hammer toe, toe cramp	10 repetitions	Daily
Big toe pull	Bunion, toe cramp	10 repetitions	Daily
Toe pull	Bunion, hammer toe, toe cramp	10 repetitions	Daily
Golf ball roll	Plantar fasciitis, arch strain, foot cramp	2 minutes	Daily
Marble pickup	Pain in ball of foot, hammer toe, toe cramp	Until all marbles have been picked up	Daily
Towel curl	Hammer toe, toe cramp, pain in ball of foot	15 to 20 repetitions	Daily

Strengthening Exercises

Calf Raise

- Stand with your weight evenly distributed over both feet. Hold on to the back of a chair or the wall for balance.
- Lift one foot so that all your weight is on the other foot.
- Then lift the heel off the floor as high as you can.
- Work up to 3 sets of 10 repetitions.
- Repeat on the other side, switching sides between sets.
- Perform the exercise 3 to 4 days per week.
- If you are unable to perform 10 repetitions on one leg, keep both feet on the ground and lift both heels simultaneously and increase the number of sets before attempting to perform with one leg as described above.

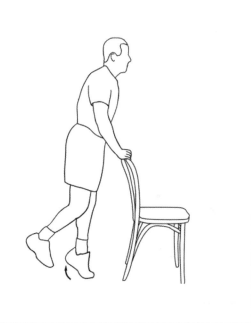

Ankle Dorsiflexion/Plantar Flexion

- Find a position in which your weight is off your feet, such as lying on a bed or on the floor with your legs straight out in front of you.
- For dorsiflexion, wrap an elastic band or tubing around your foot and anchor the other end to a door or bedpost or have someone hold it. Pull your toes toward you, then return slowly to the starting position. Repeat 10 to 15 times.
- For plantar flexion, wrap an elastic band or tubing around your foot and hold the other end in your hand. Gently point your toes, then return slowly to the starting position. Repeat 10 to 15 times.
- Perform 3 sets of 10 repetitions, 3 to 4 days per week.

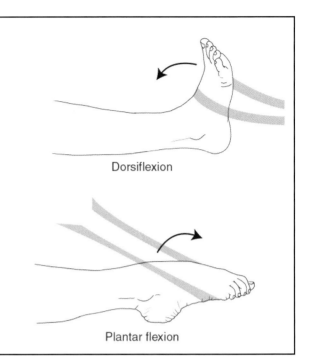

Dorsiflexion

Plantar flexion

Ankle Eversion/Inversion

- Find a position in which your weight is off your feet, such as lying on a bed or on the floor with your legs straight out in front of you.
- For inversion, wrap an elastic band or tube around the inside of your foot and anchor the other end to a door or bedpost or have someone hold it. Pull your foot inward against the resistance, then return slowly to the starting position. Repeat 10 to 15 times.
- For eversion, wrap an elastic band or tube around the outside of your foot and anchor the other end to a door or bedpost or have someone hold it. Pull your foot outward against the resistance, then return slowly to the starting position. Repeat 10 to 15 times.
- Perform 3 sets of 10 repetitions, 3 to 4 days per week.

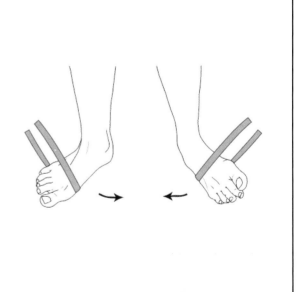

Stretching Exercise

Heel Cord Stretch

- Stand facing a wall with one foot in front and the toes of both feet pointing forward.

  Stretch with knee straight: Keep your back leg straight and your heel flat on the ground. Move your hips toward the wall until you feel a stretch in the back of the calf of your left leg.

  Stretch with knee bent: Start in the same position, but allow the back knee to bend. Move your hips toward the wall until you feel a stretch in the back of the calf of your left leg.

- Hold the stretch for 30 seconds, then relax for 30 seconds.

- Repeat 4 to 5 times.

- Perform 2 to 3 times per day.

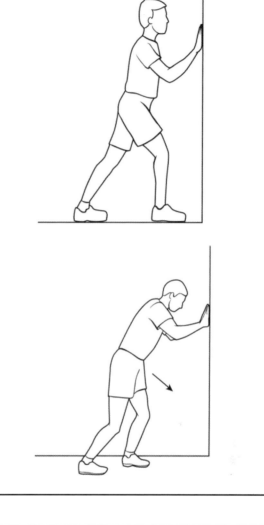

Toe Strengthening Exercises

Toe Squeeze

- Place small sponges or corks between the toes.
- Squeeze and hold for 5 seconds.
- Repeat 10 times.

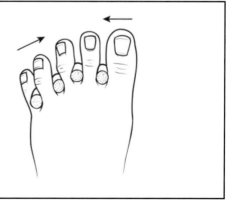

Big Toe Pull

- Place a thick rubber band around both big toes and pull the big toes away from each other and toward the small toes.
- Hold for 5 seconds.
- Repeat 10 times.

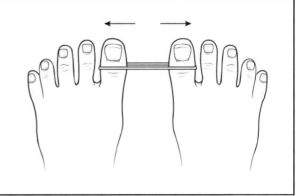

Toe Pull

- Put a thick rubber band around all your toes and spread them.
- Hold this position for 5 seconds.
- Repeat 10 times.

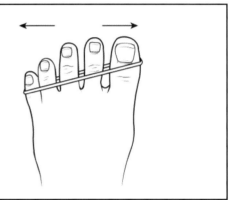

Golf Ball Roll

- Roll a golf ball under the ball of your foot for 2 minutes to massage the bottom of the foot.

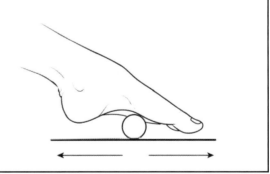

Marble Pickup

- Place 20 marbles on the floor. Using your toes, pick up one marble at a time and put each in a small bowl.
- Repeat until you have picked up all 20 marbles.

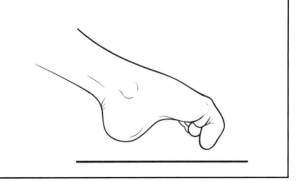

Towel Curl

- Place a small towel on the floor and curl it toward you, using only your toes. You can increase the resistance by putting weight on the end of the towel.
- Relax and repeat 15 to 20 times.

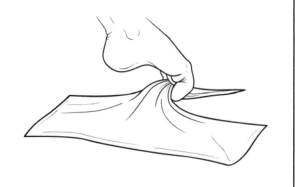

GENERAL ORTHOPAEDICS

SECTION 1

Conditioning of the Lumbar Spine

Conditioning of the lumbar spine to prevent low back pain should include strengthening and stretching exercises to improve range of motion. The focus of conditioning should be on a daily home exercise program. In general, emphasis should be placed on aerobic exercise and active treatment rather than passive treatment.

Strengthening Exercises

The four muscle groups that protect the spine from daily overuse and trauma include the abdominals, the quadratus lumborum (two groups, one on each side of the spine), and the back extensors. The back extensors are important because poor endurance of these muscle groups has been found in patients with low back pain. Isometric exercises for these muscle groups, such as the bird dog exercise, have an important stabilizing effect on the spine.

The quadratus lumborum is an important lateral stabilizer of the trunk. A strengthening exercise for this muscle is the side bridge, which should be repeated on both sides for maximum and symmetric lateral stability. The abdominals are important to stabilization of the lumbar and thoracic spine. The four major muscle groups that make up the abdominals are the transverse abdominis, the internal and external obliques, and the rectus abdominis. The transverse abdominis muscle is a stabilizer of the lumbar spine through its attachment to the thoracolumbar fascia. Traditional sit-ups have been found to greatly increase the load on the lumbar disks and therefore should be avoided by patients with low back pain. A safe exercise is abdominal bracing, which activates all the abdominal muscles, including the transverse abdominis, and does not stress the lumbar spine. This exercise does not activate the transverse abdominis if a pelvic tilt is performed.

Stretching Exercises

Stretching exercises for the trunk and pelvis are helpful for improving range of motion. The cat back stretch and the kneeling back extension exercises are excellent stretching exercises for the spine in general. Flexibility of the hamstring muscles is essential for improving the mobility of the lumbar spine and reducing stress on the lumbar spine. The seat side straddle, modified seat side straddle, sitting rotation stretch, and leg crossover are all excellent stretching exercises for the lumbothoracic spine.

www.aaos.org/essentials5/exercises

Home Exercise Program for Lumbar Spine Conditioning

- Perform the exercises in the order listed.
- If any of the exercises cause pain or increase your pain, discontinue the exercise and call your doctor.
- This exercise program may not be appropriate if back pain is severe or if substantial loss of range of motion of the spine is present.
- The following exercise program is introductory only, and progression of this program will vary based on your specific injury, symptoms, and baseline level of fitness. For further progression of this routine, your physician may recommend evaluation and treatment by a physical therapist or other exercise professional.

Strengthening and Stretching Exercises for the Lumbar Spine

Exercise Type	Muscle Group/Area Targeted	Number of Repetitions	Number of Days per Week	Number of Weeks[a]
Strengthening Exercises				
Abdominal bracing	Abdominals	5	Daily	3 to 4
Side bridges	Quadratus lumborum	5	Daily	3 to 4
Bird dog	Back extensors	5	Daily	3 to 4
Stretching Exercises				
Cat back stretch	Middle and low back	5	Daily	3 to 4
Low back extension and flexion stretch	Low back	5	Daily	3 to 4
Seat side straddle	Adductor muscles Medial hamstrings Semitendinosus Semimembranosus	5	Daily	3 to 4
Modified seat side straddle	Adductor muscles Hamstrings	5	Daily	3 to 4
Sitting rotation stretch	Piriformis External rotators Internal rotators	5	Daily	3 to 4
Leg crossover	Hamstrings	5	Daily	3 to 4

[a]These exercises can be performed indefinitely for the prevention of low back pain.

GENERAL ORTHOPAEDICS

SECTION 1

Strengthening Exercises

Abdominal Bracing
- Lie on your back on the floor with your arms at your sides, your knees bent, and your feet flat on the floor.
- Contract your abdominal muscles so that your stomach is pulled away from your waistband.
- Hold this position for 15 seconds while breathing normally. Do not hold your breath.
- Perform 5 repetitions once per day, continuing for 3 to 4 weeks.

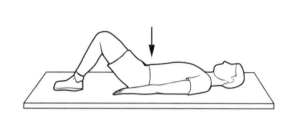

Side Bridges
- Lie on your side on the floor (for beginners, the knees may be bent 90°).
- With your elbow bent at 90°, lift your body off the floor as shown, keeping your body straight.
- Hold this position for 15 seconds and then repeat on the other side. The goal is to hold this position for 150 seconds total on each side.
- Perform 5 repetitions once per day, continuing for 3 to 4 weeks.

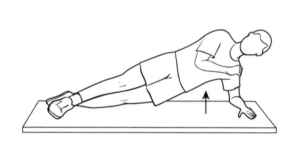

Bird Dog
- Kneel on the floor on your hands and knees.
- Lift your right arm straight out from the shoulder, level with your body, at the same time you lift your left leg straight out from the hip.
- Start by holding this position for 15 seconds. Gradually increase the hold time as tolerated, while maintaining proper body position. The goal is to hold this position for 150 seconds (30 years or older) or 170 seconds (younger than 30 years) total.
- Repeat with the opposite arm and leg.
- Perform 5 repetitions per day, continuing for 3 to 4 weeks.

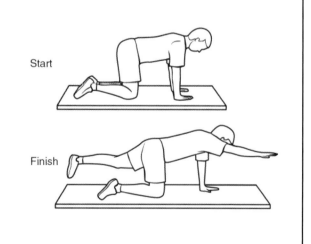

Start

Finish

Stretching Exercises

Cat Back Stretch

- Kneel on your hands and knees in a relaxed position.
- Raise your back up like a cat and hold for 30 seconds.
- Relax for 30 seconds.
- Repeat 5 times per day, continuing for 3 to 4 weeks.

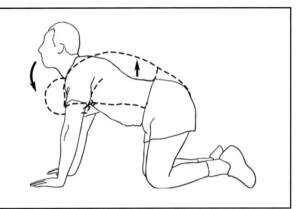

Low Back Extension and Flexion Stretch

- Lie on a firm surface, face down, and press up with your arms (position 1). Hold for 5 seconds.
- Extend your arms, rock back and sit on your bent knees, and tuck your head (position 2) until you feel a stretch in your back. Hold for 5 seconds.
- Repeat 5 times per day, continuing for 3 to 4 weeks.

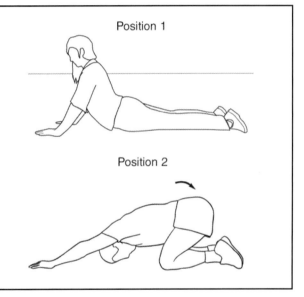

Position 1

Position 2

Seat Side Straddle

- Sit on the floor with your legs spread apart.
- Place both hands on the same ankle and bring your chin as close to your knee as possible.
- Hold the maximum stretch for 30 seconds and then relax for 30 seconds.
- Repeat on the other side.
- Repeat the sequence 5 times per day, continuing for 3 to 4 weeks.

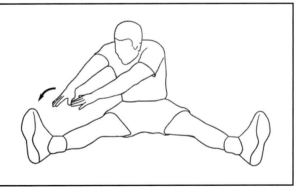

SECTION 1 **GENERAL ORTHOPAEDICS**

Modified Seat Side Straddle

- The modified seat straddle can be used if the aforementioned seat side straddle position is not tolerated. Sit on the floor with one leg extended to the side and the other leg bent as shown.
- Place both hands on the ankle of the extended leg and bring your chin as close to your knee as possible.
- Hold the maximum stretch for 30 seconds and then relax for 30 seconds.
- Reverse leg positions and repeat on the other side.
- Repeat the sequence 5 times per day, continuing for 3 to 4 weeks.

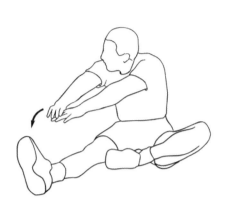

Sitting Rotation Stretch

- Sit on the floor with both legs straight out in front of you.
- Cross one leg over the other, place the elbow of the opposite arm on the outside of the thigh, and support yourself with your other arm behind you.
- Rotate your head and body in the direction of the supporting arm.
- Hold the maximum stretch for 30 seconds and then relax for 30 seconds.
- Reverse positions and repeat the stretch on the other side.
- Repeat the sequence 5 times per day, continuing for 3 to 4 weeks.

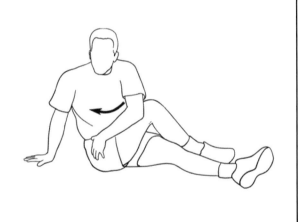

Leg Crossover

- Lie on the floor with your legs spread apart and your arms at your sides.
- Keeping the leg straight, bring your right toe to your left hand.
- Try to keep the other leg flat on the floor, but you may bend it slightly if needed for comfort.
- Hold the maximum stretch for 30 seconds and then relax for 30 seconds.
- Repeat with the left leg and the right hand.
- Repeat the sequence 5 times per day, continuing for 3 to 4 weeks.

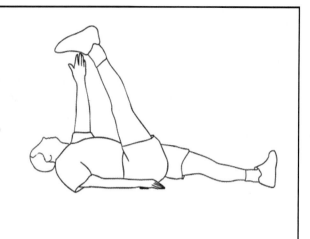

Rehabilitation: Canes, Crutches, and Walkers

Canes, crutches, and walkers (assistive devices) progressively reduce weight-bearing stresses on the lower extremities and also augment balance and stability during walking. As such, these devices are helpful in the management of arthritic conditions and lower extremity injuries.

Canes

Canes are lightweight and easily stored. For long-term use, a spade handle is easier on the hand than the standard crook handle (**Figure 1** and **Table 1**). A "quad," or four-footed cane, has four prongs at its base; it is more cumbersome than a single-tipped cane but provides a wider base of support and can be quite useful to patients after a stroke when they have only one functional upper extremity. Several new cane designs feature small, spring-loaded, pivoting platforms as the base that allows the cane to remain upright on its own. These canes may also afford slightly improved stability and slip prevention.

A cane should be used on the contralateral side from the injury to maximize stress reduction.

A cane that is too long creates excessive flexion of the elbow and increases the demand on the triceps muscle, a major stabilizer of the upper extremity when using a cane. A cane that is too short provides inadequate support and compromises walking. The optimal length of a cane will position the elbow in 20° to 30° of flexion when the tip of the cane is placed approximately 6″ in front of and 6″ lateral to the little toe.

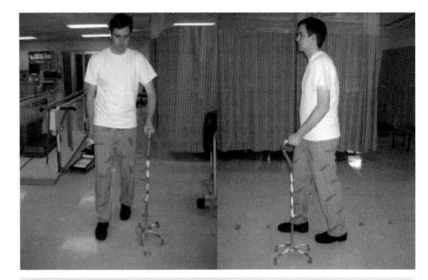

Figure 1 Photograph shows appropriate cane walking in a patient with an injured right leg.

Table 1

Patient Guide to Using a Cane

General Guidelines

Prepare the residence by removing small rugs, footstools, electrical cords, or other ground level objects that may cause falls.

Organize everyday necessities on the main level of the residence to prevent unnecessary stair climbing.

Equip the bathroom with a shower tub seat, raised toilet seat, grab bars, and nonslip bath mats.

Positioning

Height should reach the wrist crease when standing, elbow slightly bent, held in the hand opposite of the injured leg.

Walking

The cane and the injured leg strike the ground simultaneously; initiate the step with the injured leg and finish with the healthy leg.

Stairs

Grasp the handrail with the free hand, if possible.

Up: step up on the healthy leg followed by the injured leg.

Down: place the cane on the step first, followed by the injured leg and then the good leg and body weight.

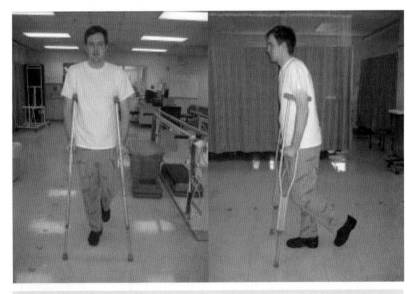

Figure 2   Photograph shows appropriate crutch walking in a patient with an injured left leg.

Crutches

Crutches offer more support than a cane (**Figure 2** and **Table 2**), but less than a walker. Crutches come in several designs:

• Wooden axillary—satisfactory for short-term use, economic

• Aluminum axillary—durable for long-term use in chronic conditions, easily adjustable (**Figure 3**)

Table 2

Patient Guide to Using Crutches

General Guidelines

Prepare the residence by removing small rugs, footstools, electrical cords, or other ground level objects that may cause falls.

Organize everyday necessities on the main level of the residence to prevent unnecessary stair climbing.

Equip the bathroom with a shower tub seat, raised toilet seat, grab bars, and nonslip bath mats.

Positioning

The crutch tip should be 4″ to 6″ in front of the little toe.

The top of the crutches should be 2″ below the armpits when standing.

Handgrips should be even with the hips.

The elbows should be slightly bent at 25°.

Weight should be absorbed with the hands so the crutch does not touch the armpit.

Do not wrap towels around the armpit pad.

Walking

Advance both crutches 1 foot.

Shift the body weight to the crutches.

Take a forward step with the healthy leg.

Stairs

Grasp the handrail in one hand and the crutch in the other hand, or use both crutches.

Up: supporting the body weight with the crutch, step up on the healthy leg while the injured leg is raised behind you, then advance crutches.

Down: advance the crutches first to the lower step followed by a body weight shift and step with the healthy leg.

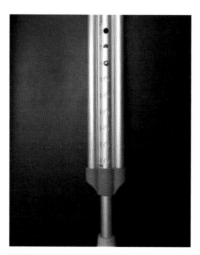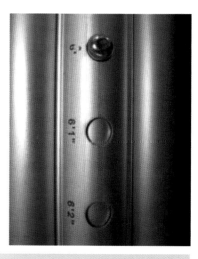

Figure 3 Photograph of adjustable aluminum crutches shows the push-button stops used to adjust for height range of generally 6 to 8 inches (eg, 5′2″ to 5′10″).

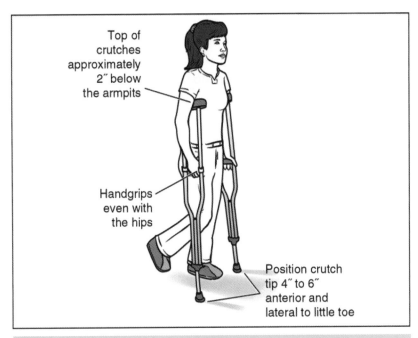

Top of crutches approximately 2″ below the armpits

Handgrips even with the hips

Position crutch tip 4″ to 6″ anterior and lateral to little toe

Figure 4   Illustration depicts properly fitted crutches. The tops of the crutches are approximately 2″ below the patient's armpits when the patient stands erect, and the handgrips are even with the patient's hips and allow 25° to 30° of flexion at the elbow.

- Hyperbaric stainless steel crutches—used by patients heavier than 280 lb
- Forearm—extend only to forearm, less bulky design for patients with chronic conditions, require better balance and upper body strength
- Platform—transmit forces through forearm, useful in patients with arthritic or traumatic conditions of hand or wrist

Patients should be properly fitted for and instructed in the use of crutches (**Figure 4**). Crutches that are too long or are used improperly can cause axillary artery or venous thrombosis or a brachial plexus compression neuropathy (primarily the radial nerve). The handgrip should be positioned to provide optimal function of the triceps and latissimus dorsi muscles. Depending on the height of the patient, position the crutch tip 4″ to 6″ anterior and lateral to the little toe. In that position, adjust the length of the crutch to allow approximately 2″ of clearance between the anterior axillary fold and the top of the crutch. Adjust the handgrip to position the elbow in 25° to 30° of flexion. As a general guideline, the length of the crutch should be 77% of the patient's height. Caution the patient against wrapping towels around the axillary pad.

Gait techniques for crutches are described in **Table 3**. Following injury to the lower extremity, the technique most commonly prescribed is a non–weight-bearing, swing-through gait. Walking on level ground using this method is easy to teach because it involves simply advancing both crutches, followed by a forward step with the uninjured leg. Ascending or descending steps is more difficult, but

Table 3

Gait Patterns Used With Crutches

Gait Pattern	Instructions
Swing-to	Advance both crutches. Lift the body to advance both feet on line with the crutches.
Swing-through	Advance both crutches. Lift the body to advance both feet beyond the crutches.
Non–weight-bearing, swing-through	Advance both crutches.
Four-point	Move one crutch forward, then advance the opposite foot, followed by the ipsilateral crutch, then the contralateral foot (three points of contact are always maintained).
Alternating two-point	Advance one crutch and the contralateral foot at the same time. Shift weight and advance the other foot and crutch (a progression of the four-point gait).

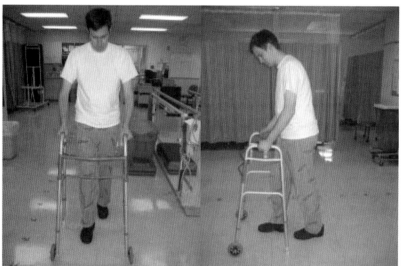

Figure 5 Photograph shows appropriate walker use in a patient with an injured right leg.

the key is to advance the crutches first when going down stairs and to advance the sound leg first when going up. A training session with a rehabilitation specialist often is helpful. Toe-touch weight bearing with crutches, if the injury permits, may be easier for the patient and demands less upper body strength than non–weight-bearing crutch walking.

Walkers

Walkers have four points of contact and provide greater support and balance than either a cane or crutch (**Figure 5** and **Table 4**). The bulkiness of a walker is its major disadvantage. Some walkers fold, making storage in cars easier, but these models are more fragile. Rolling walkers require less energy to use but are less stable. If

Table 4

Patient Guide to Using a Walker

General Guidelines

Prepare the residence by removing small rugs, footstools, electrical cords, or other ground level objects that may cause falls.

Organize everyday necessities on the main level of the residence to prevent unnecessary stair climbing.

Equip the bathroom with a shower tub seat, raised toilet seat, grab bars, and nonslip bath mats.

Positioning

Height should reach the wrist crease when standing.

Elbows should be slightly bent at 30°.

Grip with both hands to support some of your weight.

Walking

Place walker one step ahead of you.

Initiate a step with the injured leg and walk into the walker.

Do not step all the way to the front bar.

Take small steps when turning.

Stairs

Never use a walker to climb stairs.

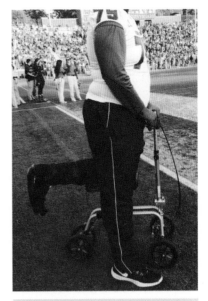

Figure 6 Photograph shows use of a rolling knee walker.

balance is adequate, a rolling walker may be advantageous for a patient with significant cardiopulmonary restrictions. Some rolling walkers incorporate a seat that can be used for the patient to easily rest between walking segments. The same principles used for fitting crutches apply for adjusting the height of a walker (that is, the handgrip should be positioned to allow 30° flexion at the elbow when the patient is in a neutral standing position). A rolling knee walker, or scooter, provides assisted mobility for patients with foot or ankle injuries (**Figure 6**). It allows the patient to rest the injured leg on a padded platform and use the uninjured leg to power the walker. Some patients may find this device easier to use than more traditional assistive devices.

GENERAL ORTHOPAEDICS

SECTION 1

Sports Medicine Evaluation and Management Principles

Definition

Sports medicine is a comprehensive term describing a branch of medicine involved in prevention, diagnosis, management, and rehabilitation of sport- and exercise-related injuries and disorders. Sports medicine is a multidisciplinary field encompassing disciplines such as rehabilitation, athletic training, nutrition, exercise physiology, and psychology. In addition, primary care, internal medicine, and medical and surgical specialties have roles in the management of sports-related problems.

Being a team physician is a complex task. The role of the team physician includes performing a preparticipation evaluation. Determining readiness for participation and implementing injury prevention programs is vital to decreasing game time injuries. Team physicians should also provide medical coverage for high-risk practices and competitions, visit the training room regularly to evaluate and monitor problems, and arrange appropriate referrals. Open lines of communication among parents, coaches, and administrators are a necessity, and injuries should be properly documented. Physicians providing care to athletes must always place the medical well-being of the athlete above the needs of the team.

General Issues of Importance in Sports Medicine

It is important for physicians responsible for covering sports practices and games to formulate administrative medical supervision plans and implement an emergency response plan that must be made available to the entire athletic and sports medicine staff. An individual who is qualified to administer cardiopulmonary resuscitation and first aid should be available at all practices and games. The emergency plan should address and designate who calls 911 in an emergency, who attends to the athlete, where the emergency response equipment is kept, and what equipment is available.

The team physician should appreciate the importance of sports and fitness participation to athlete-patients and communicate their commitment to helping them return to participation as effectively and safely as possible. Competitive athletes and serious fitness participants need a prompt diagnosis and treatment plan; they (and their parents, if applicable) also need to know the prognosis. If the athlete is part of a team, all concerned must understand the diagnosis, prognosis, and the anticipated lost playing time as soon as possible so that appropriate team planning can be initiated.

Communication plays a critical role. Prompt, authoritative, and efficient communication among parents, coaches, trainers, and involved colleagues is essential. An immediately available sports injury report form with multiple copies can help.

Personal coverage of competitions is optimal for team physicians, but is not always feasible. When not physically present, a team physician needs to be available for timely communication with coaches, trainers, parents, or athletes. The physician should provide a team approach to the care of the athlete. Coordinated involvement of all concerned with the athlete and the team (athletes, parents, coaches, trainers, colleagues, and therapists) optimizes outcomes.

Another unique aspect of sports medicine, particularly in high-profile athletes, is the public's interest in the status of the injured athlete. Treating physicians frequently are approached by the media for information about prominent athletes who are injured. It is important to protect physician-patient confidentiality. A practical, successful approach is to prepare a brief factual statement that includes no confidential details. This statement can be released upon request, with the proviso that any additional information has to come from the athlete.

Within sports medicine, more nonsurgical illnesses and injuries are encountered than surgical ones. Nonsurgical treatment does not mean "no treatment." Aggressive nonsurgical treatment, often engaging a team of specialists including internists, family physicians, rehabilitation specialists, psychologists, and nutritionists is frequently the norm in sports medicine. Understanding the injury and the necessary steps for a safe and effective return to competition is essential. Some therapeutic regimens apply to all sports and fitness activities; others are sport- or position-specific.

Any injury, even a successfully treated injury, may impact greatly on an athlete's career and life. Hence, a major focus of the sports medicine team is establishing injury prevention programs. Educating athletes on the importance of prevention should include the following:

- Good hygiene (such as not sharing towels and water bottles)
- Properly fitted and well-maintained protective equipment
- Appropriate hydration and nutrition for sport success
- The perils of using banned performance-enhancing substances (a prime responsibility of the sports medicine physician)

The sports medicine team is responsible for developing sport- and age-appropriate conditioning programs for off-season, preseason, and in-season injury prevention (**Table 1**).

Clinical Symptoms

Symptoms for athletes are exactly the same as for nonathletes in situations of sprains/strains, tendinitis, ruptures, or fractures. Certain injuries such as turf toe, myositis ossificans, knee ligament injuries, and shoulder and elbow tendinitis are more common in athletics.

Tests

A preparticipation physical evaluation (PPE) is mandated to ensure that an athlete is capable of performing in his or her sport safely and

Table 1

Prevention Strategies in Sports Medicine

Sports Injury Prevention Strategies

Preparticipation physical examination (PPE)

Perform strengthening and endurance training exercises to condition and maintain muscles used in sports

Always perform appropriate warm-up exercises

Gradually increase practice time and intensity to acclimate to full speed

Stretching should be done before and after to increase flexibility

Hydrate before, during, and after exercise

Decrease intensity during high heat/humidity periods

Rest periodically during practice and games to reduce fatigue

Gear and protective equipment should be appropriately fitted

Emphasize proper technique during practice to avoid game time injury

Take time for recovery

Special Considerations for Adolescent Athletes

Determine the young athlete's level of interest

Provide adequate adult supervision

Avoid strict and intense training to prevent early overuse injuries

Tailor rules to specific age groups

Opponents should be appropriately matched

Keep strengthening exercises light and focus on cross-training

Adjust playing field or court to accommodate for different ages

Table 2

Return to Running Program

Returning From Lower Extremity Injury

Begin with straight-line jogging

Progress from jogging to half speed, then to three-fourths speed, and then to full-speed sprinting as tolerated.

Agility drills are added in the same speed progression as with running

Jumping and plyometric activity

Sport-specific and position-specific drills

to identify those at risk for injury. History, physical examination, and appropriate laboratory studies and radiographs are needed, as indicated for specific situations. If warning signs for cardiac disease are present, additional history or physical examination should be performed, and an electrocardiogram or echocardiogram should be obtained. Cardiac studies can be added as part of the PPE, but these tests have a large false-positive rate and the cost-benefit ratio should be considered.

Treatment

Sports-oriented rehabilitation is a graduated progression, as outlined in the rehabilitation chapter of this section of the book. The final phases focus on sport- and position-specific exercises. The principles of protection, rest, ice, compression, and elevation (PRICE) should be followed. Pain-control modalities such as ice, electrical stimulation, and ultrasound are a useful adjunct. Joint range of motion, muscle flexibility, strengthening, endurance training, and functional and aerobic activities are initiated as tolerated. Pain is often useful in guiding these activities. To maintain aerobic fitness, athletes are

Table 3

Basic Interval Throwing Program

Graduated Throwing Program[a]

1. Begin with basic stretching, strengthening, and proprioceptive exercises

   After pain and inflammation subside, may continue to the next phase

2. Begin interval throwing

   Jogging/warm up

   25 throws at 45 feet for 3 sets

   Advance distance each week (45, 60, 90, 120, 150 feet)

   Perform 3 times per week at each distance

   Rest 10 min between sets

   Only advance if pain-free

3. Begin throwing off the mound (180 feet)

   Jogging/warm up

   Throwing begins at 50% maximum velocity

   Begin at 15 throws and add 15 throws each week, ending at 70 throws per session

   Advance 30, 60, 90 throws at 75% maximum velocity

   Begin adding breaking balls thrown at 50% and advance intensity weekly

   After 70 throws is reached, increase intensity to 75% maximum velocity

   Only advance if pain-free

4. Simulated game (you must meet the following criteria to move to the next level)

   No pain or stiffness while throwing

   No pain or stiffness after throwing (mild muscle soreness acceptable)

   Good throwing motion/mechanics

   Good throwing accuracy throughout the current level

   Throws are consistently on line

   Good strength throughout the current level with little fatigue

[a] Timing of beginning and advancing throwing phases will vary depending on the following factors: type of injury, surgery, and age of the athlete.

encouraged to engage in alternative activities that do not aggravate or jeopardize their injury.

Functional rehabilitation begins following adequate healing and when joint motion, muscle flexibility, strength, balance, and endurance are adequate. Examples of a gradual return to sports programs for throwing and running athletes are given in **Tables 2** and **3**.

For all athletes, a gradual return to play should include transitioning from light or partial practice to full practice as tolerated. A helpful guideline is to require at least two full practices without restriction or problems before returning to full competition. This helps the athlete, coaches, and family know that the athlete is truly ready to return to competition effectively and safely.

Team physicians should be competent in the basic evaluation and treatment of the player with a concussion. A concussion is defined as

Table 4

Signs and Symptoms of a Concussion

Headache

Nausea/vomiting

Sleep disturbances

Sensitivity to light

Disorientation

Memory abnormalities

Lack of coordination/delayed response

Confusion

Amnesia

Loss of consciousness

Poor concentration

Inappropriate emotions

Slurred speech

Dizziness

Fatigue

Irritability

Blurred vision

Empty stare

a trauma-induced complex type of neurologic and physiologic process affecting the brain. Symptoms include headaches, nausea, blurred vision, confusion, amnesia, difficulty processing information, and lack of consciousness (**Table 4**).

Evaluation of the concussed athlete should include a detailed recount of the event and symptoms, paying particular attention to the presence of amnesia and loss of consciousness. Sideline neurophysiologic function begins with a full neurologic examination and should include tests for orientation, concentration, and recall. On-the-field screening tests such as the Sport Concussion Assessment Tool 2 (SCAT2) are convenient to use on the sideline. More elaborate computerized tests such as the Immediate Post-Concussion Assessment and Cognitive Testing (ImPACT) tool can help establish baseline cognitive function. Any loss of consciousness should prompt evaluation at a medical facility. Any symptom of a concussion requires the removal of the athlete from competition followed by prompt sideline evaluation using an on-field screening test. After the diagnosis of concussion has been made, the first priority is to rest the athlete and institute a graduated stepwise progression from no activity to light aerobic activity to sport-specific exercise to noncontact drills and finally, to contact drills and return to play. The athlete must be symptom-free at each step before advancing to the next one. Return of the ImPACT score to baseline is one factor that aids in determining when to allow an athlete to return to play. A major concern with returning to play before the brain has physiologically recovered is the potential that a second impact, even a minor one, can result in severe consequences and even death (second impact syndrome).

Liability and Ethical Issues

Team physicians face many competing pressures from coaches, administrators, parents, and boosters to have athletes perform when they are injured. There also are times when athletes will want to perform when injured. It is important that the physician remains impartial and not stray from proper health care of the athlete. Ethical issues include the use of performance-enhancing drugs, and overzealous administration of corticosteroid injections or pain medications to promote playing while injured.

Sprains and Strains

Synonyms

Ligament tear
Pulled muscle
Tendon tear

Definition

Sprains and strains are common injuries that are differentiated by the tissue involved. Sprains are injuries to ligaments, the fibrous tissue that connects two bones together to provide joint stability. Strains are caused by trauma to the muscle or the musculotendinous unit.

Sprains typically occur in the ankle, knee, and wrist during sport activities. Collagen fibers that make up a ligament begin to fail as they are stretched beyond their normal limits. **Table 1** illustrates the grading scheme for sprains, which is based on the degree of injury to the ligament fibers. Classifying sprains provides useful information concerning the degree of disability, prognosis, and treatments of these injuries.

Sprains are uncommon in children with open growth plates. This is because the physis is weaker than the ligaments and the physis may fail before the ligament does, resulting in a fracture through the growth plate or physeal area. These fractures are commonly referred to as Salter-Harris fractures. Avulsion fractures are also more common in children and occur as a result of the ligament or tendon pulling off a flake of bone at the growth center. Likewise, in adults with substantial osteoporosis, the bone may fail (a fracture may occur) rather than the ligament tearing.

Strains also are common sports injuries and usually follow forceful eccentric loading of the muscle. These injuries are frequently seen in athletes who run, jump, or kick, and they typically occur at the myotendinous junction of muscles spanning two joints, such as the gastrocnemius, hamstring, and quadriceps muscles. Aging brings about collagen changes, resulting in decreased elasticity, which makes

Table 1		
Classification of Sprains		
Grade	**Degree of Injury**	**Treatment Principles**
I	Partial tear but no instability or opening of the joint on stress maneuvers	Symptomatic treatment only
II	Partial tear with some laxity indicated by partial opening of joint on stress maneuvers	Protected motion for the injured part, but full healing expected
III	Complete tear with laxity of the joint on stress maneuvers	Protected motion or possibly repair

Table 2	
Classification of Strains	
Grade	**Injury**
I	Tear of a few muscle fibers (<10%) with the fascia intact
II	Tear of moderate amount of muscle fibers (10%-50%) with the fascia intact
III	Tear of all muscle fibers (50%-100%) and intact fascia
IV	Tear of all muscle fibers (100%) and disrupted fascia

Table 3	
Ottawa Ankle Rules	

Ankle Sprains

Pain at the medial malleolus or along the distal 6 cm of the posterior/medial tibia

Pain at the lateral malleolus or along the distal 6 cm of the posterior fibula

Inability to bear weight immediately and for four consecutive steps in the emergency department

Foot Sprains

Pain in the midfoot and at the base of the fifth metatarsal

Pain in the midfoot and at the navicular bone

Inability to bear weight immediately and for four consecutive steps in the emergency department

the muscle-tendon unit susceptible to injury. Strains are graded on the amount of musculotendinous fibers torn (**Table 2**). A complete tear of a muscle, or a grade IV strain, is described as a rupture.

Clinical Symptoms

Sprains and strains typically occur acutely as a result of a traumatic event. Patients often report a popping, snapping, or tearing sensation at the time of the injury. This is typically followed by pain, swelling, stiffness, and, with lower extremity involvement, difficulty bearing weight. Injury to tendons and ligaments causes bleeding and ecchymosis, which can appear within 24 to 48 hours.

Physical Examination

The injured extremity should be examined for swelling, tenderness, and ecchymosis. These findings may not be well defined in deep muscle injuries, or in sprained joints covered by muscles. The injured area should be palpated for the site of maximal tenderness. Examination findings should always be compared with the contralateral or uninjured extremity.

With a sprain, the joint should be examined to determine stability. This may be difficult because patients will typically guard the injured extremity because of pain. Some ligamentous injuries require specific clinical maneuvers to determine injury and instability. Tests for specific joints can be found in the corresponding chapters of this text.

With strains, the examiner should gently attempt to stretch the injured muscle, palpating for a defect in the injured muscle. Distinguishing a partial from a complete rupture of the muscle is important but may be difficult initially if swelling obscures the palpable defect. The inability of the patient to actively contract the muscle to move a joint suggests a complete rupture, but pain also can limit function in grade I and II injuries. An MRI may be needed to quantify the degree of muscle injury.

Diagnostic Tests

Radiographs should be obtained if a fracture is suspected. Radiographic evaluation can demonstrate musculotendinous avulsion injuries, and so-called stress views can be used to evaluate ligamentous injury. Patients with severe sprains or strains may require further evaluation.

The Ottawa ankle rules (**Table 3**) are useful to determine if a patient with a suspected foot or ankle sprain requires radiographs on initial evaluation. Radiographs should be obtained if abnormal alignment, pain over the malleoli or midfoot areas, or any of the Ottawa findings is present.

In all suspected sprains and strains, radiographs should be obtained to rule out occult fracture if pain or swelling increases with appropriate care, or if pain and swelling persists after 7 to 10 days of appropriate management. MRI is the most sensitive test for evaluating soft-tissue injury. MRI should be used sparingly; however, it is useful when confirmation or grading is necessary. MRI also is valuable for the evaluation of suspected ruptures or severe sprains.

Differential Diagnosis
• Fracture (evident on radiographs)
• Soft-tissue contusion (swelling, no palpable defect)

Adverse Outcomes of the Disease
Chronic ligamentous laxity may lead to joint instability. Joint instability can lead to accelerated degenerative changes in the involved joint. Prolonged injury or muscle rupture can lead to muscle atrophy, weakness, loss of range of motion, and disability. Complex regional pain syndrome (CRPS) can develop after seemingly minor strains or sprains. Compartment syndrome occasionally can occur. Myositis ossificans, which is ossification in the muscle, can form in the muscle following severe strains or contusion (**Figure 1**).

Treatment
Protection, rest, ice, compression, and elevation (PRICE) is the mainstay of treatment. Cryotherapy should be instituted early. NSAIDs also are useful for analgesia and to help control inflammation.

In general, minor sprains can be treated with elastic compression bandages, bracing, or a brief period of immobilization. If necessary, strain injuries should be immobilized in a position where the muscle is stretched to help minimize bleeding from the injured muscle. Rehabilitation is often helpful in ensuring a successful recovery. An example of a treatment protocol following a substantial muscle strain of the lower extremity is illustrated in **Table 4**.

Adverse Outcomes of Treatment
Inadequate immobilization or unsupervised rehabilitation may lead to worsening of the condition. Overemphasis on treatment in the suggestible patient can lead to chronic impairment and disability, particularly in workers' compensation situations. Surgical intervention may result in scarring, infection, or postoperative arthrofibrosis.

Referral Decisions/Red Flags
Patients with grade IV strains, grade III sprains or strains, or severe grade II sprains or strains require further evaluation. Patients with chronic joint laxity may need surgical repair. Patients with symptoms disproportionate to their injury can be at risk for chronic conditions or CRPS. Equivocal radiographs should be repeated if necessary.

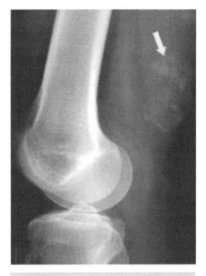

Figure 1 Lateral radiograph of the knee in a 19-year-old man obtained 4 weeks after a football injury to the posterior thigh demonstrates fluffy calcifications (arrow) in the posterior thigh musculature consistent with early myositis ossificans. (Reproduced from Lieberman JR, ed: *AAOS Comprehensive Orthopaedic Review*. Rosemont, IL, American Academy of Orthopaedic Surgeons, 2009, p 456.)

SECTION 1 GENERAL ORTHOPAEDICS

Table 4

Treatment Protocol for Hamstring Strains

Phase	Time	Goals	Treatment
I: Acute	3 to 5 days	Control pain and edema	Rest, ice, compression, elevation
	1 to 5 days	Limit hemorrhage and inflammation	Immobilization in extension, NSAIDs
	After 1 to 5 days	Prevent muscle fiber adhesions	Pain-free PROM (gentle stretching)
	Up to 1 week	Normal gait	AAROM (crutches)
II: Subacute	Day 3 to >3 weeks	Control pain and edema	Ice and compression
		Full AROM	Pain-free pool activities
		Alignment of collagen	Pain-free PROM, AAROM
		Increase collagen strength	Pain-free submaximal isometrics, stationary bike
		Maintain cardiovascular conditioning	Well-leg stationary bike, swimming with pull buoys, upper body exercise, and gentle stretching
III: Remodeling	1 to 6 weeks	Achieve phase II goals	Ice and compression
		Control pain and edema	Ice and electrical stimulation
		Increase collagen strength	Prone concentric isotonic exercises, isokinetic exercise
		Increase hamstring flexibility	Moist heat or exercise before pelvic-tilt hamstring stretching
		Increase eccentric loading	Prone eccentric exercises, jump rope
IV: Functional	2 weeks to 6 months	Return to sport without reinjury	Walk/jog, jog/sprint, sport-specific skills and drills
		Increase hamstring flexibility	Pelvic-tilt hamstring stretching
		Increase hamstring strength	Prone concentric and eccentric exercises
		Control pain	Heat, ice, and modalities; NSAIDs as needed
V: Return to competition	3 weeks to 6 months	Avoid reinjury	Maintenance stretching and strengthening[a]

AAROM = active-assisted range of motion, AROM = active range of motion, PROM = passive range of motion.

[a] Concentric high speeds at first, proceeding to eccentric low speeds.

(Adapted from Clanton TO, Coupe KJ: Hamstring strains in athletes: Diagnosis and treatment. *J Am Acad Orthop Surg* 1998;6[4]:237-248.)

Tumors of Bone

Synonyms
Bone lesion
Neoplasm

Definition
The term bone tumor is often used to describe almost any condition in which an abnormality involving bone of uncertain etiology is identified. This includes both benign and malignant neoplastic conditions, and non-neoplastic conditions such as trauma, infection, and metabolic conditions. The word tumor, however, is incorrectly used synonymously with cancer by many people, especially patients. Physicians must be careful of the manner in which they explain to patients that an abnormality has been found involving a bone. In many cases, a common benign abnormality is discovered on a radiograph or bone scan that sets off a series of additional but often unnecessary studies and concerns. It is important that when a bone tumor or bone lesion is discovered that the lesion be evaluated expediently and appropriately. In most cases, a reasonable differential diagnosis can be rendered by an experienced observer with only a thorough history, physical examination, and plain radiograph; additional advanced imaging is not needed. A critical element in interpreting an abnormality of bone on a plain radiograph involves pattern recognition. Pattern recognition aims to categorize the appearance of a bone lesion and thereby determine the next best course of action. The most basic categories that should be used when evaluating a bone lesion are benign or malignant. Characteristics or patterns that favor a benign or malignant diagnosis are listed in **Table 1**.

Clinical Symptoms
Typically, malignant bone tumors present with a history of a dull aching pain that progresses over time. It may or may not be associated with a soft-tissue mass. Symptoms are typically exacerbated with activity indicative of a lesion that has weakened the structural integrity of the bone. Benign bone tumors may or may not be symptomatic, depending on the type of tumor and the stage. Benign bone tumors are staged as follows:

- Stage 1: Latent
- Stage 2: Active
- Stage 3: Aggressive

Like malignant bone tumors, benign tumors that weaken the bone typically present with pain that is exacerbated with activity. Most benign tumors that do not weaken the bone remain asymptomatic. Important exceptions to this generalization include osteoid osteoma and osteochondroma. Constitutional symptoms such as fever, malaise, and weight loss are absent in patients with benign tumors and are

Table 1

Characteristics or Patterns of Bone Tumors

Benign
Well-defined
Nonaggressive
Without cortical destruction or periosteal reaction

Malignant
Lytic
Destructive
Permeative
Ill-defined
Aggressive
Moth-eaten
Cortical destruction
Periosteal reaction

SECTION 1 | GENERAL ORTHOPAEDICS

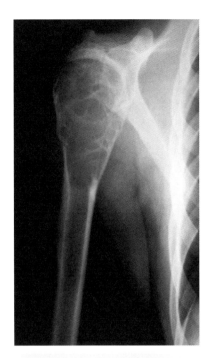

Figure 1 Radiograph of an expansile, multiloculated lesion without periosteal new bone, marked cortical thinning, and a small, nondisplaced fracture, which are essentially diagnostic for a unicameral bone cyst.

a very late presentation in patients with primary malignant bone tumors. Constitutional symptoms in patients with a bone lesion favor a diagnosis of metastatic disease, lymphoma, or infection.

Tests

History and Physical Examination

The three common clinical scenarios by which a bone tumor is discovered are as follows:

- As an incidental finding. This occurs when an imaging study is performed for an unrelated reason and a bone lesion or abnormality is discovered.
- When a patient is symptomatic and an imaging study is performed, and a bone lesion or abnormality is discovered.
- When a bone lesion is discovered as part of the evaluation of a patient with a known history of cancer.

The first scenario is the most common one; most cases will be benign, and no further tests are needed. In the second scenario, it is necessary to determine if the radiographic finding is related to the patient's symptoms or is actually an incidental finding. Obtaining a history and physical examination will direct the physician to the most logical and appropriate next step in many cases. The history should include the patient's age, past medical history, family history, location and character of symptoms, and aggravating and alleviating factors. When a metastatic lesion is suspected, the history and physical examination should include an inquiry regarding the five most common primary sites of cancer that metastasize to bone: breast, lung, kidney, thyroid, and prostate. These primary sites account for more than 85% of skeletal metastases.

Diagnostic Tests

The radiograph is the single most valuable imaging study for evaluating a bone lesion. In most cases, a determination can be made about the likelihood of the lesion being benign or malignant, and in many cases the lesion is either pathognomonic or highly suggestive of a definitive diagnosis. The need for and selection of additional imaging studies should be determined after a differential diagnosis is established from the initial radiographs. Commonly used diagnostic tests include CT and MRI. The role of CT and/or MRI in evaluating a bone lesion will depend on what specific information is being sought. MRI is superior to CT for visualizing the soft tissues and marrow infiltrative processes. CT is superior to MRI for visualizing bone detail, such as cortical continuity, erosion, or endosteal scalloping. Technetium Tc-99m bone scanning uses a radioactive technetium isotope bound to the ligand methylene-diphosphonate. In situations in which more active bone turnover exists, the bone scan will be hot, or more active than normal. Bone scans are generally sensitive for infection, trauma, and tumor, but they are not specific and do not indicate if the activity is related to trauma, infection, or tumor. Bone scans also are useful to determine if a patient with a primary cancer has skeletal metastases.

In patients older than 40 years with a suspected malignant bone tumor, the most likely diagnosis is metastatic tumor or myeloma. If a primary site cannot be found after obtaining a thorough history and physical examination, patients should undergo a CT scan of the chest, abdomen, and pelvis. A bone scan should be obtained to see if there are additional bone lesions that may be more appropriate for biopsy. Additional tests such as upper and lower endoscopy, indirect laryngoscopy, and even mammography are not necessary.

Blood Tests

In patients with aggressive bone lesions the differential diagnosis will include metastatic tumor, primary malignant bone tumor, and infection. In patients older than 40 years, the most likely diagnosis of an aggressive bone lesion will be metastases or myeloma. Serum tests that are sometimes helpful in narrowing a differential diagnosis include complete blood cell count, erythrocyte sedimentation rate, and C-reactive protein level (possible infection). In patients older than 40 years, blood tests to indicate myeloma should be performed, including serum protein electrophoresis (SPEP), urine protein electrophoresis (UPEP), quantitative serum immunoglobulin level, serum free light chain assay, and β-2-microglobulin factor. In most cases, additional blood tests will not obviate the need for a biopsy of suspected malignant bone lesions.

Biopsy

A biopsy is indicated when the diagnosis remains uncertain after appropriate history, physical examination, and review of laboratory and imaging studies. The most common methods used to biopsy bone include closed-needle biopsy and open-bone biopsy. Each method has advantages and disadvantages, but it is recommended that patients with bone tumors be evaluated by an orthopaedic surgeon before obtaining a biopsy.

Differential Diagnosis

The differential diagnosis depends on the patient's age, location of the lesion, and most importantly, the pattern appearance seen on radiographs. In most cases of benign bone tumors the diagnosis can be made based on characteristics of the plain radiograph without the need for additional imaging (**Figure 1**).

In cases of malignant tumors, age becomes a major factor in determining the differential diagnosis (**Figure 2**).

Table 2 provides a list of common benign bone tumors.

Adverse Outcomes of the Disease

Benign tumors that are latent may cause symptoms and limit function. Benign active and aggressive lesions can cause pathologic fracture and loss of function. Malignant tumors that are metastatic cause pain, disability, and loss of function. With immobility comes the risk of hypercalcemia and pneumonia.

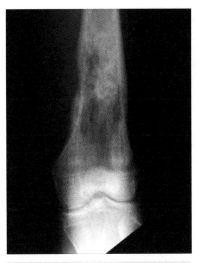

Figure 2 AP radiograph demonstrates a destructive, ill-defined lesion in the metaphysis of a skeletally immature individual with cortical breakthrough, new periosteal bone, and matrix formation (bone-forming malignant tumor). Based on the previously noted criteria, this is almost certainly an osteosarcoma.

SECTION 1 GENERAL ORTHOPAEDICS

Table 2

Benign Bone Tumors

Tumor Type	Age Range of Occurrence, in Years	Location	Characteristic Radiographic Appearance	Unique Clinical or Radiographic Feature
Osteochondroma	Childhood and young adult	Metaphysis of long bone	Bone arising from stalk or "bump" on bone	Normal-appearing bone growing from the surface of bone
Chondroblastoma	Childhood and young adult	Epiphysis of long bone	Well defined, with sclerotic border, may have cortical breakthrough	Epiphyseal location
Chondromyxoid fibroma	Adolescence	Eccentric, metaphyseal	Well defined, with internal calcifications	Favored location: tibia
Enchondroma	15-40	Hands and fingers, metaphysis of long bones	Lucent in hands and fingers; matrix calcification in long bones	Metaphysis of long bones, usually incidental finding
Osteoblastoma	10-35	Posterior elements of the spine, metaphysis of long bone	May be lytic, sclerotic, or mixed	Proclivity for the posterior elements of the spine
Osteoid osteoma	10-35	Long bones and posterior elements of the spine	Sclerotic, with small (<1 cm) lucent nidus	Distinct nidus, best seen with CT; typical night pain that is responsive to NSAIDs and/or aspirin
Eosinophilic granuloma	5-10 (rare in patient older than 30)	Vertebrae, long or flat bone	Spine lesions: vertebra plana. In long bones lytic and may appear aggressive.	Vertebra plana in a child; may involve more than one bone
Fibrous dysplasia	Late childhood through adulthood; polyostotic fibrous dysplasia present earlier	Any bone (ie, ribs, femur, tibia, maxilla, mandible, humerus)	Lytic, may expand the bone with thinning of the cortex	Ground-glass appearance on radiograph
Nonossifying fibroma	3-30	Femur and tibia are most common	Lytic, well-defined, thin, lobulated margin	Eccentric, involves cortex and expands into medullary cavity
Fibrous cortical defect	4-15	Distal femur and tibia	Radiolucent, well-defined, confined to cortex with sclerotic border	Well-defined cortical lesion with sclerotic borders <4 cm
Aneurysmal bone cyst	Younger than 30	Any bone; most commonly in vertebra, femur, and tibia	Eccentric, lytic, expansile	Fluid levels seen on CT or MRI
Giant cell tumor	20-40	Distal femur, proximal tibia, distal radius, proximal humerus, pelvis, sacrum	Eccentric, lytic epiphyseal/metaphyseal long bones	Lytic lesion extending from subchondral bone to metaphysic; may erode beyond cortex
Simple bone cyst (unicameral bone cyst)	Younger than 20	80% proximal humerus or proximal femur	Central medullary lytic lesion, may expand bone and be multicystic	Fallen-leaf sign is pathognomonic

Treatment

Many benign tumors may be observed and require no treatment. Active and aggressive lesions are managed surgically with a goal of minimizing local recurrence while maximizing function. Primary malignant tumors in children are usually treated with systemic chemotherapy and surgery. Most primary malignant bone tumors are successfully treated with limb-sparing surgery. The treatment of metastatic bone tumors includes radiation, chemotherapy, and surgery. Diphosphonates play a vital role in the management of patients with established bone metastases.

Referral Decisions/Red Flags

Further evaluation by a specialist is recommended for a suspicious bone or soft-tissue mass, unusual pain or night pain, constitutional symptoms associated with bone pain, lytic or blastic changes in bone, soft-tissue calcification, or periosteal reaction on radiographs.

GENERAL ORTHOPAEDICS

SECTION 1

PAIN DIAGRAM
Shoulder

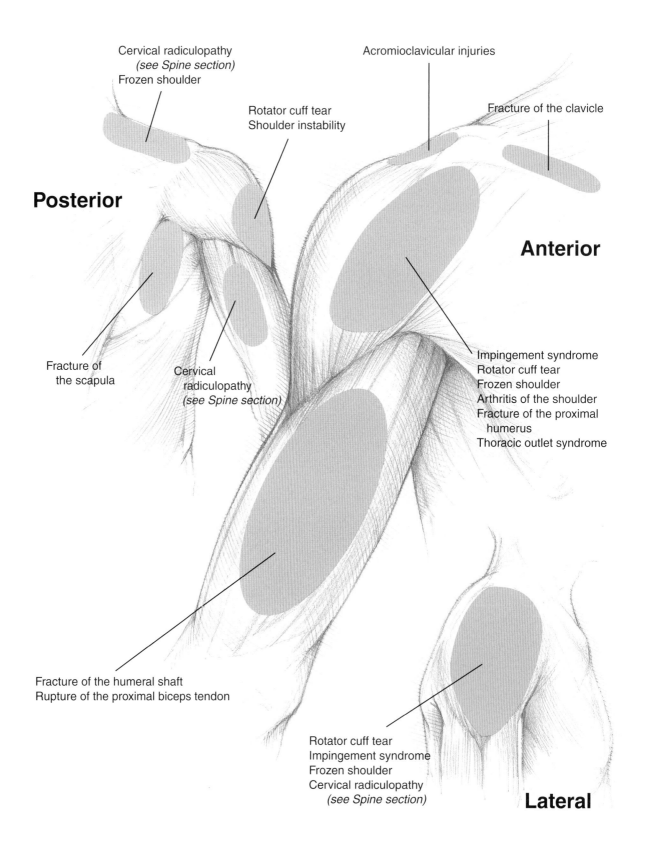

Cervical radiculopathy
(see Spine section)
Frozen shoulder

Rotator cuff tear
Shoulder instability

Acromioclavicular injuries

Fracture of the clavicle

Posterior

Anterior

Fracture of
the scapula

Cervical
radiculopathy
(see Spine section)

Impingement syndrome
Rotator cuff tear
Frozen shoulder
Arthritis of the shoulder
Fracture of the proximal
humerus
Thoracic outlet syndrome

Fracture of the humeral shaft
Rupture of the proximal biceps tendon

Rotator cuff tear
Impingement syndrome
Frozen shoulder
Cervical radiculopathy
(see Spine section)

Lateral

Shoulder

Section Editor

Robert Z. Tashjian, MD

Associate Professor
Orthopaedics
University of Utah School of Medicine
Salt Lake City, Utah

Contributor

Mark C. Hubbard, MPT

Physical Therapist
Bone and Joint Institute
Penn State Milton S. Hershey Medical Center
Hershey, Pennsylvania

ANATOMY OF THE SHOULDER

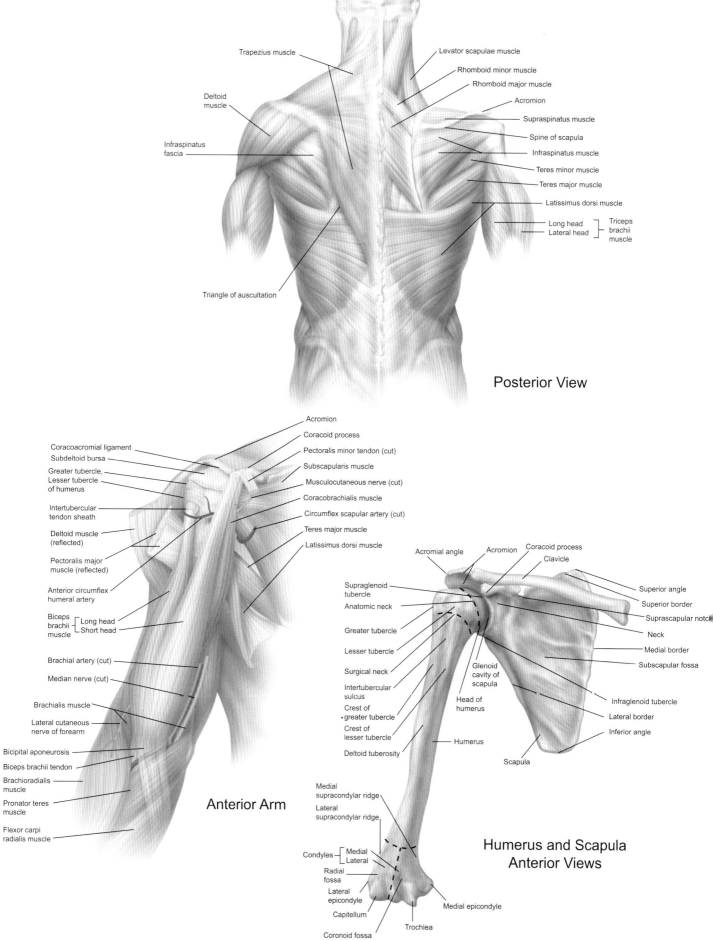

Trapezius muscle

Levator scapulae muscle

Rhomboid minor muscle

Rhomboid major muscle

Acromion

Supraspinatus muscle

Spine of scapula

Infraspinatus muscle

Teres minor muscle

Teres major muscle

Latissimus dorsi muscle

Long head
Lateral head — Triceps brachii muscle

Deltoid muscle

Infraspinatus fascia

Triangle of auscultation

Posterior View

Acromion

Coracoid process

Pectoralis minor tendon (cut)

Subscapularis muscle

Musculocutaneous nerve (cut)

Coracobrachialis muscle

Circumflex scapular artery (cut)

Teres major muscle

Latissimus dorsi muscle

Coracoacromial ligament

Subdeltoid bursa

Greater tubercle,
Lesser tubercle of humerus

Intertubercular tendon sheath

Deltoid muscle (reflected)

Pectoralis major muscle (reflected)

Anterior circumflex humeral artery

Biceps brachii muscle — Long head, Short head

Brachial artery (cut)

Median nerve (cut)

Brachialis muscle

Lateral cutaneous nerve of forearm

Bicipital aponeurosis

Biceps brachii tendon

Brachioradialis muscle

Pronator teres muscle

Flexor carpi radialis muscle

Anterior Arm

Acromial angle

Acromion

Coracoid process

Clavicle

Supraglenoid tubercle

Anatomic neck

Greater tubercle

Lesser tubercle

Surgical neck

Intertubercular sulcus

Crest of greater tubercle

Crest of lesser tubercle

Deltoid tuberosity

Superior angle

Superior border

Suprascapular notch

Neck

Medial border

Subscapular fossa

Glenoid cavity of scapula

Head of humerus

Humerus

Infraglenoid tubercle

Lateral border

Inferior angle

Scapula

Medial supracondylar ridge

Lateral supracondylar ridge

Condyles — Medial, Lateral

Radial fossa

Lateral epicondyle

Capitellum

Coronoid fossa

Medial epicondyle

Trochlea

Humerus and Scapula
Anterior Views

© 2016 American Academy of Orthopaedic Surgeons

Overview of the Shoulder

This section of *Essentials of Musculoskeletal Care* focuses on the conditions that commonly affect the shoulder in adults. These include acute injuries (fractures, dislocations, and acute tendon ruptures), chronic or repetitive injuries (impingement syndrome and most rotator cuff tears and biceps tendon ruptures), and degenerative, inflammatory, or idiopathic conditions (glenohumeral and acromioclavicular [AC] arthritis, adhesive capsulitis [frozen shoulder]). Most shoulder disorders are diagnosed using a history, a thorough physical examination, and radiographs.

A concise differential diagnosis often is achieved after evaluating the symptoms in the context of their chronicity and the patient's age. The chief symptom is usually related to pain or instability. Decreased motion, power, or function sometimes accompanies pain or instability but only rarely is the chief symptom.

Pain

Patients with acute symptoms (less than 2 weeks' duration) usually have sustained an injury such as a fracture or dislocation, a rotator cuff tear, or a biceps tendon rupture. Common physical findings include local tenderness, deformity, swelling, and ecchymosis. Determining the mechanism and magnitude of the injury and the anatomic location of the symptoms helps in making the diagnosis. For example, a football player who has severe pain and deformity at the superior aspect of the shoulder after falling directly on that shoulder most likely has an AC joint separation.

Similarly, for patients with chronic shoulder pain, knowledge of the activities related to the onset of symptoms and the location and character of symptoms often results in the correct diagnosis. Pain localized to the top of the shoulder suggests AC joint arthritis or chronic AC separation. This pain often is exacerbated by cross-body adduction in the horizontal plane. Pain from subacromial bursitis, frozen shoulder, or rotator cuff pathology is typically referred to the lateral deltoid region and may radiate to the lateral aspect of the upper arm. Overhead activities most commonly exacerbate this pain. In contrast, shoulder pain arising from cervical nerve root irritation usually follows a dermatomal distribution, is associated with numbness and/or tingling, and is often relieved by placing the forearm on top of the head. Degenerative arthritis of the glenohumeral joint may cause pain along the anterior and posterior joint lines. Both rotator cuff tears and arthritis may cause night pain, which makes sleeping on the affected side difficult.

Instability

Instability is classified by the frequency of symptomatic episodes, as well as the direction and degree of instability. An acute injury may be a first-time dislocation or a recurrent episode. The instability episode may be partial (subluxation) with spontaneous reduction, or it may be complete (dislocation). The instability can be anterior, posterior, inferior, or multidirectional. Most traumatic dislocations are anterior. Multidirectional instability should be considered when a patient presents with recurrent episodes of subluxation or dislocation and no history of significant trauma.

Range of Motion, Muscle Strength, and Function

When assessing motion, it is important to determine if a discrepancy exists between active and passive motion. Patients with rotator cuff tears lose active elevation and external rotation, although some loss of passive range of motion can occur secondary to disuse. Equal losses of active and passive range of motion may be secondary to soft-tissue contracture, as in frozen shoulder, or the result of joint incongruity from trauma or arthritis.

Muscle strength should be assessed and compared with the opposite shoulder. Tears of the rotator cuff and neurologic injury may produce weakness. Pain inhibition can affect the accuracy of muscle testing.

Functional status relates to a patient's ability to perform his or her normal activities. The level of functional disability depends on the specific type and intensity of activities the patient normally performs. Motivation and the ability to adapt to impairment also play an important role.

Patient Age

Younger Patients

Patients younger than 30 years most commonly present with traumatic injuries or instability such as glenohumeral dislocations and AC joint separations. Impingement syndrome and rotator cuff tears rarely occur in this age group.

Middle-aged Patients

Impingement syndrome and rotator cuff tears are common in this group. These must be distinguished from the early onset of adhesive capsulitis. Often it is difficult to distinguish between impingement syndrome and early adhesive capsulitis, and, adding to the confusion, the two diagnoses often coexist. Glenohumeral dislocations are much less common and must be treated with a high index of suspicion for a concomitant rotator cuff tear (50% of patients older than 40 years will have an acute tear with a dislocation).

Older Patients

Patients older than 50 years commonly have symptoms related to rotator cuff dysfunction. Rotator cuff disease can run the spectrum from acute tendinitis and chronic tendinopathy to partial-thickness and full-thickness rotator cuff tears. Rotator cuff tears and degenerative arthritis of the AC joint, the glenohumeral joint, or both also are common in this group. Acute pain following a fall in an elderly, frail patient with osteoporosis should raise suspicion for a fracture of the proximal humerus.

Musculoskeletal Conditioning of the Shoulder

A conditioning program can be separated into three basic phases: stretching exercises, to improve range of motion; strengthening, to improve muscle power; and proprioception, to enhance balance and agility. In addition, each exercise session should begin with an active warm-up, and plyometric exercises may be added for power after basic strength and flexibility goals have been achieved. Patient handouts are provided here for general stretching and strengthening exercises. Advanced proprioceptive exercises and plyometric exercises should be done under the supervision of a rehabilitation specialist or other exercise professional.

The general goal of a conditioning program is to enable people to live a more fit and healthy lifestyle by being more active. A well-structured conditioning program will prepare the individual for participation in sports and recreational activities. The greater the intensity of the activity in which the individual wishes to engage, the greater the intensity of the conditioning program that will be required. If the individual participates in a supervised rehabilitation program that provides instruction in a conditioning routine—instead of using only an exercise handout such as provided here—the focus should be on developing and committing to a home exercise fitness program. A conditioning program for the body as a whole that includes exercises for the lower extremity, the trunk, and the upper extremity is described in the chapter Musculoskeletal Conditioning: Helping Patients Prevent Injury and Stay Fit.

The shoulder is a complex structure that allows movement in many different planes. The glenohumeral and scapular rotators are important muscle groups for overhead sports activities such as tennis, baseball, and swimming. Strengthening the scapular stabilizers, as well as the rotator cuff and deltoid muscles, is important to assist with the stability of the glenohumeral joint and help prevent injury when engaging in activities that involve repetitive upper extremity motion such as gardening, housekeeping, or sports. Increased strength in these muscles can also translate to a higher velocity tennis serve or baseball pitch.

Proprioceptive and balance exercises enhance the individual's perception of the position of the body and arm in space. Scapular retraction performed while prone on a large exercise ball, push-ups performed on an air mattress, and ball rolling on a wall are examples of proprioceptive exercises for the shoulder. These exercises should be done only after adequate flexibility and strength have been achieved. Instruction and supervision in such exercises is recommended to ensure that they are performed safely.

For individuals beginning a new sport activity, a period of sport-specific training should begin only after the prescribed goals of strengthening, stretching, and proprioceptive conditioning have been met. During this period, the individual would perform the actions normally required by the sport with gradually increasing intensity and duration.

SECTION 2 SHOULDER

Forcing stretching or strengthening to the point of pain is always deleterious and should be avoided. Progress is achieved by performing these exercises frequently (2 to 3 times per day, 4 to 5 days per week) and making gradual improvement toward goals. The patient should be instructed to call the physician if any exercises cause pain.

Stretching Exercises

The capsule and muscles of the posterior shoulder may be tight, especially in individuals who participate in repetitive overhead activities, including overhead throwing sports and swimming. Horizontal adduction stretching and the sleeper stretch are helpful to relax these posterior shoulder tissues. Static stretching is performed at the end of the range of painless motion of the shoulder.

Strengthening Exercises

Exercises to strengthen the deltoid and rotator cuff muscles are often performed using commercially available elastic therapy bands. These bands are available in different thicknesses, which provide predictable levels of resistance. Similar exercises can also be performed with pulleys or free weights. It usually takes 2 to 3 weeks to progress to the next band or weight. For strength training, the patient should perform 3 sets of 8 repetitions, progressing to 3 sets of 12 repetitions. After 12 repetitions are reached, the resistance should be increased and the repetitions started over at 8. The patient should be advised not to progress to the next level of resistance if he or she still has difficulty at the current level or if pain develops. The patient should also be instructed to continue stretching exercises during this stage to maintain shoulder range of motion.

Proprioceptive Exercises

In addition to adequate strength, athletes benefit from improved control and coordination. Neuromuscular training, which improves the communication between the muscles and nervous system, includes balance and proprioceptive exercises. Balance involves the visual, vestibular, and proprioceptive systems. With balance training, the athlete may be instructed to hold a posture for 30 to 60 seconds at the limits of his or her stability.

Proprioceptive exercises for the shoulder often involve weight bearing through the arms. For example, push-ups performed with the hands on an exercise ball are an excellent advanced exercise for improving dynamic glenohumeral and scapular stability. For the novice athlete, standing push-ups done against a wall provide good proprioceptive training. This exercise can be performed with the hands directly on the wall or, to provide an additional challenge, the hands can be placed on one large or two smaller exercise balls during the push-up motion.

SECTION 2 SHOULDER

Home Exercise Program for Shoulder Conditioning

- Perform 10 minutes of general warm-up activity such as using an arm bike or elliptical before doing these exercises.
- When performing the stretching exercises, stretch slowly to the limit of motion, taking care to avoid pain. If you experience pain with the exercises, call your doctor.
- For the exercises that use a stick, you may use a yardstick or stick of similar size.
- The following exercise program is introductory only, and progression of this program will vary based on your specific injury, symptoms, and baseline level of fitness. For further progression of this routine, your physician may recommend evaluation and treatment by a physical therapist or other exercise professional.

Strengthening and Stretching Exercises for the Shoulder

Exercise	Muscle Group	Number of Repetitions/Sets	Number of Days per Week
Strengthening			
External rotation	Infraspinatus Teres minor	8 repetitions/3 sets, progressing to 12 repetitions/3 sets	3
Standing row	Middle trapezius Rhomboid	8 repetitions/3 sets, progressing to 12 repetitions/3 sets	3
Internal rotation	Pectoralis major and minor Subscapularis	8 repetitions/3 sets, progressing to 12 repetitions/3 sets	3
Bent-over horizontal abduction	Middle and lower trapezius	8 repetitions/3 sets, progressing to 12 repetitions/3 sets	3
Elbow flexion	Biceps	8 repetitions/3 sets, progressing to 12 repetitions/3 sets	3
Elbow extension	Triceps	8 repetitions/3 sets, progressing to 12 repetitions/3 sets	3
External rotation with arm abducted 90°	Infraspinatus Teres minor	8 repetitions/3 sets, progressing to 12 repetitions/3 sets	3
Stretching			
Pendulum	General	10 repetitions/2 sets, progressing to 15 repetitions/3 sets	5 to 6
Passive external rotation	Infraspinatus Teres minor	4 sets	5 to 6
Passive internal rotation	Subscapularis Pectoralis major and minor	4 sets	5 to 6
Horizontal adduction stretch	Posterior deltoid	4 sets	5 to 6
Sleeper stretch	Posterior deltoid	5 repetitions, 2 to 3 times per day, continuing for 3 to 4 weeks	5 to 6

SECTION 2 SHOULDER

Strengthening Exercises

External Rotation

- Make a 3-foot–long loop with the elastic band and tie the ends together. Attach the loop to a doorknob or other stable object.
- Standing with your side to the wall, hold the loop, as shown in the start position.
- Keeping your elbow close to your side, rotate the arm outward slowly and then slowly return to the start position.
- Perform 3 sets of 8 repetitions, progressing to 3 sets of 12 repetitions, 3 days per week.
- Repeat on the other side.

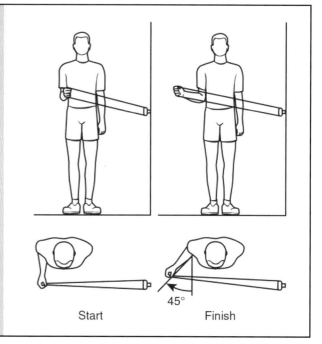

Standing Row

- Make a 3-foot–long loop with the elastic band and tie the ends together.
- Attach the loop to a doorknob or other stable object.
- Standing while facing the wall, hold the loop with both hands as shown in the start position.
- Keeping your arms close to your sides, slowly pull straight back and squeeze your shoulder blades together.
- Slowly return to the start position.
- Perform 3 sets of 8 repetitions, progressing to 3 sets of 12 repetitions, 3 days per week.
- Repeat on the other side.

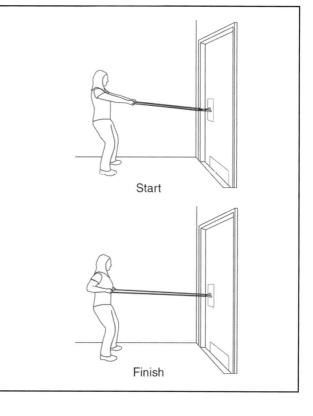

Internal Rotation

- Make a 3-foot–long loop with the elastic band and tie the ends together. Attach the loop to a doorknob or other stable object.
- Standing with your side to the wall, hold the loop as shown in the start position.
- Keeping your elbow close to your side, rotate the arm across your body slowly, and slowly return to the start position.
- Perform 3 sets of 8 repetitions, progressing to 3 sets of 12 repetitions, 3 days per week.
- Repeat on the other side.

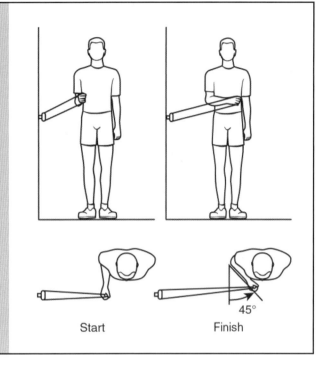

Start   Finish

Bent-Over Horizontal Abduction

- Stand next to a table.
- Bend at the waist with your side supported on the table and the other arm hanging straight down and holding a light weight (up to 5 pounds).
- Keeping the arm straight, slowly raise the hand up to eye level and then slowly lower it back to the start position.
- Perform 3 sets of 8 repetitions, progressing to 3 sets of 12 repetitions, 3 days per week.
- Repeat on the other side.

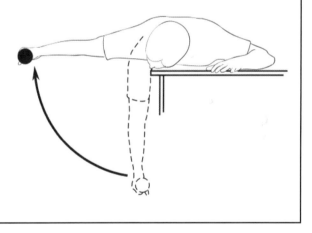

SECTION 2   SHOULDER

Elbow Flexion
- Stand with your body weight evenly distributed over both feet.
- Holding a light weight (up to 5 pounds) and keeping the arm close to the side, slowly bend the elbow up toward the shoulder as shown; hold for 2 seconds, slowly return to the starting position, and then relax.
- Perform 3 sets of 8 repetitions, progressing to 3 sets of 12 repetitions, 3 days per week.
- Repeat on the other side.

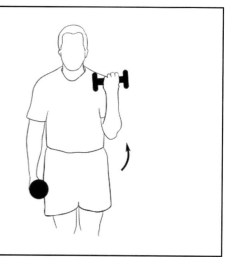

Elbow Extension
- Stand with your body weight evenly distributed over both feet.
- Holding a light weight (up to 5 pounds), raise your arm with the elbow bent and with your opposite hand supporting your elbow. Slowly straighten the elbow overhead, hold for 2 seconds, and then slowly lower the arm to the starting position.
- Perform 3 sets of 8 repetitions, progressing to 3 sets of 12 repetitions, 3 days per week.
- Repeat on the other side.

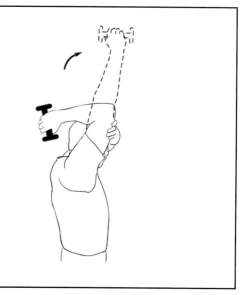

SECTION 2   SHOULDER

External Rotation With the Arm Abducted 90°

- Make a 3-foot–long loop with the elastic band and tie the ends together. Attach the loop to a doorknob or other stable object.
- Standing facing the wall, hold the loop as shown in the start position, with the arm held straight out from the shoulder and the elbow bent 90°.
- Keeping the shoulder and elbow level, slowly rotate the hand up from the elbow, and then slowly return to the start position.
- Perform 3 sets of 8 repetitions, progressing to 3 sets of 12 repetitions, 3 days per week.

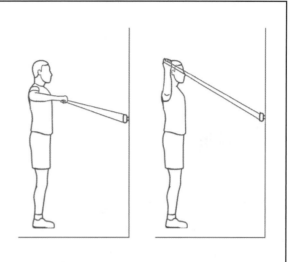

Stretching Exercises

Pendulum

- Lean forward, supporting the body with one arm and relaxing the muscles of the other arm so that it hangs freely.
- Gently move the arm in forward-and-back, side-to-side, and circular motions.
- Perform 2 sets of 10 repetitions, progressing to 3 sets of 15 repetitions, 5 to 6 days per week.
- Repeat on the other side.

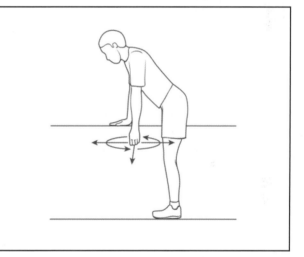

Passive External Rotation

- Grasp the stick with one hand and cup the other end of the stick with the other hand.
- Push the stick horizontally as shown, keeping the elbow against the side of the body so that the arm is passively stretched to the point of feeling a pull without pain.
- Hold for 30 seconds and then relax for 30 seconds.
- Perform 4 sets, 5 to 6 days per week.
- Repeat on the other side.

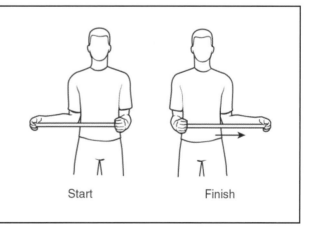

Start   Finish

SECTION 2   SHOULDER

Passive Internal Rotation

- Behind your back, grasp the stick with one hand and lightly grasp the other end of the stick with the other hand.
- Pull the stick horizontally as shown so that the arm is passively stretched to the point of feeling a pull without pain.
- Hold for 30 seconds and then relax for 30 seconds.
- Perform 4 sets, 5 to 6 days per week.
- Repeat on the other side.

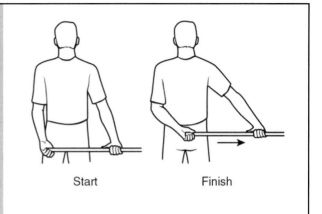

Start   Finish

Horizontal Adduction Stretch

- Gently pull the elbow of one arm across the chest as far as possible without feeling pain.
- Hold the stretch for 30 seconds and then relax for 30 seconds.
- Perform 4 sets, 5 to 6 days per week.
- Repeat on the other side.

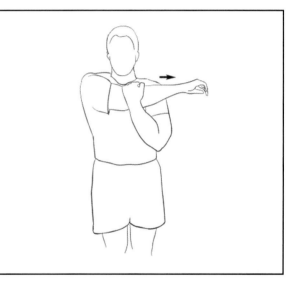

Sleeper Stretch

- Lie on your side on a firm, flat surface with the affected shoulder under you and the arm positioned as shown, keeping your back perpendicular to the surface.
- With the unaffected arm, push the other wrist down, toward the surface. Stop when you feel a stretching sensation in the back of the affected shoulder.
- Hold this position for 30 seconds, then relax the arm for 30 seconds.
- Perform 5 repetitions, 2 to 3 times per day, 5 to 6 days per week, continuing for 3 to 4 weeks.

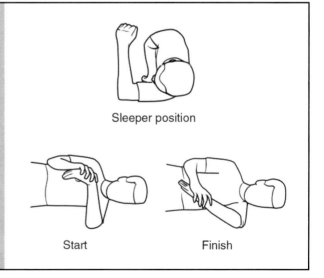

Sleeper position

Start   Finish

SECTION 2   SHOULDER

Physical Examination of the Shoulder

Inspection/Palpation

Anterior View

With the patient standing, inspect for abnormal contours and bony prominences. An acromioclavicular separation produces a "step-off" deformity with prominence of the distal clavicle. An anterior shoulder dislocation produces a prominent posterior acromion and anterior fullness of the deltoid, and the arm typically is held in slight abduction and external rotation. By contrast, with a posterior dislocation, the coracoid and anterior acromion are prominent, there is posterior fullness, and the arm is held in adduction and internal rotation.

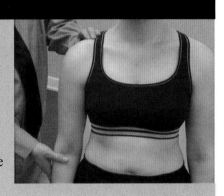

Posterior View

With the patient standing, note symmetry of shoulder heights and contours (the dominant shoulder often rests slightly lower than the opposite shoulder). Look for muscle atrophy, particularly of the trapezius, deltoid, and infraspinatus muscles. Diminished posterior contour from neck to shoulder indicates atrophy of the trapezius. With atrophy of the supraspinatus/infraspinatus muscles, loss of lateral shoulder contour occurs at the deltoid, and a prominent scapular spine can be seen. While viewing the posterior shoulder, have the patient elevate both arms in the scapular plane and evaluate both sides for any scapula dyskinesia (not shown in the video).

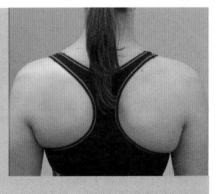

Acromioclavicular Joint

To evaluate the acromioclavicular joint, palpate the distal clavicle and the acromion for tenderness or spurs. Tenderness usually is most pronounced at the posterior joint interval and is exaggerated when the patient horizontally adducts the arm toward the opposite shoulder.

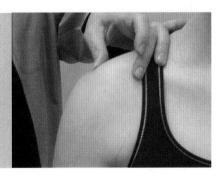

SECTION 2   SHOULDER

Subacromial Bursa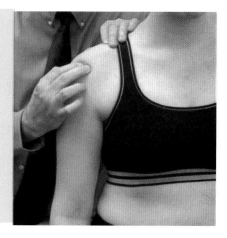

To evaluate the subacromial bursa, palpate the anterolateral portion of the acromion, moving down toward the deltoid until you feel the acromiohumeral sulcus. Tenderness in this area usually is related to subacromial bursitis or a rotator cuff tear (supraspinatus tendon).

Long Head of the Biceps Tendon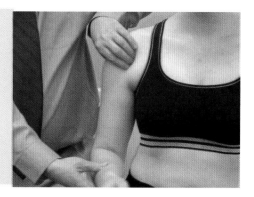

To evaluate the long head of the biceps tendon, palpate over the humeral head in the region of the bicipital groove. With tendinitis, there is tenderness and swelling, and the area of tenderness should move with the humeral head as the shoulder is rotated.

Range of Motion

Flexion

Normal shoulder motion is a composite movement that couples glenohumeral motion with movement of the scapula on the thorax. Scapular movement is derived from motion of the acromioclavicular and sternoclavicular joints. Shoulder mobility is efficiently assessed by measuring four ranges of motion: flexion, external rotation with the arm at the side, external rotation with the arm in 90° of abduction, and internal rotation.

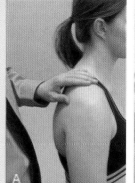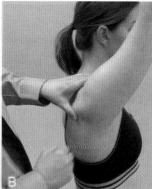

To evaluate shoulder flexion, place the patient's arm at the side (**A**). Ask the patient to raise the arm in the sagittal plane (**B**), and then measure active and passive motion in reference to the thoracic spine. Normal shoulder flexion is 160° to 170°.

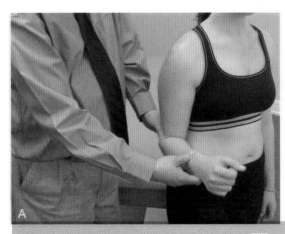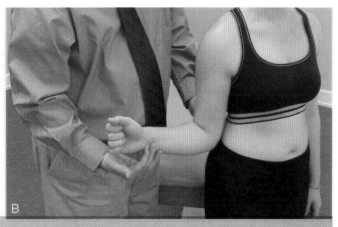

External Rotation, Arm at the Side

To evaluate external rotation, place the patient's arm at the side, held comfortably against the thorax, the elbow flexed to 90°, and the forearm parallel to the sagittal plane of the body (**A**). Measure external rotation by evaluating the maximum lateral rotation of the arm (**B**).

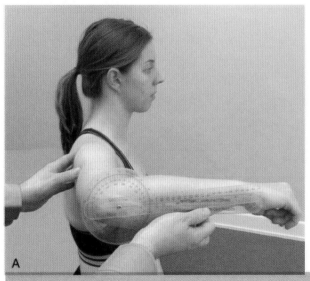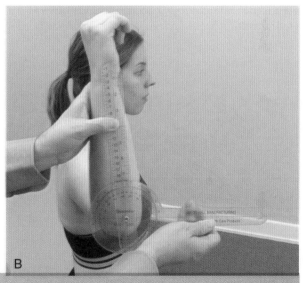

External Rotation, Arm Abducted 90°

To evaluate external rotation, a goniometer is needed. The patient's arm is abducted 90°, the arm is aligned with the plane of the scapula, the elbow is flexed 90°, and the forearm is parallel to the floor (**A**). Measure external rotation in this position by evaluating how many degrees the forearm moves away from the previous parallel position (**B**). Limited external rotation in this position is seen in some athletes who emphasize strengthening exercises without including an appropriate stretching program and in patients who have had reconstructive surgery of the shoulder.

Internal Rotation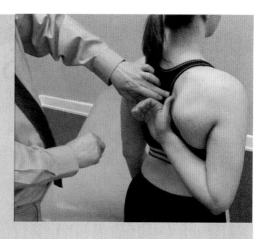

To evaluate internal rotation, ask the patient to place the arm behind the back and reach as high as possible. Note the highest midline spinous process that can be reached by the hitchhiking thumb. This maneuver is simple and easy to reproduce, but it represents a composite motion that depends on shoulder extension as well as scapular protraction and elbow, wrist, and thumb motion. Young adults typically can reach beyond the inferior tip of the scapula (approximately at the T7 level). Internal rotation may be severely limited in patients with adhesive capsulitis or degenerative arthritis. In these patients, the thumb may reach only to the sacrum, gluteal region, or greater trochanter.

Muscle Testing

Deltoid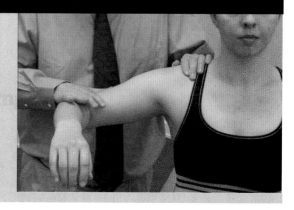

To test the deltoid muscle, place the patient's arm in 90° of abduction with the elbow flexed 90° and the forearm parallel to the floor. Push down on the distal arm as the patient resists this pressure. This position also activates the supraspinatus and, to some degree, the other rotator cuff muscles. The anterior deltoid is isolated by moving the arm forward. The posterior deltoid is isolated by moving the arm backward and then performing the muscle test.

Supraspinatus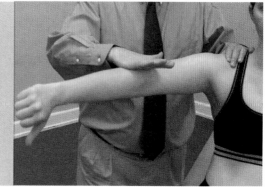

To evaluate the supraspinatus, place the patient's arm in 90° of abduction, 30° of horizontal adduction, and internal rotation with the elbow extended. Push down on the distal arm as the patient resists this pressure.

Infraspinatus and Teres Minor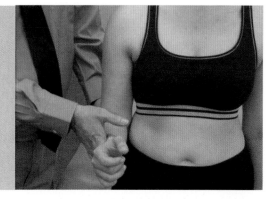

Test strength in the infraspinatus and the teres minor by placing the patient's arm at the side in neutral rotation and with the elbow flexed. Support the elbow and instruct the patient to maintain this position while you apply moderate to firm pressure at the distal forearm, attempting to internally rotate the arm.

Hornblower's Test

To evaluate the teres minor, the hornblower's test is helpful. Support the patient's arm abducted to 90° in the scapular plane with the elbow flexed to 90°. Ask the patient to rotate the arm externally 90° against resistance. A positive sign is indicated by the inability to maintain the externally rotated position, and the arm drops back to neutral position.

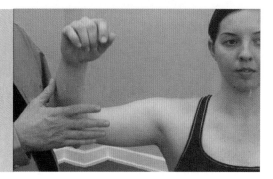

Gerber Lift-off Test

Test subscapularis strength and possible tendon rupture by asking the patient to place the hand behind the back, palm facing away from the body, and then lift it away from the back against resistance.

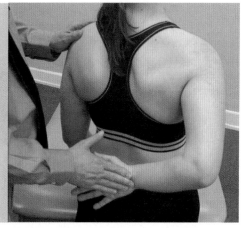

Serratus Anterior

Test serratus anterior strength by asking the patient to elevate the arm as you depress the arm with one hand and palpate the scapula with the other. With normal strength of the serratus anterior, the scapula remains in position on the chest wall. Winging and prominence of the vertebral border occurs with a weak serratus anterior muscle. Stretch or avulsion injuries of the long thoracic nerve with resultant paralysis of the serratus anterior also cause winging of the scapula and fatigue with overhead activities.

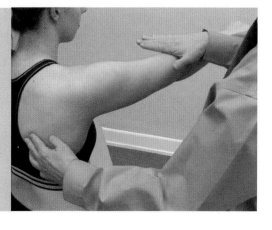

© 2016 American Academy of Orthopaedic Surgeons **Essentials of Musculoskeletal Care 5** 275

SECTION 2 SHOULDER

Rhomboid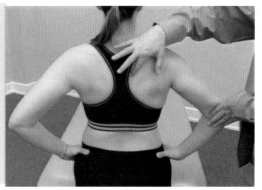

Test rhomboid function by asking the patient to place both hands on the iliac crests. Push the patient's arm forward with your hand at the elbow and palpate the vertebral border of the scapula with the other hand. An intact rhomboid maintains the scapula against the chest wall.

Special Tests

Neer Impingement Sign

The Neer impingement sign is helpful to evaluate the shoulder for impingement or rotator cuff tear. Place one hand on the posterior aspect of the scapula to maintain it in the anatomic position, and use your other hand to take the patient's internally rotated arm by the wrist and place it in full flexion. This maneuver compresses the greater tuberosity against the anterior acromion and elicits discomfort in patients who have a rotator cuff tear or rotator cuff tendinitis. It may also be painful in patients with adhesive capsulitis, anterior instability, or arthritis.

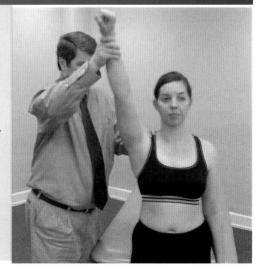

Hawkins Impingement Sign

The Hawkins impingement sign reinforces a positive Neer impingement sign. Flex the patient's shoulder to 90°, flex the elbow to 90°, and place the forearm in neutral rotation. Support the elbow and then internally rotate the humerus. Pain elicited with this test is indicative of rotator cuff tear or rotator cuff tendinitis.

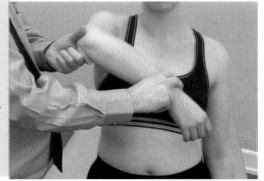

SECTION 2   SHOULDER

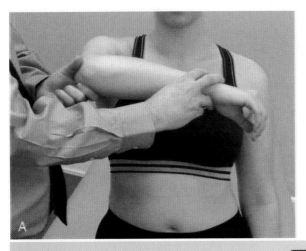
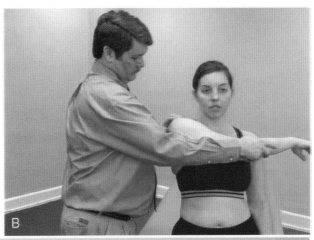

Cross-Body or Horizontal Adduction Test

To perform the cross-body adduction test, flex the patient's shoulder to 90° (**A**) and then horizontally adduct the arm across the patient's body (**B**). Pain over the acromioclavicular joint suggests arthritis of this joint but is also indicative of other acromioclavicular joint pathology, such as a sprain or separation.

Apprehension Sign for Anterior Instability

With the patient supine, place the patient's arm in 90° of abduction with the elbow flexed 90°. Gently externally rotate the forearm to 90°. Patients with anterior instability may display apprehension and report a sense of impending dislocation. A report of pain without apprehension is less specific.

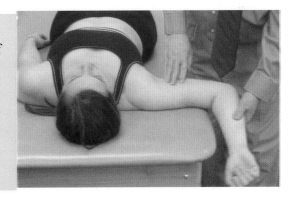

Sulcus Sign

With the patient's arm relaxed at the side, place one hand on the posterior scapula and use your other hand to apply traction to the patient's arm in an inferior direction. In patients with inferior shoulder laxity, this maneuver causes inferior subluxation of the humeral head and a widening of the sulcus between the humerus and acromion. A visible dimple is a positive sulcus sign.

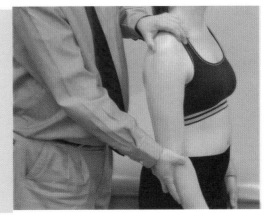

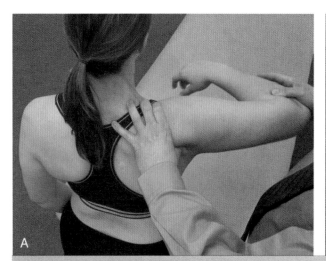
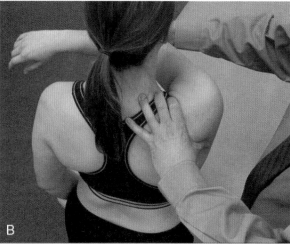

Jerk Test for Posterior Instability ▣◖

To perform the jerk test for posterior instability, place the patient's arm in 90° of flexion and maximum internal rotation with the elbow flexed 90° (**A**). Adduct the arm across the body in the horizontal plane while applying an axial load at the elbow to push the humerus in a posterior direction (**B**). If this maneuver causes a posterior subluxation or dislocation, the humeral head can be felt to "clunk" or jerk back into the joint as the arm is then horizontally abducted.

Relocation Test of Jobe ▣◖

With the patient supine, position the shoulder in 90° of abduction and 90° of external rotation. Then apply a posterior translational force to the anterior proximal humerus at the point of external rotation when the patient feels apprehensive. This application of a posteriorly directed force should prevent anterior subluxation. If this maneuver relieves the patient's apprehension and symptoms, then the test is positive and suggests anterior glenohumeral instability. Removing the posteriorly directed force will cause the patient's apprehension and pain to return.

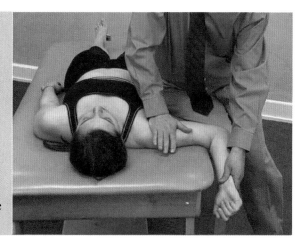

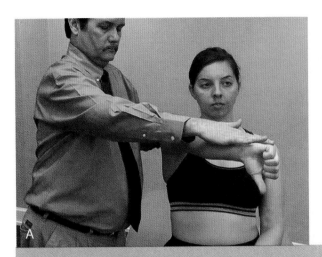
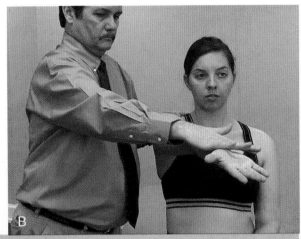

O'Brien Test

Have the seated or standing patient position the arm in 90° of flexion and 20° to 30° of horizontal adduction. Then position the shoulder in full internal rotation and the forearm fully pronated to point the thumb down (**A**). Now ask the patient to maintain this exact position as you apply a downward force to the arm. Then maintain the same position except place the arm in external rotation and the forearm in supination (**B**). Ask the patient to maintain this exact position as you again apply a downward force to the arm. Pain elicited in the first maneuver and reduced or eliminated in the second is a positive test. Pain on top of the shoulder indicates AC joint pathology, while internal shoulder pain is indicative of labral pathology.

Speed Maneuver

Stabilize the patient's arm with one hand and resist active shoulder flexion with the elbow extended and the forearm supinated. If pain occurs in the biceps groove, the test is positive for biceps tendinitis. This test may also be positive if a SLAP (superior labrum anterior to posterior) lesion is present. If profound weakness is present on resisted supination, severe second- or third-degree strain of the distal biceps should be suspected.

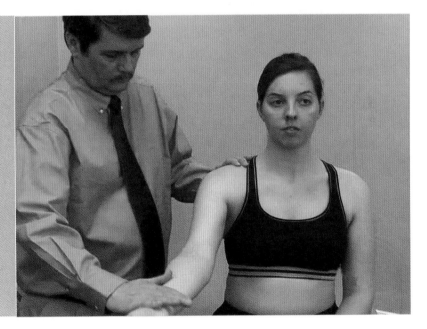

© 2016 American Academy of Orthopaedic Surgeons

Essentials of Musculoskeletal Care 5

SECTION 2   SHOULDER

Jobe Supraspinatus Test and Empty Can Test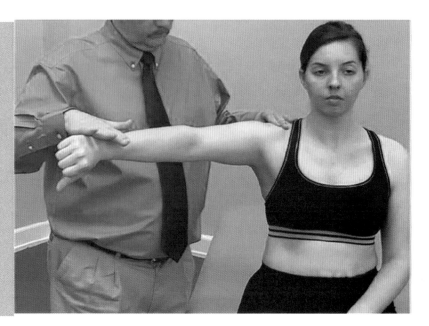

Have the patient sit or stand with the elbow in full extension and the shoulder abducted 90° and horizontally adducted 30° so that the arm is in the scapular plane. Maximally internally rotate the arm so that the thumb is pointed to the floor. Then apply downward pressure to the arm while the patient attempts to resist. Pain and/or weakness suggests supraspinatus weakness or inflammation.

Andrews Anterior Instability Test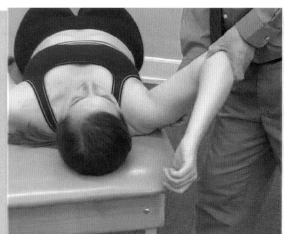

Position the patient supine with the glenohumeral joint slightly over the table edge. Grasp the distal humerus at the elbow and support the arm with the shoulder abducted 90° and externally rotated 60° to 80°. The elbow should be flexed 90°. Place the thumb of your other hand in the axilla on the anterior-inferior humeral head, with your fingers on the posterior aspect of the humeral head. While maintaining elbow flexion and neutral shoulder rotation, apply a posterior force to the humerus as the fingers of your other hand push the humeral head anteriorly. Utilize your thumb to appreciate the amount of anterior translation. Repeat the test as you increase the amount of glenohumeral abduction. As the humerus is abducted, you may feel varying amounts of anterior translation and laxity. If the capsular structures are intact, you should note a firm end point at the end of each anterior levering maneuver. Also compare bilaterally. Lack of a firm end point, patient apprehension and pain, and excessive anterior levering may indicate capsular structure compromise, leading to anterior subluxation.

SECTION 2 SHOULDER

Abdominal Compression Test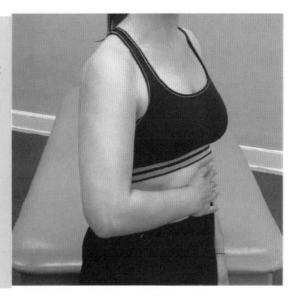

Have the patient stand with the hand on the abdomen, and bring the elbow forward such that there is a straight line from hand to elbow. Inability to maintain this position indicates a positive test.

Acromioclavicular Injuries

Synonyms

Acromioclavicular separation
Shoulder separation

Definition

Acromioclavicular (AC) injuries commonly result from a fall onto the tip of the shoulder. A common example is a fall off a bicycle. When the acromion is driven into the ground, various degrees of ligamentous disruption occur.

These injuries can be classified as one of six types based on the severity of injury and the degree of clavicular separation (**Figure 1**). In type I injuries, the AC joint ligaments are partially disrupted and the strong coracoclavicular (CC) ligaments are intact. As a result, no superior separation of the clavicle from the acromion occurs. In type II injuries, the AC ligaments are torn and the CC ligaments are intact. As a result, partial separation of the clavicle from the acromion occurs. The joint is unstable in the anterior-posterior direction and slightly unstable in the vertical direction. In type III injuries, the CC ligaments are completely disrupted, and the clavicle is completely separated from the acromion. Types IV through VI are uncommon. In these injuries, the periosteum of the clavicle and/or the deltoid and trapezius muscles also are torn, causing wide displacement.

Clinical Symptoms

Patients report pain over the AC joint and pain on lifting the arm. With type III through VI injuries, an obvious deformity is present.

Tests

Physical Examination

The patient supports the arm in an adducted position, and any motion, especially abduction, causes pain. Tenderness to palpation can be elicited over the AC joint. The distal end of the clavicle may be prominent and slightly superior to the acromion in type II injuries, and there is an obvious deformity in type III through VI injuries. Elevating the arm or depressing the clavicle will temporarily reduce the AC joint, except in type IV and V injuries, which have soft-tissue interposition. Type VI injuries are exceedingly rare.

Diagnostic Tests

AP radiographs of both shoulders will confirm type II through VI AC separations. Type I injuries are sprains; therefore, patients have pain and tenderness, but radiographs are normal.

In type II injuries, some AC joint widening can be seen on radiographs and the clavicle is typically displaced superiorly with the inferior border of the clavicle still below the superior border of the acromion. The distance between the clavicle and coracoid remains

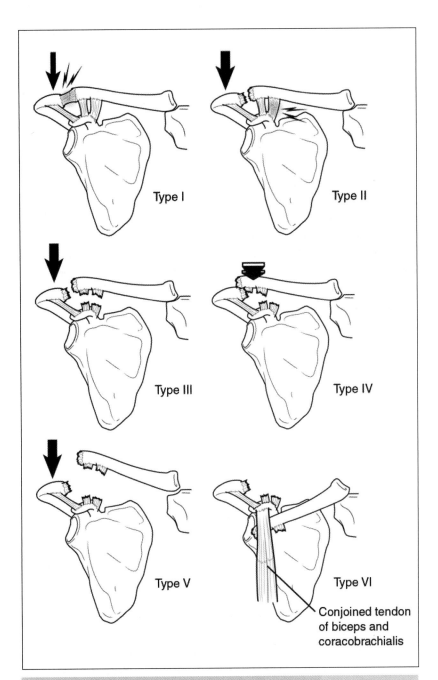

Figure 1 Illustration of classification of acromioclavicular separations. Type I, acromioclavicular (AC) ligament sprain; radiographic findings are normal. Type II, AC joint widening with less than 100% elevation of the AC joint. Type III, 100% superiorly displaced clavicle with increased coracoclavicular (CC) interspace. Type IV, superior and posterior clavicular displacement. Type V, 100% to 300% superiorly displaced clavicle with greatly increased CC interspace. Type VI, distal end of the clavicle is in the subacromial or subcoracoid space.

normal in type II injuries. In type III injuries, complete displacement of the clavicle above the superior border of the acromion is seen, as is a 30% to 100% increase in the CC interspace. These injuries can be reduced with gentle upward pressure under the elbow. In

SECTION 2 SHOULDER

type IV injuries, superior displacement of the clavicle may be seen on AP radiographs; an axillary lateral view will clearly show the predominantly posterior displacement.

In type V injuries, the CC interspace is more than twice as large as the opposite shoulder without the application of weights. These injuries are not reducible. The inferior border of the clavicle is displaced superiorly between 100% and 300% above the superior border of the acromion.

Type VI injuries are rare. With these injuries, the distal end of the clavicle lies in either the subacromial space or the subcoracoid space.

Differential Diagnosis

- Fracture of the acromion (evident on radiographs)
- Fracture of the end of the clavicle (evident on radiographs)
- Rotator cuff tear (most tenderness over the greater tuberosity, not the AC joint; no visible deformity or radiographic findings)

Adverse Outcomes of the Disease

Deformity, weakness on lifting the arm, chronic shoulder pain, and numbness in the arm are possible. Weakness is typical with forward pushing or bench-press maneuvers. Pain is noted either over the AC joint or the medial and superior border of the scapula. Arthritis of the AC joint can eventually develop.

Treatment

Nonsurgical treatment of type I and II injuries consists of wearing a sling for a few days until the pain subsides. Ice is helpful for the first 48 hours, and analgesics can be used to control severe pain. Patients may resume everyday activities as pain allows, with a full return to normal activities and sports within 4 weeks. Treatment of type III injuries is controversial. Most type III injuries can be treated nonsurgically with good functional results. However, surgical repair may be considered in a young manual laborer who does heavy overhead work. In general, type IV, V, and VI injuries require evaluation for surgical repair.

Rehabilitation Consultation

The functional goal of rehabilitation for a patient with an AC injury is to reduce the pain, protect the joint from further damage, and restore function. After the shoulder has been immobilized in a sling for an appropriate period of time (as directed by the referring practitioner), a home exercise program that includes basic pain-free exercises should be started. Exercises for the scapular rotators also are initiated, especially scapular retractions and protractions. The patient should be able to perform the exercises without pain.

Consultation with a rehabilitation professional is often recommended if the patient continues to report pain or limited mobility after performing the home exercise program for

2 to 3 weeks. The assessment should include evaluation of the strength of the glenohumeral and scapular rotators and the mobility of the AC joint. The rehabilitation specialist also should supervise the home exercise program to ensure that the patient is using proper technique and is not experiencing pain. Mobilization of the AC joint is indicated if joint motion is limited.

Adverse Outcomes of Treatment
Following prolonged immobilization in a sling, stiffness may develop; use of a sling or tape also can cause skin breakdown. AC arthritis can be a late sequela of any grade of injury, regardless of treatment.

Referral Decisions/Red Flags
Patients with type IV, V, or VI injuries; some athletes (baseball throwers and football quarterbacks on an individual basis); and laborers with type III injuries may be candidates for early surgical repair. Injuries that remain painful warrant further evaluation.

SECTION 2 SHOULDER

Home Exercise Program for Acromioclavicular Injuries

- Perform the exercises in the order listed.
- To prevent inflammation, apply a bag of crushed ice or frozen peas to the shoulder for 20 minutes after performing all the exercises.
- You should not experience any pain with the exercises. If you are unable to perform any of the exercises because of pain or stiffness, call your doctor.
- The following exercise program is introductory only, and progression of this program will vary based on your specific injury, symptoms, and baseline level of fitness. For further progression of this routine, your physician may recommend evaluation and treatment by a physical therapist or other exercise professional.

Home Exercise Program for Acromioclavicular Injuries

Exercise Type	Muscle Group	Number of Repetitions/Sets	Number of Days per Week	Number of Weeks
Active-assisted glenohumeral flexion	Deltoid and supraspinatus	10 repetitions/3 times per day	2	2 to 3
External rotation	Infraspinatus Teres minor	8 to 10 repetitions/2 sets, progressing to 15 repetitions/3 sets	3	2 to 3
Internal rotation	Subscapularis Teres major	8 to 10 repetitions/2 sets, progressing to 15 repetitions/3 sets	3	2 to 3
Scapular retraction/ protraction	Middle trapezius Serratus	8 to 10 repetitions/2 sets, progressing to 15 repetitions/3 sets	3	2 to 3

Active-Assisted Glenohumeral Flexion

- While lying on your back, interlock your fingers and slowly raise both arms over your head. Use the unaffected arm to assist in raising the affected arm.
- Range of motion likely will be limited initially (compared with the unaffected side), but should gradually improve over a number of days to weeks.
- Stretch only to the limit of comfort and hold for 5 seconds. Repeat 10 times. Perform 3 times per day.

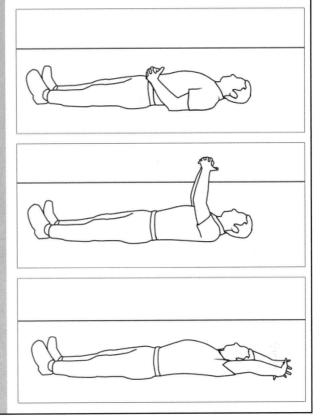

External Rotation

- Lie on your side on a firm, flat surface with the unaffected arm under you, cradling your head.
- Hold the affected arm against your side as shown, with the elbow bent at a 90° angle.
- Slowly rotate the arm at the shoulder, keeping the elbow bent and against your side, to raise the weight to a vertical position; then slowly lower the weight to the starting position to a count of 5.
- Begin with weights that allow 2 sets of 8 to 10 repetitions (approximately 1 to 2 pounds), and progress to 3 sets of 15 repetitions.
- Add weight in 1-pound increments to a maximum of 5 pounds, starting over at 2 sets of 8 to 10 repetitions each time weight is added.
- Perform the exercise 3 days per week, continuing for 2 to 3 weeks.

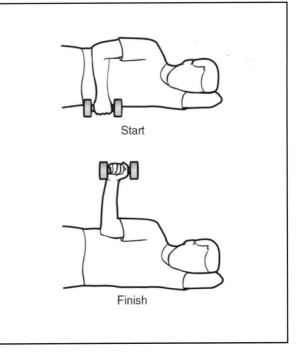

Start

Finish

SECTION 2 SHOULDER

Internal Rotation

- Lie on your side on a firm, flat surface with the affected arm under you and with a pillow or folded cloth under your head to keep your spine straight.
- Hold the affected arm against your side as shown, with the elbow bent at 90°.
- Slowly rotate the arm at the shoulder, keeping the elbow bent and against your torso, to raise the weight to a vertical position; then slowly lower the weight to the starting position.
- Begin with weights that allow 2 sets of 8 to 10 repetitions, and progress to 3 sets of 15 repetitions.
- Add weight in 1-pound increments to a maximum of 5 pounds, starting over at 2 sets of 8 to 10 repetitions each time weight is added.
- Perform the exercise 3 days per week, continuing for 2 to 3 weeks.

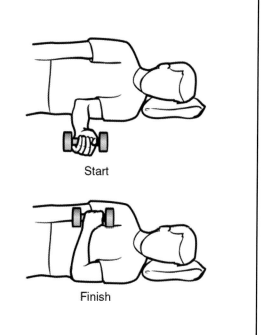

Start

Finish

Scapular Retraction/Protraction

- Lie on your stomach on a table or bed with the affected arm hanging over the side.
- Keeping the elbow straight, lift the weight slowly by moving the scapula toward the opposite side as far as possible. Do not shrug the shoulder. Then return slowly to the starting position.
- Begin with a weight that allows 2 sets of 8 to 10 repetitions without pain, and progress to 3 sets of 15 repetitions.
- Add weight in 1-pound increments to a maximum of 5 pounds, starting over at 2 sets of 8 to 10 repetitions each time weight is added.
- Perform the exercise 3 days per week, continuing for 2 to 3 weeks.

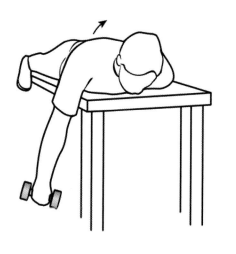

SECTION 2   SHOULDER

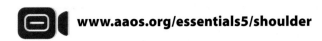
Procedure: Acromioclavicular Joint Injection

Step 1
Place the patient in the upright seated position. Stand behind the patient on the side of the shoulder to be injected. Palpate the acromioclavicular (AC) joint. The Neviaser portal, which lies at the intersection of the posterior aspect of the clavicle and the anterior aspect of the scapular spine, marks the posterior aspect of the AC joint. Use a pen to mark the location of the AC joint for injection.

Step 2
Examine the AP radiograph of the shoulder to determine the direction of the AC joint. In most patients, the joint is oriented superolateral to inferomedial.

Step 3
Wipe the top of the bottles of medication with an alcohol swab. Open a set of sterile gloves, and use the wrapper as a sterile field. Place the syringe and the needles on the wrapper.

Step 4
Prepare the AC joint with a fairly wide field. Don the gloves in sterile fashion and use one needle to draw up 3 mL of lidocaine, 3 mL of bupivacaine, and 3 mL of 40 mg/mL triamcinolone acetonide. Replace the needle, then palpate the AC joint with your nondominant hand while holding the syringe in your dominant hand.

Step 5
Place the needle into the joint in the predetermined direction (**Figure 1**). Pass the needle completely through the AC joint into the subacromial space and inject a portion of the medication into the subacromial space, then slowly withdraw the needle and inject the remaining medication into the joint.

Step 6
Dress the puncture wound with a sterile adhesive bandage.

Adverse Outcomes

Potential adverse outcomes of the procedure include infection, flare reaction to the cortisone, and fat atrophy. Infection is extremely rare, but erythema, swelling, and severe pain should be evaluated immediately, and if these presentations are concerning, the joint should be aspirated. Occasionally, patients have a temporary increase in pain for a few days after injection; this increased pain is associated

Material
- 10-mL syringe
- Two 1¼" 21-gauge needles
- Two antiseptic prepping sticks
- 3 mL of 1% lidocaine
- 3 mL of 0.5% bupivacaine
- 3 mL of 40 mg/mL triamcinolone acetonide
- Alcohol swab
- Adhesive bandage
- Sterile gloves

SECTION 2 SHOULDER

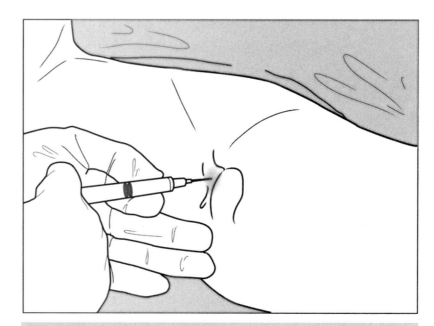

Figure 1 Illustration shows correct placement of the needle for acromioclavicular joint injection.

with a flare reaction that often settles down with the use of ice and NSAIDs. Subcutaneous injection of the steroid solution should be avoided because it may result in fat atrophy or depigmentation of the skin.

Aftercare/Patient Instructions

After injection, the patient should refrain from heavy lifting activities for 1 or 2 days, after which the patient can return to normal activities. The patient should be alert for swelling, erythema, or excessive pain.

Arthritis of the Shoulder

Synonym
Glenohumeral arthritis

Definition
Arthritis of the shoulder is characterized by destruction of joint cartilage with pain and loss of joint space and function (**Figure 1**). Like arthritis in other joints, glenohumeral arthritis generally affects patients older than 50 years and occurs as a result of many etiologies, including osteoarthritis, rheumatoid arthritis, and posttraumatic arthritis. Less common causes include osteonecrosis, infection, seronegative spondyloarthropathies, and rotator cuff tear arthropathy (a type of arthritis that results from large, long-standing rotator cuff tears) (**Figure 2**).

Clinical Symptoms
Patients report diffuse or deep-seated pain but most often localize the worst pain to the posterior aspect of the shoulder. Initially, the pain is aggravated by any strenuous activity. As the disease progresses, any movement of the shoulder causes pain, and pain at rest and at night are reported. Night pain is usually positional.

Along with pain, range of motion is progressively limited. Activities of daily living, such as dressing, combing the hair, and reaching overhead, are increasingly difficult.

Osteoarthritis involves a single joint in an older patient, whereas multiple and symmetric joint involvement and a positive rheumatoid factor suggest rheumatoid arthritis. There is no apparent relationship

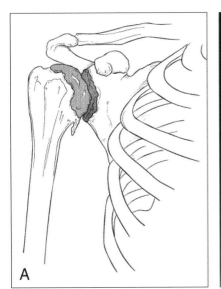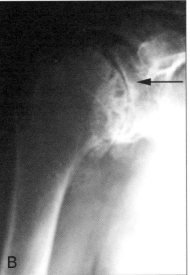

Figure 1 Illustration (**A**) and AP radiograph (**B**) show osteoarthritis of the shoulder. Note cystic changes, sclerosis, and decreased joint space (arrow).

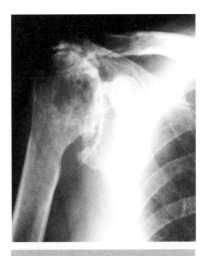

Figure 2 AP radiograph of a shoulder with end-stage rotator cuff arthropathy demonstrates superior migration of the humeral head.

SECTION 2 SHOULDER

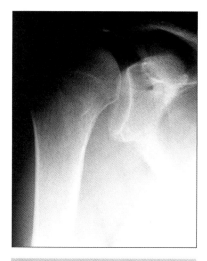

Figure 3 AP radiograph of a shoulder demonstrates superior migration of the humeral head secondary to a chronic rotator cuff tear.

between the development of osteoarthritis in the shoulder and the patient's previous level of physical activity. A history of previous fracture or dislocation, however, suggests posttraumatic arthritis or osteonecrosis. Superior migration of the humeral head (**Figure 3**) develops in association with long-standing rotator cuff tears, which results in eccentric loading of the glenoid and results in rotator cuff tear arthropathy.

Tests
Physical Examination
Examination may reveal generalized atrophy of the muscles about the shoulder. Swelling within the shoulder joint is not common; when present, it is difficult to detect. Palpation elicits tenderness over the front and back of the shoulder. Bone-on-bone crepitus is commonly present with rotation or flexion of the shoulder. Range of motion is usually decreased. Both active and passive motion are typically decreased equally. Patients with concomitant rotator cuff tears often have less active than passive range of motion.

Diagnostic Tests
AP and axillary radiographs of the shoulder are indicated. The axillary view most reliably demonstrates the joint space narrowing that indicates cartilage destruction. Other radiographic findings that support a diagnosis of osteoarthritis include flattening of the humeral head, an inferior osteophyte, and posterior erosion of the glenoid. Rheumatoid arthritis is suggested by the presence of periarticular erosions, osteopenia, and central wear of the glenoid. Superior migration of the humeral head suggests a large rotator cuff deficiency.

Differential Diagnosis
- Adhesive capsulitis (normal radiographs)
- Charcot arthropathy (gross destruction of the joint without trauma and relatively little pain)
- Fracture of the humerus (history of trauma, evident on radiographs)
- Herniated cervical disk (unilateral or bilateral radicular pain, positive Spurling test)
- Infection (acute onset, systemic symptoms, elevated white blood cell count)
- Rotator cuff tear (normal radiographs, pain mostly with overhead use)
- Tumor of the shoulder girdle (variable presentation, radiographic lesion)

Adverse Outcomes of the Disease
Chronic shoulder pain and loss of strength and motion can develop. Severe loss of strength and motion can be difficult to recover, even with joint replacement surgery.

Treatment

Nonsurgical treatment is recommended initially, including the use of NSAIDs and the application of heat and/or ice to relieve symptoms, as well as gentle stretching exercises to preserve motion. A trial of glucosamine and/or chondroitin sulfate can be considered, but their efficacy has not been definitively established. Activity modifications are beneficial in reducing pain. Corticosteroid injections may provide relief, particularly in some patients with inflammatory (rheumatoid) arthritis. Corticosteroid injections should be limited to 2 to 3 per joint because cortisone can have a detrimental effect on rotator cuff tendons. Arthroscopy with débridement and capsular release may provide improvement in patients with mild to moderate disease and relatively preserved motion.

For advanced arthritis, total shoulder replacement or hemiarthroplasty (the choice of which procedure to use remains controversial) offer a very satisfactory solution, even in younger patients (aged 30 to 50 years) who do not use their shoulders for strenuous activities. Manual laborers may be better served by glenohumeral arthrodesis because the heavy demands placed on their shoulders often result in early loosening of the prosthetic components.

Adverse Outcomes of Treatment

Addiction to narcotic pain medication is a possibility, so narcotics should be used only for short-term postoperative pain relief; alternatives should be considered when treating patients with chronic pain secondary to arthritis. NSAIDs may cause gastric, renal, and hepatic complications. In 2015, the FDA strengthened its warning linking NSAIDs with the risk of heart attack or stroke, even in the first weeks of use of an NSAID. Corticosteroid injection has a small risk of causing an infection in the joint that may preclude or compromise later joint arthroplasty. Patients who undergo shoulder replacement surgery may experience perioperative complications, including limb thrombophlebitis and possible embolus.

Referral Decisions/Red Flags

Patients with intolerable shoulder pain and/or a progressive loss of motion that does not respond to at least 3 months of nonsurgical treatment require further evaluation. In some cases, surgery may be indicated.

SECTION 2 SHOULDER

Burners and Other Brachial Plexus Injuries

Synonyms

Brachial plexopathy

Stingers

Definition

Brachial plexus injuries include a broad array of neurologic dysfunction around the shoulder, ranging from momentary paresthesias to flail upper extremity. The mechanism of injury is equally diverse, from high-energy motor vehicle crashes, falls from a height, and gunshot wounds to lower energy injuries such as athletic injuries.

Burners or stingers (transient brachial plexopathy) are transient stretch injuries to the upper trunk of the brachial plexus involving the C5 and C6 nerve roots. The most common mechanism of injury is a traction force that occurs when the shoulder is forcefully depressed and the head and neck are tilted toward the opposite side or by compression of the upper plexus between a shoulder pad and the scapula. These injuries are relatively common among college and professional athletes in contact sports, especially American football.

Brachial plexus injuries involving axonal disruption are further categorized as occurring proximal to the dorsal root ganglion in the spinal foramen (preganglionic) or anywhere distal to the ganglion (postganglionic) (**Figure 1**). This distinction is important because surgical repair is not possible and the prognosis for recovery is poor for preganglionic root avulsions.

Clinical Symptoms

Symptoms of a brachial plexus injury depend on the position of the plexus when it is injured. The mechanism of injury to the upper and middle trunks (C5, C6, and C7) involves a direct blow to the top of the shoulder accompanied by tilt of the head in the opposite direction, causing traction on the plexus with the arm adducted at the side. Lower trunk injuries (C8, T1) occur when these nerves are stretched with the arm abducted, as when grabbing onto a ledge when falling from a height. Injuries involving the entire plexus result from extreme traction from high-energy trauma.

A typical presentation is a football player injured by a direct blow to the head, neck, or shoulder. The classic symptom is sharp, burning shoulder pain that radiates down the arm in the affected nerve root distribution. Weakness is common, and the patient often is seen holding the affected arm, which often is hanging at the side. Burners last seconds to minutes, although some lasting several weeks have been reported.

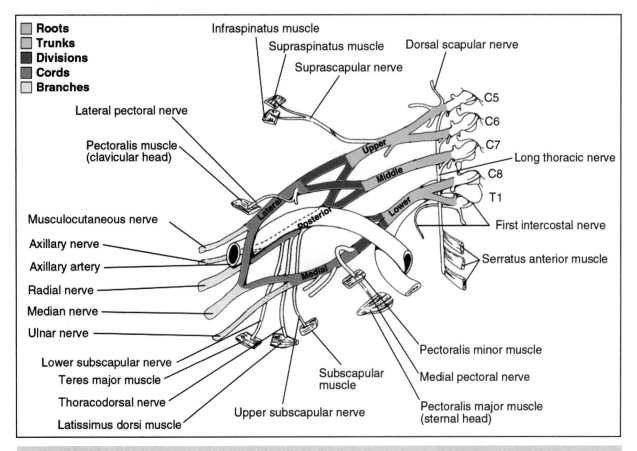

Figure 1 Illustration of the brachial plexus. (Adapted from Thompson WO, Warren RF, Barnes RP, Hunt S: Shoulder injuries, in Schenck RC Jr, ed: *Athletic Training and Sports Medicine*, ed 3. Rosemont, IL, American Academy of Orthopaedic Surgeons, 1999, pp 219-291.)

Tests

Physical Examination

A neurologic examination is the cornerstone of an accurate diagnosis. At a minimum, sensation to light touch, motor power, and deep tendon reflexes should be tested. Deficits should be mapped out by nerve root and peripheral nerve distribution. The neurologic examination also includes evaluation of the lower extremities because spasticity or weakness in the ipsilateral leg suggests a concomitant spinal cord injury.

Injuries to C8 and T1 are more likely to be preganglionic, which is confirmed by the presence of an ipsilateral ptosis, myosis, anhidrosis, and enophthalmos (Horner syndrome). Because the dorsal scapular nerve and the long thoracic nerve arise from the C5 and C5 through C7 nerve roots, respectively, intact function of the rhomboids and serratus anterior muscles in upper plexus injuries indicates that the injury is distal to these nerves and therefore postganglionic.

Examination of the neck (with cervical spine precautions if indicated) and shoulder, as well as a general examination, is indicated to rule out associated injuries such as cervical spine fractures or disk herniations; clavicle, scapula, or humerus fractures; and scapulothoracic dissociation.

As with other plexus injuries, the sideline evaluation of a burner should include the cervical spine and a neurologic examination of the extremities. Bilateral upper extremity burners or radicular symptoms into the legs should be treated as a spinal cord injury until proved otherwise.

Diagnostic Tests

Radiographs should be obtained if injury to the cervical spine or shoulder girdle is suspected. Although some controversy still exists, many experts suggest that anyone experiencing a burner or stinger should be evaluated with cervical spine radiographs, including flexion and extension lateral views, to rule out instability, congenital anomaly, or cervical stenosis (assessed by the relative width of the cervical body and the spinal canal). MRI is helpful in patients with abnormal plain radiographs or when symptoms persist.

Differential Diagnosis

- Cervical spine fracture or instability (evident on radiographs)
- Peripheral nerve injury (isolated weakness or sensory deficit confined to a specific nerve distribution)
- Transient quadriplegia (neurapraxia of the cervical spinal cord producing bilateral paresthesias and weakness)

Adverse Outcomes of the Disease

Burners resolve spontaneously, although recurrent episodes may suggest cervical stenosis and an associated increased risk for catastrophic spinal cord injury. Depending on the location and severity of a brachial plexus injury, persistent pain, sensory loss, paresthesias, and weakness, paralysis, or even amputation is possible.

Treatment

The resolution of pain and neurologic symptoms, as well as a normal neurologic examination and full range of cervical spine motion, is required before an athlete with a burner is allowed to return to play. Athletes with prolonged or bilateral symptoms or recurrent episodes should not return to play without further evaluation.

Treatment options for more severe brachial plexus injuries vary, including nonsurgical measures and several surgical repair and reconstruction procedures. Nonsurgical management is aimed at strengthening and stretching exercises and splinting to maintain passive range of motion of the joints affected by muscle paralysis or weakness, protection of anesthetic areas of skin, and pain relief. Referral to a pain clinic is often helpful in this regard.

Adverse Outcomes of Treatment

The effectiveness of therapy, splinting, and pain control must be monitored frequently. Although surgical techniques are continuously evolving, the prognosis for severe brachial plexus injuries, especially root avulsions, remains guarded.

Referral Decisions/Red Flags

Any injury that is persistent, recurrent, bilateral, or associated with other concomitant injuries requires further evaluation. Cervical spine precautions should be followed if a cervical injury is suspected.

SECTION 2 SHOULDER

Fracture of the Clavicle

Synonym
Collarbone fracture

Definition
Clavicle fractures are the most common bony injury. The most commonly used classification of clavicle fractures is based on anatomic location (middle third, distal third, proximal third) rather than treatment rationale (**Figure 1**). The most common location of injury is the middle third of the clavicle. Approximately 80% occur in this location, 15% occur in the distal third, and 5% involve the proximal third.

Clinical Symptoms
Patients typically report a history of substantial injury, such as falling on the shoulder or being struck over the clavicle with a heavy object. Shoulder motion and strength are limited by pain in the affected extremity. A bony deformity is often seen, as well as shoulder droop.

Tests
Physical Examination
Examination typically reveals an obvious deformity, or bump, at the fracture site. Gentle pressure over the fracture site will elicit pain, and a grinding sensation can be felt when the patient attempts to raise the

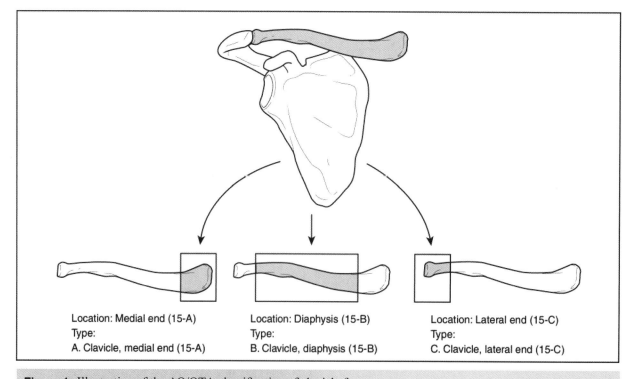

Location: Medial end (15-A)
Type:
A. Clavicle, medial end (15-A)

Location: Diaphysis (15-B)
Type:
B. Clavicle, diaphysis (15-B)

Location: Lateral end (15-C)
Type:
C. Clavicle, lateral end (15-C)

Figure 1 Illustration of the AO/OTA classification of clavicle fractures.

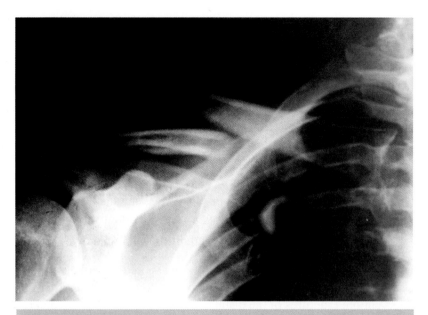

Figure 2 AP radiograph demonstrates a fracture of the middle third of the clavicle.

arm. The skin may appear tented over a fracture fragment, but the fragment rarely penetrates the skin to create an open fracture. Assess neurologic function distal to the fracture, including the axillary, musculocutaneous, median, ulnar, and radial nerves. Check the radial pulse and capillary refill.

Diagnostic Tests
AP and 10° cephalic tilt views of the clavicle will confirm most clavicle fractures (**Figure 2**). Fractures or dislocations at the medial end of the clavicle are uncommon and are often difficult to see on plain radiographs, so if there is a high index of suspicion for a clavicle fracture, CT should be performed.

Differential Diagnosis
- Acromioclavicular separation (deformity near the tip of the shoulder)
- Sternoclavicular dislocation (deformity at the sternoclavicular junction)

Adverse Outcomes of the Disease
Overall, nonunion is rare, occurring in 1% to 4% of patients. In select patient populations, including older patients with more comminuted fractures, nonunion rates can increase to 40% to 50%. Some degree of malunion is common, and a visible lump can occur, even when the fracture is well approximated. This lump may be of cosmetic concern to some patients but has little functional importance. Neurovascular complications may occur on an early or delayed basis. Rarely, clavicle fractures can result in shoulder deformity.

SECTION 2   SHOULDER

Treatment

Most midshaft clavicle fractures are treated nonsurgically. Treatment with a figure-of-8 strap should be followed closely for possible neurovascular compression or skin breakdown from strap compression overlying the fracture site. Support for 3 to 4 weeks is adequate for a child younger than 12 years, whereas 6 to 8 weeks may be required for an adult. After 2 to 3 weeks, the patient is encouraged to begin gentle shoulder exercises as pain allows. Surgical treatment should be considered for severely shortened middle third fractures, open fractures, or fractures associated with neurovascular injury or severe injury to the ipsilateral chest, such as rib fractures or flail chest. Comminuted, highly displaced fractures are also relative indications for surgery, especially in older patients, because the risk for nonunion increases in this population. Fractures with scapulothoracic dissociation or floating shoulder (ipsilateral clavicle and scapular fracture) also should be considered for surgical intervention. Fractures of the distal third of the clavicle just medial to the coracoclavicular ligaments in which the medial part of the clavicle is significantly superiorly displaced are associated with a higher rate of nonunion because the proximal fragments buttonhole through the fascia. Surgical intervention may be indicated in these cases as well.

Adverse Outcomes of Treatment

Pressure over the nerves and vessels in the armpit from a tight clavicle strap may cause numbness and paresthesias in the arm, which are usually transient but may persist. Surgical treatment of clavicle fractures is associated with a high complication rate. The particular complication depends on the type of surgery but could include infection, neurovascular injury, hardware complication, or skin breakdown.

Referral Decisions/Red Flags

Painful nonunion after 4 months of treatment requires further evaluation. Patients with widely displaced lateral or midshaft clavicle fractures or with segmental fractures have a greater risk of nonunion and should be evaluated for possible surgical treatment.

Fracture of the Humeral Shaft

Definition

Fractures of the humeral shaft often result from a direct blow to the arm, such as occurs in a motor vehicle accident, or from a fall on the outstretched hand (**Figure 1**). These fractures also can result from sports activities involving a fall or a direct blow. Most of these fractures can be treated nonsurgically, with a rate of union of almost 100%.

Clinical Symptoms

Severe pain, swelling, and deformity are characteristic of a displaced fracture of the humerus. With gentle palpation and movement of the arm, it is often possible to detect motion at the fracture site. Radial nerve injuries are associated with this fracture. If the radial nerve has been injured, patients will be unable to extend the wrist or fingers and may have loss of sensation over the back of the hand. Rarely, the nerve becomes trapped within the fracture (**Figure 2**).

Tests

Physical Examination

Examination reveals marked swelling and contusion. Look for puncture wounds in the skin near the fracture site, which indicate an open fracture. Assess neurologic function distal to the fracture, including the median, radial, and ulnar nerves. Check the radial pulse and record the color and temperature of the hand. The shoulder and elbow should be evaluated for pain, tenderness, and swelling or

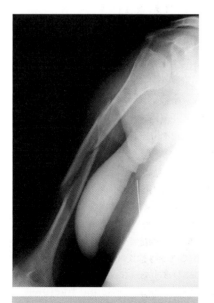

Figure 1 AP radiograph of a midshaft humeral fracture.

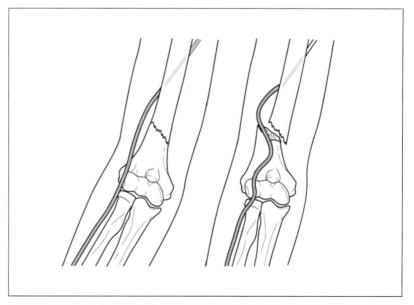

Figure 2 Illustration of radial nerve entrapment at the fracture site.

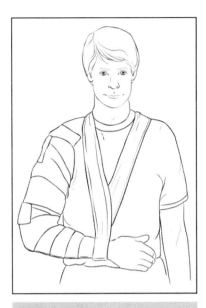

Figure 3 Illustration of a coaptation splint.

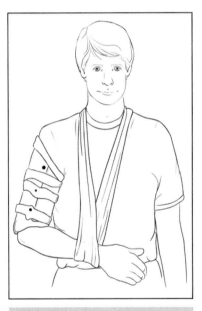

Figure 4 Illustration of a humeral fracture brace.

deformity because concomitant injury proximal or distal to the shaft fracture can be easily missed in the acute setting.

Diagnostic Tests
AP and lateral radiographs confirm the diagnosis. These views also should include both the shoulder and elbow joints.

Differential Diagnosis
• Fracture of the distal humerus (evident on radiographs)
• Fracture of the proximal humerus (evident on AP and lateral radiographs)
• Ruptured biceps tendon (swelling localized to biceps muscle)

Adverse Outcomes of the Disease
Radial nerve injury, indicated by weakness in the wrist or finger or thumb extensors and numbness in the first dorsal web space, is possible. Injury to the brachial plexus or vascular system also may occur. Healing of the fracture with angulation is common but results in minimal functional impairment unless the angulation is severe. Nonunion is possible but uncommon. Persistent stiffness in the shoulder and elbow can be a problem.

Treatment
Most humeral shaft fractures are treated nonsurgically, with up to 20° of apex anterior or apex lateral angulation being acceptable. Fractures with minimal shortening (2 cm or less) can be treated with a U-shaped coaptation splint for 2 weeks (**Figure 3**), followed by a humeral fracture brace (**Figure 4**). A coaptation splint is applied as follows: place 12 thicknesses of plaster or a commercially available prepackaged splint in a U-shaped fashion. Begin at the axilla, being careful that the medial end of the splinting material is not at the level of the fracture, and continue around the elbow, extending to the top of the shoulder. Splint material is held in place with an elastic bandage. A collar and cuff made from stockinette can be used to support the forearm and wrist. Alternatively, a simple sling can be used. Instruct the patient to exercise the fingers, wrist, and elbow at least three times per day. Allow the patient to flex the elbow as tolerated and to extend the elbow fully as pain allows. The patient may need to sleep sitting in a chair to maintain fracture alignment. The coaptation splint may need to be reapplied during these first 2 weeks. After 2 weeks, the patient is fitted with a humeral fracture brace, which is worn for at least the next 6 weeks or until radiographic evidence of healing is seen. During this time, continue to encourage range-of-motion exercises for the shoulder, elbow, wrist, and hand.

The indications for surgical treatment with open reduction and internal fixation include open fractures, fractures associated with neurovascular injury, pathologic fractures, nonunions, and fractures that cannot be controlled by closed techniques. Ipsilateral forearm and humeral fractures resulting in a "floating elbow," in which the

SECTION 2   SHOULDER

radius and ulna are fractured along with the humerus, also require surgical treatment. Multiple extremity trauma also can be an indication for open reduction and internal fixation of the humerus because it may allow earlier weight bearing through the extremity, improving patient mobility.

Radial nerve injuries associated with fractures of the humerus should be observed. Within 6 months, 95% of patients will regain nerve function. During this period of observation, the patient should be fitted with a wrist splint and receive instruction in stretching exercises to avoid flexion contractures of the wrist and fingers. Electromyography is indicated if radial nerve function does not return after 6 weeks. This provides a baseline for later comparison.

Adverse Outcomes of Treatment

Rarely, radial nerve injury occurs after manipulation. Stiffness of the shoulder and elbow, and discomfort and/or skin irritation from the splint are possible.

Referral Decisions/Red Flags

Patients who have one of the following conditions require further evaluation: associated vascular injury; an open fracture; a segmental fracture; a floating elbow; nonunion following 3 months of treatment; an associated head injury, seizure disorder, or multiple injuries; a pathologic fracture; failure to control alignment after closed reduction; or skin breakdown under the fracture brace.

SECTION 2 SHOULDER

Fracture of the Proximal Humerus

Synonyms

Humeral head fracture
Shoulder fracture
Surgical neck fracture

Definition

Fractures of the proximal humerus occur primarily in two groups: young patients, and elderly patients with osteoporosis, especially women. Most fractures are minimally displaced and can be treated with a sling and early motion.

These fractures are classified according to which segments of the proximal humerus are fractured and the amount of displacement (**Figure 1**). The four segments are the greater tuberosity (the bony prominence that provides attachment for the supraspinatus, infraspinatus, and teres minor muscles), the lesser tuberosity (the attachment site for the subscapularis), the humeral head, and the shaft. The most common two-part fracture occurs at the surgical neck (the region just distal to the tuberosities). Other two-part fractures include fracture at the anatomic neck, isolated fracture of the greater

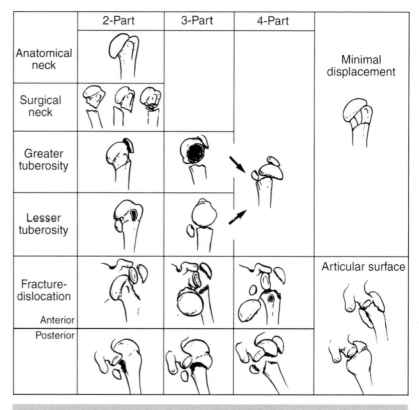

Figure 1 Illustration of the Neer classification of proximal humerus fractures.

tuberosity, and isolated fracture of the lesser tuberosity. Three-part fractures involve the humeral head, the shaft, and one of the tuberosities. Four-part fractures involve all four components of the proximal humerus. Three- and four-part fractures are severe injuries that are fortunately uncommon. In general, surgical fixation is indicated if any one of these parts is fractured with greater than 1 cm displacement or greater than 45° angulation to its normal anatomic position. Displacement of the surgical neck is well tolerated, but tuberosity displacement of even 0.5 cm may be symptomatic.

Clinical Symptoms

Patients typically have severe pain, swelling, and bruising around the upper arm, the shoulder, and even the forearm following an injury such as from a fall. The pain is worse with even the slightest movement of the arm. If the patient reports a loss of feeling in the arm, a nerve injury is more likely. If the forearm and hand appear pale, the axillary artery may have been injured.

Tests

Physical Examination

Examination reveals swelling and discoloration around the shoulder and upper arm. Assess neurologic function distal to the fracture, including the axillary, musculocutaneous, median, radial, and ulnar nerves. Check the radial pulse and capillary refill as well.

Diagnostic Tests

A trauma series of radiographs of the shoulder should include a true AP and an axillary lateral view to establish the relationship between the humeral head and the glenoid (**Figure 2**). Several techniques are available to obtain an axillary view in a patient with a painful shoulder. If the axillary view is not possible, a transscapular lateral view (also called the scapular Y view) should be obtained. Great care must be taken in interpreting the AP and the scapular Y views because errors occur more easily with these views (**Figure 3**). The most common error is missed diagnosis of an associated shoulder dislocation because of inadequate radiographs. AP views alone are insufficient to document an associated shoulder dislocation.

Differential Diagnosis

• Acromioclavicular (AC) separation (pain localized to the AC joint)
• Rotator cuff tear (weakness with elevation and external rotation, normal radiographs)
• Rupture of the long head of the biceps tendon (asymmetric bulge of arm musculature with biceps contraction)
• Shoulder dislocation (evident on AP and lateral radiographs of the glenohumeral joint)

SECTION 2 SHOULDER

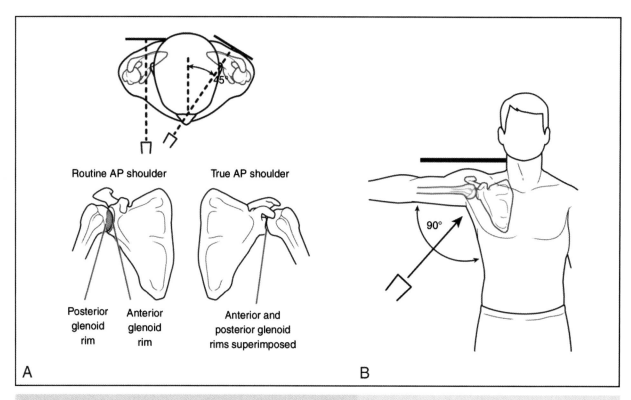

Figure 2 Illustration depicts routine and true AP (**A**) and axillary lateral (**B**) radiographic views of the shoulder.

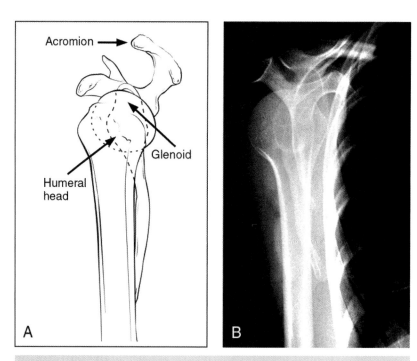

Figure 3 Transscapular lateral view of the shoulder. Illustration (**A**) and radiograph (**B**). (Panel B is reproduced from Frymoyer JW, ed: *Orthopaedic Knowledge Update 4*. Rosemont, IL, American Academy of Orthopaedic Surgeons, 1993, p 286.)

SECTION 2 SHOULDER

Adverse Outcomes of the Disease

Chronic pain, along with loss of motion, and nerve and vascular injury are possible. Nonunion or malunion can also occur. Patients may also have posttraumatic arthritis and/or osteonecrosis of the humeral head.

Treatment

Patients with minimally displaced (less than 1 cm) fractures can be treated safely with a sling and, after approximately 3 weeks, can often begin an exercise program consisting of pendulum and circumduction exercises. Isometric exercises of the deltoid and rotator cuff also are encouraged after 6 weeks when radiographic signs of healing are seen. Early range of motion is important because disabling stiffness is very common, especially in the elderly, but overaggressive exercise should be avoided because of the risk of nonunion. After 3 weeks, the sling can be worn part time, or it can be removed if pain is minimal.

Two-part fractures in which the greater tuberosity is separated more than 0.5 cm require surgical repair to restore normal function of the rotator cuff muscles. If the patient has a two-part fracture in which the lesser tuberosity is fractured, an associated posterior dislocation also is possible. Displaced two-part fractures through the humeral neck and displaced three- and four-part fractures require consideration for surgical treatment. Displaced four-part fractures disrupt the blood supply to the humeral head and in most cases require prosthetic replacement of the proximal humerus rather than internal fixation of the fracture.

Adverse Outcomes of Treatment

Nonunion and malunion are both possible. Patients often report persistent stiffness in the shoulder. Undiagnosed shoulder dislocation is also a possibility, especially if insufficient radiographs are obtained.

Referral Decisions/Red Flags

Patients with displaced two-part and all three- and four-part fractures require further evaluation. In addition, patients with associated neurovascular symptoms require further evaluation as soon as possible.

SECTION 2 SHOULDER

Fracture of the Scapula

Synonyms
Fracture of the acromion
Fracture of the coracoid process
Fracture of the shoulder blade
Glenoid fracture

Definition
Scapular fractures result from high-energy trauma such as motorcycle accidents or falls from a substantial height. These fractures may involve the body of the scapula, the glenoid, the acromion, or the coracoid process (**Figure 1**). Ninety percent of patients with scapular fractures have associated injuries, including rib fractures, which are the most common; pneumothorax; pulmonary contusion; and head, spinal cord, and brachial plexus injuries. Because of these associated injuries, scapular fractures are often missed on initial examination.

Clinical Symptoms
Pain and tenderness about the back of the shoulder are the most common symptoms. The patient typically holds the arm securely at the side, and any attempts to actively move the extremity result in pain.

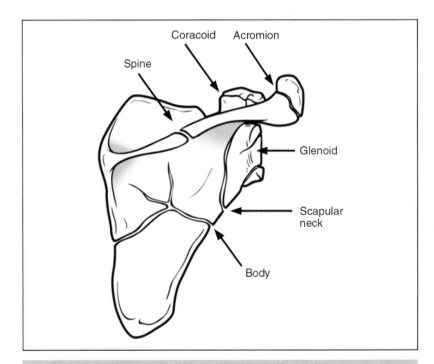

Figure 1 Illustration of fracture patterns in the scapula. (Reproduced from Zuckerman JD, Koval KJ, Cuomo F: Fractures of the scapula. *Instr Course Lect* 1993;42:271-281.)

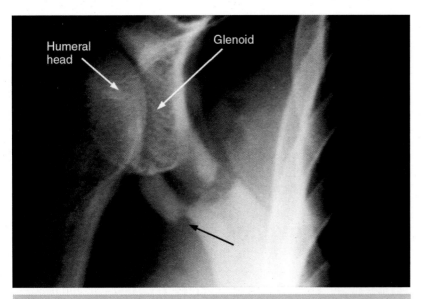

Figure 2 Oblique radiograph of the shoulder demonstrates a fracture of the body of the scapula (black arrow).

Tests

Physical Examination

Skin abrasions, swelling, and ecchymosis over the back of the shoulder are common. Tenderness to gentle palpation over the back of the shoulder or acromion suggests a possible scapular fracture.

Diagnostic Tests

Radiographic visualization of scapular fractures can be difficult. An AP view of the shoulder and a chest radiograph should be obtained. If the patient is cleared to sit upright, a transscapular lateral or oblique radiograph can help diagnose a displaced scapular body fracture (**Figure 2**). The axillary view is more useful in revealing acromial and coracoid fractures. Poorly visualized fractures and any fracture involving the glenoid should be further evaluated using CT.

Differential Diagnosis

- Acromioclavicular (AC) separation (maximum tenderness over the AC joint)
- Fracture of the proximal humerus (radiograph needed to confirm diagnosis)
- Fracture of the rib (evident on plain radiographs of the chest)
- Os acromiale (nontender, no history of trauma, incidental finding on radiographs)
- Shoulder dislocation (deformity of the anterior and lateral shoulder, evident on radiographs)

Adverse Outcomes of the Disease

Persistent loss of motion and chronic pain can occur. Malunion is common but usually asymptomatic. Complications such as suprascapular nerve injury or impingement syndrome are rare.

Treatment

Nonsurgical treatment using a sling is adequate for most patients, followed by early range of motion as tolerated, usually within 1 week of injury. Patients with scapular body fractures should be considered for hospital admission because of the risk of pulmonary contusion.

Adverse Outcomes of Treatment

Prolonged immobilization may result in shoulder stiffness.

Referral Decisions/Red Flags

Patients with displaced (>2 mm) fractures of the glenoid articular surface, fractures of the neck of the scapula with severe angular deformity (>30°), and fractures of the acromion process with impingement syndrome require further evaluation.

Frozen Shoulder

Synonyms
Adhesive capsulitis
Stiff shoulder

Definition
Adhesive capsulitis of the shoulder, commonly called frozen shoulder, is defined as an idiopathic loss of both active and passive motion. It is considered distinct from posttraumatic shoulder stiffness, a condition that is related to a substantial shoulder injury or a surgical procedure.

Frozen shoulder most commonly affects patients between the ages of 40 and 60 years, with no clear predisposition based on arm dominance or occupation. It occurs more frequently in women. Diabetes mellitus, especially type 1, is the most common risk factor. Patients with diabetes tend to be more refractory to treatment, and 40% to 50% will have bilateral involvement. Other conditions related to frozen shoulder include hypothyroidism, Dupuytren disease, cervical disk herniation, Parkinson disease, cerebral hemorrhage, and tumors.

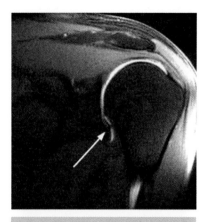

Figure 1 Coronal shoulder MRI demonstrates the contracted capsule, which is the hallmark of a frozen shoulder, and the loss of the inferior pouch (arrow).

Clinical Symptoms
Patients typically progress from an early "freezing" phase of pain and progressive loss of motion to a "thawing" phase of decreasing discomfort associated with a slow but steady improvement in range of motion. The process typically takes 6 months to 2 years or more to resolve, with most patients experiencing minimal long-term pain or functional deficit, although some motion loss may remain.

Tests
Physical Examination
Examination reveals substantial (at least 50%) reduction in both active and passive ranges of motion compared with the opposite, normal shoulder. Loss of external rotation with the arm at the side is consistent with the condition because contracture of the coracohumeral ligament, which limits external rotation, is pathognomonic for frozen shoulder. Motion is painful, especially at the extremes. Pain and tenderness at the deltoid insertion are common. Diffuse tenderness about the shoulder also may be present.

Diagnostic Tests
AP and axillary radiographs of the shoulder are indicated to ensure that smooth, concentric joint surfaces with an intact cartilage space are present and to rule out other pathology such as osteophytes, loose bodies, calcium deposits, or tumors. Other ancillary studies, such as arthrography or magnetic resonance arthrography, can substantiate a frozen shoulder diagnosis by demonstrating a contracted capsule and loss of the inferior pouch (**Figure 1**).

SECTION 2 SHOULDER

Differential Diagnosis

- Chronic posterior shoulder dislocation (evident on axillary radiographs)
- Impingement syndrome (motion preserved and pain primarily with elevation)
- Osteoarthritis (evident on radiographs)
- Posttraumatic shoulder stiffness (history of clear and substantial previous trauma)
- Rotator cuff tear (normal passive range of motion)
- Tumor (rare, but evident on shoulder or ipsilateral chest radiograph)

Adverse Outcomes of the Disease

Residual pain and/or stiffness may persist for years in some patients.

Treatment

NSAIDs, nonnarcotic analgesics, and moist heat are indicated, followed by a gentle stretching program. Often, ice is used after stretching to control swelling. Intra-articular injection of corticosteroid also should be considered, but multiple injections should be avoided. The injection should be performed under fluoroscopic or ultrasonographic guidance to ensure the injection is intra-articular. A transcutaneous electrical nerve stimulation unit (applied by a physical therapist) may help control pain. The patient should be instructed in a home stretching program to be performed within a comfortable range. Advise patients that, on average, a recovery period of 1 to 2 years is to be expected before motion is fully restored and pain is completely relieved. Nonsurgical treatment is successful approximately 80% to 85% of the time. Surgical treatment consists of arthroscopic capsular release.

Rehabilitation Consultation

The functional goal of rehabilitation for a patient with a frozen shoulder is to reduce pain and increase mobility of the glenohumeral joint and scapula. External rotation in the adducted position tends to be the most restricted range of motion associated with frozen shoulder. Pain in the subscapularis area, localized to the scapular fossa, also is very common.

The home exercise program should include stretching in external rotation with the arm at no more than 30° to 45° of abduction. A low-load prolonged shoulder stretching device may be ordered for home use to promote passive external rotation; however, the indication for this device is supported by limited research evidence. Forced stretching in any direction should be avoided. Strengthening exercises are initiated after the inflammation and painful period of frozen shoulder has subsided and should include strengthening of the glenohumeral joint and scapular rotators.

The rehabilitation assessment should include evaluation of the mobility of the glenohumeral joint and scapular mobility and posture. Research supports the effectiveness of mobilization of the glenohumeral joint to increase range of motion.

Adverse Outcomes of Treatment

NSAIDs may cause gastric, renal, and hepatic complications. In 2015, the FDA strengthened its warning linking NSAIDs with the risk of heart attack or stroke, even in the first weeks of use of an NSAID. Therapy that is too aggressive may aggravate symptoms and/or cause a fracture of the humerus.

Referral Decisions/Red Flags

If substantial improvement in pain and motion is not seen after 3 months of consistent rehabilitation, further evaluation is indicated. Indications for surgery include failure of nonsurgical treatment and patient intolerance to continued symptoms. Multiple cortisone injections should be avoided.

SECTION 2 SHOULDER

www.aaos.org/essentials5/exercises

Home Exercise Program for Frozen Shoulder

- Perform the exercises in the order listed.
- Apply moist or dry heat to the shoulder for 5 or 10 minutes before the exercises and during the external rotation passive stretch.
- If you experience pain during or after the exercises, discontinue the exercises and call your doctor.
- For the exercise that uses a stick, you may use a yardstick or stick of similar size.
- The following exercise program is introductory only, and progression of this program will vary based on your specific injury, symptoms, and baseline level of fitness. For further progression of this routine, your physician may recommend evaluation and treatment by a physical therapist or other exercise professional.

Home Exercise Program for Frozen Shoulder

Exercise Type	Muscle Group	Number of Repetitions/Sets	Number of Days per Week	Number of Weeks
Pendulum	Deltoid and rotator cuff	15 repetitions/3 times per day	Daily	3 to 4
Passive external rotation stretch	Anterior capsule	5 repetitions/3 times per day	Daily	3 to 4
Passive internal rotation stretch	Subscapularis Pectoralis major and minor	5 repetitions/3 times per day	5 to 6	3 to 4
Supine forward flexion	Inferior capsule	5 repetitions/3 times per day	Daily	3 to 4

Pendulum
- Lean forward, supporting the body with one arm and relaxing the muscles of the other arm so that it hangs freely.
- Gently move the arm in forward-and-back, side-to-side, and circular motions.
- Perform 15 repetitions in each direction 3 times per day.
- Repeat on the other side.

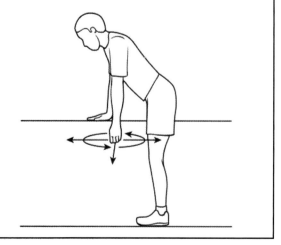

Passive External Rotation Stretch

- Stand in a doorway, facing the doorjamb.
- With the affected arm held next to your side and the elbow bent 90°, grasp the edge of the doorjamb.
- Keep the hand in place and rotate your upper body as shown in the illustration.
- Hold the stretch for 30 seconds, then return to the starting position for 30 seconds.
- Perform 5 repetitions, 3 times per day.
- Repeat on the other side.

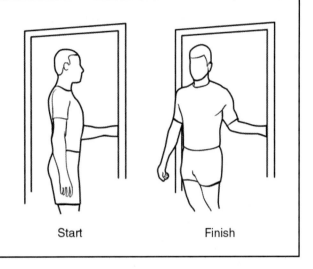

Start　　　　　Finish

Passive Internal Rotation Stretch

- Behind your back, grasp the stick with one hand and lightly grasp the other end of the stick with the other hand.
- Pull the stick horizontally as shown so that the arm is passively stretched to the point of feeling a pull without pain.
- Hold for 30 seconds and then relax for 30 seconds.
- Repeat 5 times, 3 times per day.
- Repeat on the other side.

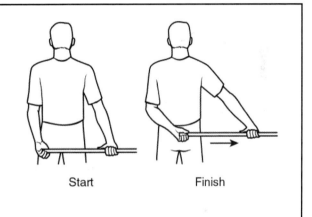

Start　　　　　Finish

Supine Forward Flexion

- Lie on your back with your legs straight.
- With the unaffected arm, grasp the affected arm at the elbow and lift the affected arm overhead until you feel a gentle stretch.
- Hold the stretch for 15 seconds and slowly lower to starting position.
- Perform 5 repetitions, 3 times per day.

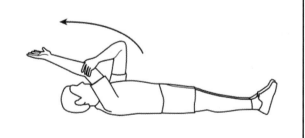

SECTION 2　SHOULDER

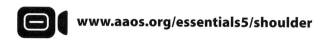

Procedure: Shoulder Joint Injection and Aspiration: Posterior

Step 1

Place the patient in the upright seated position. Stand behind the patient on the side of the shoulder to be injected. Palpate the coracoid, and outline the coracoid and the posterior corner of the acromion. The entry site for the injection should be located approximately 2 cm medial and 2 cm inferior to the posterior corner of the acromion (**Figure 1**); mark this site using a pen.

Step 2

Wipe the top of the bottles of medications with an alcohol swab. Open a set of sterile gloves, and use the wrapper as a sterile field. Place the syringe and the needles on the wrapper.

Step 3

Prepare the glenohumeral joint with a fairly wide field. Don the gloves in sterile fashion and use one needle to draw up 3 mL of lidocaine, 3 mL of bupivacaine, and 3 mL of 40 mg/mL triamcinolone acetonide. Replace the needle and, using the left thumb and grasping the shoulder with the thumb and index finger, use the left thumb to palpate the entry site for the needle that had been

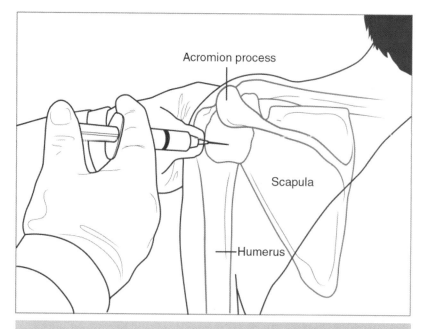

Figure 1 Illustration of needle placement for shoulder joint injection and aspiration to manage frozen shoulder.

© 2016 American Academy of Orthopaedic Surgeons

previously inserted. The thumb should lie in the posterior soft spot of the shoulder.

Step 4
Insert the needle and advance it completely, aiming for the coracoid tip. After the needle is fully advanced, deliver the medication. If resistance is met, slowly pull the needle back while injecting until resistance is not met.

Step 5
Remove the needle and place an adhesive bandage.

Adverse Outcomes
Subcutaneous injection of the steroid solution may result in fat atrophy or depigmentation of the skin and should be avoided.

Aftercare/Patient Instructions
The patient may experience increased pain for 1 or 2 days after the injection before the benefits of the steroid become apparent. Ice may be prescribed to help control discomfort in the postinjection period.

SECTION 2   SHOULDER

Impingement Syndrome

Synonyms
Rotator cuff tendinitis
Shoulder bursitis

Definition
Four muscles—the infraspinatus, supraspinatus, subscapularis, and teres minor—come together to form the rotator cuff, which covers the anterior, superior, and posterior aspects of the humeral head. Because these muscles assist in elevation of the arm, the rotator cuff, primarily the supraspinatus tendon, is pulled repetitively under the coracoacromial arch. The coracoacromial arch includes the coracoid process, the coracoacromial ligament, the acromion, and the acromioclavicular joint capsule (**Figure 1**).

Inflammation of the subacromial bursa and underlying rotator cuff tendons is a common cause of shoulder pain in middle-aged patients. Rotator cuff pathology spans a continuum from edema and hemorrhage to chronic inflammation and fibrosis to microscopic tendon fiber failure, progressing to full-thickness rotator cuff tears. The etiology is likely a combination of factors, including loss of microvascular blood supply to the tendon and repeated mechanical insult as the tendon passes under the coracoacromial arch.

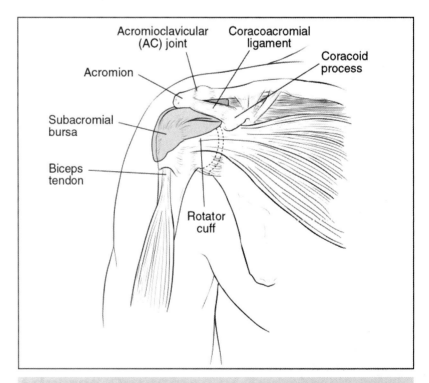

Figure 1 Illustration depicts the anatomy of the front of the shoulder. (Reproduced from Sullivan JA, Anderson SJ, eds: *Care of the Young Athlete.* Rosemont, IL, American Academy of Orthopaedic Surgeons, 2000, p 326.)

Clinical Symptoms

Gradual onset of anterior and lateral shoulder pain exacerbated by overhead activity is characteristic of impingement syndrome. Night pain and difficulty sleeping on the affected side also are common. Atrophy of the muscles about the top and back of the shoulder may be apparent if the patient has had symptoms for several months.

Tests

Physical Examination

Palpation over the greater tuberosity and subacromial bursa commonly elicits tenderness and crepitus with shoulder motion. Pain is worse between 90° and 120° of abduction and when lowering the arm. Patients with impingement generally have positive Neer and Hawkins signs. After these examinations are completed, a diagnostic injection can be performed as follows: 10 mL of 1% plain local anesthetic is injected into the subacromial space, followed by reexamination. Complete pain relief supports a diagnosis of impingement syndrome.

To evaluate weakness of the supraspinatus tendon, position the arm in 90° of elevation and internal rotation (thumb turned down). Ask the patient to resist while you push the arm down (**Figure 2**). Compare the result with that of the opposite shoulder. If the shoulder initially demonstrates weakness but is strong following subacromial injection, pain inhibition from inflammation and fibrosis rather than a full-thickness rotator cuff tear is the likely cause of the weakness. Muscle atrophy about the top and back of the shoulder usually indicates a rotator cuff tear (**Figure 3**).

Diagnostic Tests

AP and axillary radiographs of the shoulder are usually normal. Narrowing of the space between the humeral head and the undersurface of the acromion (normally greater than 7 mm) suggests a long-standing rotator cuff tear.

Differential Diagnosis

- Acromioclavicular (AC) arthritis (tenderness over the AC joint)
- Frozen shoulder (active and passive motion loss)
- Glenohumeral arthritis (pain with any motion, evident on radiographs)
- Herniated cervical disk (associated neck stiffness, deltoid weakness with absent biceps reflex, possible sensory loss)
- Rotator cuff tear (weakness of the supraspinatus that does not improve following subacromial injection of local anesthetic)
- Suprascapular nerve entrapment (atrophy of the supraspinatus and infraspinatus muscles, negative impingement sign)

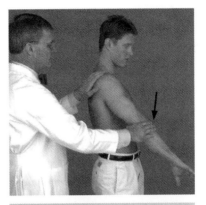

Figure 2 Photograph shows an examiner testing the strength of the supraspinatus. The patient is asked to resist as the examiner pushes the arm down (arrow).

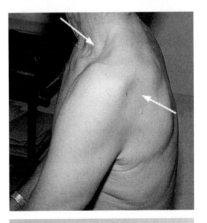

Figure 3 Photograph of a shoulder with visible muscle atrophy (arrows), which is indicative of a rotator cuff tear.

SECTION 2 SHOULDER

Adverse Outcomes of the Disease

Pain can be persistent or recurrent. Rotator cuff tendinitis may progress to a full-thickness tear.

Treatment

NSAIDs and rest from the offending activity may relieve an acute exacerbation of pain. The patient should begin a stretching program, with an emphasis on posterior capsule stretching. If a home exercise program performed three to four times per day for 6 weeks does not result in any improvement, a subacromial corticosteroid injection can be considered, followed by continued stretching. Steroid injections should not be repeated if the previous injection did not produce substantial and sustained (4 to 6 weeks) relief. Rotator cuff weakness with impingement is often the result of subacromial bursitis, rotator cuff tendinitis, or even calcific tendinitis.

A rotator cuff strengthening program should be added to the stretching program after the shoulder becomes supple and pain improves. Avoidance of repetitive overhead activities also is recommended.

Rehabilitation Consultation

The functional goal of rehabilitation for a patient with shoulder impingement should be to perform overhead activities without pain. Patients with shoulder impingement typically have a restricted glenohumeral joint capsule and weakness of the glenohumeral and scapulothoracic rotators.

A home exercise program may be initiated that includes stretching and very basic strengthening exercises. The home program should not cause more pain, although patients may report muscle soreness and a stretching sensation that may be considered uncomfortable. Ice may be used after exercise to prevent inflammation.

Formal rehabilitation should be started within 3 to 4 weeks if the home exercise program has not increased the patient's ability to perform overhead activities of daily living without pain. The assessment should include a detailed evaluation of the strength of the glenohumeral and scapulothoracic muscles as well as observation of scapulothoracic rhythm for abnormal patterns. If indicated by specific joint restrictions, mobilization of the glenohumeral and scapulothoracic joints may be an effective adjunct to a home stretching and strengthening program. The rehabilitation specialist will typically progress patients from basic strengthening exercises performed with the arms in positions of limited elevation to more advanced training with the arms above shoulder height for strengthening and advanced proprioception.

Adverse Outcomes of Treatment

NSAIDs may cause gastric, renal, or hepatic complications. In 2015, the FDA strengthened its warning linking NSAIDs with the risk of heart attack or stroke, even in the first weeks of use of an NSAID.

Tearing of the rotator cuff and rupture of the long head of the biceps tendon may occur after repeated corticosteroid injections. The latter injury is more likely to occur with more than three injections.

Referral Decisions/Red Flags

Substantial weakness of the rotator cuff or failure of 2 to 3 months of rehabilitation (with or without subacromial steroid injection) is an indication for further evaluation and surgical consideration.

SECTION 2 | SHOULDER

www.aaos.org/essentials5/exercises

Home Exercise Program for Shoulder Impingement

- Perform the exercises in the order listed.
- Apply a bag of crushed ice or frozen peas to the shoulder for 20 minutes after performing the exercises to prevent inflammation.
- These exercises should not increase the pain in your shoulder, although you may experience muscle soreness and a stretching sensation. Call your doctor if you experience increased pain or if you do not see improvement in your ability to perform overhead activities without pain after performing the exercises for 3 or 4 weeks.
- The following exercise program is introductory only, and progression of this program will vary based on your specific injury, symptoms, and baseline level of fitness. For further progression of this routine, your physician may recommend evaluation and treatment by a physical therapist or other exercise professional.

Home Exercise Program for Shoulder Impingement

Exercise Type	Muscle Group	Number of Repetitions/Sets	Number of Days per Week	Number of Weeks
Sleeper stretch	Posterior rotator cuff Posterior inferior capsule/glenohumeral ligament	5 repetitions/2 to 3 times per day	Daily	3 to 4
External rotation	Infraspinatus Teres minor	8 repetitions/2 sets, progressing to 15 repetitions/3 sets	3 to 4	6 to 8
Internal rotation	Subscapularis Teres major	8 repetitions/2 sets, progressing to 15 repetitions/3 sets	3 to 4	6 to 8

Sleeper Stretch

- Lie on your side on a firm, flat surface with the affected shoulder under you and the arm positioned as shown, keeping your back perpendicular to the surface.
- With the unaffected arm, push the other wrist down, toward the surface. Stop when you feel a stretching sensation in the back of the affected shoulder.
- Hold this position for 30 seconds, then relax the arm for 30 seconds.
- Perform 5 repetitions, 2 to 3 times per day, continuing for 3 to 4 weeks.

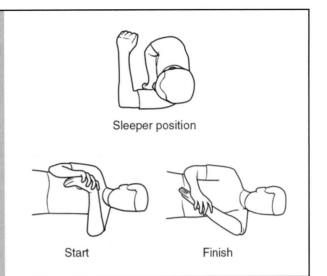

Sleeper position

Start   Finish

External Rotation

- Lie on your side on a firm, flat surface with the unaffected arm under you, cradling your head.
- Hold the affected arm against your side as shown, with the elbow bent at a 90° angle.
- Slowly rotate the arm at the shoulder, keeping the elbow bent and against your side, to raise the weight to a vertical position, and then slowly lower the weight to the starting position to a count of 5.
- Begin with approximately 1- to 2-pound weights that allow 2 sets of 8 repetitions, progressing to 3 sets of 15 repetitions.
- Add weight in 1-pound increments, starting over at each new weight level with 2 sets of 8 repetitions up to a maximum of 3 to 6 pounds, depending on your size and fitness level.
- Perform the exercise 3 or 4 days per week, continuing for 6 to 8 weeks.

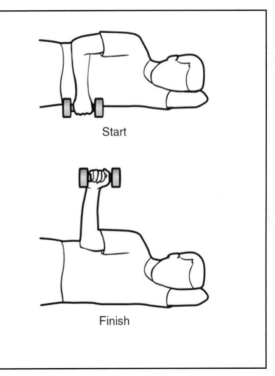

Start

Finish

SECTION 2 SHOULDER

Internal Rotation

- Lie on your side on a firm, flat surface with the affected arm under you and with a pillow or folded cloth under your head to keep your spine straight.
- Hold the affected arm against your side as shown, with the elbow bent at a 90° angle.
- Slowly rotate the arm at the shoulder, keeping the elbow bent and against your torso, to raise the weight to a vertical position, and then slowly lower the weight to the starting position.
- Begin with weights that allow 2 sets of 8 repetitions, progressing to 3 sets of 15 repetitions.
- Add weight in 1-pound increments, starting over at each new weight level with 2 sets of 8 repetitions up to a maximum of 3 to 6 pounds, depending on your size and fitness level.
- Perform the exercise 3 or 4 days per week, continuing for 6 to 8 weeks.

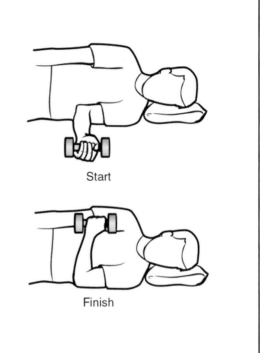

Start

Finish

SECTION 2   SHOULDER

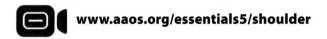
Procedure: Subacromial Bursa Injection

Note: Although this injection can be performed in the anterior or anterolateral aspect of the shoulder, the easiest way to access the subacromial space is from the posterior aspect. The posterolateral corner of the acromion is easily palpated in most patients and serves as a reliable anatomic landmark. Also, opinions differ regarding single- versus two-needle injection techniques. Proponents of the single-needle technique believe that one needle is less painful for the patient than two. Physicians who prefer the two-needle technique point out that the smaller gauge needle is easier for patients to tolerate and that the pain of the second injection is dulled by the anesthetic. A single-needle technique is shown in the video.

Step 1
Wear protective gloves during this procedure and use sterile technique.

Step 2
Seat the patient with the arm hanging down with the hand in the lap to distract the subacromial space. The injection site can be anterior, anterolateral, or straight posterior into the subacromial space.

Step 3
Palpate the acromion both posteriorly and laterally until the posterolateral corner is located.

Step 4
Cleanse this area with a bactericidal solution.

Step 5
With an index finger on the lateral acromion, insert the 25-gauge needle approximately 1 cm below the palpating finger and raise a wheal with the local anesthetic.

Step 6
Insert the syringe with the 22-gauge needle. The site of posterior injection is 1 cm medial and inferior to the posterolateral corner of the acromion (**Figure 1**). Angle the needle superiorly approximately 20° to 30° to access the subacromial space. Inject 8 to 10 mL of the 1% lidocaine solution. If resistance is encountered while attempting to inject the solution, partially withdraw the needle and reinsert. If the needle is in the proper place, little resistance to injection will be encountered. If you feel the needle hit bone, redirect it superiorly if the bony obstruction is thought to be the humerus, or inferiorly if the bone is thought to be the acromion.

Materials
- Sterile gloves
- Bactericidal skin preparation solution
- 1% lidocaine solution without epinephrine
- 2 mL of betamethasone 40 mg/mL or similar steroid
- 10-mL syringe with a 22-gauge 1¼" needle
- 3-mL syringe with a 25-gauge ¾" needle
- Adhesive bandage

SECTION 2 SHOULDER

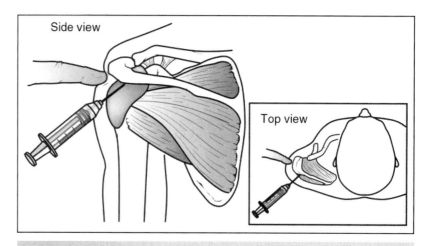

Figure 1 Illustration depicts the location for needle insertion for subacromial bursa injection using a posterior approach.

Step 7
Detach the syringe from the needle hub, leaving the needle in the correct location. Attach the second syringe with 2 mL of corticosteroid preparation and inject it into the subacromial space. The syringe can again be exchanged and local anesthetic injected as the needle is withdrawn to avoid steroid deposition subcutaneously. This reduces the risk of fat atrophy or depigmentation in dark-skinned patients.

Step 8
Dress the puncture site with a sterile adhesive bandage.

Adverse Outcomes
A temporary increase in pain is possible, and, although rare, infection can occur. Subcutaneous atrophy and depigmentation also may occur.

Aftercare/Patient Instructions
One third of patients will experience a temporary increase in pain for 24 to 48 hours after the corticosteroid injection. Advise the patient to apply ice bags to the shoulder and take an NSAID or acetaminophen if increased pain occurs the night following the injection. Instruct the patient to resume usual activities as soon as tolerated, but no later than 24 to 48 hours after the injection.

Overhead Throwing Shoulder Injuries

Synonyms
Rotator cuff tendinitis (syndrome)

Definition
The unique anatomy of the glenohumeral joint provides multiple and extreme degrees of functional motion. All overhead athletic motions (such as throwing a baseball) require the repeated systematic and sequential delivery of kinetic energy to the four rotator cuff muscle/tendon units (the infraspinatus, supraspinatus, subscapularis, and teres minor) (**Figure 1**). The primary function of these relatively small muscle/tendon units (the rotator cuff) is to precisely seat and center the humeral head in the shallow fossa of the glenoid (**Figure 2**). This working relationship between the rotator cuff and the humeral head must be operational for the larger power muscles such as the deltoid and pectoralis to function effectively, resulting in the preferred fluid motion of the shoulder. When the relationship between the rotator cuff and the humeral head malfunctions, the humeral head translocates forcefully, causing damage to surrounding structures.

Repetitive overhead throwing produces substantial dynamic stress forces on the rotator cuff–glenohumeral complex. Of the five primary phases of the optimal overhead throwing motion (**Figure 3**), late cocking, early acceleration, and follow-through are the most violent

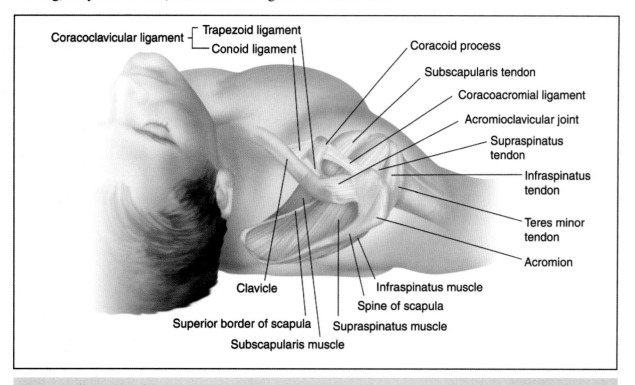

Figure 1 Illustration of the superior view of the rotator cuff muscles.

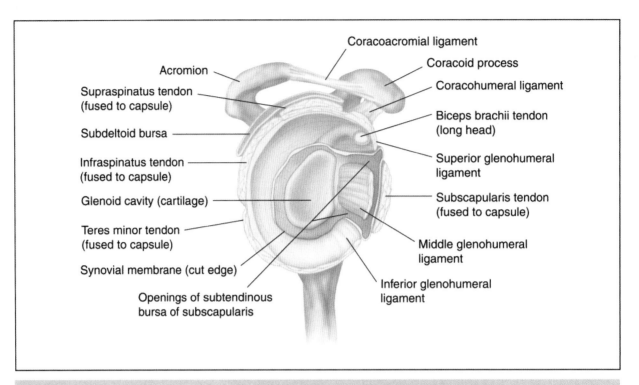

Figure 2 Illustration depicts the lateral view of the glenohumeral (shoulder) joint, opened.

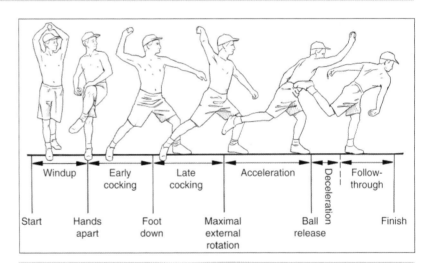

Figure 3 Illustration depicts the phases of throwing. (Reproduced from Limpisvasti O, ElAttrache NS, Jobe FW: Understanding shoulder and elbow injuries in baseball. *J Am Acad Orthop Surg* 2007;15[3]:139-147.)

and are chiefly responsible for the inflammatory tissue response. Compression forces are experienced where the humeral head contacts the glenoid and soft tissues. Tensile forces tend to stretch, irritate, and cause plastic deformation of ligaments, tendons, and capsular tissues. Therefore, excessive wear (abuse), subacute stress accumulation (overuse), and obsessive sport participation (wearout) caused by repetitive throwing will invariably damage the rotator cuff–glenohumeral complex. This damage results in malfunctioning of the rotator cuff–humeral head relationship so that the humeral head is

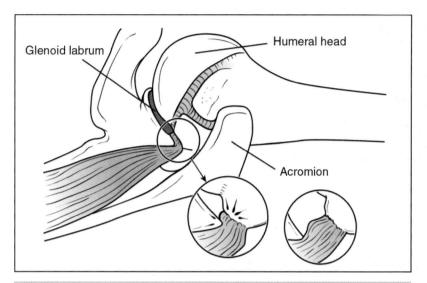

Figure 4 Illustration of the mechanism of internal impingement. The position of abduction and extreme external rotation that occurs during overhead throwing compresses the supraspinatus and infraspinatus muscles and their tendons between the posterosuperior glenoid rim, the posterior humeral head, and the greater tuberosity, causing fraying of the deep layers of the infraspinatus.

no longer firmly seated. Given the complex anatomy and mechanics of the shoulder, combining all shoulder symptoms experienced by throwers under rotator cuff tendinitis fails to appreciate the broad spectrum of rotator cuff–glenohumeral pathology. A clearer understanding of the mechanism, treatment, and prevention of these debilitating injuries is important to guide treatment.

Rotator cuff tendinitis results from various mechanisms in the thrower's shoulder. Internal impingement initially develops as a result of the throwing arm being abducted and placed in extreme external rotation. This causes the supraspinatus and infraspinatus muscles and their tendons to be compressed between the posterosuperior glenoid rim, the posterior humeral head, and the greater tuberosity (**Figure 4**). External impingement occurs with excessive superior translation of the humeral head in the glenoid fossa. Such translation decreases the space available in the subacromial area, resulting in impingement of the structures that occupy this space, most notably the subacromial bursa and the tendons of the rotator cuff.

In throwers, repetitive hyperextension combined with internal impingement (abnormal positioning of the humeral head) causes fraying of the deep layers of the infraspinatus, ultimately resulting in a partial-thickness tear. A similar situation is seen on the articular surface of the supraspinatus. With continued throwing, partial-thickness tears may proceed to full-thickness tears, but full-thickness tears are usually the result of a nonthrowing injury.

If the athlete with a dysfunctional rotator cuff–glenohumeral complex continues to pitch without resting the shoulder, the relatively unrestrained humeral head will translate (migrate) and abut the glenoid labrum, and compression and shear forces will cause

SECTION 2 SHOULDER

roughening, fraying, and tearing of the fibrocartilaginous labrum. More substantial forces can result in superior labrum anterior to posterior (SLAP) detachment with or without the biceps tendon remaining intact. The exact etiology is controversial, but some authors believe SLAP lesions develop from traction of the biceps. Others believe that the extreme external rotation that occurs during overhead throwing causes the lesion (that is, the labrum is "peeled back" by the rotating humeral head). Loss of the anchoring function of the biceps results in increased stress on the inferior glenohumeral ligament. The anterior band of the inferior glenohumeral ligament and the anterior capsule serve as static restraints to anterior translation of the humeral head. When the static restraints become dysfunctional and the dynamic muscle restraints are insufficient, anterior instability results.

Biceps tendinitis can present in the throwing athlete as anterior shoulder pain that increases with activity. Palpation of the biceps tendon in its groove on the front of the humerus typically reproduces the patient's discomfort.

Brachial plexus compression, thoracic outlet syndrome, and axillary nerve involvement should be considered when a thrower has atypical shoulder symptoms.

In a patient with substantial atrophy of the infraspinatus muscle, the possibility of suprascapular nerve entrapment should be considered. Electromyographic and nerve conduction velocity studies are diagnostic for entrapment.

Clinical Symptoms

Stage I—"Sore Shoulder" Syndrome

Initially, the athlete reports aching and soreness deep in the anterior shoulder when throwing certain pitches (usually sliders and curveballs) or after pitching a few innings. The athlete also reports a decrease in pitch velocity and accuracy and difficulties with activities of daily living. The situation improves with rest, and the athlete is able to continue to pitch.

Stage II—Profound Pathologic Pain

In this stage, the aching and soreness of stage I has gradually progressed to pain, predominantly located in the posterior shoulder, which prevents full abduction and external rotation (the throwing motion). A period of rest is no longer effective. Sleeping on the affected shoulder produces night pain, and pain medication is requested.

Tests

Physical Examination

Inspect the fully exposed trunk for muscle asymmetry, atrophy, and obvious deformity. Examine the skin for abrasion, rashes, and boils, and especially note ecchymosis or swelling. Dominant arm hypertrophy may be evident.

Palpate the shoulder area systematically, searching for tenderness in the scapular support muscles as well as the supraspinatus and infraspinatus area, posterior capsule, quadrilateral space, and posterior deltoid. Anteriorly, palpate the muscles about the humeral head, the rotator cuff attachment to the greater and lesser tuberosity, the bicipital groove, and the deltoid and pectoralis muscles. Note any tenderness of the acromioclavicular and sternoclavicular joints, clavicle, and adjacent neck structures. Similarly, palpate the upper arm, elbow, forearm, wrist, and hand.

Evaluate the full range of passive shoulder motion in forward flexion, abduction, external rotation with the arm at the side, and internal rotation (hitchhiking thumb up the back). Repeat the examination while providing active resistance, and compare the results with the opposite extremity. Active resistance to full range of motion should also be evaluated in the biceps, triceps, forearm muscles, and intrinsic muscles of the hand.

Generalized musculoskeletal laxity is indicated by the ability to actively hyperextend the elbows, wrist, and fingers. Inferior shoulder laxity is exhibited as the sulcus, or sag, sign. Perform the lift-off test bilaterally to compare subscapularis strength. With the patient supine and the elbow flexed 90°, measure external rotation at 30°, 90°, and the full overhead position. These measurements should be compared with those of the opposite extremity. Also perform the cross-body or horizontal adduction test. To evaluate anterior instability, the shoulder is abducted to approximately 150°, and pressure is applied anteriorly and then posteriorly to the humeral head to estimate the amount of translation and firmness of resistance.

Pain that limits motion, especially in forward flexion, indicates impingement. If application of anterior pressure to the humeral head relieves the pain, internal impingement should be suspected.

With the patient in the prone position, scapular protraction, tilt, and retraction are assessed. Scapular winging may be tested by having the patient perform a standing push-up against the wall. Alternatively, have the patient perform a seated press. For the seated press, the patient is seated in a chair without arms, grips the seat of the chair on either side, and attempts to lift his or her body up off the chair by extending the arms at the elbows. Axillary nerve irritation on deep palpation of the quadrilateral space indicates compression by the posterior capsule and pectoralis minor. Likewise, if pressure on the posterior capsule produces localized discomfort, capsulitis should be suspected. Also with the patient in the prone position, allow the arm to hang freely over the edge of the table and then forward flex it to 90°; pain in the anterior shoulder indicates rotator cuff tendinitis.

With the patient seated and the elbow flexed 90°, abduct the arm to 90°. While the examiner stabilizes the scapula with one hand, rotate the arm forcefully posteriorly (exteriorly). If the pain of throwing is reproduced, the pathology may be subacromial bursitis. With the arm in the same position, apply internal rotation pressure. If this maneuver produces pain, rotator cuff tendinitis should be suspected. Crepitus noted in the subacromial space with rotation of the arm in abduction is a probable indication of subacromial bursitis.

SECTION 2 SHOULDER

Provocative testing to produce pain at a specific shoulder location is very sensitive but is not specific. Impingement is indicated by positive Hawkins and Neer impingement tests.

Diagnostic Tests
Radiographs provide additional information. Evidence of sclerosis on AP internal and external rotation views represents contact erosive areas on the greater tuberosity of the humeral head and the posterior glenoid rim.

An additional diagnostic tool is the subacromial injection (9 mL lidocaine/1 mL dexamethasone). Alleviation of the patient's pain supports a diagnosis of subacromial bursitis. In addition, gadolinium-enhanced MRI may help establish a working diagnosis, especially if lateral pathology is suspected.

Differential Diagnosis
- Acromial abnormalities (radiographic findings)
- Anterior instability (apprehension with abduction and external rotation of the shoulder)
- External impingement (positive impingement test)
- Internal impingement (pain with the cocking motion of throwing)
- Labral pathology (labral defect apparent on MRI)
- Rotator cuff tendinitis (pathology) (weakness on testing, positive MRI)
- SLAP lesion (may be seen on contrast-enhanced MRI; arthroscopy is diagnostic)

Adverse Outcomes of the Disease
Athletes with the shoulder symptoms described in this chapter are usually unable to participate effectively in their sport because effective pitching requires an intact rotator cuff–glenohumeral complex and pain-free motion.

Treatment
Stage I—Sore Shoulder Syndrome
Initially, the athlete with stage I disease is placed on active rest (activity modification). No overhead weight training or throwing of any object is allowed, but daily core stability work, leg work, and running for cardiovascular endurance are encouraged. Dynamic stabilization of the humeral head by rehabilitation of the rotator cuff muscles is undertaken. Stabilization is followed by strengthening of the rotator cuff muscles with isometric exercises. Basic rehabilitation includes internal and external rotation of the shoulder with the elbow at the side, using elasticized bands of increasing stiffness. Riding a stationary bicycle or using an elliptical trainer with alternate movement of the arms also is advised. A rope-and-pulley system can be used at home to increase range of motion. Ice bags may be applied locally for pain, and rehabilitation specialists may apply electric

modalities. Initial time away from throwing should be approximately 10 days, or until the shoulder is free from soreness. Then a published protocol of interval throwing, which must be supervised and followed closely, is begun.

Stage II—Profound Pathologic Pain

In the overhead throwing athlete with stage II disease (profound pathologic pain that prevents the athlete from competing), rehabilitation must be instituted in a precise, scientific, and individualized manner. This is necessary because pain is an indication that tissue injury (inflammation) is already established.

First, upper body activity is controlled and modified to reestablish dynamic stability and muscle balance and to improve flexibility. Rehabilitation specialists, using hands-on methods, initiate the basic rotator cuff protocols, as previously outlined. The specialists also use electrical stimulation and ultrasonographic modalities and proprioception techniques. As pain permits, isotonic muscle strengthening and neuromuscular control exercises are begun. Core stabilization, which includes leg work, is coupled with a well-structured shoulder exercise program.

Referral Decisions/Red Flags

Referral is indicated if painful overhead motion persists after an initial trial of rehabilitation exercises, especially if labral pathology is suspected.

SECTION 2   SHOULDER

Rotator Cuff Tear

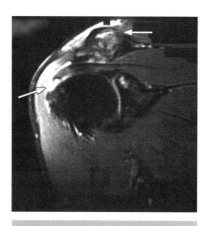

Figure 1 Coronal oblique MRI of the shoulder demonstrates a rotator cuff tear (arrows).

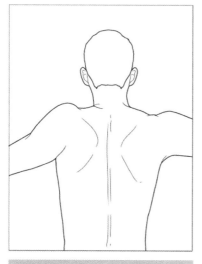

Figure 2 Illustration depicts atrophy of the supraspinatus and infraspinatus muscles and shoulder shrug with attempted abduction.

Synonyms

Musculotendinous cuff rupture
Rotator cuff rupture
Rotator cuff tendinitis

Definition

The rotator cuff is composed of four muscles: the supraspinatus, the infraspinatus, the subscapularis, and the teres minor. These muscles form a cover around the head of the humerus and rotate the arm and stabilize the humeral head against the glenoid.

Rotator cuff tears occur with acute injury, but most are the result of age-related degeneration, chronic mechanical impingement, and altered blood supply to the tendons. Tears generally originate in the supraspinatus tendon and may progress posteriorly and anteriorly (**Figure 1**). Full-thickness tears are uncommon in individuals younger than 40 years but are present in 25% of individuals older than 60 years. Most older people with rotator cuff tears are asymptomatic or have only mild, nondisabling symptoms.

Clinical Symptoms

Patients often report chronic shoulder pain for several months and a specific injury that triggered the onset of the pain. Night pain and difficulty sleeping on the affected side are characteristic of a rotator cuff tear. Common symptoms include weakness, catching, and grating, especially when raising the arm overhead.

Tests

Physical Examination

The back of the shoulder may appear sunken, indicating atrophy of the infraspinatus muscle following a long-standing cuff tear. Passive range of motion is near normal, but active range of motion may be limited. With large tears, the patient cannot raise the arm when asked to do so but can only shrug, or "hike," the shoulder (**Figure 2**).

The patient also cannot hold the arm elevated when it is lifted parallel to the floor by the examiner. Some patients, however, maintain remarkably good active motion despite large cuff tears. As the patient raises the arm, a grating sensation about the tip of the shoulder can be felt. Tenderness to palpation over the greater tuberosity is usually present as well.

Diagnostic Tests

A 30° caudal tilt radiographic view will often show a spur projecting down from the inferior surface of the acromion (**Figure 3**). Often a coracoacromial arch view (outlet view) is needed to show a hooked acromion, indicative of this spur (**Figure 4**). The presence of a spur does not necessarily indicate a rotator cuff tear, however.

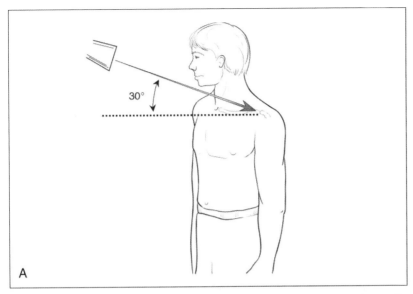

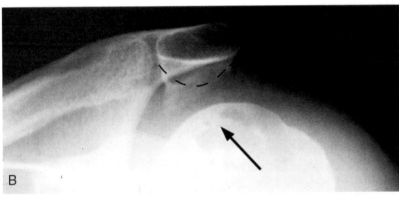

Figure 3 **A,** Illustration demonstrates the x-ray beam position for the 30° caudal tilt view. **B,** AP radiograph demonstrates a bone spur of the inferior acromion (arrow). The curved dashed line indicates the level of resection for acromioplasty.

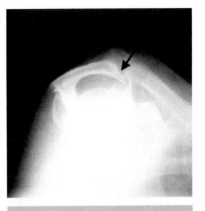

Figure 4 Outlet radiographic view demonstrates a hooked acromion (arrow).

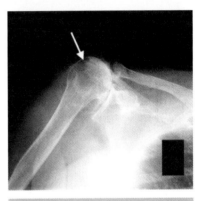

Figure 5 AP shoulder radiograph demonstrates a high-riding humeral head (arrow), which is indicative of rotator cuff arthropathy.

Soft-tissue imaging is necessary to confirm the diagnosis. With large, long-standing tears, AP radiographs may reveal a high-riding humerus relative to the glenoid, indicative of rotator cuff arthropathy (**Figure 5**).

If the diagnosis is equivocal or if surgical treatment is being considered, MRI is the imaging study of choice because it can provide additional information on the status of the muscle and on the size of full-thickness and some partial-thickness tears. Ultrasonography, in experienced hands, also is useful and accurate in evaluating the rotator cuff.

Differential Diagnosis

- Acromioclavicular joint arthritis (localized pain and tenderness and preserved motion)
- Cervical spondylosis (neck stiffness, absent biceps reflex, sensory changes)

SECTION 2 SHOULDER

- Frozen shoulder (restricted active and passive motion)
- Glenohumeral joint arthritis (evidence of arthritis on radiographs)
- Impingement syndrome/cuff tendinitis (similar pain, but preserved active motion)
- Pancoast tumor (venous distention, pulmonary changes, or bony metastases)
- Thoracic outlet syndrome (ulnar nerve paresthesias, worse with "military brace" position)

Adverse Outcomes of the Disease

Loss of shoulder motion (especially the ability to lift the arm overhead), chronic pain, and/or weakness in the affected arm is possible. Long-standing large tears sometimes result in joint degeneration.

Treatment

Nonsurgical treatment includes NSAIDs, rehabilitation with strengthening and stretching exercises, and avoiding overhead activities. Corticosteroid injections should be used judiciously. The steroid injection may decrease inflammation of an associated subacromial bursitis and provide short-term pain relief, but it also weakens the tendon. Repeated injections can ultimately accelerate propagation of the rotator cuff tear. Therefore, patients should never receive more than two or three subacromial injections. If the injections are not effective, additional injections are unlikely to help.

In general, patients with substantial symptoms and whose rehabilitation over 3 to 6 months has failed should be considered candidates for surgery. One exception to this rule is the patient who has an acute traumatic cuff tear, in which case rotator cuff repair is best performed acutely or no later than within 6 weeks of injury. If an acute tear is neglected longer than this, it may propagate and become retracted and much harder to repair. Another possible exception is a rotator cuff tear in a younger patient (younger than 55 years). Tears can enlarge with time and become more difficult to repair. Therefore, surgical repair should be considered in younger patients of working age with repairable tears.

Rehabilitation Consultation

The functional goal of rehabilitation for a patient with a rotator cuff tear is to reduce pain, increase strength, increase the range of motion of the involved shoulder, and restore function. Stiffness of the glenohumeral joint and poor scapulothoracic mobility may be present secondary to a period of immobilization. Rehabilitation should not involve forcing the shoulder into passive or active elevation. Avoiding further damage to the rotator cuff is very important. Instructions to the patient regarding a home exercise program should emphasize that the patient should experience no pain during or after the exercises. The home exercise program begins with light weights and high

SECTION 2   SHOULDER

repetitions to increase range of motion and progresses to heavier weights and fewer repetitions to strengthen the rotator cuff and the scapular rotators.

Formal rehabilitation should be prescribed immediately for athletes or if the patient does not progress on the home exercise program. Poor progress is indicated by the presence of pain and/or stiffness during or after the exercises. In addition, formal rehabilitation is indicated when, on reevaluation by the physician in 3 to 4 weeks, muscle strength or range of motion has not improved. The therapy assessment should include an evaluation of glenohumeral and scapular muscle strength, range of motion, and scapulohumeral rhythm. Treatment will include appropriate stretching exercises to restore range of motion and gentle progressive strengthening. Exercises will typically progress from training with the arms at the sides to dynamic strengthening above shoulder height if indicated by the patient's activity level and goals.

Adverse Outcomes of Treatment

NSAIDs can cause gastric, renal, or hepatic complications. In 2015, the FDA strengthened its warning linking NSAIDs with the risk of heart attack or stroke, even in the first weeks of use of an NSAID. Corticosteroid injections may result in a transient increase in pain because of the injection itself and degeneration of cuff tissue. Repair of large rotator cuff tears has a high incidence of failure, although débridement alone may relieve persistent pain.

Referral Decisions/Red Flags

Failure of 6 weeks of nonsurgical treatment is an indication for further evaluation.

SECTION 2 | SHOULDER

www.aaos.org/essentials5/exercises

Home Exercise Program for Rotator Cuff Tear

- Perform the exercises in the order listed.
- Apply a bag of crushed ice or frozen peas to the shoulder for 20 minutes after performing both exercises to prevent any further inflammation or pain.
- You should not experience pain with any of the exercises. If pain or stiffness occurs that prevents you from performing any of the exercises correctly, call your doctor.
- The following exercise program is introductory only, and progression of this program will vary based on your specific injury, symptoms, and baseline level of fitness. For further progression of this routine, your physician may recommend evaluation and treatment by a physical therapist or other exercise professional.

Home Exercise Program for Rotator Cuff Tear

Exercise Type	Muscle Group	Number of Repetitions/Sets	Number of Days per Week	Number of Weeks
Active-assisted glenohumeral flexion	Deltoid and rotator cuff	10 repetitions/3 times per day	3 to 4	6 to 8
External rotation	Infraspinatus Teres minor	8 repetitions/2 sets, progressing to 15 repetitions/3 sets	3 to 4	6 to 8
Internal rotation	Subscapularis Teres major	8 repetitions/2 sets, progressing to 15 repetitions/3 sets	3 to 4	6 to 8

SECTION 2 SHOULDER

Active-Assisted Glenohumeral Flexion

- While lying on your back, interlock your fingers and slowly raise both arms over your head. Use the unaffected arm to assist in raising the affected arm.
- Range of motion will likely be limited initially (compared with the unaffected side), but should gradually improve over a number of days to weeks.
- Stretch only to the limit of comfort and hold 5 seconds. Repeat 10 times. Perform 3 times per day.

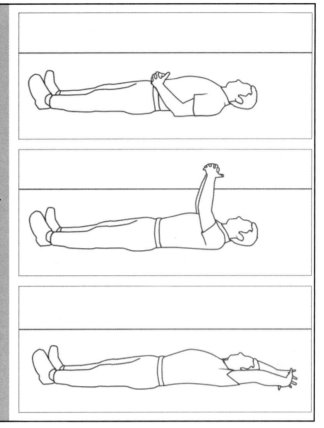

External Rotation

- Lie on your side on a firm, flat surface with the unaffected arm under you, cradling your head.
- Hold the affected arm against your side as shown, with the elbow bent at a 90° angle.
- Slowly rotate the arm at the shoulder, keeping the elbow bent and against your side, to raise the weight to a vertical position, and then slowly lower the weight to the starting position to a count of 5.
- Begin with approximately 1- to 2-pound weights that allow 2 sets of 8 repetitions, progressing to 3 sets of 15 repetitions.
- Add weight in 1-pound increments, starting over at each new weight level with 2 sets of 8 repetitions up to a maximum of 3 to 6 pounds, depending on your size and fitness level.
- Perform the exercise 3 or 4 days per week, continuing for 6 to 8 weeks.

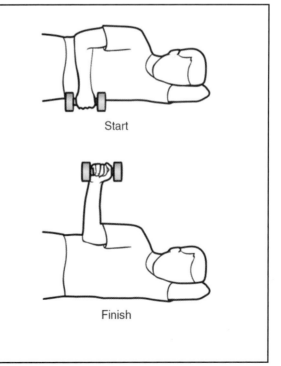

Start

Finish

SECTION 2   SHOULDER

Internal Rotation

- Lie on your side on a firm, flat surface with the affected arm under you and with a pillow or folded cloth under your head to keep your spine straight.
- Hold the affected arm against your side as shown, with the elbow bent at a 90° angle.
- Slowly rotate the arm at the shoulder, keeping the elbow bent and against your torso, to raise the weight to a vertical position, and then slowly lower the weight to the starting position.
- Begin with weights that allow 2 sets of 8 repetitions, progressing to 3 sets of 15 repetitions.
- Add weight in 1-pound increments, starting over at each new weight level with 2 sets of 8 repetitions up to a maximum of 3 to 6 pounds, depending on your size and fitness level.
- Perform the exercise 3 or 4 days per week, continuing for 6 to 8 weeks.

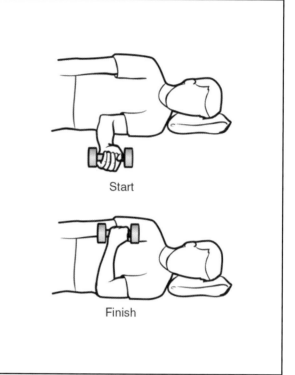

Start

Finish

SECTION 2   SHOULDER

Rupture of the Proximal Biceps Tendon

Definition

Rupture of the biceps tendon usually involves the proximal long head of the biceps. Most often, ruptures occur in older adults who have a long history of shoulder pain secondary to rotator cuff disease, either inflammation or a tear. The long head of the biceps tendon ascends in the intertubercular groove and is intra-articular for its proximal 3 cm. The shoulder capsule is continuous with the biceps tendon sheath; therefore, inflammatory changes in the shoulder can affect the tendon as well. Its anatomic position predisposes the tendon to attritional changes, and the tendon ultimately ruptures, often as a result of a trivial event.

Rupture of the proximal biceps tendon is uncommon in young adults but may occur in athletic individuals involved in weight lifting or throwing sports. Rupture of the distal biceps tendon also can occur but is less common.

Clinical Symptoms

Sudden pain in the upper arm, often accompanied by an audible snap, is often reported. Subsequently, patients notice a bulge in the lower arm. Pain in the acute stage is often mild.

Tests

Physical Examination

Examination reveals a bulge in the lower arm, which results from the muscle belly of the biceps retracting into the lower arm after the long head ruptures (**Figure 1**). A defect also can be palpated proximally. Acutely, ecchymosis can be seen tracking down the middle and lower arm.

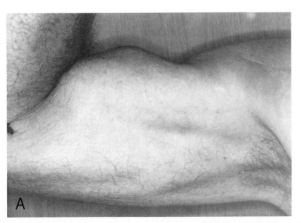
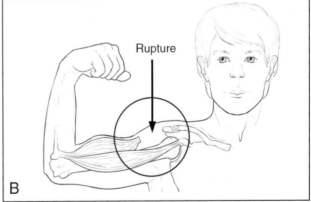

Figure 1 Images show a rupture of the proximal biceps tendon made more obvious by attempted contraction. **A,** Clinical photograph. **B,** Illustration of the underlying anatomy.

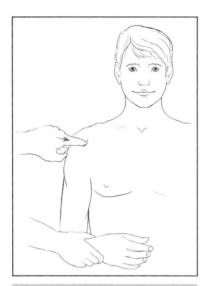

Figure 2 Illustration of palpation of the bicipital groove.

The bulge can be accentuated by having the patient contract the biceps against resistance with the elbow flexed or by performing the Ludington test. (For this test, the patient puts his or her hands behind the head and flexes the biceps muscle.) Gentle pressure over the bicipital groove of the humerus with the arm in 10° of internal rotation will elicit acute pain (**Figure 2**).

Diagnostic Tests

AP and axillary radiographs of the shoulder are useful to rule out a fracture but are not helpful in confirming a diagnosis of a ruptured biceps tendon. For patients with a previous history of disabling shoulder pain, shoulder arthrography or MRI should be considered to rule out a rotator cuff tear.

Differential Diagnosis

- Dislocated biceps tendon (tenderness over the bicipital groove, but no distal muscle bulge)
- Distal biceps rupture (pain and ecchymosis distally with high-riding muscle belly, often missed until late)
- Glenohumeral arthritis (pain in the joint exacerbated with motion, evident on radiographs)
- Impingement syndrome (can coexist with biceps tendon rupture)
- Rotator cuff tear (often coexists with biceps tendon rupture)
- Rupture of the pectoralis major muscle (abnormal muscle contour apparent in anterior axillary fold)

Adverse Outcomes of the Disease

Patients can lose approximately 10% of elbow flexion and forearm supination strength (the motion required to use a manual screwdriver). Cosmetic deformity of the arm in the form of a bulge in the lower arm also may be of concern to the patient.

Treatment

Nonsurgical treatment is effective for most patients, resulting in minimal loss of function and acceptable cosmetic deformity. Most patients regain full range of motion and normal elbow flexion strength with an exercise program consisting of range of motion and strengthening as pain allows. Patients with persistent shoulder pain and young athletes require evaluation for a concomitant rotator cuff tear.

In young athletes and in adults younger than 40 years who work as heavy laborers and need the extra strength for lifting, surgical repair of the biceps tendon should be considered.

Adverse Outcomes of Treatment

Functional improvement from surgery is often modest, and postoperative stiffness is a potential concern. Bodybuilders may trade a distal muscle bulge for a surgical scar with little subjective cosmetic improvement.

Referral Decisions/Red Flags
Young patients who perform heavy labor and older patients with a concomitant rotator cuff tear and persistent symptoms require further evaluation.

SECTION 2   SHOULDER

Shoulder Instability

Synonyms

Dislocation
Multidirectional instability
Recurrent dislocation
Subluxation

Definition

With its shallow glenoid and loose capsule, the shoulder joint has exceptional mobility. As a corollary, instability is also most common at the shoulder. Patients with shoulder instability have recurrent episodes of subluxation (the humeral head partially slips out of the socket) and/or dislocation (**Figure 1**). Instability can be anterior, posterior, inferior, or multidirectional, with anterior and multidirectional being the most common (**Figure 2**). Classically, instability is thought to lie along a spectrum, from Traumatic Unidirectional instability with a Bankart lesion (a tear of the anterior glenoid labrum) (**Figure 3**) best treated with Surgery (TUBS) to Atraumatic, Multidirectional, Bilateral signs of laxity, Rehabilitation as the preferred treatment, and Inferior capsular shift as the indicated procedure if surgery becomes necessary (AMBRI). All individuals have varying degrees of laxity (nonpathologic), which can become instability (pathologic) when affected by trauma or overuse. Posterior dislocations result from a posteriorly directed force applied when the arm is in adduction and internal rotation. This uncommon injury is associated with seizures or electric shock injuries.

Clinical Symptoms

Patients with anterior instability typically describe the sensation of the shoulder slipping out of joint when the arm is abducted and externally rotated. The initial anterior shoulder dislocation is associated with substantial trauma from a fall or forceful

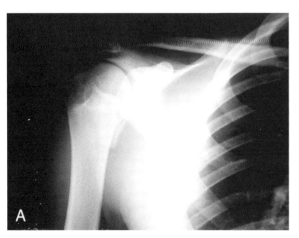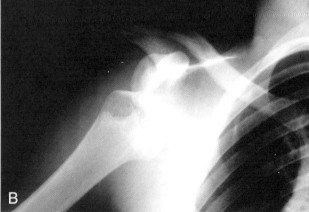

Figure 1   AP radiographs of a nondislocated shoulder (**A**) and a dislocated shoulder (**B**).

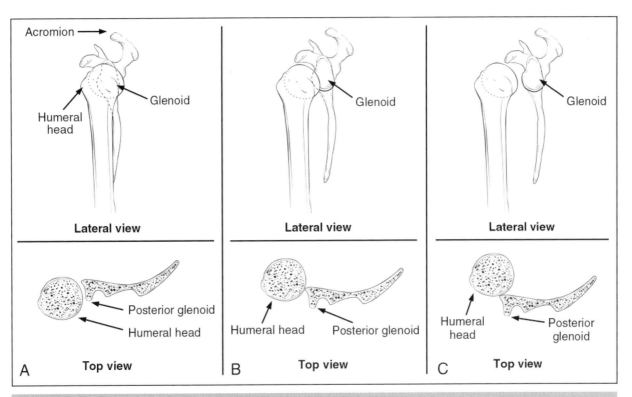

Figure 2 Illustration depicts relative positions of the humeral head and the glenoid with the humeral head reduced (**A**), subluxated anteriorly (**B**), and dislocated anteriorly (**C**).

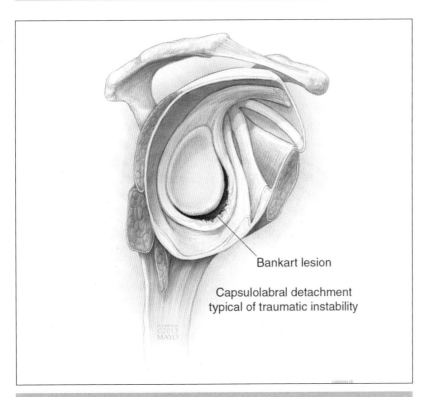

Figure 3 Illustration of a Bankart lesion. Note detachment of the labrum. (Reproduced with permission from the Mayo Foundation for Medical Education and Research, Rochester, MN.)

throwing motion, but with recurrent dislocations, the patient may experience instability by simply positioning the arm overhead. With multidirectional instability, symptoms may be vague but tend to be activity related. Ask the patient whether he or she can voluntarily dislocate the shoulder because this is an important clue. The ability to voluntarily dislocate the shoulder is quite frequently associated with a multidirectional instability component and may indicate a poor prognosis for surgical treatment. Voluntary dislocations may be associated with psychological disturbance.

Tests
Physical Examination
With an acute dislocation, any movement of the shoulder is associated with considerable pain. With an anterior dislocation, the patient supports the arm in a neutral position. Patients with a posterior dislocation hold the arm in adduction and internal rotation; external rotation is impossible. Neurovascular function, particularly function of the axillary nerve, should be carefully assessed before and after reduction.

Assessment of a patient suspected of having recurrent instability on physical examination should include the apprehension test for anterior instability, the sulcus sign test for inferior laxity (**Figure 4**), and the jerk test for posterior instability. The patient also should be assessed for generalized ligamentous laxity: Ask the patient to try to touch the thumb against the volar (flexor) surface of the forearm; also, bend the fingers back at the metacarpophalangeal joint to determine how far they extend past neutral with the finger and hand in a straight line. Patients with ligamentous laxity are more likely to have multidirectional instability, but other types of instability are possible.

Diagnostic Tests
AP and axillary radiographs of the shoulder should be obtained. The axillary view may show a bony defect at the anterior edge of the glenoid rim (**Figure 5**). A compression fracture of the posterior humeral head (a Hill-Sachs lesion) is created when the head is pressed against the anterior edge of the glenoid. A Hill-Sachs lesion is clear evidence of an anterior dislocation. Patients older than 40 years with a history of traumatic dislocation are also susceptible to rotator cuff tears at the time of dislocation. Shoulder arthrography or MRI may be indicated in these cases.

Posterior dislocation of the shoulder is easily missed if only an AP radiograph is obtained. If an axillary view cannot be obtained, request a transscapular lateral view.

Differential Diagnosis
• Glenohumeral arthritis (confirm with radiographs)
• Impingement syndrome (pain but no apprehension of instability)
• Rotator cuff tear (pain and weakness without apprehension)

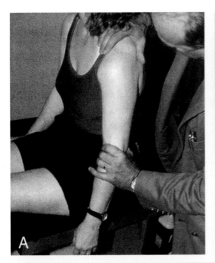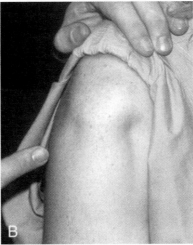

Figure 4 Photographs of the sulcus sign. **A,** With the patient's arm relaxed at the side, the examiner applies traction inferiorly. **B,** A positive sulcus sign, which indicates inferior shoulder laxity.

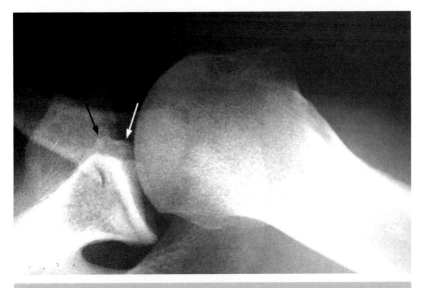

Figure 5 Axillary radiograph demonstrates erosion of the glenoid rim (arrows) associated with anterior glenohumeral instability. (Reproduced from Bigliani LU, ed: *The Unstable Shoulder.* Rosemont, IL, American Academy of Orthopaedic Surgeons, 1996, p 32.)

Adverse Outcomes of the Disease

Axillary nerve injury (deltoid dysfunction and numbness over the lateral arm) is not uncommon but usually resolves. Osteoarthritis of the glenohumeral joint, and/or persistent dislocation is possible. The risk of recurrent instability is greater in younger patients and in those with multiple episodes.

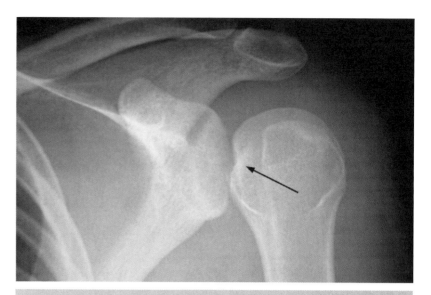

Figure 6 AP radiograph of a left shoulder demonstrates posterior dislocation of the humeral head. Note the indentation in the anterior humeral head (arrow), corresponding to a compression fracture (reverse Hill-Sachs lesion). The head may become locked on the rim, rendering the shoulder irreducible. Note the slight overlap of the humeral head on the glenoid. This view is often misread as normal; therefore, with this finding, an axillary view is required. (Reproduced from Johnson TR, Steinbach LS, eds: *Essentials of Musculoskeletal Imaging.* Rosemont, IL, American Academy of Orthopaedic Surgeons, 2004, p 200.)

Treatment

Most acute shoulder dislocations can be reduced in the emergency department. There are several ways to reduce a shoulder, two of which are described in Procedure: Reduction of Anterior Shoulder Dislocation. For patients who present with a first-time anterior dislocation, the injured arm should be immobilized in neutral rotation for 3 weeks, followed by a rehabilitation program that emphasizes strengthening the rotator cuff muscles, especially the subscapularis muscle.

Patients with atraumatic or voluntary instability (AMBRI) should be treated nonsurgically with the shoulder exercise program described in Musculoskeletal Conditioning of the Shoulder and delineated in the Home Exercise Program for Shoulder Conditioning. Educating patients to avoid voluntarily dislocating the shoulder and to avoid positions of known instability is an important part of the treatment plan.

Adverse Outcomes of Treatment

Up to 80% of posterior dislocations are missed on initial evaluation. **Figure 6** is a radiograph that demonstrates the classic signs of posterior dislocation.

Referral Decisions/Red Flags

Further evaluation is warranted in the following situations: when closed manipulation fails to reduce an acute dislocation; when recurrent dislocations (two or more) occur despite a 3-month trial of shoulder rehabilitation exercises; and in patients with multidirectional instability whose symptoms are intolerable and do not respond to a rehabilitation program.

SECTION 2 SHOULDER

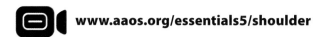

Procedure: Reduction of Anterior Shoulder Dislocation

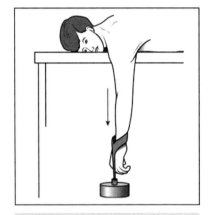

Figure 1 Illustration demonstrates the Stimson technique (gravity-assisted reduction with the patient lying on the stomach).

Prior to reduction, a neurovascular examination should be performed. Assess function of the axillary, musculocutaneous, median, radial, and ulnar nerves, with emphasis on evaluating the axillary nerve through voluntary isometric contraction of the deltoid and sensation over the lateral deltoid region. Obtain AP and axillary radiographs to document the dislocation and rule out any fractures that may displace during the reduction maneuver. Reducing a first-time dislocation is safely accomplished in the emergency department with a resuscitation cart available.

Establish an intravenous line, ensure that naloxone is available, and initiate pulse oximetry and cardiac monitoring if narcotics are used for anesthesia. Apply oxygen by mask or nasal cannula throughout the procedure. Fentanyl in a dose of 100 µg is given intravenously over 1 minute, and then repeated every 3 to 5 minutes until adequate sedation is achieved. The usual total dose of fentanyl is 3 µg/kg. Patients with recurrent dislocations may not require anesthesia. An intra-articular lidocaine injection via a posterior approach also is an effective anesthetic and may limit the need for narcotics.

Stimson Technique (Gravity-Assisted Reduction)

Step 1
Place the patient prone on a stretcher with the dislocated arm hanging off the cart. Secure the patient to the stretcher with a sheet.

Step 2
Either have an assistant sit on the floor and provide downward traction, or attach 5- to 15-lb of weight to the patient's arm (**Figure 1**). The weights should not touch the floor.

Step 3
For reduction of the left shoulder, place your left thumb on the patient's acromion and the fingers of your left hand over the front of the humeral head.

Step 4
As the muscles relax, gently push the humeral head caudally until it reduces.

SECTION 2 SHOULDER

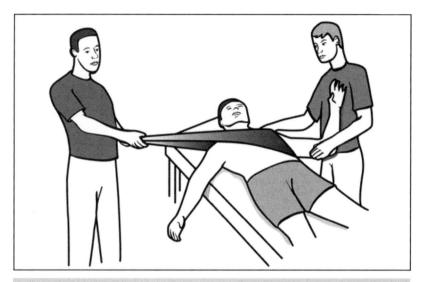

Figure 2 Illustration demonstrates the longitudinal traction technique for shoulder reduction.

Longitudinal Traction

Step 1
Place the patient supine on a stretcher with a sheet folded into a band 4 inches to 5 inches wide around the patient's chest (**Figure 2**). Stand next to the patient on the same side as the injured shoulder, at or below the level of the patient's waist.

Step 2
Position the patient's elbow in 90° of flexion to relax the biceps muscle. Have an assistant apply traction to the sheet that is wrapped around the patient's thorax while you apply steady traction to the arm.

Step 3
Reduction may be aided if you gently rotate the arm while the longitudinal traction is applied. You usually can feel and see the shoulder reduce. Occasionally, especially in large patients, the reduction may be subtle, and you may neither feel nor see it.

Adverse Outcomes
Axillary nerve palsy may develop with reduction. Be sure to test axillary nerve function (motor and sensory) before and after the reduction. General anesthesia may be required to reduce the shoulder.
  The administration of opioids such as fentanyl is associated with the risk of overdose. Fentanyl overdose is treated with naloxone. Initially, administer 0.2 to 0.4 mg intravenously, and if there is no response, administer repeated doses of up to 4 to 5 mg; doses as high as 15 to 20 mg may be administered with resistant opioids such as fentanyl. First-time dislocation in a patient older than 40 years can be associated with a rotator cuff tear, so these patients should be examined with a high index of suspicion for a tear. Humeral fracture can result with excessive force.

SECTION 2 SHOULDER

Aftercare/Patient Instructions

Obtain postreduction AP and axillary radiographs to confirm the reduction. Immobilize the arm in a sling, in neutral rotation if possible, but have the patient remove the sling and extend the elbow several times daily to prevent elbow stiffness. Begin isometric exercises for the rotator cuff.

Begin strengthening exercises for the subscapularis and infraspinatus muscles at 2 to 3 weeks postreduction in the older patient and at 6 weeks postreduction in the younger patient.

Increase shoulder external rotation to 30° or 40° and shoulder flexion to 140°. This occurs at 6 weeks postreduction in patients younger than 30 years and at 3 weeks postreduction in patients 30 years and older.

Begin vigorous shoulder motion at 6 weeks postreduction in patients 30 years and older, but delay this step to 3 months postreduction for patients younger than 30 years.

The propensity for shoulder stiffness in patients older than 40 years is an advantage in regaining stability; however, these patients are more likely to sustain a rotator cuff tear at the time of the dislocation.

In the athlete, allow return to sports activities after near-full flexion and rotation of the arm and near-normal strength of the cuff have been regained.

SECTION 2 SHOULDER

Superior Labrum Anterior to Posterior Lesions

Synonyms
Biceps tendon labral complex injuries
SLAP lesions
Superior glenoid labrum tears

Definition
Superior labrum anterior to posterior (SLAP) lesions involve an injury to the superior glenoid labrum and the biceps anchor complex. The long head of the biceps tendon originates from the superior aspect of the glenoid labrum and is confluent with the labrum in this region, also called the biceps anchor. The glenoid labrum itself, which has been likened to the shoulder equivalent of the meniscus of the knee, consists of a cartilaginous lining of the glenoid, which serves to deepen the glenoid, thereby providing increased shoulder stability. Injuries to the labrum involve either fraying (usually degenerative in nature) or frank tears (associated with acute and chronic symptoms). Injuries that involve the superior labrum are termed SLAP lesions.

Clinical Symptoms
SLAP lesions are difficult to diagnose and are often a diagnosis of exclusion, confirmed only at the time of surgery. Symptoms may include painful popping or catching in the shoulder as well as pain with overhead activities. In a throwing athlete, symptoms may be present only with maximal effort throwing, but a thorough history may reveal an insidious onset of pain while performing overhead sports that limits performance and eventually results in a persistent ache in the shoulder. The ache is often described as being deep inside the shoulder.

Tests
Physical Examination
Several tests are commonly used to detect SLAP lesions, but they have poor sensitivity and specificity. The tests include the active compression test, the crank test, the resisted supination/external rotation test, and the clunk test. They are designed to elicit pain as the lesion is compressed. Instructions on performing the active compression test (also called the O'Brien test) are delineated in Physical Examination of the Shoulder.

For the crank test, the arm is elevated to 160° in the scapular plane and loaded axially by the examiner, who then moves the arm into maximal internal and external rotation while maintaining axial loading of the shoulder. Pain or a clicking sound produced by the maneuver is a positive test.

SECTION 2 SHOULDER

The resisted supination/external rotation test attempts to mimic the "peel-back" position in an overhead thrower. For this test, the patient is placed supine with the shoulder at 90° of abduction. The elbow is flexed to 70° with the wrist in neutral rotation. The patient actively supinates against the examiner's resistance as the shoulder is slowly externally rotated to maximum external rotation. Pain at or just before maximal external rotation is a positive test.

For the clunk test, the patient is placed supine with the shoulder flexed to 180°, the elbow flexed to 90°, and the hand pointing to the floor. While holding the elbow in place, the examiner grasps the hand and uses it to internally rotate the shoulder. The clunk test is considered positive if the patient experiences a sharp pain with internal rotation.

Diagnostic Tests

Plain radiographs should be obtained because they are part of a thorough workup of any shoulder disorder, but they cannot confirm a diagnosis of a SLAP lesion. Magnetic resonance arthrography (injection of contrast medium into the shoulder before the MRI is obtained) is the gold standard to evaluate for a SLAP lesion, with a sensitivity and specificity of up to 90%. MRI without contrast has a sensitivity of less than 50%.

Differential Diagnosis

- Acromioclavicular (AC) joint arthritis (tenderness over the AC joint, positive cross-body adduction test, AC pain on bench pressing)
- Biceps tendinitis (tenderness anteriorly over the biceps tendon)
- Rotator cuff disease (pain referred to lateral deltoid)
- Shoulder instability (history of shoulder "slipping out of place," positive apprehension test)
- Subacromial impingement (positive clinical impingement signs, palpable crepitus, local tenderness over rotator cuff insertion)
- Suprascapular nerve entrapment (possible wasting of infraspinatus on examination, diagnosed using electromyography)

Adverse Outcomes of the Disease

Continued shoulder pain and some disability with activities are possible.

Treatment

Nonsurgical care should be attempted initially. This includes NSAIDs as well as rehabilitation directed at rotator cuff and periscapular stabilization, posterior capsule stretching, and strengthening with gradual return to activities. In a throwing athlete, gradual return to activities includes the use of an interval throwing program after at least 6 weeks of rest to return the athlete to a competitive level of play in a controlled manner. If nonsurgical care fails and symptoms persist, diagnostic shoulder arthroscopy is the only alternative. At the

SECTION 2 SHOULDER

time of surgery, all intra-articular pathology can be delineated and addressed.

Rehabilitation Consultation

The functional goal of rehabilitation for a patient with a SLAP lesion is to reduce pain and protect the joint from further damage. The home exercise program often includes stretching of the posterior structures.

In addition, deep bench presses, overhead presses, and biceps curls should be prohibited. Reaching behind and overhead activities should be limited to pain-free movement. If the patient does not respond to the home program of exercises, stretching, and activity modification, referral to a rehabilitation specialist is indicated. The rehabilitation specialist should evaluate the muscle strength and posterior capsule mobility and determine the appropriate exercises for the patient's condition.

Adverse Outcomes of Treatment

NSAIDs can cause gastric, renal, and hepatic complications. In 2015, the FDA strengthened its warning linking NSAIDs with the risk of heart attack or stroke, even in the first weeks of use of an NSAID. Physical therapy may not improve symptoms but has no adverse effect. The most common adverse effect following surgical repair of a SLAP lesion is shoulder stiffness.

SECTION 2 SHOULDER

Home Exercise Program for SLAP Lesions

- Perform the exercises in the order listed.
- Apply dry or moist heat to the shoulder before the exercises and during the sleeper stretch.
- To reduce inflammation, apply a bag of crushed ice or frozen peas to the shoulder for 15 to 20 minutes after performing both exercises.
- You should not experience pain during or after the exercises. If the exercises cause pain, call your doctor.
- Avoid activities that may cause additional damage to the labral tear, such as arm curls while lifting heavy objects (heavier than 5 pounds), overhead sports activities (a tennis serve or throwing a baseball), and reaching overhead or behind your body.
- The following exercise program is introductory only, and progression of this program will vary based on your specific injury, symptoms, and baseline level of fitness. For further progression of this routine, your physician may recommend evaluation and treatment by a physical therapist or other exercise professional.

Home Exercise Program for SLAP Lesions

Exercise Type	Muscle Group	Number of Repetitions/Sets	Number of Days per Week	Number of Weeks
Sleeper stretch	Infraspinatus Teres minor Posterior capsule	4 repetitions/2 to 3 sets	Daily	2 to 3
External rotation	Infraspinatus Teres minor Posterior deltoid	8 to 10 repetitions/2 sets, progressing to 15 repetitions/3 sets	3	2 to 3

Sleeper Stretch

- Lie on your side on a firm, flat surface with the affected shoulder under you and the arm positioned as shown, keeping your back perpendicular to the surface.
- With the unaffected arm, push the other wrist down, toward the surface. Stop when you feel a stretching sensation in the back of the affected shoulder.
- Hold this position for 30 seconds; then relax the arm for 30 seconds.
- Perform 2 to 3 sets of 4 repetitions daily, continuing for 2 to 3 weeks.

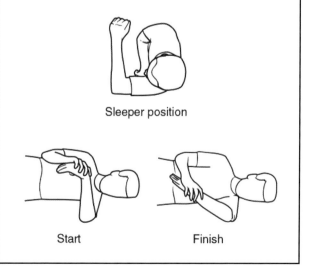

Sleeper position

Start   Finish

External Rotation

- Lie on your side on a firm, flat surface with the unaffected arm under you, cradling your head.

- Hold the injured arm against your side as shown, with the elbow bent at a 90° angle.

- Slowly rotate the arm at the shoulder, keeping the elbow bent and against your side, to raise the weight to a vertical position, and then slowly lower the weight to the starting position to a count of 5.

- Begin with weights that allow 2 sets of 8 to 10 repetitions and progress to 3 sets of 15 repetitions.

- Add weight in 1-pound increments, starting over with 8 to 10 repetitions each time weight is added.

- Perform the exercise 3 days per week, continuing for 2 to 3 weeks.

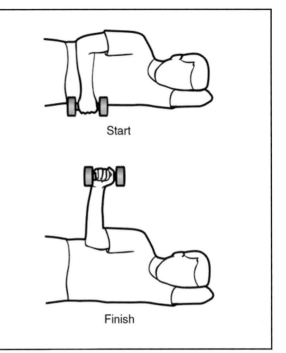

Start

Finish

SECTION 2   SHOULDER

Thoracic Outlet Syndrome

Definition

Thoracic outlet syndrome (TOS) is compression of the brachial plexus and/or subclavian vessels as they exit the narrow space between the superior shoulder girdle and the first rib (**Figure 1**). These structures may be affected individually or in combination. Women aged 20 to 50 years are most commonly affected.

TOS can be secondary to congenital anomalies such as a cervical rib or abnormally long transverse process of C7, or an anomalous fibromuscular band in the thoracic outlet. Posttraumatic fibrosis of the scalene muscles also is a possibility.

Clinical Symptoms

Symptoms are vague and varied. Compression of the brachial plexus accounts for most presenting symptoms and may mimic distal nerve entrapment, especially of the ulnar nerve, with paresthesias of the little and ring fingers. Aching pain and paresthesias can extend from the neck into the shoulder, arm, medial forearm, and fingers. Symptoms from vascular compression include intermittent swelling and discoloration of the arm. The aching fatigue and weakness are worse when the arm is in an overhead position. Psychologic disturbances such as depression are seen with TOS, but whether they contribute to the causation or are the result of a chronically painful condition is unclear.

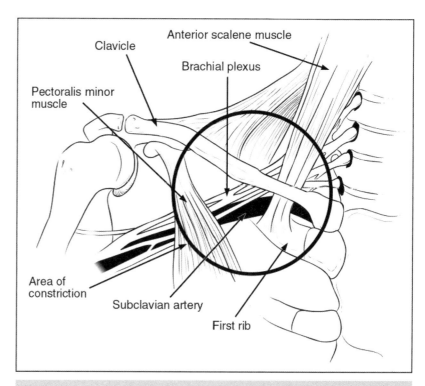

Figure 1 Illustration depicts the anatomy of the thoracic outlet.

Tests

Physical Examination

Inspect for swelling or discoloration of the arm and palpate the supraclavicular fossa to rule out a mass lesion. Auscultation over this area may reveal a bruit, especially during the provocative maneuvers described below. Compare distal pulses with those on the opposite side. Assess sensory and motor function of the axillary, musculocutaneous, medial antebrachial cutaneous, median, radial, and—most important—ulnar nerves.

Several clinical tests have been described to diagnose TOS. Perhaps the simplest and most reproducible provocative maneuver is the elevated arm stress test (**Figure 2**). With both shoulders abducted at least 90° and braced somewhat posteriorly, the patient opens and closes his or her fists at a moderate speed for 3 minutes. Reproduction of neurologic and/or vascular symptoms is a positive test. A sense of fatigue without neurologic or vascular symptoms is considered a negative or inconclusive test.

Diagnostic Tests

No laboratory studies currently exist to confirm the diagnosis of TOS. AP and lateral radiographs of the cervical spine identify cervical ribs or overly long C7 transverse processes. PA and lateral views of the chest help rule out an apical lung tumor or infection. MRI of the cervical spine may be needed if the patient has signs and symptoms of a cervical disk rupture or cervical spondylosis. AP and axillary radiographs of the shoulder are indicated if the patient has shoulder symptoms. Somatosensory-evoked potentials, nerve conduction velocity studies, and ultrasonography are not reliable in confirming the diagnosis but can be useful in ruling out alternative diagnoses (such as ulnar nerve entrapment).

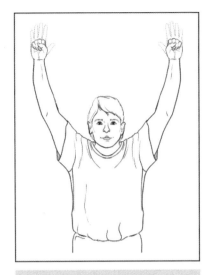

Figure 2 Illustration of the elevated arm stress test.

Differential Diagnosis

- Brachial plexus neuritis (sudden onset, severe pain, proximal muscle weakness)
- Carpal tunnel syndrome (numbness on the radial side of the hand, positive Phalen maneuver)
- Herniated cervical disk (neck pain and stiffness with unilateral or bilateral pain and neurologic findings in a radicular pattern)
- Impingement syndrome (localized shoulder pain with positive impingement signs)
- Pancoast tumor (venous congestion, lesion on apical lordotic chest radiograph)
- Ulnar nerve entrapment (positive Tinel sign at the elbow, abnormal nerve conduction velocity studies, no symptoms above the elbow)

Adverse Outcomes of the Disease

Weakness and loss of coordination of the upper extremity, chronic headaches, and the inability to work with the arm overhead are possible. Ulcerations on the arm and hand and Raynaud phenomenon are rare. Serious problems such as venous thrombosis and aneurysm of the subclavian artery are uncommon but can develop.

Treatment

Most patients can be treated nonsurgically with 3 to 6 months of a home exercise program that emphasizes muscle strengthening and posture education exercises. Strenuous activities such as carrying heavy objects should be avoided, as should placing straps over the affected shoulder, including bras, purses, and seat belts. Activities that aggravate symptoms, such as prolonged overhead activities, strenuous aerobic exercises, and sleeping on the affected shoulder, should be discouraged as well.

Maintaining proper posture is important. The patient should be taught to stand up straight with the shoulders back, not slumped forward. The use of NSAIDs, muscle relaxants, and transcutaneous electrical nerve stimulation units can help decrease the severity of the symptoms. Weight reduction, when indicated, should be encouraged as well. A multidisciplinary approach, including physical therapists, occupational therapists, and physiatrists, may be beneficial.

Because the success rate from surgery varies and the complication rate is substantial, every effort should be made to treat these patients nonsurgically.

Adverse Outcomes of Treatment

The following conditions may develop following or as a result of treatment: complex regional pain syndrome, intercostal neuroma, frozen shoulder, brachial plexus injury, or pneumothorax.

Referral Decisions/Red Flags

Vascular compromise with swelling and/or ulceration necessitates early consultation. Similarly, patients with TOS and a cervical rib or unusually long transverse process require early specialty evaluation when these findings are associated with loss of sensation, muscle atrophy, and weakness. Finally, failure of a well-supervised exercise program in a patient with disabling symptoms is an indication for further evaluation.

www.aaos.org/essentials5/exercises

Home Exercise Program for Thoracic Outlet Syndrome

- The following exercises are designed to stretch the soft-tissue structures that may be compressing the neurovascular bundle.
- Perform the exercises in the order listed.
- If any of the exercises causes an increase in your symptoms, discontinue the exercises and call your doctor.
- The following exercise program is introductory only, and progression of this program will vary based on your specific injury, symptoms, and baseline level of fitness. For further progression of this routine, your physician may recommend evaluation and treatment by a physical therapist or other exercise professional.

Home Exercise Program for Thoracic Outlet Syndrome

Exercise Type	Number of Repetitions/Sets	Number of Days per Week	Number of Weeks
Corner stretch	10 repetitions/2 sets	Daily	12
Neck stretch	10 repetitions/2 sets	Daily	12
Shoulder roll	10 repetitions/2 sets	Daily	12
Neck retraction	10 repetitions/2 sets	Daily	12

Corner Stretch
- Stand in a corner with your hands against the walls at shoulder height.
- Lean into the corner until you feel a gentle stretch.
- Hold for 5 seconds.
- Perform 2 sets of 10 repetitions daily for 12 weeks.

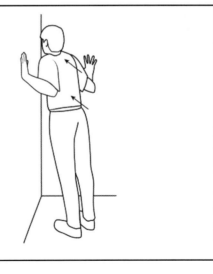

SECTION 2   SHOULDER

Neck Stretch
- Place your left hand on the far side of your head and your right hand behind your back.
- Pull your head toward your shoulder until you feel a gentle stretch.
- Hold for 5 seconds.
- Switch hand positions and repeat the exercise in the opposite direction.
- Perform 2 sets of 10 repetitions daily for 12 weeks.

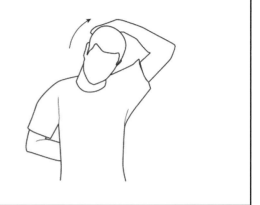

Shoulder Roll
- Roll your shoulders up, back, and then down in a circular motion.
- Perform 2 sets of 10 repetitions daily for 12 weeks.

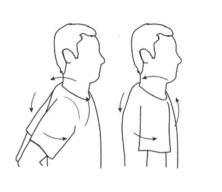

Neck Retraction
- Pull your head straight back, keeping your jaw level.
- Hold in the retracted position for 5 seconds.
- Perform 2 sets of 10 repetitions daily for 12 weeks.

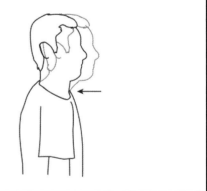

SECTION 2   SHOULDER

PAIN DIAGRAM
Elbow and Forearm

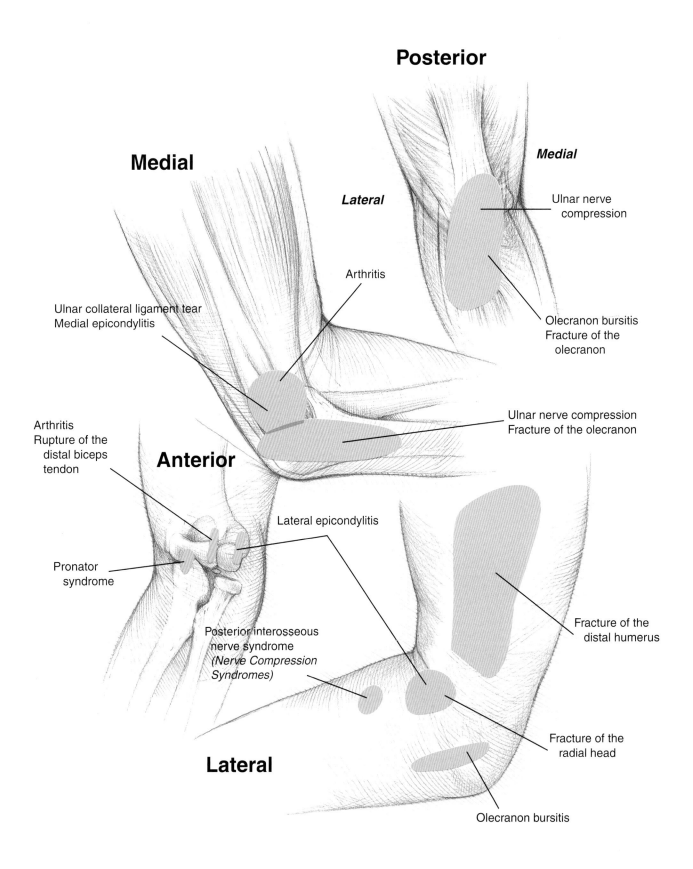

Posterior

Medial

Lateral

Medial

Ulnar nerve compression

Arthritis

Ulnar collateral ligament tear
Medial epicondylitis

Olecranon bursitis
Fracture of the olecranon

Ulnar nerve compression
Fracture of the olecranon

Arthritis
Rupture of the distal biceps tendon

Anterior

Lateral epicondylitis

Pronator syndrome

Fracture of the distal humerus

Posterior interosseous nerve syndrome
(Nerve Compression Syndromes)

Fracture of the radial head

Lateral

Olecranon bursitis

Elbow and Forearm

Section Editor

Joseph A. Abboud, MD

Orthopaedic Surgeon, Associate Professor
Shoulder & Elbow Surgery
The Rothman Institute
Philadelphia, Pennsylvania

Contributor

Mark C. Hubbard, MPT

Physical Therapist
Bone and Joint Institute
Penn State Milton S. Hershey Medical Center
Hershey, Pennsylvania

ANATOMY OF THE ELBOW AND FOREARM

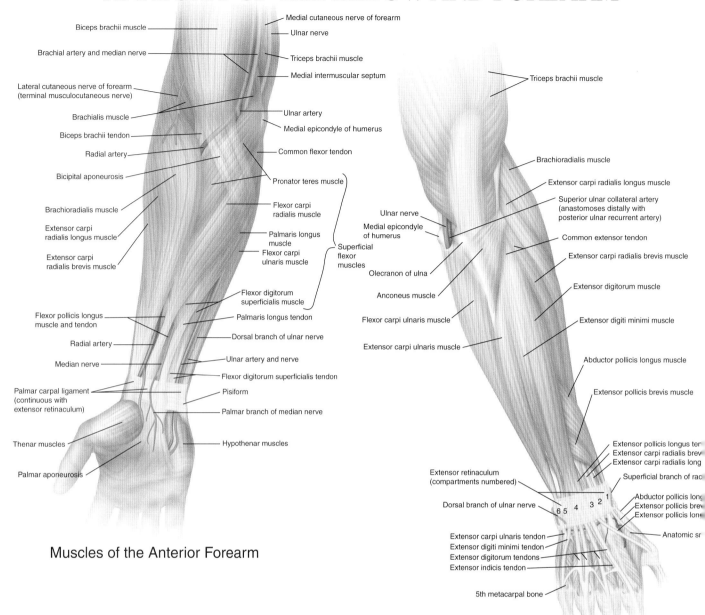

Biceps brachii muscle

Brachial artery and median nerve

Lateral cutaneous nerve of forearm (terminal musculocutaneous nerve)

Brachialis muscle

Biceps brachii tendon

Radial artery

Bicipital aponeurosis

Brachioradialis muscle

Extensor carpi radialis longus muscle

Extensor carpi radialis brevis muscle

Flexor pollicis longus muscle and tendon

Radial artery

Median nerve

Palmar carpal ligament (continuous with extensor retinaculum)

Thenar muscles

Palmar aponeurosis

Medial cutaneous nerve of forearm

Ulnar nerve

Triceps brachii muscle

Medial intermuscular septum

Ulnar artery

Medial epicondyle of humerus

Common flexor tendon

Pronator teres muscle

Flexor carpi radialis muscle

Palmaris longus muscle

Flexor carpi ulnaris muscle

Superficial flexor muscles

Flexor digitorum superficialis muscle

Palmaris longus tendon

Dorsal branch of ulnar nerve

Ulnar artery and nerve

Flexor digitorum superficialis tendon

Pisiform

Palmar branch of median nerve

Hypothenar muscles

Muscles of the Anterior Forearm

Triceps brachii muscle

Brachioradialis muscle

Extensor carpi radialis longus muscle

Superior ulnar collateral artery (anastomoses distally with posterior ulnar recurrent artery)

Ulnar nerve

Medial epicondyle of humerus

Olecranon of ulna

Anconeus muscle

Flexor carpi ulnaris muscle

Extensor carpi ulnaris muscle

Common extensor tendon

Extensor carpi radialis brevis muscle

Extensor digitorum muscle

Extensor digiti minimi muscle

Abductor pollicis longus muscle

Extensor pollicis brevis muscle

Extensor pollicis longus ter

Extensor carpi radialis brev

Extensor carpi radialis long

Superficial branch of rac

Extensor retinaculum (compartments numbered)

Dorsal branch of ulnar nerve

6 5 4 3 2 1

Abductor pollicis long

Extensor pollicis brev

Extensor pollicis lon

Anatomic sn

Extensor carpi ulnaris tendon

Extensor digiti minimi tendon

Extensor digitorum tendons

Extensor indicis tendon

5th metacarpal bone

Muscles of the Posterior Forearm

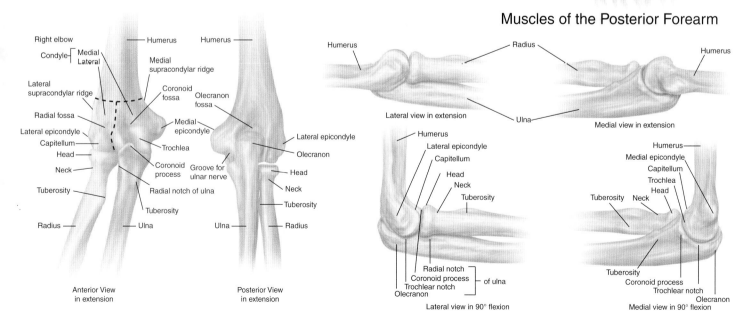

Right elbow

Condyle — Medial / Lateral

Lateral supracondylar ridge

Radial fossa

Lateral epicondyle

Capitellum

Head

Neck

Tuberosity

Radius

Humerus

Medial supracondylar ridge

Coronoid fossa

Olecranon fossa

Medial epicondyle

Trochlea

Coronoid process

Radial notch of ulna

Tuberosity

Ulna

Humerus

Lateral epicondyle

Olecranon

Head

Neck

Tuberosity

Groove for ulnar nerve

Ulna — Radius

Anterior View in extension

Posterior View in extension

Humerus

Lateral view in extension

Radius

Ulna

Medial view in extension

Humerus

Lateral epicondyle

Capitellum

Head

Neck

Tuberosity

Radial notch

Coronoid process

Trochlear notch

Olecranon

of ulna

Lateral view in 90° flexion

Humerus

Medial epicondyle

Capitellum

Trochlea

Head

Tuberosity Neck

Tuberosity

Coronoid process

Trochlear notch

Olecranon

Medial view in 90° flexion

Bones of the Elbow Joint

Essentials of Musculoskeletal Care 5

© 2016 American Academy of Orthopaedic Surgeons

Overview of the Elbow and Forearm

This section of *Essentials of Musculoskeletal Care* focuses on common and important conditions encountered in the elbow and forearm. Making a correct diagnosis of a condition in the elbow or forearm begins with clearly defining the nature and the anatomic location of the patient's chief symptom, which usually is related to pain, stiffness, swelling, or a combination of the three. Unlike the shoulder, the elbow has considerable articular congruency, and elbow instability is a much less common problem than shoulder instability.

The elbow joint has three distinct articulations: the ulnohumeral joint, the radiocapitellar joint, and the proximal radioulnar joint. The ulnohumeral and radiocapitellar joints provide flexion/extension of the elbow and pronation/supination of the forearm, and the proximal radioulnar joint works in conjunction with the distal radioulnar joint at the wrist to achieve forearm pronation and supination. Basic radiographic assessment consists of an AP view of the extended elbow and a lateral view with the elbow flexed to 90° and the forearm supinated. Oblique views can be helpful in identifying subtle fractures and when the elbow cannot be extended enough to obtain an AP view. The basic evaluation should include not only an assessment of the bony anatomy but also attention to the soft tissues; for example, the presence of a posterior fat pad may indicate an intra-articular fracture.

Acute Pain

Acute pain and swelling after an injury can be caused by a fracture, dislocation, or tendon/ligament rupture. Important physical findings include the location of the pain and any tenderness, deformity, and ecchymosis. Pain with elbow flexion/extension suggests involvement of the ulnohumeral articulation, whereas pain with forearm pronation/supination suggests involvement of the radiocapitellar and proximal radioulnar joints.

Radiographs will confirm a fracture or dislocation, although some fractures of the radial head and other articular surfaces are easily missed. Subtle radiographic signs such as bony avulsions or soft-tissue swelling seen with a fat pad sign can indicate an important bony injury. Normal radiographs do not rule out the possibility of a tendon or ligament rupture, such as a distal biceps or triceps rupture.

Acute pain or swelling over the tip of the elbow may indicate acute olecranon bursitis. Intra-articular conditions, which can cause acute synovitis of the elbow, include septic arthritis (especially in intravenous drug users), rheumatoid arthritis, or other inflammatory conditions, such as crystal deposition diseases (gout, pseudogout). A thorough evaluation of all body systems is helpful because the elbow may be only one of many joints that are involved in an inflammatory condition.

ELBOW AND FOREARM

SECTION 3

Chronic Pain

Most elbow and forearm conditions are chronic in nature (longer than 2 weeks' duration) and represent overuse injuries from work or sport. Often, a change in training habits or sports equipment (for example, a tennis racket) can be identified in the patient's history. Localization of the pain and tenderness, as well as identification of the movement or position that provokes pain, is important.

Arthritis of the elbow includes posttraumatic arthritis, inflammatory (rheumatoid or crystalline) arthritis, osteoarthritis, and septic arthritis (although septic arthritis typically presents acutely). Chronic pain resulting from inflammatory elbow arthritis can be either diffuse and poorly defined or localized to the area of greatest involvement. A patient with osteoarthritis of the elbow typically presents with pain at the extremes of motion in flexion and extension. Lateral elbow pain exacerbated by forearm rotation is likely caused by arthritis in the radiocapitellar articulation. These lateral symptoms are often the initial presentation of rheumatoid arthritis involving the elbow or of posttraumatic arthritis after a radial head fracture. Early morning pain and stiffness, and pain with weather changes are common findings in patients with any type of arthritis. Loose bodies often develop in arthritic elbows and may produce catching or locking.

Localization of Pain

Lateral Elbow

The lateral epicondyle is the common origin of the forearm extensor muscles. Pain and tenderness localized to this epicondyle and the forearm extensor muscles indicate lateral epicondylitis. This condition is commonly referred to as tennis elbow, although many patients with lateral epicondylitis have no history of playing tennis. The pain of lateral epicondylitis is exacerbated by forearm supination and wrist extension against resistance. Asking the patient with lateral epicondylitis to pick up a chair with his or her forearm pronated (the chair test) will usually elicit pain, whereas the same maneuver in the supinated position will not. When the pain and tenderness are localized approximately 5 cm distal to the lateral epicondyle, entrapment of the posterior interosseous branch of the radial nerve (radial tunnel syndrome) might be present. Because this nerve compression syndrome typically produces pain without distal motor or sensory deficits, distinguishing it from lateral epicondylitis sometimes is difficult. Some authors think the two conditions coexist in 5% of patients. Lateral ulnar collateral ligament insufficiency can also be a source of lateral elbow pain. Lateral collateral ligament tears have been reported following repeated corticosteroid injections in the elbow for lateral epicondylitis. The patient also may describe clicking or popping of the elbow and will be reluctant to fully extend the elbow, particularly with weight bearing or when pushing up from a chair.

Medial Elbow

Pain over the medial aspect of the elbow is most commonly the result of one of two conditions: ulnar nerve entrapment or medial epicondylitis (golfer's elbow). Ulnar nerve entrapment is associated with localized pain at the elbow, usually accompanied by numbness and tingling in the little finger and ulnar half of the ring finger that is exacerbated by tapping over the nerve in the ulnar groove. Patients with medial epicondylitis have pain and tenderness over and just lateral and distal to the medial epicondyle. This pain increases with wrist flexion or forearm pronation against resistance. Ulnar neuritis can complicate medial epicondylitis in up to 20% of patients. In the overhead throwing athlete with medial elbow pain, injury to the ulnar collateral ligament must be considered.

Posterior Elbow

Posterior elbow pain usually is associated with chronic olecranon bursitis. Painful spurs may develop on the posteromedial olecranon secondary to repetitive valgus strain (medial collateral ligament insufficiency) on the elbow in overhead throwing athletes during the throwing motion. Tendinitis or even frank rupture of the triceps tendon sometimes develops in weight lifters.

Anterior Elbow

Anterior elbow pain occurring acutely and associated with tenderness, ecchymosis, and change in the contour of the biceps muscle indicates a distal biceps tendon rupture. Exceedingly rare in females, this rupture typically occurs in middle-aged men who also report weak supination (screwdriver motion) following a sudden jerking movement or heavy lifting. Chronic anterior elbow discomfort can represent chronic degeneration of the biceps tendon, arthritis, synovitis, or compression of the median nerve at the elbow (pronator syndrome).

Stiffness

Normal elbow flexion/extension is from 0° (arm held out straight) to 140° to 150° of flexion. Normal forearm rotation is from 80° of pronation to 80° of supination. The elbow has a particular predisposition to develop stiffness with arthritis, trauma, or immobilization; however, mild loss of motion causes no substantial disability because most daily activities, including bringing the hand to the mouth and performing other aspects of personal hygiene, are performed in an arc of motion from 30° to 130° of flexion and 50° of pronation and supination.

SECTION 3   ELBOW AND FOREARM

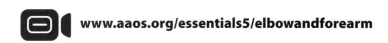

www.aaos.org/essentials5/elbowandforearm

Physical Examination of the Elbow and Forearm

Inspection/Palpation

Anterior View

Inspect the elbow for swelling and ecchymosis. Measure the carrying angle (the angle made by the intersection of the axes of the humerus and the forearm) with the elbow extended and the forearm supinated. Note that the normal carrying angle is a cubitus valgus of 5° to 8°. Cubitus varus (reverse carrying angle) usually results from a malunion of a supracondylar fracture of the humerus.

The biceps brachii tendon can be easily palpated in the middle of the antecubital fossa, especially when the patient flexes the elbow against resistance with the forearm supinated as shown. Absence of this normally palpable tendon with associated tenderness and ecchymosis suggests a complete biceps tendon rupture.

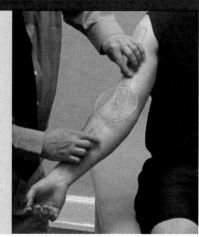

Lateral View

Check for an effusion by inspecting and palpating the area in the center of the triangle bounded by the lateral epicondyle of the humerus, the tip of the olecranon, and the radial head. Confirm the position of the radial head by feeling it move with forearm pronation/supination.

Palpate the area over the radial head to check for pain and crepitus. These findings, along with limited forearm rotation, suggest a radial head fracture (if acute) or arthritis (if chronic). Tenderness to palpation just distal to the lateral epicondyle indicates lateral epicondylitis. Tenderness 5 cm distal to the lateral epicondyle that is localized deep to the extensor muscles suggests entrapment of the posterior interosseous branch of the radial nerve.

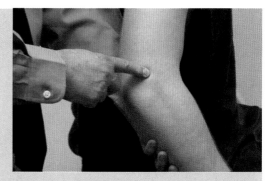

SECTION 3 ELBOW AND FOREARM

Medial View

Pain and tenderness immediately distal to the medial epicondyle suggest medial epicondylitis. The ulnar nerve lies in the ulnar groove just posterior to the medial epicondyle. Palpation and light percussion in this area may produce local pain and paresthesias in the medial forearm and ulnar two fingers (the Tinel sign), in association with ulnar nerve entrapment. Tenderness elicited with specific palpation of the sublime tubercle may indicate pathology involving the ulnar collateral ligament.

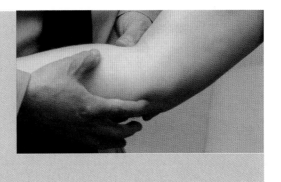

Posterior View

Inspect the area over the olecranon for focal swelling and palpate for tenderness to confirm the presence of olecranon bursitis. An olecranon fracture produces a broader area of swelling with ecchymosis and a possible skin abrasion at the point of impact. Palpate just above the olecranon to identify elbow effusion. A palpable defect, particularly with slight attempts by the patient to extend the elbow, may indicate a triceps brachii tear.

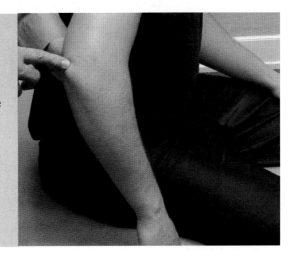

Range of Motion

Flexion and Extension: Zero Starting Position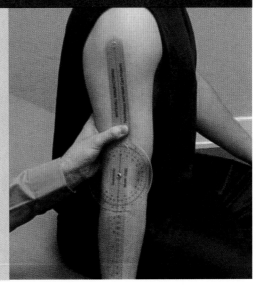

Evaluate elbow flexion and extension with the arm comfortably at the side. Observe from the lateral side. Begin the examination with the patient's elbow straight. Young children commonly hyperextend the elbow by 10° to 15°, but adults show minimal, if any, elbow hyperextension. Normal elbow range of motion is from 0° to 140° to 150° of flexion. Mild flexion contractures are of little functional consequence, as most activities of daily living are accomplished in an arc of elbow flexion from 30° to 130°. Limitation of motion may be expressed as either "The elbow flexes from 30° to 90°," or "The elbow has a flexion contracture of 30°, with further flexion to 90°."

SECTION 3   ELBOW AND FOREARM

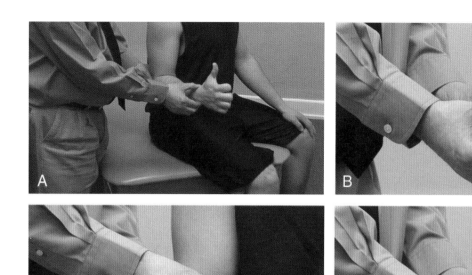

Forearm Rotation 🎥

Forearm rotation, which includes both pronation and supination, is a composite motion occurring at the proximal and distal radioulnar joints, as well as the radiohumeral joint. Measure forearm rotation by stabilizing the arm against the chest wall and flexing the elbow to 90°. Begin with the extended thumb aligned with the humerus (**A**). Palpate the radial and ulnar styloid as the forearm is rotated to estimate pronation and supination. Ask the patient to grasp a pencil or similar object (**B**) to facilitate visual estimation of forearm rotation.

Pronation is the position in which the palm is turned down (**C**), and supination is the position in which the palm is turned up (**D**). Normal pronation and supination is approximately 80° in each direction. Many activities of daily living are accomplished in an arc of motion between 50° pronation to 50° supination. A very restricted arc of forearm rotation may be of limited consequence if shoulder mobility is normal and if ankylosis of the forearm occurs in a neutral position.

Muscle Testing

Resisted Flexion 🎥

Test the strength of the flexors of the elbow, primarily the biceps brachii muscle, by resisting the patient's maximum effort to flex the supinated forearm. Weakness will be present with biceps tendinitis or rupture, dysfunction of the musculocutaneous nerve, or a lesion involving the C5 and C6 nerve roots.

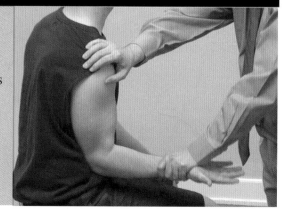

Resisted Extension 🎥

Test the strength of the extensors of the elbow, primarily the triceps brachii muscle, by resisting the patient's maximum effort to extend the elbow with the forearm in neutral position. Weakness will be present with triceps tendinitis or rupture, or a lesion involving the C7 or C8 nerve roots.

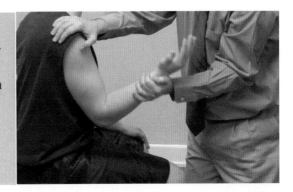

Resisted Supination 🎥

Test the strength of the forearm supinators, the most powerful of which is the biceps brachii muscle, by grasping the patient's distal forearm, supporting the elbow with your other hand, and resisting the patient's maximum effort to turn the palm up. Weakness will be evident with rupture or tendinitis of the biceps tendon at the elbow, subluxation of the biceps tendon at the shoulder, a lesion of the musculocutaneous nerve, or a lesion involving the C5 and C6 nerve roots. Patients with lateral epicondylitis also may experience pain with this maneuver.

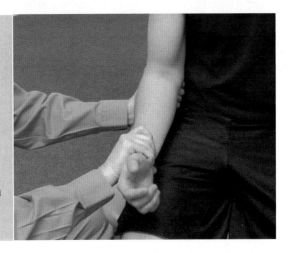

Resisted Pronation 🎥

Test the strength of the forearm pronators, the most powerful of which is the pronator teres muscle, by grasping the patient's distal forearm, supporting the elbow with your other hand, and resisting the patient's maximum effort to turn the palm down. Weakness will be evident with rupture of the pronator origin from the medial epicondyle, fracture of the medial elbow, or lesions involving the median nerve or the C6 and C7 nerve roots. Patients with medial epicondylitis also may experience pain with this maneuver.

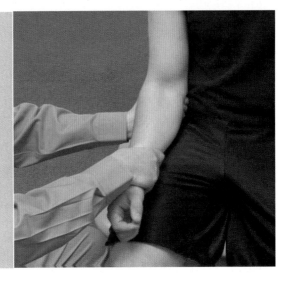

SECTION 3   ELBOW AND FOREARM

Resisted Wrist Flexion

Test the strength of the wrist flexors with the patient's arm at the side, forearm supported on a table, and elbow flexed 90°, with the wrist in flexion and the fingers extended. (This position eliminates wrist flexion activity by the finger flexors.) Ask the patient to keep the wrist flexed while you push the wrist into extension. Weakness will be evident with rupture of the muscle origin, fracture of the medial elbow, medial epicondylitis, or lesions involving the ulnar nerve (C8 and T1 nerve roots) or median nerve (C6 and C7 nerve roots).

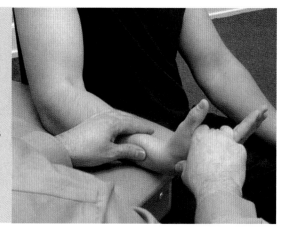

Resisted Wrist Extension

Test the strength of the wrist extensors, the most powerful of which are the extensor carpi ulnaris and extensor carpi radialis brevis muscles, with the patient's arm at the side, forearm supported on a table, and elbow flexed 90°, with the wrist in extension and the fingers in flexion. (This eliminates wrist extension activity by the finger extensors.) Ask the patient to hold the wrist in extension as you push the wrist into flexion. Weakness will be evident with rupture of the extensor origin, fracture of the lateral elbow, lateral epicondylitis, or lesions involving the radial nerve or C6 to C8 nerve roots.

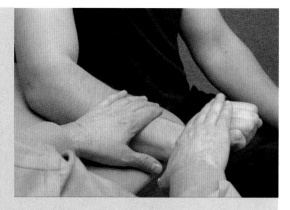

Stability Testing

Valgus Stress Test

Test the stability of the medial ligamentous structures, primarily the ulnar collateral ligament, by placing the patient in a seated or supine position. Stabilize the lateral side of the elbow with one hand and place your other hand distally on the medial aspect of the distal forearm. Place the elbow in approximately 20° of flexion to disengage the olecranon tip from the olecranon fossa of the distal humerus. While maintaining stability with your proximal hand, use your distal hand to abduct the forearm, which applies valgus stress and opens up the medial joint line of the elbow.

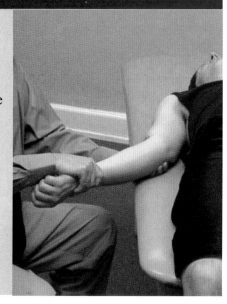

ELBOW AND FOREARM

SECTION 3

Varus Stress Test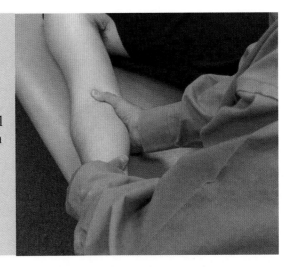

Test the stability of the lateral collateral ligament and lateral capsule by placing the patient in a seated or supine position with the forearm supinated. Stabilize the medial side of the elbow with one hand and place your other hand distally on the lateral aspect of the distal forearm. Place the elbow in approximately 20° of flexion to disengage the olecranon tip from the olecranon fossa of the distal humerus. While maintaining stability with your proximal hand, use your distal hand to adduct the forearm, which applies varus stress to the elbow and opens up the lateral joint line of the elbow.

Long Finger Test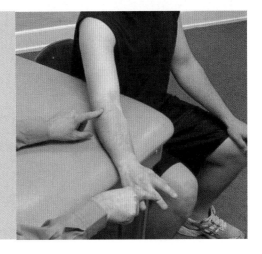

Position the patient with the forearm in pronation. Resist extension of the third digit of the hand distal to the proximal interphalangeal joint, stressing the extensor digitorum and tendon. Pain over the lateral epicondyle is a positive test for lateral epicondylitis.

Moving Valgus Stress Test (Milking Sign)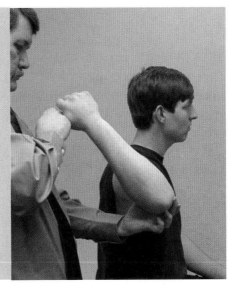

Stand behind the sitting patient on the side of the involved elbow. Place one hand on the back of the patient's shoulder and use the other hand to grasp the patient's thumb. Stabilize the shoulder and guide it into 90° of abduction and external rotation with the patient's elbow flexed generally around 90°. Additional posterior pull on the thumb further stresses the ulnar collateral ligament. Pain over the ulnar collateral ligament with stress in this position is indicative of ulnar collateral ligament pathology. The milking sign should be applied in various degrees of flexion, both greater and less than 90°.

SECTION 3   ELBOW AND FOREARM

Elbow Flexion Test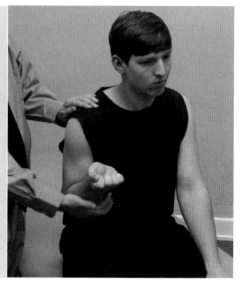

Instruct the patient to fully flex the elbow with wrist extension, shoulder girdle abduction, and depression and hold this position for 3 to 5 minutes. Tingling, numbness, and paresthesia in the ulnar nerve distribution is a positive test for cubital tunnel (ulnar nerve) syndrome.

SECTION 3 ELBOW AND FOREARM

Arthritis of the Elbow

Definition

Arthritis of the elbow can result from numerous pathologic conditions. These include rheumatoid arthritis (RA), nonrheumatoid inflammatory arthritis (including gout and pseudogout), posttraumatic arthritis, osteoarthritis (OA) (**Figure 1**), and septic arthritis. RA is the most common cause of elbow joint destruction, which almost always develops in patients with multiple joint involvement. Concomitant wrist and hand involvement occurs in 90% of patients with RA, with shoulder involvement in 80% of these patients. Active synovitis of the elbow causes periarticular erosions and symmetric joint narrowing, similar to the effect of synovitis in other joints. Further progression causes gross destruction of the bone and soft-tissue constraints. The end result is a grossly unstable elbow.

Nonrheumatoid inflammatory arthritis of the elbow generally presents as an acute crystalline synovitis (gout or pseudogout) with acute pain, swelling, stiffness, and warmth. This is often difficult to distinguish from septic arthritis. Long-standing degenerative changes of the elbow joint are unusual in these conditions.

Posttraumatic arthritis results from primary injury to the articular cartilage at the time of trauma, as well as fracture malunion. The end result is incongruity of the articular cartilage and progressive arthritis. Because posttraumatic arthritis often presents as an isolated joint impairment in an otherwise young, active patient, treatment options and the patient's expectations are often quite different from those of patients with RA.

Because the elbow is not a weight-bearing joint, OA is much less common in the elbow than it is in the hip, knee, or even the shoulder, and it may not be as symptomatic. Elbow OA is seen most often in manual laborers and weight lifters, suggesting repetitive

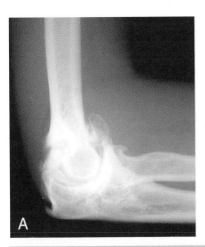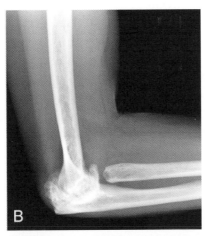

Figure 1 Radiographs demonstrate elbow arthritides. **A,** Lateral view of an elbow demonstrates radiographic changes typical of osteoarthritis. **B,** Lateral view of an elbow demonstrates erosive changes of bone typical of rheumatoid arthritis.

overuse as an underlying cause. Repetitive overuse of the elbow also commonly causes intra-articular loose bodies that can promote joint degeneration.

Septic arthritis results from infection (bacterial or nonbacterial) within the elbow joint, producing acute pain, swelling, loss of motion, and warmth. Septic arthritis is more common in patients with RA, HIV, and other immunocompromised states, as well as in intravenous drug users. Septic arthritis can result in articular cartilage destruction and ultimately joint degeneration.

Clinical Symptoms

RA of the elbow causes pain and swelling, as it does in other joints. In the early stages, the pain may be primarily localized to the lateral side of the joint and exacerbated by forearm rotation. Advanced disease causes diffuse pain and often gross instability that make even light household tasks impossible.

Symptoms of nonrheumatoid inflammatory arthritis include acute pain, swelling, effusion, loss of motion, and warmth, mimicking septic arthritis. The primary symptom reported by patients with posttraumatic arthritis is either pain or stiffness, depending on the type of injury. With malunion of a radial head fracture, the pain may be isolated to the lateral side of the joint and exacerbated by forearm rotation.

OA is characterized by pain and restricted motion. Intra-articular loose bodies are associated with symptoms of catching and locking. Posterior osteophytes typically cause limited extension and pain on terminal extension. Less commonly, anterior osteophytes can cause pain and limited flexion. Pain during midrange of motion and pain at rest are symptoms of late disease. Osteophytes on the medial side of the elbow can cause ulnar nerve irritation.

Septic arthritis generally produces acute and severe pain, stiffness, warmth, swelling, and effusion, as well as constitutional symptoms of fever, chills, and malaise.

Tests

Physical Examination

Inspection of the rheumatoid elbow demonstrates joint swelling, best seen laterally, and occasionally rheumatoid nodules over the olecranon and extensor surface of the forearm. Tenderness may occur primarily over the radial head or may be diffuse. Range of motion and varus/valgus stability also should be assessed.

An elbow with posttraumatic arthritis or OA typically does not have an effusion. The joint lines should be palpated for tenderness, and range of motion should be measured. Gently "jogging" the joint in full extension and then full flexion will elicit impingement pain from posterior and anterior osteophytes, respectively.

Synovitis resulting from nonrheumatoid inflammatory arthritis and septic arthritis typically produces severely painful range of motion, which is restricted. A substantial effusion and warmth are usually present.

Diagnostic Tests

AP and lateral radiographs of the elbow often are sufficient for diagnosis. RA produces the typical picture of osteopenia, symmetric joint narrowing, and periarticular erosions, or it may show gross joint destruction. Malunion, nonunion, and joint space narrowing are possible findings in posttraumatic arthritis. With OA, radiographs reveal osteophytes and joint space narrowing. Multiple loose bodies may be present in the anterior and posterior portions of the elbow. With nonrheumatoid inflammatory arthritis and septic arthritis, radiographs are usually normal acutely.

If an effusion is present, aspiration of the joint fluid may be helpful. Fluid should be examined for white blood cell (WBC) count (to differentiate between inflammatory and noninflammatory arthritis), crystals (present with nonrheumatoid inflammatory arthritis), Gram stain, and culture.

Differential Diagnosis

• Fracture of the distal humerus (evident on radiographs)
• Fracture of the radial head (evident on radiographs)
• Osteochondritis dissecans of the elbow (typically affects adolescent boys, capitellum usually involved, seen with repetitive overuse, may produce loose bodies)

Adverse Outcomes of the Disease

Progressive pain and stiffness are common to all arthritic conditions. RA can result in an unstable, essentially flail elbow. Septic arthritis left untreated may result in rapid joint destruction and even osteomyelitis.

Treatment

Mild limitation of elbow motion does not interfere with daily activities and is well tolerated, so treatment is often unnecessary. Modification of job or sports activities can be very helpful when symptoms warrant.

For RA, medical management should be optimized. Intra-articular corticosteroid injection and gentle rehabilitation may be beneficial. Static and hinged splints may be helpful for some patients. Synovectomy with or without radial head excision can provide pain relief in early stages of RA that are resistant to nonsurgical management. Total elbow arthroplasty is the best option for patients with RA who have advanced joint destruction.

Nonrheumatoid inflammatory arthritis is treated medically to manage the underlying pathology (such as gout or pseudogout). Intra-articular corticosteroid injections can be helpful in episodes of acute nonrheumatoid inflammatory synovitis.

For posttraumatic arthritis and OA, nonsurgical measures are limited to analgesics and gentle stretching to preserve motion. Arthroscopic débridement and removal of loose bodies can be quite

SECTION 3 ELBOW AND FOREARM

helpful. Unless the patient is elderly with a very limited activity level, total elbow arthroplasty generally is not considered beneficial because of concern about prosthesis loosening and breakage.

Prompt treatment of septic arthritis is critical and should specifically address the causal agent. Therapy generally involves a combination of appropriate antibiotics and surgical drainage.

Adverse Outcomes of Treatment

Patients with RA require regular monitoring for side effects from NSAIDs and disease-modifying agents. In 2015, the FDA strengthened its warning linking NSAIDs with the risk of heart attack or stroke, even in the first weeks of use of an NSAID. Nerve injury and infection are possible with surgery. Joint replacements can loosen or fracture with time.

Referral Decisions/Red Flags

Patients with persistent pain, locking episodes, or substantial loss of motion require further evaluation. Septic arthritis usually requires a combined medical and surgical approach.

Procedure: Elbow Joint Injection and Aspiration– Lateral Approach

This procedure can be used for either injection or aspiration of the elbow joint.

Step 1
Wear protective gloves at all times during this procedure and use sterile technique.

Step 2
Position the patient supine. Place the patient's arm against the chest or abdomen, with the elbow flexed at approximately 90° and the forearm in neutral rotation.

Step 3
Prepare the skin with a bactericidal solution.

Step 4
Palpate the soft-spot portal of the elbow that is located in the middle of the triangle formed between the lateral epicondyle, the radial head, and the olecranon tip. This soft-spot portal overlies the anconeus muscle. At this point, insert the 25-gauge needle past the muscle and through the capsule. Pull back on the syringe to confirm that intravascular injection is avoided. On injection, the needle should allow for relatively free flow of fluid without significant resistance. Next, inject the 3 mL solution of methylprednisolone acetate (2 mL) and lidocaine (1 mL) (**Figure 1**).

> **Materials**
> - Gloves
> - Bactericidal skin preparation
> - Ethyl chloride spray
> - 3- or 5-mL syringe
> - 18-gauge needle for solution preparation
> - 25-gauge needle for injection
> - 1 mL of 1% lidocaine
> - 2 mL of 40 mg/mL methylprednisolone acetate
> - Adhesive dressing

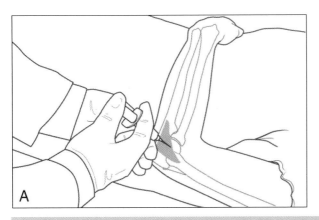 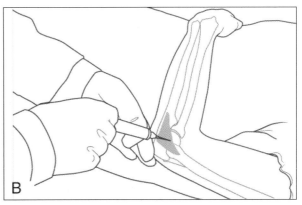

Figure 1 Images show the location for needle insertion for elbow joint injection (**A**) and aspiration (**B**) from a lateral approach.

SECTION 3   ELBOW AND FOREARM

Step 5

After injection, the elbow is taken through gentle repetitive cycles of range of motion to maximize the mixture of the fluid throughout the intra-articular portions of the joint.

Step 6

Dress the puncture site with a sterile adhesive bandage.

Adverse Outcomes

Subcutaneous infiltration of the corticosteroid preparation may cause subcutaneous fat atrophy, resulting in a waxy-appearing depression in the skin, and may cause depigmentation in dark-skinned patients. Although rare, infection is possible. Between 25% and 33% of patients will experience a "flare," which is characterized by increased pain at the injection site. Patients with diabetes may experience transient elevation of blood glucose and should be advised about this prior to injection.

Aftercare/Patient Instructions

Advise the patient that pain may increase for 24 to 48 hours after the injection. Pain often improves with the application of ice. Acetaminophen or an NSAID also is beneficial.

SECTION 3   ELBOW AND FOREARM

Dislocation of the Elbow

Definition

The elbow is the most commonly dislocated joint in children; in adults, it is second only to the shoulder and finger. Typically, a dislocated elbow is the result of a fall on an outstretched hand. More than 80% of elbow dislocations are posterior; posterolateral dislocations are the most common (**Figure 1**). A dislocation may be complete or "perched" (subluxated, with the trochlea resting on top of the coronoid process). The lateral collateral ligament is always disrupted, and other soft-tissue restraints commonly are injured as well. Concomitant fractures of the radial head/coronoid (in adults this is referred to as the terrible triad) (**Figure 2**) or medial epicondyle (in children) may be present. Neurovascular structures such as the brachial artery, median nerve, and ulnar nerve also may be injured.

Clinical Symptoms

Extreme pain, swelling, and inability to bend the elbow after a fall on an outstretched hand are characteristics of a dislocated elbow.

Tests

Physical Examination

Note areas of abnormal prominence and tenderness. The most important part of the examination is the neurovascular evaluation. Check the radial pulse and capillary refill. Assess motor and sensory function of the median, radial, and ulnar nerves.

Diagnostic Tests

AP and lateral radiographs of the elbow are adequate to make a diagnosis. Look carefully for associated fractures and bony fragments incarcerated in the joint, as these may cause widening of the joint

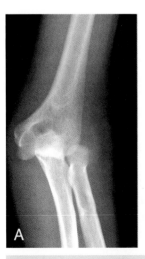
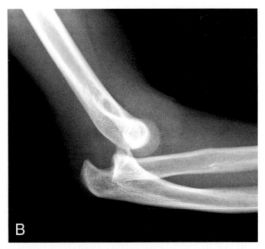

Figure 1 AP (**A**) and lateral (**B**) radiographs demonstrate posterolateral dislocation of the elbow.

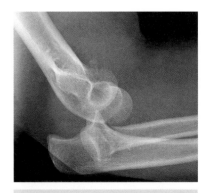

Figure 2 Lateral radiograph of an elbow demonstrates the so-called terrible triad of dislocation and fractures of the radial head and coronoid.

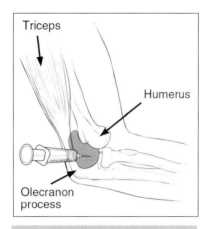

Figure 3 Illustration of the site of aspiration of hemarthrosis and injection of local anesthetic.

space. In the pediatric patient, a comparison radiograph of the contralateral elbow may help confirm the diagnosis.

Differential Diagnosis

- Fracture-dislocation of the elbow (same deformity, evident on radiographs)
- Fracture of the distal humerus (evident on radiographs)
- Fracture of the olecranon process of the ulna (evident on radiographs)
- Hemarthrosis (positive fat pad sign)
- Occult fractures (positive fat pad sign)
- Synovitis (normal radiographs, no deformity)

Adverse Outcomes of the Disease

Persistent loss of motion is common, especially in extension. Although most simple dislocations (that is, without fractures) are stable after reduction, persistent or recurrent instability is possible and should be specifically addressed rather than treated with prolonged immobilization. Heterotopic bone formation and the development of elbow joint arthritis also are possible.

Treatment

A dislocated elbow should be reduced as soon as possible after injury. Because of the possibility of occult fractures and the potential for neurovascular complications, reduction of elbow dislocations ideally should be performed by an orthopaedic surgeon unless this would result in an unacceptable delay in treatment. Reduction usually can be accomplished in the emergency department with the patient under conscious sedation. Sedation may be supplemented by aspirating the hemarthrosis and injecting 10 mL of 1% lidocaine into the joint from a lateral approach (**Figure 3**). If muscle spasm or marked swelling precludes reduction with the patient under conscious sedation, general anesthesia may be required.

Flexing the elbow tenses the triceps attachment to the olecranon and makes the reduction more difficult. The reduction should be performed by holding the elbow relatively extended (flexed approximately 45°) and applying slow, steady, downward traction on the forearm in line with the long axis of the humerus and then gently increasing elbow flexion. Gentle pressure over the olecranon tip as you are flexing the elbow also will help facilitate the reduction. The reduction usually is easily felt (as a "clunk") and, once achieved, generally is most stable with the elbow flexed and the forearm pronated. The stability of the reduction should be tested by slowly extending the elbow until the beginning of some subluxation is felt. The arm should be splinted at 90° of flexion (but avoiding more than 100° of flexion, which may contribute to vascular compromise as swelling develops).

After reduction, the neurovascular examination must be repeated.

After applying a splint to the arm, AP, lateral, and oblique radiographs should be obtained to confirm the reduction. Failure to obtain a perfectly concentric reduction suggests the possibility of a bony or cartilaginous intra-articular loose body or extensive soft-tissue injury, either of which may require surgical treatment.

Motion should begin 5 to 7 days after reduction and progress gradually during the next 3 to 6 weeks. A brace that blocks terminal extension is typically required during this time to maintain a concentric joint. The extension block may be removed at 3 to 4 weeks, with the aim of achieving full extension of the elbow 6 to 8 weeks after the dislocation, at which time use of the brace may be discontinued. At all times, radiographs must demonstrate a concentric reduction; if there is any concern, immediate referral is necessary. NSAIDs can be useful during this period and may decrease the incidence of heterotopic bone formation.

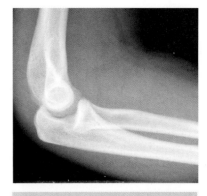

Figure 4 Lateral radiograph of an elbow with an incomplete reduction.

Adverse Outcomes of Treatment

Fracture and neurovascular injury are possible during the reduction maneuver. The ulnar nerve, because of its proximity, may become entrapped in the elbow joint. Subsequent vascular problems can result from compressive bandages or splinting with the elbow in more than 100° of flexion. Prolonged immobilization results in elbow contracture and pain and may not correct the underlying instability. Failure to identify and address persistent instability may result in the difficult situation of chronic instability. Chronic instability (especially chronic posterolateral rotatory instability of the elbow) is unusual; it may require surgical reconstruction.

Referral Decisions/Red Flags

Patients with associated neurovascular or bony injury (of the radial head/coronoid) require further evaluation, although a gentle reduction may be attempted to avoid lengthy delays. Incomplete reduction, as shown on radiographs, should never be accepted but should be referred immediately (**Figure 4**). Patients with a flexion contracture that prevents functional activities of daily living may require further evaluation.

SECTION 3 ELBOW AND FOREARM

Fracture of the Distal Humerus

Fracture Patterns
Supracondylar fracture
Transcondylar fracture
Intercondylar fracture
T condylar fracture
Lateral/medial condylar fracture

Definition
Fractures of the distal humerus are relatively uncommon, accounting for only 2% of fractures in adults. Because these fractures are often comminuted and intra-articular, the potential morbidity is high. Classification schemes used for these fractures can be quite complex, but the most important factors to consider in deciding on the best course for initial treatment are whether the fracture is displaced (**Figures 1** and **2**), whether the fracture involves the joint surface, and whether the skin and neurovascular structures are involved.

Clinical Symptoms
Marked swelling, ecchymosis, deformity, and pain about the elbow after an injury are common. Patients report increased pain with attempted flexion of the elbow.

Tests
Physical Examination
Swelling and deformity usually are clearly visible with any displaced fracture. Inspect the skin around the site to identify any open wounds.

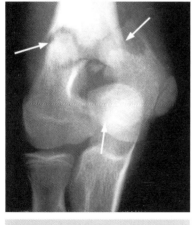

Figure 1 AP radiograph of the elbow demonstrates a displaced supracondylar fracture. (Reproduced from Beaty JH, Kasser JR: Fractures about the elbow. *Instr Course Lect* 1995;44:199-215.)

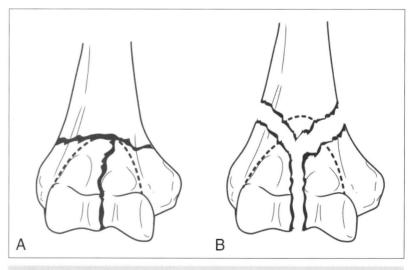

Figure 2 Illustration of distal humerus fractures. **A,** Nondisplaced T condylar fracture. **B,** Displaced intercondylar fracture.

Palpation around the joint may reveal an effusion, and crepitus may be felt with gentle flexion. Palpate the radial pulse and check capillary refill. Assess median, radial, and ulnar nerve function. Any of the peripheral nerves crossing the fracture may be injured, but ulnar nerve dysfunction is most common. Brachial artery occlusion is less common but requires early diagnosis and treatment to avoid devastating complications. Check the wrist and shoulder on the affected side for associated injuries.

Diagnostic Tests
AP and lateral radiographs of the elbow, as well as other radiographic views as clinically indicated, are adequate in most patients. In the absence of radiographic evidence of fracture, look carefully for a fat pad sign, which indicates bleeding into the joint, often from an occult fracture (**Figure 3**). In the pediatric patient, comparison views may help differentiate a true fracture from a growth plate. CT may be necessary to fully define the extent of the fracture.

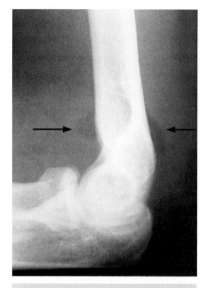

Figure 3 Lateral radiograph of the elbow. Note the anterior and posterior fat pad signs (arrows).

Differential Diagnosis
• Elbow dislocation (evident on radiographs)
• Olecranon fracture (evident on radiographs)
• Radial head fracture (evident on radiographs)
• Rupture of the distal biceps tendon (radiographs negative)

Adverse Outcomes of the Disease
Some degree of residual pain and stiffness is common. Other complications include deformity with malunion, nonunion, and ulnar neuropathy. Vascular injury can result in ischemia in the forearm and hand or compartment syndrome of the forearm muscle compartments. Prompt treatment is required to salvage function.

Treatment
The goal of treatment is to achieve and maintain a stable reduction that permits early motion. Stable, nondisplaced fractures may be treated with splinting for 10 days, followed by protected range of motion. Most distal humerus fractures are displaced to some degree, requiring open reduction and internal fixation. Other techniques, such as hinged external fixation or primary total elbow arthroplasty, might be considered under circumstances such as severe osteoporosis and/or fracture comminution. Appropriate therapy directed by a rehabilitation specialist following both surgical and nonsurgical treatment for elbow fractures can improve outcomes by ensuring appropriate exercise technique and progression, as well as proper splint selection, construction, and adjustment. Additional therapeutic techniques, including manual therapy, soft-tissue massage, and activities of daily living training, can also be beneficial.

SECTION 3 ELBOW AND FOREARM

Adverse Outcomes of Treatment

Pain and stiffness can persist after treatment. Deformity, nonunion, arthritis, and ulnar neuropathy may develop, as well as symptoms related to the prominent implants used for internal fixation. Infection, nerve damage, or hardware failure can complicate surgery.

Referral Decisions/Red Flags

Patients with displaced or open fractures of the distal humerus need further evaluation to determine whether surgical stabilization of the fracture is necessary. Likewise, patients with associated neurovascular injury need further evaluation.

Patients treated nonsurgically require close follow-up for complications such as fracture displacement and joint stiffness. Delayed vascular compromise may occur because of progressive swelling and/or tight splinting. Failure to regain motion is also an indication for referral.

SECTION 3   ELBOW AND FOREARM

Fracture of the Olecranon

Definition

The olecranon is the portion of the ulna that constitutes the bony prominence of the posterior elbow. Because of its subcutaneous location, the olecranon is easily fractured as a result of a direct blow to the elbow or a fall on an outstretched hand with the elbow flexed. As with other fractures, the most important consideration is determining whether the fracture is displaced or nondisplaced. Most of these fractures are displaced and can be further classified as noncomminuted or comminuted fractures of the olecranon or fracture-dislocations of the elbow (**Figure 1**).

Clinical Symptoms

A history of trauma followed by marked swelling and ecchymosis is typical. When an associated dislocation is present, the elbow will appear deformed as well. Because of the proximity of the ulnar nerve, the trauma itself or the resultant swelling may compress the nerve and cause numbness in the little and ring fingers.

Tests

Physical Examination

Examination usually reveals marked swelling of the entire elbow joint. Superficial abrasions at the site of impact are common and must be distinguished from deep wounds, which would make the injury an open fracture. Gentle palpation may reveal a defect if the fracture is displaced. Flexion of the elbow produces pain and is resisted. Median, radial, and ulnar nerve function should be assessed; of these,

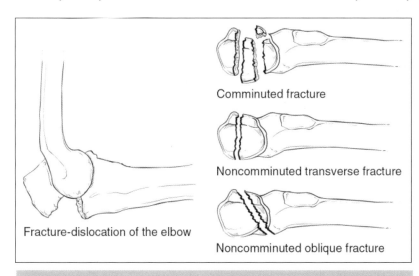

Comminuted fracture

Noncomminuted transverse fracture

Noncomminuted oblique fracture

Fracture-dislocation of the elbow

Figure 1 Illustration of types of olecranon fractures. (Adapted with permission from Jupiter JB, Mehne DK: Trauma to the adult elbow and fractures of the distal humerus, in Browner BD, Jupiter JB, Levine AM, Trafton PG, eds: *Skeletal Trauma: Fractures, Dislocations, Ligamentous Injuries*. Philadelphia, PA, WB Saunders, 1992, vol 2, pp 1125-1175.)

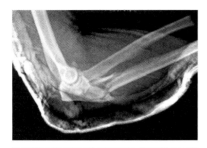

Figure 2 Lateral radiograph of an elbow demonstrates an olecranon fracture.

ulnar nerve injury is the most common. Radial and ulnar pulses and capillary refill should be assessed, but substantial vascular injury is uncommon with this fracture.

Diagnostic Tests

AP and lateral radiographs usually are adequate to confirm the diagnosis (**Figure 2**).

Differential Diagnosis

- Dislocation of the elbow (more grotesque deformity, evident on radiographs)
- Fracture of the coronoid process of the olecranon (almost always associated with an elbow dislocation)
- Fracture of the distal humerus (more proximal area of pain, evident on radiographs)
- Fracture of the radial head (lateral elbow pain increases with forearm rotation, fracture may be difficult to see on radiographs)

Adverse Outcomes of the Disease

Loss of motion and/or stability in the elbow is possible. Because the triceps inserts on the tip of the olecranon, active elbow extension can be lost with displaced fractures. Arthritis of the elbow may develop.

Treatment

Nondisplaced fractures of the olecranon can be treated with a posterior splint. To avoid excessive pull on the triceps and possible loss of reduction, the elbow should be splinted in approximately 45° of flexion. Follow-up radiographs should be obtained 7 to 10 days after the injury to ensure that the fracture has not become displaced. To avoid substantial permanent loss of motion, protected motion should begin within 2 to 3 weeks. To maintain hand strength and flexibility, instruct patients to squeeze a rubber ball or commercially available hand exerciser for 5 minutes at least twice each day.

Most olecranon fractures are displaced and are best treated surgically. Occasionally, a displaced fracture in a debilitated elderly patient who is a poor risk for surgery may be treated with a sling and early range-of-motion exercises, as pain allows. In addition to appropriate exercise selection, technique, and progression, therapy directed by a rehabilitation specialist following surgical or nonsurgical treatment for elbow fractures can improve outcomes by ensuring proper splint selection, construction, and adjustment. Additional therapeutic techniques, including manual therapy, soft-tissue massage, and activities of daily living training, may also be beneficial.

SECTION 3   ELBOW AND FOREARM

Adverse Outcomes of Treatment

Elbow stiffness, loss of motion, or arthritis may develop despite treatment. Nonunion or displacement of the fracture due to hardware failure is possible. After surgical treatment, irritation from the implants used to fix the fracture commonly occurs, necessitating a second procedure for implant removal.

Referral Decisions/Red Flags

Patients with displaced fractures or open fractures need further evaluation for possible surgical treatment.

SECTION 3   ELBOW AND FOREARM

Fracture of the Radial Head

Definition

Fractures of the radial head and neck result from falls on an outstretched hand. The most commonly used classification system, the modified Mason classification, separates these fractures into three types (**Figure 1**). Type I is a nondisplaced or minimally displaced fracture. Type II includes radial head fractures that are displaced more than 2 mm at the articular surface and angulated neck fractures that produce articular incongruity or a mechanical block. Type III fractures are severely comminuted fractures of the radial head and neck.

Clinical Symptoms

Following a fall on the outstretched hand, pain and swelling develop over the lateral aspect of the elbow. Loss of elbow motion may be related to pain inhibition and joint effusion, but a mechanical block to full forearm pronation and supination may be present in type II and III injuries. Radial head fractures also may be present in the context of an elbow dislocation (terrible triad injury). Rarely, the radial head fracture may be associated with an injury of the forearm (called an Essex-Lopresti fracture), and the forearm and wrist should be assessed.

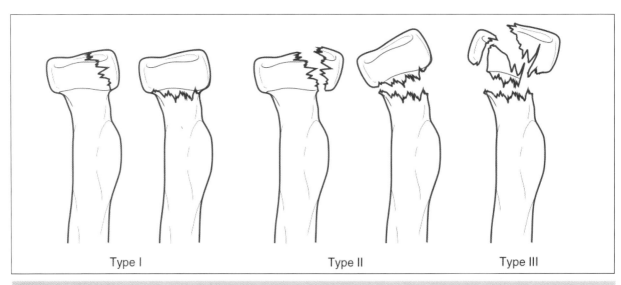

Type I   Type II   Type III

Figure 1 Illustration of the modified Mason classification of radial head fractures. Type I, nondisplaced fracture. Type II, radial head fracture that is displaced >2 mm at the articular surface and with an angulated neck fracture. Type III, severely comminuted fracture of the radial head and neck.

Tests

Physical Examination

Tenderness to palpation is localized to the lateral aspect of the joint, and a joint effusion can often be palpated. Passive forearm rotation is limited and may be associated with palpable crepitus. Elbow flexion and extension also may be limited by pain.

Tenderness over the forearm and/or wrist may indicate a more extensive soft-tissue injury involving the radioulnar interosseous membrane and the distal radioulnar joint. The presence of this type of injury makes treatment more difficult. Medial elbow tenderness and ecchymosis also may be present, indicating a medial collateral ligament strain or tear.

Diagnostic Tests

Type I fractures can be difficult to visualize radiographically but should be suspected based on positive clinical findings. Type II and III fractures are usually obvious on AP and lateral radiographs. CT is occasionally necessary to define the extent of the fracture.

Differential Diagnosis

- Elbow dislocation (clinical deformity and diffuse pain)
- Hemarthrosis of the elbow (present with radial head fracture or with other bony or soft-tissue injury)
- Olecranon fracture (pain and tenderness over the posterior tip of the elbow)
- Supracondylar fracture of the humerus (location of pain, tenderness, and deformity)

Adverse Outcomes of the Disease

Loss of motion, especially the last 10° to 15° of extension, is common, even with type I injuries. Posttraumatic arthritis of the radiocapitellar joint also may develop.

Treatment

Type I fractures should be treated with a sling or splint for comfort and early active motion as soon as pain allows. Because early motion is the key to a successful outcome, aspiration of the associated elbow hemarthrosis can be considered.

Aspiration with local anesthetic injection is useful diagnostically in type II fractures to determine whether a mechanical block to forearm rotation is present. When the fracture involves less than 2 mm articular step-off of a partial articular segment and no block to rotation, treatment should consist of early range of motion, as in type I fractures. Otherwise, open reduction and internal fixation is preferred. Open reduction and internal fixation of the radial head is most effective when there are three or fewer articular segments. More complex fractures are more amenable to prosthetic replacement.

Type III fractures usually are best treated by early open reduction

SECTION 3 ELBOW AND FOREARM

and internal fixation of the bone fragments or radial head replacement. When associated injuries of the ulnar collateral ligament or the interosseous membrane are present, excision alone of the fragments is contraindicated because this could result in persistent elbow instability.

In addition to appropriate exercise selection, technique, and progression, therapy directed by a rehabilitation specialist following surgical or nonsurgical treatment of elbow fractures can improve outcomes by ensuring proper splint selection, construction, and adjustment. Additional therapeutic techniques, including manual therapy, soft-tissue massage, and activities of daily living training, may also be beneficial.

Adverse Outcomes of Treatment
Loss of motion, instability, and wrist pain caused by proximal radial migration after radial head excision all can occur. Infection, nerve damage, hardware failure, malunion, loss of motion, and arthritis are possible following surgical intervention.

Referral Decisions/Red Flags
Type II fractures that block rotation, type III fractures, and any fracture associated with elbow dislocation or instability should be referred for surgical consideration. Failure of nonsurgical treatment, manifested by persistent pain or limited motion, also indicates the need for further evaluation.

Lateral and Medial Epicondylitis

Synonyms

Lateral epicondylitis:
    Lateral tendinosis of the elbow
    Tennis elbow
Medial epicondylitis:
    Golfer's or bowler's elbow
    Medial tendinosis of the elbow

Definition

Lateral epicondylitis and tennis elbow are the terms most commonly used to describe a condition that produces pain and tenderness at the lateral epicondyle of the humerus, the origin of the extensor carpi radialis brevis muscle. Although the term epicondylitis is commonly used, the pathology and point of maximal pain are in the tendon substance just distal and slightly anterior to the epicondyle (**Figure 1**). The term elbow tendinitis also is inaccurate because it implies an inflammatory origin. The histologic pattern of lateral epicondylitis is one of tissue degeneration with fibroblast and microvascular hyperplasia and the absence of inflammation. The term lateral tendinosis of the elbow is probably the most accurate but rarely is used.

Medial epicondylitis (also called golfer's or bowler's elbow) is similar to lateral epicondylitis in etiology and pathology and occurs in the common tendinous origin of the flexor/pronator muscles just distal to the medial epicondyle. Medial epicondylitis is much less commonly encountered than lateral epicondylitis.

Clinical Symptoms

The typical patient with lateral epicondylitis is between 35 and 50 years of age and reports a gradual onset of pain in the lateral elbow and forearm during activities involving gripping and wrist extension, such as lifting, turning a screwdriver, or hitting a backhand stroke in tennis. With time, the pain may become more severe and may occur at rest or during activities as minimal as holding a cup of coffee or using a key. Less commonly, the patient may relate the onset of symptoms to an acute event, such as a direct blow to the elbow or a sudden maximal muscle contraction.

The pain of medial epicondylitis typically occurs with active wrist flexion and forearm pronation, such as takes place during a golf swing, baseball pitching, the pull-through strokes of swimming, weight lifting, bowling, and many forms of manual labor.

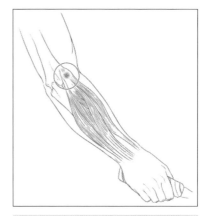

Figure 1 Illustration shows the location of pain in lateral epicondylitis.

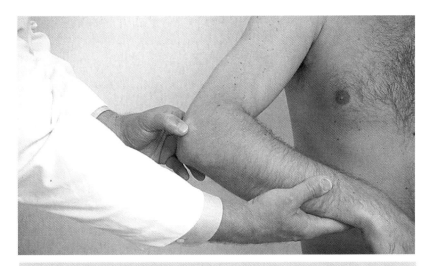

Figure 2 Photograph shows palpation of the point of maximum tenderness in lateral epicondylitis.

Tests

Physical Examination

The most consistent finding in lateral epicondylitis is localized tenderness over the common extensor origin 1 cm distal and slightly anterior to the lateral epicondyle (**Figure 2**). During the examination, it is best to have the patient's elbow flexed to 90° and the forearm pronated. Tapping lightly on the lateral epicondyle may be painful. Pain in the region also may be produced by gripping with resisted extension of the wrist when the elbow is in extension. To help differentiate lateral epicondylitis from other painful elbow conditions, ask the patient to lift a stool or chair with the palm up (using the wrist flexors) and then the palm down (using the wrist extensors). Patients with lateral epicondylitis will have pain when lifting with the palm down.

With medial epicondylitis, the area of tenderness is just distal to the medial epicondyle, and the pain is exacerbated by pronating the forearm and flexing the wrist against resistance. These patients also may have pain when lifting a chair with the palm up.

Diagnostic Tests

AP and lateral radiographs of the elbow are necessary to rule out arthritis or osteochondral loose bodies. Rarely, an area of calcification may be seen at the attachment of the extensor muscles to the lateral epicondyle or the flexor/pronator mass to the medial epicondyle of the humerus. MRI helps confirm the diagnosis and severity, but rarely helps predict treatment outcome.

Differential Diagnosis

- Cubital tunnel syndrome (compression of the ulnar nerve, paresthesias in little and ring fingers)
- Fracture of the radial head (radiographs should differentiate; pain

and tenderness over the radial head that are exacerbated by passive pronation and supination)

- Lateral plica (patient describes locking episodes and loss of elbow extension)
- Osteoarthritis of the radiocapitellar portion of the elbow joint (radiographs should differentiate; similar examination to radial head fracture but without a history of acute trauma)
- Osteochondral loose body (medial or lateral joint line pain, symptoms of locking)
- Radial tunnel syndrome (compression of the posterior interosseous nerve, tenderness typically approximately 5 cm distal to lateral epicondyle)
- Synovitis of the elbow (swelling, palpable effusion)
- Triceps tendinitis (tenderness above the olecranon)

Adverse Outcomes of the Disease

Persistent pain is the most common problem. Weakness or poor endurance with motions that involve forceful wrist flexion/extension or forearm pronation/supination, such as heavy or repetitive lifting, also is common. Inability to participate optimally in sport is common. Rupture of the flexor/pronator mass or the extensor mass from the respective epicondyle is seen occasionally.

Treatment

Modifying or eliminating the activities that cause symptoms is the most important step in treatment. In the case of tennis-related epicondylitis, this can include changing to a lighter-weight tennis racket, changing the tension of the racket strings, or overwrapping the handle to make it slightly larger or using a racket with a larger grip. For patients with severe and long-standing conditions, this activity modification may have to be permanent. NSAIDs and rub-in anti-inflammatory creams can be helpful during acute exacerbations. Use of a commercial tennis elbow strap worn just below the elbow during heavy-lifting activities may be helpful as well. Application of heat or ice may relieve pain and inflammation. After the pain has decreased, gentle stretching and forearm strengthening exercises can be initiated and are the key to successful treatment. Referral to a rehabilitation specialist is recommended if pain persists after 3 to 4 weeks. The rehabilitation specialist should determine the most effective treatment techniques for the individual patient based on the latest evidence and the patient's tolerance and response.

If symptoms persist, corticosteroid injection into the area of maximum tenderness may be helpful in lateral or medial epicondylitis. Patients should be advised that they could experience an increase in pain for 1 to 2 days after the injection. No more than three injections should be given. If the pain recurs and symptoms are severe, surgery (typically involving débridement of the area of tendinosis) can be considered. More than 95% of cases of lateral

SECTION 3   ELBOW AND FOREARM

epicondylitis and 85% of cases of medial epicondylitis will heal with nonsurgical treatment.

Rehabilitation Prescription

Treatment of the patient with humeral epicondylitis has four stages: (1) reduction of overload, pain, and inflammation; (2) promotion of total arm strength; (3) return to limited activities (those that are pain free); and (4) maintenance.

A home exercise program includes the use of ice following early attempts at exercise or unavoidable daily activities. Early submaximal exercise is initiated as signs and symptoms allow; for example, patient tolerance to a firm handshake is a criterion for determining whether a patient is ready for early exercise. Early use of submaximal isometric exercises such as squeezing a ball and manual resistive exercises for the wrist flexors, extensors, pronators, and supinators is advocated. The early goal of the home program is to promote muscle endurance and improve resistance to repetitive stress. To accomplish this goal, high repetitions per set with extremely low or no resistance are used. Three sets of 30 repetitions holding a rolled facecloth may be an appropriate early exercise target. This promotes local muscle endurance and provides a vascular response to the exercising tissues.

If the pain persists after the patient has been on the home program for 3 to 4 weeks, formal rehabilitation may be initiated. The rehabilitation specialist should perform a thorough evaluation of muscle strength, pain, and joint mobility to develop an appropriate treatment plan. No single pain-relieving modality or therapy has been found to be most effective for all patients. The rehabilitation specialist should determine the most effective modality for the individual patient based on patient tolerance and response.

Adverse Outcomes of Treatment

NSAIDs may cause gastric, renal, or hepatic complications. In 2015, the FDA strengthened its warning linking NSAIDs with the risk of heart attack or stroke, even in the first weeks of use of an NSAID. Although surgery always has a small risk of complications such as wound infection or nerve injury, the most common adverse outcome is incomplete pain relief despite adequate surgical release. Surgical failure can result from misdiagnosis, especially in cases involving nerve entrapment syndromes (of the posterior interosseous nerve with lateral epicondylitis; of the ulnar nerve with medial epicondylitis). Returning to work activities that were related to the onset of symptoms may be unlikely because of recurrence of symptoms or issues of secondary gain.

Referral Decisions/Red Flags

Failure of nonsurgical management indicates the need for further evaluation.

Home Exercise Program for Epicondylitis

- Perform the exercises in the order listed.
- To prevent inflammation, apply a bag of crushed ice or frozen peas to the painful area of the elbow for 20 minutes after performing the exercises.
- If you are unable to add weight or perform the indicated number of repetitions because of pain, call your doctor.
- The following exercise program is introductory only, and progression of this program will vary based on your specific injury, symptoms, and baseline level of fitness. For further progression of this routine, your physician may recommend evaluation and treatment by a physical therapist or other exercise professional.

Home Exercise Program for Epicondylitis

Exercise Type	Muscle Group	Number of Repetitions/Sets	Number of Days per Week	Number of Weeks
Wrist flexion (stretching)	Wrist extensor muscle group	Hold for 15 seconds; repeat 5 times. Perform on both sides.	5 to 7	3 to 4
Wrist extension (stretching)	Wrist flexor muscle group	Hold for 15 seconds; repeat 5 times. Perform on both sides.	5 to 7	3 to 4
Elbow extension	Elbow extensor muscle group	Work up to 3 sets of 10 repetitions, 2 to 3 times per day	5 to 7	3 to 4
Wrist flexion and extension	Wrist flexor and extensor muscle groups	Work up to 3 sets of 30 repetitions, 1 to 2 times per day	5 to 7	3 to 4
Forearm supination and pronation	Supinator and pronator teres	Work up to 3 sets of 10 repetitions, 1 to 2 times per day	5 to 7	3 to 4

SECTION 3 ELBOW AND FOREARM

Wrist Flexion (Stretching)

- To stretch the wrist flexors, straighten the elbow and bend the wrist back as if signaling someone to "stop."
- Use the opposite hand to apply gentle pressure across the palm and pull it as far toward the body as it will comfortably go, keeping the elbow straight. Hold for 15 seconds.
- Repeat 5 times.
- Perform on both sides, 5 to 7 days per week, for 3 to 4 weeks.

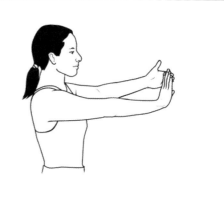

Wrist Extension (Stretching)

- To stretch the wrist extensors, straighten the elbow and bend the wrist so that the fingers are pointing down.
- Use the opposite hand to gently pull the hand as far toward the body as it will comfortably go, keeping the elbow straight. Hold for 15 seconds.
- Repeat 5 times.
- Perform on both sides, 5 to 7 days per week, for 3 to 4 weeks.

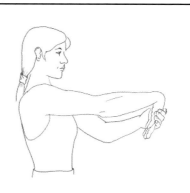

Elbow Extension

- Perform this exercise either standing with your weight evenly distributed over both feet or sitting.
- Holding a weight in the hand of the affected arm, raise the arm overhead while supporting the elbow with the opposite hand.
- Straighten the elbow overhead, hold for 5 seconds, and then bend the elbow and relax.
- Work up to 3 sets of 10 repetitions, 2 to 3 times per day.
- Perform the exercise 5 to 7 days per week, for 3 to 4 weeks.

Caution: If you do not have adequate triceps strength, do not raise the weight over your head. Bend at the waist with the elbow bent to 90°. Extend your arm back and hold this position for 5 seconds. Then bend the elbow and relax.

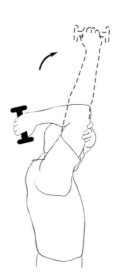

SECTION 3   ELBOW AND FOREARM

Wrist Flexion and Extension

- To exercise the wrist flexors, rest the forearm on a hard surface with the palm up.
- Flex the wrist as shown.
- Work up to 3 sets of 30 repetitions, 1 to 2 times per day.
- To exercise the wrist extensors, rest the forearm on a hard surface with the hand extending over the side.
- Extend the wrist as shown.
- Work up to 3 sets of 30 repetitions, 1 to 2 times per day.
- Perform the exercise 5 to 7 days per week, for 3 to 4 weeks.

Note: Use no weight initially; add weight in 1-pound increments to a maximum of 5 pounds. Weight can be added when target repetitions are performed without increasing pain. Always start with the elbow positioned in 90° of flexion to minimize pain with the exercises. Over time, as the pain subsides, the exercises may be performed with the elbow in a straightened position.

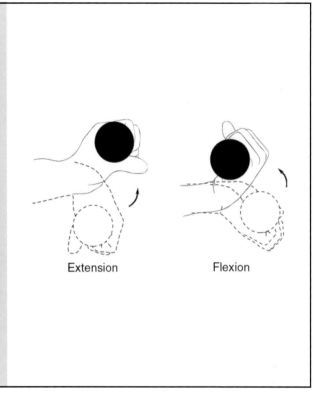

Extension   Flexion

Forearm Supination and Pronation

- Hold the forearm parallel to the ground, with the elbow bent 90°.
- To exercise the forearm supinators, pronate the forearm and then return to vertical as shown.
- Work up to 3 sets of 10 repetitions, 1 to 2 times per day.
- To exercise the forearm pronators, supinate the forearm and then return to vertical as shown.
- Work up to 3 sets of 10 repetitions, 1 to 2 times per day.
- Perform the exercise 5 to 7 days per week, for 3 to 4 weeks.

Note: Use no weight initially; add weight in 1-pound increments to a maximum of 5 pounds. Weight can be added when target repetitions are performed without increasing pain.

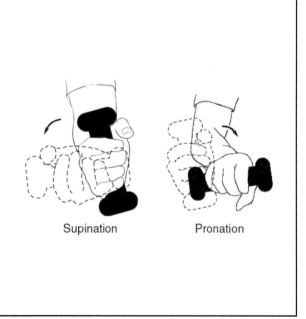

Supination   Pronation

SECTION 3 ELBOW AND FOREARM

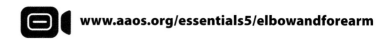
Procedure: Tennis Elbow Injection

The classic tender spot in lateral epicondylitis of the elbow (tennis elbow) is just distal to the lateral epicondyle of the humerus with the elbow in 90° of flexion.

Note: Opinions differ regarding one- versus two-needle injection techniques. A two-needle technique is shown in the video.

Materials

- Sterile gloves
- Bactericidal skin preparation solution
- 5-mL syringe with a 25-gauge, ¼″ needle
- 3 to 4 mL of a 1% lidocaine solution without epinephrine
- 2-mL syringe
- 1 mL of a corticosteroid preparation
- Adhesive bandage

Step 1

Wear protective gloves at all times during this procedure and use sterile technique.

Step 2

Place the patient's arm against the chest or abdomen, with the elbow flexed at least 90° and the forearm fully pronated.

Step 3

Prepare the skin with a bactericidal solution.

Step 4

Palpate just distal to the lateral epicondyle and locate the point of maximal tenderness. At this point, insert the 25-gauge needle, make a subcutaneous skin wheal with the local anesthetic, and advance through the tendon of the extensor carpi radialis brevis muscle to inject the remaining 2 to 3 mL of local anesthetic (**Figure 1**).

Step 5

Exchange syringes on the needle and inject the corticosteroid preparation. The syringe can again be exchanged and local anesthetic

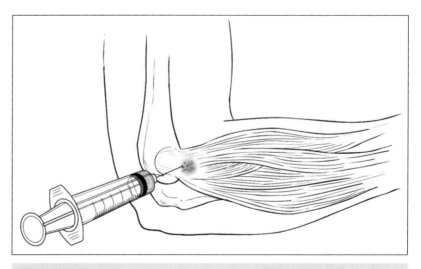

Figure 1 Illustration shows the location for needle insertion for tennis elbow injection.

injected as the needle is withdrawn to avoid steroid deposition subcutaneously. This reduces the risk of depigmentation in dark-skinned patients or fat atrophy.

Step 6
Dress the puncture site with a sterile adhesive bandage.

Adverse Outcomes
Subcutaneous infiltration of the corticosteroid preparation may cause subcutaneous fat atrophy, resulting in a waxy-appearing depression in the skin, and may cause depigmentation in dark-skinned patients. Although rare, infection is possible. Between 25% and 33% of patients will experience a "flare," characterized by increased pain at the injection site.

Aftercare/Patient Instructions
Advise the patient that pain may increase for 24 to 48 hours after the injection. Pain often improves with the application of ice. Acetaminophen or an NSAID also is beneficial.

SECTION 3   ELBOW AND FOREARM

Olecranon Bursitis

Definition

Because of its superficial location on the extensor side of the elbow, the olecranon bursa is easily irritated and inflamed (**Figure 1**). Olecranon bursitis may occur secondary to trauma, inflammation, or infection. Falls or direct blows may cause acute inflammatory bursitis. Prolonged irritation from excessive leaning on the elbow, often associated with certain occupations and avocations, may result in chronic inflammation. Olecranon bursitis also can develop in patients with chronic lung disease who lean on their elbows to aid breathing. The condition may be caused by systemic inflammatory processes, such as rheumatoid arthritis, gout, chondrocalcinosis, or hydroxyapatite crystal deposition. Infection of the olecranon bursa (septic bursitis) can occur primarily or develop as a secondary complication of aseptic bursitis.

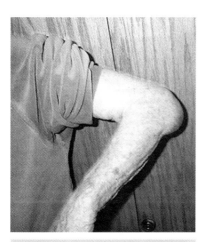

Figure 1 Photograph shows a swollen olecranon bursa. (Adapted with permission from Jupiter JB, Mehne DK: Trauma to the adult elbow and fractures of the distal humerus, in Browner BD, Jupiter JB, Levine AM, Trafton PG, eds: *Skeletal Trauma: Fractures, Dislocations, Ligamentous Injuries.* Philadelphia, PA, WB Saunders, 1992, vol 2, pp 1125-1175.)

Clinical Symptoms

The swelling associated with bursitis can develop either gradually (chronic) or suddenly (infection or trauma). Pain is variable but can be intense, and it may limit motion after an acute injury or when infection is present. Such severe swelling of the bursa may occur that patients report difficulty putting on long-sleeved shirts. As the mass diminishes in size, patients may feel firm "lumps" that are tender when the elbow is bumped. These lumps or nodules are scar tissue left as the fluid recedes.

Olecranon bursitis also occurs in patients with gout or rheumatoid arthritis. Gouty tophi (masses of monosodium urate crystals) may form in the olecranon bursa as well as along the ulnar border of the forearm, in the synovium of the elbow joint, and in numerous distant locations. Tophi are found only in patients with fairly advanced gout. As with gout, rheumatoid nodules may appear in several subcutaneous locations, such as over the olecranon and the ulnar border of the forearm. With time, these nodules may spontaneously shrink or disappear.

Tests

Physical Examination

Examination may reveal a large mass, up to 6 cm in diameter, over the tip of the elbow. The skin might be abraded or even lacerated if related to trauma. Redness and heat are not uncommon with acute bursitis and could indicate infection. Exquisite tenderness usually results from an infectious or traumatic origin. Chronic, recurrent swelling usually is less tender. The dimensions of the bursa should be measured periodically to monitor progress.

Diagnostic Tests

For large, symptomatic masses, aspiration may be both diagnostic and therapeutic. After an acute injury, bloody fluid may be found.

Fluid aspirated from the bursa should be analyzed for white blood cell (WBC) count, crystals, Gram stain, and culture. The index of suspicion for infection should be high because approximately 20% of cases of acute bursitis have a septic cause, involving either primary or secondary infection. When the origin is traumatic, radiographs should be obtained to rule out a fracture of the olecranon process of the ulna.

Differential Diagnosis
• Fracture of the olecranon process of the ulna (evident on radiographs)
• Gouty tophus or rheumatoid nodule (a tophus or nodule generally will be smaller and more discrete than an inflamed olecranon bursa)

Adverse Outcomes of the Disease
Secondary infection, chronic recurrence or drainage, and swelling or limited motion may develop.

Treatment
If the mass is small and symptoms are mild, bursitis should be left alone or treated symptomatically with activity modifications and possibly NSAIDs. Wearing an elbow pad and avoiding hyperflexion against hard surfaces may improve symptoms. Patients with more symptomatic bursitis should undergo aspiration of the bursa, followed by Gram stain and culture of any suspicious fluid. If there is no indication of septic bursitis, a compression bandage consisting of an 8-cm–diameter circular piece of foam and an elastic wrap should be applied. Reassess the patient in 2 to 7 days. If cultures are negative and fluid has reaccumulated in the bursa, repeat the aspiration and, if the fluid remains sterile, inject 1 mL of a corticosteroid preparation into the bursal sac. The bursal sac may have to be aspirated two or more times. If the elbow is at risk for repeated trauma, recommend an elbow protector.

Septic olecranon bursitis requires organism-specific antibiotic coverage based on the culture and sensitivity of the aspirate (frequently involving coverage for penicillin-resistant *Staphylococcus aureus*) and decompression by either surgical drainage or daily aspiration. Oral antibiotics may be administered if the septic bursitis is treated early and the patient is not immunocompromised. Hospitalization with intravenous antibiotics and surgical drainage and irrigation is indicated if the patient does not respond to oral antibiotics or if the patient has a more serious infection. Excision of chronically inflamed aseptic bursitis is not commonly necessary and should be avoided because a chronically draining or infected sinus may develop.

ELBOW AND FOREARM

SECTION 3

Adverse Outcomes of Treatment
Secondary infection, chronic drainage, or recurrence is possible.

Referral Decisions/Red Flags
Septic bursitis or recurrence of fluid despite repeated (three or more) aspirations indicates the need for further evaluation.

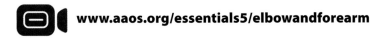

Procedure: Olecranon Bursa Aspiration

The olecranon bursa lies on the extensor aspect of the elbow, over the olecranon process of the ulna. The ulnar nerve lies adjacent to the medial face of the olecranon, behind the ulnar groove of the distal humerus. For this reason, aspiration is best done from the lateral side.

Step 1
Wear protective gloves at all times during this procedure and use sterile technique. This is important in aspirating an olecranon bursa because secondary infection can develop.

Step 2
Prepare the skin with a bactericidal solution.

Step 3
Use a 27-gauge needle to infiltrate the skin over the lateral aspect of the bursa with 1 mL of 1% lidocaine.

Step 4
Through the skin wheal, insert the 18-gauge needle attached to the 10-mL syringe into the enlarged bursa (**Figure 1**). Aspirate the contents until the bursa is flat. If there is any concern about infection, send the fluid for culture and sensitivity and do not inject the corticosteroid preparation into the cavity.

Materials
- Sterile gloves
- Bactericidal skin preparation solution
- Two 1-mL syringes
- 27-gauge, ¾" needle
- 1 mL of 1% lidocaine without epinephrine
- 10-mL syringe
- 18-gauge needle
- 1 mL of a 40 mg/mL corticosteroid preparation (optional)
- Adhesive bandage

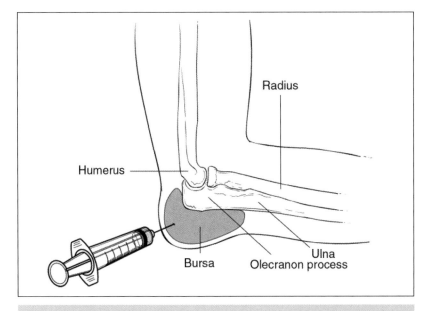

Figure 1 Illustration shows the location for needle insertion for olecranon bursa aspiration.

SECTION 3   ELBOW AND FOREARM

Step 5

If infection does not seem probable, a corticosteroid injection may be helpful. Remove the aspirating syringe and attach a 1-mL syringe containing 1 mL of a 40 mg/mL corticosteroid preparation. Inject this into the bursal cavity.

Step 6

Dress the puncture wound with a sterile adhesive bandage.

Step 7

Wrap the elbow lightly with an elastic dressing.

Adverse Outcomes

Secondary infection is possible, though not likely if sterile technique is used. Recurrence of the bursal effusion is common but can be minimized with a compressive dressing and by having the patient avoid direct trauma to the elbow, such as resting the elbow on tabletops.

Aftercare/Patient Instructions

Advise the patient to limit elbow motion for 1 or 2 days after the aspiration. If the patient has a recurrent bursitis, use a posterior plaster splint to limit elbow motion for 1 to 2 weeks after the aspiration.

SECTION 3   ELBOW AND FOREARM

Nerve Compression Syndromes

Synonyms

Cubital tunnel syndrome
Median nerve compression at the elbow
Posterior interosseous nerve compression
Pronator syndrome
Radial tunnel syndrome
Tardy ulnar palsy

Definition

Compression of the ulnar nerve at the elbow is second only to carpal tunnel syndrome as a source of nerve entrapment in the upper extremity. The nerve can be compressed at a number of sites, from 10 cm proximal to the elbow to 5 cm below the joint. The most common sites are where the ulnar nerve passes in the groove on the posterior aspect of the medial epicondyle (in the so-called cubital tunnel) and where it passes between the humeral and ulnar heads of the flexor carpi ulnaris muscle.

Ulnar nerve compression can develop acutely after a direct blow. Chronic symptoms occur in individuals who put prolonged pressure on the nerve by continuously leaning on the elbow or who keep the nerve stretched by holding the elbows flexed for long periods during work or recreation (**Figure 1**). Ulnar nerve compression also can occur after trauma that results in osteophytes or scar tissue that encroach upon the nerve. Cubitus valgus (a carrying angle greater than 10°) places the nerve on stretch and over time also may cause ulnar neuritis. Instability of the ulnar nerve with repetitive subluxation or dislocation of the ulnar nerve on elbow flexion also can cause ulnar palsy.

Compression of the posterior interosseous nerve, a deep branch of the radial nerve (radial tunnel syndrome), is a cause of lateral elbow pain and is commonly misdiagnosed as lateral epicondylitis. The posterior interosseous nerve has no sensory distribution but innervates the thumb and finger extensors and the extensor carpi ulnaris. The posterior interosseous nerve is most commonly compressed by fibrous bands between the two heads of the supinator muscle in a region termed the radial tunnel.

Pronator syndrome refers to muscular compression of the median nerve in the proximal forearm. Diagnosis is often difficult and delayed because of the vague symptoms, a lack of easily observed findings, and the frequent association with workers' compensation claims.

Clinical Symptoms

Symptoms vary depending on the duration and severity of the nerve compression. Early symptoms of ulnar nerve compression include

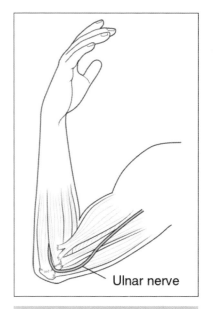

Figure 1 Illustration shows compression of the ulnar nerve during elbow flexion.

Ulnar nerve

aching pain at the medial aspect of the elbow and numbness and tingling in the ring and little fingers. The paresthesias occasionally radiate proximally into the shoulder and neck. Weakness of the intrinsic muscles is a late finding and can interfere with activities of daily living, such as opening jars or turning a key in a door. Visible muscle wasting implies ulnar nerve compression of several months or more.

Patients with radial tunnel syndrome present with symptoms similar to lateral epicondylitis but with pain that is 4 to 5 cm more distal than that of lateral epicondylitis. Because the posterior interosseous nerve contains only motor fibers, there is no numbness or tingling. Obvious muscular weakness is rarely encountered until late in the disease process.

Symptoms of pronator syndrome are often vague, consisting of discomfort in the forearm with occasional proximal radiation into the arm. Repetitive strenuous motions, such as industrial activities, weight training, or driving, often provoke the symptoms. Numbness may affect all or a part of the median nerve distribution. Women seem to be at greater risk than men for this syndrome, especially in the industrial setting.

Tests
Physical Examination

Inspect the elbow for deformity and measure the carrying angle. The nerve should be palpated for any masses or localized tenderness. Tapping lightly on the nerve may cause pain and paresthesias over the ulnar border of the hand and the ring and little fingers (Tinel sign).

Palpate the ulnar groove as the elbow is flexed and extended to determine if the nerve slips out of the groove. The elbow flexion test is a provocative maneuver. For this test, the patient flexes the elbow as far as possible, reporting any tingling or numbness in the hand as soon as it is felt. Record how quickly symptoms appear; if the symptoms do not develop within 60 seconds, the test is considered negative.

Assess sensation and muscle function of the ulnar nerve. Vibration and light touch perception are the first to be affected, and the little finger and the ulnar half of the ring finger are most likely to be involved. Two-point discrimination is affected when nerve compression has progressed to axonal degeneration.

Weakness is assessed by testing abduction and adduction of the little and index fingers, the ability to cross the index and middle fingers, and thumb-to-index pinch. The ulnarly innervated extrinsic muscles are less commonly involved. Wasting of the intrinsic muscles is a late finding and produces a hollowed-out appearance between the metacarpals on the dorsal aspect of the hand.

With posterior interosseous nerve compression, the area of tenderness is directly over the radial tunnel, which lies 4 to 5 cm distal and slightly anterior to the lateral epicondyle. With radial tunnel syndrome, pain in the proximal forearm may be elicited by extending the long (middle) finger against resistance ("middle finger test").

With pronator syndrome, physical examination findings are often subtle. The most reliable test is reproduction of pain with direct pressure over the proximal portion of the pronator teres approximately 4 cm distal to the antebrachial crease while exerting moderate resistance to pronation. Resisted pronation for 60 seconds may initiate the symptoms by contracting the flexor-pronator muscle.

Diagnostic Tests

Electromyographic/nerve conduction velocity (EMG/NCV) studies provide an objective measurement of ulnar nerve compression. A reduction in velocity of 30% or more suggests substantial compression of the ulnar nerve. EMG/NCV studies are usually normal in cases of radial tunnel and pronator syndromes. Plain radiographs of the elbow are indicated when previous elbow trauma has occurred.

Differential Diagnosis

- Carpal tunnel syndrome (numbness in thumb, index, and middle fingers; thenar muscle wasting)
- Herniated cervical disk or cervical radiculopathy (history, physical examination, and EMG/NCV should differentiate, although MRI may sometimes be necessary)
- Lateral epicondylitis (tenderness over lateral epicondyle/extensor attachment, no neurogenic symptoms)
- Medial epicondylitis (tenderness over the medial epicondyle; no distal weakness, paresthesias, or numbness)
- Thoracic outlet syndrome (normal NCV studies at the elbow; rarely, wasting in the hand)
- Ulnar nerve entrapment at the wrist (strong wrist flexors and ulnar deviators, sensation intact over the dorsomedial hand and the dorsum of the little and ring fingers)

Adverse Outcomes of the Disease

Loss of strength and sensation can be progressive and permanent in long-standing cases. Pain, tenderness, and stiffness at the elbow also can persist.

Treatment

For ulnar nerve compression, modifying activities in the workplace to limit elbow flexion and direct pressure on the ulnar nerve is the most important step in treatment. At night, an elbow splint that prevents the elbow from flexing to 90° can be worn. (A towel wrapped around the elbow is sufficient if a commercial splint is not available.) A sports elbow protector can be used at work to keep from bumping the elbow. NSAIDs may be of benefit for an acute, severe episode. Corticosteroid injections are not recommended.

ELBOW AND FOREARM

SECTION 3

Surgical decompression and transposition of the ulnar nerve should be considered for patients with bothersome symptoms or mild weakness that persists despite 3 to 4 months of nonsurgical management, or for patients with substantial or progressive weakness. There are several different methods of surgical decompression, but all involve inspecting the nerve and removing all sources of compression.

Decompression of the radial tunnel is indicated for patients with radial tunnel syndrome who have substantial discomfort that has not responded to prolonged nonsurgical care over a period of at least 3 to 6 months. Formal rehabilitation may be helpful and should include a thorough evaluation of muscle strength, pain, and joint mobility. No single pain-relieving modality or therapy technique has been found to be most effective for all patients. The rehabilitation specialist should determine the most effective modality for the individual patient based on the patient's tolerance and response.

Likewise, surgical decompression is indicated for pronator syndrome if all measures of nonsurgical treatment (including activity/job modification, anti-inflammatory medications, rehabilitation, and steroid injection) have not resulted in adequate pain relief over a period of at least 3 to 6 months.

Adverse Outcomes of Treatment

Care should be taken that any splint applied does not have straps across the medial elbow because this could increase nerve compression. NSAIDs can cause gastric, renal, or hepatic complications. In 2015, the FDA strengthened its warning linking NSAIDs with the risk of heart attack or stroke, even in the first weeks of use of an NSAID. Surgery may be complicated by infection and/or nerve damage. Symptoms are not always improved after surgery. The importance of nonsurgical care and the careful selection of surgical candidates cannot be overemphasized because these nerve compression injuries are often work related and are complicated by issues of secondary gain.

Referral Decisions/Red Flags

Substantial or progressive weakness or atrophy of the intrinsic muscles, increasing numbness despite nonsurgical treatment, or persistent symptoms that interfere with activities or work and have failed to respond to prolonged nonsurgical care indicate the need for further evaluation.

ELBOW AND FOREARM — SECTION 3

Home Exercise Program for Radial Tunnel Syndrome

- Perform the exercises in the order listed.
- To prevent inflammation, apply a bag of crushed ice or frozen peas to the painful area of the elbow for 20 minutes after performing the exercises.
- If pain steadily worsens, if the exercises increase the pain, or if the pain does not improve after you have performed the exercises for 3 to 4 weeks, call your doctor.
- The following exercise program is introductory only, and progression of this program will vary based on your specific injury, symptoms, and baseline level of fitness. For further progression of this routine, your physician may recommend evaluation and treatment by a physical therapist or other exercise professional.
- General wrist and hand strengthening exercises may be gradually added to the program after symptoms decrease and these stretching exercises are performed without aggravation of symptoms.

Home Exercise Program for Radial Tunnel Syndrome

Exercise Type	Muscle Group	Number of Repetitions/Sets	Number of Days per Week	Number of Weeks
Wrist flexion (stretching)	Wrist extensor muscle group	Hold for 15 seconds; repeat 5 times. Perform on both sides.	5 to 7	3 to 4
Wrist extension (stretching)	Wrist flexor muscle group	Hold for 15 seconds; repeat 5 times. Perform on both sides.	5 to 7	3 to 4
Wrist supination (stretching)	Wrist supinator muscle group	Hold for 15 seconds; repeat 5 times. Perform on both sides.	5 to 7	3 to 4
Nerve gliding	Median nerve	10 to 15 repetitions	6 to 7	3 to 4

Wrist Flexion (Stretching)

- To stretch the wrist flexors, straighten the elbow and bend the wrist back as if signaling someone to "stop."
- Use the opposite hand to apply gentle pressure across the palm and pull it as far toward the body as it will comfortably go, keeping the elbow straight. Hold for 15 seconds.
- Repeat 5 times.
- Perform on both sides, 5 to 7 days per week, for 3 to 4 weeks.

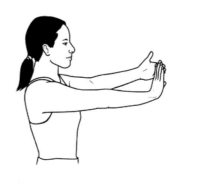

SECTION 3 ELBOW AND FOREARM

Wrist Extension (Stretching)

- To stretch the wrist extensors, straighten the elbow and bend the wrist so that the fingers are pointing down.
- Use the opposite hand to gently pull the hand as far toward the body as it will comfortably go, keeping the elbow straight. Hold for 15 seconds.
- Repeat 5 times.
- Perform on both sides, 5 to 7 days per week, for 3 to 4 weeks.

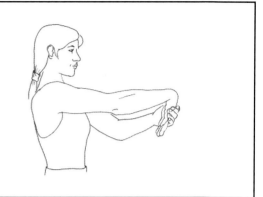

Wrist Supination (Stretching)

- To stretch the wrist into supination, keep the elbow bent at the side of the body with the palm facing up toward ceiling.
- Use the opposite hand to gently turn the forearm further into the palm up position until a stretch is felt. Hold for 15 seconds.
- Repeat 5 times.
- Perform on both sides, 5 to 7 days per week, for 3 to 4 weeks.

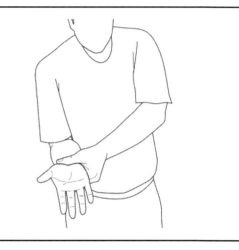

SECTION 3 ELBOW AND FOREARM

Nerve Gliding
- With the affected hand raised, make a fist with the thumb outside the fingers (1).
- Extend the fingers, keeping the thumb close to the side of the hand (2).
- Extend the hand at the wrist (bend it backward, toward the forearm), keeping the fingers straight (3).
- With the wrist straight, extend the thumb as shown (4).
- Keeping the thumb extended, extend the hand at the wrist (5).
- Reach behind your hand and grasp the thumb with the thumb and forefinger of the opposite hand. Pull the thumb downward, away from the palm of your hand (6).
- Repeat 10 to 15 times.
- Perform the exercises 6 to 7 days per week, for 3 to 4 weeks.

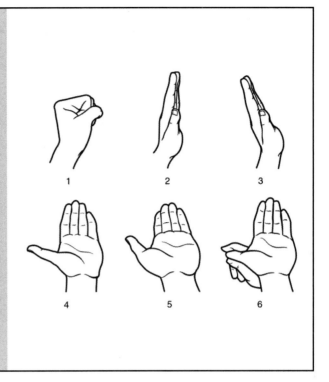

SECTION 3 ELBOW AND FOREARM

Rupture of the Distal Biceps Tendon

Definition

Rupture of the distal biceps brachii tendon is uncommon, accounting for less than 5% of biceps tendon ruptures, but when they do occur, complete tears of the distal biceps tendon cause substantially greater weakness than do tears of the proximal biceps tendon. If the lesion is not recognized and repaired in a timely fashion, elbow flexion and forearm supination strength is decreased by 30% to 50%. Most often, ruptures occur in men older than 40 years who have preexisting degenerative changes in the biceps tendon.

These ruptures typically are located at the insertion of the biceps tendon into the radius (radial tuberosity). The rupture may be incomplete or complete. With complete ruptures, the biceps aponeurosis may remain intact initially.

Clinical Symptoms

Patients often report a history of sudden, sharp pain in the anterior elbow following an excessive extension force on the flexed elbow. The pain typically is severe for a few hours (acute inflammatory response) and then is followed by a chronic, dull ache in the anterior elbow region that is made worse by lifting activities.

Tests

Physical Examination

Examination reveals tenderness and a defect in the antecubital fossa due to the absence of the usually prominent biceps tendon. Early on, ecchymosis will be present in the antecubital fossa and proximal forearm. With flexion of the elbow against resistance, the muscle belly retracts proximally (**Figure 1**). When the patient actively pronates and supinates the forearm with the elbow at 90°, the normal rise and fall of the biceps muscle belly is lost; this can be compared with the opposite arm.

If the rupture is incomplete, the defect will not be apparent, but the patient will exhibit pain and weakness on flexion and supination of the elbow against resistance. If the rupture is complete but the bicipital aponeurosis is intact, the defect is not as obvious; however, comparison with the opposite side helps to confirm the diagnosis.

Diagnostic Tests

AP and lateral radiographs of the elbow usually are normal, but they may reveal an avulsion fracture of the bicipital tuberosity. MRI is usually necessary to confirm the diagnosis. MRI will also help to distinguish between an avulsion of the tendon from the radial tuberosity and a rupture at the muscle-tendon junction (not common), which has a poorer prognosis.

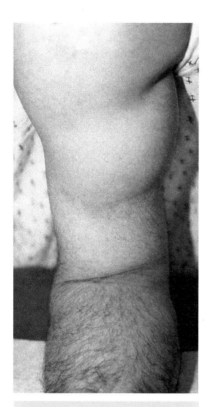

Figure 1 Photograph shows the clinical appearance of distal biceps tendon rupture. (Reproduced from Ramsey ML: Distal biceps tendon injuries: Diagnosis and management. *J Am Acad Orthop Surg* 1999;7[3]:199-207.)

Differential Diagnosis
- Bicipital tendinosis (degenerative tendon changes without rupture)
- Cubital bursitis (enlargement of the bursa between the biceps tendon and the radial tuberosity; can occur as a primary condition or secondary to other conditions)
- Entrapment of the lateral antebrachial cutaneous nerve (pain and dysesthesia at the lateral aspect of the proximal forearm)
- Pronator syndrome (no weakness or defect)

Adverse Outcomes of the Disease
Loss of elbow flexion strength is noted initially, but flexion strength improves over time; on average, only a 15% residual loss of strength is seen. Loss of forearm supination, however, is more substantial and permanent, with up to a 50% loss seen. Loss of forearm supination power (for example, turning a screwdriver) is more dysfunctional for manual laborers or individuals who perform activities that require a lot of forearm twisting. With time, the muscle retracts and becomes fibrotic. In this situation, surgical repair either is not possible or the results are compromised, with less predictable return of muscle strength.

Treatment
Most patients with complete ruptures do better with surgical repair of the tendon. Partial ruptures may be managed nonsurgically with activity modification and intermittent splinting, but if this treatment fails, surgical repair is indicated. Nonsurgical management is used with older patients who are sedentary and do not require normal elbow flexor/supinator strength and endurance. Nonsurgical treatment also may be appropriate for the nondominant arm in selected patients and in cases of delayed diagnosis.

Adverse Outcomes of Treatment
Full return of muscle strength may not occur. Injury to the radial nerve is possible. Infection, heterotopic ossification, and chronic pain may ensue.

Referral Decisions/Red Flags
Because of the adverse and progressive effect on muscle strength, rupture of the distal tendon of the biceps should be evaluated for possible surgical repair within 1 to 2 weeks of the injury. Surgical exposure and ability to repair the tendon is more difficult if referral is delayed beyond the first 2 weeks of injury.

ELBOW AND FOREARM

SECTION 3

Ulnar Collateral Ligament Tear

Definition

The ulnar collateral ligament is the primary structure resisting valgus stress at the elbow. Trauma to this ligament (including strains and tears) is relatively uncommon and rarely results in symptomatic instability or disability in the general population. The overhead throwing athlete (particularly in baseball and javelin), however, places repetitive valgus stress across the medial elbow and the ulnar collateral ligament (**Figure 1**), which can result in injury to the ligament, resulting in instability and disability that may require treatment in these athletes.

Clinical Symptoms

Onset may be acute, with the athlete experiencing a "pop" while throwing, followed by medial elbow pain. Most commonly, patients have a gradual onset of symptoms with progressive medial elbow pain with throwing. Paresthesias along the ulnar nerve distribution while throwing is a common symptom. Swelling and ecchymosis are usually minimal. This injury is being seen with increasing frequency at younger ages, especially in high school athletes. A history of abuse to the arm (excessive number of pitches per game, excessive innings per year, year-round baseball, use of breaking pitches—curve or slider—at a young age) is common.

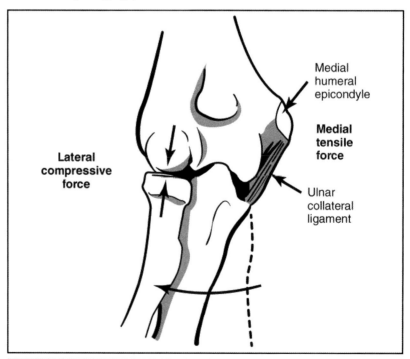

Figure 1 Illustration shows forces resulting in valgus sprain of the ulnar collateral ligament in the throwing athlete.

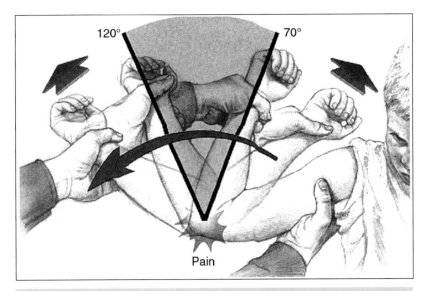

Figure 2 Illustration of the moving valgus stress test. Starting with the arm in full flexion, the examiner applies a constant valgus torque to the elbow and then quickly extends the elbow. The test is positive when pain is elicited when the elbow is flexed between 70° and 120°. (Adapted with permission from the Mayo Foundation for Medical and Education Research, Rochester, MN.)

Tests

Physical Examination

Examination generally demonstrates tenderness over the ulnar collateral ligament, and there may be some loss of terminal extension. Swelling and ecchymosis are generally absent. There is usually pain over the ulnar collateral ligament with valgus stress testing, although gross opening of the joint is uncommon. The milking maneuver and the moving valgus stress test also are useful physical examination tests. With the milking maneuver, the patient or examiner pulls on the patient's thumb to create a valgus stress with the forearm supinated and the elbow flexed to 90°. A positive test is when the patient describes pain with this maneuver. With the moving valgus stress test, this same valgus load is applied while moving the elbow into full flexion and extension (**Figure 2**). The test is positive if more intense pain at the medial elbow is reported by the patient when the elbow is flexed between 70° and 120°. Tenderness over the ulnar nerve and a positive Tinel sign also may be present and can result in an inaccurate diagnosis of primary ulnar neuritis.

Diagnostic Tests

AP and lateral radiographs are necessary to rule out fracture. Ossification within the ulnar collateral ligament may be seen in chronic cases. Posteromedial olecranon osteophytes, loose bodies, and marginal spurring also may be seen in chronic cases. MRI with intra-articular contrast is a reasonable diagnostic tool for diagnosing pathology of the ulnar collateral ligament.

SECTION 3   ELBOW AND FOREARM

Differential Diagnosis

- Cubital tunnel syndrome (stability examination, history; frequently coexists with ulnar collateral ligament injury)
- Medial epicondyle avulsion (evident on radiographs, adolescent age group)
- Medial epicondylitis (history and stability examination; typically, older age group)

Adverse Outcomes of the Disease

Persistent pain and disability in throwing sports are most common. Rarely are problems encountered with activities of daily living or in nonthrowing sports. Chronic stiffness and loss of motion may be encountered.

Treatment

Nonsurgical care, including rest, NSAIDs, rehabilitation, stretching and strengthening exercises, and activity modification, is appropriate following such an injury. Corticosteroid injections in the ulnar collateral ligament may cause weakening and attenuation of the ligament and should be avoided. A very slow return to sport (involving a detailed progressive throwing program) should be stressed. If pain relief is the main goal of the patient, nonsurgical care is likely to be successful. If a return to a highly competitive level of a throwing sport is the main goal, surgery may be necessary. If symptoms in an athlete have failed to respond to an appropriate course of nonsurgical care within 3 months, surgical reconstruction (the so-called Tommy John surgery) should be considered. The patient must realize that postoperative rehabilitation is critical and lengthy, requiring approximately 12 months before return to competition. In the properly selected athlete, surgery is over 90% successful in returning the athlete to the preinjury level of competition. With the alarming trend of ulnar collateral ligament injuries in younger baseball players, emphasis should be placed on education and prevention in youth sports (such as following pitch counts, limiting the number of innings pitched per season or per year, avoiding year-round baseball, and delaying the throwing of breaking pitches until the young athlete's body matures).

Adverse Outcomes of Treatment

Surgical risks include stiffness, nerve injury, infection, and persistent pain.

Referral Decisions/Red Flags

Failure of nonsurgical management in the high-level throwing athlete who wishes to continue to compete at this level indicates the need for further evaluation.

PAIN DIAGRAM
Hand and Wrist

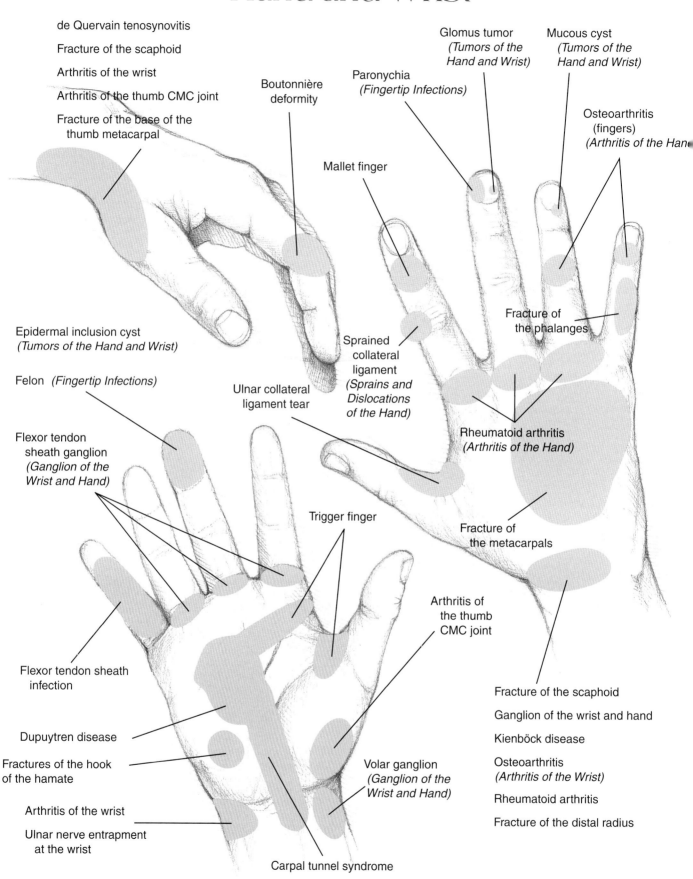

de Quervain tenosynovitis

Fracture of the scaphoid

Arthritis of the wrist

Arthritis of the thumb CMC joint

Fracture of the base of the thumb metacarpal

Boutonnière deformity

Paronychia *(Fingertip Infections)*

Glomus tumor *(Tumors of the Hand and Wrist)*

Mucous cyst *(Tumors of the Hand and Wrist)*

Osteoarthritis (fingers) *(Arthritis of the Han*

Mallet finger

Epidermal inclusion cyst *(Tumors of the Hand and Wrist)*

Felon *(Fingertip Infections)*

Flexor tendon sheath ganglion *(Ganglion of the Wrist and Hand)*

Ulnar collateral ligament tear

Sprained collateral ligament *(Sprains and Dislocations of the Hand)*

Fracture of the phalanges

Rheumatoid arthritis *(Arthritis of the Hand)*

Trigger finger

Fracture of the metacarpals

Flexor tendon sheath infection

Dupuytren disease

Fractures of the hook of the hamate

Arthritis of the wrist

Ulnar nerve entrapment at the wrist

Arthritis of the thumb CMC joint

Volar ganglion *(Ganglion of the Wrist and Hand)*

Carpal tunnel syndrome

Fracture of the scaphoid

Ganglion of the wrist and hand

Kienböck disease

Osteoarthritis *(Arthritis of the Wrist)*

Rheumatoid arthritis

Fracture of the distal radius

Hand and Wrist

Section Editor

Julie E. Adams, MD, MS

Associate Professor
Orthopaedic Surgery
Mayo Clinic
Rochester, Minnesota

Contributor

Mark C. Hubbard, MPT

Physical Therapist
Bone and Joint Institute
Penn State Milton S. Hershey Medical Center
Hershey, Pennsylvania

ANATOMY OF THE HAND AND WRIST

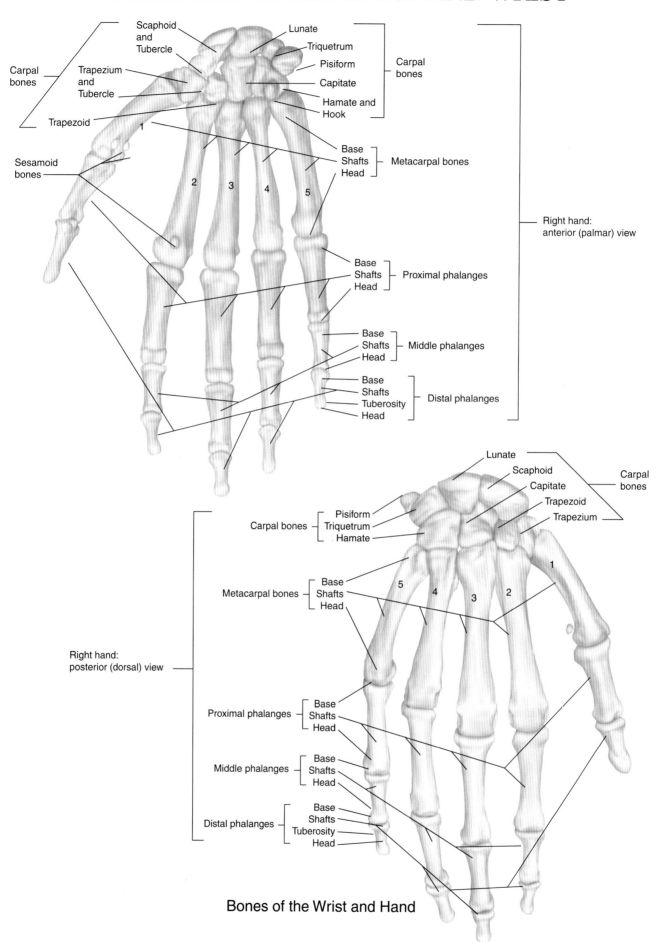

Carpal bones

Scaphoid and Tubercle

Trapezium and Tubercle

Trapezoid

Sesamoid bones

Lunate

Triquetrum

Pisiform

Capitate

Hamate and Hook

Carpal bones

Base
Shafts
Head — Metacarpal bones

1 2 3 4 5

Right hand: anterior (palmar) view

Base
Shafts
Head — Proximal phalanges

Base
Shafts
Head — Middle phalanges

Base
Shafts
Tuberosity
Head — Distal phalanges

Right hand: posterior (dorsal) view

Carpal bones
Pisiform
Triquetrum
Hamate

Lunate
Scaphoid
Capitate
Trapezoid
Trapezium

Carpal bones

Metacarpal bones
Base
Shafts
Head

5 4 3 2 1

Proximal phalanges
Base
Shafts
Head

Middle phalanges
Base
Shafts
Head

Distal phalanges
Base
Shafts
Tuberosity
Head

Bones of the Wrist and Hand

Overview of the Hand and Wrist

Carpal tunnel syndrome, trigger finger, ganglion formation, carpometacarpal (CMC) arthritis of the thumb, and radiocarpal arthritis are among the more common hand and wrist problems that bring patients to a primary care physician. Patients with chronic hand and wrist problems typically have one or more of the following symptoms: pain, instability, stiffness, swelling, weakness, numbness, or a mass.

To begin the evaluation, obtain a thorough history from the patient, including a statement of the chief complaint, a thorough history of the current condition, and a general medical history. The history of the current condition should include the duration of symptoms, the specific type and location of symptoms, factors that improve or worsen the symptoms, previous treatments, and the outcomes of those treatments on the symptoms. After obtaining the history, a physical examination should be done. With a good history and physical examination, a working diagnosis can be established in a high percentage of patients. Diagnostic testing, which often includes plain radiographs, should be done to help confirm the working hypothesis that has been synthesized from the history and physical examination or to exclude alternative conditions. Additional diagnostic evaluation commonly used for the hand includes electrophysiologic evaluation (electromyography or nerve conduction velocity tests), Doppler ultrasonography, and MRI and CT with or without arthrogram contrast.

Location of Pain

The best method of localizing the pain is to have the patient use one finger to identify the point of maximum tenderness. The pain is categorized as being in one of the following four general locations: radial, ulnar, volar, or dorsal (**Figure 1**). This localization of pain by anatomic region will help narrow the field of probable diagnoses and allow the physician to focus further diagnostic evaluations.

Radial Pain

Wrist pain in patients younger than 30 years most commonly results from trauma. Posttraumatic tenderness and pain over the radial aspect of the wrist may suggest a scaphoid fracture, which is the most commonly missed fracture in the wrist and hand. In the absence of trauma, pain associated with tenderness over the radial styloid is most likely de Quervain (wrist) tenosynovitis. Pain that is dorsal and slightly more proximal may be caused by intersection syndrome (tenosynovitis of the radial wrist extensors) or superficial radial neuritis. Pain that occurs without numbness in patients older than 40 years is likely caused by posttraumatic arthritis or osteoarthritis. Pain at the base of the thumb in women in this age group is likely to be caused by CMC arthritis.

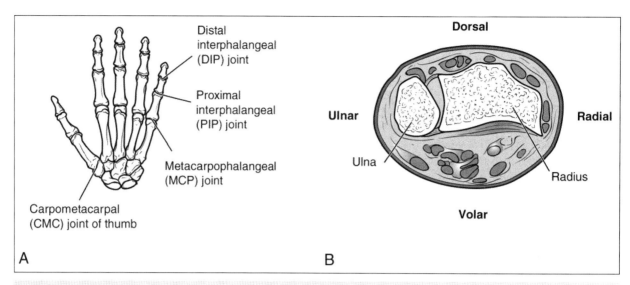

Figure 1 Illustrations of the hand and wrist. **A,** Joints of the hand: dorsal view. **B,** Localizing symptoms to one of the four quadrants of the wrist can be helpful in guiding the physical examination and for establishing a differential diagnosis.

Dorsal Pain

Generalized dorsal wrist discomfort may be associated with radiocarpal arthritis. Pain in this region associated with a well-defined mass over the dorsoradial aspect of the wrist is usually a ganglion cyst; however, an "occult" or very small ganglion cyst may be the source of pain in the absence of a defined mass. Pain and loss of motion in the wrist can also be caused by ligament injury (scapholunate ligament injury or lunotriquetral ligament injury) to the wrist or by Kienböck disease (osteonecrosis of the lunate). Plain radiographs are valuable in the initial assessment of these patients.

Ulnar Pain

Pain in this region after trauma can be caused by a tear of the triangular fibrocartilage complex, which is located distal to the ulnar styloid. In a subacute or chronic setting, ulnocarpal abutment may be the cause of discomfort. Swelling and tenderness over the dorsoulnar or volar aspects of the wrist are likely to be caused by a tendinitis of the ulnar wrist extensor (extensor carpi ulnaris) or flexor (flexor carpi ulnaris) tendons.

Volar Pain

Carpal tunnel syndrome, ganglion cyst formation, and tenosynovitis are the most common causes of volar wrist pain. Carpal tunnel syndrome is commonly associated with numbness and tingling in the radial three digits (thumb plus index and long fingers) and, often, half of the ring finger. Other causes of discomfort include a volar ganglion cyst, which should be easily palpable on the volar radial aspect of the wrist, or wrist tendinitis. Swelling over the volar region suggests inflammation of the finger flexor tendons. Patients with radiocarpal arthritis might have pain over both the dorsal and volar aspects of the wrist. Volar wrist pain also can be caused by arthritis between the pisiform and the triquetrum bones (that is, pisotriquetral arthritis).

Chronic Wrist and Finger Instability

Diagnosis of wrist instability is often complex, requiring considerable experience in history taking, physical examination, and interpretation of radiographs. Typical symptoms are sensations of slipping, snapping, or clunking with certain wrist motions after an injury. The unstable structure might be a joint (following a tear of the supporting and stabilizing ligaments that hold together the carpal bones) or a subluxating tendon (following a tear of the restraining ligaments, or retinaculum, that contain the tendon). Plain PA radiographs of the wrist might show separation between the scaphoid and the lunate (Terry Thomas sign), indicating a tear of the intrinsic ligament binding the scaphoid and the lunate (scapholunate dissociation). Chronic ligamentous instability commonly occurs in the metacarpophalangeal (MCP) joint of the thumb and can occur in any of the proximal interphalangeal (PIP) joints or MCP joints.

Stiffness

Morning stiffness is a common symptom of arthritis or tenosynovitis and may be associated with carpal tunnel syndrome or trigger finger. Patients with trigger finger often have pain, and they commonly (and erroneously) localize the problem to the PIP joint when it locks or "jumps" as the finger is flexed. In fact, the source of the problem is in the palm, where the thickened flexor tendon catches under the proximal (A1) tendon pulley at the distal palmar crease. Tenderness and palpable catching just distal to this crease confirm the diagnosis.

Swelling

Swelling in the joints of the hand and wrist is caused by synovitis, which can be secondary to osteoarthritis, infection, or a systemic inflammatory disease such as rheumatoid arthritis or gout. A history of penetrating trauma or immunocompromise in patients who present for evaluation of swelling should suggest infection as opposed to inflammatory disease. Plain radiographs are useful in diagnosing osteoarthritis and rheumatoid arthritis. Swelling around the tendons can occur in association with rheumatoid arthritis and/or overuse syndromes such as de Quervain tenosynovitis. Pain and swelling around the wrist flexor or extensor tendons suggest tendinitis; plain radiographs may show a calcific deposit close to the involved tendon in patients in whom calcific tendinitis develops.

Weakness

Weakness in the hand may be secondary to pain, as with CMC or radiocarpal arthritis or intrinsic muscle disease. Weakness without pain suggests possible peripheral nerve entrapment or central nervous system disease. Ulnar nerve entrapment at the elbow will result in decreased grip and pinch strength in addition to loss of sensation in the little and ring fingers. Wasting of the intrinsic muscles is seen on physical examination in advanced cases.

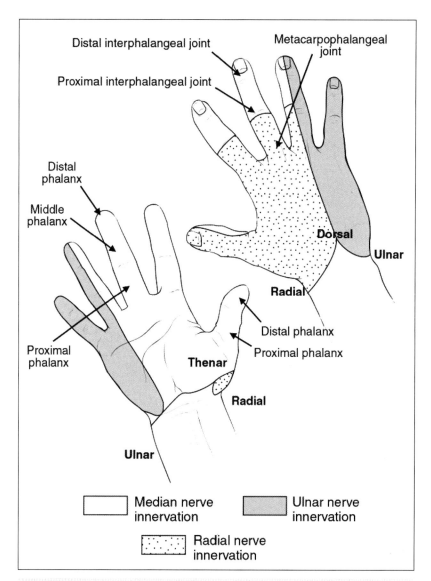

Figure 2 Illustration of the regions of and sensory distribution in the hand.

Numbness

Dysesthesias, paresthesias, and hand-based numbness and tingling are commonly caused by entrapment neuropathy. **Figure 2** shows the typical sensory distribution of the median, ulnar, and radial nerves; however, variations from this pattern can occur. Positive provocative signs (Tinel sign, Phalen maneuver, Durkan carpal compression test) and abnormal sensory test results should be considered indicative of carpal tunnel syndrome. With carpal tunnel syndrome, the numbness characteristically occurs in the thumb, the index and long fingers, and, often, the radial half of the ring finger; some patients report that the entire hand is numb.

Loss of sensation in the little and ring fingers usually is caused by entrapment of the ulnar nerve at the elbow or the wrist. Patients with thoracic outlet syndrome often report symptoms at the ulnar side of the hand and forearm, but this condition is much less common than ulnar nerve entrapment at the elbow. Both the Tinel sign and elbow flexion tests should be negative with thoracic outlet syndrome.

Neck pain associated with a positive Spurling test and with loss of sensation in the thumb and index finger suggests a common cervical radiculopathy. Electrophysiologic testing is commonly used to confirm the clinical diagnosis in patients who present for evaluation of numbness.

Masses

The most common mass in the hand and wrist is a ganglion cyst. These cysts most often occur in four locations: the dorsoradial and volar radial aspects of the wrist, the proximal finger flexor crease, and the distal interphalangeal joint. Multilobulated masses along the sides of the finger are most likely giant cell tumors. Nontender nodules in the palm and cords that cross both the MCP and PIP joints are consistent with Dupuytren contracture. A hard mass at the dorsal base of the index metacarpal is usually a carpal boss—a bony mass consisting of spurs from the second and third metacarpals, the trapezoid, and the capitate. A serpiginous mass that follows the path of the tendon sheaths is often tenosynovitis. Masses with bluish discoloration or masses that have a pulsation are usually vascular in origin.

Physical Examination of the Hand and Wrist

Inspection/Palpation

Dorsum

Observe the alignment of the fingers. Inspect the nails for pitting, discoloration, spooning, or other evidence of systemic disorders. Look for swelling, synovitis, or deformity of the finger and wrist joints. Note any osteophytes or bony prominences associated with degenerative arthritis. Muscle atrophy between the metacarpals results in weakness of the intrinsic muscles and may be caused by nerve compression or a systemic disorder.

In addition, look for skin changes or trophic changes such as altered temperature, hair growth, or sweating patterns. These may be clues to systemic disorders or localized pathology. Look for atrophy of the thenar muscles, which are innervated by the median nerve, and atrophy of the hypothenar muscles, which are innervated by the ulnar nerve. Position the patient's hands with the palms facing each other (not shown) to best visualize atrophy of the thenar muscles. Swelling in the joints of the thumb also is prominent in this position.

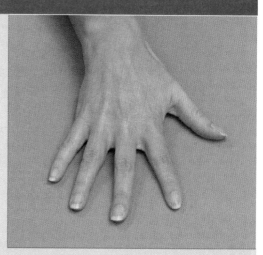

Palm

Note any thickening of the palmar fascia or contractures associated with Dupuytren disease.

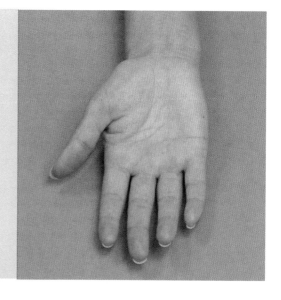

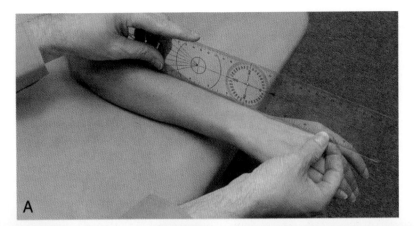

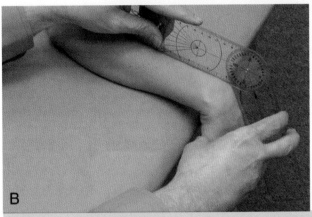

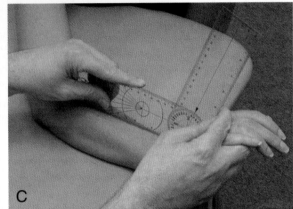

Wrist Flexion and Extension: Zero Starting Position

To measure wrist flexion and extension, a goniometer is needed. Place the patient's forearm in pronation and the carpus aligned with the plane of the forearm. Place the goniometer on the dorsum of the wrist (**A**). Aligning the goniometer on the ulnar side may falsely elevate the measurement because of the mobility of the fifth metacarpal. Wrist motion occurs at the radiocarpal and midcarpal joints. Normal wrist palmar flexion (**B**) is 75° to 80°, and normal dorsal extension (**C**) is 70° to 80°.

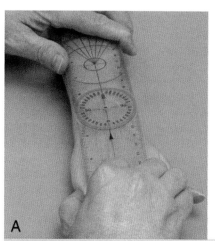 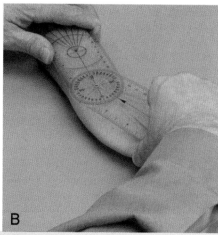 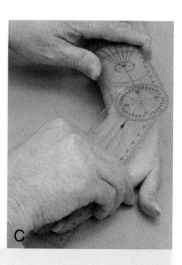

Wrist Radial and Ulnar Deviation

To measure radial and ulnar deviation, a goniometer is needed. Place the patient's forearm in pronation and the carpus aligned with the plane of the forearm. Align the goniometer with the third metacarpal and the axis of the forearm (**A**). In radial and ulnar deviation, the carpal rows move as linked segments. The buttress of the radial styloid limits radial deviation so that its arc of motion is significantly less. Normal radial deviation (**B**) is 20° to 25°, and normal ulnar deviation (**C**) is 35° to 40°.

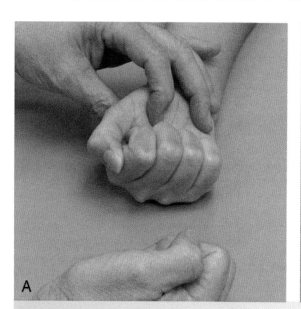 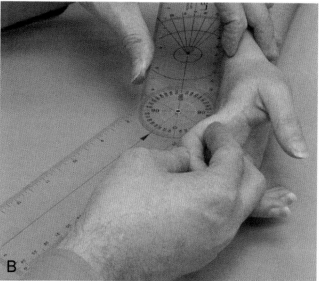

Finger Flexion and Extension

Finger joint motion occurs primarily in the flexion-extension plane, with flexion accounting for most finger joint motion. A goniometer is needed to measure finger flexion and extension. From a functional perspective, finger flexion is a composite movement of motion of the metacarpophalangeal, proximal interphalangeal, and distal interphalangeal joints. To estimate the loss of digital flexion, have the patient maximally flex the fingertip. In young and middle-aged adults, the fingertip should touch the distal palmar crease (**A**). (Loss of digital flexion can be roughly quantified by specifying that the patient lacks a certain distance [measured in centimeters] to the distal palmar crease.) Alternatively, flexion and extension also can be measured individually at the metacarpophalangeal, proximal interphalangeal, and distal interphalangeal joints (**B**). The wrist should be in neutral when measuring finger flexion. If the wrist is flexed, the extensor digitorum longus will be effectively tethered, thereby limiting finger flexion. Finally, active motion should be compared with passive motion.

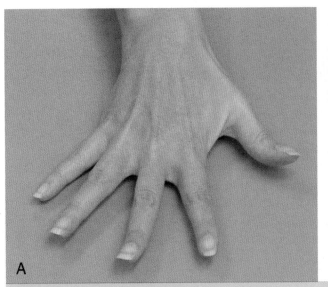
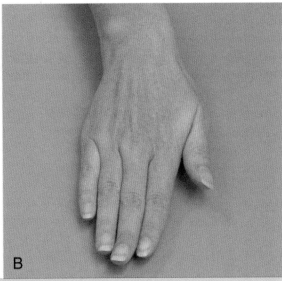

A

B

Finger Abduction and Adduction ▣❙

Abduction and adduction of the fingers occur in the plane of the palm, primarily at the metacarpophalangeal joints and centered on the long finger. Ask the patient to spread the fingers, then close them together. Abduction (**A**) is movement of the fingers away from the long finger; adduction (**B**) is movement of the other fingers toward the long finger.

Range of Motion

Thumb Opposition ▣❙

Thumb motions are complex and reflect the overall importance of the thumb to the function of the hand. The principal thumb motions are abduction, adduction, flexion, extension, and opposition. Opposition is a composite motion created by movement at the carpometacarpal, metacarpophalangeal, and interphalangeal joints and is valued as 50% to 60% of thumb function.

Measure composite thumb flexion by asking the patient to touch the tip of the thumb to the base of the little finger. Inability to do so indicates a limitation of rotation at the carpometacarpal, metacarpophalangeal, and/or interphalangeal joint. The amount of impairment can be assessed by measuring the distance from the tip of the thumb to the base of the little finger.

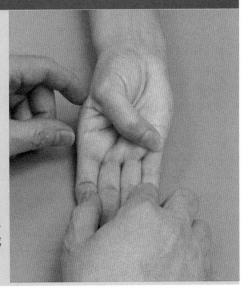

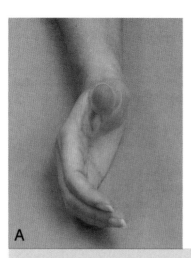
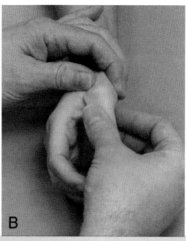
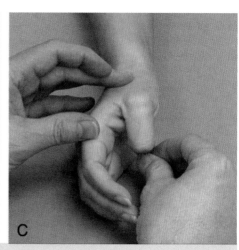

A   B   C

Thumb Flexion and Extension 📷

All thumb joints move in the plane of flexion-extension, but this movement is difficult to quantify at the carpometacarpal joint. Flexion at the thumb metacarpophalangeal joint (**A**) is typically 50° to 60°, but normal measurements are highly variable. Flexion at the interphalangeal joint (**B**) ranges from 55° to 75° and depends on age and sex. Extension beyond 0° may be observed at the metacarpophalangeal joint and may be present in the setting of thumb carpometacarpal joint arthritis and joint subluxation as a compensatory phenomenon, leading to a Z collapse pattern of the thumb (not shown). Hyperextension of 5° to 10° at the interphalangeal joint is often present and is a normal finding.

Measure thumb flexion and extension with the wrist in a neutral position (**C**). If the wrist is flexed, the extensor pollicis longus may be tethered, limiting flexion at the metacarpophalangeal and interphalangeal joints. A finger goniometer may be used to more accurately quantify the range of motion.

Wrist Extension 📷

To assess wrist extension and the loss of wrist motion, ask the patient to face you with the palms of the hands pressed together. Compare the extension of the right and left wrists when held in similar positions, as shown. Take care to position the elbows in flexion.

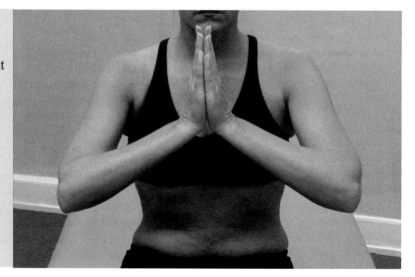

Muscle Testing

Wrist Flexion

In general, manual motor testing should be done by first asking the patient to demonstrate the primary function of a muscle and then, when possible, asking the patient to show resistance (provided by the examiner) to the opposition of that function. Responses to testing should be graded objectively, using the 0 to 5 manual muscle testing scale. To test the strength of the wrist flexors—the most powerful of which is the flexor carpi ulnaris—stabilize the patient's elbow at 90°. With the fingers extended to eliminate action of the finger flexors, resist the patient's attempt to flex the wrist. Weakness will be evident with fracture of the medial humeral condyle, medial epicondylitis, tendinitis of the medial elbow, or lesions involving the median or ulnar nerve.

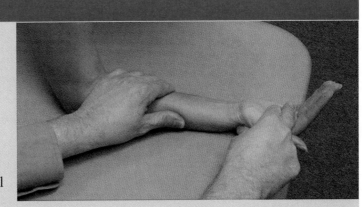

Wrist Extension

To test the strength of the wrist extensors—the most powerful of which are the extensor carpi ulnaris and extensor carpi radialis brevis—have the patient seated with the forearm supported on a table and the elbow flexed approximately 90°. Resist the patient's attempt to extend the wrist while the fingers are relaxed in a flexed position. Weakness will be evident with rupture of the extensor origin, fracture of the lateral humeral condyle, lateral epicondylitis, radial tunnel syndrome, lesions involving the radial nerve or C6-C7 nerve roots, or distal rupture of the tendon insertion.

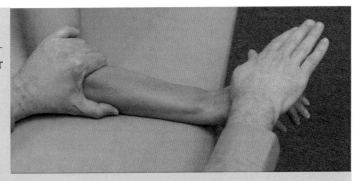

SECTION 4   HANDANDWRIST

Flexor Digitorum Profundus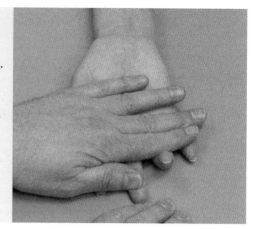

Evaluate the flexor digitorum profundus with the patient's hand palm up on the examining table and the fingers extended. Hold the proximal interphalangeal joint in extension. Ask the patient to flex the distal finger joint. Inability to flex the distal interphalangeal joint indicates an injury to the profundus tendon, injury to the median nerve or its anterior interosseous branch—which innervates the flexor digitorum profundus to the index and, often, the long finger—or injury to the ulnar nerve, which innervates the ring and little finger distal interphalangeal joints.

Flexor Digitorum Superficialis (Sublimis)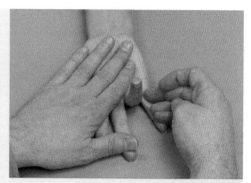

Evaluate the flexor digitorum superficialis with the patient's hand palm up on the examining table and the fingers extended. Hold the fingers in full extension except for the finger being tested. Ask the patient to flex the finger. The flexor digitorum profundus cannot independently flex the finger when it is tethered by the other fingers being held in extension. However, the flexor digitorum superficialis of each finger can work independently. A normal response is flexion at the proximal interphalangeal joint. Inability to flex this finger indicates an injury to the superficialis tendon to that finger or injury to the median nerve.

Thumb Abduction Strength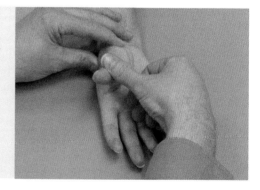

Evaluate the thumb abduction strength with the patient's hand palm up on the examination table. Ask the patient to abduct the thumb (by placing it straight up) and resist your attempt to gently push the thumb down onto the table. Weakness indicates damage to the motor branch of the median nerve, most commonly related to carpal tunnel syndrome.

Grip Strength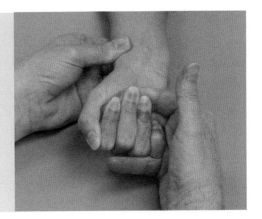

To assess grip strength, have the patient grasp three of your fingers and squeeze. A decrease in total grip strength reflects weakness of the finger flexors and/or intrinsic muscles of the hand. Grip strength testing can be easily quantified using grip meters. This objective measurement can be used to follow a patient's progress in strengthening.

Sensory Testing

Median, Ulnar, and Radial Nerves

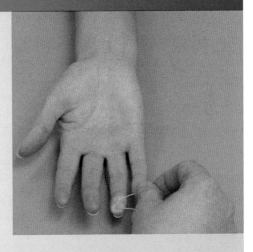

Assess median nerve sensation at the volar tip of the thumb, ulnar nerve sensation at the volar tip of the little finger, and radial nerve sensation at the dorsum of the thumb metacarpal. Check light touch and, for a more complete evaluation, assess two-point discrimination as follows. Ask the patient to close both eyes as you lightly touch two points to the fingertip. (Apply just enough pressure to blanch the skin.) A paper clip may be used for this purpose by straightening it, then bending it so that the two ends can be used to touch the patient. Determine whether the patient is able to distinguish the two points as separate points or perceives them as a single point. Two-point discrimination of 5 mm is generally considered to be normal. Inability to discriminate the two points indicates a sensory abnormality. The wider the distance required for the patient to discern two distinct points, the poorer the sensory discrimination.

Tinel Sign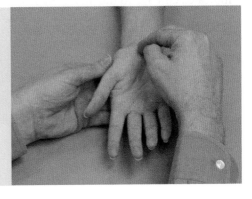

To perform Tinel testing for the median nerve, lightly percuss the median nerve at the wrist flexion crease in line with the metacarpal of the long finger. Reproduction of paresthesia into the median nerve distribution is a positive Tinel sign. This test may be performed over any peripheral nerve.

SECTION 4 HANDANDWRIST

Durkan Carpal Compression Test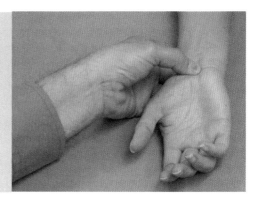

To perform the Durkan carpal compression test, compress the median nerve at the volar aspect of the wrist. Reproduction of paresthesias or numbness into the median nerve distribution is a positive sign.

Special Tests

Finkelstein Test

To perform the Finkelstein test for de Quervain tenosynovitis, have the patient make a fist with the thumb inside the fingers. Push the fist into ulnar deviation. Pain at the dorsoradial aspect of the wrist (as indicated here by placement of the examiner's forefinger) indicates a stenosing tenosynovitis of the first dorsal compartment tendons (abductor pollicis longus and extensor brevis).

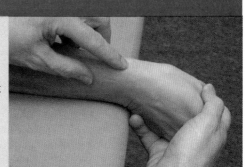

The Finkelstein test can be very painful for persons with severe de Quervain tenosynovitis, so it may be done in a staged fashion, instead (not shown). First the patient places the wrist in neutral pronosupination on a table with the ulnar aspect of the forearm resting on the table and the wrist and distal hanging over the edge of the table unsupported. Next, simple active gravity-assisted ulnar deviation is performed. A painful result indicates first dorsal extensor pathology. If that action generates a negative result, further passive ulnar deviation can be done by the examiner; pain elicited during that maneuver secures the diagnosis. If pain is not elicited by the aforementioned maneuvers, the examiner may add passive thumb flexion into the palm to assess for pain. Although commonly known as the Finkelstein test, the maneuver shown here, with the patient's thumb inside the fist, is more accurately ascribed to Eichoff. The test Finkelstein described in the literature is performed by grasping the patient's thumb and moving it into ulnar deviation. Both tests are positive when they elicit pain at the dorsoradial aspect of the wrist.

Phalen Maneuver

To perform the Phalen maneuver to assess for carpal tunnel syndrome, ask the patient to position the elbows in relaxed extension and then allow gravity flexion of the wrists. Numbness or tingling in the distribution of the median nerve within 60 seconds is a positive sign.

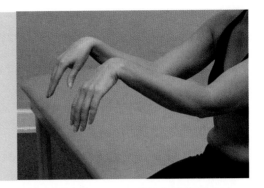

Froment Sign

To evaluate the Froment sign, ask the patient to pinch a piece of paper between the thumb and index fingertip while you apply tension to the other end of the paper. If the adductor pollicis muscle is weak (ulnar nerve paralysis), the thumb interphalangeal joint will flex. (The figure shows normal muscle function.) Compare function with that of the opposite, normal thumb.

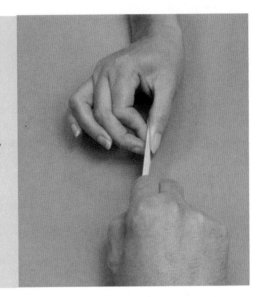

Mallet Finger Test

To assess for mallet finger (rupture of the terminal extensor tendon), isolate the extensor tendon by holding the involved finger at the middle phalanx. With the distal interphalangeal joint relaxed in flexion, instruct the patient to actively extend the distal interphalangeal joint. Inability of the patient to actively extend the distal interphalangeal joint is suggestive of an extensor tendon avulsion at its attachment on the base of the distal phalanx. A finger with this injury can be passively extended by the examiner, however.

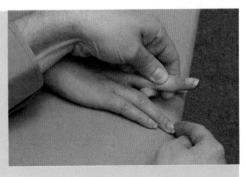

Thumb MCP Joint Ulnar Collateral Ligament Test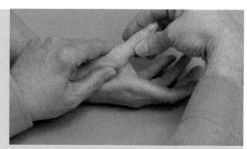

Grasp the medial and lateral aspects of the metacarpal with your thumb and index finger. Use the thumb and index finger of your other hand to grasp the medial and lateral aspects of the proximal phalanx, maintaining the joint in extension. Apply ulnar stress to the joint by abducting the proximal phalanx. While applying stress, look and feel for abnormal opening of the joint as compared to the contralateral thumb. Normally, there should be a slight opening with a firm end point. Absence of a firm end point accompanied by sensations of pain or instability indicates a sprain of the ulnar collateral ligament. By examining the thumb in full extension and 30° of flexion, you can determine if the true collateral ligament, the accessory collateral ligament, or both structures have been injured.

Thumb CMC Arthritis Tests

Grind Test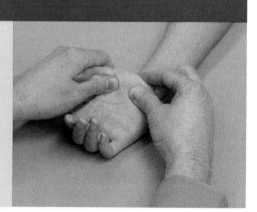

To perform the grind test for thumb carpometacarpal arthritis, ask the patient to rest the hand palm up on the examination table with the thumb in palmar abduction. Grasp the metacarpal base, apply a slight longitudinal axial load, and rotate the thumb carpometacarpal joint. This motion applied to the carpometacarpal joint is painful in patients with carpometacarpal arthritis.

Carpometacarpal Joint Relocation Test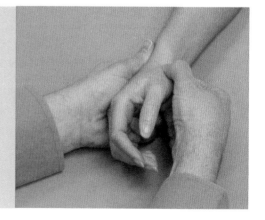

To perform the carpometacarpal joint relocation test, place dorsal to volar pressure on the thumb metacarpal, relocating the carpometacarpal joint. This is commonly painful in patients with carpometacarpal joint arthritis.

   © 2016 American Academy of Orthopaedic Surgeons

Allen Test

To perform the Allen test for arterial circulation to the hand, compress the radial and ulnar arteries at the wrist, then ask the patient to first open and close the hand three times, then make a tight fist to exsanguinate the hand (**A**) and then open the fingers (**B**).

Release the ulnar artery while keeping the radial artery compressed (**C**). If the fingers and palm fill with blood within 5 seconds, the ulnar artery is patent. Repeat these steps, keeping the ulnar artery compressed but releasing the radial artery (**D**). Note the time for refilling of the hand.

Commonly, one artery is dominant in supplying circulation to the hand.

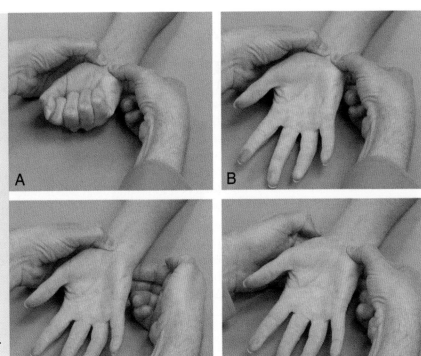

Animal Bites

Definition

Up to 3 million people in the United States sustain animal bites each year. Animal bites most commonly occur on the fingers of the dominant hand of children. Dog bites account for up to 90% of animal bites; cat bites are second most common, constituting 5% of animal bites.

The risk of infection following a dog bite is 5% to 10%; the risk of infection following a cat bite is much higher (30% to 50%) because a cat's sharp teeth create deeper puncture wounds that often seal quickly at the surface. The causative organism varies, and bite infections are typically polymicrobial. *Pasteurella multocida* is a bacterium commonly associated with dog and cat bite wounds. Other bacteria isolated in dog bite wounds include α-hemolytic streptococci, *Staphylococcus aureus*, and anaerobic organisms such as *Bacteroides* and *Fusobacterium*.

Because rabies is a concern with animal bites, it is important to be familiar with the status of rabies in your area. In the United States, more than 90% of rabies cases in humans are transmitted from wild animals, especially bats, skunks, raccoons, and foxes. Outside the United States, however, the dog is the most common vector for rabies transmission to humans. Approximately 50% of rabies cases reported to the Centers for Disease Control and Prevention in 1985 were from dog bites that occurred in countries other than the United States.

Clinical Symptoms

Pain, swelling, and redness around the puncture wound suggest an infection secondary to the bite. Loss of sensation and motion distal to the bite may indicate that a nerve or tendon has been severed. Determine whether the bite was provoked by a sudden movement toward the animal because an animal that initiates an unprovoked attack is more likely to be rabid. The animal should be found if possible and observed for 10 days for signs of rabies. If necessary, consult with an infectious disease specialist regarding the risk of rabies.

Tests

Physical Examination

Examination may reveal an irregular, jagged wound with devitalized tissue at the margins and swelling and redness around the wound. The depth and age of the wound should be determined. Purulent drainage may be present if the wound is more than 10 to 12 hours old. Sensation and tendon function should be tested in the affected hand or finger. Inspect the forearm for the presence of red streaks that indicate lymphangitis. The inner aspect of the elbow and the axilla should be palpated for the presence of enlarged lymph nodes. The patient's temperature should be checked.

Diagnostic Tests

AP and lateral radiographs of the affected part are necessary to rule out a fracture or the presence of a foreign body. These views also may reveal gas in the soft tissues. Although routine laboratory studies may not show significant abnormality for wounds seen shortly after injury, they may serve as a baseline to monitor progress of treatment. Commonly ordered laboratory studies include a complete blood cell count with differential, erythrocyte sedimentation rate (ESR), and C-reactive protein (CRP) level. With the ESR, there is a lag to elevation in the course of an infection and a slower resolution than occurs with the CRP level, which rapidly elevates and resolves following an infection. If an infection is suspected, a swab of the wound may be sent for a Gram stain as well as aerobic and anaerobic cultures. Superficial swabs likely will show nonspecific findings, however, and will grow skin flora in addition to any deep infection. If the patient undergoes a formal débridement, tissue and wound cultures should be obtained; these are of greater value to determine the causative organism or organisms. Blood cultures may be obtained to rule out systemic spread of infection.

Differential Diagnosis

• Foreign body with secondary infection (foreign body apparent on radiograph, ultrasound, or CT)

Adverse Outcomes of the Disease

Any of the following conditions could develop as a result of an untreated animal bite: sepsis in the joint, deep space infection, septic tenosynovitis, osteomyelitis, or rabies. Patients also may lose sensation and motion, and possibly the affected fingers, following an animal bite. Chronic lymphedema with hand and finger stiffness is also possible.

Treatment

Débridement, wound irrigation with 500 to 1,000 mL of saline solution or an antibiotic irrigation solution, and outpatient antibiotics are appropriate for superficial wounds that do not have a nerve, tendon, or bony injury. An anesthetic block will facilitate débridement of bite wounds on the finger. When the bite wound is on the back of the hand, 3 to 10 mL of local anesthetic should be infiltrated around the wound. Oral amoxicillin-clavulanate, 875 mg twice a day for 5 days, is one standard antibiotic regimen for the treatment of early infection.

Primary suturing of animal bite wounds is controversial and can be hazardous. Suturing should be performed only when the wound is clean following débridement and usually is best completed over a passive drain (Penrose type). Because of the higher rate of infection associated with cat bites, these wounds should not be sutured. In general, it is safest to leave animal bites open.

When signs of active infection are present, the wound should

Table 1

Summary Guide to Tetanus Prophylaxis in Routine Wound Management[a]

History of Tetanus Immunization (Doses)	Clean, Minor Wounds		All Other Wounds	
	Td[b]	TIG	Td[b]	TIG
Uncertain or <3 doses	Yes	No	Yes	Yes
3 or more doses	No[c]	No	No[d]	No

Td = tetanus and diphtheria toxoids, TIG = human tetanus immune globulin.

[a] Important details on these CDC websites: http://wwwnc.cdc.gov/travel/yellowbook/2014/chapter-3-infectious-diseases-related-to-travel/tetanus and http://www.cdc.gov/vaccines/vpd-vac/tetanus/default.htm

[b] For children younger than 7 years, DTaP or DTP (DT, if pertussis vaccine contraindicated) preferred to tetanus toxoid alone. For children age 7 years or older, Td preferred to tetanus toxoid alone. For adolescents and adults to age 64 years, tetanus toxoid as Tdap is preferred, if the patient has not previously been vaccinated with Tdap.

[c] Yes, if more than 10 years since last dose.

[d] Yes, if more than 5 years since last dose. More frequent boosters are not needed and can accentuate side effects.

(Adapted with permission from the Centers for Disease Control and Prevention.)

be managed open and allowed to close by secondary intention. Intravenous antibiotics are indicated in this situation. Empiric therapy can be started with intravenous ampicillin-sulbactam, 1.5 to 3.0 g every 6 hours, pending culture results and sensitivities. Tetracycline can be used in patients with a penicillin allergy. Antibiotic therapy should be organism specific whenever possible. The patient may be switched to oral antibiotics in 48 hours if the wound is healing satisfactorily. Tetanus prophylaxis should be given as outlined in **Table 1**. As part of standard wound management care to prevent tetanus, a tetanus toxoid–containing vaccine might be recommended for wound management in a pregnant woman if 5 years or more have elapsed since her previous tetanus and diphtheria toxoids (Td) booster. If a Td booster is recommended for a pregnant woman, healthcare providers should administer tetanus, diphtheria, and pertussis (Tdap) vaccine.

If the animal is suspected of being infected with rabies, contact local or state public health officials regarding the need for rabies prophylaxis.

Adverse Outcomes of Treatment

Infection secondary to primary wound closure can occur. Patients also may have allergic reactions to antibiotics.

Referral Decisions/Red Flags

Any patient with an animal bite that involves the tendon, nerve, joint capsule, or an underlying fracture requires further evaluation.

Arthritis of the Hand

Synonyms

Degenerative joint disease
Osteoarthritis
Rheumatoid arthritis

Definition

Osteoarthritis and secondary degenerative joint disease are the most common causes of arthritis of the hand and wrist. These conditions are characterized by progressive loss of articular cartilage, reactive bony changes at the joint margins, and subchondral cyst formation. The cause of primary osteoarthritis is unknown, but genetic predisposition is believed to be a contributing factor. Secondary arthritis develops in joints affected by trauma, mechanical problems, or preexisting lesions.

Rheumatoid arthritis is a systemic condition that affects synovial tissue. All deformities, joint destruction, and pathologic anatomy that occur in patients with rheumatoid arthritis are a result of synovial hypertrophy and inflammation. The boggy synovium stretches the joint capsule and ligaments, causing deformity and joint instability. The articular cartilage also may be destroyed. Rheumatoid synovitis may also involve the tenosynovium and invade the flexor and extensor tendons, disrupting their motion and function.

Clinical Symptoms

In osteoarthritis, the distal interphalangeal (DIP), proximal interphalangeal (PIP), and thumb carpometacarpal joints are most often involved. Patients report stiffness and loss of motion in the fingers. In rheumatoid arthritis, the wrist and metacarpophalangeal (MCP) joints are most often involved (**Figure 1**). Extensor or flexor tenosynovitis (inflammation of the tendon sheath) also is common, resulting in pain that is caused by activation, whereas patients with osteoarthritis have more pain with joint palpation. Patients with rheumatoid arthritis often have increased pain in the morning and after extended activities.

Tests

Physical Examination

Patients with rheumatoid arthritis involving the hands have fusiform swelling of multiple joints, with some joints more swollen than others. Rheumatoid arthritis commonly involves the MCP joint and the wrist joint. Boggy synovitis over the dorsum of the hand and crepitus with movement also are common, as is flexor tenosynovitis with crepitus at the wrist or in the fingers. Ulnar drift of the fingers may exist at the level of the MCP joint. Other findings include contractures of the fingers at the PIP joints (boutonnière deformity) or hyperextension at the PIP joints with flexion at the DIP joints (swan neck deformity).

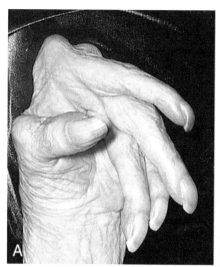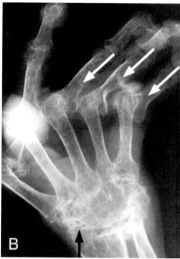

Figure 1 Clinical photograph and PA radiograph of advanced rheumatoid arthritis. **A,** Clinical appearance. Note the severe ulnar drift of the metacarpophalangeal (MCP) joint and the limited finger extension. **B,** PA radiograph demonstrates the severe ulnar drift of the MCP joints (white arrows) and the destruction of the wrist (black arrow).

Patients with osteoarthritis of the hand have bony nodules at the DIP joint (Heberden nodes). Associated mucous cyst formation over the DIP joint may be present. These nodules can be painful at first, but the pain usually resolves. Nodules also may occur at the PIP joints (Bouchard nodes). Involvement of the MCP joints is much less common with osteoarthritis. When it occurs at this location, it is often the result of previous trauma.

Diagnostic Tests

PA, oblique, and lateral radiographs with the fingers positioned in different degrees of flexion, allowing each finger to be examined in detail, are necessary. When a single digit is involved, isolated PA and true lateral radiographs of the digit also are appropriate. Serologic tests should be performed for patients who have the characteristic changes of inflammatory arthritis but for whom the diagnosis has not been established. Such tests may include erythrocyte sedimentation rate and C-reactive protein level as measures of inflammatory disease, rheumatoid factor, antinuclear antibody, and anti–cyclic citrullinated peptide antibody.

Differential Diagnosis

- Pyogenic arthritis (may resemble the swollen joints of rheumatoid arthritis) (bacteria in joint aspirate, markedly elevated white blood cell count)

Adverse Outcomes of the Disease

Rheumatoid arthritis can be slowly progressive, resulting in the typical rheumatoid hand deformity (**Figure 1**). Progressive osteoarthritis can cause joint destruction, particularly at the DIP, PIP, and wrist joints, with decreased mobility and function.

Treatment

Rheumatoid arthritis has no cure. NSAIDs and other anti-inflammatory medications should be optimized. Newer medications such as etanercept (Enbrel [Amgen]) or infliximab (Remicade [Janssen Biotech]) may be more effective in limiting symptoms but may be associated with other medical complications. Cortisone injections can be extremely helpful for a severely inflamed joint or tendon sheath. Nonsurgical treatment may include referral to an experienced occupational therapist to assist with splinting and the use of modalities. Occupational therapy and splinting can reduce deformity and limit symptoms but may not alter the natural history of the disease.

Treatment of osteoarthritis typically includes NSAIDs and, occasionally, temporary splinting of an involved joint for pain relief. Consultation with a hand therapist can be helpful to assist with hand splints and externally applied modalities such as home paraffin treatments and externally applied rub-in creams. Surgery for pain relief or stabilization may be necessary.

Adverse Outcomes of Treatment

NSAIDs can cause gastric, hepatic, and renal complications. In 2015, the FDA strengthened its warning linking NSAIDs with the risk of heart attack or stroke, even in the first weeks of use of an NSAID. Corticosteroids may adversely affect the immune system. Cortisone injections should be used very judiciously because of localized complications such as steroid atrophy (thinning or discoloration of the skin) and weakening of normal structures, such as tendons. Infection also is a risk but can be minimized with careful sterile technique.

Referral Decisions/Red Flags

When a cortisone injection for extensor tenosynovitis is not effective, surgery to excise the inflamed synovium can prevent rupture of the tendon. Particularly in the setting of rheumatoid arthritis, attritional ruptures of tendons may occur after continued abrasion of a tendon over a bony prominence. Patients who cannot flex or extend their digits, especially the little finger, ring finger, or thumb, may have ruptured the tendon, and immediate further evaluation is needed.

Patients with rheumatoid arthritis who report increasing deformity and increasing pain in the hand may need reconstructive surgery. Further evaluation is required for patients with osteoarthritis pain no longer controlled with splinting and NSAIDs and who have radiographic evidence of joint destruction.

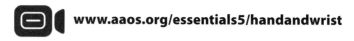
Procedure: Metacarpophalangeal or Proximal Interphalangeal Joint Injection

Materials

- Sterile gloves
- Bactericidal skin preparation solution
- Two 3-mL syringes with a 25-gauge needle
- 0.5 mL of a 1% local anesthetic solution without epinephrine
- 0.5 to 1.0 mL corticosteroid preparation
- Adhesive dressing

Note: Opinions differ regarding single- versus two-needle injection techniques. Proponents of the single-needle technique believe that one needle is less painful for the patient than two. Because the corticosteroid preparation is thicker than the local anesthetic, however, a slightly larger gauge needle is required at the outset. A two-syringe, two-needle technique is described in the video.

Injections are performed on the extensor aspect of either the metacarpophalangeal (MCP) or the proximal interphalangeal (PIP) joint.

The entry site for the MCP joint is the small sulcus just below the prominent metacarpal head that is most obvious with the finger flexed 20° (**Figure 1, A**). Identify this sulcus while moving the joint through a small amount of flexion and extension. Applying axial traction to the finger can facilitate localization of the joint. Identify the PIP joint in the same manner. Be aware, however, that the dorsal rim of the middle phalanx is often more easily palpated with this joint in extension (**Figure 1, B**).

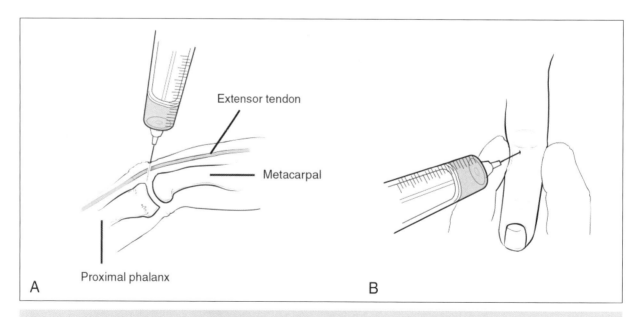

Extensor tendon

Metacarpal

Proximal phalanx

A

B

Figure 1 Illustration depicts the location for needle insertion for metacarpophalangeal joint injection (**A**) and proximal interphalangeal joint injection (**B**).

Step 1

Wear protective gloves at all times during this procedure and use sterile technique.

Step 2

Cleanse the skin with a bactericidal skin preparation solution.

Step 3

Insert the 25-gauge needle at the joint level on the dorsolateral side of the joint. Inject 0.5 mL of a 1% local anesthetic preparation into the joint, change syringes, and then, with the new syringe, inject 0.5 to 1.0 mL of corticosteroid preparation. Slight pressure against the syringe plunger should make the joint bulge slightly on either side.

Alternate method: Combine the local anesthetic medication with the corticosteroid solution into one syringe. Insert a 25-gauge needle at the joint level on the dorsolateral side of the joint and inject the preparation into the joint.

Step 4

Dress the puncture wound with a sterile adhesive bandage.

Adverse Outcomes

Although rare, infection is possible. Subcutaneous fat atrophy may occur if the corticosteroid preparation is injected external to the joint. This may produce a depressed area of thin, tender, and unsightly skin. Some patients experience changes in skin pigmentation following injection. Occasionally, these changes in skin coloration are permanent.

Aftercare/Patient Instructions

The joint might be sore for 24 to 48 hours after injection. Instruct the patient to return to your office if undue swelling, pain, or redness occurs. Ice massage and the use of acetaminophen or an NSAID will control local symptoms after injection.

Arthritis of the Thumb Carpometacarpal Joint

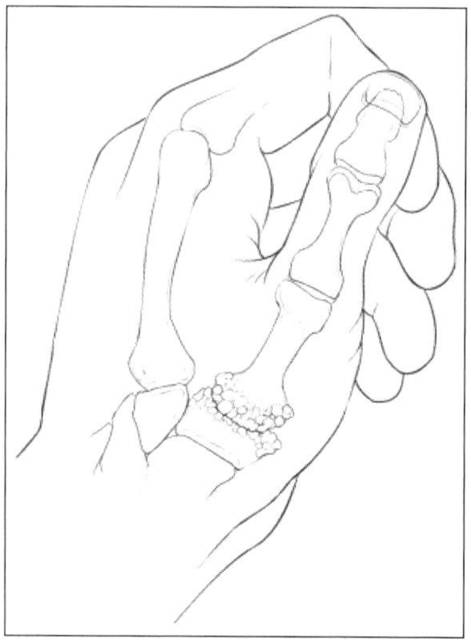

Figure 1 Illustration of carpometacarpal (CMC) arthritis of the thumb.

Synonyms

Carpometacarpal degenerative arthritis
Degenerative arthritis of the basal joint

Definition

Idiopathic degenerative arthritis of the thumb carpometacarpal (CMC) joint (**Figure 1**) most commonly occurs in women between the ages of 40 and 70 years. The idiopathic variety is caused by anatomic factors (joint configuration and ligamentous laxity) that predispose the joint to instability, shear forces, and subsequent degenerative change.

Clinical Symptoms

The most common symptom is pain at the base of the thumb that occurs with grip and pinch activities. The pain may radiate proximally into the wrist and forearm. Decreased pinch strength is a common symptom. Patients also may note instability, "catching," or "clicking" with certain movements. Late manifestations include stiffness of the CMC joint in adduction with secondary metacarpophalangeal hyperextension. Carpal tunnel syndrome may coexist with or mimic the symptoms of CMC arthritis.

Tests

Physical Examination

The hallmark of this condition is tenderness over the palmar and radial aspects of the joint in the region of the base of the thumb. Manipulation of the CMC joint with simultaneous longitudinal loading (compression) causes pain and often some crepitus or instability. The grind test for thumb CMC arthritis readily reproduces the pain of CMC arthritis. With the palm facing up and the back of the hand resting on the table, the thumb is pushed down toward the table with the metacarpophalangeal and proximal interphalangeal joints extended. The CMC joint relocation test, in which dorsal pressure is placed on the thumb metacarpal and the CMC joint is relocated by applying pressure in a palmar direction, is also useful in localizing the point of maximum discomfort.

Diagnostic Tests

PA and lateral radiographs of the thumb show joint space narrowing, subchondral sclerosis, and varying degrees of subluxation or dislocation at the CMC joint (**Figure 2**).

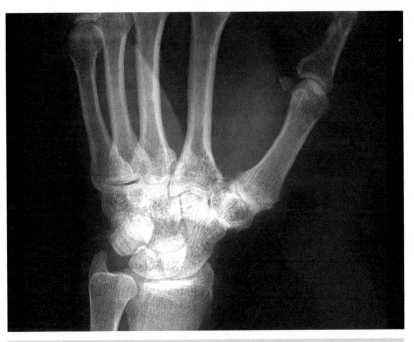

Figure 2 Radiographic appearance of CMC arthritis of the thumb.

Differential Diagnosis

- Arthritis of the wrist (evident on radiographs)
- Carpal tunnel syndrome (positive Phalen maneuver, decreased sensation in median nerve distribution)
- de Quervain tenosynovitis (positive Finkelstein test) (de Quervain tenosynovitis coexists with CMC arthritis of the thumb in many patients)
- Flexor carpi radialis tendinitis (pain with resisted wrist flexion, swelling over flexor carpi radialis tendon)
- Fracture of the scaphoid (tenderness over the anatomic snuffbox)
- Scaphotrapeziotrapezoid arthritis (tenderness over the scaphotrapeziotrapezoid joint)
- Volar radial ganglion (palpable mass over the palmar surface of the wrist)

Adverse Outcomes of the Disease

Chronic pain, loss of pinch and grip strength, adduction contracture of the thumb (thumb held against the index finger), and chronic metacarpophalangeal joint instability can occur.

Treatment

Initial treatment may consist of placing the thumb in a thumb spica splint for a few weeks, with NSAIDs for pain relief. If symptoms recur, intermittent splinting that immobilizes the entire thumb should be continued. If splinting fails, a corticosteroid preparation may be injected into the joint. Although injections do not alter the natural history of the disease, many patients report pain relief that lasts a few months with each injection. Multiple injections may be appropriate in some cases. A hand therapist may be consulted to help fabricate splints and assist with the use of externally applied modalities, such as iontophoresis, ice, heat, or rub-in creams. In addition, patients may be instructed in ergonomic changes and selective strengthening programs that result in decreased pain and functional improvement.

Adverse Outcomes of Treatment

NSAIDs can cause gastric, renal, or hepatic complications. In 2015, the FDA strengthened its warning linking NSAIDs with the risk of heart attack or stroke, even in the first weeks of use of an NSAID. Infection can develop after corticosteroid injection. Rapid progression of arthritis is possible as a result of multiple corticosteroid injections.

Referral Decisions/Red Flags

Failure of nonsurgical treatment indicates the need for further evaluation.

Procedure: Thumb Carpometacarpal Joint Injection

Note: Opinions differ regarding single- and two-needle injection techniques. Proponents of the single-needle technique believe that one needle is less painful for the patient than two. Because the corticosteroid preparation is thicker than the local anesthetic, however, a slightly larger-gauge needle is required at the outset.

Step 1

Wear protective gloves at all times during this procedure and use sterile technique.

Step 2

Before putting on the gloves, mark the level of the carpometacarpal (CMC) joint on the dorsum of the hand with your thumbnail by gently indenting the skin at the interval between the base of the thumb metacarpal and the trapezium.

Step 3

Cleanse the skin over the CMC joint at the marked site with a bactericidal skin preparation solution.

Step 4

Insert the 25-gauge needle, attached to the syringe with the anesthetic solution, at the mark on the back of the CMC joint. Inject 0.5 mL of the 1% anesthetic subcutaneously.

Step 5

Pull on the end of the thumb to open the joint space. Advance the needle into the joint and inject 0.5 to 1.0 mL of the anesthetic solution (optional) (**Figure 1**). If resistance is encountered, redirect the needle and reinsert. After the anesthetic solution is injected, leave the needle in place and change syringes.

Step 6

Inject 0.5 mL of the corticosteroid preparation through the same needle tract. The injection of fluid should meet little resistance if the needle is in the CMC joint. Alternatively, some providers simply inject the thumb CMC joint with corticosteroid rather than local anesthetic. In this case, follow steps 1, 2, and 3, then inject 0.5 mL of the corticosteroid preparation into the thumb CMC joint using a 25-gauge needle.

Step 7

Dress the puncture site with a sterile adhesive bandage.

Materials

- Sterile gloves
- Bactericidal skin preparation solution
- Two 3-mL syringes with a 25-gauge needle
- 0.5 mL corticosteroid preparation
- 2 mL of a 1% local anesthetic (optional)
- Adhesive bandage

SECTION 4 HAND AND WRIST

SECTION 4 HAND AND WRIST

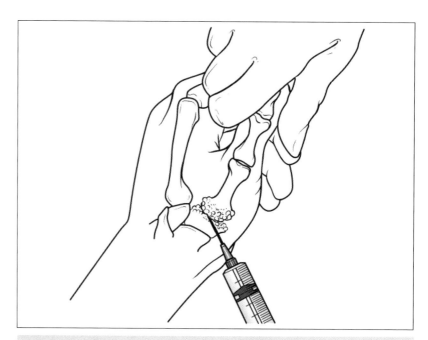

Figure 1 Illustration depicts injection into the carpometacarpal joint of the thumb.

Adverse Outcomes

Depigmentation and/or fat atrophy at the site of the injection, injury to sensory branches of the radial nerve, and joint space infection are possible.

Aftercare/Patient Instructions

Advise the patient that 33% of patients may experience a flare of discomfort, manifested by increased joint pain, for 1 to 2 days. Ice massage and the use of acetaminophen or an NSAID will facilitate control of local symptoms that stem from the injection. Also, the patient can wear a thumb spica splint for comfort for a few days after the injection. The patient should experience relief within 7 to 14 days after the injection.

Arthritis of the Wrist

Synonyms
Synovitis
Wrist joint arthritis

Definition
Arthritis in the wrist most commonly occurs secondary to previous trauma (such as fractures of the distal radius) or rheumatoid arthritis. Pseudogout and primary osteoarthritis also may affect the wrist.

Clinical Symptoms
Patients with rheumatoid arthritis typically report generalized swelling, tenderness, and limited motion. Hand function is often impaired by the synovitis and resultant instability of the carpal bones. The result is radial deviation of the wrist, ulnar deviation of the fingers, inefficient wrist and finger tendon function, decreased grip strength, and pain with daily activities. Degenerative arthritis of the wrist is associated with swelling, pain, and limited motion of the wrist.

Tests

Physical Examination
Examination reveals swelling, increased warmth, limited motion, and pain on palpation of the radiocarpal joint. Patients with rheumatoid arthritis often have associated involvement of the metacarpophalangeal joints and deformity at the wrist and fingers. The ulna may appear prominent (caput ulnae). In posttraumatic degenerative arthritis, the finger joints usually appear normal.

Diagnostic Tests
PA and lateral radiographs are helpful in distinguishing the various types of arthritis. Generalized thinning of the bone structure (osteopenia) with erosions in the area of the joint surface is characteristic of rheumatoid arthritis. Subchondral sclerosis, joint space narrowing, spur formation, and, in some cases, erosion characterize primary or secondary osteoarthritis (**Figure 1**). Early calcification of the triangular fibrocartilage complex may indicate pseudogout, which can be confirmed by the presence of calcium pyrophosphate crystals in synovial fluid aspirate.

Laboratory studies, including erythrocyte sedimentation rate and tests for rheumatoid factor, antinuclear antibodies, and uric acid, may help confirm the diagnosis. Occasionally, laboratory tests for Lyme disease may be obtained to rule out this entity as a cause of pain.

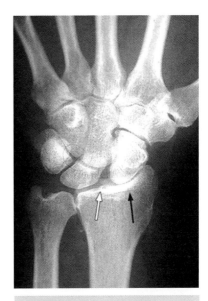

Figure 1 PA radiograph demonstrates osteoarthritis of the wrist. Note the subchondral sclerosis of the radius and the loss of radiocarpal joint space (black arrow). The scapholunate interval is also widened (white arrow).

Differential Diagnosis

• Septic arthritis of the wrist (acute onset, severe pain and restriction of wrist motion, systemic signs of infection)
• Tenosynovitis (normal radiographs, swelling over the involved tendon)

Adverse Outcomes of the Disease

Pain, loss of motion and/or strength, and impaired function in the wrist and fingers are possible.

Treatment

Medical management depends on the type of arthritis present. Temporary immobilization in a splint can help relieve pain and swelling. In the absence of infection, injection of a corticosteroid may provide temporary pain relief. Surgery is offered when hand function decreases, when the joint becomes unstable, or when nonsurgical treatment fails to relieve pain. Surgical treatment usually focuses on improving stability and limiting discomfort.

Adverse Outcomes of Treatment

Loss of motion and persistent pain can develop. NSAIDs can cause gastric, renal, or hepatic complications. In 2015, the FDA strengthened its warning linking NSAIDs with the risk of heart attack or stroke, even in the first weeks of use of an NSAID.

Referral Decisions/Red Flags

Patients with a possible wrist infection require immediate evaluation. Those with radiographic evidence of advanced disease from degenerative or rheumatoid arthritis and those who do not respond to splinting and NSAIDs also are candidates for further evaluation.

Procedure: Wrist Aspiration/Injection

Step 1
Wear protective gloves at all times during this procedure and use sterile technique.

Step 2
Cleanse the area with a bactericidal skin preparation solution.

Step 3
Palpate the Lister tubercle. Approximately 1 cm distal to the Lister tubercle, a palpable depression can be identified distal to the distal edge of the radius; this depression represents the radiocarpal joint.

Step 4
Angle your hand approximately 10° to 11° such that the needle is oriented distal to proximal 10° to 11° to replicate the dorsal-volar tilt of the radius (**Figure 1**).

Step 5
Insert the needle into the same site to aspirate the joint fluid or to inject the radiocarpal joint. The joint fluid should be submitted for

Materials
- Sterile gloves
- Ethyl chloride
- Bactericidal skin preparation solution
- 3-mL syringe with a 25-gauge needle (injection)
- 3-mL syringe with a 22-gauge needle (aspiration)
- 0.5 to 1.0 mL of 1% local anesthetic (optional [injection])
- 0.5 to 1.0 mL corticosteroid preparation (optional [injection])
- Sterile dressing

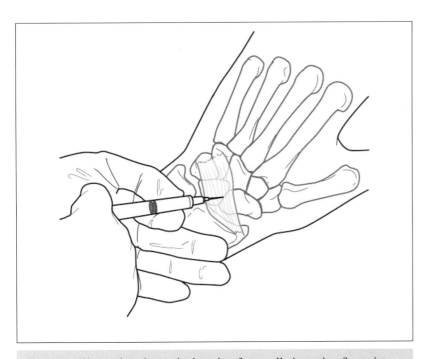

Figure 1 Illustration shows the location for needle insertion for wrist joint injection and aspiration using a dorsal approach.

crystal analysis, total cell count and differential, Gram stain, and culture and sensitivity.

If infection is not a concern, you may inject 0.5 to 1.0 mL of the corticosteroid preparation mixed with an equal amount of 1% local anesthetic for pain relief.

Step 6
Dress the puncture wound with a sterile adhesive bandage.

Adverse Outcomes
Infection is possible. The infection may progress because corticosteroids can mask the usual signs of infection.

Aftercare/Patient Instructions
Instruct the patient to watch for signs of infection, such as increasing pain, swelling, heat, or redness, and to call your office if any of these signs occur. Follow-up with the patient to review the culture results is usually appropriate.

Boutonnière Deformity

Synonyms

Central slip extensor tendon injury
Jammed finger

Definition

Boutonnière deformity occurs when the central portion of the extensor tendon ruptures at its insertion onto the middle phalanx (**Figure 1**), causing the proximal interphalangeal (PIP) joint to flex from the unopposed pull of the flexor tendon. The head of the proximal phalanx "buttonholes" between the lateral bands of the extensor tendon mechanism. As a result, the lateral bands are displaced below the axis of rotation of the PIP joint, causing it to flex further. More distally, the lateral bands are displaced dorsal to the axis of the distal interphalangeal (DIP) joint, causing it to extend or hyperextend.

Clinical Symptoms

Patients typically report a history of trauma. The finger is held partially flexed at the PIP joint and extended or hyperextended at the DIP joint. With a recent injury, the PIP joint is painful and tender. Initially, the boutonnière deformity may not be apparent, but it can develop over 7 to 21 days as the intact lateral bands of the extensor tendon slip inferiorly.

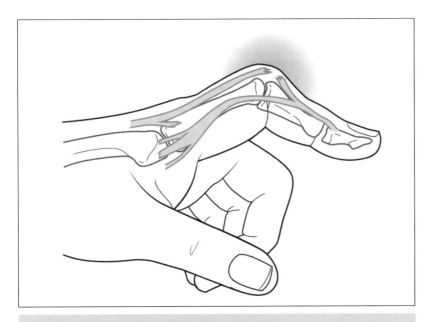

Figure 1 Illustration of boutonnière deformity.

Tests

Physical Examination

Ask the patient to extend the injured finger and observe the position of the PIP and DIP joints. The PIP joint will be flexed more than 30°, and the DIP joint will be extended or hyperextended. To demonstrate less severe deformities, hold the metacarpophalangeal and wrist joints in flexion and ask the patient to extend the PIP joint. A patient who lacks 15° to 20° of extension at the PIP joint probably has a rupture of the central slip of the extensor tendon.

Diagnostic Tests

AP and lateral radiographs will rule out a fracture or a pseudoboutonnière deformity, in which the PIP joint is fixed in flexion and radiographs show calcification at the lateral aspect of the PIP joint.

Differential Diagnosis

- Dislocation of the PIP joint (painful, locked joint following surgery)
- Fracture around the PIP joint (radiographs required to confirm)
- Pseudoboutonnière deformity (PIP joint fixed in flexion, radiographs show calcification at the lateral aspect of the PIP joint)
- Rupture of the flexor tendon sheath (annular pulley) (painful flexor tendon sheath following injury)
- Sprain of the PIP joint (may be difficult to differentiate on initial examination; sprains have isolated collateral ligament tenderness and/or instability)

Adverse Outcomes of the Disease

Flexion contracture of the PIP joint and extension contracture of the DIP joint are both possible.

Treatment

Nonsurgical treatment is usually preferable. The PIP joint should be splinted in extension for 6 weeks in a young patient or for 3 weeks in an elderly patient (**Figure 2**). The DIP joint is left free. Active and passive motion should be initiated at the DIP joint.

If the patient presents 1 to 2 weeks after injury, it may not be possible to achieve full extension at the first visit. The use of a dynamic extension splint (**Figure 2, C**) is required until full extension is achieved, followed by a static splinting program. Surgical treatment is occasionally necessary if the deformity does not correct with splinting.

Adverse Outcomes of Treatment

Failure to achieve full extension, residual PIP flexion deformity, or both are possible.

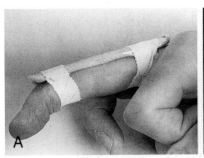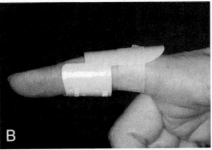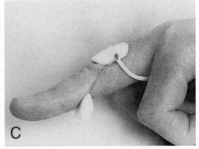

Figure 2 Clinical photographs of a static extension splint (**A**), a commercial static splint (**B**), and a dynamic extension splint (**C**) for the proximal interphalangeal joint. (Reproduced from Culver JE: Office management of athletic injuries of the hand and wrist. *Instr Course Lect* 1989;38:473-486.)

Referral Decisions/Red Flags

Failure to achieve full extension or residual deformity or both indicates the need for further evaluation.

HAND AND WRIST

SECTION 4

Carpal Tunnel Syndrome

Synonyms

Median nerve compression
Median nerve entrapment at the wrist

Definition

Carpal tunnel syndrome (entrapment of the median nerve at the wrist) is the most common compression neuropathy in the upper extremity. It most commonly affects middle-aged or pregnant women.

Any condition that reduces the size or space of the carpal tunnel (**Figure 1**) can cause compression of the median nerve, resulting in paresthesias, pain, and sometimes paralysis. Common precipitating conditions include tenosynovitis of the adjacent flexor tendons, which can occur in the setting of rheumatoid arthritis; tumors; and medical conditions such as pregnancy, diabetes mellitus, and thyroid dysfunction.

Clinical Symptoms

The symptoms most commonly reported are numbness and tingling into the radial three digits of the hand (thumb, index, and long fingers). Patients also may report a vague aching that radiates into the thenar area. Aching also may be perceived in the proximal forearm, and occasionally the pain can extend to the shoulder. The pain is

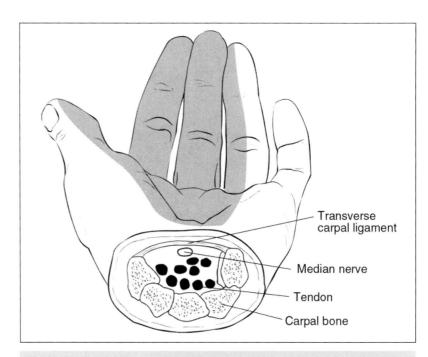

Figure 1 Illustration of the cross section of the carpal tunnel. Shading indicates the typical area of numbness with carpal tunnel syndrome. (Adapted from Szabo RM, Steinberg DR: Nerve entrapment syndromes in the wrist. *J Am Acad Orthop Surg* 1994;2[2]:115-123.)

typically accompanied by paresthesias or numbness in the median distribution (thumb and index finger, long finger, and radial half of the ring finger, or some combination thereof). Often the symptoms are worse at night.

Patients report that they frequently drop objects or that they cannot open jars or twist off lids. Pain or numbness sometimes is made worse by activities that require repetitive motion of the hand, repetitive activities, or stationary tasks performed with the wrist held flexed or extended for long periods, such as driving or reading. Patients often awaken at night with pain or numbness and typically report the need to rub or shake the hand to "get the circulation back." When the compression is severe and long-standing, persistent numbness and thenar atrophy can occur (**Figure 2**).

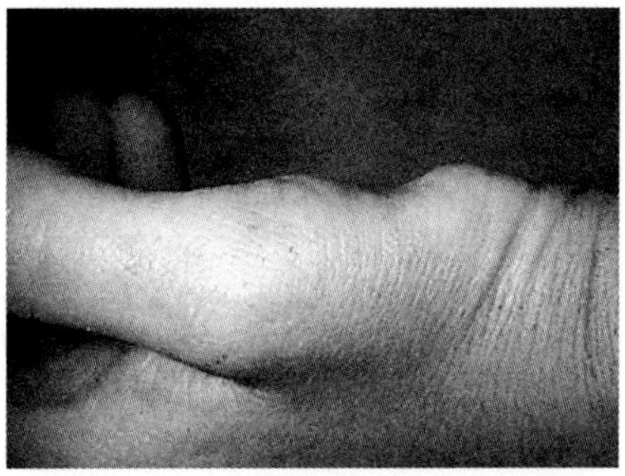

Figure 2 Clinical photograph from a patient with thenar atrophy.

Tests

Physical Examination

Inspect the hand for thenar atrophy. Testing thumb opposition against resistance may reveal weakness of the thenar muscles. Evaluate the sensation in the fingers.

The median nerve compression test is the most useful clinical test. It is performed by compressing the median nerve just proximal to the wrist crease, which, in a positive test, leads to symptoms in the median nerve distribution. The Phalen maneuver is also useful and is performed by placing the wrists in flexion. Avoid excessive elbow flexion when performing this test. Aching and numbness in the distribution of the median nerve within 60 seconds (often within 15 seconds or less) is a positive test for carpal tunnel syndrome. Tapping over the median nerve at the wrist may produce tingling in some or all of the digits in the median nerve distribution.

Patients with carpal tunnel syndrome may be unable to distinguish the two points of a caliper as separate points when they are closer together than 5 mm. Two-point discrimination of 5 mm is considered normal.

Diagnostic Tests

Radiographs of the wrist should be obtained if the patient has limited wrist motion. Most often, the diagnosis of carpal tunnel syndrome is made by clinical history and physical examination findings. Electrophysiologic testing is the most useful confirmatory test, although it is rarely required for diagnosis. These studies must be interpreted with caution, however. Some patients have no clinical signs or symptoms yet have abnormal nerve conduction velocity studies. Conversely, as many as 5% to 10% of patients with carpal tunnel syndrome have normal results.

Differential Diagnosis

- Arthritis of the carpometacarpal joint of the thumb (painful motion)
- Cervical radiculopathy affecting the C6 nerve (neck pain, numbness in the thumb and index fingers only, physical examination findings suggestive of cervical spine pathology)
- Diabetes mellitus with neuropathy (history)
- Flexor carpi radialis tenosynovitis (tenderness near the base of the thumb)
- Hypothyroidism (abnormal results on thyroid function tests)
- Pronator syndrome (median nerve compression at the elbow) (tenderness at the proximal forearm, numbness in the palmar triangle [thenar eminence], weakness in interphalangeal flexion of the thumb and/or in distal interphalangeal flexion of the index finger)
- Ulnar neuropathy (first dorsal interosseous weakness, numbness of the ring and little fingers)
- Volar radial ganglion (mass near the base of the thumb above the wrist flexion crease)
- Wrist arthritis (limited motion evident on radiographs) (may coexist with carpal tunnel syndrome)

Adverse Outcomes of the Disease

Permanent loss of sensation, hand strength, and fine motor skills are possible.

Treatment

For mild cases, splinting the wrist (in a neutral position wrist splint) may be helpful. The splint should be worn at night (at a minimum) and can be worn during the day if doing so does not interfere with the patient's work or daily activities. If these measures fail, consider injecting a corticosteroid into the carpal canal. Injection has diagnostic as well as therapeutic benefits, but improvement may be only temporary. Care must be taken to avoid direct injection into the median nerve, which may cause severe pain.

Work-related carpal tunnel syndrome may be improved with ergonomic modifications, such as using keyboard or forearm supports, adjusting the height of computer keyboards, and avoiding holding the wrist in a flexed position (as with dental hygienists).

Carpal tunnel syndrome that occurs during pregnancy usually resolves when the pregnancy terminates; therefore, treatment should consist of splinting and other nonsurgical measures, such as injection of a corticosteroid.

Surgical management is often necessary for patients who have fixed sensory loss or weakness of the thenar muscles and for those who have intolerable symptoms despite a course of nonsurgical treatment.

Rehabilitation Prescription

The purpose of nonsurgical management of carpal tunnel syndrome is to diminish the pressure on the median nerve at the wrist. In the early stages, the use of a night splint with the wrist in neutral position (0° of extension) is advocated. The wrist splint is worn for 3 to 4 weeks, during the day as well as at night. To reduce inflammation and pain, ice is used in the early stages. Heat is used to increase circulation and to promote tendon gliding. Exercises to promote tendon gliding are very important in the early stages of treatment.

   If the symptoms do not respond to the home program, the patient should be referred to a certified hand therapist. The therapist should evaluate range of motion, muscle strength, and sensory changes to determine the next stage of treatment. Strengthening exercises, continued use of a night splint, and ergonomic evaluation of the patient's job station should be part of the management of this condition. Other therapeutic modalities, such as iontophoresis, may be beneficial.

Adverse Outcomes of Treatment

NSAIDs can cause gastric, renal, or hepatic complications. In 2015, the FDA strengthened its warning linking NSAIDs with the risk of heart attack or stroke, even in the first weeks of use of an NSAID. Fluid retention, flushing of the skin, and shakiness can result from taking oral corticosteroids. Injecting corticosteroids is associated with the risk of an intraneural injection, which can have long-term adverse consequences. Prolonged nonsurgical treatment in patients with persistent sensory loss or motor weakness can result in loss of sensation and thenar atrophy.

Referral Decisions/Red Flags

Failure of nonsurgical treatment after 3 months warrants further evaluation. Persistent numbness (that is, constant numbness rather than intermittent symptoms), weakness, atrophy of the thenar muscles, or any combination of these are indications for further evaluation.

www.aaos.org/essentials5/exercises

Home Program for Carpal Tunnel Syndrome

- Apply heat to the hand for 15 minutes before performing the exercises, and apply a bag of crushed ice or frozen peas to the hand for 20 minutes after each exercise session to prevent inflammation.
- If numbness steadily worsens, if the exercises increase the pain, or if the pain does not improve after you have performed the exercises for 3 to 4 weeks, call your doctor.
- The following program is introductory only, and progression of this program will vary based on your specific injury, symptoms, and baseline level of fitness. For further progression of this routine, your physician may recommend evaluation and treatment by a physical therapist or other exercise professional.

Home Program for Carpal Tunnel Syndrome

Exercise Type	Targeted Structure	Number of Repetitions/Sets	Number of Days per Week	Number of Weeks
Nerve gliding	Median nerve	10 to 15 repetitions	6 to 7	3 to 4
Tendon gliding	Median nerve	5 to 10 repetitions/2 to 3 times per day	Progress as tolerated	Progress as tolerated

Nerve Gliding

- With the affected hand raised, make a fist with the thumb outside the fingers (1).
- Extend the fingers, keeping the thumb close to the side of the hand (2).
- Extend the hand at the wrist (bend it backward, toward the forearm), keeping the fingers straight (3).
- With the wrist straight, extend the thumb as shown (4).
- Keeping the thumb extended, extend the hand at the wrist (5).
- Reach behind your hand and grasp the thumb with the thumb and forefinger of the opposite hand. Pull the thumb downward, away from the palm of your hand (6).
- Repeat 10 to 15 times.
- Perform the exercises 6 to 7 days per week, for 3 to 4 weeks.

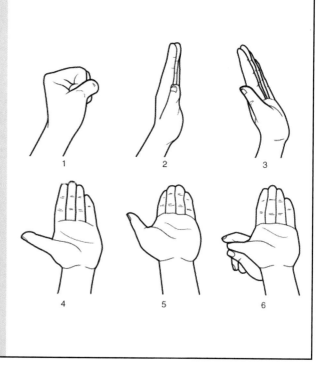

Tendon Gliding

- Perform each series below 5 to 10 times, 2 to 3 times per day.
- Proceed from position 1 through 3 in sequence; hold each position for 3 seconds.
- Movements may cause gentle pulling but should not cause increased pain.
- You may progress repetitions, frequency, and intensity of motions as tolerated.

Series A

- With your hand in front of you with your wrist straight, straighten all your fingers fully (1).
- Bend the ends of your fingers down as shown into a hook position, bending just the top two joints in each finger (2).
- Move all fingers into a tight fist position (3).

Series B

- With your hand in front of you with your wrist straight, straighten all your fingers fully (1).
- Bend your fingers down as shown, bending just the bottom joint in each finger (2).
- From position 2, bend at the middle joint, moving your fingers to your palm (3).

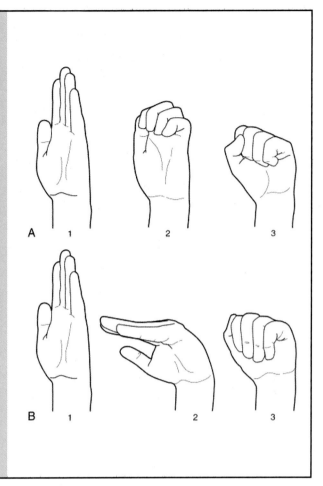

Procedure: Carpal Tunnel Injection

Note: Opinions differ regarding single- and two-needle injection techniques. Proponents of the single-needle technique believe that one needle is less painful for the patient than two.

Step 1
Wear protective gloves at all times during this procedure and use sterile technique.

Step 2
Cleanse the volar aspect of the wrist and forearm with a bactericidal skin preparation solution.

Step 3
Insert the needle 1 cm proximal to the wrist flexion crease and in line with the ring finger metacarpal. Direct the needle toward the hand or forearm (the former is shown) at an angle of 30° to 45° (**Figure 1**). If the patient reports paresthesias, redirect the needle.

Materials
- Sterile gloves
- Bactericidal skin preparation solution
- One 3-mL syringe with a 25-gauge needle
- 1 mL of a 1% local anesthetic
- 0.5 to 1 mL of a corticosteroid preparation
- Adhesive bandage

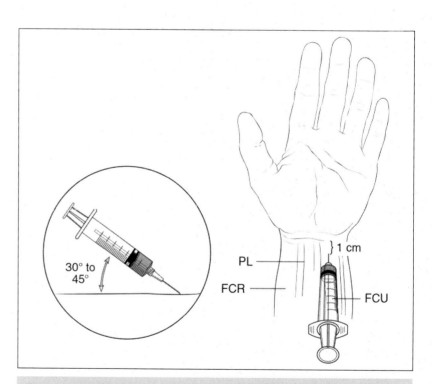

Figure 1 Illustration shows the location for needle insertion for carpal tunnel injection. FCR = flexor carpi radialis, FCU = flexor carpi ulnaris, PL = palmaris longus.

Step 4

Ask the patient if any paresthesias occurred with the introduction of the needle. If the patient reports any tingling, then the needle is too close to the nerve and must be repositioned. Aspirate to ensure that the needle is not intravascular. Inject the corticosteroid preparation with anesthetic. If resistance is encountered on attempting to inject the fluid, the tip of the needle may be embedded in the flexor tendons. Maintain some pressure on the syringe while slowly withdrawing the needle, until the fluid flows freely.

Step 5

Dress the puncture wound with a sterile adhesive bandage.

Adverse Outcomes

Infection or intraneural injection is possible.

Aftercare/Patient Instructions

Advise the patient that mild soreness may develop, that the hand and fingers may be numb for 1 to 2 hours following the injection, and that the injection could require a few days to take effect.

SECTION 4 HAND AND WRIST

de Quervain Tenosynovitis

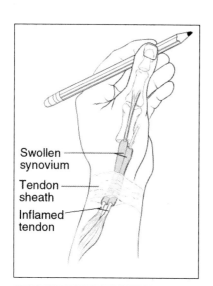

Figure 1 Illustration depicts de Quervain tenosynovitis of the first extensor compartment.

Labels on figure:
Swollen synovium
Tendon sheath
Inflamed tendon

Synonym
Stenosing tenosynovitis

Definition
de Quervain tenosynovitis is swelling or stenosis of the sheath that surrounds the abductor pollicis longus and extensor pollicis brevis tendons at the wrist (**Figure 1**). The inflammation thickens the tendon sheath (tenosynovium) and constricts the tendon as it glides in the sheath. This can cause pain, swelling, and a triggering phenomenon, resulting in locking or sticking of the tendon as the patient moves the thumb. The disorder is common in women and is often precipitated by repetitive use of the thumb. In addition, it is very common in the postpartum period, likely due to a combination of altered hormonal states and the repetitive ulnar deviation of the wrist that occurs when a mother lifts her baby.

Clinical Symptoms
Patients report swelling over the radial styloid and pain that is aggravated by attempts to move the thumb or make a fist. They also may notice creaking as the tendon moves.

Tests
Physical Examination
Examination reveals swelling and tenderness over the tendons of the first dorsal compartment in the region of the distal radius. Crepitus may be palpable as the patient flexes and extends the thumb. Full flexion of the thumb into the palm, followed by ulnar deviation of the wrist (**Figure 2**), produces pain and is diagnostic for de Quervain tenosynovitis.

Diagnostic Tests
Even though this is largely a clinical diagnosis, PA and lateral radiographs of the wrist should be considered to rule out any bony abnormality that might be a precipitating cause, such as a deformed radial styloid process resulting from trauma. Calcification associated with tendinitis occasionally can be seen on radiographs.

Differential Diagnosis
- Carpometacarpal arthritis of the thumb (swelling over the joint, pain with joint compression)
- Dorsal wrist ganglion (palpable mass)
- Flexor carpi radialis tendinitis (pain and swelling over the tendon)
- Fracture of the scaphoid (tenderness over the anatomic snuffbox)

- Intersection syndrome
- Superficial radial neuritis
- Wrist arthritis (pain with movement, evident on radiographs)

Adverse Outcomes of the Disease
Chronic pain, loss of strength, and loss of thumb motion can occur; tendon rupture is possible but rare.

Treatment
Initial treatment should consist of a 2-week course of NSAIDs and a forearm-based thumb spica splint (to immobilize both the wrist and thumb). If this initial treatment fails, the tendon sheath may be injected with a corticosteroid preparation, taking care not to inject the steroid into the tendon. The patient should have no more than three injections.

Surgical treatment should be considered if corticosteroid injections are not successful.

Adverse Outcomes of Treatment
NSAIDs can cause gastric, renal, or hepatic complications. In 2015, the FDA strengthened its warning linking NSAIDs with the risk of heart attack or stroke, even in the first weeks of use of an NSAID. The patient may experience some discomfort from wearing the splint and will stop using it. Corticosteroids can sometimes cause subcutaneous atrophy and unsightly loss of pigmentation. Infection after corticosteroid injection also is a risk, but this can be largely avoided by careful use of sterile technique. Injury to the radial sensory nerve or incomplete release is possible with surgical treatment.

Referral Decisions/Red Flags
Failure to respond to splinting and corticosteroid injections indicates the need for further evaluation.

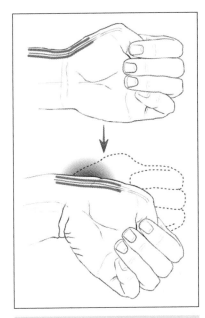

Figure 2 Illustration shows the Finkelstein test. (Note that although this test is commonly known as the Finkelstein test, Finkelstein performed it differently, and as shown here, the maneuver is more accurately attributed to Eichoff.) The arrow indicates the location of pain when the test is positive. (Adapted with permission from the American Society for Surgery of the Hand: *de Quervain's Stenosing Tenosynovitis*. Englewood, CO, 1995.)

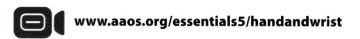

www.aaos.org/essentials5/handandwrist

Procedure: de Quervain Tenosynovitis Injection

Note: Opinions differ regarding single- and two-needle injection techniques. Proponents of the single-needle technique believe that one needle is less painful for the patient than two.

Step 1
Wear protective gloves at all times during this procedure and use sterile technique.

Step 2
Cleanse the skin with a bactericidal skin preparation solution.

Step 3
Insert the 25-gauge needle at a 45° angle to the skin in line with the two tendons (**Figure 1**). If the patient reports paresthesia into the thumb, the needle has depolarized the sensory branch of the radial nerve. Reposition the needle 2 to 3 mm dorsal or volar, to a position that does not cause paresthesia.

Step 4
This step is needed only if the two-injection technique is used. Create a skin wheal with 0.5 mL of 1% local anesthetic and advance the needle until it strikes one of the underlying tendons. Inject the remaining anesthetic while slowly withdrawing the needle, until the anesthetic flows freely. Leave the needle in place and change syringes.

Step 5
Inject 0.5 to 1 mL of corticosteroid preparation into the tendon sheath. Palpation of the tendon sheath proximal to the point of injection should reveal swelling as the corticosteroid is injected. In general, there will be some dilation of the sheath with a successful injection.

Step 6
Dress the puncture site with a sterile adhesive bandage.

Adverse Outcomes
Subcutaneous fat atrophy can follow subcutaneous infiltration of the corticosteroid preparation, leading to a waxy-appearing depression in the skin. In addition, although rare, infection is possible.

Materials
- Sterile gloves
- Bactericidal skin preparation solution
- One or two 3-mL syringes with a 25-gauge, ⅞" needle
- 0.5 to 1.0 mL of corticosteroid preparation
- 1 to 2 mL of a 1% local anesthetic

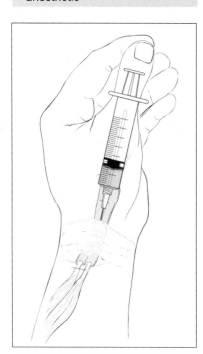

Figure 1 Illustration of the location for needle insertion for de Quervain injection.

Aftercare/Patient Instructions

Increased pain is not uncommon after the injection, especially in the first 24 to 48 hours. At least one third of patients will experience increased discomfort during this time.

Dupuytren Contracture

Synonyms
Dupuytren disease
Palmar fibromatosis
Viking disease

Definition
Dupuytren contracture is a nodular thickening and contraction of the palmar fascia (**Figure 1**). The disease has a dominant genetic component, particularly involving people of northern European descent. Dupuytren contracture most commonly affects men older than 50 years. Associated factors include epilepsy, diabetes mellitus, pulmonary disease, alcoholism, smoking, and repetitive trauma (vibration).

Clinical Symptoms
Patients initially notice one or more painless nodules near the distal palmar crease that are moderately sensitive to pressure. The nodule or nodules may gradually thicken and contract, causing the finger

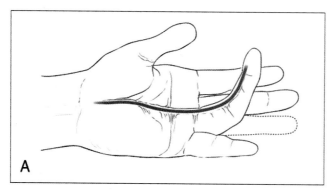

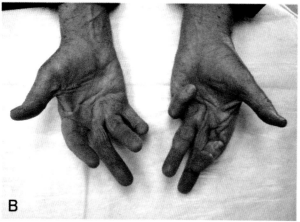
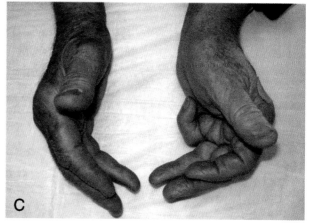

Figure 1 Images of Dupuytren contracture of the ring finger. **A,** Illustration shows the affected palmar fascial cord. **B** and **C,** Clinical appearance of the hands of a patient with bilateral Dupuytren contracture. The ring finger of the right hand, the little finger of the left hand, and both palms are affected. (Panel A adapted with permission from the American Society for Surgery of the Hand: *Dupuytren's Disease.* Englewood, CO, 1995.)

to flex at the metacarpophalangeal (MCP) joint and, occasionally as the disease progresses, the proximal interphalangeal (PIP) joint. The ring finger is most commonly involved, followed by the little finger, the long finger, the thumb, and the index finger. Although extension is limited, finger flexion is often normal. The condition is usually painless in its later stages, but as the contractures increase, patients have trouble grasping objects, pulling on gloves, and putting the hand into a pocket. Sensation in the affected fingers usually is normal.

Tests

Physical Examination

Examination reveals a palmar skin nodule that in the early stages may resemble a callus. As the disease progresses, the abnormal cords extend distally and sometimes proximally to the nodule. These bands may cross the PIP joint and commonly cross the MCP joint, holding the finger in a contracted position. The bands are seldom tender unless the patient is in the early stages of the disease.

Diagnostic Tests

Diagnosis is made on clinical examination. Radiographs are not needed.

Differential Diagnosis

- Flexion contracture secondary to joint or tendon injury (no cords or bands)
- Locked trigger finger (no associated nodules)

Adverse Outcomes of the Disease

Progressive flexion contracture of the fingers and limited function are possible.

Treatment

Splinting or other nonsurgical treatment is not curative, but night splints may slow the progression of the contractures. Percutaneous aponeurotomy may be appropriate in some cases for the treatment of isolated cords. Collagenase injection to the involved cord is an FDA-approved form of treatment. Surgery involves excising the thick cords, releasing the joint contractures, and often complex skin closure. Surgery is considered when there is a 30° fixed flexion deformity of the MCP joint or a 10° deformity of the PIP joint. More severe contractures are more difficult to correct, have a higher incidence of recurrent contracture, and require a longer course of postoperative occupational therapy.

Adverse Outcomes of Treatment

Patients may experience nerve injury, skin loss, and recurrence of the disease postoperatively.

Referral Decisions/Red Flags

Patients with significant contractures (greater than 30°) of the MCP joints who are troubled by the lack of extension are candidates for further evaluation. Likewise, patients with involvement of the PIP joint in association with Dupuytren disease require close follow-up.

Fingertip Infections

Synonyms

Felon
Paronychia

Definition

Infections of the fingertip typically occur in two locations: in the pulp, or palmar tip, of the finger (felon) and in the soft tissues directly surrounding the fingernail (paronychia) (**Figure 1**). *Staphylococcus aureus* is the most common causative organism in both conditions.

Felons usually are caused by a puncture wound and most commonly occur in the thumb or index finger (**Figure 2**). Herpetic whitlow, a virally mediated hand infection that is characterized by the formation of vesicles filled with clear fluid, also can occur in and around the fingertip (**Figure 3**). Differentiating a felon from herpetic whitlow is important because incision and drainage of a felon usually is

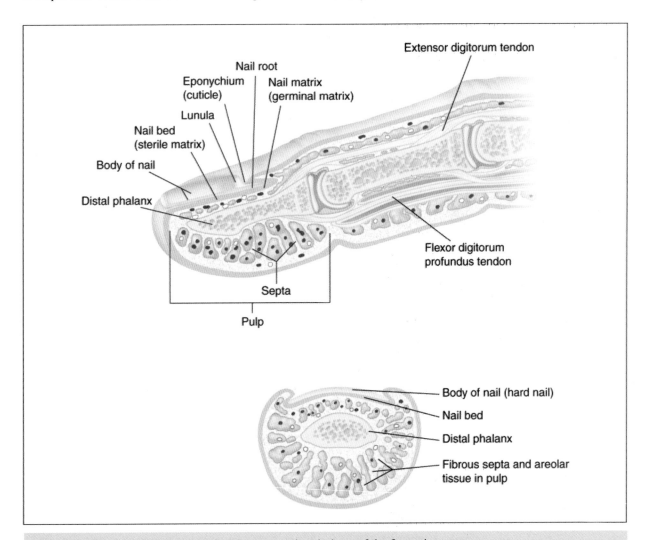

Figure 1 Illustration shows sagittal and cross-sectional views of the fingertip.

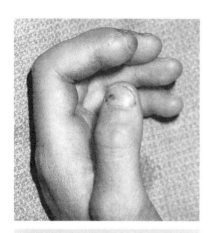

Figure 2 Clinical photograph shows felon of the index finger. (Reproduced from Stern PJ: Selected acute infections. *Instr Course Lect* 1990;39:539-546.)

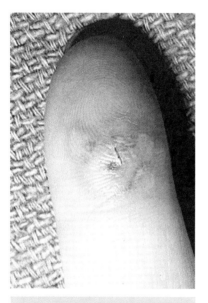

Figure 3 Clinical photograph shows herpetic whitlow. (Reproduced from Stern PJ: Selected acute infections. *Instr Course Lect* 1990;39:539-546.)

indicated, whereas incision of a whitlow is contraindicated and observation is sufficient. Healthcare workers who are frequently exposed to the herpes simplex virus from human saliva (such as respiratory therapists and dental hygienists) are at increased risk for herpetic whitlow. Paronychial infections often occur after a manicure or the development of a nail deformity, such as a hangnail or an ingrown nail.

Clinical Symptoms

A felon is characterized by severe pain and swelling in the pad of the fingertip. With a felon, the entire pulp of the fingertip is swollen, tense, red, and very tender. A puncture wound may be visible.

Paronychial infection is characterized by swelling of the tissues about the fingernail, usually along one side and about the base of the nail. Occasionally, the swelling extends completely around the nail and is then referred to as a "run-around abscess." The pain associated with a paronychia is not as intense as that with a felon.

Swelling associated with a felon or paronychia should not extend proximal to the distal flexion crease. Any such extension suggests a deeper, more complex process, such as an infection involving the flexor tendon sheath. Substantially increased pain with passive motion also may indicate flexor tendon sheath infection.

Tests
Physical Examination

The fingertip should be examined for the location and extent of the swelling. The presence of small vesicles suggests herpetic whitlow. Tenderness, redness, and fluctuance are more characteristic of a bacterial abscess (paronychia or felon).

Diagnostic Tests

Plain radiographs show soft-tissue swelling. Late in the course of infection, osteomyelitis of the distal phalanx may occur and is evident on radiographs as partial or complete resorption of the distal tuft of the phalanx. More aggressive surgical débridement is required in these cases.

Differential Diagnosis

- Chronic fungal infection (not responsive to antibiotics)
- Epidermal inclusion cyst (dorsal swelling proximal to the nail, usually not very painful)
- Septic tenosynovitis (increased pain with active and passive motion of finger)

Adverse Outcomes of the Disease

Untreated felons (**Figure 4, A**) may result in osteomyelitis of the distal phalanx. Nail deformities and progressive infection involving the distal joint and/or the flexor tendon sheath also may develop late

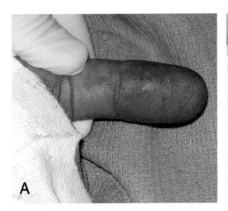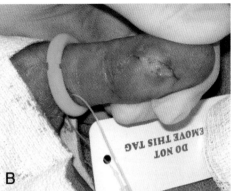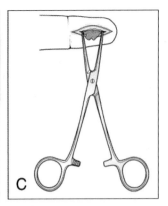

Figure 4 **A,** Clinical photograph shows a felon. **B,** Clinical photograph shows an oblique incision. **C,** Illustration of a central volar longitudinal incision shows the use of a hemostat to spread the wound and thereby release septal fluid.

in the course of these infections. Untreated felons may occasionally rupture into the flexor tendon sheath and cause septic flexor tenosynovitis.

Treatment

Most felons require surgical drainage under digital block anesthesia and tourniquet control. Either of two incisions can be used: a central volar longitudinal incision or a dorsal midaxial incision. When a puncture wound is present, the wound should be incorporated into the incision when feasible.

When a collection of pus can be seen under the skin on the pad side of the finger, use an oblique incision (**Figure 4, B**) or a central longitudinal incision extending from the flexion crease to the fingertip (**Figure 4, C**). Culture the drainage for aerobic and anaerobic organisms. It is most important to use a curved hemostat to break up the septae of the digital pulp to ensure that the abscess is completely evacuated. To allow drainage, keep the wound open, using a gauze packing strip, and remove it in 1 to 2 days. Allow the wound to close by secondary intention; never suture the wound. When no collection of pus is readily visible under the skin, use a dorsal midaxial incision (**Figure 5**). For the thumb, make the incision on the radial (noncontact) side; for the fingers, the ulnar (noncontact) side. Extend the incision to the fingertip but do not wrap it around the tip. Make the incision down to the bone where the soft-tissue attachments to the bone can be separated by blunt dissection with a small hemostat. Use open packing gauze and then remove it in 1 to 2 days.

Treatment of an early-stage paronychia is usually nonsurgical. Application of warm, moist soaks for 10 minutes four times a day, combined with an oral antibiotic for 5 days, is usually adequate. Because *S aureus* is the most likely causative organism, an oral cephalosporin such as cephalexin, 250 mg four times per day, or dicloxacillin, 250 mg four times per day, is a good initial choice. In patients at high risk for methicillin-resistant *S aureus* (MRSA), the addition of sulfamethoxazole and trimethoprim may be appropriate;

SECTION 4 **HAND AND WRIST**

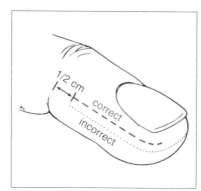

Figure 5 Illustration of midaxial incision for drainage of a felon. (Reproduced from Stern PJ: Selected acute infections. *Instr Course Lect* 1990;39:539-546.)

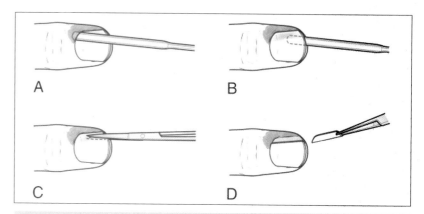

Figure 6 Illustration depicts removal of a portion of a nail for paronychia. **A,** Use an elevator to separate the nail from the dorsal skin. **B,** Use an elevator to separate the nail from the underlying nail bed. **C,** With straight scissors, divide the nail itself. **D,** Remove the nail segment with a hemostat by applying gentle traction.

alternatively, clindamycin 300 mg by mouth four times per day is used. In later stages, when a purulent collection is noted at the nail bed margin or under the nail, drainage can be performed by elevating the skin fold at the margin of the nail. More severe infections require partial or complete removal of the nail (**Figure 6**). Under digital or metacarpal block anesthesia, the nail can be carefully elevated from the underlying sterile matrix using a hemostat or blunt metal probe. The nail can be completely removed by freeing the overlying cuticle, and the nail bed protected by nonadherent gauze carefully tucked underneath the cuticle and extending to the tip of the finger. The wound should be checked in 2 to 3 days. The patient should be advised that the nail can be expected to grow out within several (up to 6) months.

Adverse Outcomes of Treatment

A painful scar may develop as a result of a misplaced incision, or a nail deformity can develop from injury to the germinal matrix. Inadequate drainage with persistent or recurrent infection may occur.

Referral Decisions/Red Flags

Persistent or progressive swelling or any evidence of an ascending hand or limb infection, despite adequate antibiotic treatment and surgical decompression, is an indication for further evaluation.

Procedure: Digital Anesthetic Block (Hand)

Note: Two techniques are shown. The dorsal web space block is preferred by some because they believe the injection is less painful for the patient. Others prefer the volar block because they believe it is more effective.

Historically, the use of local anesthesia with epinephrine was reported to be contraindicated in digits; however, recent evidence documents the safety and efficacy of 1% lidocaine with 1:100,000 epinephrine for use in the digits. In general, a digit that is warm and well perfused prior to injection will remain perfused following injection. In the case of an adverse reaction, phentolamine can be used to reverse epinephrine.

Materials
- Sterile gloves
- Bactericidal skin preparation solution
- 3-mL or 5-mL syringe with a 27-gauge needle
- 3 or 5 mL of 1% local anesthetic
- Sterile dressing

Technique 1: Dorsal Web Space Block

Step 1
Wear protective gloves at all times during this procedure and use sterile technique.

Step 2
Cleanse all surfaces of the base of the finger with a bactericidal skin preparation solution.

Step 3
Draw 3 mL of the local anesthetic into the syringe.

Step 4
Insert the 27-gauge needle into the web space alongside the extensor tendon (**Figure 1, A**). Advance the needle until it is almost at the volar skin and inject 1 mL of the local anesthetic.

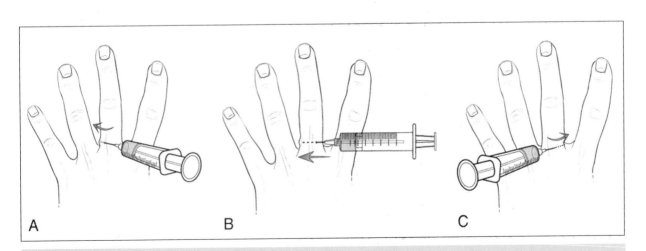

Figure 1 Illustration of injection technique 1: dorsal web space block. **A,** Dorsal location for needle insertion into the web space alongside the extensor tendon. **B,** Dorsal location for needle insertion along the top of the extensor tendon. **C,** Location for needle insertion into the web space on the opposite side of the finger.

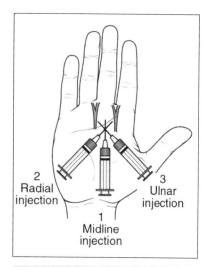

Figure 2 Illustration of injection technique 2: volar block for the long finger.

Step 5

Withdraw the needle and insert it along the top of the extensor tendon (**Figure 1, B**). Inject 1 mL of the solution.

Step 6

Repeat the procedure in the web space on the opposite side of the finger (**Figure 1, C**).

Step 7

Dress the puncture site with a sterile adhesive dressing.

Technique 2: Volar Block

Step 1

Wear protective gloves at all times during this procedure and use sterile technique.

Step 2

Cleanse all surfaces of the base of the finger with a bactericidal skin preparation solution.

Step 3

Draw 5 mL of the local anesthetic into the syringe.

Step 4

Insert the 27-gauge needle into the palmar midline of the digit near the distal palmar crease. The first injection (approximately one third of the anesthetic) should be made at the midline. The needle should then be repositioned and another one third of the anesthetic injected toward the radial digital nerve. Reposition the needle again and inject the remainder of the anesthetic toward the ulnar digital nerve (**Figure 2**).

Step 5

Dress the injection site with a sterile adhesive dressing.

Adverse Outcomes

Although rare, infection is possible. Never inject circumferentially around the base of a digit because this could cause circumferential hydrostatic pressure that can reduce circulation to the finger.

Aftercare/Patient Instructions

Advise the patient that local swelling at the site of the block should resolve in a few hours. Instruct the patient to call your office if the finger becomes dusky or completely white and to avoid touching hot surfaces or using sharp objects until all sensation has returned.

Fingertip Injuries/ Amputations

Definition

Fingertip injuries and amputations are common. Some apparent amputations are actually crush injuries or lacerations. In addition to the soft tissue of the pulp, the distal phalanx and nail may be involved.

Clinical Symptoms

Patients report a history of a crush injury or a knife injury to the fingertip. Knife injury usually involves a finger in the nondominant hand.

Tests

Physical Examination

The fingertip should be inspected carefully to determine the vascularity and sensation of the skin flaps and whether bone is exposed. The orientation of the amputation also should be noted (**Figure 1**) because the level and angle of amputation may determine appropriate treatment. The nail bed should be carefully examined for a painful subungual hematoma that should be drained and for lacerations of the nail bed that should be repaired. The vascularity of the tip, as well as sensation, should be noted.

Diagnostic Tests

If bone is exposed or if the finger is markedly swollen, AP and lateral radiographs of the finger should be obtained.

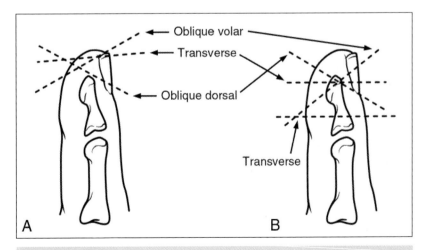

Figure 1 Illustration of the varied orientations of fingertip injuries/ amputations. **A,** Levels of soft-tissue amputations that can be treated open and allowed to close by secondary intention. **B,** Levels of amputation that require shortening of the bone.

Differential Diagnosis

- Amputation with injury to the nail matrix (evident on clinical examination)
- Amputation with open fracture (evident on radiographs)

Adverse Outcomes of the Disease

A painful amputation stump, dystrophic nail, loss of motion in the finger, and loss of grip and pinch strength are possible. Cold sensitivity/Raynaud phenomenon, a painful neuroma, or an epidermal inclusion cyst also can develop. Complex regional pain syndrome also is possible.

Treatment

The goals of treatment are to provide the fingertip with good soft-tissue coverage and adequate sensation, and to preserve as much length as is consistent with good function. Whether or not bone is exposed and the angle of the amputation relative to the long axis of the finger often dictate the appropriate treatment options (**Figure 1**).

When no bone is exposed, the physician must decide if the skin can be closed without excess tension. If not, the wound should be allowed to close by secondary intention. Fingertip wounds of 1 cm or less almost always heal well without closure. Initial treatment consists of thorough débridement and irrigation of the finger under a digital block and application of sterile dressings and a distal splint for comfort and contact protection. The initial dressings should be changed after 24 to 72 hours. Wet to dry dressings using normal saline solution twice a day are then applied. The patient should be taught how to apply these dressings and how to put on the removable splint at home. The dressing changes are continued until the tip has healed. Finger range-of-motion exercises should begin after 48 hours. After the wound has healed, tip desensitization techniques can be started in occupational therapy. In most cases, allowing the wound to heal by secondary intention provides good function and acceptable cosmetic results and retains maximum finger length. Almost all fingertip injuries involving an area less than 1 cm square can be managed with débridement and the application of a dressing.

If bone is exposed, a decision must be made whether to shorten the bone or to provide skin coverage by a reconstructive flap procedure. As a general guide, the exposed phalanx of any of the fingers can be shortened to provide soft-tissue coverage without sacrificing function. Shortening the thumb is more controversial. Associated nail bed injuries require special attention.

Treatment of amputation in children younger than 6 years differs somewhat from the treatment in adults. Most children experience rapid healing and can be treated with local care and serial dressings. For some patients, "composite" grafting, or reapplication of the amputated fingertip as a full-thickness skin graft, is desirable. After thorough débridement and defatting, the skin of the amputated fingertip is sutured to the finger as a composite graft. Even if this graft does not survive (approximately 50% do survive), it serves as a biologic dressing until reepithelialization of the fingertip occurs. For fingertip injuries in children, always use absorbable sutures, such as 4-0 or 5-0 chromic or plain gut, in the skin to limit the anxiety that occurs in follow-up visits.

The tetanus immunization status of the patient must be checked and updated if necessary. If the wound is grossly contaminated and/or crushed, or if the patient has diabetes mellitus, antibiotics may be used.

Replantation may be considered if the thumb is amputated at or proximal to the interphalangeal (IP) joint, if a finger is amputated proximal to the middle of the middle phalanx, or if multiple fingers are amputated. A replantation center should be contacted for specific instructions. The amputated part is wrapped in sterile gauze soaked in normal saline solution and placed in a plastic bag, and then the bag is placed on ice. The replantation team will usually make the determination whether replantation is possible and recommended.

Most patients function well with single-finger amputations. Some patients are concerned with cosmesis, in which case a cosmetic finger prosthesis can be fitted.

Referral Decisions/Red Flags

Patients with thumb amputations proximal to the IP joint and multiple finger amputations are suitable candidates for specialty evaluation.

Flexor Tendon Injuries

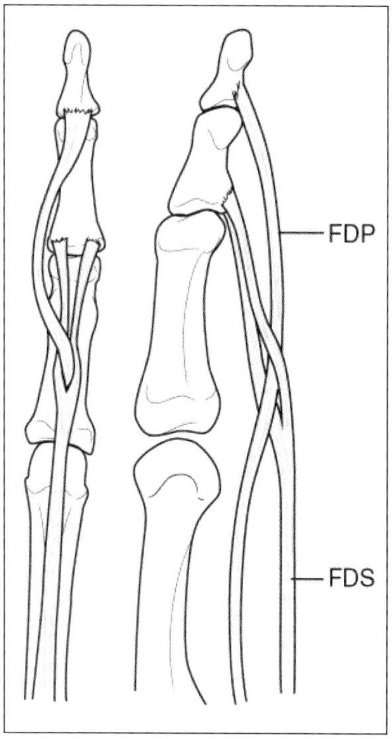

Synonyms
Jersey finger
Rugger jersey finger
Tendon laceration or rupture

Figure 1 Illustration of the extrinsic flexor tendons of the finger. FDP = flexor digitorum profundus, FDS = flexor digitorum sublimis.

Definition
The flexor tendons of the hand are vulnerable to laceration and rupture. Complete lacerations of both the flexor digitorum sublimis (FDS) and flexor digitorum profundus (FDP) cause immediate loss of flexion at the proximal interphalangeal (PIP) and distal interphalangeal (DIP) joints. Incomplete or partial lacerations can be missed on initial examination, only to present several days later as a complete rupture in the weakened tendon.

Ruptures of flexor tendons also can occur in patients with osteoarthritis, in patients with rheumatoid arthritis or other inflammatory arthritides, or as a result of trauma. Patients with rheumatoid arthritis may experience tendon rupture from direct synovial invasion of the tendon or from chronic wear over bony osteophytes. Tendon rupture caused by chronic wear over bony osteophytes usually occurs during athletics (such as football, wrestling, or rugby) when a player grabs another's jersey (thus the name "jersey finger"). When the fingers flex, the ring finger is most prominent and, therefore, the profundus tendon of the ring finger is most commonly ruptured during this activity.

Clinical Symptoms
Each finger is supplied with two flexor tendons: the FDP inserts onto the distal phalanx, and the FDS inserts onto the middle phalanx (**Figure 1**). Therefore, if the FDP is cut but the FDS is intact, patients can flex the PIP and metacarpophalangeal (MCP) joints but not the DIP joint. If the FDS is cut but the FDP is intact, patients can flex the DIP, PIP, and MCP joints (**Figure 2**). Because of the close proximity of the digital nerves to the flexor tendons, open injuries to the flexor tendons are commonly associated with injuries to the digital nerves as well. In this situation, patients may report numbness on one or both sides of the finger; the examiner should conduct a detailed examination of two-point discrimination.

With traumatic rupture of the FDP, the ring finger becomes caught, as in a sports jersey (**Figure 3**), and the profundus tendon is avulsed from its insertion, possibly accompanied by a bony fragment. This injury can be missed or diagnosed late because it is often considered to be a jammed finger.

Level of cut tendon	(1)	(2)	(3)
Tendon(s) cut	FDP	FDP and FDS	FDS
Loss of flexion joint(s)	DIP	PIP and DIP	None
Retained flexion joint(s)	MCP and PIP	MCP	MCP, PIP, and DIP

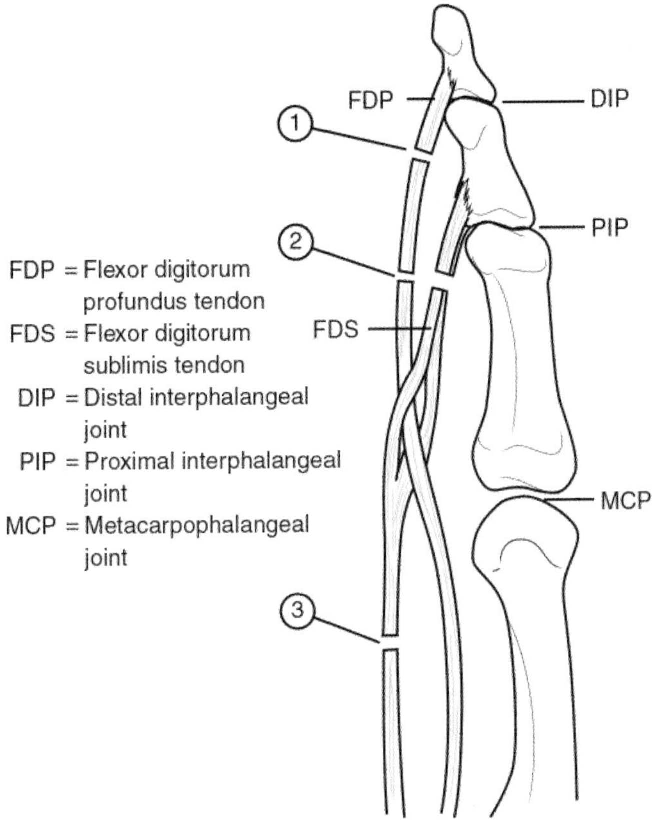

FDP = Flexor digitorum profundus tendon
FDS = Flexor digitorum sublimis tendon
DIP = Distal interphalangeal joint
PIP = Proximal interphalangeal joint
MCP = Metacarpophalangeal joint

Figure 2 Table and illustration depict the effects of flexor tendon injuries on flexion of the finger joint.

Tests

Physical Examination

First, test for active flexion; then test for strength of flexion. If the peritendinous structures are intact, the patient may retain flexion even in the presence of a complete laceration; however, flexion will be weak. Test flexion strength at both the DIP and PIP joints by asking the patient to flex the injured finger against your finger as you apply resistance.

Check flexion of the FDP by asking the patient to flex the fingertip at the DIP joint while the PIP joint is held in extension. To test the integrity of the FDS, hold the fingers straight, then have the patient flex each finger individually at the PIP joint. With a lacerated FDS

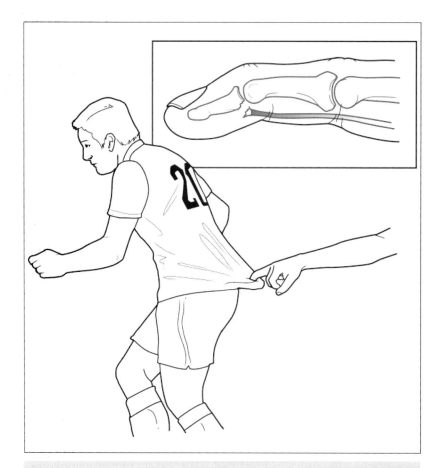

Figure 3 Illustration of the typical mechanism of injury in rupture of the flexor digitorum profundus tendon (jersey finger).

but an intact FDP, PIP flexion will not occur when the other fingers are held extended. This is because the FDP tendons cannot function independently. This test is not reliable at the little finger because 20% to 30% of the population has a band connecting the ring and little fingers that prevents independent function of the sublimis to the little finger. In addition, in some patients, the FDP of the index finger can weakly flex the finger with the other fingers held extended.

Partial lacerations can pose a diagnostic challenge. Patients typically have full range of motion, but they have more pain with active flexion than would be expected. When the diagnosis is unclear, evaluation for possible surgical exploration should be considered.

Patients with a tendon rupture may have mild swelling over the flexion surface of the DIP joint and tenderness along the palmar surface of the finger. Test the strength of flexion at the DIP joint. When flexion is weak, rupture of the FDP must be considered. Patients with rheumatoid arthritis may not remember the point at which the tendon ruptured; they usually report only that the finger will not flex.

Sensation in the finger also should be evaluated with assessment of two-point discrimination in the radial and ulnar aspect of the affected digits because open tendon injuries are often accompanied by injuries to the nearby digital nerves. The vascular status of injured fingers should be checked and documented as well.

Diagnostic Tests

PA and lateral radiographs of the involved finger may show a small avulsed fragment from the distal phalanx in an FDP rupture. These views also may identify a fracture.

Differential Diagnosis

- Anterior interosseous nerve paralysis (no laceration)
- Partial tendon laceration (full flexion with pain and weakness)
- Stenosing tenosynovitis ("trigger finger") with the finger locked in extension (no visible wound, tenderness over the proximal flexor pulley)

Adverse Outcomes of the Disease

Loss of flexion and loss of grip and pinch strength in the involved and adjacent fingers are possible.

Treatment

The principal goal of initial treatment is to correctly identify the condition and ensure that the patient is evaluated for surgical repair. Patients with flexor tendon injuries should be referred for consultation and surgical repair; initial treatment consists of cleaning and repairing superficial wounds and splinting the hand in the position shown in **Figure 4**. Ideally, surgical exploration and repair should be performed within 1 week after injury.

Adverse Outcomes of Treatment

Postoperative infection or failure of the repair is possible.

Referral Decisions/Red Flags

Patients with any type of suspected flexor tendon injury (rupture or laceration) require further evaluation for surgical repair.

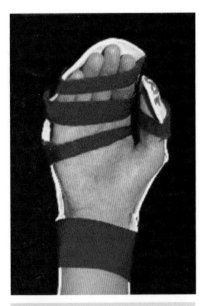

Figure 4 Clinical photograph shows a flexor tendon splint.

Flexor Tendon Sheath Infections

Synonym
Septic tenosynovitis

Definition
The flexor tendons of the fingers and thumb are enclosed in a specialized tenosynovial sheath that extends from the distal palm to the area of the distal interphalangeal (DIP) joint (**Figure 1**). Inoculations of this space from a puncture wound can cause severe finger infections. Infections within this space can develop from a puncture wound or can spread to the sheath from more superficial infection. These bacterial infections can be progressive and require both prompt diagnosis and treatment.

Clinical Symptoms
Patients typically present with a history of a recent puncture wound to the flexor surface of the finger or thumb. Progressive swelling of the entire digit and significant pain develop 24 to 48 hours after injury (**Figure 2**).

Tests
Physical Examination
Signs of a well-established septic flexor tenosynovitis are characterized by the Kanavel signs: (1) fusiform swelling of the finger, (2) significant tenderness along the course of the tendon

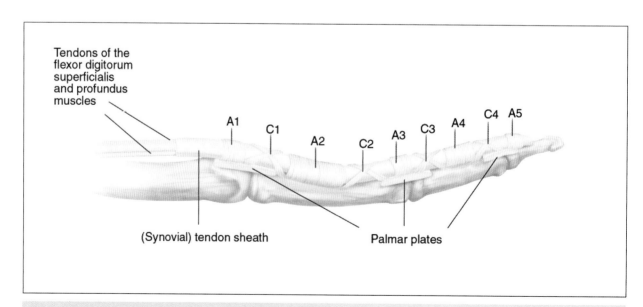

Figure 1 Illustration of the oblique palmar view of a finger shows the tendons lying in their sheath.

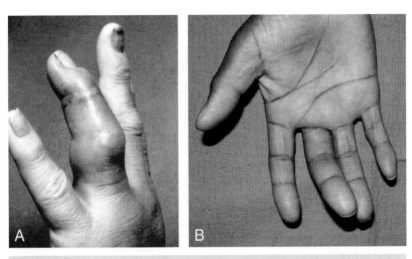

Figure 2 Clinical photographs of septic tenosynovitis of the ring finger (**A**) and the long finger (**B**). Note the flexed position of the affected finger at rest. (Panel A reproduced from Stern PJ: Selected acute infections. *Instr Course Lect* 1990;39:539-546.)

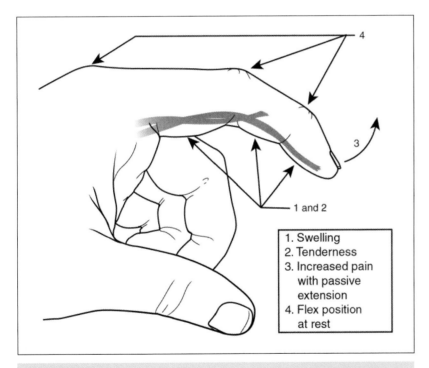

1. Swelling
2. Tenderness
3. Increased pain with passive extension
4. Flex position at rest

Figure 3 Illustration of the Kanavel signs, which are indicative of well-established septic tenosynovitis.

sheath, (3) a marked increase in pain on passive extension, and (4) a flexed position of the finger at rest (**Figure 3**).

Diagnostic Tests

Radiographs may show soft-tissue swelling or, rarely, a foreign body or subcutaneous air.

Differential Diagnosis

- Aseptic flexor synovitis (negative bacterial cultures as might be seen in rheumatoid arthritis)
- Cellulitis (little or no pain with active motion of the finger)

Adverse Outcomes of the Disease

These infections can progress rapidly; therefore, complications such as skin loss or loss of the entire finger are possible. Further, these infections can progress to the deep spaces of the hand and ultimately gain access to the forearm. Late problems include significant stiffness from adhesions and involvement of the bone and joint.

Treatment

If septic tenosynovitis is suspected but the swelling is not severe, parenteral antibiotics should be initiated, and the patient should be reevaluated in 12 to 24 hours. Both *Staphylococcus* and *Streptococcus* should be covered. If the patient responds to parenteral antibiotics, these should be continued for 24 to 72 hours and then switched to oral antibiotics for an additional 7 to 14 days. If the patient has an established purulent flexor tenosynovitis or if the infection progresses or does not respond to antibiotic treatment, urgent referral for surgical drainage is indicated.

Adverse Outcomes of Treatment

Finger stiffness can persist, despite successful treatment of septic tenosynovitis.

Referral Decisions/Red Flags

Patients with well-established septic tenosynovitis and those who do not respond to antibiotic treatment require evaluation for possible surgery.

Fracture of the Base of the Thumb Metacarpal

Synonyms
Bennett fracture
Rolando fracture

Definition
A Bennett fracture is an oblique fracture of the base of the thumb metacarpal that enters the carpometacarpal (CMC) joint. This fracture has two pieces, one large and one small. The small volar fragment remains attached to the volar oblique ligament of the carpus, and the major metacarpal fragment displaces at the CMC joint (**Figure 1**). A Rolando fracture, which is less common than a Bennett fracture, is a Y-shaped intra-articular fracture at the base of the thumb metacarpal. A comminuted intra-articular fracture at the base of the thumb metacarpal also occurs.

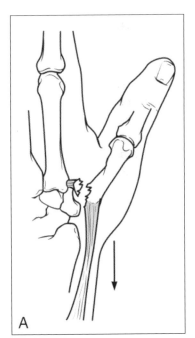
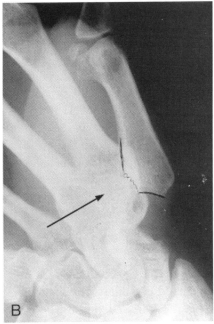

Figure 1 Fracture-subluxation of the base of the thumb metacarpal (Bennett fracture). **A,** Illustration shows the mechanism of injury. The medial fragment of the thumb metacarpal is stabilized by the intact volar oblique ligament. The arrow indicates the proximal pull of the abductor pollicis longus tendon. **B,** Radiograph demonstrates a Bennett fracture (arrow).

Clinical Symptoms

Patients report pain and limited motion. Swelling and ecchymosis about the base of the thumb are common and are indicative of a metacarpal fracture or CMC dislocation.

Tests

Physical Examination

The thumb is painful to palpation at the base of the metacarpal. Examination also shows that, when the tip of the thumb is held into the palm, the base of the thumb metacarpal is displaced radially and posteriorly. The patient cannot move the thumb without pain.

Diagnostic Tests

AP, lateral, and oblique radiographs of the thumb will demonstrate these fractures.

Differential Diagnosis

- Arthritis of the CMC joint (narrow joint space evident on radiographs)
- Dislocation of the CMC joint (evident on radiographs)
- Fracture of the scaphoid (evident on radiographs)
- Synovitis of the CMC joint (swollen joint, normal radiographs)

Adverse Outcomes of the Disease

Posttraumatic arthritis of the CMC joint is possible, resulting in pain at the base of the thumb, along with loss of motion and pinch strength.

Treatment

The goal of treatment is to restore the axial length of the thumb and to replace the metacarpal shaft fragment against the smaller volar lip fragment. Although anatomic reduction of the fracture is the goal, even with some offset a good functional outcome is possible. A Bennett fracture almost always requires some form of surgical fixation to achieve stability in the joint. Nondisplaced two-part fractures of the base of the thumb metacarpal can be treated in a thumb spica cast for 4 weeks.

Adverse Outcomes of Treatment

After surgery, pin tract irritation and infection can occur, as can tenderness around the surgical plates and screws. Displacement of the fracture (loss of position) and posttraumatic arthritis also are possible.

Referral Decisions/Red Flags

Intra-articular base of the thumb metacarpal fractures often require surgical treatment. These patients should be considered for early referral.

Fracture of the Hook of the Hamate

Synonyms

Fracture of the hamate
Fracture of the hamular process

Definition

A fracture of the hook of the hamate involves the palmarmost aspect of the hamate bone of the wrist (**Figure 1**). Fractures of the hook of the hamate most commonly occur in players of racquet sports, golf, and baseball.

Clinical Symptoms

Patients most commonly present with a history of either repetitive trauma or direct trauma, as from grounding a golf club inadvertently or hitting a baseball, with resultant pain in the base of the ulnar side of the hand.

Tests

Physical Examination

Pressure over the hook of the hamate will elicit pain, and swelling may be observed. Resisted flexion of the little finger with the wrist in ulnar deviation often increases the pain. Numbness along the ulnar nerve distribution (little finger and ulnar half of the ring finger) may

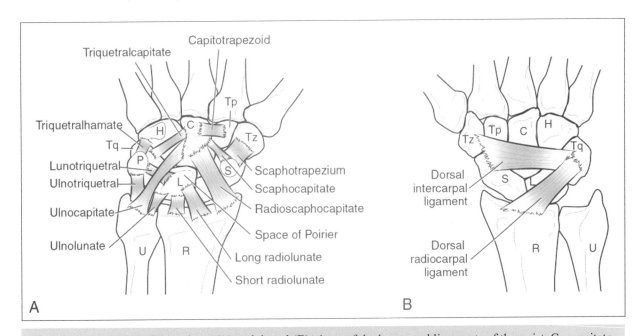

Figure 1 Illustration of the palmar (**A**) and dorsal (**B**) views of the bones and ligaments of the wrist. C = capitate, H = hamate, L = lunate, P = pisiform, R = radius, S = scaphoid, Tp = trapezoid, Tq = triquetrum, Tz = trapezium, U = ulna.

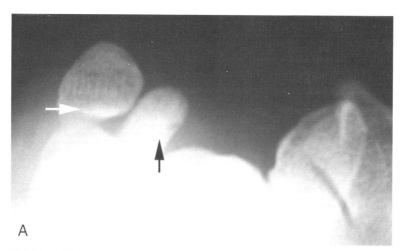
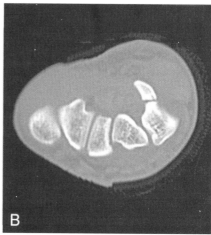

Figure 2 **A,** Fracture of the hook of the hamate (black arrow) seen on the carpal tunnel radiographic view. Note the relationship of the pisiform (white arrow) to the hamate. **B,** CT scan demonstrates the fracture. (Panel A reproduced from Johnson TR, Steinbach LS, eds: *Essentials of Musculoskeletal Imaging.* Rosemont, IL, American Academy of Orthopaedic Surgeons, 2003, p 344.)

be present. The hook is located 1 to 2 cm distal to and 1 to 2 cm radial to the pisiform and is readily palpable in the palm.

Diagnostic Tests
Plain radiographs are often interpreted as normal. A semisupinated oblique view or a carpal tunnel view may show the hook fracture (**Figure 2, A**). Often a CT scan is necessary to demonstrate the fracture (**Figure 2, B**).

Differential Diagnosis
- Flexor carpi ulnaris tendinitis (tenderness with wrist flexion)
- Little finger carpometacarpal joint fracture (tenderness more distal and dorsally, increases with wrist flexion)
- Pisiform fracture (tender more proximally, over the pisiform)
- Pisotriquetral arthritis (painful pisotriquetral compression)
- Ulnar artery thrombosis (abnormal Allen test)

Adverse Outcomes of the Disease
If left untreated and, often, if treated, hook of the hamate fractures progress to nonunion. The nonunion is usually painful and may require additional treatment. If the nonunion is long-standing, tendon rupture to the little finger may occur as the tendon abrades over the roughened edge of the nonunion, resulting in an attritional rupture.

Treatment
If hook of the hamate fracture is identified early, the wrist should be immobilized in a neutral position with a splint or cast. Usually in the course of the process, excision of the hook of the hamate is offered to control symptoms of wrist discomfort and reduce the risk of tendon rupture.

Adverse Outcomes of Treatment

Excision of the hook of the hamate can be associated with some loss of little finger flexion and power grip, but more typically patients note little or no adverse sequelae.

Referral Decisions/Red Flags

Hook of the hamate fractures should be referred for early evaluation and treatment.

Fracture of the Distal Radius

Synonyms

Barton fracture
Chauffeur's fracture
Colles fracture
Die-punch fracture
Smith fracture

Definition

Fractures involving the distal radius are among the most frequently occurring fractures in adults (**Figure 1**). The most common type is the Colles fracture (**Figure 2**), in which the distal radius fracture fragment is tilted upward, or dorsally. The articular surface of the radius may or may not be involved, and the ulnar styloid is usually fractured. A Smith fracture is the opposite of a Colles fracture: the distal fragment is tilted downward, or volarly. A Barton fracture (**Figure 3**) is an intra-articular fracture associated with subluxation of the carpus, either dorsally or volarly, along with the displaced articular fragment of the radius. A chauffeur's fracture is an oblique fracture through the base of the radial styloid. A die-punch fracture is a depressed fracture of the articular surface opposite the lunate or scaphoid bone. The most important concepts for classifying distal radius fractures are whether they are open or closed and whether they are displaced or nondisplaced.

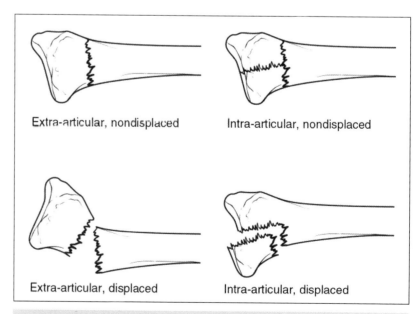

Extra-articular, nondisplaced

Intra-articular, nondisplaced

Extra-articular, displaced

Intra-articular, displaced

Figure 1 Types of fractures of the distal radius. The illustration depicts a lateral view of the radius.

Clinical Symptoms

The usual history is a fall on an outstretched hand. Patients have acute pain, tenderness, swelling, and deformity of the wrist.

Tests

Physical Examination

Look for swelling, deformity, and discoloration around the wrist and distal radius. Observe for skin injury and bleeding (usually with fat droplets in the blood) that would suggest an open fracture. Test for sensation in the hand over the median, radial, and ulnar nerve distribution. Also check the circulation to the fingertips. Examine the elbow for swelling and tenderness.

Diagnostic Tests

AP and lateral radiographs of the distal forearm, including the wrist, are necessary. Radiographs of the elbow should be obtained when elbow swelling and tenderness are present because some patients will have combined injuries to the distal end of the radius, the forearm, and the elbow.

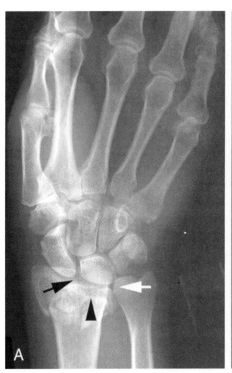
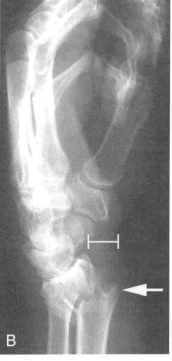

Figure 2 Radiographs of the Colles fracture. **A,** PA radiograph demonstrates loss of ulnar inclination (black arrow), shortening of the radius (white arrow), and the intra-articular extent of the fracture (arrowhead). **B,** Lateral radiograph demonstrates dorsal translation of the radius (lines) and dorsal angulation of approximately 30° (arrow). (Reproduced from Johnson TR, Steinbach LS, eds: *Essentials of Musculoskeletal Imaging.* Rosemont, IL, American Academy of Orthopaedic Surgeons, 2003, pp 339-340.)

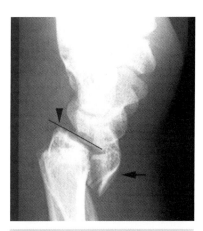

Figure 3 Lateral radiograph of a reverse (volar) Barton fracture. Note the volarly displaced distal radius fragment (black arrow), the increased volar angulation (line), and the volar subluxation of the carpus (arrowhead). (Reproduced from Johnson TR, Steinbach LS, eds: *Essentials of Musculoskeletal Imaging.* Rosemont, IL, American Academy of Orthopaedic Surgeons, 2003, p 340.)

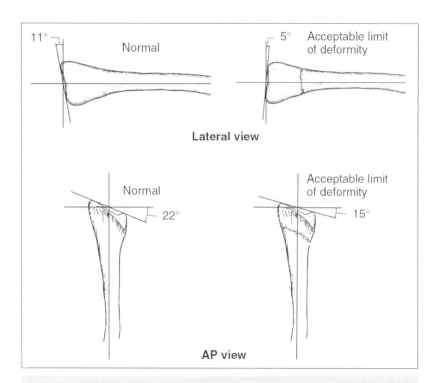

Figure 4 Illustration of the general guidelines for radiographic alignment of distal radius fractures following reduction.

Differential Diagnosis

• Carpal fracture-dislocation (evident on radiographs)
• Fracture of the scaphoid (tenderness over the anatomic snuffbox, possibly evident on radiographs)
• Tenosynovitis of the wrist (normal radiographs)

Adverse Outcomes of the Disease

Malunion, loss of wrist motion, loss of finger motion, complex regional pain syndrome, decreased grip strength, posttraumatic arthritis, or (uncommonly) compartment syndrome can occur when a fracture of the distal radius is not treated.

Treatment

Open fractures require irrigation and débridement and antibiotics. Initial treatment usually focuses on reduction and splinting of the fracture. For most fractures, a sugar tong splint is appropriate. Anatomic reduction is ideal, but less-than-perfect bone alignment can be associated with a good functional outcome. Older, less active persons are more tolerant of residual deformity than are younger individuals. There is considerable controversy in the orthopaedic literature as to what constitutes an acceptable reduction.

General guidelines for acceptable radiographic alignment after reduction of distal radius fractures are as follows (**Figure 4**): (1) On the lateral view, no more than 5° of dorsal angulation is acceptable. (2) On the AP view, no less than 15° of radial inclination is acceptable. (3) A step-off in the articular surface greater than 2 mm should be reduced. If these parameters are not met, early referral to an orthopaedic surgeon should be considered.

AP and lateral radiographs of the fracture should be repeated each week for several weeks after the fracture to determine if the alignment is satisfactory.

For nondisplaced and minimally displaced extra-articular fractures, a sugar tong splint should be applied for 2 to 3 weeks and a short arm cast for an additional 2 to 3 weeks. It is important to obtain interval radiographs every 7 to 10 days for the first approximately 3 weeks to ensure that displacement does not occur. The patient should be encouraged to move the shoulder and elbow of the injured arm through a full range of motion twice a day to prevent shoulder stiffness. Likewise, active and passive finger motion (five sets, four times per day) should be encouraged.

Displaced fractures often are unstable and require additional internal and/or external fixation techniques.

The presence of a distal radius fracture may be an indicator of osteopenia, osteoporosis, or vitamin D deficiency; patients should be asked about prior fractures and known or suspected diagnosis of osteopenia, osteoporosis, or vitamin D deficiency. In older patients or those at risk, a dual-energy x-ray absorptiometry (DEXA) scan can be considered. In addition, vitamin D supplementation may be considered at 1,000 to 2,000 IU daily. Obtaining serum vitamin D levels may be considered in the evaluation and workup if the patient is deemed to be at high risk, such as those with comorbidities such as celiac disease, diabetes mellitus, and eating disorders, as well as in the patient with a special diet. In 2009, the American Academy of Orthopaedic Surgeons recommended the use of vitamin C (500 mg daily) to reduce the risk of complex regional pain syndrome in the setting of distal radius fractures.

Adverse Outcomes of Treatment

Recurrence of deformity, malunion, loss of wrist motion (flexion, extension, pronation, and supination), posttraumatic wrist arthritis, carpal tunnel syndrome, loss of finger motion, compartment syndrome, or paresthesias of the radial sensory nerve all can result following treatment.

Referral Decisions/Red Flags

Displaced fractures that exceed the aforementioned parameters and intra-articular fractures require further evaluation. Fractures that initially are nondisplaced but that show progressive collapse on radiographic follow-up require further evaluation. Clinical examination that demonstrates any neurologic dysfunction necessitates urgent referral.

Fracture of the Metacarpals and Phalanges

Synonyms
Boxer's fracture
Fighter's fracture

Definition
Metacarpal fractures are among the most common fractures in adults (**Figure 1**). The most common fracture in the hand is a boxer's fracture, an injury of the distal metaphysis of the fifth metacarpal that results when the closed fist strikes an object (**Figure 2**). In phalangeal fractures in adults, the distal phalanx is the most commonly injured (**Figure 3**), followed by the proximal and then the middle phalanx. Approximately 20% of these fractures are intra-articular.

Phalangeal fractures are more common than metacarpal fractures in children. The most common fracture involves the physis of the little finger. Growth disturbances from physeal injuries of the phalanges are rare.

Clinical Symptoms
Patients typically have a history of trauma. Local tenderness, swelling, deformity, or decreased range of motion are common findings.

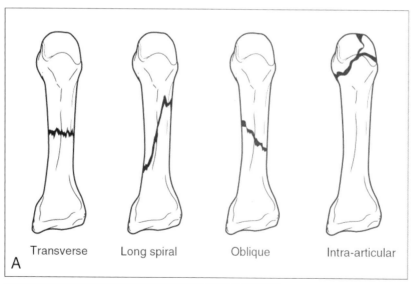
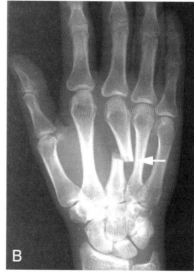

Transverse   Long spiral   Oblique   Intra-articular

A   B

Figure 1 A, Illustration of types of metacarpal fractures. **B,** PA radiograph of a right hand demonstrates a displaced transverse fracture of the middle metacarpal (arrow). (Panel B reproduced from Johnson TR, Steinbach LS, eds: *Essentials of Musculoskeletal Imaging.* Rosemont, IL, American Academy of Orthopaedic Surgeons, 2003, p 347.)

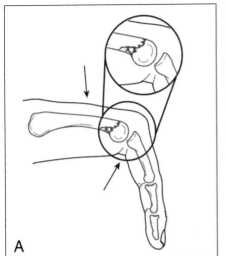
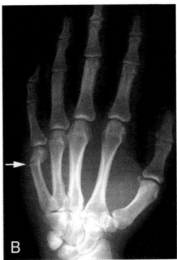

Figure 2 Boxer's fracture. **A,** Illustration depicts the direction of force that causes the fracture. **B,** PA radiograph of a left hand demonstrates an angulated fracture of the neck of the fifth metacarpal (arrow). The degree of angulation shown here is well tolerated without loss of function. (Panel B reproduced from Johnson TR, Steinbach LS, eds: *Essentials of Musculoskeletal Imaging.* Rosemont, IL, American Academy of Orthopaedic Surgeons, 2003, p 347.)

Tests

Physical Examination
Examination reveals swelling over the fracture site. The involved finger may appear shortened, or the knuckle may be depressed. The distal fragment may be rotated in relation to the proximal fragment. This is not easy to see with the fingers extended; however, when the patient makes a partial fist, the rotated fragments cause the involved finger to overlap onto the neighboring finger (**Figure 4**). In general, assess the bones of the involved finger for angulation, rotation, and the potential for digital crossover in flexion. Assess sensory function of the digital nerves.

Diagnostic Tests
Radiographs are always indicated for suspected fractures. For fractures of the phalanges, PA and true lateral views of the individual digits should be obtained. For metacarpal fractures, PA, lateral, and oblique views of the hand are indicated.

Differential Diagnosis
- Metacarpophalangeal (MCP) and interphalangeal (IP) joint dislocations (evident on clinical examination)
- MCP and IP joint sprains (instability and joint tenderness)

Adverse Outcomes of the Disease
Malunion, nonunion, posttraumatic arthritis, and loss of finger motion are all possible.

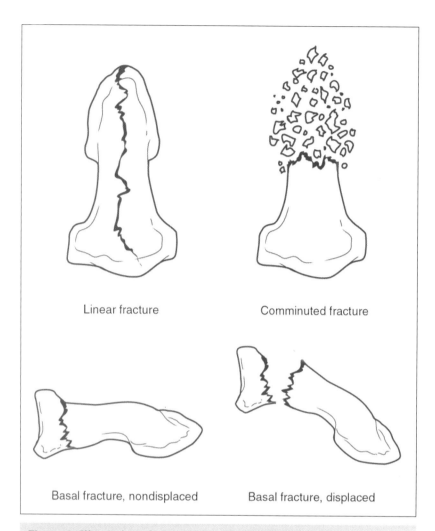

Linear fracture

Comminuted fracture

Basal fracture, nondisplaced

Basal fracture, displaced

Figure 3 Illustration of types of distal phalanx fractures.

Treatment

Metacarpal Neck Fracture

For a boxer's fracture with 10° to 15° of angulation, apply an ulnar gutter splint for 2 to 3 weeks with the PIP and DIP joints free. This treatment also is appropriate with more than 15° of angulation but no extensor lag (the patient can fully extend the finger). Advise the patient that although this fracture will not result in any functional deficit, there could be a loss of prominence of the metacarpal head dorsally and prominence of the metacarpal head volarly. If this is unsatisfactory to the patient, further evaluation is indicated.

With an extensor lag, or with more than 40° of angulation, referral for reduction is appropriate. Similar guidelines are appropriate for fractures of the metacarpal neck of the ring finger, although slightly less angulation is accepted because of prominence of the metacarpal head. The second and third metacarpals have less mobility, and therefore less angulation is acceptable in these injuries. Use of a radial gutter splint is appropriate with less than 10° of angulation, but with greater angulation, functional loss could result, and referral for reduction is appropriate.

Nondisplaced Fractures of the Metacarpal and Phalangeal Shafts

Casting or splint immobilization for 3 weeks is indicated for phalangeal fractures and for 4 weeks for metacarpal fractures. When casting or splinting, consider including the joint above and below the fracture and the adjacent digits. To avoid fixed contracture formation, the safe position of immobilization is with the MCP joints held in approximately 70° of flexion and the proximal interphalangeal (PIP) and distal interphalangeal (DIP) joints held in extension (0° to 10° of flexion). When loss of position is a possible problem, radiographs should be repeated 1 week after the injury.

Immobilization of phalangeal fractures for more than 3 to 4 weeks will result in stiffness. Do not wait for radiographic evidence of healing to begin exercises because full healing may not be apparent on plain radiographs for 2 to 5 months. If the fracture seems clinically stable and pain is minimal after cast removal, motion should be started.

Displaced Fractures of the Metacarpal and Phalangeal Shafts

Because of pull by the flexor tendons, displaced transverse fractures of the metacarpals and phalanges tend to angulate (**Figure 5**), spiral fractures tend to rotate, and oblique fractures tend to shorten. Patients with these types of fracture need further evaluation on initial presentation.

Intra-articular Fractures

Splint nondisplaced intra-articular fractures with the MCP joints in flexion and the PIP and DIP joints in extension. Repeat radiographs in 1 week to assess for continued articular congruity, and then initiate active range of motion at 3 weeks. Displacement of intra-articular fractures greater than 1 mm is unacceptable because of loss of joint congruity; therefore, patients with displaced intra-articular fractures require further evaluation.

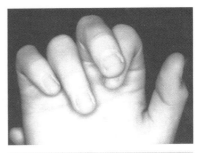

Figure 4 Malrotation of a finger associated with a phalangeal fracture is more apparent with the fingers in flexion, as seen in this clinical photograph. In normal alignment, the nail plates of the fingers would be parallel, with no crossover of the fingers. Note the malrotation of the index finger. (Reproduced with permission from Breen TF: Sport-related injuries of the hand, in Pappas AM, Walzer J, eds: *Upper Extremity Injuries in the Athlete*. New York, NY, Churchill Livingstone, 1995, pp 451-496.)

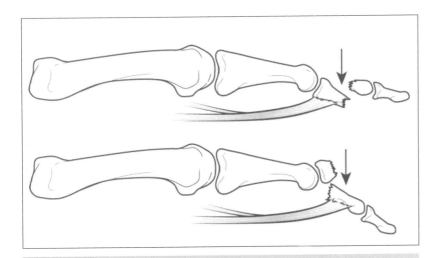

Figure 5 Illustration depicts angulation of phalangeal fractures caused by pulling of the flexor tendons.

Adverse Outcomes of Treatment

Joint stiffness is the most common problem with hand fractures and is directly related to prolonged immobilization. Malunion caused by inadequate reduction also is possible.

Referral Decisions/Red Flags

Displaced fractures and intra-articular fractures often require surgical treatment. Patients with these types of fracture should be considered for early referral.

Fracture of the Scaphoid

Definition

The scaphoid spans the distal and proximal rows of the carpus; in that position it is vulnerable to falls on the outstretched hand. The scaphoid is the most commonly fractured carpal bone, and young men are most commonly affected. These fractures are not common in children and older adults because the distal radius is the weak link in patients in these age groups; thus, these patients are more likely to sustain a fracture of the distal radius than fracture of the scaphoid. Of all scaphoid fractures, approximately 20% occur in the proximal pole, 60% in the middle or waist, and 20% in the distal pole (**Figure 1**).

Fractures of the scaphoid are important because of their frequency and because their diagnosis is often delayed or missed. Patients may think they have a simple sprain and fail to seek medical attention. At the time of initial injury, routine radiographs may not demonstrate the fracture, and, as a result, the fracture is inadequately treated.

Scaphoid fractures also have a significant incidence of nonunion and osteonecrosis. The blood supply to this bone is limited because articular cartilage covers 80% of the scaphoid, and the major blood supply, which enters the bone in the distal third at the dorsal ridge, might be disrupted by the injury. Because of these anatomic features, fractures of the scaphoid that are displaced more than 1 mm have a relatively high rate of nonunion.

Clinical Symptoms

Patients usually present with a history of a dorsiflexion wrist injury. Pain about the radial (thumb) side of the wrist in the anatomic snuffbox, defined by the abductor and long thumb extensor tendons just distal to the radial styloid (**Figure 2**), is characteristic. Patients have pain on palpation of the snuffbox, and any type of wrist motion, such as gripping, is painful. Swelling about the back and radial side of the wrist also is common. If the patient reports a history of a high-energy injury, such as a car accident, ligamentous injuries

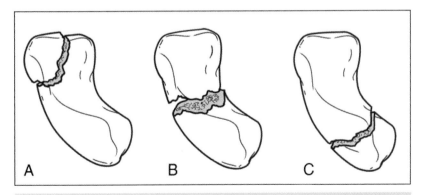

Figure 1 Illustration of types of scaphoid fracture. **A,** Distal tubercle fracture. **B,** Waist fracture. **C,** Proximal pole fracture.

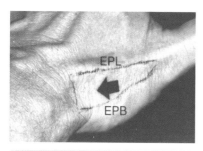

Figure 2 The triangular area outlined on the hand shown in this clinical photograph is the anatomic snuffbox.
EPB = extensor pollicis brevis, EPL = extensor pollicis longus.

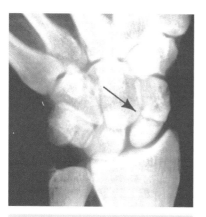

Figure 3 PA radiograph with the wrist in ulnar deviation demonstrates a scaphoid fracture (arrow).

and resultant carpal instability (perilunar instability) are possible in addition to the scaphoid fracture.

Tests

Physical Examination

Palpation over the anatomic snuffbox reveals marked tenderness. Likewise, pressure over the scaphoid tubercle on the underside of the wrist will produce pain. In addition, the patient may have decreased motion and grip strength. An intra-articular effusion is not uncommon for patients who present with an acute scaphoid fracture. Assess function of the median, ulnar, and radial nerves, as well as circulatory status.

Diagnostic Tests

Scaphoid fractures may not be visible on PA and lateral radiographs of the wrist obtained at the time of initial injury. Therefore, if these radiographs appear normal, obtain a PA view with the wrist in ulnar deviation and an oblique view to help visualize the fracture (**Figure 3**). If this series of initial radiographs is normal but the pain persists for 2 to 3 weeks, the PA and oblique views should be repeated. If the radiographs are still normal, an MRI should be ordered.

Differential Diagnosis

- de Quervain tenosynovitis (positive Finkelstein test)
- Fracture of the distal radius (evident on plain radiographs)
- Scapholunate dissociation (increased gap between scaphoid and lunate [**Figure 4**])
- Wrist arthritis (narrowing of joint space, evident on radiographs)

Adverse Outcomes of the Disease

Nonunion, decreased grip strength and range of motion, and osteoarthritis of the radiocarpal joint are possible.

Treatment

Patients with marked snuffbox tenderness (even with normal radiographs) should be treated initially as though they have a scaphoid fracture and placed in a forearm-based thumb spica splint or cast with the thumb interphalangeal joint free. Close follow-up with additional radiographs or MRIs will identify occult scaphoid fractures. Because the interval to treatment can be important in minimizing the risk of nonunion, patients should be immobilized in a forearm-based thumb spica splint or cast with the thumb interphalangeal joint free at the time of initial presentation until a definitive diagnosis can be reached. Typically, either an MRI or repeat radiographs may then be obtained and clinical examination done in 7 to 14 days. After the diagnosis of an acute nondisplaced fracture of the scaphoid has been confirmed, treatment is controversial because agreement is lacking on the optimal type of immobilization for these fractures. Data are conflicting regarding the optimal position of the wrist, whether the elbow should be immobilized, and whether the thumb should be included in the cast. However, most practitioners agree that a short arm-thumb spica cast with the interphalangeal joint free provides adequate immobilization; this cast is left in place for 6 weeks. If radiographs obtained after this time show that the fracture is healing, immobilization is continued until clinical and radiographic evidence of union is noted. If the fracture line appears to be getting wider, however, indicating resorption at the fracture site, or if the fracture shows any displacement, then further evaluation for possible surgery is indicated.

If the patient has pain over the region of the snuffbox but the initial radiographs are normal, place the hand and wrist in a thumb spica splint for 1 to 2 weeks and then obtain repeat radiographs. If the radiographs are still normal but tenderness over the scaphoid persists, order an MRI. If the image is positive, treat the hand as for an acute nondisplaced scaphoid fracture.

It may be difficult to determine on routine radiographs whether a scaphoid fracture has healed, and immobilization may be discontinued too soon. As a general rule, the closer the fracture line is to the proximal pole, the longer the time for healing. For fractures of the distal pole, the average time to healing is 6 to 8 weeks. Fractures of the middle third require 8 to 12 weeks to heal, and fractures of the proximal pole can take 12 to 24 weeks or longer. If plain radiographs do not clearly reveal that the fracture has healed, a thin-cut CT scan in the plane of the scaphoid can be obtained to better visualize the fracture site.

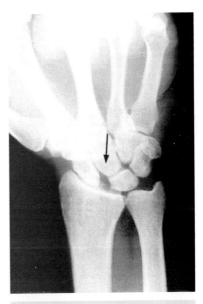

Figure 4 Clenched-fist radiograph shows scapholunate dissociation (arrow) with increased gap between the scaphoid and the lunate.

Adverse Outcomes of Treatment
Loss of motion from prolonged immobilization and/or loss of grip strength can result.

Referral Decisions/Red Flags
All patients with nondisplaced fractures of the proximal pole and those with displaced fractures of the scaphoid require early further evaluation for possible surgical treatment. All patients with scaphoid fractures in association with other wrist ligament injuries (perilunar instability) require urgent referral to a hand surgeon. Patients who show cystic absorption at the fracture site or displacement of the fracture after immobilization, or those with nondisplaced fractures that have not healed after 2 months of immobilization, require further evaluation for possible surgical treatment.

Ganglion of the Wrist and Hand

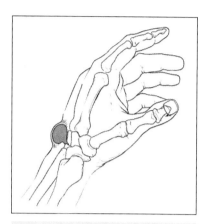

Figure 1 Illustration of a wrist ganglion.

Synonyms

Flexor tendon sheath ganglion
Mucous cyst
Synovial cyst
Volar retinacular ganglion

Definition

A ganglion is a cystic structure that arises from the capsule of a joint or a tendon synovial sheath (**Figure 1**). The cyst contains a thick, clear, mucinous fluid identical in composition to joint fluid. Through degeneration or tearing of the joint capsule or tendon sheath, a connection to the joint or tendon sheath with a one-way valve is established. Thus, synovial fluid can enter the cyst but cannot flow freely back into the synovial cavity. Ganglions vary in size, and significant symptoms may result from increased pressure on surrounding structures.

Ganglions are the most common soft-tissue tumors of the hand, generally affecting persons between the ages of 15 and 40 years. These benign tumors typically develop, and sometimes disappear, spontaneously. Common locations include the dorsum of the wrist, the volar radial aspect of the wrist, and the base of a finger. Ganglia at the base of a finger typically arise from the proximal annular ligament (A1 pulley) of the flexor tendon sheath. These also are known as volar retinacular ganglia.

Mucous cysts are a type of ganglion that develops from an arthritic interphalangeal joint, most commonly in women between the ages of 40 and 70 years. These cysts may compress the underlying germinal matrix of the nail, resulting in pitting or indentations on the nail plate.

Clinical Symptoms

Wrist

Patients typically present with a lump, which may or may not be painful (**Figure 2**). The pain, if present, is typically described as aching and is aggravated by activities that require frequent movement of the wrist. Ganglia in the wrist often vary in size, with an increase in size associated with times of increased activity. A history of variation in size is a key factor to distinguish a ganglion from other soft-tissue tumors. Occasionally, a ganglion will occur in an area of the wrist where it may result in compression of the median or ulnar nerve. In this situation, sensory symptoms in the fingers and/or weakness of the intrinsic muscle may develop.

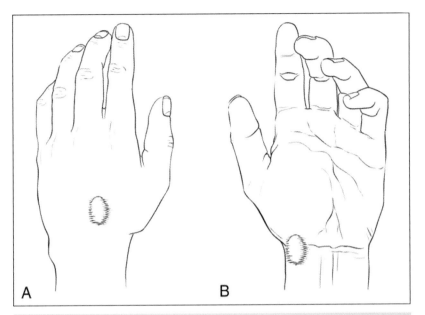

Figure 2 Illustration of the clinical appearance of dorsal (**A**) and volar (**B**) wrist ganglia. (Adapted with permission from the American Society for Surgery of the Hand: *Ganglion Cysts.* Englewood, CO, 1995.)

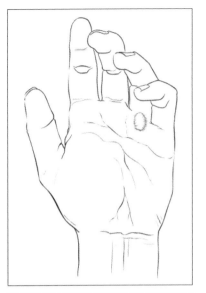

Figure 3 Illustration of the flexor tendon sheath ganglion. (Adapted with permission from the American Society for Surgery of the Hand: *Ganglion Cysts.* Englewood, CO, 1995.)

Hand and Finger

Patients with flexor tendon sheath cysts report tenderness when grasping and have a bump at the base of the finger (usually at the level of the proximal flexion crease) (**Figure 3**).

A tender mass in this area usually is a flexor tendon sheath ganglion. Patients with mucous cysts have swelling on the dorsum of the finger distal to the distal interphalangeal (DIP) joint (**Figure 4**). They also may report a cycle of the cyst breaking open, draining a clear, jellylike fluid, and healing. Treatment often is sought when the cyst becomes painful, ulcerated, or infected or is cosmetically displeasing. Patients also may have furrowing of the fingernail because of pressure of the cyst on the nail matrix.

Tests

Physical Examination: Wrist

A dorsal ganglion is typically a smooth, round or multilobulated structure on the dorsoradial aspect of the wrist that becomes more prominent with flexion. It usually is positioned directly over the scapholunate joint but can occur more distally, even though its stalk usually emanates from the scapholunate joint.

A volar radial ganglion usually is a less well-defined mass situated between the flexor carpi radialis tendon and the radial styloid. It may extend underneath the radial artery and, in some cases, may adhere to the radial artery. On palpation, the ganglion may appear to pulsate and can be confused with an aneurysm. Symptoms also become more pronounced with extreme flexion or extension.

A ganglion is mildly tender with pressure. A prominent ganglion

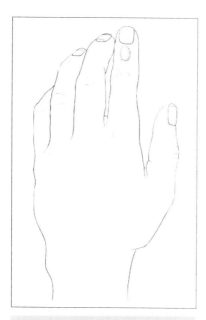

Figure 4 Illustration of a mucous cyst on the dorsum of the finger distal to the distal interphalangeal joint. (Adapted with permission from the American Society for Surgery of the Hand: *Ganglion Cysts.* Englewood, CO, 1995.)

often will transilluminate when a penlight is shined through it from the side. Solid tumors will not transilluminate.

If a definite mass is not visible, the possibility of an occult ganglion, which is characterized by more subtle swelling, should be considered. Palpation must be especially thorough and careful to identify a small tender mass that is different from what is felt on the opposite wrist. MRI may be necessary to determine if an occult ganglion is present.

Physical Examination: Hand and Finger

A volar retinacular ganglion of the flexor tendon sheath is characterized by a small, firm, tender mass at the base of the finger in the area of the metacarpophalangeal flexion crease, most often at the long or ring fingers (**Figure 3**). These ganglions are sometimes difficult to detect because of their small size. They rarely affect motion and do not move with excursion of the tendon.

Mucous cysts usually lie to one side of the extensor tendon at the DIP joint (**Figure 4**). Initial clinical findings include a mass or a blister. Periarticular arthritic nodules may contain mucous cysts.

Diagnostic Tests

PA, lateral, and oblique radiographs of the hand or PA and lateral radiographs of the wrist or the involved finger should be obtained to rule out bony pathology. In most cases, ganglia are not associated with radiographic changes. With a mucous cyst, degenerative changes and a small bony spur usually are seen rising from the dorsum of the distal phalanx at the DIP joint.

Differential Diagnosis
Wrist

- Arthritis (evident on radiographs)
- Bone tumor (evident on radiographs)
- Intraosseous ganglion (evident on radiographs)
- Kienböck disease (collapse of the lunate)
- Soft-tissue tumor, benign or malignant (solid mass on palpation, rare; ganglia transilluminate, but solid masses do not)

Hand and Finger

- Dupuytren disease (presence of cords or bands)
- Epidermal inclusion cyst (history of laceration and repair)
- Giant cell tumors (different locations, but usually about the phalanges)
- Lipoma (larger in size, often in the palm)
- Soft-tissue tumor, benign or malignant (solid mass on palpation, rare)

Adverse Outcomes of the Disease
Wrist

Patients may experience a decrease in grip strength and painful wrist motion; they also may complain about the unsightly bump. On rare occasions, a ganglion will cause substantial compression on the median nerve.

Hand and Finger
Patients often have pain in the hand and finger and an obvious deformity at the fingernail. Infection also can occur in association with a mucous cyst.

Treatment
Wrist
When the patient has significant symptoms, immobilizing the wrist will relieve symptoms and may cause the ganglion to decrease in size. However, immobilization is rarely a permanent solution. Occasionally, aspiration of a dorsal wrist ganglion will lead to resolution. Because of the proximity of the radial artery, volar wrist ganglions should be aspirated with great care.

When the patient has significant symptoms or is seriously bothered by the appearance of the wrist ganglion, then surgical excision is indicated.

Hand and Finger
Treatment of a ganglion of the tendon sheath consists of needle rupture followed by massage to disperse the contents of the cyst or injection with 1% or 2% local anesthetic until the cyst pops. Exercise caution when performing a needle rupture because of the proximity of the neurovascular bundle. Surgical management is occasionally required for painful flexor sheath ganglia.

Aspiration and/or rupture of a mucous cyst is not recommended because of the danger of introducing an infection into the DIP joint. If infection occurs, the patient should be started on a first-generation cephalosporin (unless allergic), tetanus immunization status should be updated if necessary, and a specialist should be consulted.

Adverse Outcomes of Treatment
Wrist
Recurrence of wrist ganglia occurs in 10% to 15% of patients after surgical excision and in 85% to 90% after needle aspiration. Injury to the radial artery can occur as a result of aspiration of a volar wrist ganglion.

Hand and Finger
Recurrence of hand and finger ganglia is common. Skin loss is possible, as is injury to the digital nerve.

Referral Decisions/Red Flags
Wrist
Any mass with atypical findings should be evaluated with additional diagnostic tests or either incisional or excisional biopsy. Recurrence after aspiration also is an indication for further evaluation.

Hand and Finger

Persistence of a painful or bothersome cyst after one or two attempts at needle rupture or aspiration indicates that surgical excision should be considered. Increased erythema and pain in a mucous cyst suggests infection that may require surgical treatment.

www.aaos.org/essentials5/handandwrist

Procedure: Dorsal Wrist Ganglion Aspiration

Materials

- Gloves
- Bactericidal skin preparation solution
- 5- or 10-mL syringe
- Large-bore needle, such as an 18-gauge needle
- Sterile bandage

Step 1
Wear protective gloves at all times during this procedure and use sterile technique.

Step 2
Cleanse the area with a bactericidal skin preparation solution.

Step 3
Optional: Spray the skin with ethyl chloride to decrease pain.

Step 4
Penetrate the ganglion with the large-bore needle and attempt to withdraw as much fluid as possible (**Figure 1**). With your free hand, compress the ganglion and displace the thick fluid toward the needle. As you compress the mass, you may need to move the needle to the right or left slightly to break small cavities within the ganglion. Injecting corticosteroid has not been shown to influence the recurrence rate and is not recommended.

Step 5
Apply a sterile dressing.

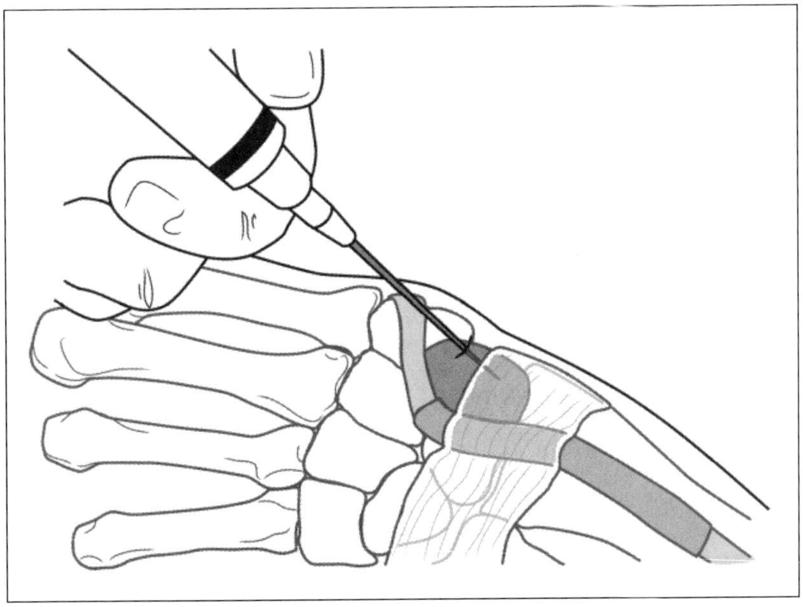

Figure 1 Illustration depicts the location for needle insertion for dorsal wrist ganglion aspiration.

Adverse Outcomes

Infection and recurrence of the ganglion are possible. Injury to the radial artery also can occur following attempts to aspirate volar wrist ganglia.

Aftercare/Patient Instructions

The patient may remove the dressing within a few hours.

Human Bite Wounds

Synonyms

Clenched-fist injury
Fight bite

Definition

Human bite wounds to the hand occur either directly, from a bite (usually to the fingers), or indirectly, when the hand strikes a tooth (clenched-fist injury). Few infections of the hand can progress more quickly or result in more significant complications. Both early recognition and appropriate treatment are important.

Human bite wounds result in greater concentrations of bacteria, especially anaerobic species, than most animal bite wounds. *Eikenella corrodens* can cause infections in human bite wounds, but the most common organisms causing these infections are α-hemolytic streptococci and *Staphylococcus aureus*.

Clinical Symptoms

The history of the injury and a laceration is diagnostic but may be difficult to elicit. Warmth, swelling, pain, and a purulent discharge are often present (**Figure 1**). Examination may reveal evidence of damage to underlying structures, including lack of extension or flexion as a result of tendon damage or a loss of sensation over the tip of the finger as a result of nerve injury.

Tests

Physical Examination

Measure and record the location of the laceration. A small laceration over the ring or little finger is a sign of a possible clenched-fist injury. Be alert for a tooth wound that is proximal to the

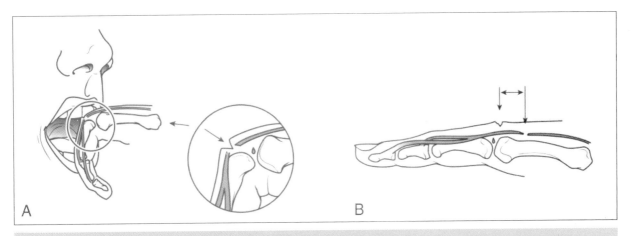

Figure 1 A, Illustration of the mechanism of tendon laceration and intra-articular contamination by saliva in a human bite. **B,** An injury to a tendon that is cut in flexion will retract as the joint extends, as shown in this illustration.

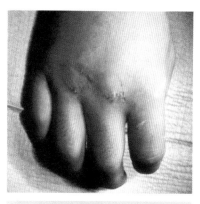

Figure 2 Clinical photograph of a possible tooth injury over the metacarpophalangeal joint of the long finger. (Reproduced from Pollak AN, Barnes L, Ciotola JA, Gulli B, eds: *Emergency Care and Transportation of the Sick and Injured*, ed 10. Rosemont, IL, American Academy of Orthopaedic Surgeons, 2010, p 822.)

metacarpophalangeal (MCP) joint when the finger is extended but lies over the knuckle when the fist is clenched (**Figure 2**). Document the location and severity of swelling, erythema, and any purulent discharge. When the injury is on the dorsum of the hand, significant swelling may occur quickly (within 2 to 3 hours). Assess function of the flexor and extensor tendons and sensory nerves distal to the laceration. Examine the forearm for signs of ascending infection (such as lymphangitic streaks or enlarged epitrochlear nodes).

Diagnostic Tests
PA, lateral, and oblique radiographs of the hand should be obtained to rule out an underlying fracture or the presence of a foreign body. Aerobic and anaerobic cultures should be obtained when any drainage is present. White blood cell count, erythrocyte sedimentation rate, and C-reactive protein level can serve as a baseline for following the clinical course, but these tests may be within normal limits in the early phases after injury.

Differential Diagnosis
• Laceration from a sharp object (accurate history)
• Septic joint caused by a retained foreign body (possibly evident on radiographs)

Adverse Outcomes of the Disease
Tendon rupture and/or laceration can occur as a result of the bite. An abscess involving the deep palmar space, osteomyelitis, joint sepsis, joint stiffness, and possibly septic tenosynovitis can develop with a delay in treatment.

Treatment
Bite wounds can be treated on an outpatient basis if the joint has not been penetrated, if there has been no tendon or bony injury, and when medical treatment is sought within 8 hours of the injury.

Anesthetize the wound with a 1% lidocaine solution and carefully examine and débride the skin edges and any underlying necrotic tissue. The extensor mechanism over the MCP joints should be examined with the finger flexed to assess for damage to the tendons or penetration of the underlying joint. It is important to explore the wound with the patient's fingers both flexed and extended. If the possibility of joint infection exists, an arthrotomy is necessary to irrigate the joint. Irrigate the wound with a large amount of an antibiotic irrigation solution and apply saline-soaked gauze or a nonadherent dressing. Human bites should not be closed primarily.

Immobilize the hand in a bulky dressing that incorporates a dorsal plaster splint that holds the hand in a safe position (with the MCP joint at 60° to 90° of flexion and the interphalangeal joints in a resting, extended position). Appropriate tetanus prophylaxis should be given as outlined in **Table 1**, followed by antibiotics. Penicillin and a first-generation cephalosporin provide adequate coverage in most

Table 1

Summary Guide to Tetanus Prophylaxis in Routine Wound Management[a]

History of Tetanus Immunization (Doses)	Clean, Minor Wounds		All Other Wounds	
	Td[b]	TIG	Td[b]	TIG
Uncertain or <3 doses	Yes	No	Yes	Yes
3 or more doses	No[c]	No	No[d]	No

Td = tetanus and diphtheria toxoids, TIG = human tetanus immune globulin.

[a] Important details on the CDC website: http://wwwnc.cdc.gov/travel/yellowbook/2010/chapter-2/tetanus.aspx.

[b] For children <7 years, DTaP or DTP (DT, if pertussis vaccine contraindicated) preferred to tetanus toxoid alone. For children ≥7 years, Td preferred to tetanus toxoid alone. For adolescents and adults to age 64 years, tetanus toxoid as Tdap is preferred, if the patient has not previously been vaccinated with Tdap.

[c] Yes, if more than 10 years since last dose.

[d] Yes, if more than 5 years since last dose. More frequent boosters are not needed and can accentuate side effects.

(Adapted with permission from the Centers for Disease Control and Prevention.)

instances. Tetracycline can be used for patients who are allergic to penicillin. If cultures obtained from specimens taken at the time of initial wound care are positive, antibiotic type and dosage should be adjusted accordingly. As part of standard wound management care to prevent tetanus, a tetanus toxoid–containing vaccine might be recommended for wound management in a pregnant woman if 5 years or more have elapsed since her previous tetanus and diphtheria toxoids (Td) booster. If a Td booster is recommended for a pregnant woman, healthcare providers should administer tetanus, diphtheria, and pertussis (Tdap) vaccine.

Advise patients who present soon after injury and without an established abscess to return within 24 hours for a recheck to confirm that infection has not developed. After the first 24 hours, daily whirlpool treatment or twice-daily dressing changes can be started. The wound should be allowed to close by secondary intention. For established infections, urgent surgical débridement and intravenous antibiotics are usually necessary. Early referral is necessary in these cases.

Adverse Outcomes of Treatment

Inadequate evaluation or treatment can lead to significant complications, including the need for amputation in advanced cases. Infection may develop with primary wound closure. Patients may experience sensitivity to antibiotics.

Referral Decisions/Red Flags

Wounds that involve the joint, tendon, nerve, or bone require further evaluation. A bite wound that becomes infected despite treatment with antibiotics also requires further evaluation.

SECTION 4 HAND AND WRIST

Kienböck Disease

Synonym

Osteonecrosis of the carpal lunate

Definition

Kienböck disease—osteonecrosis of the carpal lunate—most commonly affects men between the ages of 20 and 40 years (**Figure 1**). Patients may have a history of trauma, but the cause of the disrupted blood supply is frequently difficult to establish. With progression of the disease, the lunate collapses and fragments, which ultimately results in end-stage arthritis of the wrist.

Clinical Symptoms

Pain, stiffness, and diffuse swelling over the dorsal-central aspect of the wrist are common. Patients often report weakness or an inability to grasp heavy objects.

Tests

Physical Examination

Examination typically reveals tenderness directly over the lunate bone (mid-dorsal wrist area, just distal to the radius). Grip strength usually is decreased. With progression of the disease, dorsal swelling and limited wrist motion are common.

Diagnostic Tests

PA and lateral radiographs of the wrist are indicated. In the early phase of Kienböck disease, radiographs show increased density (whiteness) of the lunate bone compared with the surrounding carpal bones. In later stages, the dead bone will fragment and collapse, resulting in generalized degenerative arthritis of the wrist (**Figure 2**).

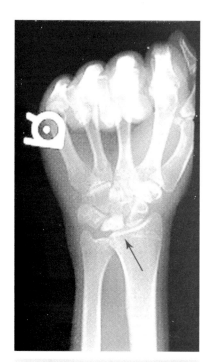

Figure 1 PA clenched-fist radiograph of the left hand of a patient with Kienböck disease shows significant sclerosis of the lunate (arrow) and possible early collapse.

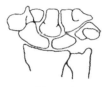 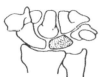 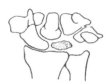 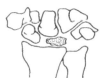 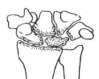

Stage 1: No visible change in the lunate

Stage 2: Sclerosis of the lunate

Stage 3A: Sclerosis and fragmentation of the lunate

Stage 3B: Stage 3A with proximal migration of the capitate or fixed rotation of the scaphoid

Stage 4: Stage 3A or 3B combined with degenerative changes at adjacent joints

Figure 2 Illustration of the radiographic classification of Kienböck disease according to the method of Lichtman and associates, modified by Weiss and associates. (Reproduced with permission from the American Society for Surgery of the Hand: *Hand Surgery Update*. Rosemont, IL, American Academy of Orthopaedic Surgeons, 1994, p 86.)

Differential Diagnosis

- Fracture of the distal radius (evident on radiographs)
- Fracture of the scaphoid (evident on radiographs)
- Ganglion (discrete mass, normal radiographs)
- Scapholunate dissociation (increased distance between the scaphoid and lunate on radiographs)
- Tenosynovitis of the extensor tendon (diffuse swelling over extensor tendon extending onto the hand)
- Wrist arthritis (narrowing of joint space but normal contour of lunate)

Adverse Outcomes of the Disease

Untreated Kienböck disease can result in progressive arthritis.

Treatment

If radiographs are normal, or if the lunate shows significant sclerosis, splint the wrist in a neutral position for 3 weeks. Wrist radiographs should be obtained with the shoulder abducted 90° and the elbow flexed 90° to obtain a true measure of the relationship between the radius and the ulna at the wrist (ulnar variance). NSAIDs may make the patient more comfortable. If pain persists after 3 weeks, further evaluation is indicated. In general, MRI is necessary to complete staging of the disease.

Adverse Outcomes of Treatment

Loss of motion, chronic pain, and decreased grip strength are possible. If NSAIDs are used to control pain, the treating physician should prescribe them with the awareness that in 2015, the FDA strengthened its warning linking NSAIDs with the risk of heart attack or stroke, even in the first weeks of use of an NSAID.

Referral Decisions/Red Flags

If plain radiographs show any abnormality of the lunate, further evaluation is indicated. Persistent dorsal wrist pain, despite 3 weeks of immobilization, also is an indication for further evaluation.

Mallet Finger

Synonyms
Baseball finger
Terminal extensor tendon rupture

Definition
A mallet finger deformity is caused by rupture, laceration, or avulsion of the insertion of the extensor tendon at the base of the distal phalanx. Sometimes, instead of the tendon tearing, the injury avulses a fragment of the distal phalanx at the tendinous attachment (**Figure 1**).

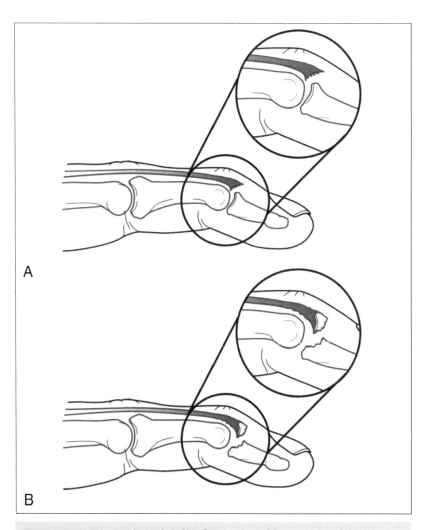

A

B

Figure 1 **A,** Illustration of mallet finger caused by rupture of the extensor tendon at its insertion. **B,** Illustration of mallet finger caused by avulsion of a piece of distal phalanx.

Clinical Symptoms

Patients report pain and an inability to straighten the finger at the distal interphalangeal (DIP) joint. In addition to an extension lag at the DIP joint, patients may report a compensatory change of hyperextension in the proximal interphalangeal (PIP) joint (referred to as swanning).

Tests

Physical Examination

Examination reveals that the DIP joint is in flexion and that the patient is unable to actively extend the joint although it can be passively extended. The dorsal area of the DIP joint initially is tender and slightly swollen, but approximately 2 weeks after the injury occurs, the fingertip usually is not painful.

Diagnostic Tests

A lateral radiograph may reveal a small bony avulsion from the dorsal side of the distal phalanx. With large dorsal avulsion fragments, the distal phalanx may displace in a palmar direction from the unopposed pull of the flexor tendon.

Differential Diagnosis

• Fracture of the distal phalanx (evident on radiographs)
• Fracture-dislocation of the DIP joint (evident on radiographs)

Adverse Outcomes of the Disease

Permanent extensor lag of the DIP joint is possible. Persistent deformity associated with flexion of the fingertip is also possible, despite treatment.

Treatment

Continuous splinting of the DIP joint in extension is done to restore full function of the extensor tendon. The splint can be applied on either the volar or the dorsal surface of the finger (**Figure 2**). With acute injuries, the splint should be worn for 6 to 8 weeks. If the injury is more than 3 months old, a splint should be worn for at least 8 weeks. If prolonged splinting is required, the patient should be instructed carefully in how to monitor for skin problems, because excessive skin pressure can result in skin breakdown.

Advise patients to maintain the DIP joint in extension when the splint is removed for cleaning. If the fingertip droops at any time after the splint is applied, the healing process is disrupted and the period of splinting must be extended. Four or 5 days after the splint is applied, check the dorsal skin for maceration or pressure spots. If the joint does not come into full extension by the second visit, the patient should be evaluated for possible surgical pinning.

Visits every 2 to 3 weeks with the provider or with a hand therapist are helpful to monitor progress and usually lead to a better outcome

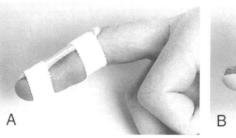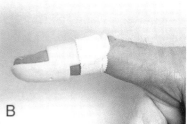

Figure 2 Clinical photographs of types of splints used in the treatment of mallet finger. **A,** Dorsal aluminum splint. **B,** Commercial splint. (Reproduced from Culver JE Jr: Office management of athletic injuries of the hand and wrist. *Instr Course Lect* 1989;38:473-482.)

than if the splint is applied and the patient is not seen again until 6 to 8 weeks later; in some cases, the splint will need to be adjusted over time to maintain full digital extension. At the end of the splinting period, if no extensor lag is evident, guarded active flexion is started, with splinting continued at night or during sporting activities for an additional 2 to 4 weeks.

Certain occupations, such as cooking, dishwashing, and typing, make splint wear difficult, and patients whose lifestyle requires doing these tasks repeatedly should be evaluated for possible surgical pinning.

Adverse Outcomes of Treatment
Prolonged splinting can result in skin breakdown.

Referral Decisions/Red Flags
Patients with volar subluxation of the distal phalanx and/or an avulsed bony fragment that involves more than one third of the joint surface may require further evaluation. Patients with compensatory hyperextension at the PIP joint (that is, swanning) may benefit from an anti-swanning splint to prevent full extension and hyperextension of the PIP joint for 3 to 4 weeks, followed by a DIP immobilization splint alone.

SECTION 4　HAND AND WRIST

Nail Bed Injuries

Synonyms
Smashed finger
Subungual hematoma

Definition
Many injuries to the fingertip are crushing in nature, resulting in various degrees of injury to the fingernail, nail bed, and distal phalanx (**Figure 1**). The types of nail bed injury include simple lacerations, stellate lacerations, severe crush injuries, and avulsions. Most are associated with fractures of the distal phalanx.

Clinical Symptoms
Patients usually have pain and obvious injury to the fingertip.

Tests
Physical Examination
Determine the extent of the injury, noting any subungual hematoma and its extent, avulsion or laceration of the nail, and whether an associated fracture of the distal phalanx is displaced or nondisplaced. When the fingernail is avulsed, note the extent of injury to the nail bed (both germinal and sterile matrices). Examine the fingernail for attached remnants of the nail bed. An avulsion of the fingernail in a child or infant may be associated with a physeal injury, in which case referral to a specialist is indicated.

Diagnostic Tests
PA and lateral radiographs of the finger are necessary when a fracture of the distal phalanx is suspected.

Differential Diagnosis
• Mallet finger (unable to fully extend the distal interphalangeal joint)

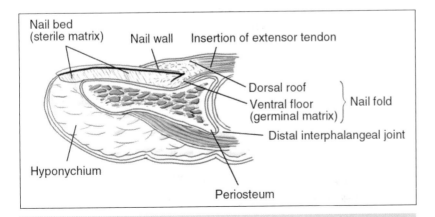

Figure 1 Illustration of the anatomy of the nail bed of the finger: sagittal cross-sectional view.

Adverse Outcomes of the Disease

If the patient has sustained damage to the nail bed, particularly the germinal matrix, a permanent nail deformity may result.

Treatment

Subungual Hematomas

Painful subungual hematomas can be treated with decompression. After scrubbing the finger and applying a disinfectant, create a hole in the fingernail over the hematoma, using battery-operated microcautery, if available, or a heated paper clip or 18-gauge needle. The hole must be large enough to allow continued drainage. Penetrate only through the nail and avoid perforating too deeply into the nail bed, because this is extremely painful and may result in scarring of the nail bed.

Nail Bed Lacerations

For lacerations of the nail bed with injury to the nail plate, the nail plate should be removed only if the nail is "floating" and ready to come off of the digit. Although historically it was believed that all nail bed lacerations require repair, more recent data suggest that repair is not required in most cases. If the nail is in place and not floating, it may be left intact and the nail bed left unrepaired, with few anticipated adverse sequelae. Should the nail bed require repair, this should be done with adequate anesthesia, with sterile preparation of the finger and the use of a finger tourniquet if 1% lidocaine with 1:100,000 epinephrine does not supply adequate hemostasis. Elevate all or part of the nail plate using a blunt Freer elevator and small scissors. The entire nail can be removed or just enough to allow visualization of the laceration and suture placement. Irrigate the wound, remove the hematoma, and meticulously suture the nail bed using No. 6-0 or 7-0 bioabsorbable gut suture. After repair, stent the nail fold open by placing some xeroform gauze or a piece of a red rubber catheter into the nail fold. This gauze can be left in place because it will grow out with the new nail. An associated minimally displaced or nondisplaced fracture usually will be stabilized with the repair.

Nail Avulsions

The proximal portion of the nail bed (germinal matrix) may be avulsed and lying on top of the nail fold (**Figure 2**). This must be replaced underneath the nail fold and sutured in place. The sutures should be placed through the proximal fold to pull the nail bed into the fold. If the nail avulsion is associated with a fracture, the distal phalanx may need to be stabilized. Any nail bed tissue adherent to the fingernail should be gently removed with a scalpel and sewn in place in the nail bed defect using small bioabsorbable suture. A large fragment of nail or the whole nail itself, when it has a large amount of nail bed still attached to it, should not have the tissue removed; rather, the entire fragment should be sewn anatomically in place. Any injuries to the nail fold should be repaired with No. 5-0 gut, nylon, or monofilament suture. Injuries in children should be repaired with bioabsorbable sutures.

Wound Care
The finger should be dressed with antibacterial ointment, nonadherent gauze, sterile gauze, and an outer wrap. The finger should be splinted for protection.

Adverse Outcomes of Treatment
Abnormal growth and subsequent deformity of the nail can occur.

Referral Decisions/Red Flags
Nail bed injuries with complex lacerations or loss of tissue or injury to the germinal matrix may require more involved surgical treatment. Associated open fractures of the distal phalanx require further evaluation.

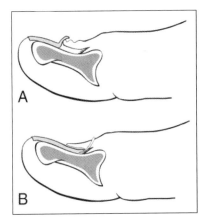

Figure 2 Illustration of nail avulsion. **A,** The proximal portion of the nail bed (germinal matrix) is avulsed and is lying on top of the nail fold. **B,** Replacement of the germinal matrix into the nail fold.

Materials

- Sterile gloves
- Bactericidal skin preparation solution
- 3-mL syringe with a 27-gauge needle
- 3 mL of a 1% local anesthetic
- Wire cutter
- Hemostat
- No. 15 blade

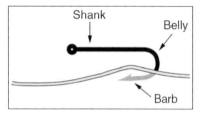

Figure 1 Illustration of an embedded fishhook with parts of the hook labeled.

Procedure: Fishhook Removal

Retrograde extraction of a fishhook is difficult because of the barb (**Figure 1**). Most fishhook injuries involve the skin and subcutaneous tissues only. Although many techniques of fishhook removal have been described, only two are discussed here (**Figures 2** and **3**). Remember to wear protective gloves at all times during this procedure and use sterile technique.

Technique 1

Step 1
Cleanse the skin with a bactericidal skin preparation solution.

Step 2
Use a 27-gauge needle to infiltrate the skin with 2 to 3 mL of 1% local anesthetic.

Step 3
Grasp the exposed end of the hook (shank) with the thumb and index finger and rotate the hook to force the barb out through the skin.

Step 4
Cut the barbed end of the hook with a wire cutter.

Step 5
Remove the rest of the hook retrograde. It will back out easily after the barb is gone.

Step 6
Apply a topical antibiotic and a sterile bandage to the wound.

Technique 2
These instructions were written to guide a right hand–dominant healthcare provider.

Step 1
Cleanse the skin with a bactericidal skin preparation solution.

Step 2
Inject 2 to 3 mL of 1% local anesthetic about the hook.

Step 3
Using a hemostat, grasp the belly of the hook at the point at which it penetrates the skin.

Step 4
Grasp the shank of the hook with your left thumb and long finger and press against the skin. At the same time, press gently downward on the belly of the hook with the left index finger to disengage the barb from the surrounding tissues.

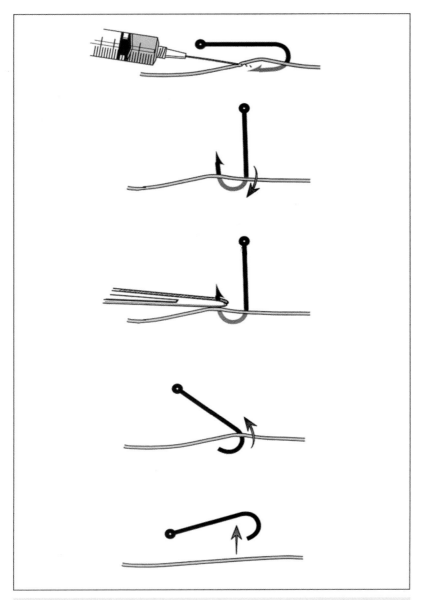

Figure 2 Illustration of technique 1 for removing a fishhook, in which the barb is pushed out through the skin.

Step 5
With your right hand, pull sharply on the hemostat to remove the hook. You may need to make a small incision with a No. 15 blade over the embedded portion of the hook to facilitate removal.

Step 6
Dress the site with a sterile adhesive bandage.

Adverse Outcomes
Use of the first technique may inflict further soft-tissue damage by pushing the barb through the skin. Breakage of the hook or infection is possible. Fishhook injuries usually occur in a marine environment

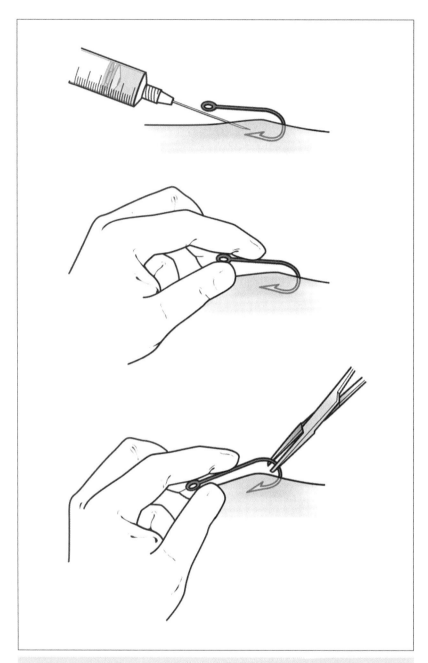

Figure 3 Illustration of technique 2 for removing a fishhook, in which the barb is pulled out.

and can be associated with unusual infections (*Vibrio* species, atypical mycobacterial organisms).

Aftercare/Patient Instructions

Check whether the patient has current tetanus prophylaxis. Advise the patient to keep the wound clean until it is healed, usually in 3 to 4 days. Instruct the patient to return to your office if redness, fever, or proximal swelling occurs. Consider the prophylactic administration of an oral cephalosporin.

Sprains and Dislocations of the Hand

Synonyms

Gamekeeper's thumb
Jammed finger
Skier's thumb
Sprain

Definition

Sprains of the fingers are common injuries characterized by a partial or complete tear of a collateral ligament and/or volar capsular ligament (**Figure 1**). Most sprains of the fingers are relatively straightforward injuries that can be managed effectively without surgery. The exception is a complete rupture of the ulnar collateral ligament of the thumb metacarpophalangeal (MCP) joint, which usually requires surgical treatment.

The ulnar collateral ligament of the thumb MCP joint is an important stabilizer of the thumb. When this ligament is torn, the thumb deviates outward when the thumb is stressed radially (**Figure 2**). The name gamekeeper's thumb derives from the chronic injury observed in English gamekeepers as a result of their method of killing rabbits. Currently, a frequent cause of this injury in the acute

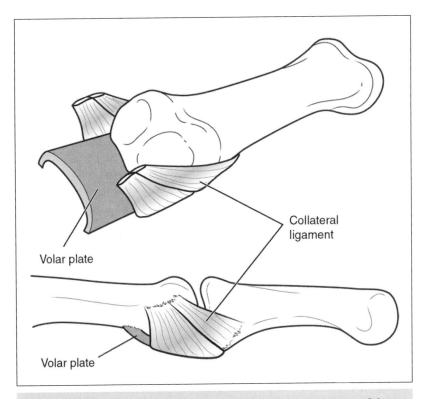

Volar plate

Collateral ligament

Volar plate

Figure 1 Illustration of the collateral ligaments and volar plates of the proximal interphalangeal (PIP) joint.

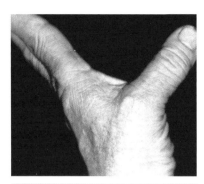

Figure 2 Clinical photograph of an ulnar collateral ligament tear.

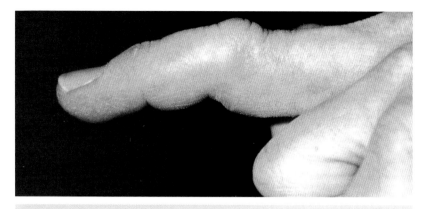

Figure 3 Clinical photograph of a dislocation at the PIP joint. (Copyright Science Source.)

setting is forced abduction of the thumb against a ski pole (skier's thumb); however, the injury also occurs during ball-playing sports or from a fall.

Most dislocations in the hand are hyperextension injuries that result from a complete tear of the volar capsule that usually results in dorsal displacement of the distal element. Dislocation is most common at the proximal interphalangeal (PIP) joint (**Figure 3**). Dorsal dislocations of the MCP joint are either simple or complex. Complex dislocations are associated with interposition of the volar plate between the metacarpal head and the proximal phalanx (**Figure 4**). Complex dislocations (involving any of the fingers or thumb) may not be reducible by closed methods and may require open reduction.

Clinical Symptoms

Patients almost always report a history of trauma and acute onset of pain. With an acute thumb ulnar collateral ligament injury, pain and swelling is localized to the inside (ulnar aspect) of the thumb MCP joint; in the chronic setting, pain may be minimal but instability is a problem. With a dislocation, patients describe a deformity that developed immediately after the injury. The patient or another individual may have reduced or attempted to reduce a dislocation before the patient sought medical attention.

Tests
Physical Examination

If the joint is swollen but not grossly deformed, palpate both sides of the joint for tenderness over the collateral ligaments (**Figure 5**). Radiographs should be obtained to rule out fractures. If there is no fracture, then joint stability should be tested by applying radial and ulnar stresses to the joint (**Figure 6**). If the finger angulates easily while held in full extension under stress, it likely indicates a complete tear of the collateral ligament. If the patient has pain with stress testing but no instability, the ligament injury is likely incomplete.

Dislocations are often obvious on inspection. Complex dislocations of the MCP joint are characterized by fixed displacement of the distal

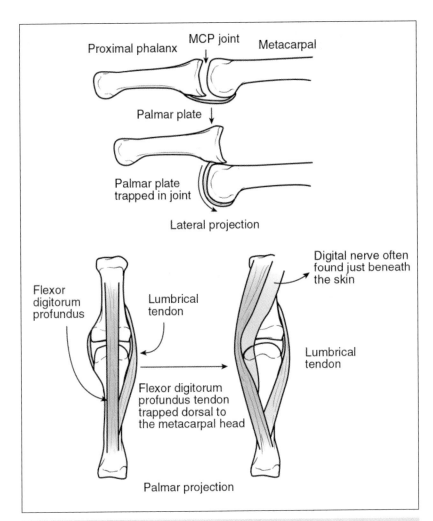

Figure 4 Illustration of complex dislocation of the metacarpophalangeal (MCP) joint. The lateral projection shows the palmar (volar) plate trapped in the joint. The palmar projection shows the flexor digitorum profundus tendon trapped dorsal to the metacarpal head.

segment. Usually, complex dislocations occur at the MCP joint and are characterized by a palmar prominence of the metacarpal head and angulation and dorsal displacement of the proximal phalanx. Patients with complex MCP dislocations have limited active flexion.

Diagnostic Tests
AP and lateral radiographs of the digit (rather than the entire hand) are necessary to rule out a fracture or a fracture-dislocation (**Figure 7**).

Differential Diagnosis
• Extensor tendon rupture (boutonnière deformity, inability to extend the PIP joint)
• Fracture (evident on radiographs)

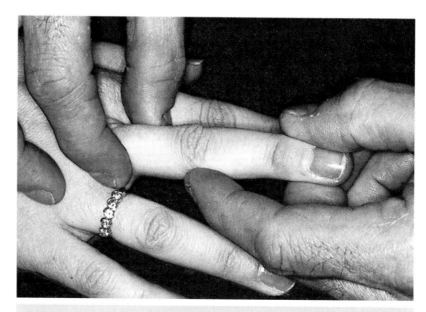

Figure 5 Clinical photograph shows palpation of the collateral ligaments.

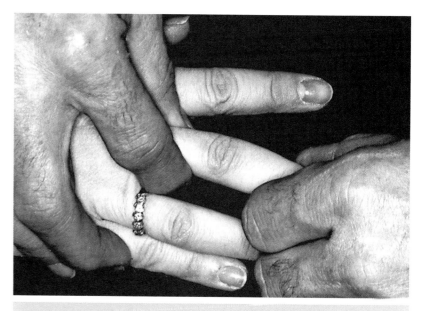

Figure 6 Clinical photograph shows application of radial and ulnar stresses to the PIP joint.

Adverse Outcomes of the Disease

Limited motion, stiffness, chronic pain, and swelling may persist. Chronic hyperextension of the PIP joint or flexion contracture can occur.

Treatment

Most sprains of the collateral ligaments can be treated with splinting. The exception is an unstable, complete rupture of the ulnar collateral ligament of the thumb MCP joint. These injuries may require surgical stabilization because interposition of the adductor pollicis tendon between the end of the ulnar collateral ligament and the base of the proximal phalanx prevents adequate repair of the avulsed ligament.

Nonsurgical treatment of sprains and dislocations focuses on relocation of the joint and protection of the reduction with splinting. Reduction of a dorsal dislocation of the PIP joint is usually performed with axial traction and flexion of the proximal phalanx (see below). Buddy taping to an adjacent finger is effective treatment of collateral ligament injuries in the finger joints (**Figure 8**). Complete rupture of the volar plate, associated with dorsal dislocation, is treated by splinting the joint in 20° to 30° of flexion for 2 to 3 weeks or using buddy taping and early motion. Incomplete tears of the ulnar collateral ligament of the thumb MCP joint can be treated in a thumb spica cast with the thumb slightly flexed for 2 to 4 weeks. The duration of treatment is based on subsequent clinical examination and radiographs.

Closed reduction of a PIP or distal interphalangeal (DIP) joint dislocation should be performed under a digital block anesthetic. To reduce the dislocation, grasp the distal portion of the finger and apply longitudinal traction while stabilizing the finger or hand proximal to the dislocation. Apply gentle pressure over the dorsum of the deformity to guide the reduction. After reduction, move the finger through a range of motion and then assess collateral ligament stability. If the joint seems stable, the finger can be buddy taped. If the joint has full range of motion after the reduction but tends to dislocate during the last 20° of extension, apply a dorsal extension block splint to limit terminal extension (**Figure 9**). This type of splint blocks the last 20° to 30° of extension. Use the splint for 2 to 3 weeks, then buddy tape the finger to an adjacent finger for an additional 3 weeks.

The relocation of MCP joint dislocations may require a regional nerve block. If the dislocation cannot be reduced with adequate anesthesia, soft tissue could be interposed, and open reduction may be necessary (**Figure 10**).

DIP dislocations are typically dorsal or dorsolateral. With open injuries, an associated tear of the extensor tendon should be suspected. After adequate digital block anesthesia, longitudinal traction should be applied to reduce the dislocation. Open dislocations need appropriate irrigation and débridement but tend to be stable after reduction. Next, a dorsal aluminum splint should be applied over the middle and distal phalanges for 1 to 2 weeks. If the fingertip droops after the reduction and the patient cannot actively extend the distal phalanx, the injury should be treated as a mallet finger. The flexor digitorum profundus tendon should be carefully examined after relocation for discomfort on DIP flexion. Some patients have a substantial partial flexor digitorum profundus injury following dorsal dislocation of the DIP joint.

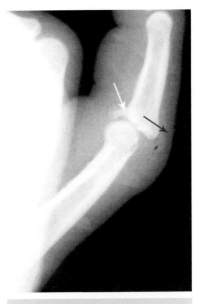

Figure 7 Lateral radiograph of a finger shows fracture-dislocation of the PIP joint: dorsal translation of the middle phalanx (black arrow) associated with a complex fracture of the base of the middle phalanx (white arrow).

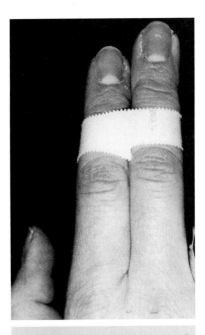

Figure 8 Clinical photograph of buddy taping.

▣◀ Buddy Taping

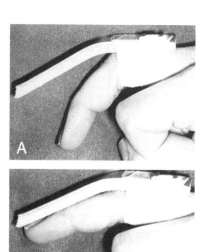

Figure 9 Clinical photographs of a dorsal extension block splint for PIP dislocations. The splint allows flexion (**A**) but blocks the last 20° to 30° of extension (**B**), preventing excessive motion of the volar plate.

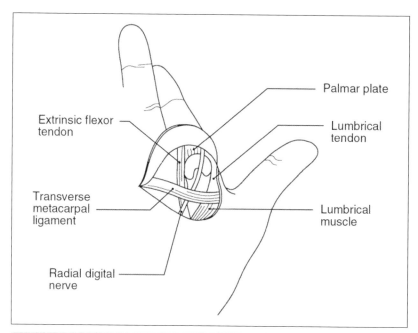

Figure 10 Illustration of entrapment of the metacarpal head between the lumbrical and extrinsic flexor tendons. (Reproduced with permission from the American Society for Surgery of the Hand: *Hand Surgery Update*. Rosemont, IL, American Academy of Orthopaedic Surgeons, 1994, p 22.)

Adverse Outcomes of Treatment

Instability, joint stiffness, persistent hyperextension deformity, and/or residual flexion deformity can develop. Arthritis also may develop with an inadequate reduction or as a sequela of the injury.

Referral Decisions/Red Flags

Patients with an unstable thumb MCP joint (suggestive of complete ulnar collateral ligament injury) require further evaluation for possible surgical stabilization. Patients whose dislocations cannot be reduced easily with digital anesthesia are candidates for open reduction. In addition, patients with fracture-dislocations and open dislocations require further evaluation. Open dislocations are best treated surgically to achieve adequate débridement and repair.

Trigger Finger

Synonyms
Locked finger
Stenosing tenosynovitis of the flexor tendons

Definition
The flexor tendons of the fingers glide back and forth under four annular and three cruciform pulleys that keep the tendons from bowstringing. The flexor tendon or first annular pulley may become thickened from chronic inflammation and irritation. Any thickening can limit the amount of effective tendon excursion. In addition, the tendons may develop changes, thereby limiting motion through the pulleys. As a result of the limited motion, the finger may snap or lock during flexion, or digital motion may become limited (**Figure 1**). The long and ring fingers are most commonly affected, but any digit may be involved.

Trigger finger is commonly seen in association with rheumatoid arthritis, diabetes mellitus, and hypothyroidism. It is often observed in middle-aged women. A higher prevalence of trigger finger is observed in patients with carpal tunnel syndrome and de Quervain stenosing tenosynovitis. Triggering may occur in young children, usually in the thumb. Triggering in the lesser digits in children is unusual and may be associated with a metabolic disorder.

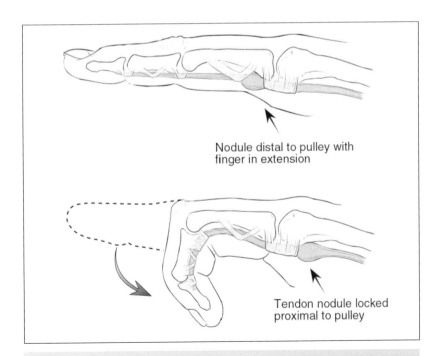

Nodule distal to pulley with finger in extension

Tendon nodule locked proximal to pulley

Figure 1 Illustration of trigger finger. A nodule or thickening in the flexor tendon becomes trapped proximal to the pulley, making finger extension difficult.

Clinical Symptoms

Patients typically report pain and catching when they flex the finger and may describe the finger as going "out of joint." They may awaken with the finger locked in the palm, although the finger gradually unlocks during the day. The proximal interphalangeal (PIP) joint may be identified as the source of the pain, but the pathology is at the level of the metacarpophalangeal (MCP) joint. Some patients have a painful nodule in the distal palm, usually at the level of the distal flexion crease, with no history of triggering. In other patients, the only symptoms are swelling and/or stiffness in the fingers, particularly in the morning.

Tests

Physical Examination

Examination reveals tenderness in the palm at the level of the distal palmar crease, usually at the level of the MCP joint. A nodule also may be palpable at this site. The nodule moves, and the finger may lock when the patient flexes and extends the affected finger. This maneuver is almost always painful. Full flexion of the finger may not be possible. With long-standing triggering, lack of terminal PIP extension may develop.

Diagnostic Tests

This is a clinical diagnosis; radiographs are not needed.

Differential Diagnosis

- Anomalous muscle belly in the palm (swelling more proximal in the palm)
- Diabetes mellitus (single and multiple trigger fingers)
- Dupuytren disease (palpable cord)
- Extensor tendon subluxation (visible subluxation of the extensor apparatus into the valley between the digits)
- Ganglion of the tendon sheath (tendon mass at the base of the finger that does not move with flexion)
- Partial tendon injury
- PIP joint injury
- Rheumatoid arthritis (multiple joint involvement)

Adverse Outcomes of the Disease

Flexion contracture of the PIP joint or stiffness in extension may develop.

Treatment

Initial treatment may involve an injection of corticosteroid into the tendon sheath. Care must be exercised to avoid injecting the tendon. Patients may also consider splinting or therapy programs aimed at differential gliding of the superficial and deep flexor tendons. If symptoms persist, a second injection in 3 to 4 weeks is permissible. However, because patients with rheumatoid disease are already at increased risk for tendon rupture, multiple injections should be done only after careful consideration, and surgical release may be considered. If two injections fail to resolve the trigger finger, surgical release is often offered.

Adverse Outcomes of Treatment

Repeated corticosteroid injections might lead to rupture of the flexor tendon and also may injure the digital sensory nerve. Infection also is a risk. In patients with diabetes mellitus, steroid injections may increase blood glucose levels. Rarely, injury to the digital nerve may occur at surgery.

Referral Decisions/Red Flags

Failure of nonsurgical treatment, development of contractures in the PIP joint, and/or a locked finger (in flexion or extension) indicate a need for further evaluation. Patients with rheumatoid arthritis in whom the problem does not resolve after a single injection also may need additional evaluation. Patients with type 1 diabetes mellitus should be counseled regarding the effect of the steroid injection on their blood glucose levels; you may elect to refer such patients for specialty evaluation.

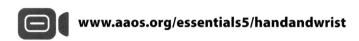
Procedure: Trigger Finger Injection

Materials

- Gloves
- Bactericidal skin preparation solution
- 1 to 2 mL of a 1% local anesthetic
- One or two 3-mL syringes with a 25-gauge needle
- 0.5 to 1 mL of a corticosteroid preparation
- Adhesive dressing

The flexor tendons pass beneath a pulley situated just distal to the distal palmar crease. Palpating this area as the patient flexes and extends the finger reveals a click or snapping sensation as the enlarged tendon passes beneath the pulley.

Note: Opinions differ regarding single- and two-needle injection techniques. Proponents of the single-needle technique believe that one needle is less painful for the patient than two. In addition, it is not specifically necessary to enter the tendon sheath with the injection. In the single-syringe technique, both the local anesthetic and the corticosteroid mixture are drawn up in a single syringe. This preparation is aseptically injected just over the A1 pulley level (at the distal palmar crease) in the subcutaneous tissue. The video shows a two-needle, two-syringe technique. A single-needle, single-syringe technique is described here.

Step 1
Wear protective gloves at all times during this procedure and use sterile technique.

Step 2
Cleanse the palm with a bactericidal skin preparation solution.

Step 3
Identify the lump on the tendon.

Step 4
Inject 1 mL of a 1% anesthetic solution and 0.5 mL of a corticosteroid preparation into the subcutaneous tissue at the distal palmar crease (**Figure 1**).

Step 5
Dress the puncture site with a sterile adhesive bandage.

Adverse Outcomes
Injection of a corticosteroid in patients with insulin-requiring diabetes mellitus may lead to transient elevation of blood glucose levels.

Aftercare/Patient Instructions
Advise the patient of possible significant discomfort for 1 to 2 days following any injection of a corticosteroid. Also, the finger may be

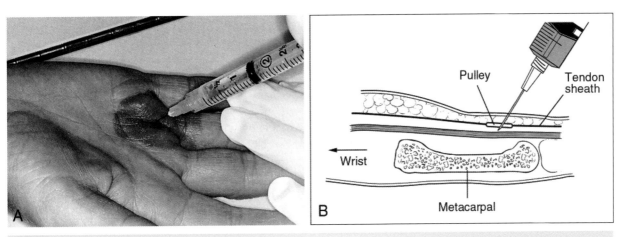

Figure 1 **A,** Clinical photograph of the location for needle insertion for trigger finger injection. **B,** Illustration of proper positioning of the needle through the pulley and into the tendon sheath.

numb for 1 to 2 hours until the local anesthetic wears off. Instruct the patient to return to your office if swelling, redness, or inordinate pain occurs. The patient should be able to use the finger in a normal fashion after the injection.

SECTION 4   HAND AND WRIST

Tumors of the Hand and Wrist

Definition

Most tumors in the hand and wrist are benign. Primary malignant tumors and skeletal metastases account for less than 1% of hand tumors. Ganglia are the most common benign soft-tissue tumors, followed by giant cell tumors and epidermal inclusion cysts. Enchondromas are the most common benign neoplasm of the bones of the hand, accounting for 90% of all cases. Squamous cell carcinomas are the most common malignant neoplasm of the hand, and chondrosarcomas are the most common primary malignant bone tumor in the hand. Malignant melanomas are frequently seen in the upper extremity because of exposure of the arm to the sun.

Clinical Symptoms

Many tumors of the hand are painless. The exception is a glomus tumor, which characteristically is extremely painful to pressure and sensitive to cold. Enchondromas frequently present with pain after a patient sustains a pathologic fracture through the weakened bone. Lipomas can cause pain and numbness in the fingers if the lesion is compressing an adjacent nerve. Masses located near joints can cause loss of motion.

Tests

Physical Examination

Note the position, size, and characteristics of the mass (**Figures 1** and **2**). These factors help to narrow the diagnostic possibilities.

A ganglion cyst is characterized as a mass located over the dorsal or volar radial aspect of the wrist, over the flexion crease of the finger at the level of the web space, or over the top of the distal interphalangeal joint of a finger.

Epidermal inclusion cysts typically occur around the end of a digit or at the end of an amputation stump. Pressing a small flashlight against an inclusion cyst will not transilluminate the mass, but this same maneuver will transilluminate a ganglion cyst.

A giant cell tumor is characterized by a multinodular, firm, nontender mass located around an interphalangeal joint, usually of the thumb or the index or long finger.

A blue or red area visible under the fingernail could be a glomus tumor, subungual hematoma, or foreign body. However, subungual discoloration in the absence of trauma should raise a suspicion of melanoma. Likewise, a mole (nevus) that changes shape or color can indicate a malignant melanoma.

Lipomas typically are superficial, soft, reasonably well defined, and nontender on palpation. A frequent location in the hand is the thenar

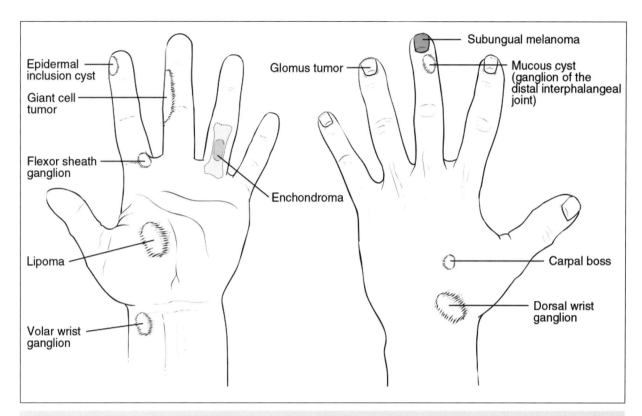

Epidermal inclusion cyst

Giant cell tumor

Flexor sheath ganglion

Lipoma

Volar wrist ganglion

Glomus tumor

Enchondroma

Subungual melanoma

Mucous cyst (ganglion of the distal interphalangeal joint)

Carpal boss

Dorsal wrist ganglion

Figure 1 Illustration of typical locations and types of benign hand tumor.

eminence. When lipomas are located on the palmar surface of the wrist, compression of the median or ulnar nerve may occur.

Recurrent paronychia infections and chronic nail deformities can be caused by underlying squamous cell carcinoma. A diagnosis of Kaposi sarcoma should be suspected in a patient with AIDS in whom skin nodules or red-brown plaques develop.

A symptomatic enchondroma is characterized by tenderness and swelling over the involved phalanx (usually the proximal). A pathologic fracture may be present.

A carpal boss is a dorsal prominence at the base of the third metacarpal or second metacarpal at the carpometacarpal joints. These dorsal osteophytes may be confused with a neoplasm. A ganglion is sometimes associated with a carpal boss.

Diagnostic Tests
PA and lateral radiographs of the involved finger or PA, lateral, and oblique views of the hand should be obtained.

Differential Diagnosis
See **Table 1** and **Figure 1** for a complete listing.

Adverse Outcomes of the Disease
Ganglions can result in limited joint motion. Nail changes, skin atrophy, and infection can develop as a result of a mucoid cyst. Drainage is a problem associated with epidermal inclusion cysts

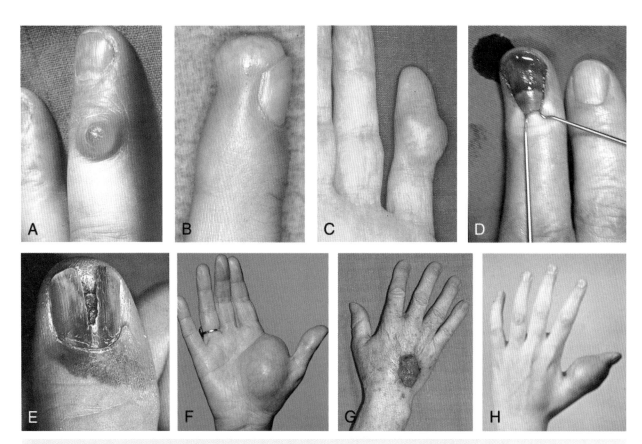

Figure 2 Photographs of the clinical appearance of various hand tumors. **A,** Ganglion (mucous) cyst. **B,** Epidermoid cyst. **C,** Giant cell tumor. **D,** Glomus tumor. **E,** Melanoma. **F,** Lipoma. **G,** Squamous cell carcinoma. **H,** Enchondroma. (Reproduced from Evers B, Klammer HL: Tumors and tumorlike lesions of the hand: Analysis of 424 surgically treated cases. *J Am Acad Orthop Surg* 1997;1[1]:34-43.)

(whitish or cream colored) mucoid cysts (clear drainage). Patients with giant cell tumors may have limited tendon function because of peritendinous adhesions. Nerve compression can develop as a result of lipoma. An enchondroma can result in a weak portion of the bone, and fracture can occur. Squamous cell carcinomas and malignant melanoma can metastasize and result in death.

Treatment

Treatment is based on the diagnosis. For some tumors, MRI will add significant additional information regarding the nature of the mass. Surgical excision and histologic examination are required for most expanding or symptomatic masses.

Adverse Outcomes of Treatment

Ganglions recur at the same site following aspiration in 85% to 90% of patients and recur following surgery in 10% to 15% of patients. The recurrence rate of giant cell tumors is relatively high after surgical excision. Joint stiffness can develop after treatment of pathologic fractures caused by enchondromas.

Table 1

Common Benign Tumors of the Hand and Wrist

Type of Tumor[a]	Common Location(s)	Patient Age and Sex	Signs and Symptoms	Radiographic Findings
Ganglion cyst[b]				
Epidermal inclusion cyst	Fingertip or anywhere from penetrating injury	Teens to middle age; more common in men	Painless, slow growing; does not transilluminate	Round soft-tissue mass, also in distal phalanx
Giant cell tumor of tendon sheath	Digits on palmar surface	>30 years; ratio of men to women, 2:3	Slowly enlarging painless mass	20% show cortical erosion
Glomus tumor	50% occur under fingernail	30 to 50 years; ratio of women to men, 2:1	Triad of symptoms: marked pain, cold intolerance, very tender, blue discoloration of nail	Some show erosion on lateral view
Lipoma	Thenar area in palm and first web space	30 to 60 years; slight predominance in women	Painless, slow growing; might cause nerve entrapment	No bony involvement, soft-tissue mass
Enchondroma	In proximal phalanges or metacarpals	10 to 60 years; affects men and women equally	Might become painful after trauma because of fracture	Radiolucent expansive lesion, cortex thin, fracture and areas of calcification possibly visible

[a] See Figure 1.

[b] See the chapter Ganglion of the Wrist and Hand.

Referral Decisions/Red Flags

Patients with a painful or expanding mass, one that interferes with function, or one believed to be malignant require further evaluation. Pigmented subungual lesions should be referred for evaluation.

Ulnar Nerve Entrapment at the Wrist

Synonym
Ulnar tunnel syndrome

Definition
Entrapment of the ulnar nerve at the wrist usually is caused by a space-occupying lesion such as a lipoma, ganglion, ulnar artery aneurysm, or muscle anomaly (**Figure 1**). Repetitive trauma, such as operating a jackhammer or using the base of the hand as a hammer, also may cause ulnar neuropathy at the wrist. Ulnar nerve entrapment at the wrist is less common than ulnar nerve entrapment at the elbow.

Clinical Symptoms
Patients may or may not have pain, but they often report weakness and numbness.

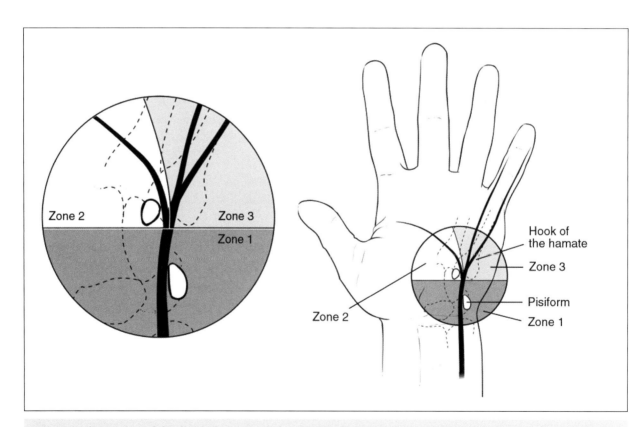

Figure 1 Illustration of the distal ulnar tunnel showing the three zones of entrapment. Lesions in zone 1 cause both motor and sensory symptoms, lesions in zone 2 cause motor deficits, and lesions in zone 3 create sensory deficits.

Tests

Physical Examination

Inspect the hypothenar eminence for atrophy. Assess sensory and motor function of the ulnar nerve. In some patients, only the motor branch of the ulnar nerve may be affected, sparing the sensory branches; however, with sensory involvement, tapping over the ulnar nerve in the hypothenar region will produce tingling in the ring and little fingers (Tinel sign). Sensation over the dorsal and ulnar aspects of the hand is normal. When the ulnar nerve is involved at the elbow, almost all patients will have both sensory and motor involvement and numbness over the dorsal and ulnar sides of the hand. Motor weakness is detected by atrophy of the hypothenar and intrinsic muscles or weakness of the intrinsic muscles (muscles that spread the finger) (**Figure 2**).

Diagnostic Tests

Results of electrophysiologic studies may be abnormal and may differentiate ulnar entrapment at the wrist from the more common entrapment at the elbow.

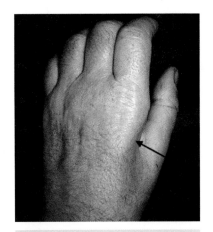

Figure 2 Clinical photograph shows intrinsic muscle wasting (arrow) indicative of ulnar nerve entrapment at the wrist.

Differential Diagnosis

- Carpal tunnel syndrome (usually involves the thumb and the index, long, and ring fingers)
- Cervical (C7-C8) radiculopathy (more proximal muscle involvement, numbness on the dorsum of the hand)
- Peripheral neuropathy (from diabetes, alcoholism, or hypothyroidism; more generalized numbness)
- Thoracic outlet syndrome (symptoms more diffuse)
- Ulnar artery thrombosis in the hand (abnormal Allen test, firm cord on the ulnar side of the hand, sometimes cold intolerance or vascular changes in the hand or digits)
- Ulnar neuropathy at the elbow or cubital tunnel syndrome (sensory changes on the dorsum of the hand)
- Wrist arthritis (pain, limited motion, evident on radiographs)

Adverse Outcomes of the Disease

Loss of intrinsic muscle function causes decreased grip strength and pinch. Sensory loss, when present, involves the ring and little fingers. In advanced disease, clawing of the ring and little fingers can develop.

Treatment

Because the usual cause of ulnar entrapment at the wrist is extrinsic compression (because of lipoma, ganglion, or tumor, for example), treatment is usually surgical. When the obvious cause is external pressure, such as resting the hypothenar area on a keyboard or desk, then the use of padding or a change in position could help.

Adverse Outcomes of Treatment
Postoperative infection, persistent symptoms, or both are possible.

Referral Decisions/Red Flags
Patients with ulnar weakness and neuropathy need further evaluation.

PAIN DIAGRAM
Hip and Thigh

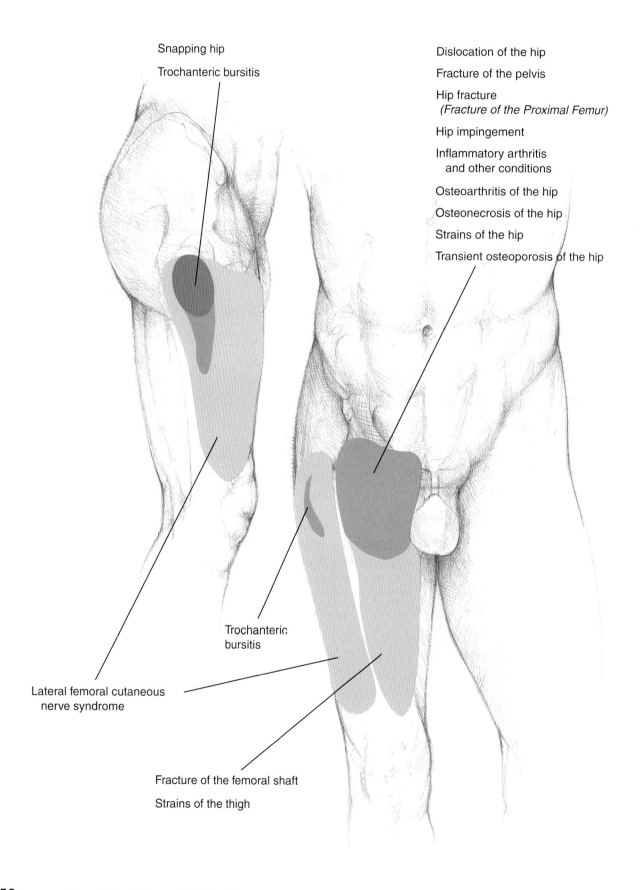

Snapping hip

Trochanteric bursitis

Dislocation of the hip

Fracture of the pelvis

Hip fracture
(Fracture of the Proximal Femur)

Hip impingement

Inflammatory arthritis
and other conditions

Osteoarthritis of the hip

Osteonecrosis of the hip

Strains of the hip

Transient osteoporosis of the hip

Trochanteric
bursitis

Lateral femoral cutaneous
nerve syndrome

Fracture of the femoral shaft

Strains of the thigh

Hip and Thigh

Section Editor

Kathleen Weber, MD, MS

Assistant Professor
Midwest Orthopaedics at Rush
Rush University Medical Center
Chicago, Illinois

Contributor

Mark C. Hubbard, MPT

Physical Therapist
Bone and Joint Institute
Penn State Milton S. Hershey Medical Center
Hershey, Pennsylvania

ANATOMY OF THE HIP AND THIGH

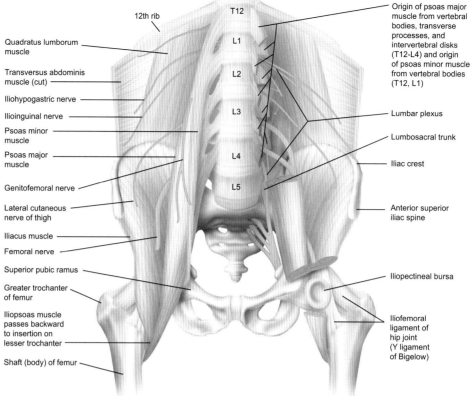

12th rib

T12

L1

L2

L3

L4

L5

Quadratus lumborum muscle

Transversus abdominis muscle (cut)

Iliohypogastric nerve

Ilioinguinal nerve

Psoas minor muscle

Psoas major muscle

Genitofemoral nerve

Lateral cutaneous nerve of thigh

Iliacus muscle

Femoral nerve

Superior pubic ramus

Greater trochanter of femur

Iliopsoas muscle passes backward to insertion on lesser trochanter

Shaft (body) of femur

Origin of psoas major muscle from vertebral bodies, transverse processes, and intervertebral disks (T12-L4) and origin of psoas minor muscle from vertebral bodies (T12, L1)

Lumbar plexus

Lumbosacral trunk

Iliac crest

Anterior superior iliac spine

Iliopectineal bursa

Iliofemoral ligament of hip joint (Y ligament of Bigelow)

Anterior Muscles of the Pelvis

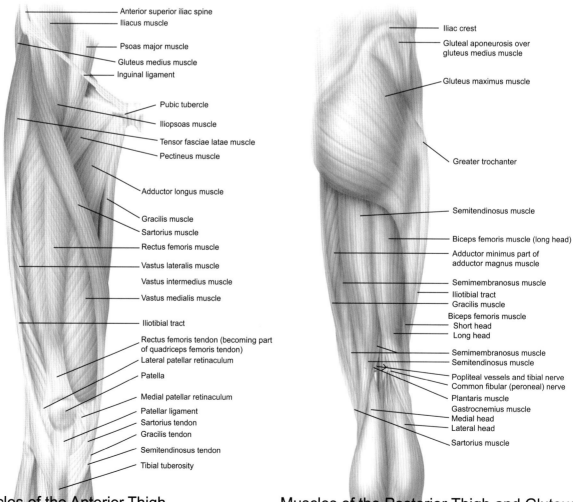

Anterior superior iliac spine
Iliacus muscle
Psoas major muscle
Gluteus medius muscle
Inguinal ligament
Pubic tubercle
Iliopsoas muscle
Tensor fasciae latae muscle
Pectineus muscle
Adductor longus muscle
Gracilis muscle
Sartorius muscle
Rectus femoris muscle
Vastus lateralis muscle
Vastus intermedius muscle
Vastus medialis muscle
Iliotibial tract
Rectus femoris tendon (becoming part of quadriceps femoris tendon)
Lateral patellar retinaculum
Patella
Medial patellar retinaculum
Patellar ligament
Sartorius tendon
Gracilis tendon
Semitendinosus tendon
Tibial tuberosity

Iliac crest
Gluteal aponeurosis over gluteus medius muscle
Gluteus maximus muscle
Greater trochanter
Semitendinosus muscle
Biceps femoris muscle (long head)
Adductor minimus part of adductor magnus muscle
Semimembranosus muscle
Iliotibial tract
Gracilis muscle
Biceps femoris muscle
  Short head
  Long head
Semimembranosus muscle
Semitendinosus muscle
Popliteal vessels and tibial nerve
Common fibular (peroneal) nerve
Plantaris muscle
Gastrocnemius muscle
  Medial head
  Lateral head
Sartorius muscle

Muscles of the Anterior Thigh

Muscles of the Posterior Thigh and Gluteus

Overview of the Hip and Thigh

Hip or proximal thigh pain generally comes from one of the following sources: (1) the hip joint itself, (2) the soft tissues around the hip and pelvis, (3) the pelvic bones, or (4) referred pain from the lumbar spine. Diagnosing pathology involving the hip joint and pelvis is often possible with a careful history and physical examination combined with plain radiographs; in some cases, however, advanced imaging studies such as MRI, CT, or nuclear medicine scans may be required.

The hip joint, consisting of the articulation between the cartilaginous surfaces of the femoral head and the pelvic acetabulum, is a diarthrodial, synovial ball-and-socket joint (**Figure 1**). The acetabulum is formed by the confluence of the ilium, the ischium, and the pubis, and the articular surface that is created is horseshoe shaped. The proximal femur consists of the femoral head and neck and the greater and lesser trochanters. The greater trochanter is a large bony prominence found at the lateral base of the femoral neck; it serves as the attachment site for the abductor musculature (the gluteus medius and minimus). The lesser trochanter is a smaller bony prominence located on the medial aspect of the proximal femur; it serves as the attachment site for the iliopsoas tendon (a powerful hip flexor).

Radiographic examination of the hip should include an AP radiograph of the pelvis and either a frog-lateral view of the pelvis

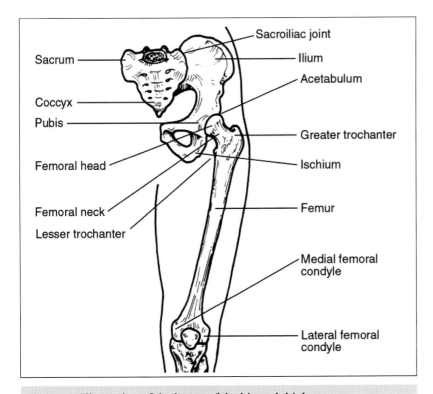

Figure 1 Illustration of the bones of the hip and thigh.

or AP and lateral radiographs of the involved hip. Radiographs should be evaluated carefully for displaced or nondisplaced fractures, degenerative changes of the hip joint (including joint space narrowing), hip dysplasia, and changes in bony architecture, such as lytic or blastic lesions that could suggest a primary or metastatic tumor.

Type of Pain

Pain arising from the hip joint may be secondary to osteoarthritis, osteonecrosis, inflammatory conditions such as rheumatoid arthritis, septic arthritis, fractures of the proximal femur or pelvis, or dislocations of the femoral head. Patients with these conditions usually report pain in the groin or the anterior aspect of the proximal thigh, but pain may be present in the buttock or lateral aspect of the thigh or may be referred to the supracondylar region of the knee. Hip joint pathology is often associated with a decrease in range of motion that in degenerative conditions is associated with difficulty in activities such as putting on shoes. A limp also may be present, and patients with traumatic injuries (such as proximal femoral or pelvic fractures) are typically unable to bear weight on the extremity and are unable to perform a straight leg raise.

Problems involving the bony pelvis include traumatic high-energy fractures, insufficiency fractures associated with osteoporosis, stress fractures, avulsion fractures from attached tendons, and primary or metastatic tumors. Problems involving both the hip joint and bony pelvis often manifest as pain in the groin, buttock, or lateral thigh.

Conditions that affect the soft tissues around the hip, such as trochanteric bursitis, lateral femoral cutaneous nerve impingement, and snapping hip syndrome, typically cause pain on the lateral or anterolateral aspect of the proximal thigh. Patients with an injury of the adductor muscles will note pain in the groin; hamstring injuries are associated with pain in the buttock or posterior aspect of the thigh.

The sacroiliac (SI) joint is relatively immobile. Some individuals have been found to experience more SI mobility than others and may experience SI pain. High-energy injuries such as high-energy pelvic ring disruption can lead to significant SI pain. Other conditions that involve the SI joint, such as scronegative arthritides or traumatic arthritis, can cause buttock and posterior thigh pain but are unlikely to restrict function.

Pathology in the lumbar spine may present as referred pain to the buttock and posterior thigh or as pain that radiates down the ipsilateral extremity in a radicular pattern. Patients with degenerative problems of the lumbar spine or strains of the lumbar musculature may have pain limited to the buttock, whereas disorders that cause entrapment of the spinal nerves (such as disk herniations) will cause pain that radiates in a dermatomal pattern. With these conditions, patients typically do not have symptoms referable to the groin, significant discomfort with rotation of the hip, or limited range of motion of the hip joint, although they often present with what they describe as "pain in the hip."

Nonmusculoskeletal pathology may present as groin or hip pain and should be considered in the differential diagnosis, especially if the source of pain is found not to be the hip. Constitutional symptoms such as fever, chills, and weight loss suggest the possibility of malignancy or infection. Inguinal or abdominal hernias and rectus abdominis strains may present with pain in the groin or anterior thigh and may be difficult for the patient to distinguish from hip pathology. Gastrointestinal disorders such as inflammatory bowel disease, diverticulosis, diverticulitis, or appendicitis may mimic hip pain. Pain from abdominal aortic aneurysms may mimic groin pain. Urinary tract infections or nephrolithiasis may refer pain to the hip region.

Pathology of the reproductive system also may present as pain in the groin or hip area. Prostatitis, epididymitis, hydroceles, varicoceles, testicular torsions, and testicular neoplasms have been known to cause groin pain in men. Ectopic pregnancy, dysmenorrhea, endometriosis, and pelvic inflammatory disease may cause pain in the hip or groin area in women. Pelvic floor muscles that are weak or too tight can produce hip, buttock, or groin pain. The patient should be referred to the appropriate specialist if any of these disorders is suspected.

Gait

A brief examination of the patient's gait can be very helpful in making a diagnosis. Ask the patient to walk up and down the hall several times at a brisk pace. An abductor or gluteus medius lurch is manifested by a lateral shift of the body to the weight-bearing side with ambulation. This type of gait often occurs in patients who have intra-articular hip pathology (osteoarthritis, inflammatory arthritis, or osteonecrosis of the hip). Pain associated with a limp suggests pathology around the pelvis or hip and requires further investigation.

Musculoskeletal Conditioning of the Hip

A conditioning program consists of three basic phases: stretching exercises, to improve range of motion; strengthening, to improve muscle power; and proprioception, to enhance balance and agility. The exercise session should begin with an active warm-up. Plyometric exercises may be added for power after basic strength and flexibility have been achieved. Patient handouts can be provided for the stretching and strengthening exercises. Advanced proprioceptive exercises and plyometric exercises should be done under the supervision of a rehabilitation specialist or other exercise professional.

The goal of a conditioning program is to improve overall function, thus enabling a more fit and healthy lifestyle. A well-structured conditioning program will prepare the individual for participation in sports and recreational activities. The greater the intensity of the activity that the individual wishes to engage in, the greater the

SECTION 5   HIP AND THIGH

intensity of the conditioning required. If the individual participates in a supervised rehabilitation program, the focus should be on proper exercise technique, advancing conditioning as tolerated, and developing a comprehensive home exercise fitness program. A well-rounded conditioning program should include shoulder, hip, knee, foot, back, and core exercises and is described in Musculoskeletal Conditioning: Helping Patients Prevent Injury and Stay Fit in the General Orthopaedics section.

An exercise program for conditioning of the hip should include an active warm-up; stretching, strengthening, and proprioceptive exercises; and, after basic stretching and strengthening have been achieved, plyometrics for power.

Active Warm-Up
The hip muscle groups are large and require an adequate warm-up, such as riding on a stationary bicycle or jogging for 10 minutes to raise the core body temperature. In addition, dynamic stretching exercises such as leg swings can be used to warm up the synovial fluid in the hip joint and actively stretch the muscles before activity.

Strengthening Exercises
Exercises that isolate muscle contraction and do not stimulate co-contractions are important for strengthening the hip muscles. In general, weight-bearing exercises produce co-contractions, and non–weight-bearing exercises do not. Co-contractions are important for stabilizing the joint that is being strengthened. Strengthening of the large hip muscle groups requires heavier weights and few (6 to 12) repetitions. After beginning with a weight that allows the patient to perform 6 to 8 repetitions initially, working up to 12 repetitions should be the goal of the strengthening phase. The exercises described below isolate the gluteus medius (posterior fibers), the gluteus maximus, and the internal and external rotators, which often are weak and can contribute to hip pathology.

Static Stretching Exercises
Static stretching should be done to increase the flexibility of the muscles surrounding the hip. A static stretch is performed at the end of the available range of painless motion of the muscle and joint.

Neuromuscular and Proprioceptive Conditioning
Conditioning programs should enhance neuromuscular control, balance, and functional performance. The program should consist of balance exercises, dynamic joint stability exercises, jump and landing training/plyometric exercises, agility drills, and sport-specific exercises. Neuromuscular training improves the ability to generate fast and optimal muscle firing patterns to improve dynamic joint stability and relearn or improve movement patterns necessary for

sports and activities of daily living. Proprioception training improves the awareness of the limb/joint position and joint movement. Training includes balance and perturbation exercises. Balance involves the visual, vestibular, and proprioceptive systems. With balance training, the athlete consciously attempts to hold a posture for 30 to 60 seconds. These exercises might include balancing on one leg or balancing on one leg while touching the other foot to different points within reach on the ground. With perturbation training, the athlete stands on an unstable surface such as a balance board while it is being perturbed by an outside force. Jumping exercises, such as jumping forward and backward over a barrier, are a basic form of plyometrics. These should be attempted only by individuals with full range of motion and adequate strength in the hip, pelvic and abdominal, and back muscles. These types of plyometric and proprioceptive exercises should be supervised by a rehabilitation specialist or other exercise professional.

SECTION 5 HIP AND THIGH

www.aaos.org/essentials5/exercises

Home Exercise Program for Hip Conditioning

- Before beginning the conditioning program, warm up the muscles and the hip joint by riding a stationary bicycle or jogging for 10 minutes and performing leg swings as follows: While standing, swing one leg forward and backward 10 times and then side-to-side 10 times. Repeat with the opposite leg. Place one hand against a wall for balance if needed.
- When performing the stretching exercises, stretch slowly to the limit of motion, taking care to avoid pain. If you experience pain with the exercises, call your doctor.
- After performing the active warm-up and strengthening exercises, perform static stretching exercises to maintain or increase flexibility.
- The following exercise program is introductory only, and progression of this program will vary based on your specific injury, symptoms, and baseline level of fitness. For further progression of this routine, your physician may recommend evaluation and treatment by a physical therapist or other exercise professional.

Home Exercises for Hip Conditioning

Exercise	Muscle Group	Number of Repetitions/Sets	Number of Days per Week
Strengthening			
Hip extension (prone)	Gluteus maximus	6 to 8 repetitions, progressing to 12 repetitions	3 to 4
Side-lying hip abduction	Gluteus medius	6 to 8 repetitions, progressing to 12 repetitions	3 to 4
Internal hip rotation	Medial hamstrings	6 to 8 repetitions, progressing to 12 repetitions	3 to 4
External hip rotation	Piriformis	6 to 8 repetitions, progressing to 12 repetitions	3 to 4
Stretching			
Seat side straddle	Adductor muscles Medial hamstrings Semitendinosus Semimembranosus	4 repetitions/2 to 3 sets	Daily
Modified seat side straddle	Hamstrings Adductor muscles	4 repetitions/2 to 3 sets	Daily
Hamstring stretch	Hamstrings	4 repetitions/2 to 3 sets	Daily
Sitting rotation stretch	Piriformis External rotators Internal rotators	4 repetitions/2 to 3 sets	Daily
Knee to chest	Posterior hip muscles	4 repetitions/2 to 3 sets	Daily
Leg crossover	Hamstrings	4 repetitions/2 to 3 sets	Daily
Crossover stand	Hamstrings	4 repetitions/2 to 3 sets	Daily
Iliotibial band stretch	Tensor fascia	4 repetitions/2 to 3 sets	Daily
Foam roller for iliotibial band	Iliotibial band	Once per side, for 2 to 3 minutes each	Daily
Quadriceps stretch (prone)	Quadriceps	4 repetitions/2 to 3 sets	Daily

Strengthening Exercises

Hip Extension (Prone)

- Lie face down with a pillow under your hips and one knee bent 90°. Elevate the leg off the floor, lifting the leg straight up with the knee bent.
- Lower the leg to the floor slowly, to a count of 5. Ankle weights should be used, starting with a weight light enough to allow 6 to 8 repetitions and working up to 12 repetitions.
- Repeat on the other side.
- Perform the exercise 3 to 4 days per week.
- After you have worked up to 12 repetitions, add as much weight as can be lifted only 8 times and work up to 12 repetitions again. Continue this cycle of adding weight and increasing repetitions.

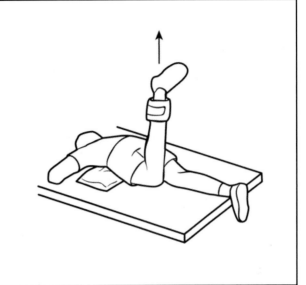

Side-Lying Hip Abduction

- Lie on your side while cradling your head in your arm. Bend the bottom leg for support.
- Slowly move the top leg up and back to 45°, keeping the knee straight. Lower the leg slowly, to a count of 5, and relax it for 2 seconds. Ankle weights should be used, starting with a weight light enough to allow 6 to 8 repetitions and working up to 12 repetitions.
- Repeat on the other side.
- Perform the exercise 3 to 4 days per week.
- After you have worked up to 12 repetitions, add as much weight as can be lifted only 8 times and progress to 12 repetitions again. Continue this cycle of adding weight and increasing repetitions.

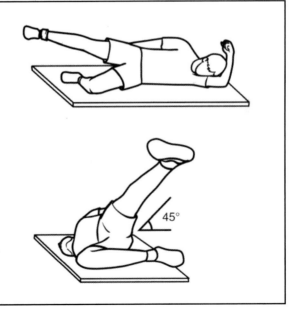

SECTION 5   HIP AND THIGH

SECTION 5 HIP AND THIGH

Internal Hip Rotation

- Lie on your side on a table with a pillow between your thighs. Bend the top leg 90° at the hip and 90° at the knee.
- Start with the foot of the top leg below the level of the top of the table; lift to the finish position, which is rotated as high as possible.
- Lower the leg slowly, to a count of 5. Ankle weights should be used, starting with a weight light enough to allow 6 to 8 repetitions, working up to 12 repetitions.
- Repeat on the other side.
- Perform the exercise 3 to 4 days per week.
- After you have worked up to 12 repetitions, add as much weight as can be lifted only 8 times and progress to 12 repetitions again. Continue this cycle of adding weight and increasing repetitions.

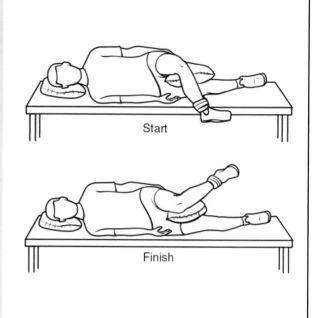

Start

Finish

External Hip Rotation

- Lie on your side on a table with the bottom leg bent 90° at the hip and 90° at the knee.
- Start with the foot below the level of the top of the table; lift to the finish position, which is rotated as high as possible.
- Lower the leg slowly, to a count of 5. Ankle weights should be used, starting with a weight light enough to allow 6 to 8 repetitions and working up to 12 repetitions.
- Repeat on the other side.
- Perform the exercise 3 to 4 days per week.
- After you have worked up to 12 repetitions, add as much weight as can be lifted only 8 times and progress to 12 repetitions again. Continue this cycle of adding weight and increasing repetitions.

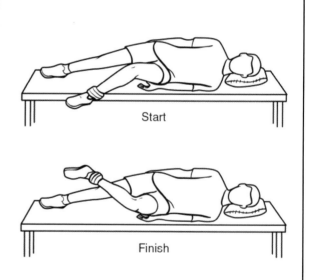

Start

Finish

Stretching Exercises

Seat Side Straddle

- Sit on the floor with your legs spread apart.
- Place both hands on the same knee and slide your hands down the shin toward the ankle until a stretch is felt in the back of the leg. Hold the stretch for 30 seconds and then relax for 30 seconds.
- Attempt to keep your back straight and bend from the hips.
- Repeat on the other side.
- Repeat the sequence 4 times, performing 2 to 3 sets per day.

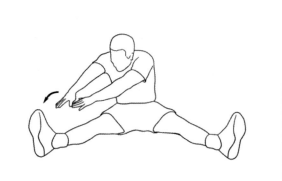

Modified Seat Side Straddle

- Sit on the floor with one leg extended to the side and the other leg bent as shown.
- Place both hands on the knee of your straight leg and slide the hands down the shin toward the ankle until a stretch is felt in the back of the leg. Hold the stretch for 30 seconds and then relax for 30 seconds.
- Attempt to keep your back straight and bend from the hips.
- Reverse leg positions and repeat on the other side.
- Repeat the sequence 4 times, performing 2 to 3 sets per day.

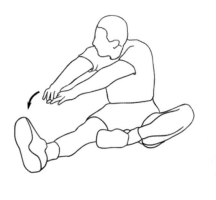

Hamstring Stretch

- Lie on your back with one leg straight and with a strap around your other foot.
- Keeping your knee straight, pull the strap until a gentle stretch is felt in the back of the leg. Hold the stretch for 30 seconds and then return the leg to the resting position on the table or floor and relax for 30 seconds.
- Repeat with the other leg.
- Repeat the sequence 4 times per leg.
- Perform 2 to 3 sets per day.

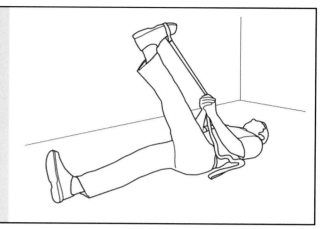

Sitting Rotation Stretch

- Sit on the floor with both legs straight out in front of you.
- Cross one leg over the other, place the elbow of the opposite arm on the outside of the thigh, and support yourself with your other arm behind you.
- Rotate your head and body in the direction of the supporting arm. A gentle stretch will be felt in the outside of the buttock or thigh. Hold the stretch for 30 seconds and then relax for 30 seconds.
- Reverse positions and repeat the stretch on the other side.
- Repeat the sequence 4 times.
- Perform 2 to 3 sets per day.

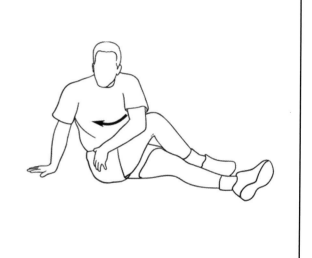

Knee to Chest

- Lie on your back on the floor with your legs straight.
- Grasp one knee and slowly bring it toward your chest as far as it will go. You will feel a stretch in the buttock or back of the leg. Hold the stretch for 30 seconds and then relax for 30 seconds.
- Repeat with the other leg; then do both legs together.
- Repeat the sequence 4 times.
- Perform 2 to 3 sets per day.

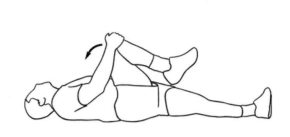

Leg Crossover

- Lie on the floor with your legs spread and your arms at your sides.
- Keeping the leg straight, bring your right toe to your left hand.
- Try to keep the other leg flat on the floor, although you may bend it slightly if needed for comfort. Hold the stretch for 30 seconds and then relax for 30 seconds.
- Repeat with the left leg and the right hand.
- Repeat the sequence 4 times.
- Perform 2 to 3 sets per day.

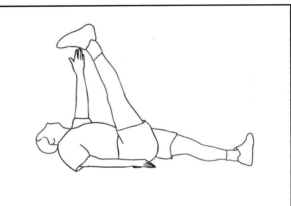

Crossover Stand

- Stand with your legs crossed, with your feet close together and your legs straight.
- Slowly bend forward and try to touch your toes. You will feel the stretch in the back of the leg that is positioned behind. Hold the stretch for 30 seconds and then relax for 30 seconds.
- Repeat with the position of the legs reversed.
- Repeat the sequence 4 times.
- Perform 2 to 3 sets per day.

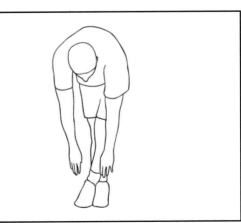

SECTION 5   HIP AND THIGH

Iliotibial Band Stretch

- Stand next to a wall for support.
- Begin with your weight distributed evenly over both feet, and then cross one leg behind the other.
- Lean the hip of the crossed-over leg toward the wall until you feel a stretch on the outside of the leg. Hold the stretch for 30 seconds and then relax for 30 seconds.
- Repeat on the opposite side.
- Repeat the sequence 4 times.
- Perform 2 to 3 sets per day.

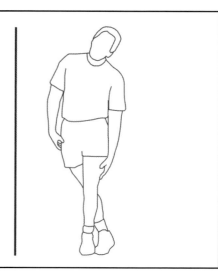

Foam Roller for Iliotibial Band

- Position the foam roller under the outside of your thigh.
- Use your arms to slowly move the lateral or outside portion of your thigh over the foam roller.
- The foam roller should move slowly. Stop and hold the position for 5 to 10 seconds at areas of tightness or discomfort, then proceed up and down the outer thigh.
- Avoid rolling over the bony prominence of the outer hip (arrow) or the knee (double arrow).
- Mild to severe discomfort may be present but should improve with consistent daily use of the foam roller. If the discomfort does not improve within 1 to 2 weeks, seek the advice of your sports medicine physician.
- Perform every day, for 2 to 3 minutes on each leg.

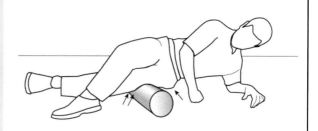

SECTION 5 | **HIP AND THIGH**

Quadriceps Stretch (Prone)

- Lie on your stomach with your arms at your sides and your legs straight.
- Bend one knee to bring your foot up toward your buttocks and grasp the ankle with the hand on the same side.
- Pull on the ankle. The stretch will be felt on the front of the thigh. Hold the stretch for 30 seconds and then relax for 30 seconds.
- Repeat on the opposite side.
- Repeat the sequence 4 times.
- Perform 2 to 3 sets per day.

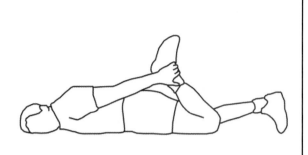

Physical Examination of the Hip and Thigh

Inspection/Palpation

Anterior View

With the patient standing, look for atrophy of the anterior thigh musculature and note the overall alignment of the hip, knee, and ankle.

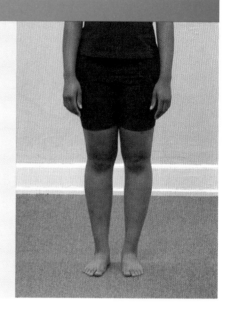

Posterior View

With the patient standing, look for atrophy of the buttock and posterior thigh musculature. Note any pelvic obliquity (one iliac crest lower than the opposite side). Limb-length discrepancy will cause one iliac crest to be lower than the other, but this apparent obliquity can be corrected by placing blocks under the shorter limb. Fixed pelvic obliquity from a spinal deformity cannot be corrected by this maneuver. Palpate the iliac crests, the posterior iliac spine (deep to the dimples of Venus), and the greater trochanter. A Trendelenburg test can be conducted at this time to determine gluteus medius weakness. For the Trendelenburg test, the patient is instructed to stand first on one leg and then the other for comparison. With normal hip abductor strength, the pelvis will stay level or the side opposite the stance leg will elevate slightly. With abductor weakness in the stance leg, the contralateral iliac crest will drop. This is a positive Trendelenburg test.

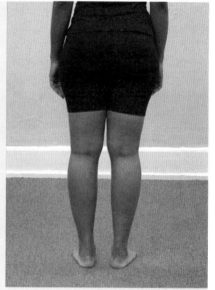

Gait

To assess gait, observe the patient walk across the room. Hip deformities often cause a limp that can range in severity from barely detectable to a marked swaying of the trunk and slowing of gait. Patients with a painful hip joint may have an antalgic gait; that is, they shorten the stance phase on the affected side to avoid placing weight across the painful joint. A Trendelenburg gait, characterized by a lateral shift of the body weight, is seen in patients with weakness of the abductor musculature and can be seen in degenerative disorders of the hip. As the hip joint degenerates and friction within the hip joint increases, it becomes more difficult for the abductor musculature to level the pelvis during gait.

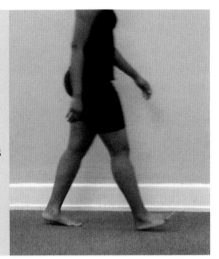

Anterior View, Supine

With the patient supine, palpate to identify any masses, abnormal adenopathy, or tenderness in the region of the anterior superior iliac spine (ASIS) or greater trochanter. (The examiner is palpating the ASIS in the photograph.) Patients with avulsion of the sartorius or rectus femoris will report tenderness at or directly inferior to the ASIS. Patients with meralgia paresthetica (entrapment of the lateral femoral cutaneous nerve) will report tenderness immediately medial to the ASIS and hypoesthesia over the distal lateral thigh.

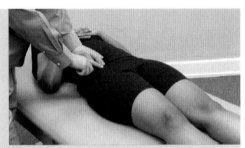

Patients who report a popping sensation in the hip while ambulating most likely have a thickened or tight iliotibial band that snaps over the greater trochanter as the hip moves into flexion and internal rotation. Have the patient re-create the snapping, and palpate the iliotibial band as it snaps over the greater trochanter. This may be visible (and at times can be seen from across the room).

Lateral View, Side-Lying

Place the patient in a side-lying position on the unaffected side to facilitate the examination. Structures in the region of the greater trochanter may be palpated with the patient in the supine position, but examination of this area is easier with the patient lying on the unaffected side. Tenderness to palpation directly over the greater trochanter reproduces pain with greater trochanteric bursitis. Tenderness at the proximal tip of the trochanter may indicate gluteus medius tendinitis. Tenderness at the posterior margin of the trochanter may indicate external rotator tendinitis.

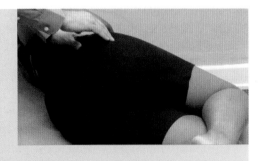

SECTION 5 HIPANDTHIGH

Range of Motion

Flexion: Zero Starting Position

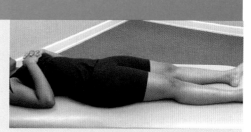

To evaluate hip flexion, the patient is supine on a firm, flat surface with the opposite hip held in enough flexion to flatten the lumbar spine. Flattening the lumbar spine prevents excessive lordosis, which may camouflage a hip flexion contracture. Avoid positioning the opposite hip in excessive flexion, as this will rock the pelvis into abnormal posterior inclination, thereby creating a false-positive hip flexion contracture. Instead, flex the opposite hip to a position where the lumbar spine just starts to flatten or, more precisely, to a position where the inclination of the pelvis is similar to that of a normal standing posture (that is, the anterior superior iliac spine is inferior to the posterior iliac spine by only 2° to 3°).

Maximum Flexion

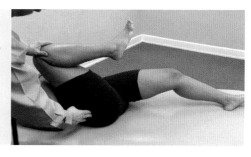

Maximum hip flexion is the point at which the pelvis begins to rotate. Normal hip flexion in adults is 110° to 130°.

Hip Flexion Contracture—Thomas Test

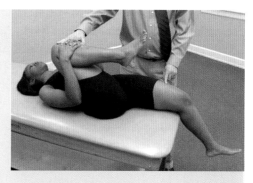

The Thomas test is used to evaluate for hip flexion contracture or psoas tightness. Begin with the patient sitting at the end of the examination table with the legs extending far enough that when the patient lies supine, the table edge will not contact the posterior aspect of the calves. Have the patient then assume a supine position, with the legs hanging off the end of the table. Instruct the patient to pull one hip into maximum flexion. Observe the contralateral hip to see if it also flexes off the surface of the table. A normal hip will remain on the table or flex very slightly. Greater flexion indicates psoas tightness or a flexion contracture.

Abduction and Adduction: Zero Starting Position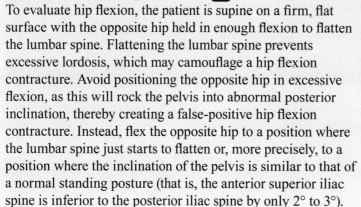

The zero starting position is with the pelvis level; the limbs are at a 90° angle to a transverse line across the anterior superior iliac spines.

SECTION 5   HIPANDTHIGH

Abduction

To assess hip abduction, a goniometer is needed. Start with the patient supine and the limbs at a 90° angle to a transverse line across the anterior superior iliac spines. Abduct the leg until maximum abduction is reached, which is when the pelvis begins to tilt, a movement that you can detect by keeping your hand on the patient's opposite anterior superior iliac spine when moving the leg. Normal hip abduction in adults is 35° to 50°.

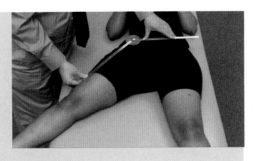

Adduction

To measure adduction, a goniometer is needed. Start with the patient supine. Flex the opposite extremity to allow adduction of the affected extremity (**A**). Maximum adduction is reached when the pelvis starts to rotate. If flexing the opposite extremity is impractical, measure adduction by moving the affected extremity over the top of the opposite limb (**B**). Normal hip adduction in adults is 25° to 35°.

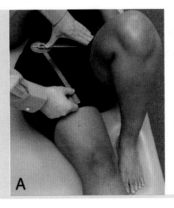
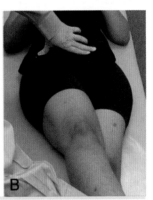

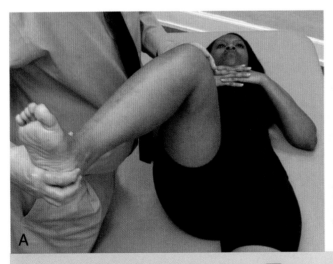
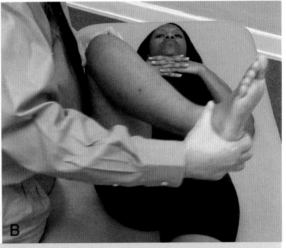

Internal-External Rotation in Flexion

In adults, measure hip rotation with the hips in flexion; however, this technique should not be used in children or when assessment of femoral torsion or a more precise measurement of hip rotation in a "walking" position is required.

To evaluate hip rotation in flexion, with the patient supine, flex the hip and knee to 90°, with the thigh held perpendicular to the transverse line across the anterior superior iliac spines. Measure internal rotation by rotating the tibia away from the midline of the trunk, thus producing inward rotation of the hip (**A**). Measure external rotation by rotating the tibia toward the midline of the trunk, thus producing external rotation at the hip (**B**).

SECTION 5   HIPANDTHIGH

Hamstring Flexibility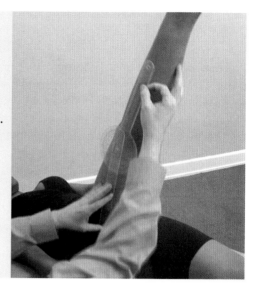

With the patient supine and the contralateral hip and knee maintained in full extension, instruct the patient to flex the hip to 90° and then, while maintaining this position, actively extend the knee fully. Patients unable to obtain within 10° of full knee extension are considered to have hamstring tightness.

Muscle Testing

Hip Flexors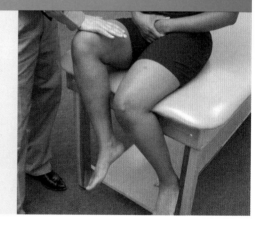

To assess the hip flexor muscles, ask the seated patient to flex the hip upward as you resist the effort with your hand by pushing down on the distal thigh just above the knee.

Hip Extensors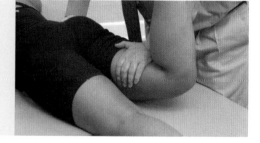

To assess the hip extensor muscles, with the patient prone, place the patient's knee in approximately 90° of flexion and ask the patient to extend the hip as you resist the effort with your hand by pushing against the distal thigh.

Hip Abductors

To assess the hip abductors, have the patient lie on the unaffected side. Ask the patient to abduct the hip as you resist the effort with your hand on the lateral aspect of the distal thigh. Note that hip abductor strength also can be assessed using the Trendelenburg test.

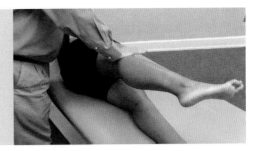

Hip Adductors

To assess the hip adductors, with the patient supine, place your hand on the medial aspect of the distal thigh and ask the patient to adduct the hip as you resist the effort.

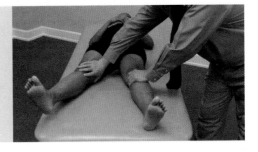

Special Tests

Trendelenburg Test

The Trendelenburg test is used to evaluate hip abductor strength, primarily the gluteus medius. Stand behind the patient to observe the level of the pelvis. Ask the patient to stand on one leg. With normal hip abductor strength, the pelvis will remain level. If hip abductor strength is inadequate on the stance limb side, the pelvis will drop below level on the opposite side, indicating a positive test.

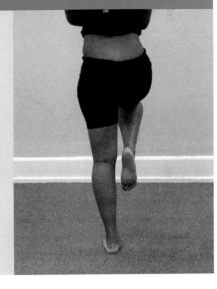

SECTION 5 HIPANDTHIGH

FABER Test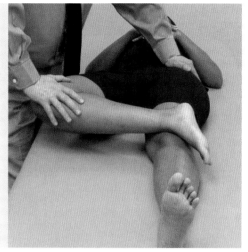

The FABER (flexion-abduction-external rotation) test, sometimes called the figure-of-4 test, Patrick test, or Jansen test, is a stress maneuver to detect hip and sacroiliac pathology. With the patient supine, place the affected hip in flexion, abduction, and external rotation with the patient's foot on the opposite knee. Stabilize the pelvis with your hand on the contralateral anterior superior iliac spine and press down on the thigh of the affected side. If the maneuver is painful, the hip or sacroiliac region may be affected. Increased pain with this test also may be a nonorganic finding.

Log Roll Test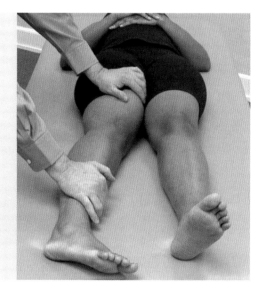

With the patient supine, internally and externally rotate the relaxed lower extremity. Pain in the anterior hip or groin, particularly with internal rotation, is considered a positive result. A positive test may indicate acetabular or femoral neck pathology, such as in osteoarthritis or femoral head osteonecrosis.

Piriformis Test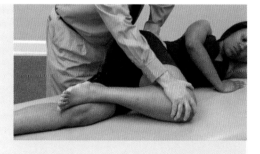

With the patient lying on the unaffected side and the hip and knee flexed to approximately 90°, stabilize the pelvis with one hand and use your other hand to apply flexion, adduction, and internal rotation pressure at the knee, pushing it to the examination table. If a tight piriformis is impinging on the sciatic nerve, pain may be produced in the buttock and even down the leg.

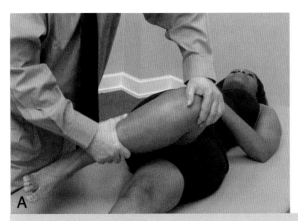
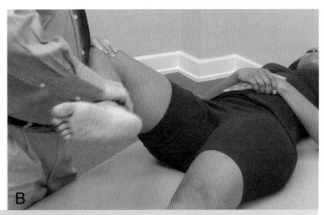

Scouring Test 📹

With the patient supine and the hip flexed and adducted, use the patient's knee and thigh to apply a posterolateral force through the hip as the femur is rotated in the acetabulum. **A,** Passively flex, adduct, and internally rotate the hip while longitudinally compressing to scour the inner aspect of the joint. **B,** To scour the outer aspect, abduct and externally rotate the hip while maintaining flexion during longitudinal compression. Pain or a grating sound or sensation is a positive result and may indicate labral pathology, a loose body, or other internal derangement.

SECTION 5 HIPANDTHIGH

Dislocation of the Hip (Acute, Traumatic)

Definition

Dislocation of the hip occurs when the femoral head is displaced from the acetabulum. Because of its strong capsule and deep acetabulum, the hip is rarely dislocated in adults. The causative injury usually is high-energy trauma, such as a motor vehicle accident or a fall from a height. Posterior dislocations (femoral head posterior to the acetabulum) are far more common than anterior dislocations, accounting for more than 90% of these injuries.

Clinical Symptoms

Dislocation of the hip is a severe injury. Patients have pain and are typically unable to move the lower extremity. Patients often have other associated musculoskeletal injuries, and there is a high prevalence of associated head, intra-abdominal, and chest injuries.

Tests

Physical Examination

A posterior dislocation results in the affected limb being short, with the hip fixed in a position of flexion, adduction, and internal rotation (**Figure 1**). The status of the distal pulses and the function of the sciatic and femoral nerves should be assessed. Sciatic nerve palsies are common (8% to 20% incidence), with the peroneal division of the sciatic nerve most commonly affected.

With an anterior dislocation, the hip assumes a position of mild flexion, abduction, and external rotation. Femoral nerve palsy may be present, but nerve injuries are less frequent with anterior dislocations.

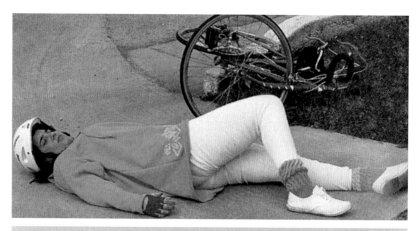

Figure 1 Photograph of the clinical appearance of an individual with a posterior dislocation of the right hip. (Reproduced with permission from Pollak AN, Barnes L, Cioltola JA, Gulli B, eds: *Emergency Care and Transportation of the Sick and Injured*, ed 10. Rosemont, IL, American Academy of Orthopaedic Surgeons, 2010, p 1042.)

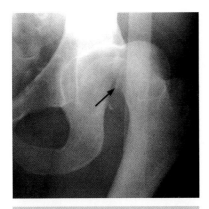

Figure 2 AP radiograph demonstrates posterior dislocation of the left hip with an associated fracture of the femoral head (arrow).

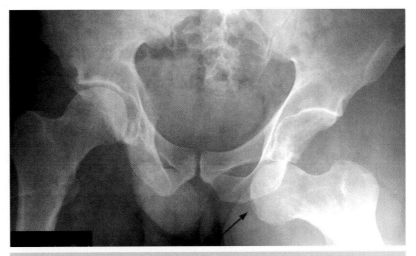

Figure 3 AP radiograph of the pelvis demonstrates an anterior dislocation of the left hip (arrow).

Inspect the extremity for abrasions about the anterior aspect of the knee or for a knee effusion. Significant knee ligament injuries are commonly associated with hip dislocations because most hip dislocations typically occur from a direct blow to the flexed hip and knee. An associated fracture of the ipsilateral femur or acetabulum may be present.

Diagnostic Tests

Radiographs should include an AP view of the pelvis and AP and lateral views of the femur, including the knee. In the normal pelvis, the size of the femoral heads and joint spaces will be symmetric on AP radiographs. With a posterior hip dislocation (**Figure 2**), the affected femoral head appears smaller than the contralateral, normal femoral head; with an anterior hip dislocation (**Figure 3**), the affected femoral head appears larger. Associated fractures of the acetabulum (particularly fractures of the posterior wall) are common; in these cases, a CT scan should be obtained to fully define the fracture pattern (**Figure 4**). Following reduction of the dislocation, it is imperative to ensure that the reduction is completely concentric without interposition of associated bony fragments or residual subluxation; if there are any questions regarding these parameters, a CT scan should be obtained.

Differential Diagnosis

• Fracture of the acetabulum or pelvis (pain in the groin and/or buttock)
• Fracture of the hip or shaft of the femur (pain in the groin, buttock, and thigh)

SECTION 5   HIP AND THIGH

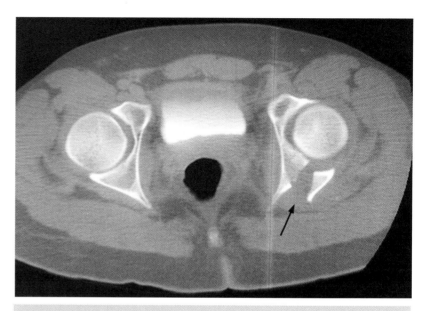

Figure 4 CT scan of the pelvis demonstrates a displaced fracture of the posterior wall of the acetabulum (arrow).

Adverse Outcomes of the Disease

Osteonecrosis of the femoral head is the most common early complication and occurs in approximately 10% of patients. Dislocation of the hip joint tears the hip capsule and disrupts the blood supply to the femoral head; a delay in reduction or incomplete reduction increases the risk of osteonecrosis. Osteonecrosis may not be apparent for as long as 2 or 3 years after the injury; therefore, these patients require follow-up over several years. Posttraumatic arthritis (secondary to the severe impact to the cartilaginous surfaces), sciatic or femoral nerve injury, and chronic pain can occur.

Treatment

An acute traumatic hip dislocation is an emergency. A reduction should be performed as soon as possible to decrease the risk of osteonecrosis. The reduction should be performed in an atraumatic fashion to avoid damage to the articular cartilage or fracture of the femoral head or acetabulum. Associated fractures of the femoral head or intra-articular loose bodies should be ruled out before the reduction is performed. Repeat radiographs and, frequently, a postreduction CT scan are necessary to identify unrecognized intra-articular bony fragments and to confirm a perfectly concentric reduction; if bony fragments are identified within the joint, they must be surgically removed. Nerve and vascular function should be carefully evaluated and documented both before and after the reduction. Postreduction treatment of an uncomplicated dislocated hip is early crutch-assisted ambulation with weight bearing as tolerated until the patient is pain free, usually 2 to 4 weeks after the injury. Patients should then begin hip abduction and extension exercises and use a walking aid in the hand opposite the involved hip until they can walk without a limp. Associated fractures of the acetabulum often require surgical treatment to ensure that adequate stability has been restored to the joint; small retained bony fragments often can be removed arthroscopically.

Adverse Outcomes of Treatment

Despite a rapid closed reduction, osteonecrosis can still occur. The impact of the injury itself may cause severe damage to the cartilaginous surfaces of the femoral head or the acetabulum, resulting in posttraumatic arthritis. A delay in time to reduction or incomplete reduction increases the risk of osteonecrosis of the femoral head. Even when a rapid, closed complete reduction is performed, osteonecrosis can occur. Articular cartilage damage or femoral head and acetabulum fractures can occur during reduction.

Referral Decisions/Red Flags

All traumatic dislocations of the hip are serious injuries requiring immediate attention.

SECTION 5   HIP AND THIGH

Fracture of the Femoral Shaft

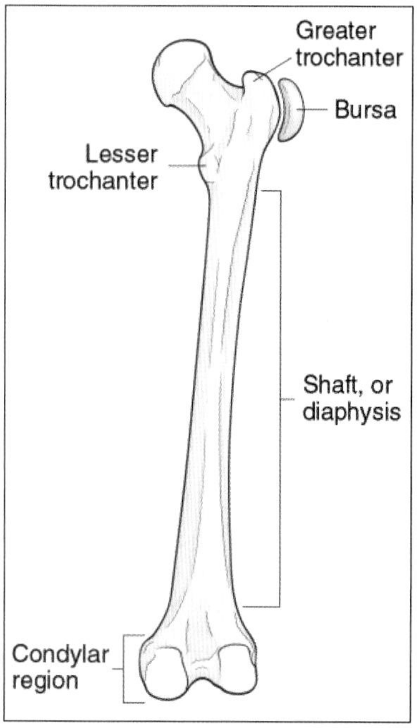

Figure 1 Illustration of the anatomy of the femur.

Definition

The shaft, or diaphysis, of the femur is defined as the portion of the femur from the subtrochanteric region to the supracondylar area (**Figure 1**). In most adults, fractures of the femoral shaft are caused by high-energy trauma, such as a motor vehicle accident. As such, this injury is severe and is potentially associated with life-threatening pulmonary, intra-abdominal, and head injuries. Pathologic fractures of the femoral shaft are less common, occur in bone weakened by osteopenia or tumors, result from low-energy injuries such as a simple fall, and have a much lower incidence of associated complications.

Clinical Symptoms

Patients with femoral shaft fractures present with severe pain in the thigh along with an obvious deformity and are typically unable to move, let alone bear weight on the extremity. Patients who have sustained the injury as a result of high-energy trauma are likely to have multisystem injuries and may not be alert or able to respond to questioning.

Tests

Physical Examination

Inspect for deformity, swelling, and open injuries. It is important to recognize that a femoral shaft fracture can act as a distracting injury, causing the examiner to overlook other associated musculoskeletal injuries; thus, a thorough examination of the entire extremity is mandatory to rule out associated injuries. Ligamentous injuries of the ipsilateral knee are common; however, often the knee cannot be examined until the patient is anesthetized for surgical treatment. Evaluate and document the vascular status of the limb distal to the fracture. Assess function of the femoral, peroneal, and posterior tibial nerves. In the presence of deformity and vascular compromise, simple manual longitudinal traction should be applied to determine whether the deformity is the cause of the ischemia. Because these are typically high-energy injuries, standard Advanced Trauma Life Support (ATLS) protocols should be applied to evaluate for and potentially treat associated life-threatening injuries.

Diagnostic Tests

The fracture is confirmed by AP and lateral radiographs of the femur (**Figure 2**). High-energy trauma can disrupt adjacent joints; therefore, radiographs of the hip, knee, and pelvis must be obtained. It is particularly important to identify an ipsilateral fracture of the femoral neck because treatment options differ and failure to identify a concomitant femoral neck fracture can lead to nonunion of the femoral neck fracture or osteonecrosis of the femoral head (**Figure 3**). If vascular compromise is identified, arterial studies are required.

Differential Diagnosis
- Fracture of the pelvis, acetabulum, or proximal femur (evident on radiographs)
- Malignant or metastatic lesion of the femur (pain in the thigh with activity or at rest, evident on radiographs)
- Osteomyelitis with bone destruction (pain in the thigh, evident on radiographs)
- Soft-tissue injury without fracture (pain, swelling, ecchymosis of the thigh, pain with hip and/or knee motion)
- Stress fracture of the femur (pain in the thigh that increases with weight bearing; may be evident on plain radiographs, but MRI may be needed to confirm the diagnosis)

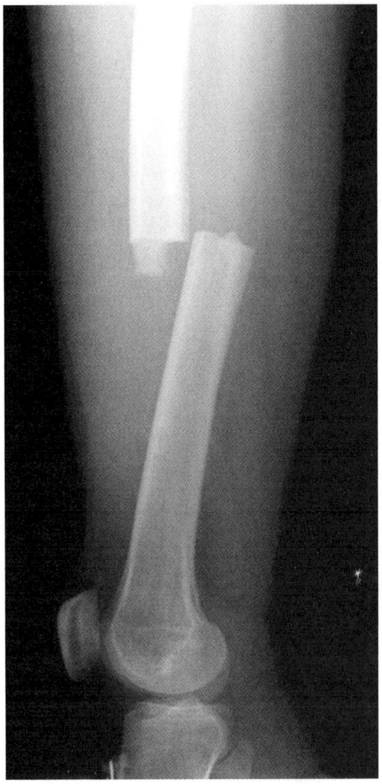

Adverse Outcomes of the Disease
The most significant adverse outcomes are those associated with high-energy trauma or long bone fractures, such as fat embolism, adult respiratory distress syndrome, and multisystem organ failure. An acute arterial injury may be life threatening and requires immediate recognition and treatment. Complications of open fractures, such as infection, may result in chronic osteomyelitis. Even if uneventful healing occurs, the high energy associated with these injuries may have long-lasting effects on associated soft tissues. Persistent pain, limp, and difficulty returning to jobs that require manual labor are not uncommon.

Treatment
Immediate, temporary splinting may be applied for comfort and to provide stabilization during transfers, followed by the application of skeletal traction until surgical intervention is undertaken. Skeletal traction pins can be applied to the distal femur or the proximal tibia. These provide patient comfort and prevent shortening of the extremity, which can be difficult to overcome after the fracture has been treated surgically. Surgical treatment is indicated for most patients to lessen the risk of pulmonary and other systemic complications related to recumbency. Patients with open fractures should receive appropriate tetanus prophylaxis along with immediate systemic antibiotic treatment, followed by emergent surgical débridement of the soft-tissue injury as soon as the patient is medically stabilized.

Adverse Outcomes of Treatment
Nonunion, malunion, and infection are potential problems with any fracture treated surgically.

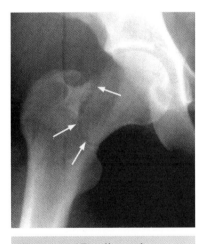

Figure 2 Lateral radiograph demonstrates a femoral shaft fracture.

Figure 3 AP radiograph demonstrates a femoral neck fracture (arrows) in a patient with a femoral shaft fracture in the same extremity caused by high-energy trauma.

SECTION 5 HIP AND THIGH

Referral Decisions/Red Flags

Femoral shaft fractures are markers of a high-energy traumatic injury and thus require appropriate evaluation and treatment of associated musculoskeletal, head, thoracic, and intra-abdominal injuries. Open injuries require special attention to ensure that appropriate tetanus prophylaxis and intravenous antibiotics are administered, along with prompt surgical débridement and fracture fixation.

SECTION 5   HIP AND THIGH

Fracture of the Pelvis

Definition

Pelvic fractures include fractures of the pelvic ring and the acetabulum. Pelvic injuries range in severity from stable, low-energy fractures (typically seen in older patients) that heal readily when treated nonsurgically to unstable, high-energy fractures that are associated with massive blood loss and resultant hemodynamic instability that can lead to death if not stabilized emergently. Stable pelvic ring fractures generally involve only one side of the pelvic ring. For example, a unilateral fracture of the superior and inferior pubic ramus is a stable injury. Unstable pelvic ring fractures disrupt the ring at two sites. For example, a fracture of a superior and inferior pubic ramus combined with a fracture of the sacrum or ilium is considered an unstable pelvic fracture. Another unstable pattern is disruption of the symphysis pubis combined with a fracture of the sacrum or disruption of one or both sacroiliac ligaments (**Figure 1**). Acetabular fractures are, by definition, intra-articular injuries that, if displaced, can lead to posttraumatic arthritis. Acetabular fractures usually are high-energy injuries.

Clinical Symptoms

Low-energy pelvic fractures are often seen in elderly patients. Presenting symptoms are similar to those in patients with a fracture

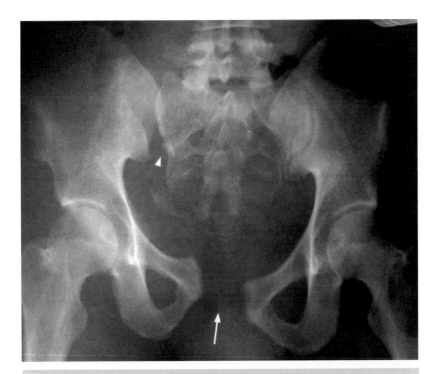

Figure 1 AP radiograph of the pelvis demonstrates an unstable pelvic fracture with disruption of the symphysis pubis (arrow) and sacroiliac joint (arrowhead).

of the proximal part of the femur, including pain in the groin with attempts at weight bearing or an inability to bear weight on the extremity. Pain is typically localized to the groin, the lateral hip, or the buttock area. Most pelvic and acetabular fractures are high-energy injuries and are associated with other musculoskeletal injuries as well as traumatic injuries to the head, chest, and abdomen.

Tests

Physical Examination

Low-energy pelvic fractures are associated with pain on attempted range of motion of the hip and on attempted straight leg raise. Patients who are able to ambulate have an antalgic gait pattern.

Patients with high-energy pelvic fractures require treatment in a trauma center with the application of standard trauma protocols, including an initial evaluation of the airway, breathing, and circulatory status. The cervical spine should be examined to ensure that there is no pain with attempted range of motion. The pelvic area should be inspected for swelling, ecchymosis, and obvious deformity as well as for lacerations, which may represent an open fracture of the pelvis. Palpation and gentle compression of the pelvis often will localize the area of injury. The neurovascular status of the lower extremities should be evaluated carefully because peripheral nerve injuries are not uncommon and pelvic fractures that involve the sacrum can directly damage the spinal nerve roots. Unstable fractures also may be associated with genitourinary injuries of the prostate and bladder. If blood is present in the perineal area, a urologic consultation should be obtained before placing a Foley catheter. A thorough history should be obtained, with special attention paid to any history of chest pain, palpitation, syncope, loss of consciousness, or shortness of breath that may have resulted in a fall. Appropriate referral is indicated if there is concern for associated medical conditions.

Diagnostic Tests

Standard trauma protocols include an AP radiograph of the chest, a lateral view of the cervical spine, and an AP view of the pelvis. The AP pelvis view typically identifies most pelvic fractures. If a pelvic fracture is seen on this view, pelvic inlet and outlet views (**Figure 2**) should be obtained to assist with identification of the injury pattern. If an acetabular fracture is demonstrated, oblique views of the pelvis are required to fully define the extent of the fracture. CT scans are often needed to define these complex injuries and plan for appropriate surgical intervention (**Figure 3**).

Differential Diagnosis

- Hip arthritis (pain in the groin or buttock, limited hip motion, evident on radiographs)
- Hip fracture (pain in the groin or buttock, shortened and externally rotated leg)

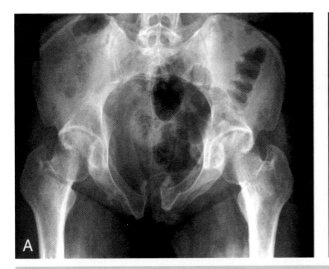 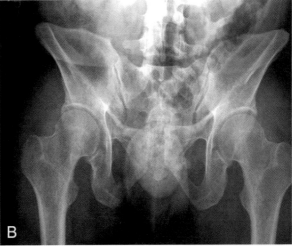

Figure 2 Pelvic inlet (**A**) and outlet (**B**) views are useful for determining rotational and vertical displacement of the pelvis. Note the displacement and rotation of the left pubic ramus on these radiographs.

- Hip strain (pain in the groin or buttock)
- Stress fracture of the pelvis or sacrum (MRI may be necessary for diagnosis)
- Tumors involving the bony pelvis or sacrum (pain in the low back, groin, rectum, and/or buttock; evident on radiographs)

Adverse Outcomes of the Disease

High-energy injuries are associated with a significant prevalence of associated musculoskeletal, head, chest, and abdominal trauma. These injuries may result in serious sequelae, including death. Associated genitourinary injuries are common and can lead to pain and/or sexual dysfunction. Neurologic injuries may be permanent, leading to abnormal motor and/or sensory dysfunction of the ipsilateral lower extremity. Although nonunion of these fractures is uncommon, malunion of the pelvis sometimes occurs and can lead to deformity of the pelvis and/or limb-length discrepancy with persistent pain. Acetabular fractures, classified as intra-articular injuries, can result in posttraumatic arthritis secondary to chondral injury that occurs when the femoral head strikes the acetabulum. This may occur even if the fracture is fixed anatomically with rigid internal fixation. Patients with pelvic ring and acetabular fractures are at substantial risk for thromboembolic complications. Even if these injuries proceed to uneventful bony union, the psychosocial implications of these injuries are substantial because many patients have persistent pain that can result in an occupation change.

Treatment

The treatment of pelvic fractures is determined by the degree of pelvic instability and the presence of associated injuries. Pelvic fractures associated with minor injuries, such as falls in the elderly patient, are common and typically have a stable pattern. Treatment

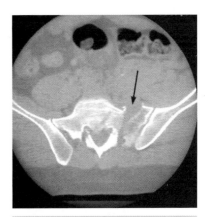

Figure 3 CT scan of the pelvis demonstrates an unstable fracture of the left side of the sacrum (arrow).

of these low-energy stable fractures consists of analgesics, relative rest, and gait training for protected weight bearing with a walker. It is important to monitor the patient and implement prophylactic measures to help prevent potential complications related to immobility, such as venous thromboembolism and skin breakdown. Most patients require protected weight bearing for approximately 6 weeks, until the pain has subsided and the fracture demonstrates early healing. These patients should also undergo evaluation and treatment of osteoporosis to prevent the occurrence of future fragility fractures.

High-energy pelvic fractures often are life threatening. Initial treatment focuses on hemodynamic resuscitation along with identification and treatment of associated injuries. As a temporizing measure, a sheet can be tautly and carefully applied around the patient's pelvis to decrease pelvic volume and effect a temporary reduction, thereby potentially reducing pelvic bleeding. After the patient is hemodynamically stable, skeletal traction may be used for patient comfort and to effect a temporary reduction of the fracture until definitive surgical treatment is performed.

Adverse Outcomes of Treatment

Degenerative arthritis of the sacroiliac joint or the hip joint, heterotopic ossification, malunion, nonunion, or neurovascular injury may occur. Sexual dysfunction is a known sequela of these injuries, along with problems associated with concomitant musculoskeletal injuries.

Referral Decisions/Red Flags

High-energy displaced pelvic fractures and open pelvic fractures are best managed at a level I trauma center, where a multidisciplinary approach can be used to optimize patient survival. Fractures involving the acetabulum or the sacroiliac joint require evaluation for possible surgical reduction and fixation.

Fracture of the Proximal Femur

Synonym
Hip fracture

Definition
Hip fractures (proximal femur fractures) are a common injury in elderly individuals with osteoporosis. These fractures generally involve either the femoral neck or the intertrochanteric region. Both types occur with approximately the same frequency and affect a similar patient population; however, surgical treatment of the two injuries differs. Femoral neck fractures also are known as intracapsular hip fractures and thus by definition occur in the region of the proximal femur that is within the hip capsule itself (**Figure 1**). Intracapsular hip fractures often lead to a disruption of the blood supply to the femoral head; thus, nonunion and osteonecrosis are common complications of this injury. Intertrochanteric hip fractures are extracapsular, occurring in the region of the proximal femur between the base of the femoral neck and the distal aspect of the lesser trochanter (**Figure 2**), and they require more robust fixation than do femoral neck fractures. They are associated with lower rates of osteonecrosis or nonunion, as the blood supply to the femoral head is not typically disrupted; however, implant failure is a much more common problem with these injuries.

Advanced age is the most important risk factor for a proximal femur fracture. The frequency of hip fractures generally doubles with each decade beyond age 50 years. There are several reasons for this. Decreased proprioceptive function and loss of protective responses increase the likelihood that elderly individuals will fall. Also, because elderly individuals walk slowly, when they fall they tend to fall to the side as opposed to forward, so the lateral thigh and hip region often strikes the ground first. Dizziness, stroke, syncope, peripheral neuropathies, and medications are other factors that can compromise balance and predispose elderly patients to hip fractures.

White women are two to three times more likely than African American or Hispanic women to sustain a hip fracture. Other risk factors include sedentary lifestyle, smoking, alcoholism, use of psychotropic medication, dementia, osteoporosis, and living in an urban area.

Clinical Symptoms
Most patients report a fall followed by pain in the groin and the inability to bear weight on the extremity or ambulate. A few patients will be able to walk with crutches, a cane, or a walker but have groin or buttock pain on weight bearing that worsens with ambulation. Occasionally, patients report pain referred to the supracondylar

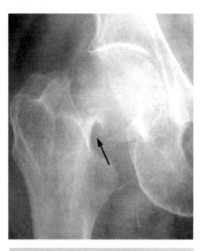

Figure 1 AP radiograph demonstrates a displaced femoral neck fracture (arrow).

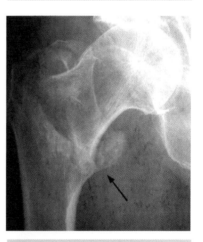

Figure 2 AP radiograph demonstrates an intertrochanteric fracture of the hip (arrow).

SECTION 5   HIP AND THIGH

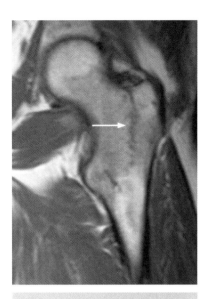

Figure 3 T1-weighted MRI demonstrates a nondisplaced intertrochanteric hip fracture (arrow).

region of the knee. Elderly patients with hip pain after a fall should be treated as if they have a hip fracture until proven otherwise.

Tests

Physical Examination

A patient with a displaced femoral neck or intertrochanteric fracture, when supine, lies with the limb externally rotated and abducted; if the fracture is displaced, the leg will also be shortened. A patient with a stress fracture or a nondisplaced fracture of the femoral neck may have no obvious deformity. Attempts by the examiner to gently rotate the limb while the hip is extended elicit pain, and the patient will be unable to perform a straight leg raise (lift the heel on the affected side off the examination table while keeping the knee straight).

Diagnostic Tests

An AP view of the pelvis and cross-table lateral views of the involved hip reveal most fractures of the proximal femur. It is important to avoid a frog-lateral radiograph in a patient with a suspected proximal femur fracture because that patient positioning will cause severe pain and may cause displacement of a nondisplaced fracture. An MRI should be obtained if the history and physical examination are suggestive of a fracture but plain radiographs are negative (**Figure 3**).

Differential Diagnosis

- Pathologic fracture (underlying or associated tumor, benign or malignant)
- Pelvic fracture (normal hip joint motion, pain on external rotation)
- Stress fracture of the femoral neck or pelvis (normal but painful hip motion)

Adverse Outcomes of the Disease

Proximal femur fractures are generally markers of poor health, and medical complications frequently accompany these injuries, including thromboembolic events, pneumonia, decubitus ulcers, and urinary tract infections. The 1-year mortality rate following proximal femur fractures in elderly patients has been reported to be 10% to 30%, and patients often lose both ambulatory capacity and functional independence. Complications directly related to the fracture include nonunion and osteonecrosis.

Treatment

Most proximal femur fractures are treated surgically because the risks of nonsurgical treatment (primarily related to the extended period of bed rest required, with the associated risk of thromboembolic events, pneumonia, decubitus ulcers, and general deconditioning) generally outweigh the risks of surgical treatment of all except the most medically unstable patients and patients who are nonambulatory and/or who have dementia with minimal pain associated with transfers.

Patients in whom a proximal femur fracture has been diagnosed should be evaluated by an orthopaedic surgeon, an internist, and an anesthesiologist in a timely manner to expedite surgical treatment. Patients should undergo a thorough evaluation to determine if medical comorbidities are present that can be optimized preoperatively to decrease the risk of perioperative morbidity and mortality. Thromboembolic prophylaxis (mechanical, pharmacologic, or both in combination) should be instituted immediately because these patients are at extraordinarily high risk for thromboembolic events. Numerous studies have suggested that a delay of more than 48 hours from the time of injury to surgical intervention is associated with increased mortality. Therefore, surgical intervention should not be delayed longer than 48 hours unless some other intervention will substantially decrease the patient's perioperative risk from surgical treatment. Although skin traction has been commonly used in the past to relieve preoperative discomfort, recent prospective randomized studies have shown that it is less effective than a pillow placed beneath the patient's knee.

The form of surgical treatment selected is determined primarily by fracture location (femoral neck versus intertrochanteric), displacement, and patient activity level. Intertrochanteric fractures are treated with either a screw and side plate (**Figure 4, A**) or an intramedullary nail (**Figure 4, B**). Nondisplaced or valgus impacted femoral neck fractures are treated by percutaneous fixation with multiple (typically three) screws (**Figure 4, C**). Displaced fractures in elderly patients are typically treated with prosthetic replacement (arthroplasty) (**Figure 4, D**) (either hemiarthroplasty for minimal ambulators or nonambulators or total hip arthroplasty for patients who are able to ambulate before surgery) because the risks of nonunion and osteonecrosis approach 50% if fracture fixation is performed. Femoral neck fractures in patients younger than 60 years are typically associated with high-energy trauma and constitute a surgical emergency because anatomic surgical fixation in a timely manner is required for optimal outcomes. Bone mineral density measurement should be part of the evaluation of patients who present with fractures of the femoral neck or intertrochanteric area of the femur. If low bone mineral density is found, appropriate treatment should be instituted.

Adverse Outcomes of Treatment

Femoral neck fractures treated with internal fixation are associated with osteonecrosis of the femoral head and fracture nonunion. In hips treated with either hemiarthroplasty or total hip arthroplasty, prosthetic dislocation can occur. The most common complications of surgical treatment of an intertrochanteric fracture are posttraumatic arthritis and/or failure of fixation with nonunion (**Figure 5**). All patients with proximal femur fractures should undergo evaluation for osteoporosis and treatment as appropriate because they are at

SECTION 5   HIP AND THIGH

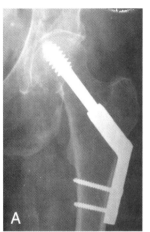 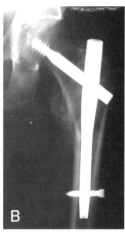 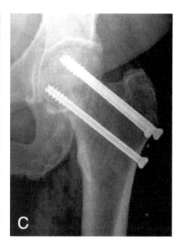 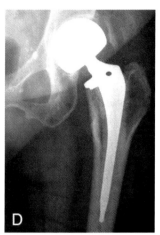

Figure 4 Postoperative AP radiographs. **A,** Intertrochanteric hip fracture treated with a screw and side plate. **B,** Intertrochanteric hip fracture treated with an intramedullary nail. **C,** Nondisplaced femoral neck fracture treated with three cannulated screws. **D,** Displaced femoral neck fracture treated with cemented arthroplasty of the hip.

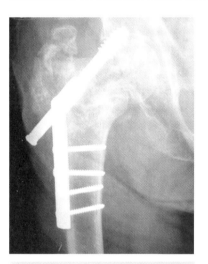

Figure 5 AP radiograph demonstrates a failed fixation following an intertrochanteric hip fracture.

substantial risk for fracture of the contralateral hip and other fragility fractures, such as distal radius and vertebral compression fractures.

Referral Decisions/Red Flags

A femoral neck fracture in a patient younger than 60 years constitutes a surgical emergency because the risk of osteonecrosis and fracture nonunion is substantial. Prompt surgical fixation and an anatomic reduction decrease the risk of these complications. In a patient with a history and physical examination suggestive of a fracture but with negative plain radiographs, an MRI should be obtained to definitively diagnose or rule out a proximal femur fracture. All proximal femur fractures should be considered for surgical treatment given the high risk of complications associated with nonsurgical treatment.

Hip Impingement

Synonym

Femoral acetabular impingement (FAI)

Definition

Hip impingement, or femoral acetabular impingement (FAI), occurs when areas of osseous deformities on the acetabular rim, the femoral head-neck junction, or both abut at extremes of hip motion and cause injury to the acetabular labrum and cartilage. Studies have demonstrated that most labral tears occur after repetitive microtrauma as a result of these subtle structural deformities.

Clinical Symptoms

Patients with hip impingement can range in age from teenagers to middle-aged weekend athletes. Pain secondary to hip impingement may occur after an acute event, but more often the patient reports an insidious onset of pain that becomes more severe with time. The location of the pain is important because intra-articular hip pathology is classically associated with groin pain. With hip impingement, patients may place a hand over the side of the hip and report that they feel a deep pain located between their fingers and thumb; this is known as the "C sign." Some patients also may report pain on the lateral aspect of the hip over the greater trochanter, with associated hip abductor weakness. Associated catching, locking, or clicking also may be present. Many patients describe worsening pain with prolonged sitting or pain with stair climbing, getting in and out of a car, putting on shoes or socks, or activities that require rotational movement.

Tests

Physical Examination

Decreased hip flexion and internal rotation compared with the opposite extremity may be observed in patients with hip impingement. The classic provocative maneuver is to place the hip in maximum flexion, adduction, and internal rotation (FADDIR); pain with this maneuver is a positive impingement sign (**Figure 1**).

Diagnostic Tests

AP and lateral radiographs of the hip are indicated for patients with pain and limited internal rotation of the hip. The classic radiographic features are a loss of femoral head-neck offset on either the AP or lateral view (cam impingement), a crossover sign (pincer impingement), or both, in the setting of normal joint space (**Figure 2**).

In pure femoral cam impingement, the anterior femoral neck loses its normal concave anatomy and instead has a "bump" that impinges on the anterosuperior labrum with flexion, causing labral tears and delamination of the adjacent cartilage.

In pincer impingement, the acetabulum either has focal overcoverage (focal retroversion) or global overcoverage (coxa profunda or protrusio). The morphology of a normal acetabulum is anteverted, in that the posterior rim is more lateral than the anterior rim. Pincer acetabular impingement arises when the anterior acetabular rim is prominent relative to the posterior rim, resulting in a radiographic appearance in which the anterior wall is more lateral than the posterior wall. This is known as the crossover sign. Either MRI or CT with three-dimensional constructions can provide further

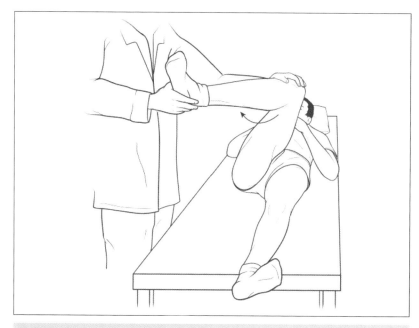

Figure 1 Illustration of the FADDIR (flexion, adduction, internal rotation) maneuver.

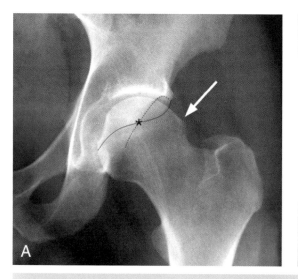
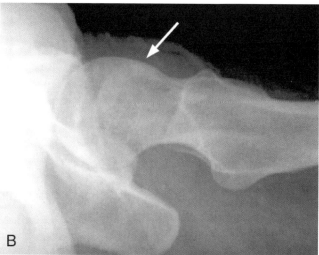

Figure 2 Radiographs from a patient with hip impingement. **A,** AP view of the left hip demonstrates a preserved joint space with a cam deformity (arrow) of the femur and crossover sign (*) on the acetabulum. The solid line indicates the anterior wall; the dashed line indicates the posterior wall. **B,** Cross-table lateral view also demonstrates the loss of femoral head concavity (arrow).

information on the three-dimensional anatomy of the hip. MRI may be falsely negative for evidence of labral tears or articular cartilage injury because of variable technique or interpretation. Magnetic resonance arthrography of the hip is the most accurate modality for demonstrating associated labral tears and osseous abnormalities (**Figure 3**).

Differential Diagnosis
- Athletic pubalgia/sports hernia (pain over rectus insertion and adductor tendons)
- Developmental dysplasia of the hip (evident on radiographs)
- Femoral cutaneous nerve entrapment (sensory changes, burning pain, normal hip range of motion)
- Groin strains (normal radiographs)
- Osteoarthritis (narrow joint space on radiographs with associated osteophytes, subchondral sclerosis and cystic changes)
- Osteonecrosis of the femoral head (evident on plain radiographs or MRI)
- Psoas impingement or snapping psoas tendon (audible snap in groin reproducible with flexion, circumduction, and extension)
- Trochanteric bursitis (local tenderness of the greater trochanter, pain with resisted hip abduction, normal motion)
- Tumor of the pelvis or spine (back pain, night pain, normal hip range of motion)

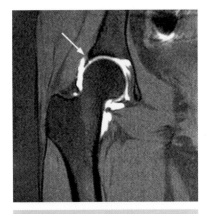

Figure 3 T2-weighted coronal magnetic resonance arthrogram of a right hip demonstrates a labral tear (arrow).

Adverse Outcomes of the Disease
Hip impingement and other hip deformities may be the etiology for 60% to 80% of cases of osteoarthritis of the hip. The assertion that hip impingement can potentially cause osteoarthritis has not been scientifically proved, but long-term prospective natural history studies may provide strong support for this idea. If hip impingement is a major contributor to hip osteoarthritis, it is thought that surgical intervention for hip pain secondary to hip impingement may delay the onset or potentially even prevent hip osteoarthritis.

Treatment
The initial treatment of all patients is nonsurgical and consists of a combination of acetaminophen, NSAIDs, and activity modification. A rehabilitation specialist familiar with nonarthroplasty hip joint dysfunction should be consulted for hip range of motion and strength training, with the goal of restoring muscular balance to the hip. Modalities such as deep tissue massage or active release therapy may be helpful in patients with associated tendinitis or stiffness about the hip secondary to long-standing hip impingement. Fluoroscopically guided intra-articular hip injections with a combination of a local anesthetic and a corticosteroid are both diagnostic and therapeutic, and complete pain relief is the most accurate test to determine an

SECTION 5   HIP AND THIGH

intra-articular etiology for hip pain. Pain relief occurs in many patients after a course of nonsurgical treatment.

Patients with hip impingement that has been refractory to nonsurgical treatment are candidates for surgical intervention. Hip impingement was originally treated with open surgical hip dislocation to safely provide exposure to the femoral head-neck junction and the acetabular rim. More recently, arthroscopic techniques have been developed to perform surgery for hip impingement. Early postoperative mobilization and range of motion with a continuous passive motion machine and a stationary bicycle are important for motion recovery. Postoperative rehabilitation is important for restoration of motion and the return to functional as well as sporting activities.

Adverse Outcomes of Treatment

Adverse outcomes of nonsurgical treatment include complications related to the chronic use of NSAIDs, such as gastric, renal, or hepatic problems. Extended treatment with acetaminophen in large doses can lead to hepatic toxicity. In 2015, the FDA strengthened its warning linking NSAIDs with the risk of heart attack or stroke, even in the first weeks of use of an NSAID. Postoperative complications associated with hip arthroscopy can include temporary numbness in the groin or the dorsal aspect of the foot secondary to nerve palsy. A small number of patients have long-standing numbness over the lateral thigh secondary to surgery near the lateral femoral cutaneous nerve. Other potential postoperative complications with either open or arthroscopic surgery include heterotopic ossification, deep vein thrombosis, and stiffness. In rare cases, postoperative femoral neck fracture and joint instability can occur. The long-term result of untreated hip impingement is the development of early osteoarthritis.

Referral Decisions/Red Flags

Patients who have persistent hip or groin pain, especially with flexion and internal rotation of the hip, that is refractory to nonsurgical treatment should be referred for further evaluation and potential surgical intervention. Hip pain in a young patient can be difficult to diagnose, and early referral is appropriate.

Inflammatory Arthritis

Synonym
Synovitis of the hip

Definition
Most inflammatory conditions that involve the hip are local manifestations of systemic disorders; however, these conditions may first present with hip symptoms. Although any of the inflammatory arthritides listed in the differential diagnosis may involve the hip, the prevalence of hip involvement is highest in rheumatoid arthritis and ankylosing spondylitis. End-stage arthritis of the hip also is commonly observed in patients with systemic lupus erythematosus, but this is often secondary to osteonecrosis.

With few exceptions, the pathophysiology of inflammatory arthropathies results from an immunologic host response to antigenic challenge. The exact cause remains unclear, but epidemiologic and genetic evidence supports a genetic component to many inflammatory arthritides.

Clinical Symptoms
Inflammatory arthritis of the hip is characterized by a dull, aching pain in the groin, lateral thigh, or buttock region. The pain is often episodic, with patients experiencing morning stiffness, improvement with moderate activity, and increased pain and stiffness following vigorous activity. Patients often will note a progressive limp as well as limited range of motion, which can manifest as difficulty with dressing or putting on shoes. With increasing time and disease progression, symptoms are indistinguishable from osteoarthritis of the hip.

Tests
Physical Examination
Gait abnormalities such as an antalgic gait (short stance phase on the affected side) are common in the earlier phases of the disease, whereas a Trendelenburg gait develops with progressive loss of articular cartilage. Hip range of motion is often restricted, with a loss of internal rotation the most sensitive finding in adults with hip joint disease. Synovial inflammation can be detected by placing the patient in a prone position with the knee flexed and applying gentle rotation to the extremity (as if rolling a rolling pin), moving the hip only. If synovial inflammation is present, this maneuver will cause pain.

Diagnostic Tests
An AP view of the pelvis as well as AP and frog-lateral radiographs of the involved hip are obtained. In the early stages of inflammatory conditions, radiographs may show subtle osteopenia and/or a joint

Essentials of Musculoskeletal Care 5

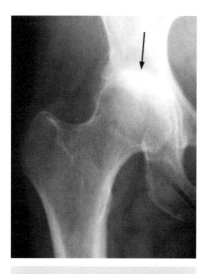

Figure 1 AP radiograph of the hip demonstrates inflammatory arthritis of the hip with concentric joint space narrowing (arrow), minimal osteophytes, and generalized osteopenia.

effusion. In later stages of inflammatory arthritis, symmetric joint space loss and periarticular bone erosions are typical (**Figure 1**).

For a patient with a history and physical examination consistent with acute synovitis of the hip, laboratory studies should include complete blood count, acute phase reactants (erythrocyte sedimentation rate or C-reactive protein), rheumatoid factor, anti–cyclic citrullinated peptide, and antinuclear antibody tests. When an effusion is present, aspiration performed under fluoroscopic guidance can be considered. The aspirate should be sent for culture, cell count with differential analysis, and inspection for crystalline deposits.

Differential Diagnosis

- Ankylosing spondylitis (stiffness of the spine and hips, low back pain, evident on radiographs)
- Calcium pyrophosphate deposition disease (uncommon in the hip)
- Gout (rare in hip, previous diagnosis of gout most probable, pain in the groin or buttock)
- Hemophilic arthropathy (previous diagnosis of hemophilia, pain with motion, evident on radiographs)
- Infection (acute onset, pain in the groin, fever, marked restriction of motion)
- Inflammatory bowel disease (previous diagnosis of bowel disease most probable, groin and buttock discomfort)
- Osteoarthritis of the hip (pain in the groin or buttock, limited range of motion)
- Osteonecrosis (dull ache in the groin or buttock, evident on radiographs and/or MRI)
- Reiter syndrome (arthritis, conjunctivitis, pain in the hip, urethritis)
- Rheumatoid arthritis (pain in the groin or buttock, decreased range of motion, evident on radiographs, other joint involvement, evidence of synovitis)
- Stress fracture (pain in the groin or buttock with activity, evident on MRI)
- Systemic lupus erythematosus (pain in the groin or buttock, limited range of motion, other joint involvement)
- Trochanteric bursitis (pain in the lateral aspect of the thigh)

Adverse Outcomes of the Disease

Adverse outcomes of the disease include persistent pain, progressive gait abnormalities, and joint contractures, which may lead to decreased ambulatory capacity and loss of functional independence.

Treatment

For noninfectious inflammatory arthritis, a nonsurgical treatment plan administered in conjunction with a rheumatologist may include NSAIDs, disease-modifying agents, acetaminophen or other analgesics, the use of an assistive device held in the hand contralateral to the affected hip, and activity modification. Intra-articular corticosteroid injections can be considered, but they generally require fluoroscopic or ultrasound guidance for accurate placement. A rehabilitation program emphasizing range-of-motion exercises and pain-free strengthening can be helpful but may exacerbate the patient's symptoms. Total hip arthroplasty is the treatment of choice for patients with advanced symptoms in whom nonsurgical treatment has failed.

Adverse Outcomes of Treatment

Adverse outcomes of nonsurgical treatment include complications related to the chronic use of NSAIDs, such as gastric, renal, or hepatic problems. In 2015, the FDA strengthened its warning linking NSAIDs with the risk of heart attack or stroke, even in the first weeks of use of an NSAID. Extended treatment with acetaminophen in large doses can lead to hepatic toxicity. Corticosteroids are often used as part of the treatment algorithm and can lead to osteonecrosis of the femoral head. The most common short-term complications related to total hip arthroplasty include neurovascular injury, thromboembolic events, infection, leg-length inequality, and prosthetic dislocation. Wear-related complications are unusual because this patient population is typically inactive; however, prosthetic loosening requiring revision surgery can still occur.

Referral Decisions/Red Flags

For noninfectious arthritis, symptoms recalcitrant to nonsurgical treatment that lead to persistent pain and functional disability indicate the need for further evaluation.

SECTION 5   HIP AND THIGH

Lateral Femoral Cutaneous Nerve Syndrome

Synonym
Meralgia paresthetica

Definition
Compression or entrapment of the lateral femoral cutaneous nerve is characterized by pain, burning (dysesthesia), or hypoesthesia over the lateral thigh. Motor nerve dysfunction does not occur, because the lateral femoral cutaneous nerve is a sensory nerve. The nerve is most susceptible to compression where it exits the pelvis just medial to the anterior superior iliac spine. This syndrome can be caused by several factors, including obesity, compression from tight clothing or straps around the waist (such as a tool belt or backpack), scar tissue from previous surgical procedures, significant trauma (especially involving hip extension), or mild repetitive trauma over the course of the nerve. The nerve also can be injured during anterior surgical approaches to the hip, pelvis, or acetabulum. Rarely, pathologic intrapelvic or abdominal processes (cecal tumors) cause compression of the lateral femoral cutaneous nerve.

Clinical Symptoms
Symptoms associated with this condition include pain and dysesthesia in the anterolateral or lateral thigh that sometimes extends to the lateral knee. Uncommonly, patients report aching in the groin area and, if the condition is acute, pain radiating to the sacroiliac joint area. Joggers describe the pain as an "electric jab" each time the affected hip extends, usually after running a short distance.

Tests
Physical Examination
Hypoesthesia or dysesthesia in the distribution of the lateral femoral cutaneous nerve is typical, with the most reproducible spot of hypoesthesia above and lateral to the knee (**Figure 1**). Burning is most consistent in this area. Pressure or tapping over the nerve where it exits the pelvis just medial to or directly over the anterior superior iliac spine can produce tenderness or reproduce paresthesias along the distribution of the nerve. Muscle weakness and reflex changes are absent. Abdominal and pelvic examinations are needed to exclude intra-abdominal pathology.

Diagnostic Tests
An AP radiograph of the pelvis will rule out any bony abnormality, and AP and lateral radiographs of the hip may be appropriate when

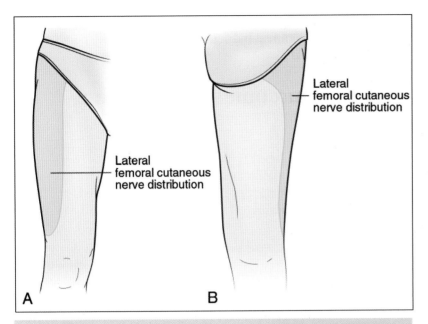

Figure 1 Illustrations of anterior (**A**) and posterior (**B**) views of the leg show the location of hypoesthesia or dysesthesia associated with lateral femoral cutaneous nerve entrapment.

the patient has restricted internal rotation of the hip and groin pain. CT or MRI is appropriate to investigate a suspected intrapelvic mass.

Differential Diagnosis

- Diabetes mellitus or other causes of peripheral neuropathy (numbness in the feet)
- Hip arthritis (limited internal rotation, limp)
- Intra-abdominal tumor (pelvic or abdominal mass, hematochezia, weight loss)
- Lumbar disk herniation (L1 through L4 motor and sensory changes, positive prone rectus femoris stretch test)
- Trochanteric bursitis (tenderness over the trochanter, stiffness when rising)

Adverse Outcomes of the Disease

Pain and dysesthesia will continue if the patient is not treated.

Treatment

Numbness is often well tolerated, but burning dysesthesia can become intolerable. Removing the source of compression, such as a tight waistband, a weight-lifting belt, or mild repetitive trauma to the nerve, can relieve the symptoms of burning. In patients with obesity, significant weight loss often relieves symptoms. Infiltration of the area around the nerve where it exits the pelvis near the anterior superior iliac spine with a corticosteroid preparation may reduce symptoms. Neuropathic pain medications, such as gabapentin, can be

SECTION 5   HIP AND THIGH

useful in appropriate patients. Surgical release of the nerve is rarely required; its most common indication is in patients with persistent burning dysesthesia.

Adverse Outcomes of Treatment

In some instances, symptoms persist despite treatment.

Referral Decisions/Red Flags

A suspected pelvic or abdominal mass signals the need for immediate further evaluation. The presence of intolerable symptoms that have failed to respond to nonsurgical treatment also indicates the need for further evaluation.

Osteoarthritis of the Hip

Synonyms
Degenerative arthritis of the hip
Osteoarthrosis of the hip

Definition
Osteoarthritis of the hip is characterized by a loss of articular cartilage in the hip joint. The osteoarthrosis may be primary (idiopathic) or secondary to hip diseases during childhood, trauma, osteonecrosis, previous joint infection, or other conditions.

Clinical Symptoms
The classic presentation is a gradual onset of anterior thigh or groin pain. Some patients have pain in the buttock or the lateral aspect of the thigh. The pain may be referred to the distal thigh (knee) and may be perceived only in the knee. Initially, pain occurs only with activity, but gradually the frequency and intensity of the pain increase to the point that pain occurs at rest and at night. As osteoarthritis progresses, decreased range of motion develops, which may manifest as a limp and difficulty putting on trousers or shoes. Ambulatory capacity gradually decreases as pain increases. Occasionally, patients will have a severe limp and stiffness but little pain.

Careful questioning may reveal a history of hip problems as an infant or toddler (indicative of developmental dysplasia of the hip), as a small child (indicative of Legg-Calvé-Perthes disease), or as an adolescent (suggestive of slipped capital femoral epiphysis). Patients with osteoarthritis of the hip may have other coexisting conditions, as listed in the differential diagnosis.

Tests
Physical Examination
The earliest sign of osteoarthritis of the hip is a loss of internal rotation as determined by range-of-motion testing. Gradually, global decreases in range of motion occur, and a fixed external rotation and flexion contracture develops in many patients. Flexion contractures are particularly problematic because they greatly affect gait patterns, as the patient must compensate by increasing lumbar spine extension to afford hip extension. In addition, an antalgic gait (short stance on the painful leg) and an abductor lurch (swaying the trunk far over the affected hip) develop as the body tries to compensate for the pain and secondary weakness in the hip abductor muscles.

Diagnostic Tests
AP and lateral radiographs of the hip are indicated for patients with pain and limited internal rotation of the hip. The classic radiographic features of osteoarthritis of the hip are joint space narrowing,

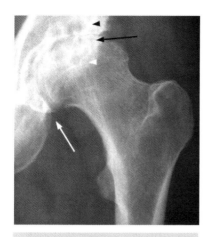

Figure 1 AP radiograph demonstrates degenerative joint disease of the hip with joint space narrowing (black arrow), osteophyte formation (white arrow), subchondral cyst formation (black arrowhead), and subchondral sclerosis (white arrowhead).

osteophyte formation, subchondral cyst formation, and subchondral sclerosis (**Figure 1**).

Differential Diagnosis

- Degenerative lumbar disk disease (normal hip motion)
- Femoral cutaneous nerve entrapment (sensory changes, burning, normal motion)
- Herniated lumbar disk (diminished knee reflex, sensory changes)
- Inflammatory arthritis of the hip (rheumatoid arthritis, systemic lupus erythematosus, ankylosing spondylitis)
- Osteonecrosis of the femoral head (evident on radiographs)
- Trochanteric bursitis (local tenderness, normal motion)
- Tumor of the pelvis or spine (back pain, night pain, normal motion)

Adverse Outcomes of the Disease

Osteoarthritis of the hip is a progressive condition with a natural history of increasing pain and a subsequent decrease in function associated with progressive gait abnormality. In the end stages of the disease, pain is severe, occurring at night and at rest and severely limiting ambulation, and large fixed contractures of the hip develop secondarily. Progressive bone loss of the femoral head or the acetabulum may occur but is uncommon.

Treatment

Initial treatment of all patients is nonsurgical and consists of a combination of acetaminophen, NSAIDs, activity modification, and the use of an assistive device held in the hand contralateral to the affected hip. Non–weight-bearing exercise (such as the use of a stationary bicycle or swimming/aquatic therapy) and hip strengthening are occasionally helpful but can exacerbate symptoms. Intra-articular injections with corticosteroids are used occasionally; they generally require fluoroscopic or ultrasound guidance for accurate placement.

Vigorous, young patients in whom nonsurgical treatment fails and who have a biomechanical derangement of the hip may be candidates for a realignment osteotomy of the proximal femur or the acetabulum. Hip fusion is a potential surgical option for a young patient who either must return to work as a manual laborer or who leads a vigorous lifestyle. Most patients in whom nonsurgical treatment fails, however, are most appropriately treated with total hip arthroplasty (**Figure 2**). Total hip arthroplasty is associated with dramatic decreases in pain as well as increases in function and is among the most cost-effective medical interventions available when quality-adjusted years of life are considered. Metal-on-metal hip resurfacing (**Figure 3**), which uses a cap on the femoral head rather than the stemmed femoral component used in a conventional total hip arthroplasty, may be an appropriate alternative for young, active patients. It has the potential benefits of preserving proximal femoral bone stock (should revision surgery be required in the future) and allowing the return to higher level activities, such as running sports, that are not typically recommended following conventional total hip arthroplasty with a stemmed femoral component.

Adverse Outcomes of Treatment

Adverse outcomes of nonsurgical treatment include complications related to the chronic use of NSAIDs, such as gastric, renal, or hepatic problems. Extended treatment with acetaminophen in large doses can lead to hepatic toxicity. In 2015, the FDA strengthened its warning linking NSAIDs with the risk of heart attack or stroke, even in the first weeks of use of an NSAID. The most common short-term complications related to total hip arthroplasty include neurovascular injury, thromboembolic events, infection, leg-length inequality, and prosthetic dislocation. Long-term complications of total hip arthroplasty are more common in young, active patients and relate primarily to wear of the bearing surface and loosening of the components that may require revision surgery. Patients who are treated with osteotomy or hip fusion may require further surgical intervention in the form of total hip arthroplasty if the surgery is unsuccessful, subsequent arthritis develops, or pain relief is incomplete.

Referral Decisions/Red Flags

Patients who have persistent pain despite nonsurgical treatment including acetaminophen, multiple different NSAIDs, activity modification, and/or the use of an assistive device require appropriate referral for further evaluation of potential surgical intervention. Young patients may be referred earlier to determine if an alternative to conventional total hip arthroplasty (such as redirectional osteotomy, hip fusion, or hip resurfacing) is appropriate.

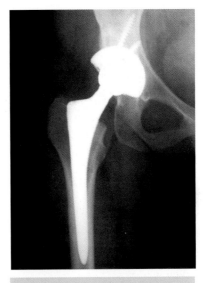

Figure 2 AP radiograph of the hip of a patient with osteoarthritis following total hip arthroplasty.

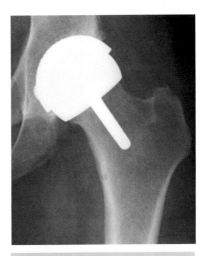

Figure 3 AP radiograph of a hip following metal-on-metal hip resurfacing.

SECTION 5   HIP AND THIGH

Osteonecrosis of the Hip

Synonym
Aseptic necrosis of the hip

Definition
Osteonecrosis of the hip results from the death of varying amounts of bone in the femoral head. The causative event may be traumatic disruption of the vascular supply to the femoral head or deficient circulation from other causes (such as microvascular thrombosis in patients with sickle cell anemia). Initially, only the osteocytes and other cells are affected, but with time the bone structure fragments and collapses. As a result, the overlying articular surface collapses and progressive arthritis develops.

Osteonecrosis affects 10,000 to 20,000 new patients per year in the United States, occurs with greater frequency in the third through fifth decades of life, and often is bilateral. Risk factors include trauma (hip dislocation or femoral neck fracture), history of corticosteroid use, alcohol abuse, sickle cell disease, rheumatoid arthritis, and systemic lupus erythematosus. Of note, the association with corticosteroids generally is related to the amount and duration of medication; however, osteonecrosis sometimes develops after only one or two exposures to corticosteroids.

Clinical Symptoms
Patients usually report the indolent onset of a dull ache or a throbbing pain in the groin, lateral hip, or buttock area. Patients may report severe pain during the initial phases of the disease when bone death occurs. Secondary arthritis develops with progressive collapse of the femoral head, and symptoms may be indistinguishable from osteoarthritis. Limited range of motion may occur, and patients often report a progressive limp. The history should focus on the following risk factors for the disease:

- Alcohol abuse
- Caisson disease (scuba diving)
- Chronic pancreatitis
- Corticosteroid use
- Crohn disease
- Gaucher disease
- HIV infection
- Myeloproliferative disorders
- Radiation treatment
- Rheumatoid arthritis
- Sickle cell disease
- Smoking

- Systemic lupus erythematosus
- Trauma

Tests
Physical Examination
Patients have pain with attempted straight leg raising (lifting the heel of the affected extremity off the examination table with the knee held straight) as well as with range of motion of the hip. Range of motion may be decreased (particularly internal rotation) in addition to being painful. Patients often have an antalgic gait (short stance phase), but a Trendelenburg gait may occur after secondary arthritis develops.

Diagnostic Tests
An AP view of the pelvis and AP and frog-lateral radiographs of the hip should be obtained. In the earliest stages of the disease, plain radiographs may be normal. With time, patchy areas of sclerosis and lucency may be present. With disease progression, a "crescent sign" appears, which is a well-defined sclerotic area just beneath the articular surface that represents a subchondral fracture. The femoral head typically becomes progressively more aspherical with time, leading to secondary degenerative changes of the acetabulum, which may appear indistinguishable from degenerative arthritis (**Figure 1**).

In patients in whom osteonecrosis is suspected but radiographic findings are normal or equivocal, MRI is indicated (**Figure 2**). Patients with unilateral atraumatic osteonecrosis may benefit from an MRI of the contralateral hip to diagnose asymptomatic disease on that side that may benefit from surgical treatment to prevent disease progression.

Differential Diagnosis
- Fracture of the femoral neck (evident on radiographs and MRI)
- Lumbar disk disease (back pain, reflex changes, radiation below the knee)
- Muscle strain or groin pull (normal radiographs, intermittent limp)
- Osteoarthritis of the hip (no risk factors, absence of sclerosis within the femoral heads on radiographs)
- Septic arthritis of the hip (fever, constitutional symptoms)
- Transient osteoporosis of the hip (disabling pain without previous trauma, osteopenia, female patient in the third trimester of pregnancy, or a middle-aged man)

Adverse Outcomes of the Disease
The natural history of osteonecrosis is not well understood. In general, in patients with smaller lesions in non–weight-bearing areas and limited exposure to vascular insult, symptoms tend to resolve without femoral head collapse and development of arthritis. In patients with larger lesions and/or sustained insult to the vascular supply of the femoral head, however, femoral head collapse and

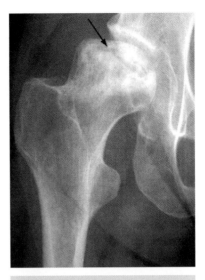

Figure 1 AP radiograph of the hip demonstrates osteonecrosis of the femoral head with collapse (arrow).

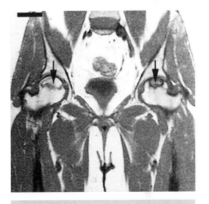

Figure 2 Coronal T1-weighted MRI of the hip demonstrates areas of low signal intensity consistent with osteonecrosis of the femoral heads (arrows). (Reproduced from Johnson TR, Steinbach LS, eds: *Essentials of Musculoskeletal Imaging.* Rosemont, IL, American Academy of Orthopaedic Surgeons, 2004, p 470.)

SECTION 5   HIP AND THIGH

secondary degenerative arthritis develop. End-stage degenerative changes also develop in these patients, including progressive pain, decreased range of motion, decreased ambulatory capacity, and limp.

Treatment

Treatment options before collapse are controversial. A myriad of different treatment options have been attempted, including protected weight bearing, pulsed magnetic electrical fields, and surgical interventions, but few studies have adequate randomization or statistical power to provide guidance with regard to selecting among these options. Surgical choices for the patient without collapse aimed at maintaining the native femoral head include core decompression (removing a core of bone from the femoral head and neck to decrease bone marrow pressure and encourage blood flow) with or without bone grafting, vascularized fibular grafting (harvesting a portion of the ipsilateral fibula with a vascular pedicle and transplanting it to the femoral head and neck to stimulate revascularization), and fresh osteochondral allografting of the femoral head. The former two options aim to relieve pressure in the femoral head that may be causing pain and stimulate healing of the lesion. After femoral head collapse has occurred, most physicians recommend arthroplasty, although some have advocated core decompression for short-term pain relief.

Adverse Outcomes of Treatment

If attempts to preserve the femoral head fail, degenerative arthritis may develop subsequently, requiring further surgical intervention in the form of total hip arthroplasty. A unique complication of core decompression is a fracture of the femoral shaft if the core biopsy tract is placed below the level of the lesser trochanter. The results of total hip arthroplasty in this patient population are often inferior because patients may be young and vigorous and bone metabolism may be altered, placing higher demands on the prosthesis and increasing the risk of prosthetic loosening.

Referral Decisions/Red Flags

Plain radiographic evidence of or clinical suspicion for osteonecrosis requires further evaluation to determine if surgical intervention to preserve the femoral head is indicated.

Snapping Hip

Definition

Snapping hip is characterized by a snapping or popping sensation that occurs as tendons around the hip move over bony prominences. The most common cause is the iliotibial band snapping over the greater trochanter. Snapping also can occur when the iliopsoas tendon slides over the pectineal eminence of the pelvis or from intra-articular tears of the acetabular labrum (the fibrocartilage rim at the periphery of the acetabulum).

Clinical Symptoms

Iliotibial band subluxation usually occurs with walking or rotation of the hip. When asked to localize their symptoms, patients will point to the trochanteric area (**Figure 1**). Some patients notice the snapping when they lie on their side with the affected side up and rotate the leg. If a trochanteric bursitis subsequently develops, patients will report increased pain when first rising in the morning, pain at night, and difficulty lying on the affected side.

Snapping caused by subluxation of the iliopsoas tendon usually is felt in the groin as the hip extends from a flexed position, as when rising from a chair. Many patients feel the snapping but have no disability. In a few patients, the snapping is either annoying or painful.

Snapping from intra-articular causes is more disabling and more likely to cause patients to reach for support.

Tests

Physical Examination

Iliotibial band subluxation can be re-created by having the patient stand and then rotate the hip while holding it in an adducted position. A snap can be palpated as the iliotibial band slides over the greater trochanter. Snapping of the iliopsoas tendon may be palpated as the hip extends from a flexed position and the tendon moves over the pectineal eminence of the pelvis. Restricted internal rotation of the involved hip, a limp, or shortening of the limb suggests problems within the hip joint. The Ober test is used to evaluate the tightness of the iliotibial band. For this test, the patient lies on the uninvolved side. The examiner flexes the patient's knee to 90°, then abducts the involved hip approximately 40° and extends it to its limit. While the hip extension and knee flexion are maintained and the pelvis is stabilized, the hip is allowed to adduct passively. If the hip fails to adduct to at least the midline of the body or the patient experiences pain along the iliotibial band, the test is positive.

Diagnostic Tests

AP radiographs of the pelvis and lateral hip can exclude bony pathology or intra-articular hip disease. Radiographs typically are normal for patients with a snapping hip. A CT arthrogram may

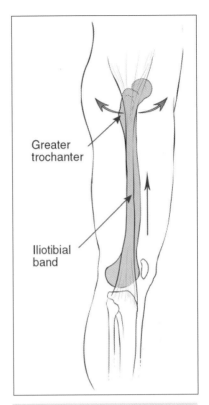

Figure 1 Illustration shows how the iliotibial band slips anteriorly and posteriorly over the prominent greater trochanter.

SECTION 5   HIP AND THIGH

be necessary to rule out intra-articular loose bodies. MRI with gadolinium may be necessary to rule out a tear of the acetabular labrum. A diagnostic, fluoroscopically or ultrasound-guided anesthetic injection may be useful to distinguish between intra-articular and extra-articular sources of symptoms.

Differential Diagnosis
- Osteoarthritis of the hip (limited internal rotation)
- Osteochondral loose body (fragment of bone and cartilage within the joint, pain with hip motion)
- Osteonecrosis of the femoral head (compromised blood supply to the femoral head, groin pain)
- Tear of the acetabular labrum (pain, catching, or instability with hip motion)

Adverse Outcomes of the Disease
Pain and annoyance are commonly reported.

Treatment
Snapping hip is often painless, and after the diagnosis is made with certainty, patients often require only an explanation of the source of the symptoms for reassurance. Patients who are significantly bothered by the symptoms should be advised to avoid provocative maneuvers and activities so that the symptoms can subside. Treatment consists of exercises to stretch and strengthen the iliotibial band, hip abductors, hip adductors, and hip flexors. A short course of NSAIDs may reduce the discomfort associated with tendon snapping and secondary bursitis. Corticosteroid injection into the greater trochanteric bursa (for snapping iliotibial band) or into the psoas tendon sheath (for snapping iliopsoas tendon) may reduce pain.

Surgery is reserved for the uncommon cases that are disabling and fail to resolve with nonsurgical management.

Rehabilitation Prescription
The functional goal of rehabilitation for a patient with a snapping hip is to reduce pain and increase the ability of the patient to return to functional activities, such as walking and running. Stretching exercises for tight muscles around the hip should be performed in conjunction with strengthening exercises. Weakness of the hip abductors is very commonly associated with tightness of the iliotibial band.

The home exercise program for snapping hip should include stretching and strengthening exercises. If the pain does not diminish within 2 or 3 weeks on a home program, formal rehabilitation may be ordered. The prescription should include a complete evaluation of hip strength and the flexibility of the soft-tissue structures, including the iliotibial band, the hamstrings, and the hip flexors. Increasing the endurance of the trunk muscles should be part of the rehabilitation prescription.

Adverse Outcomes of Treatment

NSAIDs can cause gastric, renal, or hepatic complications. In 2015, the FDA strengthened its warning linking NSAIDs with the risk of heart attack or stroke, even in the first weeks of use of an NSAID. Postoperative infection or persistent pain is possible if surgical intervention is undertaken.

Referral Decisions/Red Flags

Unclear diagnosis, intra-articular pathology, or failure of nonsurgical measures indicates the need for further evaluation.

Home Exercise Program for Snapping Hip

- Perform the exercises in the order listed.
- Apply dry or moist heat to the hip for 5 to 10 minutes before exercising to prepare the tissues. Alternatively, riding a stationary bicycle for 10 minutes also will prepare the tissues for stretching.
- Apply a bag of crushed ice or frozen peas to the hip for 20 minutes after exercising to help reduce inflammation.
- If you experience pain in the hip during or after exercising, discontinue the exercises and call your doctor.
- The following exercise program is introductory only, and progression of this program will vary based on your specific injury, symptoms, and baseline level of fitness. For further progression of this routine, your physician may recommend evaluation and treatment by a physical therapist or other exercise professional.

Home Exercises for Snapping Hip

Exercise Type	Muscle Group	Number of Repetitions/Sets	Number of Days per Week	Number of Weeks
Piriformis stretch	Piriformis	4 repetitions/2 to 3 sets	5 to 7	2 to 3
Iliotibial band stretch	Tensor fascia latae	4 repetitions/2 to 3 sets	5 to 7	2 to 3
Hip abduction	Gluteus medius	10 repetitions/2 sets, progressing to 15 to 20 repetitions/3 sets	3 to 5	2 to 3
Foam roller for iliotibial band	Iliotibial band	Once per side for 2 to 3 minutes each	Daily	2 to 3
Hip flexor stretch	Hip flexors	4 repetitions per side/2 to 3 sets	5 to 7	2 to 3

SECTION 5   HIP AND THIGH

Piriformis Stretch

- Lie on your back and bend both knees so that your feet are flat on the floor.
- Place the ankle of the affected leg on the opposite knee and clasp your hands behind the thigh as shown.
- Pull the thigh toward you until you feel a stretch in the hip. To increase the intensity of the stretch, apply pressure to the affected leg, pushing away from the body.
- Hold the stretch for 30 seconds and then relax for 30 seconds.
- Perform 2 to 3 sets of 4 repetitions 5 to 7 days per week, continuing for 2 to 3 weeks.
- Perform the stretch on both sides.

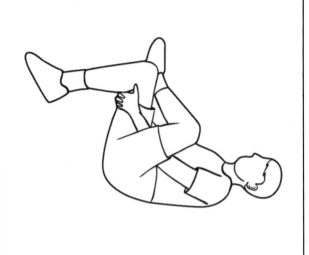

Iliotibial Band Stretch

- Stand approximately 2 feet away from a wall with the affected side to the wall.
- Fully extend your arm and place your hand on the wall for support.
- Cross the unaffected leg (the leg farther from the wall) over the opposite leg.
- Lean your hips toward the wall until you feel a stretch on the outside of the affected leg.
- Hold the maximum stretch for 30 seconds and then relax for 10 seconds.
- Perform 2 to 3 sets of 4 repetitions on each side, 5 to 7 days per week, continuing for 2 to 3 weeks.

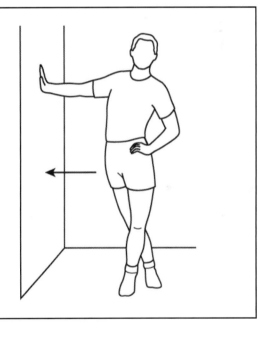

Hip Abduction

- Lie on your side with the affected hip on top. Cradle your head in your arm and bend your bottom leg to provide support.
- Slowly move the top leg up and back to 45°, keeping the knee straight. Hold this position for 5 seconds.
- Slowly lower the leg to a count of 5 and relax it for 2 seconds.
- Ankle weights should be used, starting with a weight light enough to allow 2 sets of 10 repetitions and progressing to 3 sets of 15 to 20 repetitions.
- Then return to 2 sets of 10 repetitions and add weight in 2- to 3-pound increments, progressing each time to 3 sets of 15 to 20 repetitions.
- Perform the exercise 3 to 5 days per week, continuing for 2 to 3 weeks.

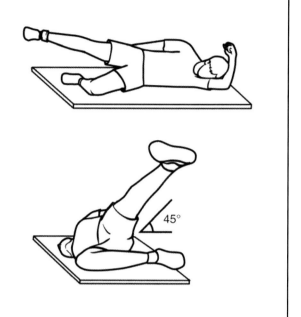

Foam Roller for Iliotibial Band

- Position the foam roller under the outside of your thigh.
- Use your arms to slowly move the lateral or outside portion of your thigh over the foam roller.
- The foam roller should move slowly. Stop and hold the position for 5 to 10 seconds at areas of tightness or discomfort, then proceed up and down the outer thigh.
- Avoid rolling over the bony prominence of the outer hip (arrow) or the knee (double arrow).
- Mild to severe discomfort may be present but should improve with consistent daily use of the foam roller. If the discomfort does not improve within 1 to 2 weeks, seek the advice of your sports medicine physician.
- Perform every day, for 2 to 3 minutes on each leg. Continue for 2 to 3 weeks.

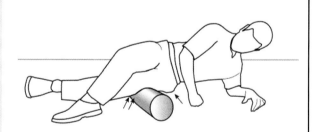

SECTION 5   HIP AND THIGH

Hip Flexor Stretch

- Kneel on the affected knee, with the opposite foot forward as shown in the diagram.
- Shift your body forward until a pull is felt in the front of the affected hip. Keep your upper body straight, and avoid arching your back.
- Hold the stretch for 30 seconds and then relax for 10 seconds.
- Perform 2 to 3 sets of 4 repetitions, 5 to 7 days per week, continuing for 2 to 3 weeks.
- The stretch should be performed on each side unless directed differently by your healthcare provider.

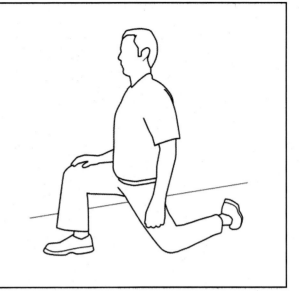

Strains of the Hip

Definition

Hip strain is a general term applied to injuries of the muscle-tendon units around the hip. Several muscles, including the abdominals, the hip flexors (iliopsoas, sartorius, and rectus femoris), and the hip adductors, should be considered when a patient has pain around the hip after an acute or overuse injury (**Figure 1**). Vigorous muscular contraction while the muscle is on stretch frequently causes the injury. For example, forceful hip flexion can strain the iliopsoas muscle, as when a soccer player forcibly flexes the hip to kick a ball and the leg is blocked or forcefully extended by an opponent. Overuse injuries are a common cause of hip strains.

Clinical Symptoms

The most common presenting symptom is pain over the injured muscle that is exacerbated when that area continues to be used during strenuous activities.

Tests

Physical Examination

The deep location of the hip muscles compromises the examination, and precise localization of the injured muscle is not always possible. A strain of the hip adductors is identified by tenderness in the groin and increased pain with passive abduction. Additionally, resistive strength testing of the muscle typically elicits pain. Injury to the abdominal muscles is identified by increased pain when the patient flexes the trunk. When a hip flexor is injured, the pain is worse with

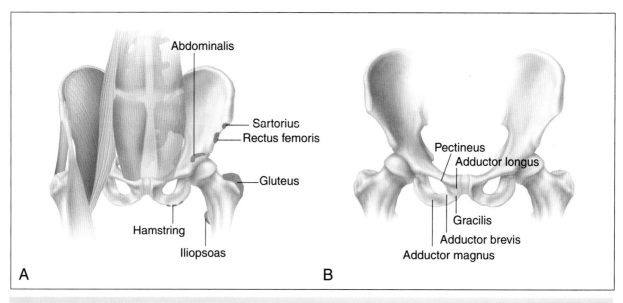

Figure 1 **A,** Illustration of the anterior pelvis shows muscle origins and insertions. **B,** Illustration of the anterior pelvis shows adductor muscle insertions.

flexion of the hip against resistance or with passive extension of the hip. Strain of the rectus femoris is delineated by increased pain when putting the rectus femoris on stretch. Injury to the iliopsoas typically causes pain in the deep groin or inner thigh, whereas pain from a proximal sartorius strain is more superficial and lateral.

Diagnostic Tests

AP radiographs of the pelvis and a frog-lateral view of the involved hip can rule out a fracture or other bony lesion. A bone scan or MRI can contribute useful information to help the physician arrive at the correct diagnosis, but these studies are rarely necessary except in the elite athlete (**Figure 2**).

Differential Diagnosis

- Athletic pubalgia (sports hernia) (pain in groin, may have vague symptoms)
- Hip avulsion fractures (may be seen with strains of the sartorius [avulsion fracture of the anterior superior iliac spine] or rectus femoris [avulsion fracture of the anterior inferior iliac spine])
- Osteonecrosis of the hip (chronic dull ache in the groin, inner thigh, or buttock; evident on radiographs, MRI)
- Pelvic or proximal femoral tumors (pain at rest or at night, increased pain with weight bearing)

Adverse Outcomes of the Disease

Chronic injury can be debilitating and threaten athletic performance. If pain persists, the patient's gait may be altered, resulting in secondary injuries.

Treatment

Rehabilitation enhances full recovery and should be initiated after confirmation of the injury. For most patients, activity modification, followed by a home exercise program, is sufficient. Elite athletes usually are treated with a more aggressive and costly regimen (**Table 1**). Rehabilitation can be divided into five phases that generally are completed within approximately 6 weeks. Phase I (48 to 72 hours) includes rest, ice, compression, and protected weight bearing with crutches if needed. Phase II (72 hours up to 1 week) includes passive range-of-motion exercises, accompanied by heat, electrical stimulation, or ultrasound. The final three phases include different isometric exercises and sport-specific training. The purpose of the final phases is to increase strength and flexibility and focus on returning the patient to the preinjury level of activity. If pain is exacerbated during the rehabilitation process, the patient should return to the phase of treatment that preceded the recurrence of symptoms. NSAIDs can be a useful adjunct to a rehabilitation program to reduce pain and inflammation.

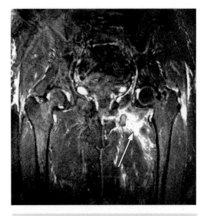

Figure 2 Coronal short tau inversion recovery (STIR) sequence MRI of the pelvis demonstrates high signal intensity (arrow), indicating edema, at the origin and proximal muscle belly of several of the adductor muscles. This finding is consistent with a muscle strain.

HIP AND THIGH

SECTION 5

Table 1

Rehabilitation Guidelines for Muscle Injuries in Elite Athletes

Phase	Goals	Treatment	Time Frame
I	Reduce pain, inflammation, and bleeding	Rest, ice, and compression; crutches if needed	48 to 72 h
II	Regain range of motion	Passive range of motion, heat, ultrasound, electrical muscle stimulation	72 h to 1 week
III	Increase strength, flexibility, and endurance	Isometrics, well-leg cycling	Weeks 1 to 3
IV	Increase strength and coordination	Isotonic and isokinetic exercises	Weeks 3 to 4
V	Return to competition	Sport-specific training	Weeks 4 to 6

(Reproduced with permission from DeLee JC, Drez D Jr, eds: *Orthopaedic Sports Medicine: Principles and Practice.* Philadelphia, PA, WB Saunders, 1994, vol 2, pp 1063-1085.)

Rehabilitation Prescription

Strains of the hip are usually secondary to overuse and/or muscle imbalances. For example, running long distances can result in muscle fatigue. The hip abductors, extensors, and internal and external rotators are among the weakest muscle groups in the hip, so a home exercise program that attempts to strengthen these muscles is appropriate, provided there is no pain with the exercise.

If pain persists after the patient has been on a home program for 3 to 4 weeks, formal rehabilitation may be ordered. The evaluation should include a detailed assessment of the trunk and hip muscles, including testing of the quadratus lumborum, abdominals, and back extensors. After the deficits are determined, an extensive strengthening program should be initiated.

Adverse Outcomes of Treatment

Recalcitrant pain may indicate a more serious injury or tendinous disruption that requires further evaluation. Recurrent injuries also are possible and are more likely to occur in competitive or weekend athletes who fail to maintain flexibility of the affected muscle. NSAIDs can cause gastric, renal, or hepatic complications. In 2015, the FDA strengthened its warning linking NSAIDs with the risk of heart attack or stroke, even in the first weeks of use of an NSAID.

Referral Decisions/Red Flags

Symptoms that do not respond to treatment require further evaluation to ensure that a more serious injury has not occurred and that a malignancy or osteonecrosis of the hip is not responsible for the symptoms.

www.aaos.org/essentials5/exercises

Home Exercise Program for Strains of the Hip

- Perform the exercises in the order listed.
- After each set of exercises, apply a bag of crushed ice or frozen peas to the hip for 20 minutes.
- If pain in the hip is aggravated by exercising or does not go away within 3 to 4 weeks, call your doctor.
- The following exercise program is introductory only, and progression of this program will vary based on your specific injury, symptoms, and baseline level of fitness. For further progression of this routine, your physician may recommend evaluation and treatment by a physical therapist or other exercise professional.

Home Exercises for Strains of the Hip

Exercise Type	Muscle Group	Number of Repetitions/Sets	Number of Days per Week	Number of Weeks
Hip abduction	Gluteus medius	10 repetitions/2 sets, progressing to 15 to 20 repetitions/3 sets	3 to 5	3 to 4
Hip adduction	Adductors	10 repetitions/2 sets, progressing to 15 to 20 repetitions/3 sets	3 to 5	3 to 4
Straight leg raise	Quadriceps	10 repetitions/2 sets, progressing to 15 to 20 repetitions/3 sets	3 to 5	3 to 4
Hip extension	Gluteus maximus	10 repetitions/2 sets, progressing to 15 to 20 repetitions/3 sets	3 to 5	3 to 4
Hip rotation	*External*: Piriformis *Internal*: Medial hamstring	10 repetitions/2 sets, progressing to 15 to 20 repetitions/3 sets	3 to 5	3 to 4

Hip Abduction

- Lie on your side with the affected hip on top. Cradle your head in your arm and bend your bottom leg to provide support.
- Slowly move the top leg up and back to 45°, keeping the knee straight.
- Hold this position for 5 seconds.
- Slowly lower the leg and relax it for 2 seconds.
- Ankle weights should be used, starting with a weight light enough to allow 2 sets of 10 repetitions, progressing to 3 sets of 15 to 20 repetitions. After that becomes easy, add weight in 1-pound increments and return to 2 sets of 10 repetitions, progressing to 3 sets of 15 to 20 repetitions.
- Perform the exercise 3 to 5 days per week, continuing for 3 to 4 weeks.

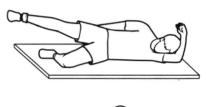
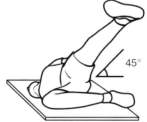

Hip Adduction

- Lie on the floor on the side of the affected leg with both legs straight.
- Cross the unaffected leg in front of the affected one.
- Raise the affected (bottom) leg 6 to 8 inches off the floor.
- Hold this position for 5 seconds.
- Lower the leg and rest for 2 seconds.
- Perform 2 sets of 10 repetitions.
- Work up to 3 sets of 15 to 20 repetitions.
- Perform the exercise 3 to 5 days per week, continuing for 3 to 4 weeks.

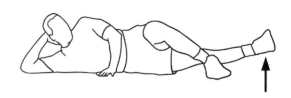

SECTION 5 HIP AND THIGH

© 2016 American Academy of Orthopaedic Surgeons

Straight Leg Raise

- Lie on the floor on your back.
- Keep the affected leg straight and bend the unaffected leg at the knee so that the foot is flat on the floor.
- Tighten the thigh muscle of the straight leg and slowly raise it 6 to 10 inches off the floor.
- Hold this position at peak height for 5 seconds, then slowly return the leg to the starting position.
- Perform 2 sets of 10 repetitions, 3 to 5 days per week, progressing to 3 sets of 15 to 20 repetitions, 3 to 5 days per week.
- After the exercise becomes easy, add 1-pound ankle weights and begin again with 2 sets of 10 repetitions, 3 to 5 days per week, progressing to 3 sets of 15 to 20 repetitions, 3 to 5 days per week.
- Continue for 3 to 4 weeks.

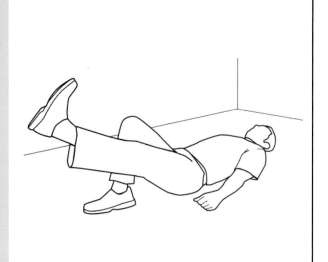

Hip Extension

- Lie face down with a pillow under your hips and the knee on the affected side bent 90°.
- Elevate the leg off the floor to a count of 5, lifting the leg straight up with the knee bent.
- Ankle weights should be used, starting with a weight light enough to allow 2 sets of 10 repetitions, progressing to 3 sets of 15 to 20 repetitions. After that becomes easy, add weight in 1-pound increments and return to 2 sets of 10 repetitions, progressing to 3 sets of 15 to 20 repetitions.
- Perform the exercise 3 to 5 days per week, continuing for 3 to 4 weeks.

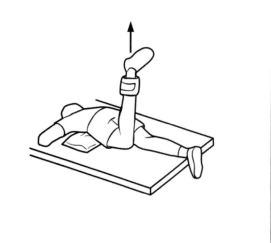

SECTION 5   **HIP AND THIGH**

Hip Rotation

- Lie face down with a pillow under your hips and the knee on the affected side bent 90°.
- Rotating from the hip, move the ankle slowly from side to side, attempting to touch the floor.
- Ankle weights should be used, starting with a weight light enough to allow 2 sets of 10 repetitions, progressing to 3 sets of 15 to 20 repetitions. After that becomes easy, add weight in 1-pound increments and return to 2 sets of 10 repetitions, progressing to 3 sets of 15 to 20 repetitions.
- Perform the exercise 3 to 5 days per week, continuing for 3 to 4 weeks.

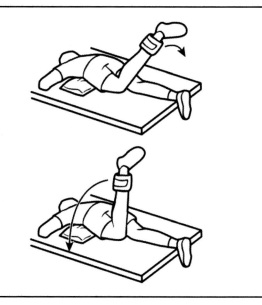

SECTION 5   HIP AND THIGH

Strains of the Thigh

Definition

Injury to the thigh muscles can be temporarily painful and devastating to the avid elite or weekend athlete. The posterior thigh muscles (hamstring muscles) are injured more often than the anterior thigh muscles (quadriceps). Most hamstring strains occur when one of these muscles (biceps femoris, semimembranosus, or semitendinosus) is put on stretch during an active contraction. The strain or tear usually occurs at the musculotendinous junction. The quadriceps may sustain a similar injury; however, the quadriceps is more often injured by a direct blow.

Clinical Symptoms

A patient with a hamstring strain typically reports a sudden onset of posterior thigh pain that occurred while running, water skiing, or some other rapid movement. A "pop" may have been perceived at the onset of pain. Quadriceps contusions are associated with a direct blow during contact sports.

Tests

Physical Examination

Physical examination reveals local tenderness at the site of the injured muscle. With time, the inflammation spreads and the tenderness can become less localized. Muscle injury and associated hemorrhage may be evident by ecchymosis located in the region of the affected muscle. The hamstrings span two joints, originating above the hip on the ischial tuberosity and inserting below the knee on the tibia and fibula. Placing the hamstring on stretch to confirm the diagnosis requires flexion of the hip followed by extension of the knee. Three components of the quadriceps muscle (vastus medialis, vastus intermedius, and vastus lateralis) span only one joint. Therefore, pain associated with strain or contusion of this part of the quadriceps muscle is exacerbated by flexion of the knee and is not related to the position of the hip. The fourth component of the quadriceps muscle, the rectus femoris, spans two joints—the hip and the knee. To put this muscle on stretch, perform the prone rectus femoris test by flexing the knee with the hip in extension.

Diagnostic Tests

Radiographs or other specialized imaging studies usually are not needed in patients with a typical history and physical examination. If there is a suspicion of a fracture or bony avulsion injury, plain radiographs can be obtained. MRI can confirm a strain of the thigh (**Figure 1**), but this is rarely indicated because the history and physical examination can adequately provide a correct diagnosis.

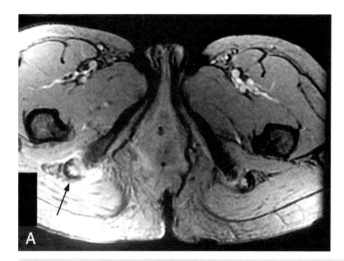
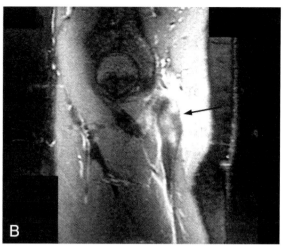

Figure 1 **A,** Axial MRI of the pelvis of a 39-year-old woman who sustained an acute injury while water skiing. Area of signal change (arrow) indicates an acute hamstring injury. **B,** Sagittal MRI of the hip and thigh of the same patient also demonstrates the hamstring injury (arrow).

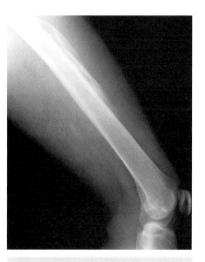

Figure 2 Radiograph demonstrates myositis ossificans of the thigh.

Differential Diagnosis

- Adductor injuries (pain in the groin and inner thigh; ecchymosis; occasional sharp, stabbing pain)
- Iliopsoas strains (pain in the groin with hip flexion)
- Muscle strain of other pelvic/hip muscles (pain with ambulation)
- Pelvic avulsion fractures (pain and ecchymosis over the anterior superior iliac spine, evident on radiographs)
- Proximal femoral tumor (pain in the groin or thigh at rest or at night, pain with weight bearing, evident on radiographs)

Adverse Outcomes of the Disease

Chronic hamstring injuries are debilitating and can end an elite athlete's career. Contusion (hemorrhage) in the quadriceps muscle may progress to myositis ossificans (**Figure 2**), with a resulting restriction of knee flexion and a possible diagnostic dilemma because the clinical appearance may simulate a malignant tumor.

Treatment

Initial treatment includes the prevention of further swelling and hemorrhage by having the patient rest and elevate the limb while applying ice and compressive wraps as needed. As time passes, the patient should begin a program of rehabilitation with stretching and strengthening of the injured muscle. The degree of rehabilitation necessary depends on the patient's general activity level and the severity of the injury. Most patients can be treated with a home exercise program. Elite athletes usually are treated with a more aggressive and costly regimen. The long-term results are generally similar. If myositis ossificans develops in the quadriceps muscle, the rehabilitation process is typically longer, but surgical excision of the ossific mass is rarely needed. NSAIDs may be used as an adjunct to a rehabilitation program to reduce pain and inflammation.

Rehabilitation Prescription

The hamstrings, adductors, and quadriceps muscle groups of the thigh are commonly injured. Sometimes a muscle imbalance of the hip and trunk is responsible for strains of these muscle groups. Early treatment consists of rest, ice, compression, and elevation (RICE) of the affected limb. In addition to RICE treatment, quadriceps injuries should be initially treated with active pain-free stretching, not passive stretching, in an attempt to prevent the development of myositis ossificans.

Depending on the severity of the injury, 1 to 3 weeks of rest may be required. Following the period of rest, early mobilization of the muscle is important to the healing process. Gentle stretching of the involved muscle group is important to regain flexibility, and strengthening is important to prevent a recurrence of the injury. An early home exercise program might include gentle stretching of the hamstrings and strengthening of the hip muscles, especially the abductors.

If pain and stiffness persist, formal rehabilitation may be ordered. The evaluation should include a detailed assessment of the trunk and hip muscle strength, a flexibility assessment of the involved muscle, and pain-relieving modalities to promote healing of the muscle.

Adverse Outcomes of Treatment

NSAIDs can cause gastric, renal, or hepatic complications. In 2015, the FDA strengthened its warning linking NSAIDs with the risk of heart attack or stroke, even in the first weeks of use of an NSAID. Failure to rehabilitate the injury adequately can result in chronic problems.

Referral Decisions/Red Flags

Patients with symptoms that fail to respond to appropriate rehabilitation require further evaluation.

SECTION 5   HIP AND THIGH

Home Exercise Program for Strains of the Thigh

- Perform the exercises in the order listed.
- Apply dry or moist heat to the thigh for 5 to 10 minutes before exercising to prepare the tissues.
- Apply a bag of crushed ice or frozen peas for 20 minutes after exercising to prevent inflammation.
- If exercising increases pain or the pain does not go away after adhering to the program for 3 to 4 weeks, call your doctor.
- The following exercise program is introductory only, and progression of this program will vary based on your specific injury, symptoms, and baseline level of fitness. For further progression of this routine, your physician may recommend evaluation and treatment by a physical therapist or other exercise professional.

Home Exercises for Strains of the Thigh

Exercise Type	Muscle Group	Number of Repetitions/Sets	Number of Days per Week	Number of Weeks
2-person hamstring stretch *or* hamstring stretch	Hamstrings	4 repetitions/2 to 3 sets	Daily	3 to 4
Hip abduction	Gluteus medius	10 repetitions/2 sets, progressing to 15 to 20 repetitions/3 sets	3 to 5	3 to 4
Hamstring curl (standing)	Hamstrings	10 repetitions/3 sets, progressing to 15 to 20 repetitions/3 sets	3 to 5	3 to 4
Straight leg raise	Quadriceps	10 repetitions/3 sets, progressing to 15 to 20 repetitions/3 sets	3 to 5	3 to 4
Straight leg raise (prone)	Gluteus maximus	10 repetitions/3 sets, progressing to 15 to 20 repetitions/3 sets	3 to 5	3 to 4
Wall slide	Quadriceps Hamstrings	10 repetitions/3 sets, progressing to 15 to 20 repetitions/3 sets	3 to 5	3 to 4

2-Person Hamstring Stretch

- Lie on the floor on your back with your legs straight or with one leg bent slightly at the knee if that is more comfortable.
- Your partner raises one of your legs just to the point of tightness and applies light resistance for 30 seconds while you attempt to resist by trying to lower the leg.
- Do the same with the other leg.
- Repeat the cycle 4 times.
- Perform 2 to 3 sets of 4 repetitions per day, continuing for 3 to 4 weeks.

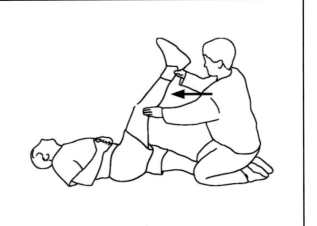

Hamstring Stretch

- Lie on your back on a table or the floor with one leg straight and a strap around your other foot.
- Keeping your knee straight, pull the strap until a gentle stretch is felt in the back of the leg. Hold the stretch for 30 seconds and then return the leg to the resting position on the table or floor; relax for 30 seconds.
- Repeat with the other leg.
- Repeat the sequence 4 times per leg.
- Perform 2 to 3 sets per day, continuing for 3 to 4 weeks.

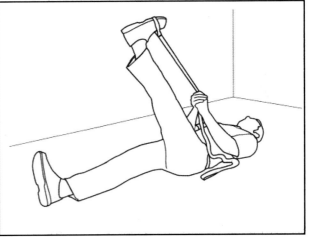

SECTION 5   HIP AND THIGH

Hip Abduction

- Lie on your side with the affected hip on top. Cradle your head in your arm and bend your bottom leg to provide support.
- Slowly raise the top leg up and back to 45°, keeping the knee straight.
- Slowly lower the leg to a count of 5 and relax it for 2 seconds.
- Ankle weights should be used, starting with a weight that allows 2 sets of 10 repetitions and progressing to 3 sets of 15 to 20 repetitions.
- After the exercise becomes easy, add weight in 2- to 3-pound increments and perform 2 sets of 10 repetitions, progressing each time to 3 sets of 15 to 20 repetitions.
- Perform the exercise 3 to 5 days per week for 3 to 4 weeks.

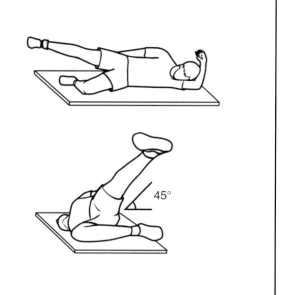

Hamstring Curl

- Stand on a flat surface with your weight evenly distributed on both feet.
- Hold on to the back of a chair or the wall for balance.
- Bend the affected knee, raising the heel of the affected leg toward the ceiling as far as you can without pain.
- Hold this position for 5 seconds and then relax.
- Perform 3 sets of 10 repetitions, 3 to 5 days per week, progressing to 3 sets of 15 to 20 repetitions, 3 to 5 days per week. Continue for 3 to 4 weeks.

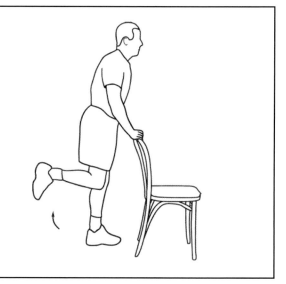

Straight Leg Raise

- Lie on the floor on your back.
- Keep the affected leg straight and bend the unaffected leg at the knee so that the foot is flat on the floor.
- Tighten the thigh muscle of the straight leg and slowly raise it 6 to 10 inches off the floor.
- Hold this position at the peak height for 5 seconds, then slowly return the leg to the starting position.
- Perform 3 sets of 10 repetitions, 3 to 5 days per week, progressing to 3 sets of 15 to 20 repetitions, 3 to 5 days per week. Continue for 3 to 4 weeks.
- After the exercise becomes easy, add 1-pound ankle weights and begin again with 2 sets of 10 repetitions, 3 to 5 days per week, progressing to 3 sets of 15 to 20 repetitions, 3 to 5 days per week.

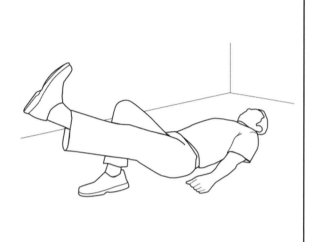

Straight Leg Raise (Prone)

- Lie on the floor on your stomach with your legs straight.
- Tighten the hamstrings of the affected leg and raise the leg toward the ceiling approximately 6 inches. Keep your stomach muscles tight, and avoid arching your back.
- Hold the position for 5 seconds.
- Lower the leg and rest it for 2 seconds.
- Perform 3 sets of 10 repetitions, 3 to 5 days per week, progressing to 3 sets of 15 to 20 repetitions, 3 to 5 days per week. Continue for 3 to 4 weeks.

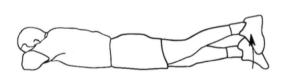

SECTION 5   HIP AND THIGH

Wall Slide

- Lie on your back with the unaffected leg extending through a doorway and the affected leg extending against the wall.
- Let the foot gently slide down the wall.
- Hold the position for a maximum flexion of 5 seconds and then slowly straighten the leg.
- Perform 3 sets of 10 repetitions, 3 to 5 days per week, progressing to 3 sets of 15 to 20 repetitions, 3 to 5 days per week. Continue for 3 to 4 weeks.

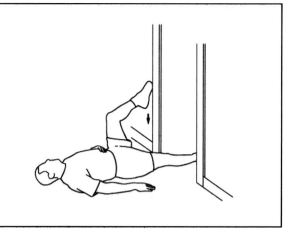

Stress Fracture of the Femoral Neck

Synonym
Stress fracture of the hip

Definition
Femoral neck stress fractures are often misdiagnosed or missed. A failure to identify this injury may be catastrophic. Stress fractures are usually the result of a dynamic, continuing process rather than a single acute, traumatic event. Stress fractures of the femoral neck occur most commonly in military recruits and athletes, especially runners. These fractures can be classified based on the anatomic location of the fracture. Tension stress fractures, which tend to occur in older patients, are usually transverse and occur on the superior aspect of the proximal femoral neck. These injuries have a strong tendency to displace. Fractures on the inferior medial side of the femur (compression side) occur more commonly in younger athletes and usually do not displace.

Clinical Symptoms
Patients usually present with vague pain in the groin, anterior thigh, or knee that is associated with activity or weight bearing and usually subsides after cessation of activity. Athletes usually report an increase in exercise intensity or activity level in the few weeks preceding symptoms.

Tests
Physical Examination
Examination of the hip may reveal pain at extreme range of motion or a limited range of motion, most notable in internal rotation. Occasionally, the patient will walk with an antalgic gait. Tenderness at the proximal thigh or groin may be present, related to soft-tissue irritation in the area. A resisted straight leg raising maneuver (lifting the heel of the affected side off the examination table with the knee held straight) may reproduce the groin or thigh pain.

Diagnostic Tests
Although plain radiographs are the first diagnostic test ordered, they are not diagnostic in most patients. Classic radiographic signs of stress fracture, including radiolucent lines, sclerosis, or periosteal new bone formation, usually are not apparent until 2 to 4 weeks after the onset of symptoms. Bone scans, however, can detect stress fractures as soon as 24 to 48 hours after the injury (**Figure 1**).

MRI is extremely sensitive for identifying stress fractures of the femoral neck (and useful for differentiating compression-side from tension-side involvement) and should be considered in all patients

SECTION 5 HIP AND THIGH

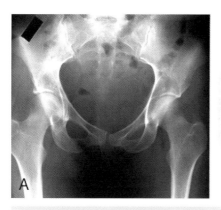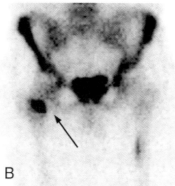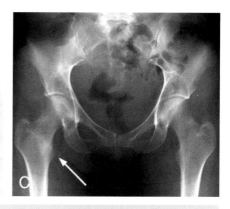

Figure 1 Images of stress fracture at the base of the femoral neck. **A,** Initial AP radiograph demonstrates no apparent sign of fracture. **B,** Bone scan demonstrates markedly increased uptake at the site of femoral neck fracture (arrow). **C,** AP radiograph following a period of rest from impact activities demonstrates increased osseous density at the site of fracture healing (arrow).

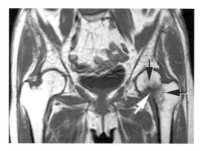

Figure 2 Coronal T1-weighted MRI reveals a linear stress fracture along the medial left femoral neck (white arrow) surrounded by reactive edema (black arrows). (Reproduced from Johnson TR, Steinbach LS, eds: *Essentials of Musculoskeletal Imaging.* Rosemont, IL, American Academy of Orthopaedic Surgeons, 2004, p 451.)

with clinical evidence of a stress fracture but negative radiographs (**Figure 2**).

Differential Diagnosis

- Acute fracture of the femoral neck (evident on radiographs and MRI, history of trauma)
- Muscle strain or groin pull (normal radiographs, intermittent limp)
- Osteoarthritis of the hip (no risk factors, absence of sclerosis within the femoral heads on radiographs)
- Osteonecrosis (dull ache in groin or buttock, evident on radiographs and/or MRI)
- Pathologic fracture (underlying or associated benign or malignant tumor; evident on bone scan, MRI, or radiographs)
- Pelvic fracture (normal hip joint motion, pain on external rotation)
- Tear of the acetabular labrum (pain or instability with hip motion)

Adverse Outcomes of the Disease

Unlike patients with acute femoral neck fractures, patients with stress fractures are usually healthy and active. Adverse outcomes are associated with fracture displacement and include nonunion, osteonecrosis, and progressive varus deformity.

Treatment

The treatment of stress fractures is usually guided by the type and the presence of fracture displacement. Displaced fractures in the young patient are treated as a surgical emergency, and immediate anatomic reduction and internal fixation is mandatory.

Nondisplaced compression-side (medial-side) stress fractures are treated with cessation of activity and crutches with no weight bearing until the fracture is healed. Healing usually takes 6 to 8 weeks. During this time period, serial radiographs are essential to monitor for fracture displacement or widening. Internal fixation may be necessary if the fracture progresses or the symptoms persist despite appropriate nonsurgical treatment.

All tension-side stress fractures are treated surgically whether the fracture is displaced or nondisplaced. These injuries have a high tendency to displace, and an aggressive approach is necessary. Internal fixation is the treatment of choice in these patients.

Adverse Outcomes of Treatment

Osteonecrosis of the femoral head and fracture nonunion are potential complications of internal fixation of femoral neck stress fractures.

Referral Decisions/Red Flags

A displaced femoral neck fracture in a patient younger than 60 years constitutes a surgical emergency because the risks of osteonecrosis and fracture nonunion are significant, and prompt surgical fixation decreases the risk of these complications. All stress fractures require consideration for surgical treatment given the high risk of displacement of tension-side fractures.

Femoral stress fractures may be associated with osteopenia or osteoporosis. Consider evaluation for bone density deficits in these patients.

SECTION 5 HIP AND THIGH

Transient Osteoporosis of the Hip

Synonym
Bone marrow edema syndrome

Definition
Transient osteoporosis of the hip is an uncommon idiopathic condition characterized by spontaneous onset of hip pain associated with radiographic osteoporosis of the femoral head and neck. The condition is most common in middle-aged men and in women during the third trimester of pregnancy. Resolution is spontaneous, usually within 6 to 12 months.

Clinical Symptoms
Patients typically have spontaneous onset of pain in the anterior thigh (groin), the lateral hip, or the buttock. Pain is usually worse with weight bearing and better at rest. Symptoms typically worsen for the first several months and then gradually abate.

Tests
Physical Examination
Patients usually have an antalgic gait and pain at the limits of hip motion.

Diagnostic Tests
Plain radiographs of the hip typically demonstrate diffuse osteoporosis of the femoral head and neck, although signs may not be evident in the early phase of the disease. MRI is helpful to rule out other diagnoses and help confirm the diagnosis of transient osteoporosis. The typical MRI findings include bone marrow edema of the femoral neck with diffuse decreased signal intensity on T1-weighted images and diffuse increased signal intensity on T2-weighted images. The signal change usually extends into the intertrochanteric region (**Figure 1**).

Differential Diagnosis
- Infections involving the proximal femur or hip joint (pain, constitutional symptoms)
- Osteonecrosis of the femoral head (pain in the groin or buttock, sclerosis on radiographs)
- Pigmented villonodular synovitis of the hip (pain in the groin or buttock, evident on MRI and biopsy)

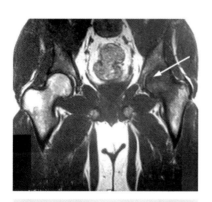

Figure 1 Coronal T1-weighted MRI of the pelvis demonstrates diffuse decreased signal intensity (arrow), indicating transient osteoporosis of the hip.

- Stress fracture of the femoral neck (pain in the groin or buttock, evident on radiographs or MRI)
- Tumors involving the proximal femur (pain in the groin, buttock, or thigh; evident on radiographs or MRI)

Adverse Outcomes of the Disease

Fracture of the femoral neck can occur during the time the bone is weakened by osteoporosis. Pregnant women with the disease appear to be at higher risk for femoral neck fracture.

Treatment

The disease is a self-limited process that typically resolves spontaneously within 6 to 12 months after the onset of symptoms. After other diseases have been excluded and a firm diagnosis is established (usually by the characteristic MRI appearance), supportive treatment is begun. Patients are provided with mild analgesics and placed on crutches to limit weight bearing until symptoms resolve and radiographs demonstrate reconstitution of normal bone density.

Referral Decisions/Red Flags

The diagnosis may be difficult to make with certainty. In pregnant women, decisions regarding imaging studies and the choice of analgesics should be made in consultation with the patient's obstetrician. Pregnant women with the disease appear to be at greater risk for femoral neck fracture.

HIP AND THIGH

SECTION 5

Trochanteric Bursitis

Synonym
Greater trochanteric bursitis

Definition
Inflammation and hypertrophy of the greater trochanteric bursa may develop without apparent cause or in association with lumbar spine disease, intra-articular hip pathology, significant limb-length inequalities, inflammatory arthritis, or previous surgery around the hip (particularly when internal fixation devices are placed in or near the greater trochanter) (**Figure 1**).

Clinical Symptoms
Patients usually have pain and tenderness over the greater trochanter. The pain may radiate distally to the knee or ankle (but not to the foot) or proximally into the buttock. The pain is worse when the patient first rises from a seated or recumbent position, lessens somewhat after a few steps, and recurs after walking for 30 minutes or more. Patients report night pain and are unable to lie on the affected side. Inflammation (tendinitis) of the gluteal tendons may cause a similar pain pattern.

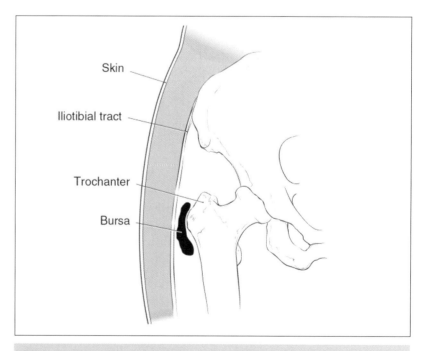

Figure 1 Illustration shows the location of the trochanteric bursa, between the iliotibial band and the greater trochanter.

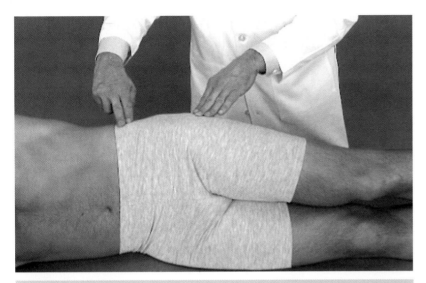

Figure 2 Photograph shows palpation of the greater trochanter with the patient in the lateral decubitus position. With trochanteric bursitis, there is point tenderness over the lateral greater trochanter.

Tests

Physical Examination

With the patient in the lateral decubitus position, palpate the greater trochanter (**Figure 2**). Point tenderness over the lateral greater trochanter is the essential finding. Pain is often exacerbated with active hip abduction. Tenderness above the trochanter suggests tendinitis of the gluteus medius tendon. Patients report increased discomfort with hip adduction or adduction combined with internal rotation.

Diagnostic Tests

AP radiographs of the pelvis and lateral radiographs of the hip are necessary to rule out bony abnormalities and intra-articular hip pathology. Occasionally, rounded or irregular calcific deposits may be seen above the trochanter at the attachment of the gluteus medius. Bone scans and MRI rarely are needed to make the diagnosis but occasionally may be helpful to rule out uncommon conditions such as occult fractures, tumors, or osteonecrosis of the femoral head.

Differential Diagnosis

- Metastatic tumor (evident on radiographs, weight loss, constitutional symptoms)
- Osteoarthritis of the hip (painful internal rotation, evident on radiographs)
- Sciatica (pain posteriorly, pain radiating to the foot, motor and sensory changes, reflex changes)
- Septic arthritis of the hip (fever, severe pain with motion)
- Snapping hip (obvious snap of the iliotibial band)
- Trochanteric fracture (evident on radiographs, persistent limp when walking, positive Trendelenburg sign)

Adverse Outcomes of the Disease

Chronic pain, a limp, or sleep disturbances are possible.

Treatment

NSAIDs, activity modifications, iliotibial band stretching, ice, and short-term use of a cane are sufficient for most patients. It is important to incorporate hip abduction strengthening as part of a comprehensive program. Injection of a local anesthetic and corticosteroid preparation into the greater trochanteric bursa can be helpful in relieving symptoms. Occasionally, repeat injections are required for symptomatic relief. Surgery is indicated only rarely, for refractory cases.

Rehabilitation Prescription

The pathology underlying trochanteric bursitis can be difficult to identify. Regardless, the muscles surrounding the hip joint can play an important role in the management of pain and flexibility with this condition. Regular stretching of the piriformis and tensor fascia latae may reduce pain over the greater trochanter. A home exercise program that attempts to stretch these muscles is appropriate provided the physician has identified no contraindications.

Adverse Outcomes of Treatment

NSAIDs can cause gastric, renal, or hepatic complications. In 2015, the FDA strengthened its warning linking NSAIDs with the risk of heart attack or stroke, even in the first weeks of use of an NSAID. In some patients, pain may persist. Rarely, infection from the injection can develop, but this can be largely avoided by the careful use of sterile technique.

Referral Decisions/Red Flags

Failure of treatment, diagnostic uncertainty, and/or suspected fracture are indications for further evaluation.

Home Exercise Program for Trochanteric Bursitis

- Perform the exercises in the order listed.
- Apply dry or moist heat to the hip for 5 to 10 minutes before exercising to prepare the tissues.
- Alternatively, riding a stationary bicycle for 10 minutes also will prepare the tissues for stretching.
- Apply a bag of crushed ice or frozen peas to the hip for 20 minutes after exercising to help reduce inflammation.
- If you experience pain in the hip during or after exercising, discontinue the exercises and call your doctor.
- The following exercise program is introductory only, and progression of this program will vary based on your specific injury, symptoms, and baseline level of fitness. For further progression of this routine, your physician may recommend evaluation and treatment by a physical therapist or other exercise professional.

Home Exercises for Trochanteric Bursitis

Exercise Type	Muscle Group	Number of Repetitions/Sets	Number of Days per Week	Number of Weeks
Piriformis stretch	Piriformis	4 repetitions/2 to 3 sets	5 to 7	2 to 3
Iliotibial band stretch	Tensor fascia latae	4 repetitions/2 to 3 sets	5 to 7	2 to 3
Foam roller for iliotibial band	Iliotibial band	Once per side, for 2 to 3 minutes each	Daily	2 to 3
Hip abduction	Gluteus medius	10 repetitions/2 sets, progressing to 15 to 20 repetitions/3 sets	3 to 5	2 to 3

Piriformis Stretch

- Lie on your back and bend both knees so that your feet are flat on the floor.
- Place the ankle of the affected leg on the opposite knee and clasp your hands behind the thigh as shown.
- Pull the thigh toward you until you feel a stretch in the hip.
- Hold the stretch for 30 seconds and then relax for 30 seconds.
- Perform 2 to 3 sets of 4 repetitions, 5 to 7 days per week, continuing for 2 to 3 weeks.
- Perform the stretch on both sides.

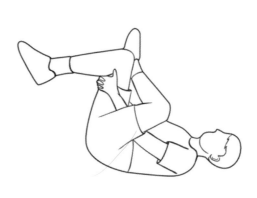

Iliotibial Band Stretch

- Stand approximately 2 feet away from a wall with the affected side to the wall.
- Fully extend your arm and place your hand on the wall for support.
- Cross the affected leg (the leg farther from the wall) over the opposite leg.
- Lean your hips toward the wall until you feel a stretch on the outside of the affected leg.
- Hold the maximum stretch for 30 seconds and then relax for 10 seconds.
- Repeat the sequence 4 times on each side.
- Perform 2 to 3 sets of 4 repetitions, 5 to 7 days per week, continuing for 2 to 3 weeks.
- Perform the stretch on both sides.

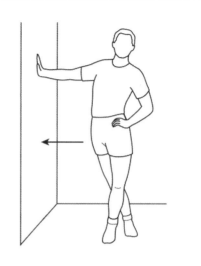

Foam Roller for Iliotibial Band

- Position the foam roller under the outside of your thigh.
- Use your arms to slowly move the lateral or outside portion of your thigh over the foam roller.
- The foam roller should move slowly; stop and hold the position for 5 to 10 seconds at areas of tightness or discomfort, then proceed up and down the outer thigh. Avoid rolling directly over the bony prominence on the outside of your hip (arrow) because doing so may irritate the trochanteric bursa.
- Mild to severe discomfort may be present but should improve with consistent daily use of the foam roller. If the discomfort does not improve within 1 to 2 weeks, seek the advice of your sports medicine physician.
- Perform every day, for 2 to 3 minutes on each leg. Continue for 2 to 3 weeks.

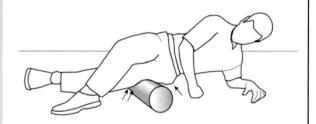

Hip Abduction

- Lie on your side with the affected hip on top. Cradle your head in your arm and bend your bottom leg to provide support.
- Slowly move the top leg up and back to 45°, keeping the knee straight. Hold this position for 5 seconds.
- Slowly lower the leg to a count of 5 and relax it for 2 seconds.
- Ankle weights should be used, starting with a weight light enough to allow 2 sets of 10 repetitions and progressing to 3 sets of 15 to 20 repetitions.
- Add weight in 2- to 3-pound increments and return to 2 sets of 10 repetitions, progressing each time to 3 sets of 15 to 20 repetitions.
- Perform the exercise 3 to 5 times per week, continuing for 2 to 3 weeks.

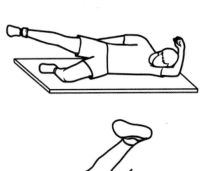
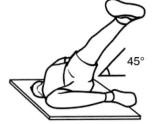

SECTION 5 HIP AND THIGH

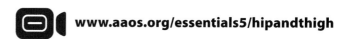
Procedure: Trochanteric Bursitis Injection

Note: Opinions differ regarding single- versus two-needle injection techniques. Proponents of the single-needle technique believe that one needle is less painful for the patient than two. Because the corticosteroid preparation is thicker than the local anesthetic, however, a slightly larger gauge needle is required at the outset. Physicians who prefer the two-needle technique point out that the smaller gauge needle is easier for patients to tolerate and that the pain of the second injection is dulled by the anesthetic. A two-syringe, two-needle technique is described in the video.

Step 1
Wear protective gloves at all times during the procedure and use sterile technique.

Step 2
Ask the patient to lie in the lateral decubitus position with the affected hip upward. Place a pillow between the patient's knees to relax the iliotibial band and reduce the pressure required to inject the solution.

Step 3
Cleanse the skin with a bactericidal skin preparation.

Step 4
Draw lidocaine into a 10-mL syringe.

Step 5
Draw the chosen dose of corticosteroid preparation into the same syringe and mix the two solutions.

Step 6
Palpate the greater trochanter and identify the point of maximum tenderness.

Step 7
Insert the needle until it contacts bone, then withdraw it 1 or 2 mm so that the tip is in the bursa and not in the bone (**Figure 1**). Usually, a 1½″ needle is sufficient, but for larger patients a spinal needle might be needed to reach the trochanteric bursa. Do not withdraw the needle too far or it will be outside the trochanteric bursa.

Step 8
Aspirate to ensure that the needle is not in an intravascular position; then inject one 1- to 2-mL aliquot of the corticosteroid preparation/local anesthetic mixture.

Materials
- Sterile gloves
- Bactericidal skin preparation solution
- 10-mL syringe
- 20-gauge or 22-gauge 1½″ needle (use a spinal needle in larger patients)
- 3 to 5 mL of 1% lidocaine
- 40 to 80 mg of a corticosteroid preparation
- Sterile adhesive sponge
- Adhesive dressing

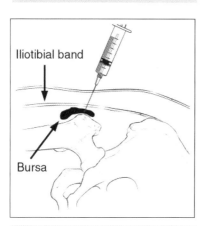

Figure 1 Illustration of trochanteric bursitis injection. The location for needle insertion is shown with anatomic landmarks. (Adapted with permission of the Mayo Foundation for Medical Education and Research.)

Step 9
Partially withdraw the needle; then redirect and reinsert it and inject another 1- to 2-mL aliquot. Continue this to infiltrate the entire bursa, an area of several square centimeters around the point of maximum tenderness.

Step 10
Withdraw the needle completely and apply gentle pressure over the injection site with a sterile dressing sponge.

Step 11
Dress the puncture wound with a sterile adhesive bandage.

Adverse Outcomes
Although rare, infection or allergic reactions to the local anesthetic or corticosteroid preparation are possible. Always query the patient about medication and latex allergies before the procedure. In some patients with diabetes mellitus, poor control of blood glucose levels can occur, but this is usually temporary. Deposition of the corticosteroid subcutaneously may cause fat atrophy or depigmentation at the injection site. A minority of patients will require a series of injections to achieve lasting pain relief; however, repeated injections with corticosteroids should be avoided.

Aftercare/Patient Instructions
Advise the patient that as the local anesthetic wears off, pain often persists or becomes worse for a few days until the corticosteroid takes effect. Instruct the patient to attempt weight bearing as tolerated and contact you if symptoms recur or if redness, fever, immobilizing pain, or any other evidence of a local problem related to the injection occurs.

SECTION 5   HIP AND THIGH

PAIN DIAGRAM
Knee and Lower Leg

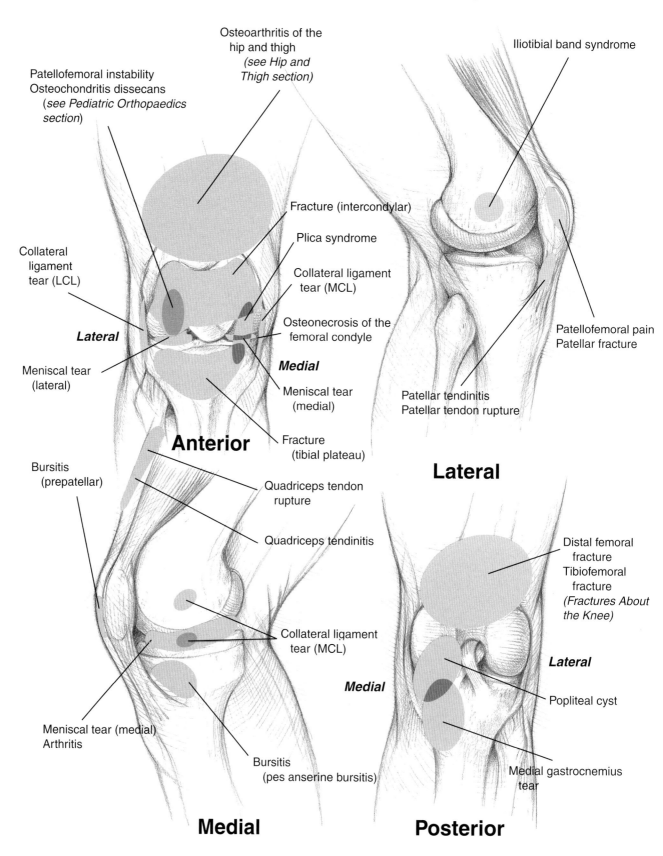

Patellofemoral instability
Osteochondritis dissecans
(*see Pediatric Orthopaedics
section*)

Osteoarthritis of the
hip and thigh
(*see Hip and
Thigh section*)

Iliotibial band syndrome

Collateral
ligament
tear (LCL)

Fracture (intercondylar)

Plica syndrome

Collateral ligament
tear (MCL)

Osteonecrosis of the
femoral condyle

Lateral

Medial

Meniscal tear
(lateral)

Meniscal tear
(medial)

Fracture
(tibial plateau)

Anterior

Patellofemoral pain
Patellar fracture

Patellar tendinitis
Patellar tendon rupture

Lateral

Bursitis
(prepatellar)

Quadriceps tendon
rupture

Quadriceps tendinitis

Distal femoral
fracture
Tibiofemoral
fracture
(*Fractures About
the Knee*)

Lateral

Collateral ligament
tear (MCL)

Medial

Popliteal cyst

Meniscal tear (medial)
Arthritis

Bursitis
(pes anserine bursitis)

Medial gastrocnemius
tear

Medial

Posterior

Knee and Lower Leg

Section Editor

Robert A. Gallo, MD
Associate Professor
Orthopaedic Surgery
Hershey Medical Center
Hershey, Pennsylvania

Contributor

Mark C. Hubbard, MPT
Physical Therapist
Bone and Joint Institute
Penn State Milton S. Hershey Medical Center
Hershey, Pennsylvania

ANATOMY OF THE KNEE AND LOWER LEG

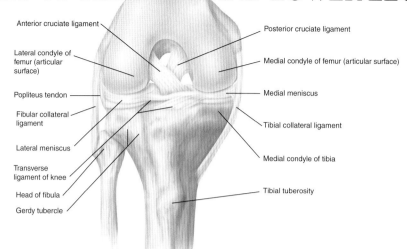

Anterior cruciate ligament

Lateral condyle of femur (articular surface)

Popliteus tendon

Fibular collateral ligament

Lateral meniscus

Transverse ligament of knee

Head of fibula

Gerdy tubercle

Posterior cruciate ligament

Medial condyle of femur (articular surface)

Medial meniscus

Tibial collateral ligament

Medial condyle of tibia

Tibial tuberosity

**Knee: Cruciate and Collateral Ligaments
(Anterior View, Right Knee in Flexion)**

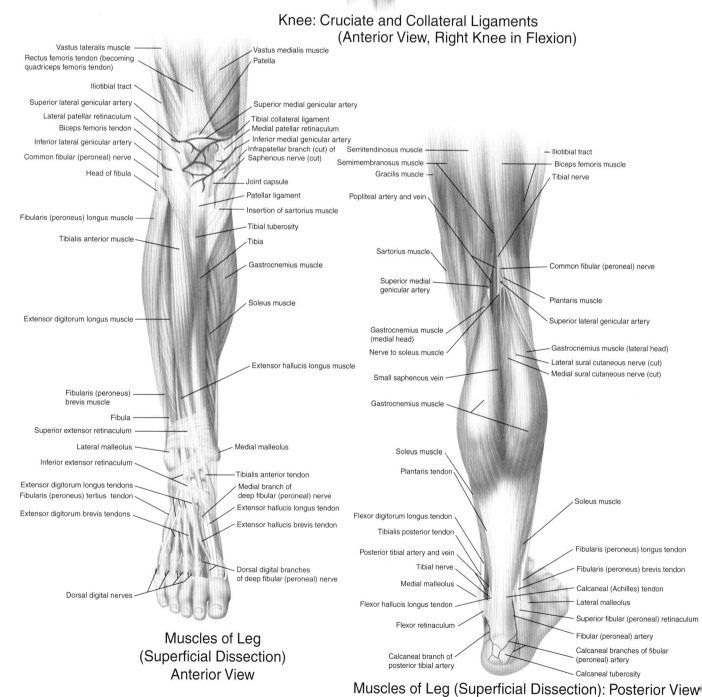

Vastus lateralis muscle

Rectus femoris tendon (becoming quadriceps femoris tendon)

Iliotibial tract

Superior lateral genicular artery

Lateral patellar retinaculum

Biceps femoris tendon

Inferior lateral genicular artery

Common fibular (peroneal) nerve

Head of fibula

Fibularis (peroneus) longus muscle

Tibialis anterior muscle

Extensor digitorum longus muscle

Fibularis (peroneus) brevis muscle

Fibula

Superior extensor retinaculum

Lateral malleolus

Inferior extensor retinaculum

Extensor digitorum longus tendons

Fibularis (peroneus) tertius tendon

Extensor digitorum brevis tendons

Dorsal digital nerves

Vastus medialis muscle

Patella

Superior medial genicular artery

Tibial collateral ligament

Medial patellar retinaculum

Inferior medial genicular artery

Infrapatellar branch (cut) of Saphenous nerve (cut)

Joint capsule

Patellar ligament

Insertion of sartorius muscle

Tibial tuberosity

Tibia

Gastrocnemius muscle

Soleus muscle

Extensor hallucis longus muscle

Medial malleolus

Tibialis anterior tendon

Medial branch of deep fibular (peroneal) nerve

Extensor hallucis longus tendon

Extensor hallucis brevis tendon

Dorsal digital branches of deep fibular (peroneal) nerve

**Muscles of Leg
(Superficial Dissection)
Anterior View**

Semitendinosus muscle

Semimembranosus muscle

Gracilis muscle

Popliteal artery and vein

Sartorius muscle

Superior medial genicular artery

Gastrocnemius muscle (medial head)

Nerve to soleus muscle

Small saphenous vein

Gastrocnemius muscle

Soleus muscle

Plantaris tendon

Flexor digitorum longus tendon

Tibialis posterior tendon

Posterior tibial artery and vein

Tibial nerve

Medial malleolus

Flexor hallucis longus tendon

Flexor retinaculum

Calcaneal branch of posterior tibial artery

Iliotibial tract

Biceps femoris muscle

Tibial nerve

Common fibular (peroneal) nerve

Plantaris muscle

Superior lateral genicular artery

Gastrocnemius muscle (lateral head)

Lateral sural cutaneous nerve (cut)

Medial sural cutaneous nerve (cut)

Soleus muscle

Fibularis (peroneus) longus tendon

Fibularis (peroneus) brevis tendon

Calcaneal (Achilles) tendon

Lateral malleolus

Superior fibular (peroneal) retinaculum

Fibular (peroneal) artery

Calcaneal branches of fibular (peroneal) artery

Calcaneal tuberosity

Muscles of Leg (Superficial Dissection): Posterior View

Essentials of Musculoskeletal Care 5   *© 2016 American Academy of Orthopaedic Surgeons*

Overview of the Knee and Lower Leg

Knee and lower leg problems are diagnosed by obtaining an appropriate medical history, performing a physical examination, and obtaining appropriate imaging studies. Radiographs are the initial imaging study of choice. Patients with knee problems report pain, instability, stiffness, swelling, locking, or weakness. These findings may occur in or around any aspect of the knee. Careful localization of the pain and tenderness will substantially narrow the differential diagnosis. The examination of patients with knee problems also includes a screening evaluation of the hip, spine, and back; some patients with problems intrinsic to the hip present with distal thigh pain and other symptoms that mimic knee disorders, whereas lumbar radiculopathy can produce thigh, knee, or leg pain.

Radiographic examination of the adult knee includes AP, 30° weight-bearing, lateral, and axial patellofemoral (Merchant or sunrise) views (**Figure 1**). Because of a higher incidence of osteochondritis dissecans and reduced likelihood of osteoarthritis, tunnel views obtained with the knee at 40° of flexion should replace the 30° weight-bearing views in patients younger than 20 years. If the patient is able to stand, weight-bearing AP radiographs of both knees should be obtained to allow comparison of the injured knee with the opposite, uninjured knee. A 30° weight-bearing view has been shown to demonstrate arthritis and joint space loss more readily than the AP view obtained in full extension. An axial patellofemoral view helps visualize the patellofemoral joint. Radiographs should be inspected

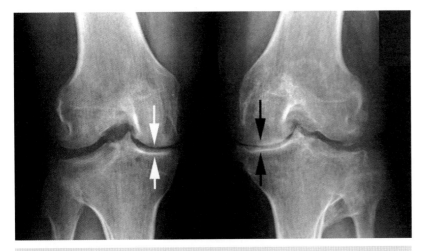

Figure 1 A 30° weight-bearing radiograph demonstrates joint space narrowing in the medial compartment of the left knee (black arrows). Note the more subtle joint space narrowing in the medial compartment of the right knee (white arrows) with less obvious degenerative change. (Reproduced from Johnson TR, Steinbach LS, eds: *Essentials of Musculoskeletal Imaging.* Rosemont, IL, American Academy of Orthopaedic Surgeons, 2004, p 532.)

Table 1

**Possible Causes of Acute
Leg and Knee Pain**

Musculotendinous strains or
   contusions

Fractures

Dislocations

Compartment syndrome

Ligamentous injuries

Extensor mechanism injuries
   (patellar fracture, quadriceps
   or patellar tendon rupture)

Meniscal injuries

for changes in bony architecture, including lytic lesions, blastic lesions, and other areas of radiolucencies and opacities.

Weight-bearing AP radiographs obtained with the knee in full extension and 30° of flexion are used to evaluate medial and lateral compartment arthritis, fractures of the distal femur and proximal tibia, and tibiofemoral alignment. Lateral radiographs are helpful in assessing the patella for fractures and malposition (patella alta and patella baja). Axial patellofemoral views are used to assess patellar alignment within the trochlea and arthritis of the patellofemoral joint.

With the exception of an acute traumatic effusion and no apparent radiographic fracture, MRI is rarely indicated in the initial diagnostic workup. However, MRI often plays an important role as an advanced diagnostic tool or in surgical planning.

Acute Pain

Acute pain in the leg and knee often occurs secondary to an injury. Possible diagnoses fall into several categories, any of which can be associated with acute pain (**Table 1**).

Prompt diagnosis of unreduced fractures, unreduced dislocations, or acute compartment syndrome is required to prevent permanent residual sequelae, including substantial loss of limb function. Deformity and acute effusions often indicate the presence of a substantial injury.

Fractures can involve any of the periarticular osseous structures; dislocations can affect the tibiofemoral, patellofemoral, or rarely, the tibiofibular joint. The location of swelling, deformity, and tender areas can narrow the differential diagnosis, and radiographs can often confirm the presence of a fracture or dislocation. Patellar fractures can result from direct or indirect forces, such as rapid deceleration during falls, whereas fractures of the proximal tibia and distal femur often stem from major trauma. Knee dislocations are rare and result from low- or high-energy events. A high index of suspicion should be reserved for these injuries because knee dislocations often spontaneously reduce and can be associated with occult vascular injuries. The ankle-brachial index of the affected extremity should be determined in any patient suspected of sustaining a knee dislocation. In this setting, an ankle-brachial index less than 0.9 should prompt further vascular imaging. Patellar dislocations are often reduced at the scene when a patient or helper extends the knee. Compartment syndrome results from fractures or crush injuries and represents a surgical emergency. Clinically, the predominant early findings are paresthesia and excessive pain as the pressure increases within the tight fascial compartment. Although compartment syndrome is a clinical diagnosis, compartment pressure measurements are the definitive method to confirm a diagnosis. To minimize myonecrosis, fasciotomies should not be delayed in persons with suspected compartment syndrome.

Although these injuries are not as urgent, isolated ligamentous disruptions, musculotendinous strains and tears, and meniscal tears are other structural causes of acute pain. Patients with ligamentous injuries often recall a "pop" that occurred at the time of injury and present with acute pain, substantial swelling, and instability. Patients with injuries to the extensor mechanism (such as quadriceps or patellar tendon rupture) report sudden collapse and an inability to actively straighten the knee. Meniscal injury should be suspected in persons with a history of a twisting injury sustained with the foot planted on the ground and localized pain and tenderness along the joint. Some patients with meniscal tears describe a locking sensation that prevents full extension and is relieved by gentle manipulation, which reduces or "unlocks" the meniscus. Contusions result from direct blows and cause localized pain and tenderness; musculotendinous strains are indirect causes of pain and swelling.

Acute pain without obvious injury can be caused by infection or crystalline arthropathy. Septic arthritis within the knee joint is rare in adults. More commonly, the prepatellar bursa is the source. Inspection and palpation of the involved area can help localize the infection. Infection in the prepatellar bursa causes swelling superficial to the patella; joint sepsis produces a substantial effusion within the knee joint deep to the patella. Although presentation is similar, infection is often distinguished from an acute crystalline arthropathy flare using knee aspiration for cell count, crystal, Gram stain, and culture. A cell count greater than 50,000 cells per mL suggests infection, and prompt irrigation and débridement of the joint should be considered.

Chronic Pain

Chronic knee and leg pain conditions are defined as those that have been present for more than 2 weeks. Conditions that cause chronic knee pain include osteoarthritis, overuse syndromes (including bursitis, tendinitis, and patellofemoral-related disease), tumors, chondral injuries, and meniscal tears. Inflammatory or crystalline arthropathies such as gout are chronic conditions that can sometimes manifest as an acute flare with an effusion and minimal radiographic change. The etiology of calf pain includes a spectrum of disorders. In addition to the unique ailments discussed in this section, chronic pain in the calf region also can be secondary to less common conditions such as infection (such as osteomyelitis or pyomyositis) and tumor (soft-tissue or bone).

Osteoarthritis and degenerative meniscal tears have similar presenting symptoms and often occur simultaneously. Although both are characterized by symptoms localized to the joint line and can be associated with loss of motion and radiographic changes, isolated degenerative meniscal tears can cause pain without radiographic changes. Bursitis, tendinitis, patellofemoral syndromes, and chondral injuries have similar characteristics; they are often bilateral, associated with increased activity, and worsen with rising or walking after sitting. Primary tumors involving the bone and joint are uncommon but important to recognize. Night sweats and unrelenting night pain are concerning signs and symptoms that should prompt further investigation for the presence of a tumor, which can usually

SECTION 6   KNEE AND LOWER LEG

be identified on radiographs. The most common malignant primary bone tumors are osteosarcoma in adolescents and chondrosarcoma in adults, whereas the most common benign tumor involving the knee is the giant cell tumor, which typically occurs in persons aged 20 to 30 years. Metastatic disease in the knee region is uncommon.

Location of Pain

Anterior Knee Pain

Anterior knee pain is a common presenting symptom and suggests the presence of chondromalacia patella. Usually, patients describe a diffuse, dull, achy pain deep to the patella. In contrast, pain and focal tenderness at the upper and lower poles of the patella indicate tendinitis or partial tear of the patellar insertions of the quadriceps and patellar tendons, respectively.

Medial Knee Pain

Pain along the medial joint line is the hallmark finding associated with a torn meniscus. When the tear involves a large or unstable segment of the meniscus, patients may report a sensation of catching or locking. However, pain and tenderness in this region also can be secondary to arthritis or a focal chondral defect involving the medial compartment of the knee. When the medial joint line is associated with localized swelling and recent injury, a sprain or tear of the midsubstance of the medial collateral ligament should be considered. Alternatively, the medial collateral ligament can be injured near its femoral or tibial attachments with pain localized to the medial epicondyle or a region several centimeters distal to the joint line, respectively. Because of its proximity, injuries to the distal medial collateral ligament are often confused with pes anserinus pathology. The pes anserinus is composed of the insertion of the sartorius, gracilis, and semitendinosus tendons and is named as such because it resembles a goose's foot. Pain in this area in the absence of trauma suggests inflammation of the bursa beneath the pes anserine tendons.

Lateral Knee Pain

Pain along the lateral aspect of the knee is usually caused by iliotibial band syndrome, a lateral meniscal tear, lateral compartment arthritis, or a focal chondral defect affecting the lateral femoral condyle or tibial plateau. Although iliotibial band syndrome, presumably caused by friction between the tendon and the underlying lateral epicondyle, can cause pain anywhere along its course from the lateral epicondyle to the Gerdy tubercle, meniscal tears and chondral pathology are usually localized to the lateral joint line.

Posterior Knee Pain

Posterior knee pain is relatively uncommon. Meniscal tears involving the meniscal root and those associated with the formation of a Baker cyst are common causes of posterior knee pain. In addition, patients with knee effusions may perceive popliteal pain from the distention of the joint capsule. Because of the posterior location of the popliteal neurovascular bundle, abnormalities of the neurovascular system should be considered in patients presenting with posterior knee pain. Popliteal artery aneurysms present as painful, pulsatile masses in the popliteal space and can result in catastrophic consequences if left unrecognized.

Instability

The knee joint can be divided into three compartments: medial tibiofemoral, lateral tibiofemoral, and patellofemoral. The tibiofibular joint, the articulation between the tibia and fibula, is rarely a source of knee symptoms and therefore is not commonly mentioned as a compartment.

Instability refers to a phenomenon in which an articulation has periods in which its components are incongruent, such as the patella subluxating laterally within the femoral trochlea during patellar subluxation or the tibia shifting anteriorly on the femur in the anterior cruciate ligament–deficient knee. Some patients present with feelings of instability, and others describe a sensation of giving way, slipping, or buckling. Buckling can also be caused by collapse of the knee secondary to pain causing reflex inhibition of the quadriceps mechanism.

Tibiofemoral

In the acute setting, muscle guarding by the patient often limits ligamentous evaluation. An ideal examination of the cruciate (anterior and posterior) and collateral (medial and lateral) ligaments is performed with the patient relaxed. Patient relaxation can often be gauged by the amount of tension palpated within the hamstring tendons posteriorly on the medial and lateral aspects of the knee.

Chronic knee instability can occur with severe arthritis; the loss of articular cartilage and the narrowing of the compartment are results of the ligaments not being fully tensioned. In these instances, the knee may have increased laxity when the ligament is tested; however, if the ligament is intact, there will be a firm end point when the ligament eventually tightens.

Patellofemoral

Instability within the patellofemoral joint usually manifests laterally with patellar subluxation or dislocation over the lateral trochlear ridge. Medial subluxation is seen almost exclusively in patients who have undergone a previous "lateral release" in which the lateral retinaculum is surgically divided to release a theoretical lateral tether to the patella. In most cases of patellar instability, the patella transiently subluxates or dislocates and spontaneously reduces. Occasionally, the patella will remain dislocated and the patient's knee will appear deformed and locked in approximately 45° of flexion. In either case, the patient usually exhibits apprehension when lateral displacement of the patella is attempted.

SECTION 6   KNEE AND LOWER LEG

Stiffness

Stiffness generally refers to difficulty obtaining full range of motion. Stiffness has many acute causes (ligamentous injuries, fractures, infection, postoperative) and chronic causes (osteoarthritis, previous trauma or surgery). Stiffness is often associated with an effusion (an accumulation of fluid within the joint) and is an indicator that pathology is present. Distention of the knee joint capsule prevents full flexion. Although an effusion can be a subtle finding, especially in patients with obesity, stiffness can be the finding that alerts both patient and provider that intra-articular pathology exists.

Swelling

Swelling can occur intra-articularly (as an effusion) or extra-articularly. An effusion can be difficult to appreciate on examination. Distention occurs in regions where the osseous structures do not obscure the capsule from the skin. Therefore, an effusion is usually most noticeable above the patella in the suprapatellar pouch and posteriorly within the popliteal fossa. Conversely, extra-articular swelling is superficial to the joint capsule and is often more apparent. Prepatellar bursitis is the most common cause of extra-articular swelling around the knee. The swollen bursa is found superficial to the extensor mechanism and just inferior to the patella.

Locking

Locking of the knee occurs when a fragment, usually a loose body or a portion of a torn meniscus, gets caught between the femoral condyle and the tibial plateau and prevents the knee from extending fully. The knee can typically flex from the locked position, but the end range of flexion is also restricted. Patients "unlock" the knee by forcefully flexing, extending, or twisting, or making a "trick" movement.

"Pseudolocking" is a phenomenon that can present in patients with osteoarthritis or, less commonly, medial synovial plica syndrome. In osteoarthritis, pseudolocking occurs when adjacent irregular articular surfaces stick momentarily as they glide on one another, whereas with medial synovial plica syndrome, the thickened synovial tissue (plica) becomes momentarily caught beneath the patella as the knee extends. Most patients report that pseudolocking happens most commonly when the knee has been immobile, such as rising after prolonged sitting.

Weakness

Weakness of the muscles around the knee can occur acutely or chronically. Acute catastrophic weakness most often involves a complete disruption of the extensor mechanism at the insertion of the quadriceps or patellar tendon into the patella or a displaced patellar fracture. With partial ruptures, the extensor mechanism may remain functional, but without proper protection and a period of activity modification, the tear may become complete. Weakness of knee flexion may be related to a hamstring strain, or rarely, a tear of the proximal hamstring insertion into the ischial tuberosity. Alternatively, weakness can be secondary to a reflex inhibition from knee pain or a knee effusion. An effusion with as little as 30 mL of synovial fluid can cause this inhibition.

Musculoskeletal Conditioning of the Knee

A conditioning program consists of three basic phases: stretching exercises to improve range of motion; strengthening exercises to improve muscle power; and proprioception (joint position sense) exercises to enhance balance and agility. In addition, the exercise session should begin with an active warm-up. Plyometric exercises (high-intensity explosive exercises) may be added for power only after basic strength and flexibility have been achieved. Patient handouts are provided here for the strengthening and stretching exercises. Advanced proprioception exercises and plyometric exercises should be performed under the supervision of a rehabilitation specialist or other exercise professional.

The goal of a conditioning program is to enable people to live a more fit and healthy lifestyle by being more active. A well-structured conditioning program also will prepare the individual for participation in sports and recreational activities. The greater the intensity of the activity in which a person wishes to engage, the greater the intensity of the conditioning that will be required. If the individual participates in a supervised rehabilitation program that provides instruction in a conditioning routine instead of using only an exercise handout such as provided here, the focus should be on developing and committing to a home exercise fitness program. A conditioning program for the body as a whole that includes exercises for the shoulder, hip, foot, and spine, as well as the knee, is described in the chapter Musculoskeletal Conditioning: Helping Patients Prevent Injury and Stay Fit, found in the General Orthopaedics section.

The knee has both dynamic and static stabilizers. Muscles provide dynamic stability to the knee joint and the patellofemoral articulation. Strengthening the quadriceps and hamstrings muscle groups provides dynamic stability to the knee. In addition, the hip muscles such as the gluteus maximus, the gluteus medius, and the internal and external rotators help to control the movements of the femur and the position of the patellofemoral articulation. Conditioning of the knee should focus on three phases: strengthening, stretching, and neuromuscular (proprioceptive) training. Plyometric exercises (power training) would be added for the competitive athlete after basic strength and flexibility have been achieved. Advanced proprioception exercises and plyometric exercises should be performed under the supervision of a rehabilitation specialist or other exercise professional.

Strengthening Exercises

Exercises to strengthen the quadriceps and hamstrings can be performed conveniently with progressively heavier ankle weights.

The resistance training must be progressive so that the muscle is constantly stimulated to grow. Forward lunges (for the quadriceps), hamstring curls, side-lying hip abductions, and hip extensions are good strengthening exercises. The patient should begin with a weight that allows 6 to 8 repetitions and should work up to 12 repetitions. After reaching 12 repetitions with a given weight, the patient should add weight and drop back to 6 to 8 repetitions.

Stretching Exercises

The effectiveness of strengthening exercises for the quadriceps muscle group can be compromised if the range of motion of the knee is limited. Stretching the soft tissues, especially after trauma or periods of immobilization, can be very effective in increasing range of motion. Hamstring stretching exercises such as leg crossovers and crossover standing increase the range of motion at the knee and hip during functional activities such as walking and running.

  After the patient has achieved normal range of motion and strength, sport-specific or work-specific training should begin. The knee musculature needs to be strong and powerful, and protective reflexes need to be optimized to reduce the risk of injury during athletic maneuvers such as sudden changes in direction while running.

Proprioceptive Training

Proprioceptive training is important for balance. Balance, or postural control, is the result of the integration of visual, vestibular, and proprioceptive afferent inputs. The goal of proprioceptive training is to enhance the activity of the proprioceptors, thereby improving their ability to protect the ligaments of the knee. Several commercial devices, such as tiltboards and proprioceptive disks, are available for proprioceptive training. Advanced balance training should be performed under the supervision of a physical therapist, athletic trainer, or other exercise specialist.

Plyometric Exercises

Explosive power of the lower leg is necessary for a high level of athletic performance. Plyometrics and explosive weight training facilitate the development of power in the quadriceps, hamstrings, and gluteal muscles. Examples of plyometric exercises are jumping rope and jumping from side to side over a 6-inch–high barrier. More advanced exercises should be performed under the supervision of a physical therapist, athletic trainer, or other trained professional.

Home Exercise Program for Knee Conditioning

- Before beginning the conditioning program, warm up the muscles by riding a stationary bicycle or jogging for 10 minutes.
- After the active warm-up and the strengthening exercises, stretching exercises should be performed to maintain or increase flexibility. When performing the stretching exercises, you should stretch slowly to the limit of motion, taking care to avoid pain.
- If you experience pain with exercising, call your doctor.
- The following exercise program is introductory only, and progression of this program will vary based on your specific injury, symptoms, and baseline level of fitness. For further progression of this routine, your physician may recommend evaluation and treatment by a physical therapist or other exercise professional.

Strengthening and Stretching Exercises for the Knee

Exercise	Muscle Group	Number of Repetitions/Sets	Number of Days per Week	Number of Weeks
Strengthening				
Forward lunge	Quadriceps	Work up to 3 sets of 10 repetitions	3	6 to 8
Hamstring curl	Hamstrings	10 repetitions/3 sets	3	6 to 8
Side-lying hip abduction	Gluteus medius	6 to 8 repetitions, progressing to 12 repetitions	3	6 to 8
Hip extension (prone)	Gluteus maximus	6 to 8 repetitions, progressing to 12 repetitions	3	6 to 8
Straight leg raise	Quadriceps	6 to 8 repetitions, working up to 12 repetitions	3	6 to 8
Straight leg raise (prone)	Gluteus maximus	6 to 8 repetitions, working up to 12 repetitions	3	6 to 8
Wall slide	Quadriceps Hamstrings	Work up to 3 sets of 10 repetitions	3	6 to 8
Stretching				
Hamstring stretch	Hamstrings	3 to 6 repetitions/3 sets	Daily	6 to 8
Leg crossover	Hamstrings	3 to 6 repetitions/3 sets	Daily	6 to 8
Standing crossover	Hamstrings	3 to 6 repetitions/3 sets	Daily	6 to 8

SECTION 6 KNEE AND LOWER LEG

Strengthening Exercises

Forward Lunge

- Stand up with the feet approximately 3 to 4 feet apart and with the forward foot pointing forward and the back foot angled to provide support.
- Lunge forward, bending the forward knee and keeping the back and the back leg straight. You should feel a slight stretch in the left groin area. Do not let the forward-lunging knee pass beyond the toes.
- Hold the stretch for 5 seconds.
- Repeat with the opposite leg.
- Work up to 3 sets of 10 repetitions, 3 days per week. Continue for 6 to 8 weeks.

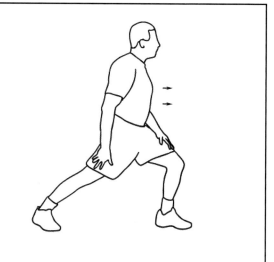

Hamstring Curl

- Stand on a flat surface with your weight evenly distributed over both feet. Hold on to the back of a chair or the wall for balance.
- Raise the heel of one leg toward the ceiling. Hold this position for 5 seconds and then relax.
- Perform 3 sets of 10 repetitions, 3 days per week. Continue for 6 to 8 weeks.

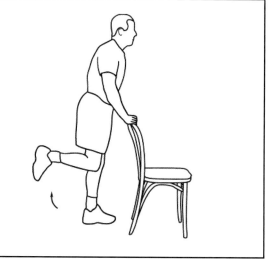

SECTION 6 KNEE AND LOWER LEG

Side-Lying Hip Abduction

- Lie on your side, cradling your head in your arm. Bend the bottom leg for support.
- Slowly move the top leg up and back to 45°, keeping the knee straight. Hold this position for 5 seconds.
- Slowly lower the leg and relax it for 2 seconds.
- Ankle weights should be used, starting with a weight light enough to allow 6 to 8 repetitions, progressing to 12 repetitions. Then add weight and return to 6 to 8 repetitions.
- Repeat on the opposite leg.
- Perform the exercise 3 days per week. Continue for 6 to 8 weeks.

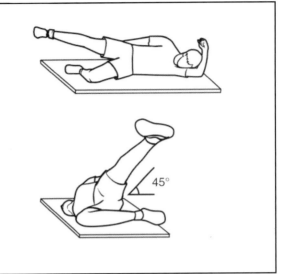

Hip Extension (Prone)

- Lie face down with a pillow under your hips and one knee bent 90°.
- Elevate the leg off the floor approximately 4 inches for a count of 5, lifting the leg straight up with the knee bent.
- Ankle weights should be used, starting with a weight light enough to allow 6 to 8 repetitions, working up to 12 repetitions. Then add weight and return to 6 to 8 repetitions.
- Repeat on the opposite leg.
- Perform the exercise 3 days per week. Continue for 6 to 8 weeks.

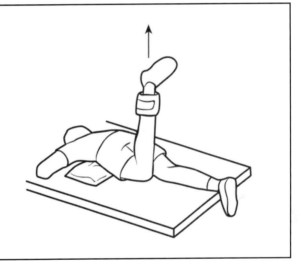

SECTION 6 KNEE AND LOWER LEG

Straight Leg Raise

- Lie on the floor supporting your torso with your elbows as shown, with one leg straight and the other leg bent.
- Tighten the thigh muscle of the straight leg and slowly raise it 6 to 10 inches off the floor. Hold this position for 5 seconds. Repeat with the opposite leg.
- Ankle weights may be used, starting with a weight light enough to allow 6 to 8 repetitions, working up to 12 repetitions. Then add weight and return to 6 to 8 repetitions.
- Perform the exercise 3 days per week, for 6 to 8 weeks.

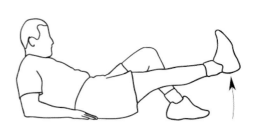

Straight Leg Raise (Prone)

- Lie on the floor on your stomach with your legs straight.
- Keeping the leg straight, tighten the hamstrings of one leg and raise the leg approximately 6 inches. Keep your stomach muscles tight and avoid arching the back.
- Repeat with the opposite leg.
- Ankle weights may be used, starting with a weight light enough to allow 6 to 8 repetitions, working up to 12 repetitions. Then add weight and return to 6 to 8 repetitions.
- Perform the exercise 3 days per week. Continue for 6 to 8 weeks.

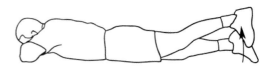

Wall Slide

- Stand with your back against a wall and your feet approximately 1 foot from the wall.
- Tighten your stomach muscles so that your lower back is flat against the wall.
- Stop when your knees are bent 90°. The knees should not pass beyond the toes.
- Hold for 5 seconds and then return to the starting position. Work up to 3 sets of 10 repetitions.
- Perform the exercise 3 days per week, for 6 to 8 weeks.

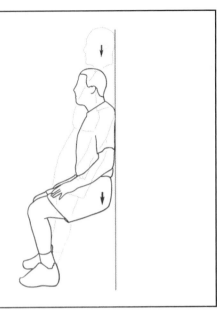

Stretching Exercises

Hamstring Stretch

- Sit on the floor with your legs straight in front of you, and place your hands on the backs of your calves. For comfort, you may slightly bend the leg not being stretched.
- Slowly lift and pull one leg toward your ear, keeping your back straight. Hold the stretch for 5 seconds.
- Alternate from side to side.
- Repeat the exercise with each leg 3 to 6 times. Perform 3 sets per day for 6 to 8 weeks.

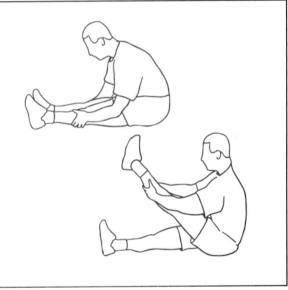

SECTION 6 KNEE AND LOWER LEG

Leg Crossover
- Lie on the floor with your legs spread and your arms out to the sides.
- Bring your right toe to your left hand, keeping the leg straight.
- Hold the stretch for 5 seconds.
- Alternate from side to side.
- Repeat the exercise with each leg 3 to 6 times. For comfort, you may slightly bend the leg not being stretched. Perform 3 sets per day for 6 to 8 weeks.

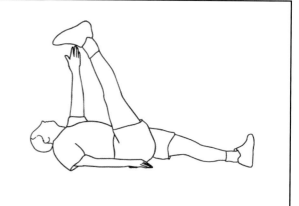

Standing Crossover
- Stand with your legs crossed.
- Keeping your feet close together and your legs straight, slowly bend forward toward your toes.
- Hold the stretch for 5 seconds.
- Repeat with the opposite leg crossed in front for 3 to 6 repetitions. Perform 3 sets per day for 6 to 8 weeks.

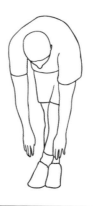

SECTION 6 | KNEE AND LOWER LEG

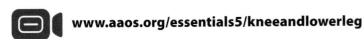

Physical Examination of the Knee and Lower Leg

Inspection/Palpation

Anterior View

With the patient standing, inspect alignment and muscle symmetry, especially of the medial portion of the quadriceps muscles. Valgus malalignment is characterized by an ankle-to-ankle distance wider than the distance between the knees (knock knees). Conversely, varus malalignment is characterized by a knee-to-knee distance wider than the distance between the ankles. Persons with genu varum are referred to as being bowlegged. Internal femoral torsion, usually caused by the femoral neck leaning forward on the femoral shaft (femoral anteversion), aligns the knees with the patellae pointed inward when the feet are pointing straight ahead.

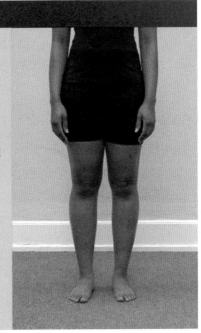

Posterior View

With the patient standing, assess for asymmetry of the posterior thigh and calf musculature, including the hamstrings and calf muscles.

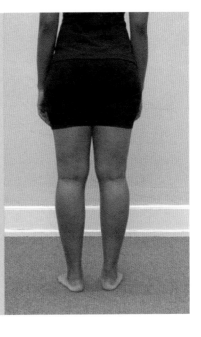

SECTION 6   KNEEANDLOWERLEG

Gait

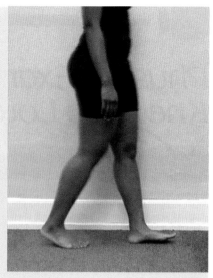

Watch the patient walk. Gait observation provides information on function and may be helpful in developing a differential diagnosis. With arthritic and other knee conditions that produce pain with weight bearing, the patient will limit motion and shorten the duration of weight bearing on the affected side (antalgic gait pattern).

Persons with primary hip pathology may demonstrate a Trendelenburg gait in which the patient leans over the affected leg to compensate for hip abductor weakness. Patients with insufficiency of the lateral knee ligamentous structures, either from trauma or severe medial compartment osteoarthritis, may walk with a varus thrust, which involves normal alignment when standing but in which the knee falls into varus malalignment when the foot strikes the ground during ambulation. Footdrop or inability to dorsiflex the ankle can indicate a peroneal nerve injury, which can be seen in association with an injury to the lateral collateral ligament.

Squat

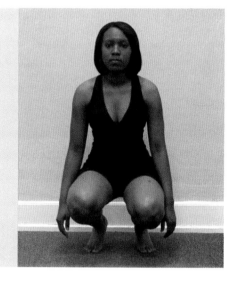

To assess knee flexion, ask the patient to squat. The patient should be able to flex both knees symmetrically. Pain with squatting may indicate meniscal injury or patellofemoral arthritis.

Knee Effusion

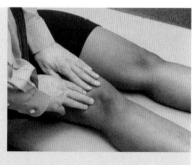

To assess for the presence of an effusion, with the patient supine and the knee extended, inspect the suprapatellar region. If a large knee effusion is present, fullness of the suprapatellar region and loss of the normal dimpling on either side of the patella will be apparent. Subtle knee effusions can be demonstrated by "milking down" joint fluid from the suprapatellar pouch. To perform the milking maneuver, apply downward pressure to the patella with one hand while using the other hand to hold the fluid wave in place. Excess fluid will create a "spongy" feeling as the patella is pushed down.

Patella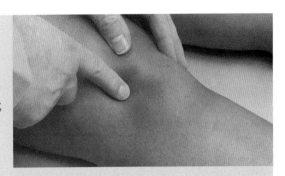

To assess for pathology within the extensor mechanism, palpate the superior and inferior poles of the patella. Quadriceps and patellar tendinitis produce tenderness at the superior and inferior poles of the patella, respectively; complete rupture of these tendons creates a palpable defect at their respective locations. The defect becomes more prominent with increasing knee flexion and is associated with the patient's inability to actively straighten the knee.

Patellar tenderness can be elicited by placing the patient supine, ensuring relaxation of the extensor mechanism, and displacing the patella laterally and medially to allow palpation of the edges and undersurface of the patella. To perform a sensitive test for patellofemoral crepitus, place the patient supine with the hip flexed to 90°, and then place a hand on the patella as the knee is moved through a range of motion. A sensation of crepitus with this maneuver suggests articular cartilage damage within the patellofemoral joint.

Joint Line Tenderness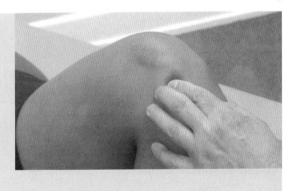

Assess joint line tenderness with the patient supine and the knee flexed 90°. Identify the joint line within the soft spot between the femur and the tibia, then palpate the joint line along the entire joint margin on both the medial and lateral sides of the knee. An area of focal tenderness directly at the joint line supports the diagnosis of a torn meniscus. Joint line tenderness remains the most sensitive and specific physical examination test for the diagnosis of a meniscal tear.

Infrapatellar Bursa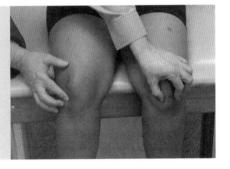

The swollen infrapatellar bursa is usually visible as a dumbbell-shaped swelling on either side of the patellar tendon. In addition, the infrapatellar bursa can be palpated inferior to and on either side of the patella. Swelling of the infrapatellar bursa associated with erythema is concerning for a septic bursitis.

SECTION 6   KNEEANDLOWERLEG

Patellar Tracking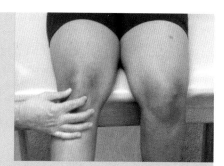

To assess patellar tracking within the trochlea, place one hand on the patella and palpate the patella while the patient flexes and extends the knee. As the knee moves from extension to flexion, the patella normally moves in a gentle arc from a relatively lateral position when the knee is extended to a more central position during early flexion, and then back to a relatively lateral position as flexion continues. With patellar instability, this arc of movement is exaggerated and may make an inverted J-shaped motion (the "J sign"), a sudden lateral movement of the patella as the knee nears full extension.

Range of Motion

Knee motion consists primarily of flexion and extension and can be accurately measured using a goniometer. In adults, knee flexion normally ranges from 135° to 145°, and extension reaches at least 0°. Substantial knee hyperextension (> 5°) is more often seen in young children or in persons with hyperelasticity (loose joints).

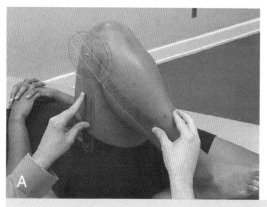
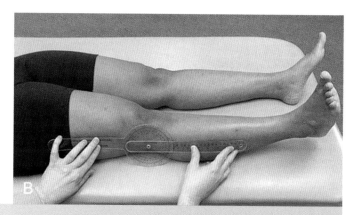

Active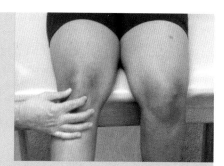

Active flexion may be measured with a goniometer while the patient squats, using the straight knee as the starting position, or, more traditionally, with the patient supine (**A**). Extension (**B**) or hyperextension is motion opposite to flexion, which is measured relative to full extension and compared with the contralateral knee.

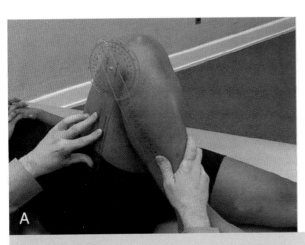
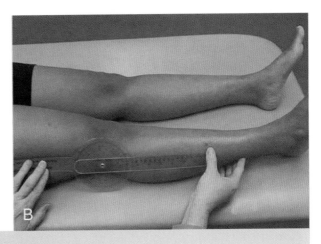

Passive 🎞

Using a goniometer, obtain measurements of passive knee flexion (**A**) and extension (**B**) with the patient supine or prone and with the examiner's hands placed on the ankle and knee to flex and extend the patient's knee. Passive extension can also be measured with the patient supine and the heel resting on a support that elevates the leg 5 cm above the examination table.

Muscle Testing

Quadriceps 🎞

Assess quadriceps muscle strength by asking the seated patient to extend the knee. Apply resistance by pushing down on the tibia after the knee is fully extended.

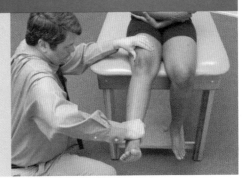

Hamstrings 🎞

Hamstring strength testing is best measured with the patient placed prone. Place the knee in approximately 90° of flexion, and then ask the patient to flex the knee against resistance applied to the distal tibia.

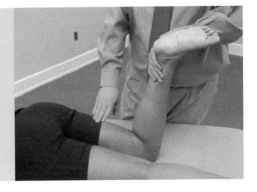

Special Tests

Patellar Apprehension Sign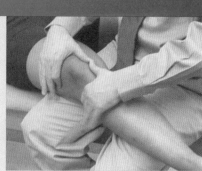

Assess patellar instability with the patient supine and the knee relaxed in approximately 30° of flexion and draped across your thigh. Using your thumbs, apply gentle, laterally directed pressure to displace the patella laterally. Normally, the patella eventually reaches a firm end point laterally after being displaced. In cases of patellar instability, often you will appreciate the absence of a firm end point. Furthermore, the patient often anticipates or perceives pain associated with patellar subluxation over the lateral trochlear ridge, becomes apprehensive, and contracts the quadriceps muscle to avoid further lateral displacement of the patella (apprehension sign).

Patellar Grind Test (Clarke Sign)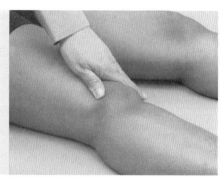

Assess for cartilage degeneration on the undersurface of the patella with the patient supine, the knee extended, and the quadriceps muscle relaxed. Place one hand superior to the patella and push the patella inferiorly. Ask the patient to tighten the quadriceps muscle against this patellar resistance. A grinding sound and/or pain may indicate patellofemoral chondromalacia. However, this test is often positive for grinding and/or pain in patients with normal knees.

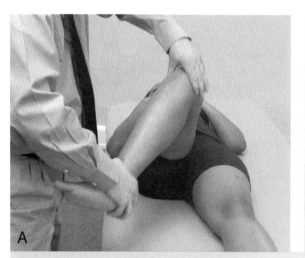
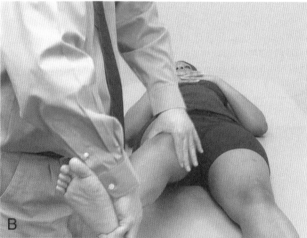

A

B

McMurray Test

The McMurray test is used to evaluate the knee menisci. With the patient supine, flex the knee to the maximum pain-free position (**A**). Hold the leg in that position while externally rotating the foot and then gradually extend the knee while maintaining the tibia in external rotation (**B**). This maneuver stresses the medial meniscus and often elicits a localized medial compartment click and/or pain in patients with a tear of the posterior horn of the medial meniscus. The same maneuver performed while rotating the foot internally stresses the lateral meniscus. To be useful, this test requires pain-free flexion beyond 90°.

Essentials of Musculoskeletal Care 5 *© 2016 American Academy of Orthopaedic Surgeons*

Valgus Stress Test

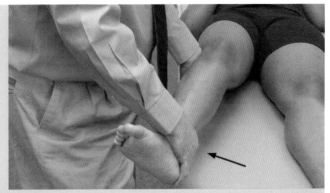

Assess medial collateral ligament stability by applying valgus stress to both knees, once with the knee extended and once with the knee in 30° of flexion. With the patient supine and the thigh supported to relax the quadriceps, place one hand on the lateral side of the knee, grasp the medial distal tibia with the other hand, and abduct the knee (arrow). If the affected knee exhibits increased medial joint space opening under a valgus stress and with the knee flexed to 30°, an isolated injury of the medial collateral ligament likely exists. The additional finding of medial laxity with valgus stress in full extension indicates a more severe injury that involves not only the medial collateral ligament, but also likely the posterior cruciate ligament and/or other posteromedial structures of the knee.

Varus Stress Test

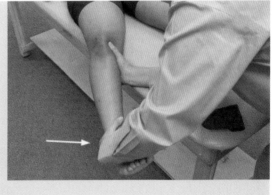

Assess the integrity of the lateral collateral ligament by applying varus stress with the knee in extension and in 30° of flexion and comparing the degree of lateral opening with that of the opposite knee. Many patients, especially those with global hyperlaxity, have physiologic varus laxity. With the patient supine, place one hand on the medial side of the knee, grasp the lateral distal tibia with the other hand, and adduct the knee (arrow). At 30° of knee flexion, if the affected knee has increased excursion compared with the opposite knee in a varus direction, the patient likely has an injury involving only the lateral collateral ligament. If the knee also exhibits asymmetric varus laxity in full extension, the patient has an injury involving the entire posterolateral corner, including but not limited to the lateral collateral ligament, popliteus tendon, and popliteofibular ligament.

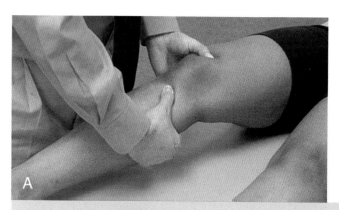

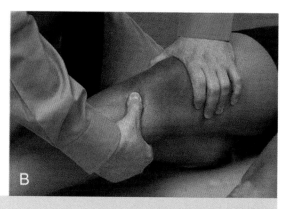

Lachman Test 📹

The Lachman test is used to assess the ability of the anterior cruciate ligament to resist anterior translation of the tibia relative to the femur. With the patient supine, the thigh supported, and the thigh muscles relaxed, flex the patient's knee to 30° and then, after you stabilize the distal femur from the lateral side of the knee with one hand, with your other hand grasp the proximal tibia from the medial side and translate it directly anteriorly (**A**). Alternatively, in the cases of larger patients, you may rest the patient's thigh on your flexed knee on the examination table (**B**). Keep the knee in neutral rotation, then lift the proximal tibia anteriorly while stabilizing the femur. Focus on the amount of bony translation of the tibia relative to the femur and on the presence or absence of a firm end point on reaching full anterior translation. Increased anterior tibial translation and/or the absence of a firm end point suggests a tear of the anterior cruciate ligament. The Lachman test is the best maneuver for assessing the integrity of the anterior cruciate ligament.

Pivot Shift Test 📹

The pivot shift test is used to assess the integrity of the rotatory function of the anterior cruciate ligament. With the patient supine, place the knee in full extension and then slowly flex the knee while applying a simultaneous valgus stress and internal rotation stress. Conversely, the pivot shift can also be elicited by holding the leg in external rotation and flexion, applying a valgus force throughout the range of motion, and slowly extending the knee. In both cases, anterior subluxation of the lateral femoral condyle greater than that of the medial femoral condyle occurs between 20° and 40° of knee flexion.

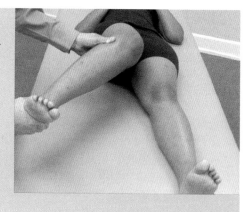

SECTION 6   KNEEANDLOWERLEG

Anterior Drawer Test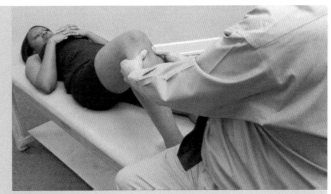

The anterior drawer test is done to determine the ability of the anterior cruciate ligament to provide sagittal stability when damage to secondary restraints exists. The anterior drawer test differs from the Lachman test only in the degree of knee flexion in which the test is performed. Although the anterior drawer test is easier to perform than the Lachman test, it lacks the sensitivity of the Lachman test. The anterior drawer test is performed with the patient supine and the knee flexed to 90° and in neutral rotation. Stabilize the leg by sitting on the patient's foot and palpating the hamstring tendons to ensure that the secondary restraints to anterior tibial translation are relaxed. Grasp the proximal tibia with both hands and thrust the tibia anteriorly. Compare the results with the unaffected knee, which should always be examined first.

Posterior Drawer Test (Gravity Sag Sign)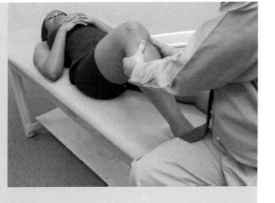

The posterior drawer test assesses the function of the posterior cruciate ligament as a restraint to posterior tibial translation. With the patient supine and the foot supported on the table, flex the knee to 90°. Grasp the proximal tibia with both hands and place your thumbs on the top of the medial and lateral tibial plateaus. In the normal knee, the anterior tibial plateaus are located 10 mm anterior to the femoral condyles at rest. Push the tibia posteriorly; translation of the tibial plateaus to be flush with the femoral condyles indicates at least 10 mm of posterior laxity. This amount of posterior tibial translation is consistent with a complete tear of the posterior cruciate ligament. In many cases of posterior cruciate ligament injury, a positive posterior drawer test may not be apparent because the tibia rests at a level equal to or posterior to that of the femoral condyles (the gravity sag sign). In this instance, no further posterior displacement may be noted when pushing the tibia posteriorly, but the anterior drawer test may exhibit a false-positive response because of the anterior force used to reduce the knee to a normal position.

SECTION 6 KNEEANDLOWERLEG

Noble Test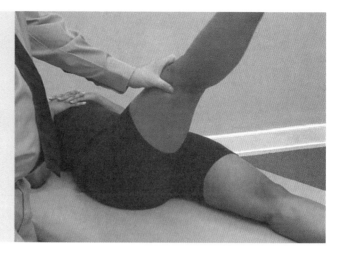

The Noble test assesses for the presence of iliotibial band friction syndrome. With the patient supine and the knee flexed to 90°, apply pressure with your thumb to the iliotibial band over the lateral femoral condyle and then extend the knee. Tenderness elicited between 30° and 40° of knee flexion is a positive sign.

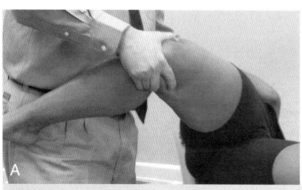
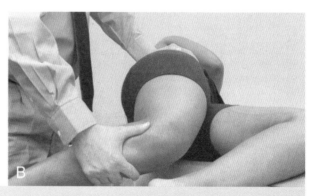

Ober Test

The Ober test can be used to determine the degree of tightness in the tensor fascia lata and iliotibial band. Position the patient lying on the unaffected side with the unaffected knee and hip flexed. Flex the affected knee to 90° and abduct and extend the ipsilateral hip while stabilizing the pelvis (**A**). Then slowly lower the affected thigh as far as possible (**B**). Inability of the extremity to drop below horizontal to the level of the table indicates tightness in the tensor fascia lata and iliotibial band. This tightness may contribute to patellofemoral pain or iliotibial band syndrome.

Fibular Collateral Ligament Palpation in Figure-of-4 Position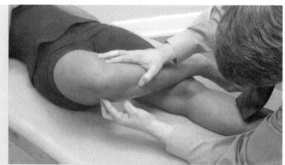

With the knee in the figure-of-4 position, the fibular collateral ligament can be palpated to evaluate its integrity. With the patient supine, flex the affected knee and place the ipsilateral hip in flexion, abduction, and external rotation with the patient's foot placed on the opposite knee (the figure-of-4 position). Palpate the fibular collateral ligament directly in line with the fibula and lateral epicondyle. An intact fibular collateral ligament should be readily palpable in this position; the absence of a cordlike structure may indicate a loss of integrity of the ligament.

External Rotation Recurvatum Test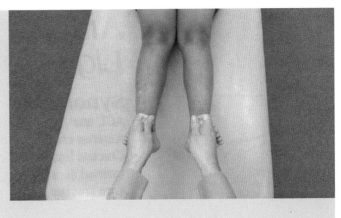

Injuries to the posterolateral corner of the knee can be demonstrated by performing the external rotation recurvatum test. With the patient supine, grasp the great toe of both feet and lift up slightly so that the knees elevate off the table. Asymmetric recurvatum (hyperextension), varus, and knee external rotation greater than 10° compared with that of the opposite limb suggests substantial injury to the posterolateral structures of the knee.

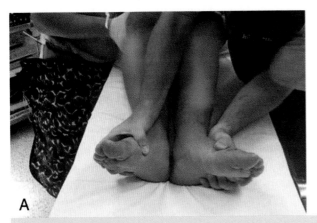

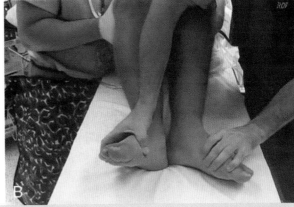

A

B

Dial Test

The Dial test is another test used to determine injury to the posterolateral structures of the knee. The test can be performed with the patient supine or prone. With the patient's hips and thighs in neutral rotation, grasp the heels and flex the knees to 30° (the thighs should remain on the table) (**A**). Apply an external rotation force to each leg. A difference in external rotation between legs of greater than 10° indicates an injury to the posterolateral structures of the knee. Repeat the test with the knees flexed to 90° (**B**). Increased external rotation at 90° suggests a combined posterolateral corner and posterior cruciate ligament injury. If the Dial test is positive only at 30°, an isolated injury to the posterolateral corner structures is likely.

SECTION 6   KNEEANDLOWERLEG

Anterior Cruciate Ligament Tear

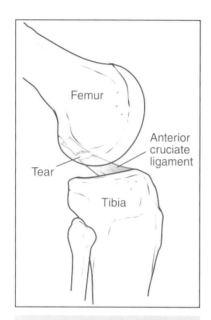

Figure 1 Illustration of the lateral view of the knee depicts a complete anterior cruciate ligament tear.

Synonyms
ACL tear
Anterior cruciate insufficiency
Cruciate ligament tear
Internal derangement of knee
Torn cruciate

Definition
The anterior cruciate ligament (ACL) is a primary stabilizer of the knee against anterior translation (**Figure 1**). A tear of the ACL results from a rotational (twisting) or hyperextension force applied to the knee joint that overcomes the strength of the ligament. Although partial tears can occur, injuries involving the ACL more often result in complete tears. Most ACL tears are from noncontact injuries. An ACL tear is often accompanied by a substantial meniscal tear, a tear of the medial collateral ligament, or, more rarely, tears of the lateral ligamentous complex or the posterior cruciate ligament. Knee injuries that disrupt multiple ligaments are uncommon, but they result in gross knee instability and can be associated with damage to the popliteal artery; this constitutes a limb-threatening emergency.

Clinical Symptoms
Patients with ACL tears usually report sudden pain and giving way of the knee from a twisting or hyperextension-type injury. One third of patients report an audible "pop" as the ligament tears. A patient who sustains an ACL tear during athletic activity usually is unable to continue participating because of pain and/or instability. The pain increases because an effusion, caused by edges of the torn ligament bleeding into the joint (hemarthrosis), develops rapidly.

As the swelling resolves over the course of days to weeks, the patient may have minimal difficulty moving the knee; however, if the tear is left untreated, recurrent instability often develops, particularly with attempts to return to agility sports involving pivoting, running, or jumping. Chronic knee instability from an untreated ACL tear can result in further meniscal and articular cartilage damage resulting in degenerative arthritis.

Tests
Physical Examination
The most sensitive test for ACL insufficiency is the Lachman test, in which the knee is flexed to 30° and the tibia is gently pulled forward while the femur is stabilized (**Figure 2**). It is critical that the patient's leg, especially the hamstrings, be relaxed. Otherwise, the contraction of the hamstrings, which are dynamic stabilizers to anterior tibial

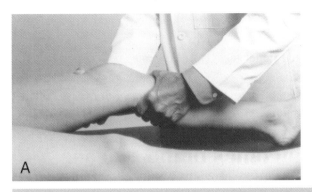
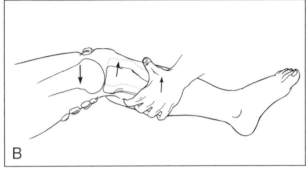

Figure 2 Images of the Lachman test. **A,** Photograph shows the knee flexed approximately 30°. The examiner gently pulls the tibia forward with the medial hand while stabilizing the distal femur with the lateral hand. In a relaxed patient, increased anterior translation of the tibia (compared with the unaffected knee) with a soft end point constitutes a positive test. **B,** Illustration shows movement of the tibia relative to the femur.

translation, precludes an accurate examination. Because of the subcutaneous location of the medial tibia, the tibia is easier to grasp on the medial side (right hand for the right knee, left hand for the left knee) while the femur is stabilized from the lateral side with the opposite hand. If the thigh is large, it may be difficult to support the thigh with one hand. In this situation, the examiner may place his or her knee under the patient's thigh. The examiner uses one hand to stabilize the patient's thigh in this position. The examiner's other hand gently elevates the tibia from the supported femur. Increased motion of the tibia with no solid end point indicates an ACL tear. Because of the effect of other secondary stabilizers such as the medial meniscus, the anterior drawer test, which is performed with the knee flexed to 90°, can be negative in 50% of acute ACL tears and thus is less helpful than the Lachman test. The pivot shift test, which assesses the ability of the ACL to resist rotation, can be difficult to perform, especially acutely after the injury, because this test requires complete relaxation and can be uncomfortable for patients with knee subluxation.

Diagnostic Tests

AP, lateral, and tunnel radiographs of the knee should be obtained for persons with a suspected ACL tear. Usually, these radiographs are positive only for an effusion; occasionally, they may demonstrate an avulsion fracture of the tibial eminence or lateral capsular margin of the tibia (lateral capsular sign or Segond fracture). Tibial eminence fractures are more common in persons with open physes. Although radiographs and MRIs are both helpful in ruling out other causes of an acute effusion, MRI is sensitive and specific for the detection of ACL tears and can help the examiner visualize associated pathology.

Differential Diagnosis

- Meniscal tear (continued tenderness along the joint line, pain or trapping with circumduction) (can occur with an ACL tear)
- Patellar dislocation/subluxation (positive apprehension sign when displacing the patella laterally)

- Patellar tendon or quadriceps rupture (inability to perform straight leg raise)
- Periarticular fracture (tenderness over the bone, evident on radiographs)
- Posterior cruciate ligament tear (positive posterior drawer test, firm end point on Lachman test)

Adverse Outcomes of the Disease

If left untreated, the recurring instability resulting from an ACL tear may cause subsequent meniscal tears and degenerative disease. Because of its role as a secondary stabilizer to anterior tibial translation, the posterior horn of the medial meniscus is particularly susceptible to injury with chronic ACL insufficiency. The resultant instability often makes it difficult to successfully return to participation in agility sports such as soccer, American football, or basketball.

Treatment

Initial treatment of an acute ACL injury includes rest, ice, and the use of crutches until the patient can ambulate without a limp. If the knee effusion (hemarthrosis) is tense, aspiration can be considered to relieve symptoms. A knee immobilizer or range-of-motion brace may be used for comfort when necessary until acute pain subsides.

Early range-of-motion exercises should be initiated promptly. With the patient sitting, the injured knee should be actively extended and flexed as comfort allows. Exercises should be performed repeatedly for several minutes four or five times daily. Full extension and flexion should be regained as soon as pain and swelling permit.

Definitive treatment of an ACL injury depends on the patient's age and desired activity level and any associated injuries. For young, active patients, ACL reconstruction offers the best chance for a successful return to agility sports and limits potential injury to menisci. Older or less active individuals may be treated with physical therapy aimed at controlling the instability. ACL functional bracing also may be helpful with older or less active patients, but this has not been definitively shown to provide sufficient stability for most younger patients to return to sports participation. Younger patients, especially those who hope to return to sporting activities, typically require surgical reconstruction.

In most surgical cases, the ACL is reconstructed using a graft and not repaired. Previous attempts at repair yielded successful results in only 50% of patients, whereas reconstructions generally produce a 90% rate of good and excellent results. Reconstructions can be performed by using a portion of the patient's own patellar tendon, hamstrings, or quadriceps tendon or by using cadaver tissue.

Rehabilitation Prescription

The goal of initial treatment of a torn ACL is to control the inflammation and pain with rest, ice, compression, and elevation of the leg. In addition, maintaining the range of motion and regaining muscle strength are important to rehabilitation. Strengthening of the quadriceps and particularly the hamstring muscle group, as in balance training, is critical for knee stability following an ACL injury. Excessive anterior shearing forces during knee extension from 60° to 0°, especially from 30° to 10°, can cause damage, as can varus and valgus stress in full knee extension. Therefore, exercises that protect the ACL injury by avoiding these ranges of motion and positions, such as hamstring curls to strengthen the hamstring muscle group and isometric quadriceps contraction and straight leg raises to strengthen the quadriceps, are used initially.

If instability, pain, and inflammation continue after 2 to 3 weeks, a formal rehabilitation program may be ordered. The evaluation should include assessment of the strength of the hip and trunk muscles, especially the hip external rotators and abductors, as well as the knee, hamstring, and quadriceps muscles. Outpatient rehabilitation for an ACL-deficient knee should emphasize strengthening of these muscle groups as well as neuromuscular training such as plyometrics and perturbation training, added at the appropriate phase of recovery. In addition, the rehabilitation specialist's evaluation might identify structural deviations that sometimes contribute to ACL injury, such as a large Q angle, excessive foot pronation, hip anteversion, and genu recurvatum and valgum, to help determine the appropriate treatment.

Adverse Outcomes of Treatment

Nonsurgical treatment is associated with the risk of recurrent instability, meniscal tears, and degenerative joint disease. Scarring of the knee joint (arthrofibrosis) with loss of motion can occur after ACL injury or postoperatively after ACL reconstruction, especially when full range of motion has not been restored prior to surgical intervention. Surgical reconstruction is associated with several risks: the usual risks of surgery, such as infection, phlebitis, pulmonary emboli, neurovascular insult, and scarring; the possibility that the ACL can retear; or failure of the ACL graft to incorporate or successfully remodel, resulting in recurrence of laxity. Fracture of the tibial or patellar graft site or rupture of the patellar tendon also can occur after ACL reconstruction when a portion of the patellar tendon is used for the ACL graft. More commonly, patients treated with reconstruction using autogenous patellar tendon or hamstrings tendons report anterior knee pain or posterior thigh pain, respectively. Most patients report numbness lateral to the incision; this results from injury to the infrapatellar branch of the saphenous nerve and often resolves spontaneously.

Referral Decisions/Red Flags

Patients with suspected ACL tears and/or posttraumatic knee effusions require further evaluation and treatment. Even patients who are not candidates for ACL reconstruction can benefit from regular monitoring of the ACL tear, which, when left untreated, can result in a medial meniscal tear.

Home Exercise Program for ACL Tear

- Perform all six exercises in the order listed.
- After each exercise session, apply a bag of crushed ice or frozen peas to the knee for 20 minutes or until numb, keep the leg elevated, and apply a compression bandage to the knee.
- If pain or swelling increases at any time or if it does not improve after you have adhered to the program for 3 to 4 weeks, call your doctor.
- The following exercise program is introductory only, and progression of this program will vary based on your specific injury, symptoms, and baseline level of fitness. For further progression of this routine, your physician may recommend evaluation and treatment by a physical therapist or other exercise professional.

Home Exercises for ACL Tear

Exercise Type	Muscle Group	Number of Repetitions/Sets	Number of Days per Week	Number of Weeks
Hamstring curl (standing)	Hamstrings	20 repetitions/3 sets	4 to 5	3 to 4
Straight leg raise	Quadriceps	20 repetitions/3 sets	4 to 5	3 to 4
Hip abduction	Gluteus medius	20 repetitions/3 sets	4 to 5	3 to 4
Hip adduction	Adductor group	20 repetitions/3 sets	4 to 5	3 to 4
Straight leg raise (prone)	Gluteus maximus	20 repetitions/3 sets	4 to 5	3 to 4
Wall slide	Quadriceps, hamstrings	20 repetitions/3 sets	4 to 5	3 to 4

Hamstring Curl (Standing)

- Stand on a flat surface with your weight evenly distributed on both feet.
- Hold on to the back of a chair or the wall for balance.
- Bend the affected knee, raising the heel of the affected leg toward the ceiling as far as possible without pain.
- Hold this position for 5 seconds and then relax.
- Perform 3 sets of 20 repetitions, 4 to 5 days per week, continuing for 3 to 4 weeks.

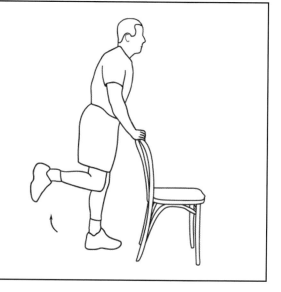

Straight Leg Raise

- Lie on the floor, supporting your torso with your elbows as shown.
- Keep the affected leg completely straight and bend the other leg at the knee so that the foot is flat on the floor.
- Tighten the thigh muscle of the affected leg and slowly raise it 6 to 10 inches off the floor, keeping the knee as straight as possible.
- Hold this position for 5 seconds and slowly return to the starting position.
- Perform 3 sets of 20 repetitions, 4 to 5 days per week, continuing for 3 to 4 weeks.

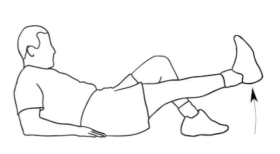

Hip Abduction

- Lie on your side with the affected side on top and with the bottom leg bent to provide support.
- Slowly raise the top leg to 45°, keeping the knee straight.
- Hold this position for 5 seconds.
- Slowly lower the leg and relax it for 2 seconds.
- Perform 3 sets of 20 repetitions, 4 to 5 days per week, continuing for 3 to 4 weeks.

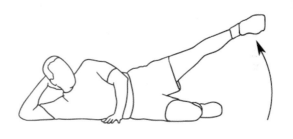

Hip Adduction

- Lie down on the floor on the side of your affected leg with both legs straight.
- Cross the unaffected leg in front of the affected leg.
- Raise the affected leg 6 to 8 inches off the floor.
- Hold this position for 5 seconds.
- Lower the leg and rest for 2 seconds.
- Perform 3 sets of 20 repetitions, 4 to 5 days per week, continuing for 3 to 4 weeks.

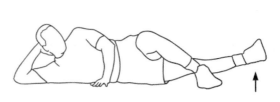

SECTION 6 KNEE AND LOWER LEG

Straight Leg Raise (Prone)
- Lie on the floor on your stomach with your legs straight.
- Tighten the hamstrings of the affected leg and raise the leg toward the ceiling approximately 6 inches. Tighten your stomach muscles to avoid arching your back.
- Hold this position for 5 seconds.
- Lower the leg and rest it for 2 seconds.
- Perform 3 sets of 20 repetitions, 4 to 5 days per week, continuing for 3 to 4 weeks.

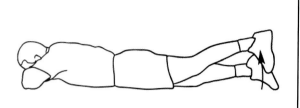

Wall Slide
- Lie on your back with the unaffected leg extending through a doorway and the affected leg extended against the wall.
- Let the foot gently slide down the wall.
- Hold this position of maximum flexion for 5 seconds and then slowly straighten the leg.
- Perform 3 sets of 20 repetitions, 4 to 5 days per week, continuing for 3 to 4 weeks.

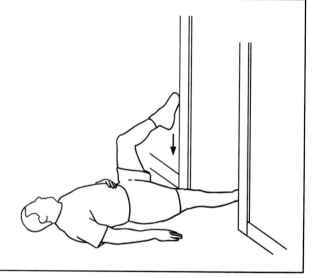

SECTION 6 KNEE AND LOWER LEG

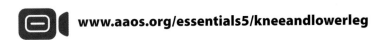

Procedure: Knee Joint Aspiration/Injection

Aspiration of the knee joint can serve both diagnostic and therapeutic purposes. Traumatic injuries such as single- or multiple-ligament injuries, chondral or osteochondral injuries, or other intra-articular fractures may produce large effusions around the knee. Pain can be relieved by draining a tense hemarthrosis. Aspiration also can help identify the etiology of an effusion. Gram stain, culture, and crystal analysis help differentiate infectious from inflammatory processes. With an injury, fat droplets from the bone marrow will accumulate on the surface of bloody aspirate placed in a small cup if an intra-articular fracture (of the distal femur, patella, or tibial plateau) is present.

Injection into the knee joint is the method commonly used to administer corticosteroids or other medications to an inflamed joint. Patients with an arthritic condition of the knee may experience improvement of symptoms for substantial periods with the appropriate administration of an intra-articular corticosteroid or viscosupplement preparation (hyaluronic acid).

> **Materials**
> - Sterile gloves
> - Bactericidal skin preparation solution
> - 25-gauge needle
> - 10-mL syringe with an 18-gauge, 1½″ needle
> - 30-mL or 60-mL syringe with an 18-gauge, 1½″ needle
> - 5 mL of a local anesthetic
> - Corticosteroid or viscosupplement preparation (optional)
> - Adhesive dressing

Step 1
Wear protective gloves at all times during this procedure and use sterile technique.

Step 2
With the patient supine on the examination table and with the abdominal and lower extremity muscles as relaxed as possible, maintain the knee extended.

Step 3
Palpate the landmarks for entry into the joint. Understand that the knee joint will extend almost one handwidth above the superior aspect of the patella, especially when a joint effusion is present. Typical entry will occur via the lateral aspect of the knee 1 cm superior and 1 cm lateral to the superolateral aspect of the patella (**Figure 1**).

Step 4
Spray an ethyl chloride solution to anesthetize the skin at the desired location.

Step 5
Prepare the skin with a bactericidal solution.

Step 6
Using an 18-gauge, 1½″ needle attached to a 10-mL syringe, enter the knee joint at the anesthetized site. Alternately, a 30- or 60-mL syringe

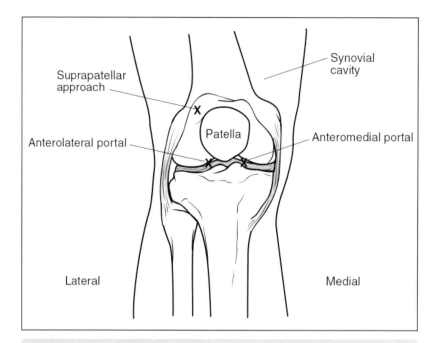

Figure 1 Illustration demonstrates the location for needle insertion for knee joint aspiration or injection. Although aspiration typically is performed via the superolateral parapatellar approach to avoid interference from the infrapatellar fat pad, injection also may be performed via the anteromedial or anterolateral portal approaches.

can be used for larger effusions. Penetration of the joint capsule will be felt as a give or "pop." Withdraw the plunger of the syringe to aspirate the fluid; in a large effusion, the flow should be easy. If establishing flow is difficult, try changing the path of the needle slightly—the needle could be within a fat pad or thick synovium. Using a needle smaller than an 18-gauge size during aspiration increases the likelihood the needle tip will become clogged. Manual pressure can be applied to the suprapatellar region to milk more fluid out of the knee. As fluid is withdrawn, the needle may become blocked with synovium; again, a slight change in direction, with the application of forward pressure to the plunger, will usually free the needle tip and allow flow to continue unimpeded.

Step 7
After the aspiration is complete, inject the medication or local anesthetic into the joint, if indicated. The aspirating syringe may be removed from the needle while maintaining the needle within the knee, and a syringe with the solution to be injected can be attached.

Step 8
When the aspiration and/or injection is complete, apply a sterile dressing.

Adverse Outcomes
As with any invasive procedure, extreme care should be taken to use sterile technique. Because of skin penetration, bacteria can be

introduced into the knee and cause an infection; however, infection is rare following injections. Any areas of erythema or compromised skin should be avoided during passage of the needle through the skin and joint. Other common side effects include increased pain at the injection site that can last 24 to 48 hours after the injection or aspiration. If corticosteroid is injected subcutaneously, depigmentation can occur.

Aftercare/Patient Instructions

After removing a large effusion, apply a compression wrap to minimize the reaccumulation of fluid. Rest and elevation of the lower extremity are recommended for the first 24 to 48 hours following the procedure. Instruct the patient to notify you immediately at any sign of infection, rapid reaccumulation of fluid, or severe pain.

SECTION 6   KNEE AND LOWER LEG

Arthritis of the Knee

Synonyms
Degenerative joint disease
Osteoarthritis
Rheumatoid arthritis
"Wear and tear" arthritis

Definition
Osteoarthritis (OA) is the most common form of knee arthritis. Knee OA can involve each of the three compartments of the knee, individually or in combination: the medial compartment, including the medial tibial plateau and the medial femoral condyle; the lateral compartment, including the lateral tibial plateau and lateral femoral condyle; and the patellofemoral joint, including the patella and the femoral trochlear groove. The medial compartment of the knee is the area most frequently involved in OA. When medial compartment degeneration is predominant, a bowlegged (genu varum) deformity results. Conversely, knock-knee (genu valgum) deformity occurs when the destructive arthritic process primarily involves the lateral compartment. Isolated patellofemoral OA can exist, especially in patients with patellar subluxation or patella baja; however, it is most frequently associated with concomitant tibiofemoral OA.

Secondary knee arthropathy usually occurs in individuals with a history of intra-articular trauma (such as tibial plateau or patellar fractures) or meniscal tears requiring extensive meniscectomy, or those with chronic ligament insufficiencies such as anterior cruciate ligament–deficient knees. Knee OA also can occur secondary to inflammatory arthritides such as rheumatoid arthritis or crystalline arthropathies. Rheumatoid (inflammatory) arthritis, which is less common than OA, typically involves the joint symmetrically but often results in genu valgum because of ligamentous laxity. Crystalline arthropathies typically involve a single joint at a time and are caused by uric acid (gout) or calcium pyrophosphate (pseudogout) that precipitates into crystals and become an intra-articular irritant.

Clinical Symptoms
OA most commonly affects patients older than 55 years, particularly those who have obesity and those who are genetically predisposed to the condition. Insidious onset and periodic exacerbations of pain are common. As OA progresses, the patient will have increasing and more consistent pain with weight bearing, irrespective of the initial cause. Common symptoms include buckling or giving way, which is thought to be caused by reflex quadriceps inhibition or laxity from joint erosion. The patient usually reports a history of difficulty climbing and descending stairs. Stiffness and intermittent joint swelling can limit motion at the extremes of flexion and extension. Symptoms of locking or catching, often mimicking a meniscal

tear, can result from the impingement or sticking of rough joint surfaces and reflexive dysfunction of the quadriceps muscle or the impingement of inflamed synovial tissue between the joint surfaces. As the disease evolves into severe OA, pain can occur during periods of rest or even awaken the patient from sleep. With the crystalline arthropathies, the symptoms are more episodic, ranging from periods of minimal symptoms to those of excruciating pain.

Tests

Physical Examination

Examination can reveal an angular (varus or valgus) knee deformity, which can be visually confirmed by a weight-bearing examination and often corroborated by the patient noticing a worsening deformity. Especially in cases of posttraumatic arthritis, the opposite knee can be used for comparison; however, it is not uncommon for a patient to have windswept deformities (one knee valgus, one knee varus). The osteoarthritic knee often will have a mild effusion and diffuse tenderness along the joint line that may extend into the pes anserinus insertion on the anteromedial tibia. In persons with arthritis affecting the medial and lateral compartments, careful palpation may reveal thickening and osteophytes along the articular margin of the femur, whereas crepitus around the patellofemoral joint can usually be elicited in persons with patellofemoral arthritis. Loss of range of motion often parallels progression of the arthritis and can be pronounced in individuals with genu valgum.

Diagnostic Tests

Weight-bearing AP radiographs of both knees in full extension will demonstrate the true degree of joint space narrowing and deformity within the knee (**Figure 1**). Common radiographic findings of degenerative arthritis include asymmetric joint space narrowing, sclerosis within the subchondral bone, periarticular cysts, and

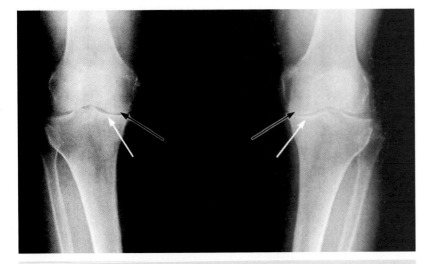

Figure 1 Weight-bearing AP radiograph of both knees demonstrates substantial collapse of the medial joint space (black arrows) and subchondral sclerosis (white arrows).

osteophytes. The hallmark radiographic features of inflammatory arthritis are symmetric joint space narrowing, periarticular osteopenia, and bony erosions at the articular margins. Further information can be obtained from lateral and axial patellofemoral radiographs such as Merchant and sunrise views, which optimize visualization of the patellofemoral joint. In addition, weight-bearing AP radiographs with the knee in approximately 40° of flexion can visualize narrowing of the articular surface because these views profile different weight-bearing areas of the tibia and femur. These weight-bearing images provide optimal visualization of the posterior aspect of the weight-bearing femoral condyle and can be more sensitive for arthritis, especially in cases in which the posterior femoral condyles are involved.

Differential Diagnosis

- Herniated L3 or L4 disk with radiculopathy (diminished knee reflex, numbness)
- Meniscal tear (history of trauma and/or locking and catching) (may be concomitant)
- Osteonecrosis of the femur or tibia (patient older than 50 years, female, history of steroid use, blood dyscrasia)
- Pigmented villonodular synovitis (unexplained recurring hemarthrosis)
- Primary hip pathology (dermatomal referred pain to the knee, limited range of hip motion)
- Septic arthritis (fever, malaise, abnormal joint fluid)
- Tendinitis/bursitis (tenderness directly over a tendon or bursa)

Adverse Outcomes of the Disease

Chronic pain may occur and result in substantial loss of knee function. Walking and other weight-bearing activities may produce substantial discomfort. The overall physical condition of the patient declines because a high level of activity cannot be maintained. Weight gain often occurs.

Treatment

Nonsurgical management may include NSAIDs and activity modification. Selective use of intra-articular injections (corticosteroids or viscosupplementation) can be a useful adjunct treatment, although evidence on their efficacy remains equivocal. Other treatment options including ice, heat, and liniments also may temporarily relieve stiffness and aching. Mechanical aids such as knee sleeves and elastic bandages can help control swelling that occurs with activity and have been shown to improve gait partly by keeping the joint warm. Shock-absorbing shoe insoles or heels decrease impact on the knee with heel strike, and a lateral heel wedge helps unload the medial compartment in persons with varus gonarthrosis; however, clinical evidence of the success of these devices is lacking.

Physical therapy to improve leg strength, flexibility, gait, and balance has been demonstrated to be as effective as NSAIDs for improved pain relief and function. Nonimpact exercises such as water aerobics and recumbent cycling help maintain muscle tone while minimizing pain. Progressive resistance exercises (weight training) in pain-free arcs of motion help diminish muscle atrophy and improve muscle endurance. Using a cane or a single crutch on the side opposite the painful limb (so that the painful limb can be protected during the heel-strike phase) may help decrease pain while ambulating. A patient with poor balance or a history of falling should use an ambulatory assistive device, such as a walker, and may be a candidate for physical therapy. Severe functional limitations and pain at rest or at night indicate the failure of nonsurgical management and the need for surgical treatment.

Arthroscopic management is generally not advocated in the treatment of advanced OA. In mild to moderate cases of OA associated with varus or valgus deformity, an unloading tibial or femoral osteotomy can be successful in improving alignment and decreasing pain. Osteotomies can be expected to result in 5 to 10 years of improved symptoms. Eventually, surgical management of advanced cases involves a total knee replacement.

Rehabilitation Prescription

Rest and ice can control acute inflammation in the arthritic knee. In more chronic cases, a home exercise program of active flexion and extension range-of-motion exercises for the knee and isometric exercises for the quadriceps muscle can be useful. If a formal rehabilitation program is necessary, the assessment should include an evaluation of gait, hip and knee strength, range of motion, and balance. Weak muscles should be targeted.

Adverse Outcomes of Treatment

NSAIDs can cause gastric, renal, or hepatic complications. Although cyclooxygenase-2 (COX-2)–specific NSAIDs are more gastroprotective, they are not immune from causing these adverse effects. In 2015, the FDA strengthened its warning linking NSAIDs with the risk of heart attack or stroke, even in the first weeks of use of an NSAID. Chronic acetaminophen use can result in hepatic and renal dysfunction. Repeated intra-articular injections of corticosteroids typically provide only temporary relief and can result in iatrogenic sepsis and/or accelerated destruction of cartilage. Depending on the preparation of the hyaluronic acid, the active component in most viscous injections, viscosupplementation can cause a severe transient synovitic reaction, especially after repeated injection.

SECTION 6 KNEE AND LOWER LEG

Referral Decisions/Red Flags

Any patient with pain at rest, decreased range of motion, or substantial functional limitations requires further evaluation.

Home Exercise Program for Arthritis

- Perform all six exercises, in the order listed.
- After each exercise session, apply a bag of crushed ice or frozen peas to the knee for 20 minutes or until numb, keep the leg elevated, and apply a compression bandage to the knee.
- If pain or swelling increases at any time or if it does not improve after you have adhered to the program for 3 to 4 weeks, call your doctor.
- The following exercise program is introductory only, and progression of this program will vary based on your specific injury, symptoms, and baseline level of fitness. For further progression of this routine, your physician may recommend evaluation and treatment by a physical therapist or other exercise professional.

Home Exercises for Arthritis

Exercise Type	Muscle Group	Number of Repetitions/Sets	Number of Days per Week	Number of Weeks
Hamstring curl (standing)	Hamstrings	20 repetitions/3 sets	4 to 5	3 to 4
Straight leg raise	Quadriceps	20 repetitions/3 sets	4 to 5	3 to 4
Hip abduction	Gluteus medius	20 repetitions/3 sets	4 to 5	3 to 4
Hip adduction	Adductor group	20 repetitions/3 sets	4 to 5	3 to 4
Straight leg raise (prone)	Gluteus maximus	20 repetitions/3 sets	4 to 5	3 to 4
Wall slide	Quadriceps, hamstrings	20 repetitions/3 sets	4 to 5	3 to 4

Hamstring Curl (Standing)

- Stand on a flat surface with your weight evenly distributed on both feet.
- Hold on to the back of a chair or the wall for balance.
- Bend the affected knee, raising the heel of the affected leg toward the ceiling as far as possible without pain.
- Hold this position for 5 seconds and then relax.
- Perform 3 sets of 20 repetitions, 4 to 5 days per week, continuing for 3 to 4 weeks.

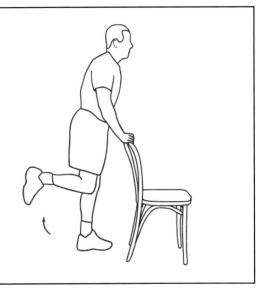

SECTION 6   KNEE AND LOWER LEG

Straight Leg Raise

- Lie on the floor, supporting your torso with your elbows as shown.
- Keep the affected leg straight and bend the other leg at the knee so that the foot is flat on the floor.
- Tighten the thigh muscle of the affected leg and slowly raise it 6 to 10 inches off the floor.
- Hold this position for 5 seconds and then relax.
- Perform 3 sets of 20 repetitions, 4 to 5 days per week, continuing for 3 to 4 weeks.

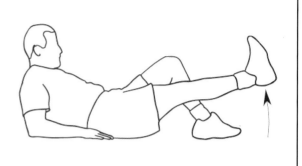

Hip Abduction

- Lie on your side with the affected side on top and with the bottom leg bent to provide support.
- Slowly raise the top leg to 45°, keeping the knee straight.
- Hold this position for 5 seconds.
- Slowly lower the leg and relax it for 2 seconds.
- Perform 3 sets of 20 repetitions, 4 to 5 days per week, continuing for 3 to 4 weeks.

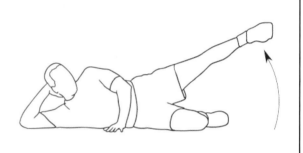

Hip Adduction

- Lie down on the floor on the side of your affected leg with both legs straight.
- Cross the unaffected leg in front of the affected leg.
- Raise the affected leg 6 to 8 inches off the floor.
- Hold this position for 5 seconds.
- Lower the leg and rest for 2 seconds.
- Perform 3 sets of 20 repetitions, 4 to 5 days per week, continuing for 3 to 4 weeks.

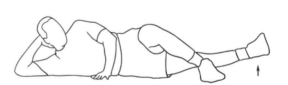

Straight Leg Raise (Prone)

- Lie on the floor on your stomach with your legs straight.
- Tighten the hamstrings of the affected leg and raise the leg toward the ceiling approximately 6 inches. Tighten your stomach muscles to avoid arching your back.
- Hold this position for 5 seconds.
- Lower the leg and rest it for 2 seconds.
- Perform 3 sets of 20 repetitions, 4 to 5 days per week, continuing for 3 to 4 weeks.

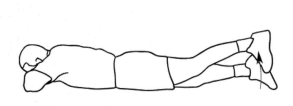

Wall Slide

- Lie on your back with the unaffected leg extending through a doorway and the affected leg extended against the wall.
- Let the foot gently slide down the wall.
- Hold this position of maximum flexion for 5 seconds and then slowly straighten the leg.
- Perform 3 sets of 20 repetitions, 4 to 5 days per week, continuing for 3 to 4 weeks.

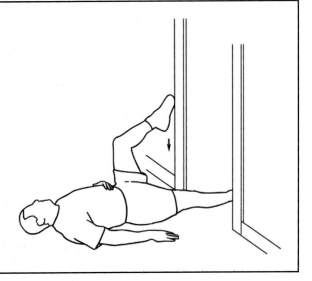

SECTION 6   KNEE AND LOWER LEG

Bursitis of the Knee

Synonyms

Pes anserine bursitis
Prepatellar bursitis

Definition

Bursae are sacs located between the skin and bony prominences or between tendons, ligaments, and bone. Bursae are lined with synovial tissue, which produces a small amount of fluid to decrease friction between adjacent structures. Chronic pressure or friction (overuse) causes thickening of this synovial lining and subsequent excessive fluid formation and can provoke localized swelling and pain.

The prepatellar bursa on the anterior aspect of the knee is superficial and lies between the skin and the bony patella. This bursa can become inflamed (bursitis) or infected (septic bursitis) as a result of trauma to the anterior knee, such as a direct blow, or from chronic irritation from activities that require extensive kneeling, such as wrestling, praying, or carpet installation (housemaid's knee). Bacterial infections typically result from direct penetration, which may be an unrecognized event in patients with dry skin and/or who kneel extensively, or may be iatrogenic following aspiration of a noninfected, swollen bursa. Skin flora, such as *Staphylococcus aureus* and *Streptococcus* species, are the most common infecting organisms.

The pes anserinus bursa lies beneath the insertion site of the sartorius, gracilis, and semitendinosus muscles on the medial flare of the tibia and several centimeters distal to the tibial plateau. Although pes anserine bursitis may result from overuse, it more commonly occurs in patients with early osteoarthritis in the medial compartment of the knee.

Clinical Symptoms

Initially, pain is present only with activity or direct pressure and tends to be more severe after the patient has been sedentary for some time and attempts to walk. Patients also note localized swelling over the involved structure. This swelling is more pronounced with prepatellar bursitis, which often manifests as a dome-shaped swelling over the anterior aspect of the knee when inflamed and fluid filled. Because of its more subtle presentation, pes anserine bursitis can be confused with medial meniscal pathology because the bursitis pain is located along the anteromedial aspect of the proximal tibia (**Figure 1**). Unlike meniscal pain, however, pes anserine bursitis pain is distal to the joint line.

Symptoms from bursitis, which, if infected, can be treated with antibiotics alone, must be differentiated from those of septic joint arthritis. The patient with septic knee arthritis usually demonstrates

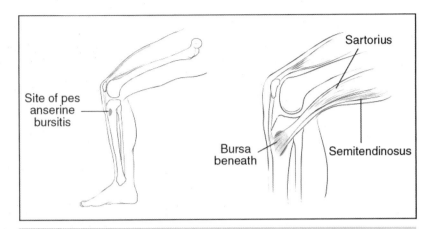

Figure 1 Illustration of the medial view of the region of pes anserine tenderness.

intense joint pain, a large effusion, erythema, guarding with attempted motion, limited range of motion, and a low-grade fever.

Tests

Physical Examination

Areas of potential swelling are inspected and gait observed. The pes anserine insertion and the prepatellar regions should be palpated for localized tenderness, and range of motion should be recorded. Patients with acute prepatellar bursitis typically have swelling superficial to the patella such that the patella may not be palpable in its subcutaneous position. Because of swelling of the pes anserine bursa, the saphenous nerve and its infrapatellar branch can become compressed and cause numbness distal to the patella.

A patient with septic bursitis often presents with increased pain, warmth, and erythema over the patella. With noninfectious traumatic bursitis, the area may be warm but is typically not painful or erythematous. Systemic signs of infection, such as fever and elevated white blood cell count, usually are not as dramatic with an infected prepatellar bursa as they are with septic arthritis of the knee; however, the clinical appearance of infectious and noninfectious bursitis may be the same.

Diagnostic Tests

AP and lateral radiographs should be obtained in patients with chronic pain to rule out bony conditions. Radiographs demonstrate diffuse anterior soft-tissue swelling in persons with prepatellar bursitis, whereas those with septic arthritis usually have an effusion that is most pronounced in the suprapatellar pouch. If septic bursitis is suspected, aspiration should be performed to rule out septic arthritis. This aspiration should be performed in such a manner as to limit potential contamination of the joint, and, if possible, the needle should not be inserted through an area of erythematous skin. The fluid should be sent for Gram stain and culture, cell count, crystal analysis, and synovial fluid analysis.

SECTION 6   KNEE AND LOWER LEG

Differential Diagnosis

- Inflammatory arthritis (multiple joint involvement, abnormal laboratory studies)
- Medial meniscal tear (catching, locking, tenderness over joint line)
- Osgood-Schlatter disease (preadolescent patients, tender over tibial tuberosity apophysis)
- Osteoarthritis of the knee (intra-articular effusion, osteophytes)
- Patellar fracture (intra-articular hemarthrosis, history of trauma)
- Patellar tendinitis (jumper's knee) (tenderness at the inferior pole of the patella)
- Saphenous nerve entrapment (numbness over the medial shin, dysesthesia)
- Septic arthritis of the knee (fever, intra-articular effusion, knee held in more flexion, elevated serum inflammatory markers)
- Tumor (pain, mass, night sweats)

Adverse Outcomes of the Disease

Chronic bursitis may result in continued pain and thickening of the bursal wall. Pressure from continued swelling may cause weakening of overlying ligaments and/or tendons. Progression of a septic bursitis may result in chronic drainage or spread to the knee joint.

Treatment

Most patients with noninfected bursitis respond to nonsurgical treatment, including a short-term course of NSAIDs, ice, and activity modification. Therapeutic modalities such as ultrasound and phonophoresis may help. Patients with identifiable musculotendinous tightness may benefit from quadriceps, hamstring, or iliotibial band stretching exercises to prevent atrophy and maintain flexibility. Injection of a corticosteroid preparation into the bursal sac may be appropriate in recalcitrant cases but can potentially predispose toward septic bursitis. Surgical treatment of knee bursitis is the exception rather than the rule. Early-onset, mild septic bursitis can be managed with oral antibiotics. More severe infections require initial treatment with intravenous antibiotics and close monitoring. Repeat aspiration has been advocated by some to decompress the bursa. Surgical drainage and excision of the bursa may be necessary but often is not required.

Adverse Outcomes of Treatment

NSAIDs can worsen hypertension and cause gastric, renal, or hepatic complications, especially if taken in supratherapeutic doses and for prolonged periods. In 2015, the FDA strengthened its warning linking NSAIDs with the risk of heart attack or stroke, even in the first few weeks of use of an NSAID. Infection from corticosteroid injection or any needle puncture of the bursa (including aspiration attempts) is possible. Another potential side effect from corticosteroid injection is tendon or ligament weakening, especially when the injection is placed deep to the bursa and adjacent to the patellar tendon, and may result in spontaneous rupture. Chronic or recurrent infection, septic arthritis, or the emergence of resistant organisms may occur.

Referral Decisions/Red Flags

Any patient whose symptoms do not respond to nonsurgical treatment, who has septic bursitis, or who has signs of ligament or tendon insufficiency, requires further evaluation. Associated osteoarthritis in recurrent pes anserine bursitis requires evaluation. Prepatellar bursa infections may require surgical treatment when they do not respond to antibiotics or become recurrent.

SECTION 6   KNEE AND LOWER LEG

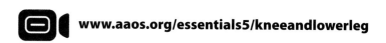

Procedure: Pes Anserine Bursa Injection

For patients with tenderness and pain over the pes anserine bursa, an injection of steroid preparation may provide temporary relief. The injection is performed with a small-gauge needle.

Materials
• Sterile gloves
• Bactericidal skin preparation
• Ethyl chloride spray
• Syringe
• Needle for solution preparation
• Needle for injection
• Local anesthetic as needed
• Steroid solution as needed
• Adhesive dressing

Step 1
Wear protective gloves at all times during this procedure and use sterile technique.

Step 2
Seat the patient with the leg hanging freely.

Step 3
To begin the injection procedure, have the patient indicate the location of maximal tenderness. Medial to the patellar tendon and the tibial tuberosity, the bursa lies between the conjoint tendon of the sartorius gracilis and semitendinosus muscles and the medial collateral ligament.

Step 4
Spray an ethyl chloride solution to anesthetize the skin at the desired location.

Step 5
Prepare the skin with a bactericidal solution.

Step 6
Advance the needle until the tibial periosteum is met, retract 1 to 2 mm, and inject (**Figure 1**). Always aspirate to verify that the needle is not inside a vessel. The fluid should flow easily.

Step 7
Following injection, apply a sterile dressing to the injection site.

Adverse Outcomes
Subcutaneous injection of the steroid solution may result in fat atrophy or depigmentation of the skin and should be avoided.

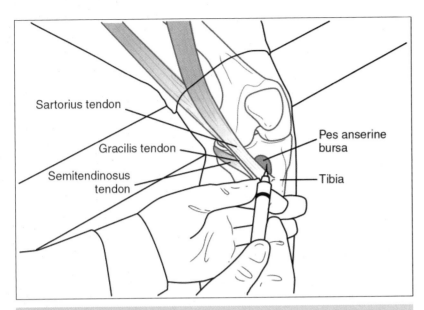

Figure 1 Illustration shows the proper location for pes anserine bursa aspiration and injection.

Aftercare/Patient Instructions

The patient may experience increased pain for 1 or 2 days after the injection before the benefits of the steroid become apparent. Ice may be prescribed to help control any discomfort in the postinjection period.

Claudication

Definition

Claudication is activity-associated discomfort in the legs with a neurogenic or vascular etiology. Neurogenic claudication is associated with spinal stenosis. Ischemia to the cauda equina is the underlying pathology and is induced by postures that mechanically compress the nerve roots with resultant paresthesias and dysesthesias. Vascular claudication is secondary to peripheral vascular disease and compromised arterial blood flow with walking activities. Both entities can result in presentations with a similar type of leg pain.

Clinical Symptoms

Patients with neurogenic claudication experience vague pain that begins in the buttocks and spreads to the legs while walking. Walking down inclines substantially increases symptoms secondary to the associated increased lordotic posture. Symptoms typically improve when the patient sits or lies supine. Pain and paresthesias do not resolve immediately on cessation of walking in patients with neurogenic claudication. This differs from the pain associated with vascular claudication, which typically subsides when walking stops. Another distinguishing characteristic is that riding a stationary bicycle often improves pain from neurogenic claudication but exacerbates vascular claudication. In general, the pain of neurogenic claudication tends to radiate from proximal to distal in the lower extremity, whereas the pain of vascular claudication tends to start distally and progress proximally. In either scenario, claudication can result in paresthesias and/or dysesthesias.

Tests

Physical Examination

Patients with neurogenic claudication may have no abnormal physical findings at rest, but weakness and reflex changes can develop after activities that provoke leg pain. Patients with arterial insufficiency may have diminished or absent pulses below the waist, distal extremities that are cool to the touch, skin ulcerations in the tips of the toes, and increased erythema and pallor changes with elevation.

Diagnostic Tests

AP and lateral radiographs of the spine in patients with neurogenic claudication show degenerative changes such as narrowing of disk space and the spinal canal. MRI and CT results can help further define the pathology, although neither imaging study is necessary as a primary screening tool. The ankle-brachial index (ABI) can be used as an initial screening tool in persons with suspected arterial insufficiency. The ABI is a vascular flow study that measures the ratio of systolic pressure at the ankle to systolic pressure in the arm; a ratio of less than 0.9 is considered abnormal. Doppler ultrasonographic studies and arteriography can visualize any areas of narrowing within the arterial system in patients with vascular claudication.

Differential Diagnosis

- Calf muscle strain (focal tenderness, pain worse with specific motion or activity)
- Chronic exertional compartment syndrome (in athletes, pain following or during exercise, abnormal compartment pressures at rest and with activity)
- Herniated L3 or L4 disk with radiculopathy (diminished knee reflex, numbness, focal neurologic deficit)
- Tibial stress fracture (in athletes, pain following or during exercise)

Adverse Outcomes of the Disease

Patients with either vascular or neurogenic claudication may experience substantial compromise in quality of life because of their inability to walk. Cases of unrecognized or untreated arterial insufficiency can result in progressive ischemia and loss of the distal extremity.

Treatment

Patients with neurogenic claudication can be treated with over-the-counter analgesic medications, intermittent NSAIDs, epidural corticosteroid injections, flexion exercises for the lumbar spine, and, in severe cases, surgical decompression. Therapeutic options for vascular claudication include supportive measures and pharmacologic treatment initially, and surgery such as bypass grafting for patients with more advanced, limb-threatening claudication. Supportive measures include meticulous foot care, well-fitting and protective shoes, and the avoidance of elastic support hose, which are typically used for venous insufficiency.

Adverse Outcomes of Treatment

NSAIDs can worsen hypertension and cause gastric, renal, or hepatic complications, especially if taken in supratherapeutic doses and for prolonged periods. In 2015, the FDA strengthened its warning linking NSAIDs with the risk of heart attack or stroke, even in the first weeks of use of an NSAID.

Referral Decisions/Red Flags

Any patient with neurogenic claudication whose symptoms do not respond to nonsurgical measures may benefit from a consultation with a spine surgeon. Patients with vascular claudication require evaluation by a vascular surgeon.

SECTION 6 KNEE AND LOWER LEG

Collateral Ligament Tear

Definition

The stability of the knee joint largely depends on its ligaments and the muscles that span the joint. Four major ligaments provide primary stabilization of the knee. The medial collateral ligament (MCL) and lateral collateral ligament (LCL) are extra-articular (outside the joint) and stabilize the knee against valgus and varus stresses (**Figure 1**). The anterior cruciate ligament (ACL) and posterior cruciate ligament (PCL) are intra-articular (inside the joint) and stabilize the knee against anterior and posterior tibial translation.

The mechanism of injury in an MCL tear (or sprain) is commonly a valgus (abduction) force, such as a clipping injury in football. LCL injury is less common than MCL injury, results from a varus (adduction) force to the knee, and is often combined with injuries to other structures within the posterolateral aspect of the knee. These structures include the popliteus tendon, the popliteofibular ligament, and in extreme cases, the peroneal nerve and biceps femoris tendon. Injuries to the collateral ligaments can occur alone or in association with a meniscal tear or an injury to the ACL and/or PCL.

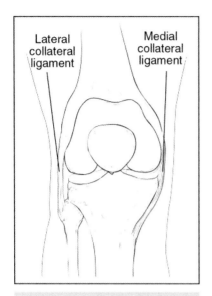

Figure 1 Illustration depicts the medial and lateral knee structures.

Clinical Symptoms

Many patients are able to ambulate after an isolated acute collateral ligament injury and may be able to return to play for the remainder of the game. Patients often report localized swelling or stiffness and medial or lateral pain and tenderness along the course of the ligament. Pain may increase and motion may become limited during the first 6 to 8 hours following injury. Within 24 to 48 hours, localized ecchymosis and a small effusion may develop. A large, acute hemarthrosis usually indicates a tear to one of the cruciate ligaments. Instability and mechanical symptoms such as locking or popping are infrequent after an isolated collateral ligament injury. However, because of the valgus force and impact of the lateral femoral condyle against the lateral tibial plateau, lateral meniscal tears can occur when the MCL is injured. The presence of mechanical symptoms and lateral joint line tenderness in the setting of an MCL injury should increase suspicion for the presence of a possible lateral meniscus tear.

Tests

Physical Examination

Amount of physiologic laxity differs substantially between patients, especially on varus stress tests. Therefore, the uninjured knee should be examined to help the examiner understand the normal ligamentous excursion for the individual patient and to reduce the patient's fears about the examination of the painful limb. Swelling adjacent to the injured ligament is common, but the presence of a large knee effusion often indicates an associated intra-articular injury.

The MCL may be tender either focally or along its entire course from the medial epicondyle of the medial femoral condyle to its broad tibial insertion, just distal to the pes anserinus. Isolated tenderness at the most proximal or distal extent of the MCL may indicate an avulsion-type injury. An LCL injury may be tender from the lateral femoral epicondyle to its insertion on the fibular head. The MCL is best palpated with the knee in slight flexion, whereas the LCL is best examined with the leg in the figure-of-4 position (**Figure 2**).

Both knees should be examined by applying varus stress and then valgus stress with the knee first in full extension and then in 30° of flexion. Varus and valgus stress tests performed at 30° of knee flexion isolate the LCL and MCL, respectively, because the cruciate ligaments and posterior capsule are relaxed. Varus or valgus laxity in full extension indicates a more extensive injury that includes an ACL and/or PCL tear plus disruption of the posterior capsule. These injuries should be considered knee dislocations with spontaneous reduction, and therefore should prompt a thorough neurovascular examination, including an ankle-brachial index of the affected extremity.

With laxity testing, a joint space opening increase of less than 5 mm compared with the unaffected knee is considered a grade I (interstitial) tear, whereas an increase of more than 10 mm is considered a grade III (complete) tear. A grade II (partial) tear falls between these parameters. The degree of instability may be masked in a patient who guards against knee manipulation because of substantial pain and involuntary muscle contraction. Therefore, false-negative stress test results are not uncommon acutely after the injury.

Diagnostic Tests

AP and lateral radiographs should be obtained and evaluated for congruency of the tibiofemoral articulation and evidence of an avulsion fracture at the femoral origin of the MCL or the fibular insertion of the LCL. Widening of the medial or lateral compartment should prompt further investigation into an MCL or LCL injury, respectively. MRI is sensitive for the detection of collateral ligament injuries, can define the location and severity of injury, and can help identify other pathology.

Differential Diagnosis

- ACL tear (moderate to marked knee effusion, positive Lachman test result)
- Meniscal tear (mild to moderate knee effusion, joint line tenderness)
- Osteochondral fracture (radiographic evidence of loose osteochondral fragment)
- Patellar subluxation or dislocation with spontaneous reduction (positive apprehension sign)
- PCL tear (positive posterior drawer test, posterior sag of the tibia)
- Physeal fracture of the distal femur (children and adolescents, tenderness at the epiphyseal plate, evident on radiographs, especially stress radiographs)

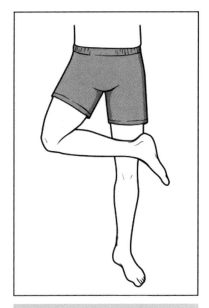

Figure 2 Illustration of the figure-of-4 position.

SECTION 6 KNEE AND LOWER LEG

• Tibial plateau fracture (moderate to marked effusion, bony tenderness, radiographic evidence of fracture, difficulty bearing weight)

Adverse Outcomes of the Disease

Instability after isolated injury to the collateral ligaments is rare. However, when combined with a cruciate ligament injury or malalignment that accentuates the function of the LCL or MCL (genu valgum for the MCL, genu varum for the LCL), collateral ligament injuries may cause feelings of instability.

Treatment

Because of their extra-articular locations and adequate blood supply, generally, the collateral ligaments usually heal and can be managed nonsurgically with a hinged knee brace for protection. For isolated grade I and II sprains of the MCL and LCL, treatment is largely supportive and consists of rest, ice, compression, and elevation (RICE), coupled with a short-term course of crutches and NSAIDs as needed acutely. Range-of-motion exercises are initiated early in the treatment period, and weight bearing is advanced as tolerated. Return to play with a hinged brace is usually permitted within 1 month and based on resolution of the symptoms.

For grade III collateral ligament injuries, treatment can be more varied. Owing to a robust blood supply and propensity to heal, grade III MCL injuries that occur proximally and within the midsubstance of the ligament can be treated nonsurgically with a hinged brace. Stiffness tends to develop with these injuries, and therefore, long-term immobilization should be avoided. Gradual return to full weight bearing ensues over the course of 4 to 6 weeks. Often, 3 to 4 months of protective bracing is required before the patient can return to unrestricted activity. Typically, surgery is required to manage isolated grade III LCL injuries, which often involve injury to the posterolateral capsular complex and popliteus tendon, and tibial avulsions of the MCL. Depending on the location and quality of the torn tissue, the ligament is either repaired or reconstructed. Avulsions directly off the bone are more likely to be repaired. Repairs are optimally performed within 7 days of injury.

Rehabilitation Prescription

Mild to moderate collateral ligament tears are initially treated with RICE to control inflammation and pain. In mild to moderate cases, early protected movement (7 days postinjury) that avoids varus or valgus stress is very important in reestablishing tensile strength and mobility of the ligament. Healing of the collateral ligament is enhanced with movement and delayed with immobilization. A hinged knee brace can protect the healing ligament. A home exercise program should consist of active flexion and passive extension range-of-motion exercises for the knee and isometric exercises for the quadriceps muscle.

If pain, inflammation, and restricted motion continue after 3 to 4 weeks, formal physical therapy may be ordered. The evaluation should include an assessment of hip and knee muscle strength and exercises targeting the weak muscles.

Adverse Outcomes of Treatment

Although chronic instability is uncommon after an isolated collateral ligament injury, recurrence of the injury is possible. Patients are vulnerable to recurrence for 6 months; therefore, bracing for high-risk activities (contact sports) is recommended. Missed associated diagnoses, such as those of meniscal and ACL tears, can produce persistent pain, swelling, or a sense of instability. These injuries may require surgical intervention. In 2015, the FDA strengthened its warning linking NSAIDs with the risk of heart attack or stroke, even in the first weeks of use of an NSAID.

Referral Decisions/Red Flags

Patients with hemarthrosis, substantial joint effusion, subjective instability, or a grade III injury require further evaluation, including an MRI and referral to an orthopaedic surgeon. Failure to respond to nonsurgical treatment could indicate a missed diagnosis, such as an associated cruciate ligament or posterior capsule rupture or a meniscal tear.

Home Exercise Program for Collateral Ligament Tear

- Perform the exercises in the order listed.
- These exercises should be performed with the knee braced for a grade II or III injury, as informed by your doctor using criteria for tests.
- Follow your doctor's instructions as to whether the knee should be in a brace while performing these exercises.
- Dry or moist heat may be applied to the back of the knee during the passive knee extension.
- To prevent additional inflammation, after completing the exercises apply a bag of crushed ice or frozen peas to the affected side of the knee for up to 20 minutes.
- If pain increases at any time or does not improve after performing these exercises for 3 to 4 weeks, call your doctor.
- The following exercise program is introductory only, and progression of this program will vary based on your specific injury, symptoms, and baseline level of fitness. For further progression of this routine, your physician may recommend evaluation and treatment by a physical therapist or other exercise professional.

Home Exercises for Collateral Ligament Tear

Exercise Type	Muscle Group	Number of Repetitions/Sets	Number of Days per Week	Number of Weeks
Hamstring curl (standing)	Hamstrings	25 to 50 repetitions/2 to 3 sets	5 to 6	3 to 4
Hamstring curl (seated)	Hamstrings	25 to 50 repetitions/2 to 3 sets	5 to 6	3 to 4
Passive knee extension (prone)	Hamstrings	One repetition/2 to 3 times per day	5 to 6	3 to 4
Passive knee extension (seated)	Hamstrings	25 to 50 repetitions/2 to 3 sets	5 to 6	3 to 4
Quadriceps setting	Quadriceps	10 to 20 repetitions/2 to 3 sets	5 to 6	3 to 4
Straight leg raise	Quadriceps	10 to 20 repetitions/2 to 3 sets	5 to 6	3 to 4

Hamstring Curl (Standing)

- Stand on a flat surface with your weight evenly distributed on both feet. Hold on to the back of a chair or the wall for balance.
- Bend the affected knee, raising the heel of the affected leg toward the ceiling as far as possible without pain.
- Hold this position for 5 seconds and then relax. Straighten the knee fully between repetitions.
- Perform 2 to 3 sets of 25 to 50 repetitions, 5 to 6 days per week, continuing for 3 to 4 weeks.

Hamstring Curl (Seated)

- Sit on a chair with your feet flat on the floor.
- Slide the foot on the affected side back and hold the position for 5 seconds.
- Perform 2 to 3 sets of 25 to 50 repetitions, 5 to 6 days per week, continuing for 3 to 4 weeks.

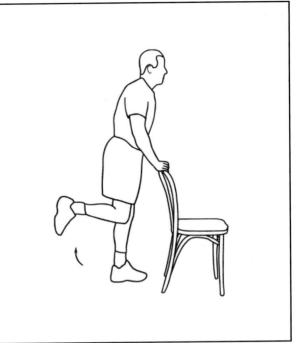

Passive Knee Extension (Prone)

- Lie face down on a table or bed with your thighs supported just above the knee.
- Relax your legs and let gravity pull the knees down (into extension).
- Stay in this position for 5 to 10 minutes.
- Repeat this 2 to 3 times per day, 5 to 6 days per week, continuing for 3 to 4 weeks.

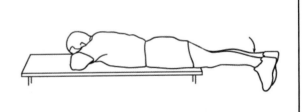

Passive Knee Extension (Seated)

- Sit in a chair with the affected leg propped up on another chair of equal height, as shown.
- Relax your leg and let gravity pull the knee down (into extension).
- Hold this position for 10 seconds.
- Perform 2 to 3 sets of 25 to 50 repetitions, 5 to 6 days per week, continuing for 3 to 4 weeks.

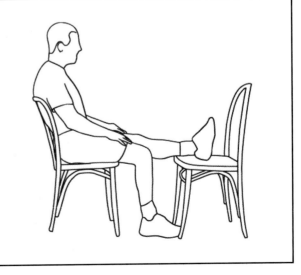

SECTION 6   KNEE AND LOWER LEG

Quadriceps Setting

- Lie on the floor with the affected leg straight out and the other bent.
- Squeeze the thigh muscle of the straight leg for 10 seconds and then release it.
- Perform 2 to 3 sets of 10 to 20 repetitions, 5 to 6 days per week, continuing for 3 to 4 weeks.

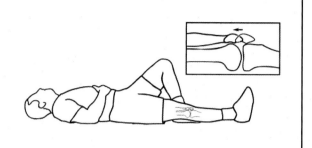

Straight Leg Raise

- Add in the straight leg raise exercise after 1 to 2 weeks and only if the leg can be kept fully straight when lifted.
- Lie on the floor with the affected leg straight and the unaffected leg bent.
- Tighten the thigh muscle of the straight leg and slowly raise it 6 to 10 inches off the floor.
- Hold this position for 5 seconds. Relax the leg completely between repetitions.
- Work up to 3 sets of 10 to 20 repetitions. Perform the exercise 5 to 6 days per week, continuing for 3 to 4 weeks.

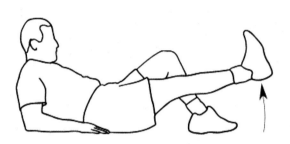

Compartment Syndrome

Definition

The muscles of the leg are divided by fibrous septae into four compartments: anterior, lateral, superficial posterior, and deep posterior (**Figure 1**). Compartment syndromes are characterized by an elevation of intracompartmental pressure to a degree that compromises blood flow to the involved muscles and nerves. Although acute compartment syndromes are most common after tibial fractures, especially proximal fractures, any condition that can potentially cause substantial swelling, such as contusions, muscle strains, or crush injuries, can result in this limb-threatening condition. Acute compartment syndrome is an emergency requiring fasciotomy, a surgical procedure in which the fascia is split to allow the muscle to expand and decompress. Compartment syndrome of the leg may affect one or more of the four compartments. The anterior compartment, located just lateral to the tibial crest, is the most frequently involved.

Exertional compartment syndrome of the leg, sometimes called chronic compartment syndrome, is an exercise-induced pathologic increase in tissue pressure (typically greater than 40 mm Hg) that usually involves the anterior and lateral compartments. Although the exact cause is unknown, this condition produces leg pain and

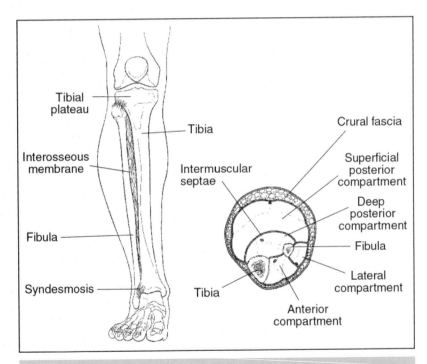

Figure 1 Illustration of the frontal and cross-sectional views of the leg shows compartmental anatomy. (Reproduced from Sullivan JA, Anderson SJ, eds: *Care of the Young Athlete.* Rosemont, IL, American Academy of Orthopaedic Surgeons, 1999, p 406.)

occasionally episodic footdrop and paresthesia radiating into the foot during exercise.

Clinical Symptoms

The hallmark of an acute compartment syndrome is severe leg pain that is out of proportion to what would otherwise be expected. As the condition progresses, patients also may experience paresthesia or numbness on the dorsum of the foot (with anterior or lateral compartment involvement) or on the plantar aspect of the foot (with involvement of the deep posterior compartment). In advanced cases, the dorsalis pedis and tibialis posterior pulses may become diminished or absent.

Exertional compartment syndrome is associated with exercise. Symptoms develop gradually and progress with exercise and usually begin at a predictable time after initiation of activity. With cessation of the activity, the compartment tissue pressures return to normal (less than 15 mm Hg), and symptoms gradually resolve within 30 minutes. Patients with an exertional compartment syndrome do not experience pain at rest. Because the anterior compartment is most commonly involved, patients may note paresthesia in the dorsum of the first web space and weakness with ankle dorsiflexion. This weakness can manifest as a sensation of the foot slapping the ground and increasing clumsiness while running.

Tests

Physical Examination

Acute compartment syndromes are characterized by increased pain with passive stretching of the muscles of the involved compartment. For example, with an anterior compartment syndrome, passive stretch of the extensor hallucis longus (such as flexing the great toe) causes marked pain, whereas inversion of the foot passively stretches the peroneus longus and peroneus brevis and is painful in persons with elevated lateral compartment pressures. Deep and superficial posterior compartment syndromes can be detected by extending the great toe and dorsiflexing the ankle, respectively. Altered sensation of the nerves in the involved compartments is often present at the onset of the syndrome. Paralysis and loss of dorsalis pedis and tibialis posterior pulses are late findings.

Most patients with exertional compartment syndrome have no abnormal physical findings when they are not exercising. Some will have a fascial defect at the inferior aspect of the anterior compartment. If the leg is examined during or immediately after exercise, the involved compartment musculature often appears swollen and may be tender to palpation.

Diagnostic Tests

Acute compartment syndrome is a clinical diagnosis and is best confirmed by history and physical examination. In equivocal cases, compartment pressures (anterior, lateral, superficial posterior, and deep posterior) may be measured using an indwelling catheter, a needle attached to a pressure monitor, or a commercially available portable compartment pressure monitor. An acute compartment syndrome is present when the compartment pressure is elevated to within 30 mm Hg of the diastolic blood pressure. The diagnosis of exertional compartment syndromes is confirmed with a resting compartment pressure greater than 15 mm Hg, compartment pressure greater than 30 mm Hg immediately after exercise, and compartment pressure greater than 20 mm Hg 5 minutes after exercise.

Differential Diagnosis

Chronic compartment syndrome

• Shin splints (tenderness along tibia)

• Stress fracture (pain at rest, radiographic findings)

Acute compartment syndrome

• Claudication (diminished pulse)

• Contusion (clinical differentiation, low compartment pressure)

Adverse Outcomes of the Disease

Tissue necrosis from compromised blood flow to muscles and nerves with acute compartment syndrome may be limb threatening and can result in infection or acute kidney failure as the kidneys filter the breakdown products of the dead muscle. Although patients with exertional compartment syndrome do not have the potential for myonecrosis and loss of limb, they may experience substantial compromise in quality of life because of their inability to exercise.

Treatment

Treatment of an acute compartment syndrome is immediate fasciotomy, or "opening" the compartment by incising longitudinally the fascial tissues that form the compartment. Nonsurgical treatment of exertional compartment syndrome requires discontinuing an activity or decreasing its intensity to an asymptomatic level. Because exertional compartment syndrome typically involves only one or two compartments rather than all four, surgical treatment is fasciotomy of the involved compartments.

Adverse Outcomes of Treatment

Incomplete fasciotomy can result in continued tissue necrosis following treatment of acute compartment syndrome.

Referral Decisions/Red Flags

Acute compartment syndromes are surgical emergencies. Failure to diagnose and immediately treat a compartment syndrome can result in tissue necrosis and permanent muscle contracture, pain, weakness, neurologic injury, and acute renal failure. Loss of pulse and sensation occurs relatively late in the course of acute compartment syndrome; therefore, if these are present, substantial muscle damage has already

SECTION 6 KNEE AND LOWER LEG

occurred. In rare situations, acute compartment syndrome will develop in a patient with chronic exertional compartment syndrome. Presumably, this occurs when the swelling and pressure increase to such an extent that they do not return to normal after cessation of exercise. This condition requires emergent treatment.

Contusions

Synonym
Bruise

Definition
Contusions are injuries to the leg sustained from a direct, blunt blow. Although the resulting disability usually is minor, some contusions are quite painful and produce substantial swelling and tenderness. Excessive swelling may result in a compartment syndrome, which therefore should be considered in the clinical evaluation.

Clinical Symptoms
Contusions cause swelling, tenderness, and ecchymosis of the involved muscle. Active muscle contraction and passive stretch may be painful.

Tests
Physical Examination
Physical examination reveals a tense, swollen, and tender extremity, which can be larger in circumference than the contralateral leg. Ecchymosis may be present immediately after the injury or, in cases in which a deep muscle group is contused, may surface several days after the injury.

Diagnostic Tests
AP and lateral radiographs should be obtained to rule out a fracture about the knee in patients involved in high-energy trauma or with severe pain. Weeks after a severe quadriceps contusion, a faint radiodense mass may appear adjacent and parallel to the femur. This calcific mass, myositis ossificans traumatica, matures and becomes more radiodense.

Differential Diagnosis
- Compartment syndrome (disproportionate pain with passive movement, elevated compartment pressures)
- Fracture about the knee (evident on radiographs)
- Knee dislocation (evident on radiographs)

Adverse Outcomes of the Disease
Heterotopic ossification is the formation of mature bone in areas generally reserved for soft tissues. Myositis ossificans traumatica, a type of heterotopic ossification, results from direct injury to the muscles. Myositis ossificans traumatica can follow any contusion, but it is most common following thigh contusions. With myositis ossificans, a firm mass develops at the site of injury 3 to 4 weeks after the injury. Radiographic changes begin at 3 to 4 weeks and mature

as a bony mass by 3 to 6 months. Although often concerning for a tumor, myositis ossificans is a benign condition and only requires treatment if symptomatic.

Muscle contusions can be problematic for persons with bleeding disorders, either congenital (von Willebrand disease, hemophilia) or acquired (those receiving anticoagulants, such as warfarin or aspirin). Because of an inability of these individuals to effectively form blood clots, large intramuscular hematomas can develop after seemingly minimal trauma. These patients should be closely monitored for signs and symptoms of acute compartment syndrome. Administration of factor replacement or fresh-frozen plasma may be necessary in severe cases.

Treatment

Contusions are treated with minor analgesics, rest, ice, elevation, range-of-motion exercises, stretching, and strengthening exercises (bilateral heel raise, heel raise with weights, single-leg heel raise). In severe quadriceps contusions, the knee can be acutely wrapped in hyperflexion using an elastic bandage. This treatment maintains the quadriceps in stretch and may hasten recovery and return to play. In the rare case in which a patient has myositis ossificans and persistent loss of motion and a painful bony mass, the heterotopic bone, which is deep to the quadriceps muscle, can be surgically excised.

Adverse Outcomes of Treatment

In addition to its potential for gastric, renal, or hepatic complications, NSAID use, especially ketorolac, can inhibit platelet function and result in increased intramuscular bruising, worsen symptoms, and in rare cases, result in compartment syndrome. Therefore, caution should be used when administering these medications in this setting. In 2015, the FDA strengthened its warning linking NSAIDs with the risk of heart attack or stroke, even in the first weeks of use of an NSAID.

Referral Decisions/Red Flags

Contusions must not be confused with fractures about the knee or knee dislocations, which require immediate referral and treatment. Persons with underlying hypocoagulation conditions or those with impending compartment syndrome must be identified, closely monitored, and treated immediately.

Fractures About the Knee

Definition

Distal femur fractures may be classified as supracondylar or intercondylar, as involving the medial or lateral femoral condyle or both (**Figure 1**), and account for 4% to 7% of all femoral fractures. Fractures of the proximal tibial metaphysis are called tibial plateau fractures and often extend into the articular surface (**Figure 2**). Tibial plateau fractures usually occur after a valgus force causes the lateral femoral condyle to impact the less dense lateral tibial plateau. These fractures may be associated with meniscal and collateral ligament injuries. These injuries tend to occur in two populations: in young patients as a result of high-energy trauma and in association with other injuries; and in elderly patients with osteoporosis and as a result of a low-energy force. Periprosthetic supracondylar fractures can occur after a knee replacement and usually are adjacent to the proximal portion of the femoral component. These fractures occur more commonly when the anterior femoral cortex is notched during the replacement surgery.

Clinical Symptoms

Patients report an injury with immediate onset of pain and swelling. In some patients with nondisplaced fractures, substantial pain may

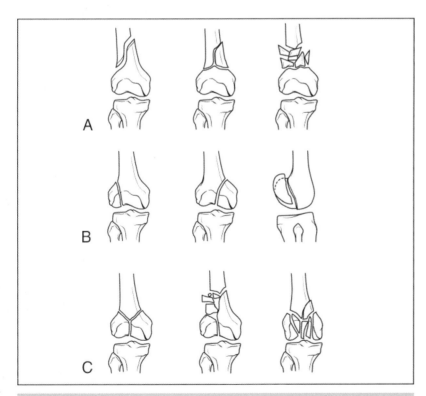

Figure 1 Illustration shows supracondylar and intercondylar fracture patterns of the distal femur. **A,** Distal shaft fractures (extra-articular). **B,** Unicondylar fractures. **C,** Intercondylar/bicondylar fractures.

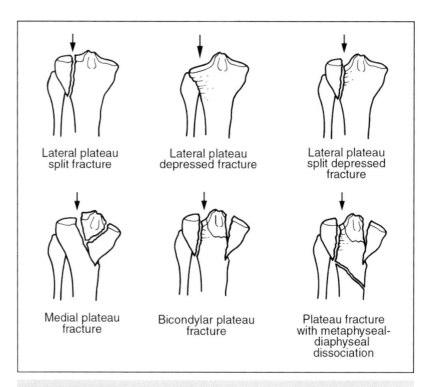

Lateral plateau
split fracture

Lateral plateau
depressed fracture

Lateral plateau
split depressed
fracture

Medial plateau
fracture

Bicondylar plateau
fracture

Plateau fracture
with metaphyseal-
diaphyseal
dissociation

Figure 2 Illustration shows tibial plateau fracture patterns. (Adapted from Perry CR: Fractures of the tibial plateau. *Instr Course Lect* 1994;43:119-126.)

be present only with weight bearing. However, most patients have constant pain and cannot bear any weight on the injured extremity.

Tests

Physical Examination

Some patients sustain open fractures in association with apex-anterior angulated supracondylar fractures, whereas skin compromise and fracture blisters from the intense swelling may develop in other patients with this fracture. Swelling of the knee is often marked because the intra-articular extension of the fracture allows bleeding from the vascular metaphysis into the joint. Because of the proximity of neurovascular structures and the propensity for acute compartment syndrome, especially in patients who sustain high-energy tibial plateau fractures, a thorough distal neurovascular examination including motor and sensory testing and evaluation of pulses should be performed. Ankle-brachial index should be obtained if substantial deformity exists or if vascular injury is suspected.

Diagnostic Tests

Initial radiographic examination should include AP and lateral views of the knee. Oblique radiographs and CT scans are usually obtained to further assess the fracture configuration and the amount of displacement of the joint surface. MRI can help identify nondisplaced fractures and evaluate for the presence of concomitant meniscal and ligamentous injury. When distal pulses are diminished or absent or ankle-brachial index is less than 0.9, further imaging to assess the lower extremity arterial flow should be performed emergently. At most trauma centers, CT angiography is readily available and can be performed at the same time as the knee CT.

Differential Diagnosis

- Cruciate ligament disruption (no fracture evident on radiographs)
- Knee dislocation (evident on radiographs)
- Patellar fracture (evident on radiographs)
- Quadriceps or patellar tendon rupture (palpable defect, inability to actively extend the knee against gravity, full passive extension)
- Thigh contusion and/or compartment syndrome (negative radiographs, compartment pressure measurements if in question)

Adverse Outcomes of the Disease

Posttraumatic arthritis will eventually develop in most intra-articular fractures involving a weight-bearing joint. Fractures with an intra-articular step-off (articular surface displacement) are more likely to result in accelerated posttraumatic arthritis than those that are anatomically reduced. Nondisplaced, intra-articular fractures may become displaced with articular incongruency if appropriate weight-bearing precautions are not followed. Because of the high shear forces associated with muscular insertions, supracondylar fractures are prone to nonunion if left untreated.

Treatment

Nonsurgical treatment can be considered for nondisplaced or minimally displaced fractures. Weight bearing should be partial and crutch assisted to avoid displacement until healing occurs (typically 6 weeks). Displaced fractures usually require open reduction and internal fixation. With intra-articular fractures, the goal of surgical treatment is restoration of joint alignment and congruity. Emergent treatment is required for open fractures, vascular injuries requiring repair, and compartment syndrome. Anticoagulation using chemoprophylaxis should be considered in most cases because of the risk of thromboembolic events in the setting of trauma and limited weight bearing.

Adverse Outcomes of Treatment

Early complications of treatment typically involve soft-tissue structures and include skin breakdown, compartment syndrome, thromboembolic disease, knee arthrofibrosis (stiffness), and injury to adjacent neurovascular structures. Late complications, occurring several months later, usually involve the bony structures. Nonunion, malunion, failure of fixation, and prominent hardware typically manifest several weeks after the injury. Infection can present early or late postoperatively and is more common following open fractures.

SECTION 6 KNEE AND LOWER LEG

Referral Decisions/Red Flags

Periarticular fractures require prompt evaluation by an orthopaedic surgeon. Even seemingly inconsequential nondisplaced fractures in this region are at increased risk for displacement.

Iliotibial Band Syndrome

Synonyms
Iliotibial band tendinitis
Runner's knee

Definition
The iliotibial band (ITB) is a dense, fibrous band of tissue that originates from the anterior superior iliac spine region, extends down the lateral portion of the thigh, and inserts on the anterolateral tibia at the Gerdy tubercle. When the knee is extended, the ITB sits anterior to the lateral femoral epicondyle. When the knee is flexed beyond 30°, the ITB moves posterior to the lateral femoral epicondyle (**Figure 1**). ITB syndrome develops when the distal portion of the ITB rubs against the lateral femoral epicondyle. The friction between the ITB and the lateral epicondyle causes irritation and subsequent inflammation of the ITB. Secondary to the repetitive flexion and extension of the knee, ITB syndrome is seen most commonly in long-distance runners and cyclists. However, this syndrome can develop in any athlete, especially those with predisposing factors, such as genu varum, internal tibial rotation, and excessive foot pronation.

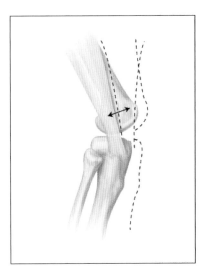

Figure 1 Illustration demonstrates movement of the iliotibial band over the prominence of the lateral femoral epicondyle with flexion and extension of the knee.

Clinical Symptoms
Patients with ITB syndrome usually describe pain at the anterolateral aspect of the knee that worsens with running (especially downhill) or cycling. This pain is usually most intense at heel strike. Occasionally, patients report an audible popping laterally within the knee with walking or running. The patient is usually asymptomatic at rest before activity but may have some residual discomfort after activity.

Tests

Physical Examination
Tenderness to direct palpation is most evident directly over the lateral femoral epicondyle, a prominence palpated 2 to 3 cm proximal to the lateral joint line. This tenderness is usually maximal at 30° of knee flexion when the ITB contacts the lateral epicondyle. The Ober test may help confirm the diagnosis. Functional testing, such as eliciting lateral knee pain when the patient hops with a flexed knee, suggests the presence of ITB syndrome.

Diagnostic Tests
AP and lateral radiographs are usually negative with ITB syndrome, but they should be obtained to exclude other pathology presenting as lateral knee pain.

Differential Diagnosis

- Hamstring strain
- Lateral collateral ligament sprain (opening with varus stress)
- Meniscal injury (joint line tenderness, mechanical symptoms, positive McMurray test)

Adverse Outcomes of the Disease

Continued lateral knee pain may result in decreased activity and associated lowered fitness level.

Treatment

Most patients respond to nonsurgical treatment, including physical therapy, a short-term course of NSAIDs, ice, and activity modifications. Physical therapy interventions must address the entire lower limb. A program to improve hamstring, tensor fasciae latae, and hip external rotator flexibility and hip abductor weakness should be initiated. Acute management may include modalities to decrease inflammation, such as phonophoresis or iontophoresis and cryotherapy. NSAIDs may help control the acute inflammatory process.

Following the initial period of inflammation control, alterations in training may help with long-term prevention. Runners can alter their duration or pace of training, adjust their stride length, or reverse direction if they run on a circular track. Runners can also consider changing the side of the road they run on because most roads are crowned to facilitate drainage. Persons who exhibit excessive pronation or excessive lateral wear may benefit from a custom-made orthosis. Cyclists can adjust their seat height or foot position on the pedals.

Local injection with corticosteroids may be administered only when the symptoms do not respond to stretching, physical therapy, and exercise modification. Surgical interventions such as ITB lengthening are rarely required.

Adverse Outcomes of Treatment

NSAIDs can worsen hypertension and cause gastric, renal, or hepatic complications, especially if taken in supratherapeutic doses and for prolonged periods. In 2015, the FDA strengthened its warning linking NSAIDs with the risk of heart attack or stroke, even in the first weeks of use of an NSAID. Infection, ITB weakening, and subcutaneous fat or skin atrophy are rare complications following corticosteroid injections into the ITB.

Referral Decisions/Red Flags

Symptoms that do not respond to nonsurgical treatment require further evaluation and possible surgical intervention.

Gastrocnemius Tear

Synonym
Tennis leg

Definition
Acute strains or ruptures of the medial head of the gastrocnemius muscle usually occur at the musculotendinous junction. The injury often occurs while playing tennis, running on a hill, or jumping. These injuries are most common in athletes older than 30 years.

Clinical Symptoms
The patient typically describes a pulling or tearing sensation in the calf. Most of the pain is located proximally and medially at the musculotendinous junction. This injury can result in diffuse calf pain, swelling, and tenderness.

Tests
Physical Examination
The patient typically has tenderness and swelling over the medial gastrocnemius just distal to the muscle bulk. The patient holds the ankle in plantar flexion to avoid placing tension on the injured muscle and typically ambulates with the ankle in a plantarflexed position. The patient is unable to perform a single-leg toe raise. Ecchymosis can develop in the calf over 24 hours. In severe cases, a palpable defect can be appreciated at the musculotendinous junction. Because the lateral gastrocnemius and soleus are intact, the patient has a negative Thompson test result, that is, passive plantar flexion of the foot on squeezing the calf. This test is positive with an Achilles tendon rupture.

Diagnostic Tests
Usually, no specific diagnostic tests are necessary to evaluate a medial gastrocnemius tear. In recalcitrant cases, MRI may be considered to further define the injury.

Differential Diagnosis
- Achilles tendinitis (more distal localization)
- Achilles tendon rupture (positive Thompson test)
- Popliteal cyst rupture (no trauma, no plantar flexion)

Adverse Outcomes of the Disease
Scar tissue can form and result in chronic pain, dysfunction, or reinjury because of musculotendinous shortening. Another potential complication of a medial gastrocnemius tear is deep vein thrombosis resulting from inactivity and trauma.

SECTION 6 KNEE AND LOWER LEG

Treatment

Medial gastrocnemius tears are treated nonsurgically initially with such measures as NSAIDs, rest, ice, elevation, a controlled ankle motion (CAM) walker boot and/or 0.5-inch heel lift, a calf sleeve or compression hose, and crutches. Crutches are discontinued when ambulation is pain free. Therapeutic activities include isometric calf contractions in plantar flexion and gentle range-of-motion stretching and strengthening exercises (bilateral heel raise, heel raise with weights, single-leg heel raise). Most of these injuries heal, and most patients return to their previous functional level within 6 to 8 weeks after injury.

Rehabilitation Prescription

The initial treatment goal is to control the pain and inflammation with the use of rest, ice, compression, and elevation (RICE). A home exercise program should include early movement; within 7 to 21 days postinjury, gentle active and passive range-of-motion exercises should be initiated. The passive exercises should include gentle stretching of the gastrocnemius muscle group, and the active exercises should include calf raises.

If pain and limited function continue for more than 3 to 4 weeks, formal rehabilitation may be ordered. The evaluation should include an assessment of the entire lower extremity, and the rehabilitation specialist should design a program to increase the range of motion and improve muscle strength as indicated, taking into consideration the activities to which the individual will be returning.

Adverse Outcomes of Treatment

NSAIDs can worsen hypertension and cause gastric, renal, or hepatic complications, especially if taken in supratherapeutic doses and for prolonged periods. In 2015, the FDA strengthened its warning linking NSAIDs with the risk of heart attack or stroke, even in the first weeks of use of an NSAID. Loss of dorsiflexion and atrophy of the calf can occur if range-of-motion and strengthening exercises are not encouraged.

Referral Decisions/Red Flags

A large palpable defect or persistent symptoms despite appropriate therapeutic measures indicates the need for further evaluation.

Home Exercise Program for Medial Gastrocnemius Tear

- Perform the exercises in the order listed.
- Apply moist or dry heat to the affected area before and during the heel cord stretch.
- Progress gently to the calf raises.
- To prevent further inflammation, apply a bag of crushed ice or frozen peas to the affected area for 20 minutes or until numb after performing the calf raises.
- If the exercises increase the pain or if the pain does not improve after you have performed the exercises for 3 to 4 weeks, call your doctor.
- The following exercise program is introductory only, and progression of this program will vary based on your specific injury, symptoms, and baseline level of fitness. For further progression of this routine, your physician may recommend evaluation and treatment by a physical therapist or other exercise professional.

Home Exercises for Medial Gastrocnemius Tear

Exercise Type	Muscle Group	Number of Repetitions/Sets	Number of Days per Week	Number of Weeks
Heel cord stretch	Gastrocnemius/soleus	4 repetitions/2 to 3 sets	Daily	3 to 4
Calf raise	Gastrocnemius/soleus	10 repetitions/3 sets	3 to 4	3 to 4

Heel Cord Stretch

- Stand facing the wall with the affected leg straight and the knee of the unaffected leg bent, as shown.
- The foot of the affected leg should be turned in slightly, and the heel should not come off the ground.
- Hold the stretch for 30 seconds with the knee straight and then relax for 30 seconds.
- Perform 4 repetitions, 2 to 3 times per day, continuing for 3 to 4 weeks.

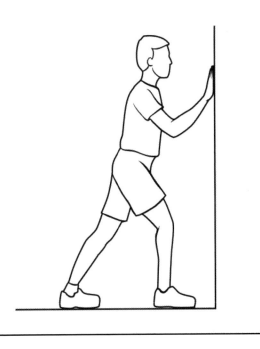

Calf Raise

- Stand on a flat surface with your weight evenly distributed on both feet.
- Hold on to the back of a chair or the wall for balance and lift the foot on the unaffected side.
- Keeping the knee of the affected leg straight, raise the heel off the floor as high as you can, using your body weight as resistance. (If this causes pain or discomfort, perform the exercise keeping the toes of both feet on the floor at first.)
- Work up to 3 sets of 10 repetitions, 3 to 4 days per week, continuing for 3 to 4 weeks.

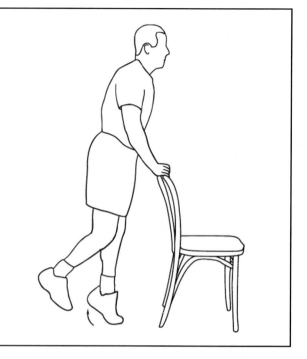

SECTION 6   KNEE AND LOWER LEG

Meniscal Tear

Synonyms

Internal derangement of knee
Locked knee
Torn cartilage

Definition

The medial and lateral menisci are fibrocartilaginous pads that function as shock absorbers between the femoral condyles and tibial plateaus. These gasket-like structures facilitate the efficient transfer of forces from the femoral condyles to the tibial plateau. Meniscal tears disrupt the normal mechanics of the knee; therefore, various degrees of symptoms result and the knee is predisposed to degenerative arthritis because of the concentration of weight-bearing forces (**Figure 1**, **Table 1**). Meniscal tears occur alone or in

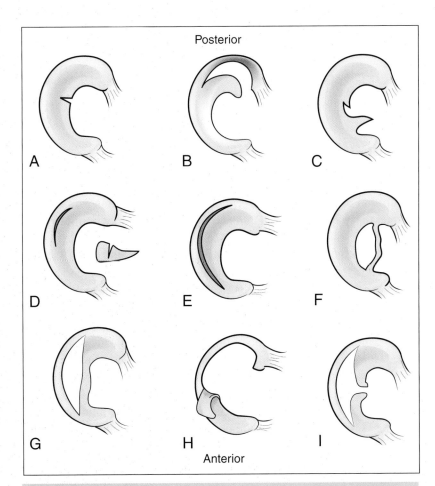

Figure 1 Illustration of common patterns of meniscal tears. **A,** Radial tear. **B,** Flap tear. **C,** Parrot beak tear. **D,** Incomplete longitudinal tear. **E,** Complete longitudinal tear. **F,** Bucket-handle tear. **G,** Displaced bucket-handle tear. **H,** Displaced flap tear. **I,** Double flap tear.

Table 1	
Classification of Meniscal Tears	
Tear Type	**Characteristics**
Vertical longitudinal	Common, especially in the setting of anterior cruciate ligament tears; can be repaired if located in the peripheral third of the meniscus
Bucket handle	A vertical longitudinal tear displaced into the notch
Radial	Starts centrally and proceeds peripherally; not reparable because of loss of circumferential fiber integrity
Flap	Begins as a radial tear and proceeds circumferentially; may cause mechanical locking systems
Horizontal cleavage	Occurs more frequently in the older population and may be associated with meniscal cysts
Complex	A combination of tear types; more common in the older population

(Reproduced from Lieberman JR, ed: *Comprehensive Orthopaedic Review.* Rosemont, IL, American Academy of Orthopaedic Surgeons, 2009, vol 2, p 1133.)

association with ligament injuries such as anterior cruciate ligament tears.

Clinical Symptoms

Patients with traumatic tears typically report a twisting injury to the knee. Older patients with degenerative tears may have a history of minimal or no trauma and recall a seemingly insidious painful episode that happened during an activity such as simply rising from a squatting position. Patients usually can ambulate after an acute injury and frequently are able to continue to participate in athletics.

Traumatic tears can be followed by delayed knee effusion and stiffness over 2 to 3 days. Mechanical symptoms such as locking, catching, and popping may develop as the acute inflammation resolves and the patient resumes normal activities. Patients usually report pain along the joint line of the medial or lateral side of the knee. This pain worsens with twisting or squatting activities. In some cases, large, unstable fragments of meniscal tissue become incarcerated in the knee joint and cause a locked knee, one that is unable to achieve full passive extension. Patients with an incarcerated fragment often describe a period of locking that is resolved by gently manipulating the knee. More frequently, motion is limited by a feeling of tightness in the knee secondary to the effusion. The mechanical symptoms and degree of pain tend to wax and wane.

Occasionally, patients will describe a "pop" followed by a sharp pain in the posterior aspect of the knee following an innocuous episode. In patients with obesity, this history should alert the examiner to the presence of a tear of the posterior medial meniscal root, the posterior attachment site of the medial meniscus. This particular injury renders the meniscus nonfunctional and can result in a more rapidly progressive degeneration of the affected medial compartment.

Tests

Physical Examination

The most common finding on physical examination is point tenderness over the medial or lateral joint line. Young patients who have traumatic tears that occur within 5 mm of the meniscal attachment sites to the capsule typically present with a large effusion or hemarthrosis. In degenerative tears or tears that involve the avascular central body of the meniscus, effusions are typically small or absent. Knee motion may be limited secondary to pain, an incarcerated fragment, or an effusion. During provocative testing, forced flexion and circumduction (internal and external rotation of the foot) frequently elicit pain on the side of the knee with the meniscal tear. The McMurray test is positive when the flexion-circumduction maneuver is associated with a painful click.

Diagnostic Tests

Although MRI is specific and sensitive for meniscal pathology, each patient with a meniscal tear should undergo weight-bearing radiography prior to MRI. Radiography is a cost-effective imaging modality that provides information on the degree of osteoarthritis, which has been correlated with outcomes after meniscal surgery. A weight-bearing AP view with the knees in 45° of flexion is sensitive for early osteoarthritis and is recommended in patients older than 40 years (**Figure 2**).

Differential Diagnosis

- Anterior cruciate ligament tear (hemarthrosis, positive Lachman test)
- Crystalline disease (crystals in aspirate)
- Loose body (fragment may be evident on radiographs, but purely cartilaginous loose body may not)
- Medial collateral ligament tear (pain and instability with valgus stress)
- Osteoarthritis (joint space narrowing may be evident on weight-bearing radiographs)
- Osteochondritis dissecans (evident on radiographs, especially of the medial femoral condyle)
- Osteonecrosis of the femoral condyle (patient older than 50 years, pain, evident on radiographs or MRIs)
- Patellar subluxation or dislocation (tender medial patella, apprehension sign)
- Pes anserine bursitis (tender distal to medial joint line)

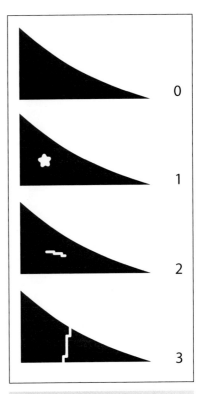

Figure 2 Illustration of a grading scale for meniscal tears seen on MRI. 0 = no intrameniscal signal, 1 = focal intrameniscal signal that does not communicate to a meniscal surface, 2 = intrameniscal line/band that does not communicate to a meniscal surface, 3 = intrameniscal line/band that communicates with at least one meniscal surface.

SECTION 6   KNEE AND LOWER LEG

- Saphenous neuritis (tender to palpation along the course of the saphenous nerve)
- Tibial plateau fracture (bony tenderness, evident on radiographs)

Adverse Outcomes of the Disease

Any injury that compromises the meniscal capability to effectively transfer force from the femur to the tibia can result in accelerated degeneration of the articular cartilage of the weight-bearing portion of the knee. Because the meniscus has a relatively poor blood supply, most tears are not amenable to repair and must be excised. However, in some instances, especially in persons with a peripheral tear (close to the meniscocapsular junction), tears may be reparable. Failure to recognize and treat these injuries can result in further damage to the torn segment and a lost opportunity to restore the function of the meniscus.

Treatment

A locked knee with loss of range of motion should be managed surgically to reduce pain and restore motion. In the absence of mechanical symptoms, and particularly when a degenerative tear is present, initial treatment should consist of rest, ice, compression, and elevation (RICE). A short course of oral analgesics, such as acetaminophen or ibuprofen, may facilitate return to normal activity. Traumatic tears in younger patients should be evaluated and treated aggressively. Sports activity should be restricted until MRI evaluation is performed or symptoms resolve. Arthroscopic surgical débridement or repair is indicated in younger patients with substantial tears, in patients with a locked knee, and in older patients whose symptoms do not respond to nonsurgical treatment.

Rehabilitation Prescription

Initial treatment should consist of RICE to control soft-tissue edema, joint effusion, and pain. Early controlled movement is generally effective in improving mobility and reducing pain. The type of meniscal injury called a bucket-handle tear, in which the posterior fragment flips anteriorly, can cause locking and is beyond the scope of rehabilitation.

A home exercise program should include early, pain-free movement such as hamstring curls and straight leg raises. In addition, using a stationary bicycle can help reduce pain and increase range of motion. If the pain continues for more than 3 to 4 weeks, formal rehabilitation is an option. The evaluation should include a thorough assessment of lower extremity flexibility and strength, as well as core muscle function around the hip and trunk. In addition, exercises to promote healing should be initiated.

Adverse Outcomes of Treatment

NSAIDs can worsen hypertension and cause gastric, renal, or hepatic complications, especially if taken in supratherapeutic doses and for prolonged periods. In 2015, the FDA strengthened its warning linking NSAIDs with the risk of heart attack or stroke, even in the first weeks of use of an NSAID. Meniscal repair has a 10% to 30% failure rate and, in symptomatic cases of retear of incomplete healing, requires subsequent re-repair or partial meniscectomy. Persistent pain after a partial meniscectomy can occur secondary to concomitant pathology, such as osteoarthritis or saphenous neuritis. Traumatic osteoarthritis can be a late complication in the involved compartment after partial meniscectomy. The rate and degree of osteoarthritic progression can be correlated to the amount of meniscus remaining following resection. The more of the meniscus that remains, the more efficient the load transfer will be, and the slower the rate of joint degeneration. Although postoperative infection is rare, deep vein thrombosis is not uncommon postoperatively, and appropriate chemoprophylaxis should be considered in patients at increased risk of thromboembolism.

Referral Decisions/Red Flags

Not all patients with a meniscal tear identified on advanced imaging require surgical intervention to alleviate pain. However, patients with a traumatic effusion, mechanical symptoms, or ligamentous instability may have a reparable tear and should be referred to an orthopaedic surgeon early in treatment. Patients whose injuries do not respond to nonsurgical management, such as intra-articular steroid injections, NSAIDs, or physical therapy, and who have persistent joint line tenderness or effusions may benefit from surgical intervention and should be referred for further evaluation.

SECTION 6 KNEE AND LOWER LEG

Home Exercise Program for Meniscal Tear

- Perform the exercises in the order listed.
- To prevent inflammation, after completing the exercises apply a bag of crushed ice or frozen peas to the affected side of the knee for 20 minutes or until numb.
- If the exercises increase the pain in your knee or if the pain does not improve after performing the exercises for 3 to 4 weeks, call your doctor.
- The following exercise program is introductory only, and progression of this program will vary based on your specific injury, symptoms, and baseline level of fitness. For further progression of this routine, your physician may recommend evaluation and treatment by a physical therapist or other exercise professional.

Home Exercises for Meniscal Tear

Exercise Type	Muscle Group	Number of Repetitions/Sets	Number of Days per Week	Number of Weeks
Hamstring curl	Hamstrings	25 repetitions/3 sets	4 to 5	3 to 4
Straight leg raise	Quadriceps	10 repetitions/3 sets	4 to 5	3 to 4

Hamstring Curl

- Stand on a flat surface with your weight evenly distributed on both feet.
- Hold on to the back of a chair or the wall for balance.
- Bend the affected knee, raising the heel toward the ceiling as far as possible without pain.
- Hold this position for 5 seconds and then relax.
- Perform 3 sets of 25 repetitions, 4 to 5 days per week, continuing for 3 to 4 weeks.

Seated version

- Sit on a chair with your feet flat on the floor.
- Slide the foot on the affected side back and hold the position for 5 seconds.
- Perform 3 sets of 25 repetitions, 4 to 5 days per week, continuing for 3 to 4 weeks.

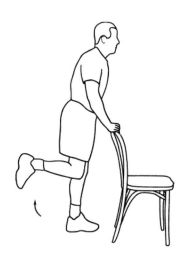

Straight Leg Raise

- Lie on the floor, supporting your torso with your elbows as shown.
- Keep the affected leg completely straight and bend the other leg at the knee so that the foot is flat on the floor.
- Tighten the thigh muscle of the affected leg and slowly raise it 6 to 10 inches off the floor.
- Hold this position for 5 seconds and then relax.
- Perform 3 sets of 10 repetitions, 4 to 5 days per week, continuing for 3 to 4 weeks.

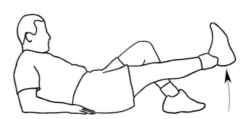

Osteonecrosis of the Femoral Condyle

Synonym
Avascular necrosis

Definition

Osteonecrosis literally means "bone death." It occurs in the femoral condyle when a segment of bone loses its blood supply. The etiology remains unknown, but osteonecrosis may begin as a stress fracture and probably involves some combination of trauma and altered blood flow. The weight-bearing surface of the medial femoral condyle is the most commonly involved region. The osteonecrotic subchondral bone is susceptible to microfracture and, when subjected to weight bearing, can result in segmental collapse of the subchondral bone and articular surface. Ultimately, progression to osteoarthritis is likely.

Osteonecrosis of the femoral condyle can be idiopathic or associated with chronic steroid therapy, renal transplantation, systemic lupus erythematosus, sickle cell anemia, and Gaucher disease. The typical patient is a woman (the female-to-male ratio is 3:1) older than 60 years.

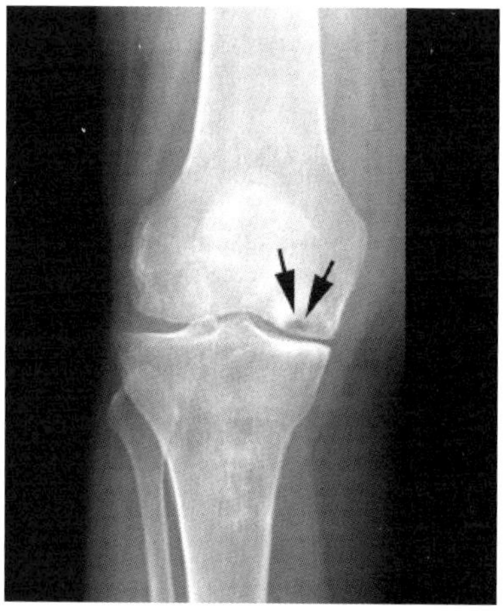

Figure 1 AP radiograph demonstrates subchondral sclerosis in the medial femoral condyle with subchondral lucency (arrows), which suggests spontaneous osteonecrosis. (Reproduced from Johnson TR, Steinbach LS, eds: *Essentials of Musculoskeletal Imaging.* Rosemont, IL, American Academy of Orthopaedic Surgeons, 2004, p 544.)

Clinical Symptoms

Although chronic osteonecrosis can become asymptomatic, especially when the weight-bearing surfaces are not involved, patients typically describe a sudden, sharp pain localized to the medial compartment. The pain is not typically associated with a known trauma but likely develops when a shear force causes a subchondral fracture or disruption of the articular surface. The pain is often constant, worsens with activity, and is sharper than that associated with osteoarthritis. Bilateral symptoms occur in less than 20% of patients.

Tests

Physical Examination

Physical examination may reveal a mild effusion, loss of motion as a result of patient guarding, and in prolonged, unrecognized cases, a flexion contracture. Many patients demonstrate focal tenderness to palpation directly over the medial femoral condyle.

Diagnostic Tests

Radiographically, osteonecrosis can be difficult to identify. However, the secondary signs of osteonecrosis of the medial femoral condyle can be seen on radiographs. Early radiographic indicators of osteonecrosis include sclerosis (**Figure 1**) and flattening of the normal convexity of the condyle, whereas later stages demonstrate the typical radiographic features of osteoarthritis such as joint space narrowing and osteophyte formation.

Imaging such as MRI and bone scanning (**Figure 2**) can help identify the lesion and provide information that may predict lesions susceptible to subchondral collapse and eventual progression to osteoarthritis. Location of the lesion within the weight-bearing zone and a larger involvement of the condyle portend a poorer outcome and likelihood of progression.

Differential Diagnosis

- Meniscal tears (joint line tenderness, pain worsens with circumduction, evident on MRI)
- Osteoarthritis (tricompartmental involvement)
- Osteochondritis dissecans (sex and age predilection, location)
- Pes anserine bursitis (location)

Adverse Outcomes of the Disease

Unrecognized or untreated symptomatic osteonecrosis can result in subchondral collapse with incongruity of the joint surface and will progress to osteoarthritis. Although no "cure" exists for osteonecrosis, current treatment seeks to prevent collapse of the articular surface.

Treatment

Nonsurgical management includes limiting weight bearing and use of an unloading brace to protect the affected subchondral bone from collapse, NSAIDs and corticosteroid injection to provide analgesia, and a conditioning program to restore quadriceps strength and endurance with modifications as necessary to avoid pain when exercising. Aquatherapy and other water exercises are excellent options that can allow for motion and strengthening without painful weight bearing. Surgical intervention may be indicated when symptoms persist despite a prolonged course of nonsurgical treatment. Surgical options include débridement with drilling or microfracture of the lesions, osteotomy (bone-cutting procedures) to alter the weight-bearing axis and unload the affected compartment, and, in advanced cases, total knee replacement.

Adverse Outcomes of Treatment

NSAIDs can worsen hypertension and cause gastric, renal, or hepatic complications, especially if taken in supratherapeutic doses and for prolonged periods. In 2015, the FDA strengthened its warning linking NSAIDs with the risk of heart attack or stroke, even in the first weeks of use of an NSAID. Surgical procedures to alleviate the symptoms of osteonecrosis have mixed outcomes. Although arthroscopic procedures are relatively safe, osteotomies that alter the weight-bearing axis increase risk to neurovascular structures during surgery and can result in nonunion and overcorrection or undercorrection. Total knee replacement can potentially provide pain relief and

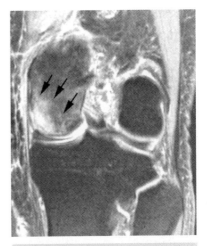

Figure 2 Coronal T2-weighted, fat-suppressed MRI demonstrates extensive edema in the medial femoral condyle (arrows), which is characteristic of spontaneous osteonecrosis. (Reproduced from Johnson TR, Steinbach LS, eds: *Essentials of Musculoskeletal Imaging.* Rosemont, IL, American Academy of Orthopaedic Surgeons, 2004, p 545.)

improved function, but results are generally less successful in persons with osteonecrosis than in persons with osteoarthritis.

Referral Decisions/Red Flags

Failure to improve with nonsurgical treatment warrants consideration of surgical intervention. Disproportionate pain, which can indicate complex regional pain syndrome, also indicates the need for further evaluation.

Patellar/Quadriceps Tendinitis

Synonyms
Extensor mechanism tendinitis
Jumper's knee

Definition
Extensor mechanism tendinitis is an overuse or overload syndrome involving either the quadriceps tendon at its insertion on the superior pole the patella or the patellar tendon at the inferior pole of the patella or at its insertion at the tibial tuberosity. Younger adults (younger than 40 years) with this condition often engage in jumping or kicking sports (jumper's knee) or have erratic exercise habits. Patellar or quadriceps tendinitis also sometimes develops in older patients after a lifting strain, noticeable change in exercise level, or substantial weight gain.

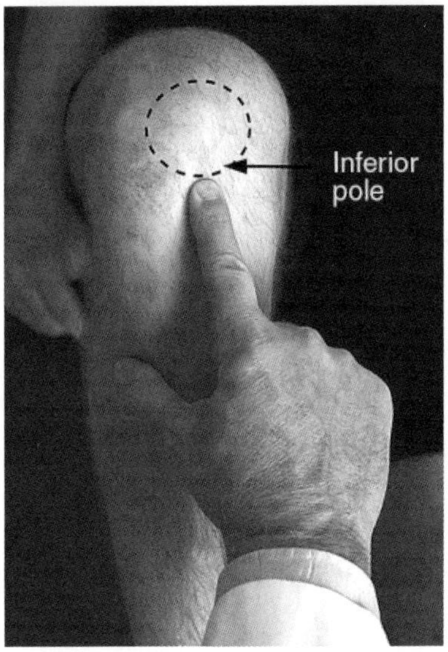

Clinical Symptoms
Anterior knee pain is the hallmark symptom. Patients often identify a tender spot where symptoms concentrate. The pain often commences immediately after exercise or after sitting that has been preceded by exercise. Climbing or descending stairs, running, jumping, or squatting often exacerbates the pain.

Figure 1 Photograph of palpation of the infrapatellar bursa.

Tests
Physical Examination
Patients' knees are usually tender to palpation at the bony attachments of the quadriceps tendon or patellar tendon. Increased heat, mild swelling, and soft-tissue crepitus may also be palpated in the tender region. Examination around the infrapatellar bursa (below the patella and behind the patellar tendon) often reveals "puffiness" (**Figure 1**). Knee motion is often normal but is frequently painful with resisted full extension and extreme degrees of passive flexion. With a long-standing condition, quadriceps atrophy, especially of the vastus medialis obliquus, can develop.

Diagnostic Tests
AP and lateral radiographs of the knee are often normal. However, lateral views may show small enthesophytes (calcifications of the tendinous insertions) or heterotopic ossification at the upper or lower pole of the patella. Additionally, a large ossicle from an unhealed tibial tuberosity apophysis (**Figure 2**) may be identified in persons with a history of Osgood-Schlatter disease in adolescence. These findings are often incidental and do not routinely cause symptoms. The tibial tuberosity fibrous union can become painful, especially after a seemingly innocuous injury. In these rare cases, surgical

SECTION 6 KNEE AND LOWER LEG

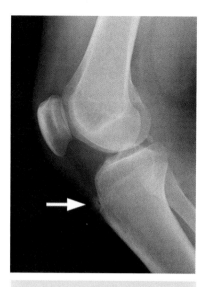

Figure 2 Lateral radiograph demonstrates a tibial tuberosity fibrous union (arrow), which persists in persons with a history of Osgood-Schlatter disease in adolescence.

intervention to excise the fragment may alleviate symptoms. MRI is reserved for recalcitrant cases and can define the severity of the disease and identify other sources of pain.

Differential Diagnosis

- Anterior or posterior cruciate ligament injury (positive Lachman or posterior drawer test)
- Inflammatory conditions (multisystem findings, elevated serum inflammatory markers)
- Partial rupture of the extensor mechanism (weakness, palpable defect, difficulty with straight leg raise test)
- Patellofemoral syndrome (anterior knee pain, abnormal patellofemoral signs other than superior or inferior pole tenderness)
- Septic arthritis of the knee (fever, warmth, painful motion, elevated serum inflammatory markers)

Adverse Outcomes of the Disease

Prolonged pain and, rarely, spontaneous rupture of the quadriceps or patellar tendon may occur.

Treatment

Treatment is directed primarily at relieving symptoms and involves three critical aspects: relative rest and pain control, restoring pain-free motion and strength, and resuming activities.

First, there should be a period of relative rest from aggravating activities. Depending on the severity of the condition, this period of rest can range from 3 days to 6 weeks or more. In some instances, intermittent use of a knee immobilizer can be helpful. NSAIDs can help control symptoms, but local injections of corticosteroids should be avoided because they substantially increase the risk of extensor mechanism rupture. Analgesic creams, application of ice to the knee after activity, and heat applied to the knee before activity can be helpful.

The second phase of treatment focuses on regaining pain-free range of motion, flexibility of the quadriceps and hamstrings, and strength. Exercises focusing on pain-free quadriceps strengthening and flexibility should be initiated and include eccentric loading exercises often in conjunction with other rehabilitation techniques or modalities. Using a knee sleeve with a patellar window or a compression strap at the level of the patellar tendon (infrapatellar strap) can be helpful to unload the force. If improvement does not occur, treatments such as platelet-rich plasma injections into the tendon or surgical débridement of the tendon or, if present, excision of a nonunited tibial tuberosity ossicle, may be beneficial.

The third phase of treatment is gradual resumption of the activities that precipitated the symptoms while continuing the exercises that restored strength and flexibility. Applying heat to the knee before activity and applying ice to the knee after exercising can be helpful.

Rehabilitation Prescription

The early rehabilitation of patellar tendinitis includes rest, ice, and compression of the patellar tendon area. The home exercise program should include pain-free activities that promote range of motion, provide gentle stretching, return normal muscle strength to the quadriceps, and reduce any muscle weakness in the hip. Straight leg raises, knee flexion, and stretching the quadriceps are important to early rehabilitation. If pain persists after 3 to 4 weeks, formal rehabilitation may be ordered. The evaluation should include assessment of the hip and trunk muscles and patellar mobility, as well as further strengthening of the quadriceps and hamstring muscle groups. Gradual resumption of eccentric loading has been demonstrated to be effective in treating patellar tendinitis. Closed-chain exercises such as partial squats and lunges should be added and progressed when they can be performed pain free.

Adverse Outcomes of Treatment

NSAIDs can worsen hypertension and cause gastric, renal, or hepatic complications, especially if taken in supratherapeutic doses and for prolonged periods. In 2015, the FDA strengthened its warning linking NSAIDs with the risk of heart attack or stroke, even in the first weeks of use of an NSAID. Occasionally, spontaneous rupture of the tendon occurs and may be precipitated by a steroid injection adjacent to the patellar tendon. Quadriceps and patellar tendinitis is often recalcitrant to treatment, even surgical treatment, and it may take longer than anticipated for the patient to return to normal, pain-free activity. Therefore, persistent functional impairment is the most common disability and does not necessarily resolve with surgical intervention.

Referral Decisions/Red Flags

Patients with a possible rupture of the extensor mechanism require prompt referral to an orthopaedic surgeon. Typically, ruptures involving the extensor mechanism are surgically repaired within 1 week of injury. Patients with tendinitis that does not respond to nonsurgical management also require further evaluation.

SECTION 6 KNEE AND LOWER LEG

Home Exercise Program for Patellar/Quadriceps Tendinitis

- Perform the exercises in the order listed.
- To prevent inflammation, apply a bag of crushed ice or frozen peas just below the kneecap after completing all the exercises.
- If the pain continues or gets worse, call your doctor.
- The following exercise program is introductory only, and progression of this program will vary based on your specific injury, symptoms, and baseline level of fitness. For further progression of this routine, your physician may recommend evaluation and treatment by a physical therapist or other exercise professional.

Home Exercises for Patellar/Quadriceps Tendinitis

Exercise Type	Muscle Group	Number of Repetitions/Sets	Number of Days per Week	Number of Weeks
Straight leg raise	Quadriceps	10 repetitions/3 sets	Daily	3 to 4
Hamstring curl	Hamstrings	15 repetitions/3 sets, progressing to 25 repetitions/3 sets	Daily	3 to 4
Prone quadriceps stretch	Quadriceps	4 repetitions/2 to 3 times per day	Daily	3 to 4
Supine hamstring stretch	Hamstrings	4 repetitions/2 to 3 times per day	Daily	3 to 4

Straight Leg Raise
- Lie on the floor, supporting your torso with your elbows as shown.
- Keep the affected leg straight and bend the other leg at the knee so that the foot is flat on the floor.
- Tighten the thigh muscle of the affected leg and slowly raise it 6 to 10 inches off the floor. Keep the knee completely straight.
- Hold this position for 5 seconds, slowly lower the leg, and then relax.
- Perform 3 sets of 10 repetitions per day, continuing for 3 to 4 weeks.

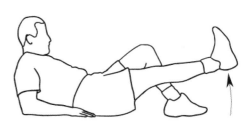

Hamstring Curl

- Stand on a flat surface with your weight evenly distributed on both feet.
- Hold on to the back of a chair or the wall for balance.
- Bend the affected knee, raising the heel of the affected leg toward the ceiling as far as possible without pain.
- Hold this position for 5 seconds and then relax.
- Perform 3 sets of 15 repetitions per day, progressing to 3 sets of 25 repetitions per day, continuing for 3 to 4 weeks.

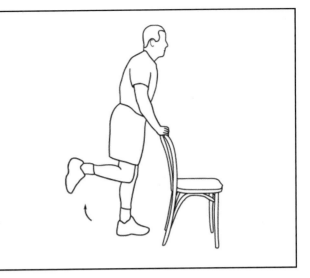

Prone Quadriceps Stretch

- Lie face down on a flat surface with your arms at your sides and your legs straight.
- Bend the affected knee and grasp the ankle with your hand (or use a towel or rubber tubing).
- Keeping your thigh flat on the surface, pull gently and hold for 30 seconds. The stretch should be felt in the front of the thigh. Relax for 30 seconds between repetitions.
- Perform 4 repetitions, 2 to 3 times per day, continuing for 3 to 4 weeks.

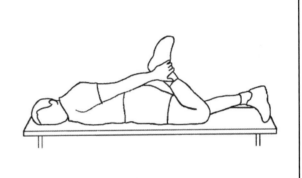

Supine Hamstring Stretch

- Lie on the floor with one leg straight and one leg bent. Clasp your hands behind the thigh of the bent leg, near the knee.
- Straighten the leg and then pull it gently toward your head, until you feel a stretch. (If you have difficulty clasping your hands behind your leg, loop a towel around your thigh. Grasp the ends of the towel and pull the leg toward you.)
- Hold this position for 30 to 60 seconds.
- Repeat with the opposite leg. Perform 4 times on each leg, 2 to 3 times per day for 3 to 4 weeks.

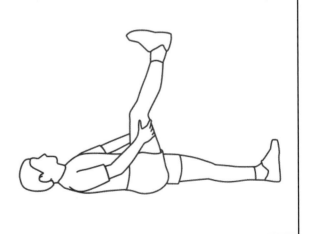

SECTION 6   KNEE AND LOWER LEG

Patellar/Quadriceps Tendon Ruptures

Definition

A displaced patellar fracture or rupture of the quadriceps or patellar tendon can disrupt the extensor mechanism of the knee, resulting in an inability to actively extend the knee fully. Quadriceps and patellar tendon disruptions typically occur with a fall on a knee that is partially flexed. When the quadriceps muscle forcibly contracts to break the impact of the fall, the quadriceps or patellar tendon may be overwhelmed and rupture. Patellar fractures stem from a direct blow such as from a motor vehicle accident or a fall from a standing height, or by the indirect mechanism of a fall similar to that described for patellar/quadriceps tendon ruptures.

Although patellar fractures can occur in any age group, white men between ages 40 and 60 years have a predilection for quadriceps tendon ruptures, and middle-aged African American men have a predilection for patellar tendon rupture. Persons with simultaneous bilateral tendon ruptures and persons who are neither middle-aged African American men with a patellar tendon tear nor middle-aged white men with a quadriceps tendon tear should be assessed for endocrinopathy or prolonged use of fluoroquinolones. A history of quadriceps or patellar tendinitis is uncommon.

Clinical Symptoms

Patients report immediate onset of pain and swelling after an acute injury. Walking is usually limited, but in persons who are able to ambulate, usually with an incomplete rupture, a sense of instability or "giving way" is invariably present.

Tests

Physical Examination

A large effusion and a palpable defect in the area of the rupture is pathognomic for an extensor mechanism disruption (**Figure 1**). Displaced fractures of the patella are usually apparent, but ruptures of the quadriceps or patellar tendon may be missed because the examiner is afraid to adequately palpate the painful torn region. The hallmark of a clinically substantial extensor mechanism disruption is the inability to extend the knee against gravity or perform a straight leg raise.

Diagnostic Tests

Combining physical examination with AP and lateral radiography of the knee can mitigate the need for more advanced imaging. The lateral projection demonstrates a patellar fracture or patella alta or baja. Patella alta (the patella is higher than usual) can indicate rupture of the patellar tendon, whereas patella baja (the patella is lower than usual) may be present with a rupture of the quadriceps tendon. On

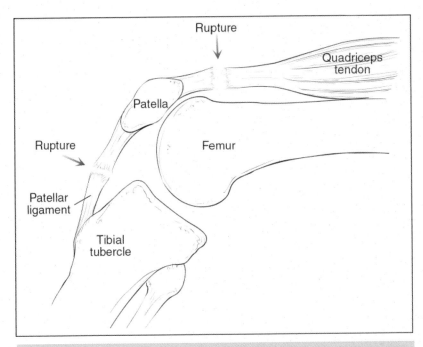

Figure 1 Illustration shows common areas of patellar and quadriceps tendon ruptures. These areas should be palpated during the physical examination.

a standard lateral radiograph, the image is obtained at 30° of knee flexion. At this angle, the inferior pole of the patella should be in line with the Blumensaat line. MRI will confirm a tendon rupture but is rarely necessary in the presence of the clinical triad of palpable defect, inability to actively extend the knee, and patella alta or patella baja.

Differential Diagnosis

- Collateral ligament tear (varus or valgus injury, medial or lateral tenderness and instability)
- Cruciate ligament disruption (effusion may be similar, but the patient can extend the knee)
- Gout (synovial crystals, elevated serum inflammatory markers)
- Meniscal tear (relatively small effusion, joint line tenderness, circumduction pain)

Adverse Outcomes of the Disease

Marked disability will develop secondary to the deficient extensor mechanism unless the rupture is surgically repaired. Persons with an extensor mechanism disruption will be unable to actively fully extend the knee. Delay in treatment substantially increases the difficulty of surgery and may compromise the outcome.

SECTION 6 KNEE AND LOWER LEG

Treatment

Surgical repair is the treatment of choice for a complete rupture of the quadriceps or patellar tendon and for a displaced patellar fracture. Partial tendon tears and nondisplaced fractures can be treated with a period of immobilization, including either a cylinder cast or knee immobilizer.

Adverse Outcomes of Treatment

Postoperative infection and thromboembolism can occur following surgical intervention, and appropriate prophylaxis should be considered. In addition, pain and weakness of the extensor mechanism can persist for 6 months to 1 year after surgery. Retears usually occur within the first 6 months of treatment.

Referral Decisions/Red Flags

All patients who present with the clinical triad of palpable defect, inability to actively extend the knee, and patella alta or patella baja require prompt evaluation for surgery. Ruptures involving the extensor mechanism are surgically repaired within 1 week of injury.

SECTION 6   KNEE AND LOWER LEG

Patellofemoral Maltracking

Synonyms

Miserable malalignment syndrome
Patellar dislocation
Patellofemoral malalignment
Patellar subluxation

Definition

Patellofemoral maltracking encompasses a spectrum of pathologic conditions that are defined by abnormal motion of the patella as it glides over the distal femur. Patellofemoral maltracking includes entities such as lateral patellar overload syndrome from excessive lateral patellar tilt and recurrent patellar instability. Patellofemoral instability usually occurs in a lateral direction as the patella glides over the lateral trochlea and ranges from subluxation to dislocation (**Figure 1**). Medial patellar instability is rare but can occur in the setting of a previous surgical lateral retinacular release. The term "patellofemoral malalignment" is synonymous with patellar maltracking and indicates that the patella is tilted laterally or predisposed to lateral subluxation. Patellar subluxation and dislocation can occur with minimal trauma (such as a minor twist with a foot planted) in individuals with one or more anatomic predisposing factors such as patella alta, a shallow trochlear groove, a relatively flat patellar undersurface, excessive anterior version of the femoral neck in relation to the femoral shaft, external rotation of the tibia, and overall ligamentous laxity that predisposes to patellar hypermobility. In persons with normal patellofemoral mechanics, subluxation or dislocation may be caused by direct trauma or, more frequently, by an indirect mechanism of injury. In these cases, the primary restraint to lateral patellar translation, the medial patellofemoral ligament, is either torn or stretched and rendered incompetent.

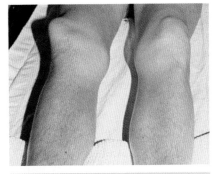

Figure 1 Photograph depicts acute lateral patellar dislocation of a right knee. (Reproduced from Crosby LA, Lewallen DG, eds: *Emergency Care and Transportation of the Sick and Injured,* ed 10. Rosemont, IL, American Academy of Orthopaedic Surgeons, 2010, p 1045.)

Clinical Symptoms

Patellar dislocations can present in two ways: obvious dislocation or transient dislocation with a spontaneous reduction. Patients with an obvious dislocation describe a knee stuck in flexion with an unusual prominence of the medial femoral condyle from a laterally dislocated patella that is no longer covering the trochlea. More commonly, the patella reduces spontaneously. In both scenarios, patients usually report hearing a "pop" at the time of injury, an acute hemarthrosis, and loss of motion. In persons who cannot recall a dislocation, the symptoms mimic those of an anterior cruciate ligament tear. Recurrent episodes of instability tend to be less traumatic than the initial episode, and, with each subsequent episode, symptoms are milder.

In contrast to patients with patellar instability, the primary symptom in patients with symptomatic malalignment is retropatellar pain. This type of anterior knee pain usually is exacerbated when the patient uses stairs, especially when descending. Patients also may report pain with prolonged sitting (movie theater sign) or during squatting. With long-standing maltracking, excessive pressure on the lateral facet of the patella and lateral trochlea can result in progressive degenerative changes involving the lateral patellofemoral joint.

Tests

Physical Examination

Patients with patellar instability demonstrate apprehension with attempts to manually translate the patella laterally (apprehension sign). Range of motion may be limited because of pain or effusion. The medial patellofemoral ligament is invariably injured in patellar instability cases, and it can be tender anywhere along its course from the adductor tubercle to the superior two thirds of the medial patella. Patients with chronic instability exhibit the apprehension sign but may not have tenderness.

The signs of malalignment are more subtle. During gait, the patellae may tend to point inward (femoral anteversion, tibial torsion) or assume a knock-knee alignment (genu valgum). A high-riding patella (patella alta) and abnormal lateral tracking (positive J sign) can contribute to lateral patellar instability. The patella may have excessive lateral excursion (lateral translation greater than one half the width of the patella) or tightness of the lateral retinaculum (inability to elevate the lateral edge of the patella to a horizontal position), which can cause lateral patellar instability or lateral patellar tilt, respectively.

Diagnostic Tests

Standard radiographic views to assess the patellofemoral articulation include AP, lateral, and axial patellofemoral views. An axial patellofemoral view, such as the Merchant or Laurin view, demonstrates the relationship of the patella to the femoral trochlea. Normally, the patella is centered within the trochlea. Malalignment can manifest as lateral patellar subluxation or lateral patellar tilt (**Figure 2**). Occasionally, radiographs will define an avulsion injury to the medial patellofemoral ligament. A shallow trochlear groove with a relatively flat patellar undersurface or a patella with an acutely slanted lateral facet may be evident on radiographs and predispose to patellar instability. In patients with excessive lateral pressure syndrome, disease can progress to lateral patellofemoral arthrosis. Radiographs reveal joint space narrowing and other degenerative changes, especially in the lateral articulation. Although axial CT can help delineate the exact nature of the patellar and trochlear articulations, MRI can provide a more detailed assessment of the articular surfaces and the medial patellofemoral ligament. In cases of patellar instability, MRI can confirm the presence of a transient patellar dislocation based on typical bone bruising patterns (edema

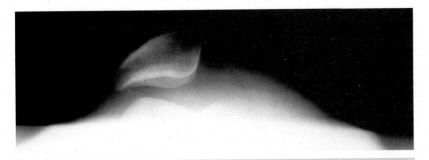

Figure 2 Axial patellofemoral radiograph (Laurin view) of the knee demonstrates patellar tilt and subluxation.

within the lateral femoral trochlea and medial patella) and injury seen within the medial patellofemoral ligament.

Differential Diagnosis

- Anterior cruciate ligament tear (increased anterior laxity with Lachman test)
- Medial collateral ligament tear (pain and laxity with valgus testing)
- Medial meniscal tear (medial joint line tenderness)
- Patellofemoral pain syndrome (pain without malalignment or instability)

Adverse Outcomes of the Disease

Anterior knee pain secondary to patellar instability or maltracking can result in secondary quadriceps weakness, which further compromises stability and exacerbates the underlying problem. In cases of chronic patellar instability or lateral patellar overload, patellofemoral chondrosis can develop because of abnormal stresses on the articular cartilage. With continued dislocations, the lateral trochlea may become deficient and the patella may shear off a fragment of articular cartilage, which can cause locking.

Treatment

Treatment for patellar maltracking depends on the chronicity of the disease. Chronic patellar instability and excessive lateral tilt require less aggressive initial treatment than do acute, traumatic patellar dislocations. The initial treatment of an acute patellar subluxation or dislocation includes application of a protective brace with the knee in extension, oral analgesics, frequent application of ice in the first 24 to 48 hours, and modified weight bearing. Patients are instructed in isometric exercises of the quadriceps that are performed initially with the splint intact. When tenderness has resolved over the medial structures (the medial patellofemoral ligament), range-of-motion and more vigorous strengthening exercises are initiated. The total duration of immobilization varies depending on symptoms, but should not exceed 4 weeks. Quadriceps exercises may begin during this early stage of immobilization. Further imaging should be considered in first-time patellar dislocations or high-energy dislocations to determine whether there is pathology, such as a bony avulsion of the medial patellofemoral ligament or osteochondral fracture that may warrant urgent surgical intervention.

Initial treatment of patients with chronic recurrent maltracking or instability should include exercises that emphasize quadriceps strengthening and flexibility. An elastic brace with a lateral buttress (such as a lateral J-brace) can facilitate the return to occupational or recreational activities. Physical therapy modalities such as electrical stimulation or taping can be useful.

When nonsurgical measures fail, anatomic factors should be carefully considered prior to any surgical intervention. For example, in patients with recurrent patellofemoral instability, a repair or reconstruction of the medial patellofemoral ligament with or without realignment of the extensor mechanism may be indicated to restore a normal patellofemoral relationship. Realignment procedures are usually osteotomies that involve shifting the tibial tuberosity medially and anteriorly.

Adverse Outcomes of Treatment

NSAIDs can worsen hypertension and cause gastric, renal, or hepatic complications, especially if taken in supratherapeutic doses and for prolonged periods. In 2015, the FDA strengthened its warning linking NSAIDs with the risk of heart attack or stroke, even in the first weeks of use of an NSAID. The most common adverse outcome of treatment is residual instability or patellofemoral pain. Poor outcomes can result from failure of realignment or reconstruction technique to provide the desired change in patellofemoral mechanics, incorrect use of isolated lateral release for instability, or articular cartilage damage that remains untreated. Even when successful stabilization and alignment of the patella is achieved, patellofemoral pain may persist secondary to the presence of degenerative articular cartilage.

Referral Decisions/Red Flags

Patients with a substantial effusion after a traumatic knee injury and an osteochondral fracture from an acute patellar dislocation require further evaluation. Patients with patellofemoral malalignment or pain that does not respond to nonsurgical measures may benefit from surgery.

Patellofemoral Pain

Synonyms

Anterior knee pain
Patellofemoral (pain) syndrome

Definition

Patellofemoral syndrome refers to a constellation of problems characterized by diffuse, aching anterior knee pain that increases with activities that place additional loads across the patellofemoral joint, such as running, ascending or descending stairs, kneeling, and squatting. Forces on the articular surface of the patella can vary from three to eight times body weight in activities ranging from walking to running. The etiology of this syndrome is multifactorial and, in many situations, is related to overuse and overloading of the patellofemoral joint. Although patellar maltracking sometimes causes anterior knee pain, it is not a necessary component.

The term chondromalacia should not be used to describe this condition because chondromalacia indicates that pathologic changes exist in the articular surface of the patella; this may not necessarily be true. Conversely, many patients who undergo arthroscopy are found to have degenerative changes on the undersurface of the patella consistent with chondromalacia, yet they have no symptoms referable to the patellofemoral joint. For this reason, the terms patellofemoral pain syndrome or anterior knee pain are preferable.

Clinical Symptoms

Patients most commonly report diffuse, aching anterior knee pain that is worse after prolonged sitting (movie theater sign), climbing stairs, jumping, or squatting. Some patients report a sense of instability or a retropatellar catching sensation, but there is usually no history of swelling. The pain often develops after an increase in activity level or weight training. Occasionally, there is a history of a direct blow to the patella, but in most instances, patients recall no preexisting trauma.

Tests
Physical Examination

When the patellofemoral joint is thought to contribute to the patient's pain, evaluation should be deferred until the end of the examination; otherwise, the patient is likely to resist the entire examination.

Examination should be performed while the patient is bearing weight. Gait should be assessed for evidence of patellar "squinting," that is, when the patellae point toward each other during ambulation (a sign of increased femoral anteversion or weakness of the gluteus medius). Alignment should be inspected for genu valgum ("knock knees") and foot pronation (flatfoot), which can result in a functional increase in genu valgum. The girth of the vastus medialis obliquus

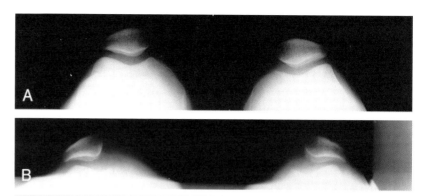

Figure 1 Bilateral axial patellofemoral radiographs obtained to evaluate for patellofemoral pain syndrome. **A,** Patellae are well aligned in their respective femoral grooves. **B,** Bilateral patellar subluxation.

muscle (the musculature of the medial distal thigh) should be compared with the contralateral limb. Any deficiency could represent weakness of this muscle, which can contribute to patellofemoral pain.

With the patient sitting, patellar tracking should be observed throughout the entire range of motion. The patella should be palpated as it moves within the trochlea to determine whether crepitus occurs and, if so, at what position. As the knee nears full extension, the patella may move laterally more than 1 cm (J sign) or may subluxate over the lateral trochlear ridge. Soft-tissue restraints to medial and lateral patellar translation can be evaluated by placing the patella between the thumb and index finger and shifting the patella directly laterally and medially. At 30° of flexion, the examiner should be able to translate the patella at least one quadrant medially and no more than two quadrants laterally. The patellar apprehension sign, a sign of patellar instability, occurs when the patient feels nervous and asks the examiner to stop attempting to laterally translate the patella.

Patellar tilt indicates lateral retinacular tightness. Patellar tilt is evaluated by grasping the patella and attempting to evert the lateral edge of the patella. Inability to bring the lateral edge up to neutral suggests lateral retinacular tightness. Hamstring muscle tightness can be gauged by assessing resistance to passive knee extension with the hip flexed to 90° in the supine position. Conversely, quadriceps muscle tightening can be evaluated by observing resistance to knee flexion with the hip fully extended.

Diagnostic Tests

AP, lateral, and bilateral axial patellofemoral radiographs are necessary. The axial patellofemoral view is particularly beneficial in assessing alignment and any evidence of arthritic change (**Figure 1**).

Differential Diagnosis

- Meniscal tear (joint line tenderness, possible locking)
- Patellar malalignment (malalignment seen clinically and on radiographs)

- Patellar osteoarthritis (seen in older patients) (effusion, crepitus, and evidence on axial radiograph)
- Patellar tendinitis (jumper's knee) (inferior patellar pole tenderness, local tenderness at patellar tendon)
- Pathologic plica (medial parapatellar pain and tenderness, palpable cord in the medial parapatellar region)
- Quadriceps tendinitis (local tenderness at insertion)

Adverse Outcomes of the Disease

Pain and dysfunction are the principal problems. Often, pain limits the patient's ability to exercise, which is a vital component of any rehabilitation protocol.

Treatment

Nonsurgical management, including physical therapy, is the hallmark treatment for patellofemoral pain. Activity should be adjusted to a pain-free level. A program of quadriceps strengthening and quadriceps and hamstring flexibility should be initiated. Quadriceps exercises need to be individually modified to include short-arc, closed-chain, or isometric exercises as necessary to avoid causing knee pain, shear forces, or excessive pressure on the patella. A patellar pad or knee sleeve with a patellar cutout, patellar taping to decrease lateral pressure (McConnell taping), or an infrapatellar strap can potentially help decrease the pain to tolerable levels. Some patients benefit from intermittent, short-term use of acetaminophen or NSAIDs. Weight loss is recommended for patients with obesity, and its analgesic effects are independent of exercise. Patients with persistent pain despite an extensive course of nonsurgical treatment may be candidates for surgery.

Rehabilitation Prescription

A home exercise program should include exercises to strengthen the quadriceps, gain full flexion range of motion, and strengthen the hamstrings. If pain persists after 3 to 4 weeks, formal rehabilitation by a rehabilitation specialist may be recommended. The evaluation should include an assessment of the hip and trunk muscles, patellar mobility, and quadriceps/hamstring muscle group strength. In addition to exercises, manual therapy techniques are often used in the management of patellofemoral pain.

Adverse Outcomes of Treatment

NSAIDs can worsen hypertension and cause gastric, renal, or hepatic complications, especially if taken in supratherapeutic doses and for prolonged periods. In 2015, the FDA strengthened its warning linking NSAIDs with the risk of heart attack or stroke, even in the first weeks of use of an NSAID. Aggressive full-arc and open-chain quadriceps exercises can aggravate the symptoms and generally should either be avoided or used late in the rehabilitation period.

SECTION 6 KNEE AND LOWER LEG

Referral Decisions/Red Flags

Persistent symptoms, including pain or recurrent effusions, or findings suggestive of patellar instability indicate the need for further evaluation if an extensive course of supervised physical therapy has failed to alleviate the symptoms.

Home Exercise Program for Patellofemoral Pain

- Perform the exercises in the order listed. Gentle quadriceps and hamstring stretches should be performed first.
- If symptoms allow, 5 to 10 minutes of gentle stationary cycling with low resistance can be performed as a warm-up before performing the following exercise program.
- To prevent inflammation, after completing the exercises apply a bag of crushed ice or frozen peas along the sides of the kneecap for 20 minutes or until numb.
- If the pain worsens or does not improve, call your doctor.
- The following exercise program is introductory only, and progression of this program will vary based on your specific injury, symptoms, and baseline level of fitness. For further progression of this routine, your physician may recommend evaluation and treatment by a physical therapist or other exercise professional.

Home Exercises for Patellofemoral Pain

Exercise Type	Muscle Group	Number of Repetitions/Sets	Number of Days per Week	Number of Weeks
Standing quadriceps stretch	Quadriceps	4 repetitions, 2 to 3 times per day	Daily	3 to 4
Supine hamstring stretch	Hamstrings	4 repetitions, 2 to 3 times per day	Daily	3 to 4
Hamstring curl	Hamstrings	15 repetitions, progressing to 15 repetitions/3 sets	4 to 5	3 to 4
Straight leg raise	Quadriceps	10 repetitions/3 sets	4 to 5	3 to 4
Straight leg raise (prone)	Quadriceps	10 repetitions/3 sets	4 to 5	3 to 4

SECTION 6　KNEE AND LOWER LEG

Standing Quadriceps Stretch

- Bend your knee up toward your buttock and grasp your ankle. (If you cannot comfortably reach your ankle, a looped belt or towel can be used around the ankle.)
- Pull up gently and hold this position for 30 to 60 seconds. A gentle stretch should be noted in the front of the thigh or hip of the leg being stretched.
- Repeat with the opposite leg.
- Perform 4 repetitions, 2 to 3 times per day, continuing for 3 to 4 weeks.

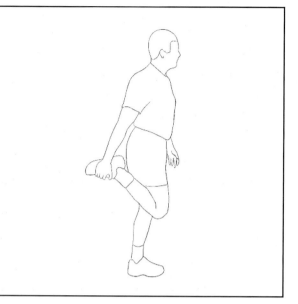

Supine Hamstring Stretch

- Lie on the floor with one leg straight and one leg bent. Clasp your hands behind the thigh of the bent leg, near the knee.
- Straighten the leg and then pull it gently toward your head, until you feel a stretch. (If you have difficulty clasping your hands behind your leg, loop a towel around your thigh. Grasp the ends of the towel and pull the leg toward you.)
- Hold this position for 30 to 60 seconds.
- Repeat with the opposite leg.
- Perform 4 repetitions, 2 to 3 times per day, continuing for 3 to 4 weeks.

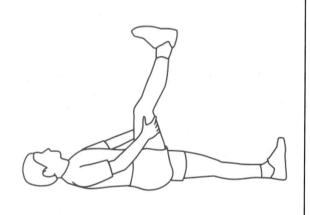

Hamstring Curl

- Stand on a flat surface with your weight evenly distributed on both feet.
- Hold on to the back of a chair or the wall for balance.
- Bend the affected knee, raising the heel of the affected leg toward the ceiling as far as possible without pain.
- Hold this position for 5 seconds and then relax.
- Perform 15 repetitions, progressing to 3 sets of 15 repetitions.
- Perform the exercise 4 to 5 days per week, continuing for 3 to 4 weeks.

Seated version

- Sit on a chair with your feet flat on the floor.
- Slide the foot on the affected side back and hold the position for 5 seconds.

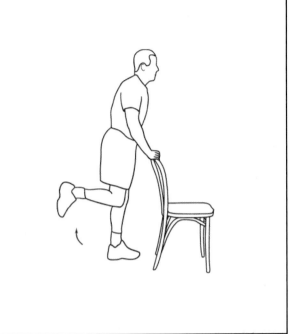

Straight Leg Raise

- Lie on the floor, supporting your torso with your elbows as shown.
- Keep the affected leg straight and bend the other leg at the knee so that the foot is flat on the floor.
- Tighten the thigh muscle of the affected leg and slowly raise it 6 to 10 inches off the floor.
- Hold this position for 5 seconds and then relax.
- Perform 3 sets of 10 repetitions 4 to 5 days per week, continuing for 3 to 4 weeks.

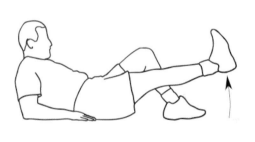

Straight Leg Raise (Prone)

- Lie face down on the floor with your legs straight.
- Keeping the affected leg straight, raise the leg approximately 8 inches off the floor.
- Hold this position for 5 seconds.
- Lower the leg and rest it for 2 seconds.
- Perform 3 sets of 10 repetitions, 4 to 5 days per week, continuing for 3 to 4 weeks.

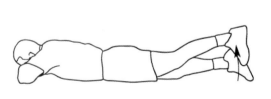

SECTION 6 KNEE AND LOWER LEG

Plica Syndrome

Definition

A plica is a fold of the synovium of the knee. The synovium of the knee joint has five basic plicae, which are usually asymptomatic. Three (suprapatellar, medial, and infrapatellar) are distinct structures, whereas two others are less pronounced and are considered to be minor folds. The suprapatellar plica extends from the undersurface of the quadriceps tendon to the medial or lateral capsule of the knee. The medial plica extends from the medial joint capsule to the medial anterior fat pad. The infrapatellar plica (ligamentum mucosa) extends anterior to, and may sometimes cover, the anterior cruciate ligament.

A plica that becomes inflamed and thickened from trauma or overuse may interfere with normal joint motion because the pathologic structure "bowstrings" over the femoral condyle or other structures. Plica syndromes usually result from a combination of trauma and mechanical malalignment and can occur at any age, although adolescents have a predisposition for development of symptoms. The medial plica is the plica that most often becomes pathologic.

Clinical Symptoms

The onset of pain is often insidious but may be related to a fall or injury. Patients most often describe activity-related aching in the anterior or anteromedial aspect of the knee. Some patients describe a painful snapping or popping in the knee. Buckling or a sense of instability may occur, but true giving way, locking, or obvious effusion is uncommon.

Tests

Physical Examination

The knee is palpated for areas of tenderness. With a pathologic medial plica, tenderness is localized to the medial aspect of the patella and can be palpated. With the knee flexed, a pathologic plica may be palpated as a thickened band with the anteromedial "soft spot" adjacent to the patellar tendon. To palpate the medial plica, the knee is placed in 90° of flexion and then extended. With a pathologic plica, a "pop" may occur at approximately 60° of flexion, when the plica presumably glides over the edge of the medial femoral condyle. Other conditions, such as patellofemoral disorders, may present with similar symptoms.

Diagnostic Tests

AP, lateral, and axial patellofemoral radiographs and MRI studies are usually normal in persons with plica syndrome but should be obtained to rule out other conditions.

Differential Diagnosis

- Meniscal tear (giving way, joint line tenderness, pain with circumduction)
- Osteochondritis dissecans (spontaneous onset, evident on radiographs)
- Patellofemoral instability (positive apprehension sign)
- Prepatellar bursitis (location)
- Quadriceps or patellar tendinitis (tenderness at tendon insertion sites)
- Septic arthritis (severe pain, fever, effusion, diagnostic joint aspiration)

Adverse Outcomes of the Disease

Persons with medial plica syndrome have continued discomfort and interference with running activities. As the disease progresses, erosive changes in the femoral condyle cartilage can develop, because of the snapping of the thickened plica over the condyle.

Treatment

Initial management aims to decrease the inflammation and thickening of the plica. Activity modifications and NSAIDs should be considered. An injection of local anesthetic and corticosteroid preparation into the medial plica can be both diagnostic and therapeutic. An appropriate flexibility and strengthening program should be tailored based on the physical examination. With persistent symptoms, a palpable and painful plica, and no other evidence of other intra-articular disorders, arthroscopic resection of the plica should be considered.

Rehabilitation Prescription

Early rehabilitation should include rest, ice, compression, and elevation (RICE) of the affected knee. The home exercise program should include quadriceps strengthening exercises to reduce pain and prevent joint stiffness. Atrophy of the quadriceps muscle can be prevented with early isometric exercises such as straight leg raises.

If symptoms do not respond to the home exercise program after 1 month, a more complex problem involving abnormal patellofemoral mechanics may be present, and formal rehabilitation should be recommended. The evaluation should include an assessment of foot mechanics, patellofemoral mobility, and strength of the hip and trunk muscles. After determining the extent of the muscle imbalances and mechanics, the rehabilitation specialist will develop, implement, and progress the treatment plan.

Adverse Outcomes of Treatment

NSAIDs can worsen hypertension and cause gastric, renal, or hepatic complications, especially if taken in supratherapeutic doses and for prolonged periods. In 2015, the FDA strengthened its warning linking NSAIDs with the risk of heart attack or stroke, even in the first weeks of use of an NSAID. Repeated intra-articular corticosteroid injections can result in accelerated destruction of articular cartilage and/or iatrogenic sepsis. Surgical resection may be ineffective or, in rare cases, complicated by thromboembolism, infection, and stiffness.

Referral Decisions/Red Flags

Continued discomfort and symptoms of instability indicate the need for further evaluation.

Home Exercise Program for Plica Syndrome

- Perform the exercises in the order listed.
- If symptoms allow, 5 to 10 minutes of gentle stationary cycling with low resistance can be performed as a warm-up before performing the following exercise program.
- Gentle quadriceps and hamstring stretching should be performed first.
- To prevent inflammation, after completing the exercises apply a bag of crushed ice or frozen peas to the affected side of the knee for 20 minutes or until numb. You should experience improved range of motion and less pain in your knee.
- If the pain does not change or becomes worse, call your doctor.
- The following exercise program is introductory only, and progression of this program will vary based on your specific injury, symptoms, and baseline level of fitness. For further progression of this routine, your physician may recommend evaluation and treatment by a physical therapist or other exercise professional.

Home Exercises for Plica Syndrome

Exercise Type	Muscle Group	Number of Repetitions/Sets	Number of Days per Week	Number of Weeks
Standing quadriceps stretch	Quadriceps	4 repetitions, 2 to 3 times per day	Daily	3 to 4
Supine hamstring stretch	Hamstrings	4 repetitions, 2 to 3 times per day	Daily	3 to 4
Straight leg raise	Quadriceps	Work up to 10 repetitions/3 sets	Daily	3 to 4

Standing Quadriceps Stretch

- Bend your knee up toward your buttock and grasp your ankle. (If you are unable to grasp the ankle comfortably, a looped belt or towel can be used to lift the ankle.)
- Pull up gently and hold this position for 30 to 60 seconds.
- Repeat with the opposite leg.
- Perform 4 repetitions, 2 to 3 times per day, continuing for 3 to 4 weeks.

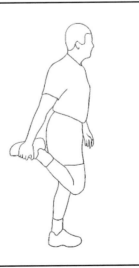

SECTION 6   KNEE AND LOWER LEG

Supine Hamstring Stretch

- Lie on the floor with one leg straight and one leg bent. Clasp your hands behind the thigh of the bent leg, near the knee.
- Straighten the leg and then pull it gently toward your head until you feel a stretch. (If you have difficulty clasping your hands behind your leg, loop a towel around your thigh. Grasp the ends of the towel and pull the leg toward you.)
- Hold this position for 30 to 60 seconds.
- Repeat with the opposite leg.
- Perform 4 repetitions, 2 to 3 times per day, continuing for 3 to 4 weeks.

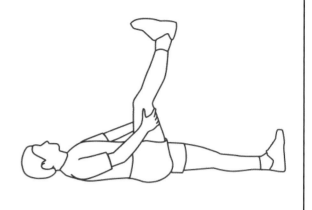

Straight Leg Raise

- Lie on the floor, supporting your torso with your elbows as shown.
- Keep the affected leg straight and bend the other leg at the knee so that the foot is flat on the floor.
- Tighten the thigh muscle of the affected leg and slowly raise it 6 to 10 inches off the floor. Be sure to keep the knee completely straight.
- Hold this position for 5 seconds and then relax.
- Work up to 3 sets of 10 repetitions per day, continuing for 3 to 4 weeks.

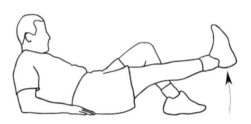

SECTION 6   KNEE AND LOWER LEG

Popliteal Cyst

Synonyms
Baker cyst
Synovial cyst

Definition
A popliteal cyst, commonly known as a Baker cyst, is the most common benign synovial cyst in the knee. A popliteal cyst develops in the popliteal bursa located at the posteromedial aspect of the knee joint. This normally thin bursa communicates with the knee joint and becomes more prominent (cystic) when synovitis or trauma creates excessive joint fluid that then tracks into the popliteal bursa. Popliteal cysts are associated with degenerative meniscal tears and systemic inflammatory conditions such as rheumatoid arthritis.

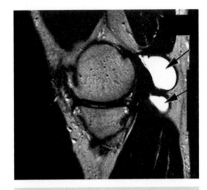

Figure 1 T2-weighted sagittal MRI demonstrates a popliteal cyst. Areas of high signal intensity (arrows) indicate fluid, which indicates a cyst.

Clinical Symptoms
Patients describe a sensation of fullness or swelling in the posterior aspect of the knee without a known history of trauma. This subjective feeling may be accompanied by pain or tenderness. Occasionally, a larger cyst can cause a "mass effect" and produce symptoms (such as numbness of the plantar surface of the foot) consistent with tibial nerve neuropathy. Cysts increase and decrease in size depending on activity levels. Cysts can enlarge and dissect down the posterior calf and eventually rupture. When these cysts rupture, symptoms produced can mimic a deep vein thrombosis. Ruptures of popliteal cysts usually occur in patients older than 40 years who have degenerative arthritis or rheumatoid arthritis.

Tests
Physical Examination
With the patient prone or standing, the popliteal fossa should be inspected and compared with the opposite leg and any asymmetry should be noted. If a cyst is identified, it should be palpated to determine the size and consistency of the cyst, the amount of tenderness produced, and the presence of a pulsatile mass. Most cysts are located between the medial head of the gastrocnemius muscle and the semimembranosus muscle. Effusion and accompanying mechanical signs indicate an intra-articular irritant generating the excessive joint fluid.

Diagnostic Tests
Radiographs of the knee are usually negative but may show the outline of the cyst or show calcification present in the cyst or within the knee. MRI usually is not necessary but can demonstrate the location and character of the cystic fluid and delineate any associated intra-articular pathology (**Figure 1**).

Ultrasonography is becoming an increasingly useful modality for imaging popliteal cysts. In addition to its role in characterizing the location and extent of the cyst, ultrasonography is useful in localizing needle placement for cyst aspiration. Cyst aspiration without ultrasonographic guidance should be approached with caution because of the proximity of neurovascular structures in the popliteal fossa. Cyst fluid may be gelatinous and not easily retrievable with a standard-bore needle.

Differential Diagnosis

- Deep vein thrombosis (evident on ultrasonogram or venogram)
- Exertional compartment syndrome (evident on physical examination)
- Inflammatory arthritis (positive serologic studies)
- Medial gastrocnemius strain (evident on physical examination)
- Popliteal artery aneurysm (pulsatile mass)
- Soft-tissue tumor (evident on MRI)
- Superficial phlebitis (superficial tenderness, negative ultrasonogram or venogram)

Adverse Outcomes of the Disease

Other than producing a sensation of fullness, most popliteal cysts are relatively asymptomatic. Rarely, a cyst will impinge on the tibial nerve and cause numbness on the plantar surface of the foot or will rupture and cause pain in the posterior calf that, with the swelling, may mimic a deep vein thrombosis.

Treatment

The benign nature of this condition should be emphasized to each patient. Aspiration has been suggested but may provide only transient relief because the cyst lining remains intact and the fluid often reaccumulates. In addition, the cyst contents may be gelatinous and quite difficult to aspirate. Treatment should be directed at the cause of increased synovial fluid. When intra-articular lesions that increase production of synovial fluid can be successfully treated (usually by arthroscopic excision of a torn medial meniscus), the cyst usually resolves spontaneously and excision is unnecessary. Cysts associated with severe arthritis typically resolve after knee replacement. Rarely, cyst excision may be required in some patients. Ruptured popliteal cysts are treated symptomatically with minor analgesics, rest, and elevation.

Adverse Outcomes of Treatment

NSAIDs can worsen hypertension and cause gastric, renal, or hepatic complications, especially if taken in supratherapeutic doses and for prolonged periods. In 2015, the FDA strengthened its warning linking NSAIDs with the risk of heart attack or stroke, even in the first weeks of use of an NSAID. Open excision is associated with the risk of injury to neighboring nerves and blood vessels; dissection should be performed with caution. The recurrence rate when excision is combined with resolution of any internal derangement is low (approximately 5%).

Referral Decisions/Red Flags

Night pain, weight loss, fever and/or chills, or other constitutional symptoms indicate the possibility of a neoplastic process and therefore the need for further evaluation. A pulsatile mass within the popliteal cyst may represent a popliteal artery aneurysm that requires evaluation by a vascular surgeon.

SECTION 6 KNEE AND LOWER LEG

Posterior Cruciate Ligament Tear

Synonym
PCL sprain

Definition
The posterior cruciate ligament (PCL) is a critical ligament in the knee and serves as the primary restraint to posterior translation of the tibia relative to the femur. Anatomically, the PCL originates on the medial intercondylar wall of the femur, runs obliquely behind the anterior cruciate ligament, and inserts on the posterior aspect of the tibia below the joint line. Injury to the PCL ranges in severity from a stretch injury to a complete rupture. Most PCL injuries result from a direct blow to the tibia, such as when the leg strikes a dashboard during a motor vehicle collision or on a fall to the ground with the foot plantarflexed. PCL injuries are less common than injuries to the anterior cruciate ligament (ACL) and are often overlooked because many people with an isolated PCL injury can function at a near-normal level.

Clinical Symptoms
Four injury patterns suggest a possible PCL injury:

- A dashboard injury during a motor vehicle collision (a posteriorly directed force to the anterior knee with the knee in flexion)
- A fall onto a flexed knee with the foot in plantar flexion (results in direct posteriorly directed impact to the tibial tuberosity; in comparison, the foot in dorsiflexion results in a direct blow to the patella and often causes a patellar fracture)
- A pure hyperflexion injury to the knee
- A hyperextension injury to the knee. (Typically, the ACL ruptures first; then, with sufficient force, injury to the PCL follows. This combination most commonly occurs in contact sports, secondary to a direct load on the anteromedial proximal tibia with the knee in extension. This mechanism of injury frequently results in a knee dislocation with or without spontaneous reduction.)

An effusion commonly develops within the first 24 hours after injury, and range of motion usually is limited. Patients also may report pain and feelings of instability with weight bearing, especially with combined ligamentous injuries.

Tests
Physical Examination
Examination begins with inspection of the knee. In injuries incurred in a motor vehicle collision or during contact sports, abrasions or ecchymosis adjacent to the tibial tuberosity suggests an anterior blow

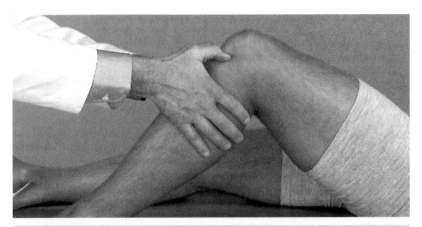

Figure 1 Photograph shows the examiner's thumb palpating the position of the tibial plateau relative to the femoral condyles. With a normal posterior cruciate ligament, the tibial plateau is 1 cm anterior to the femoral condyles.

to the knee and should alert the examiner to the possibility of a PCL injury. Because of its intra-articular location, a substantial effusion and decreased range of motion often accompany the injury and, unless a meniscal tear is present, tenderness to palpation does not.

The most sensitive test is the posterior drawer test. However, ligamentous examination within the first few days after injury may be limited by patient guarding. Furthermore, if the tibia is subluxated posteriorly because of gravity, results of the posterior drawer test can be easily misinterpreted as an ACL tear when the tibia is pulled back to the anterior position. This misinterpretation can be further complicated by the frequent coexistence of an ACL tear. To facilitate an accurate assessment, the resting position of the tibial plateau relative to the femoral condyles should be identified prior to drawer testing. With a PCL injury, the tibia can be posterior relative to the femur because of gravity, and there will be no place for an examiner's thumbs on the anterior tibial plateaus (**Figure 1**). Comparison with the other knee is helpful. If the tibia sags behind the femur, a PCL injury likely is present.

Because PCL injuries often occur as part of a multiligamentous injury, examination of the ACL and collateral ligaments is mandatory. In acute multiligamentous injuries, distal neurovascular status should be carefully assessed and recorded because limb-threatening vascular injury or severe neurologic deficits may be present. An ankle-brachial index less than 0.9 should prompt further imaging of the arterial system to rule out an intimal tear that can thrombose and cause a complete arterial occlusion.

Diagnostic Tests

AP and lateral radiographs of the knee obtained in the acute setting can aid in diagnosis and identify bony avulsions, which may be amenable to acute surgical repair. Lateral radiographs obtained with the patient contracting his or her hamstring can reveal abnormal posterior tibial translation. MRI can further define a PCL tear,

SECTION 6 KNEE AND LOWER LEG

including its severity and location. Furthermore, MRI can delineate concomitant injuries to the ligaments, menisci, and articular cartilage.

Differential Diagnosis

- ACL tear (positive Lachman test, positive pivot shift test)
- Articular cartilage injury (pain on palpation, evident on radiographs or MRI)
- Combined ligament injury (laxity in multiple directions, evident on MRI)
- Medial or lateral collateral ligament tear (pain on palpation and varus/valgus laxity)
- Meniscal tear (joint line tenderness)
- Patellar or quadriceps tendon rupture (inability to achieve straight leg raise)
- Patellar or tibial plateau fracture (evident on radiographs)
- Patellofemoral dislocation (apprehension with lateral patellar displacement)

Adverse Outcomes of the Disease

Limb-threatening vascular injury may be overlooked if a dislocated or hyperextended knee that has spontaneously reduced is not identified and fully evaluated. Substantial permanent peroneal or tibial nerve injury and severe knee instability can occur. Recurrent instability, subsequent meniscal tears, and osteoarthritis of the knee are all possible long-term consequences of an untreated PCL injury.

Treatment

Isolated PCL injuries typically are treated with a rehabilitation program that initially concentrates on resolving swelling and restoring range of motion. After these goals have been achieved, progression to strengthening exercises may be initiated, with an emphasis on the quadriceps (short-arc terminal extension exercises from 30° to 0° of flexion). Functional bracing may be helpful when the patient returns to contact sports.

Failure of nonsurgical treatment typically manifests as recurrent instability and/or subsequent meniscal tears. PCL reconstruction is required to restore functional stability in these patients. After reconstructive procedures, instability is improved, but increased translation relative to the normal side may persist. Patients with combined injuries to the PCL and other ligaments, with or without knee dislocation, usually require surgical reconstruction.

Rehabilitation Prescription

A patient with a PCL injury who is not a candidate for surgery should start an intense rehabilitation program designed to improve range of motion and muscle strength of the quadriceps and hamstrings, including neuromuscular training and hip and trunk strengthening.

Early rehabilitation should include rest, ice, compression, and elevation (RICE). After the initial healing stage of 1 to 5 days, range-of-motion exercises and quadriceps muscle strengthening should be started. The patient should avoid activities that involve a high knee flexion angle until the hamstrings and quadriceps muscles become stronger. Wall slides are a safe exercise to promote increased mobility. Both prone and supine straight leg raises help prevent quadriceps atrophy. Initially, hamstring curls should not be performed to avoid a posterior subluxation force. The rehabilitation evaluation should include an assessment of quadriceps, hip, and trunk muscle strength.

Adverse Outcomes of Treatment

Osteoarthritic changes involving the medial and patellofemoral compartments are well-documented sequelae to both nonsurgical and surgical management, although a recent study questions the validity of this statement. Surgical reconstruction may be complicated by iatrogenic injury to the popliteal artery or tibial nerve, infection, thromboembolism, or graft loosening and recurrent instability.

Referral Decisions/Red Flags

Neurovascular compromise or deficits indicate the possibility of a knee dislocation. An ankle-brachial index should be obtained acutely on any patient suspected of having a PCL injury. An index less than 0.9 can indicate vascular injury and should prompt further investigation. Any patient with a PCL injury and the possibility of damage to other ligamentous structures requires evaluation by a specialist.

SECTION 6 KNEE AND LOWER LEG

Home Exercise Program for PCL Injury

- Perform the exercises in the order listed.
- If symptoms allow, 5 to 10 minutes of gentle stationary cycling with low resistance can be performed as a warm-up before performing the following exercise program.
- To prevent inflammation, after completing all the exercises apply a bag of crushed ice or frozen peas to the back of the knee for 20 minutes or until numb.
- If pain does not improve, if it worsens, or if the knee joint becomes inflamed, call your doctor.
- The following exercise program is introductory only, and progression of this program will vary based on your specific injury, symptoms, and baseline level of fitness. For further progression of this routine, your physician may recommend evaluation and treatment by a physical therapist or other exercise professional.

Home Exercises for PCL Injury

Exercise Type	Muscle Group	Number of Repetitions/Sets	Number of Days per Week	Number of Weeks
Straight leg raise	Quadriceps	10 repetitions/3 sets	6 to 7	3 to 4
Straight leg raise (prone)	Quadriceps	10 repetitions/3 sets	6 to 7	3 to 4

Straight Leg Raise

- Lie on the floor, supporting your torso with your elbows as shown.
- Keep the affected leg straight and bend the other leg at the knee so that the foot is flat on the floor.
- Tighten the thigh muscle of the affected leg and slowly raise it 6 to 10 inches off the floor. Be sure to keep the knee completely straight.
- Hold this position for 5 seconds and then relax.
- Perform 3 sets of 10 repetitions, 6 to 7 days per week, continuing for 3 to 4 weeks.

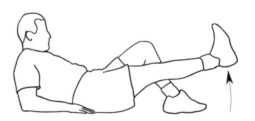

Straight Leg Raise (Prone)

- Lie face down on the floor with your legs straight.
- Keeping the knee of the affected leg straight, raise the leg approximately 6 to 8 inches.
- Hold this position for 5 seconds.
- Lower the leg and rest it for 2 seconds.
- Perform 3 sets of 10 repetitions, 6 to 7 days per week, continuing for 3 to 4 weeks.

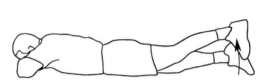

SECTION 6 KNEE AND LOWER LEG

Shin Splints

Definition

Shin splints (medial tibial stress syndrome) is a condition characterized by the gradual onset of pain in the posteromedial aspect of the distal third of the leg. This condition commonly develops as a response to increased exercise or activity level and probably represents inflammation of the tibial periosteum secondary to repetitive muscle contraction.

Clinical Symptoms

Shin splints are generally associated with prolonged walking or running activity. Symptoms develop gradually with exercise, such as running on hard surfaces or early-season hill training, or with increased training intensity, pace, or distance. Pain is localized to the distal third of the medial tibia, the site of the origin of the tibialis posterior muscle. The patient may demonstrate pes planus associated with overpronation.

Tests

Physical Examination

The hallmark of examination for shin splints is tenderness along the posterior medial crest of the tibia in the middle or distal third of the leg. Some patients have pain with resisted plantar flexion.

Diagnostic Tests

AP and lateral radiographs should be obtained to rule out a stress fracture. An MRI or bone scan may demonstrate inflammation diffusely along the posteromedial tibia.

Differential Diagnosis

- Exertional compartment syndrome (no symptoms at rest, elevated compartment pressure)
- Stress fracture (findings on imaging studies)

Adverse Outcomes of the Disease

No adverse outcomes of shin splints are known, except continued pain and inability to walk or run.

Treatment

Mild shin splints may be relieved by limiting activity to soft surfaces, decreasing training, and avoiding hills. NSAIDs, ice massage, and analgesic creams also may be helpful. Further measures include cushioned antipronation shoe inserts, local ultrasound with phonophoresis, foot and ankle stretching and strengthening exercises, and a calf sleeve. Moderate shin splints may require replacing running with nonprovocative exercise, and severe shin splints may respond only to restricting all but non–weight-bearing sports. Rarely, surgery such as excision of the inflamed tibial periosteum may be indicated, but its results are mixed.

Adverse Outcomes of Treatment
NSAIDs can worsen hypertension and cause gastric, renal, or hepatic complications, especially if taken in supratherapeutic doses and for prolonged periods. In 2015, the FDA strengthened its warning linking NSAIDs with the risk of heart attack or stroke, even in the first weeks of use of an NSAID.

Referral Decisions/Red Flags
Conditions such as stress fractures and exertional compartment syndromes must be ruled out before a diagnosis of shin splints is definitively made.

SECTION 6   KNEE AND LOWER LEG

Stress Fracture

Synonym

Dreaded black line

Definition

A stress fracture is a hairline or microscopic break in a bone caused by microtraumatic, cumulative overload on bone. Several factors, including overtraining, incorrect biomechanics, fatigue, hormonal imbalance, poor nutrition, vitamin D deficiency, and osteoporosis, have been implicated as contributing causes. Anterior tibial stress fractures have a poor prognosis and may require surgery.

Clinical Symptoms

Stress fractures of the tibia and fibula typically follow a relatively rapid increase in exercise intensity. The pain initially occurs only in association with exercise, but with continued activity, the pain is elicited with normal walking or even at rest or at night. Patients usually describe a focal area of pain within the tibia or fibula. Anterior (tension side) tibial stress fractures are tender on the subcutaneous anterior tibial crest; posterior medial (compression side) stress fractures are tender at the posterior border.

Tests

Physical Examination

Tenderness is usually localized to the affected area of bone. Impact as well as varus, valgus, anterior, and posterior stress on the bone can cause pain. In bones that lie deep within muscle and cannot be easily palpated (for example, the femoral neck), eliciting pain by placing stress across the area of injured bone is a critical part of the examination. Six or more weeks after the onset of symptoms, a bony callus may be palpable in areas where subcutaneous tissues are thin, such as the anterior tibia.

Diagnostic Tests

AP and lateral radiographs of the tibia should be obtained (**Figure 1**). However, stress fractures may not be visible on plain radiographs for 3 weeks or longer after injury. When the pain is not severe, the patient is not involved in an occupation or athletic activity that puts him or her at risk for further injury, and the patient can keep his or her activity level below the pain threshold, radiographs may be repeated 3 to 4 weeks after the initial examination. When immediate confirmation of the suspected diagnosis is necessary, however, a bone scan may be ordered because it will show increased uptake at the location of the stress fracture (**Figure 2**). Correlating these findings with the area of pain and tenderness is important because bone scans of athletes who place repetitive stresses on the legs often demonstrate areas of increased uptake in asymptomatic locations. Alternatively,

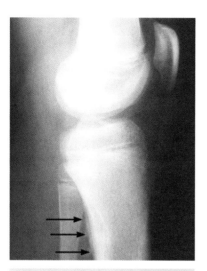

Figure 1 Lateral radiograph demonstrates sclerosis and periosteal reaction in the posterior tibia (arrows), consistent with a stress fracture. (Reproduced from Johnson TR, Steinbach LS, eds: *Essentials of Musculoskeletal Imaging.* Rosemont, IL, American Academy of Orthopaedic Surgeons, 2004, p 517.)

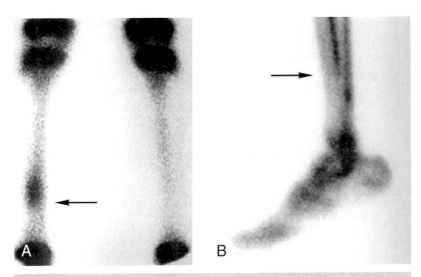

Figure 2 Bone scans of stress fractures. **A,** Bilateral AP view demonstrates stress fracture with focal uptake (arrow). **B,** Lateral view demonstrates medial tibial stress syndrome with more diffuse uptake along the posteromedial shaft of the tibia. (Reproduced from Sullivan JA, Anderson SJ, eds: *Care of the Young Athlete.* Rosemont, IL, American Academy of Orthopaedic Surgeons, 1999, p 408.)

MRI may confirm the diagnosis; however, false-negative results can occur with MRI.

Differential Diagnosis
- Exertional compartment syndrome (no radiographic findings, elevated compartment pressures)
- Shin splints (no radiographic findings)

Adverse Outcomes of the Disease
In most situations, the pain of a stress fracture limits participation in competitive or recreational activities and thus prevents further injury. Some patients continue activity and may cause a displaced fracture. Fractures of the anterior tibial cortex are at higher risk for complete fracture. Although complete fracture may occur, prolonged healing time is a more likely outcome of delayed diagnosis of a painful stress fracture.

Treatment
When diagnosed early, most stress fractures of the tibia and fibula respond well to a period of relative rest. Mild pain may respond to activity modifications. Bone stimulators and long-leg pneumatic splints or other removable fracture braces have been proposed to expedite the healing process and alleviate some pain for patients with moderate pain. When substantial pain occurs with walking, initial treatment is cast immobilization and limited weight bearing. Low-impact exercises such as bicycling and swimming may be substituted to maintain cardiovascular conditioning. Predicted time to return to

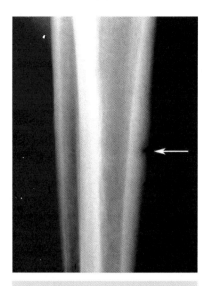

Figure 3 Lateral radiograph of the tibia demonstrates delayed union of an anterior cortex tibial stress fracture (arrow), the "dreaded black line." (Reproduced from Boden BP, Osbahr DC: High-risk stress fractures: Evaluation and treatment. *J Am Acad Orthop Surg* 2000;8[6]:344-353.)

◉◀ Synovial Injection-Animation

◉◀ Synovial Injection

activity depends on the severity and duration of symptoms before diagnosis. Resumption of normal activities commences after pain has completely resolved.

Anterior tibial stress fractures (tension side of the tibia) can occur at multiple sites on the same limb. Anterior fractures have a poorer prognosis, less likelihood of resolution, and a higher chance of progression to a complete, displaced fracture of the tibia. These patients must be followed closely, and if unresponsive to nonsurgical measures, may require surgical treatment with intramedullary nailing.

Adverse Outcomes of Treatment

NSAIDs can worsen hypertension and cause gastric, renal, or hepatic complications, especially if taken in supratherapeutic doses and for prolonged periods. In 2015, the FDA strengthened its warning linking NSAIDs with the risk of heart attack or stroke, even in the first weeks of use of an NSAID. Nonsurgical management of stress fractures, especially anterior tibial stress fractures, may fail. Surgical treatment with intramedullary nailing can result in permanent anterior knee pain.

Referral Decisions/Red Flags

Patients whose symptoms do not substantially improve after 2 to 3 weeks of rest require further evaluation. Menstrual cycle frequency, calcium and vitamin D intake, and potential eating disorders should be discussed with women. An unusual and difficult stress injury to diagnose is a fatigue fracture of the anterior cortex of the midshaft of the tibia, referred to as the "dreaded black line" because of its radiographic appearance (**Figure 3**). Treatment of this injury is controversial and ranges from cast immobilization with no weight bearing to intramedullary rod insertion.

PAIN DIAGRAM
Foot and Ankle

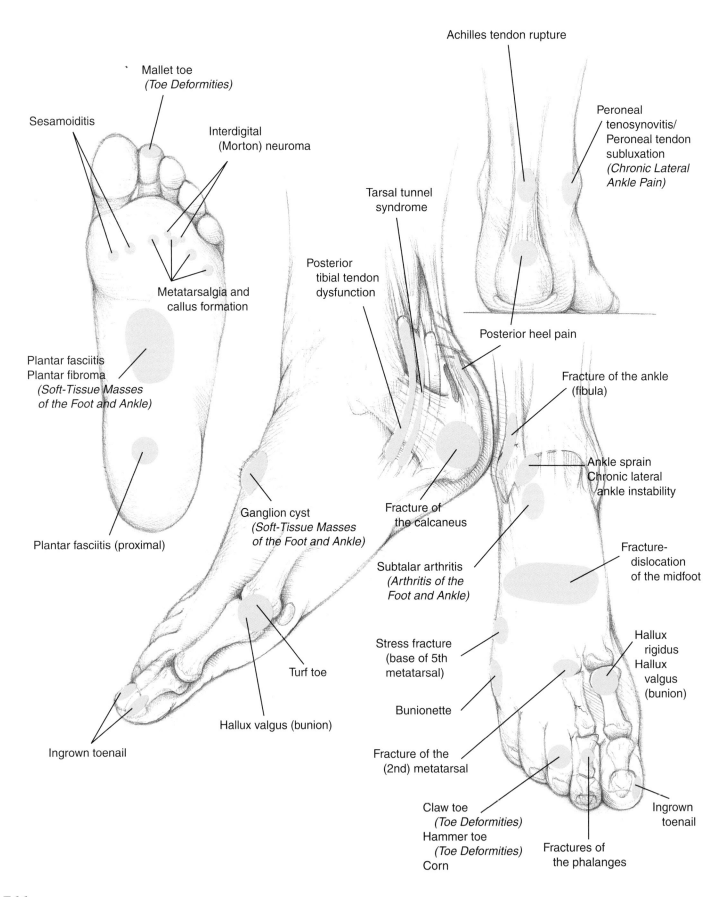

Mallet toe
(Toe Deformities)

Sesamoiditis

Interdigital
(Morton) neuroma

Achilles tendon rupture

Peroneal
tenosynovitis/
Peroneal tendon
subluxation
*(Chronic Lateral
Ankle Pain)*

Tarsal tunnel
syndrome

Metatarsalgia and
callus formation

Posterior
tibial tendon
dysfunction

Posterior heel pain

Plantar fasciitis
Plantar fibroma
*(Soft-Tissue Masses
of the Foot and Ankle)*

Fracture of the ankle
(fibula)

Plantar fasciitis (proximal)

Ganglion cyst
*(Soft-Tissue Masses
of the Foot and Ankle)*

Fracture of
the calcaneus

Ankle sprain
Chronic lateral
ankle instability

Fracture-
dislocation
of the midfoot

Subtalar arthritis
*(Arthritis of the
Foot and Ankle)*

Hallux
rigidus
Hallux
valgus
(bunion)

Turf toe

Stress fracture
(base of 5th
metatarsal)

Hallux valgus (bunion)

Bunionette

Ingrown toenail

Fracture of the
(2nd) metatarsal

Ingrown
toenail

Claw toe
(Toe Deformities)
Hammer toe
(Toe Deformities)
Corn

Fractures of
the phalanges

Foot and Ankle

Section Editor

Umur Aydogan, MD

Assistant Professor of Orthopaedics
Foot and Ankle Surgery
Bone and Joint Institute
Penn State Milton S. Hershey Medical Center
Hershey, Pennsylvania

Contributor

Mark C. Hubbard, MPT

Physical Therapist
Bone and Joint Institute
Penn State Milton S. Hershey Medical Center

ANATOMY OF THE FOOT AND ANKLE

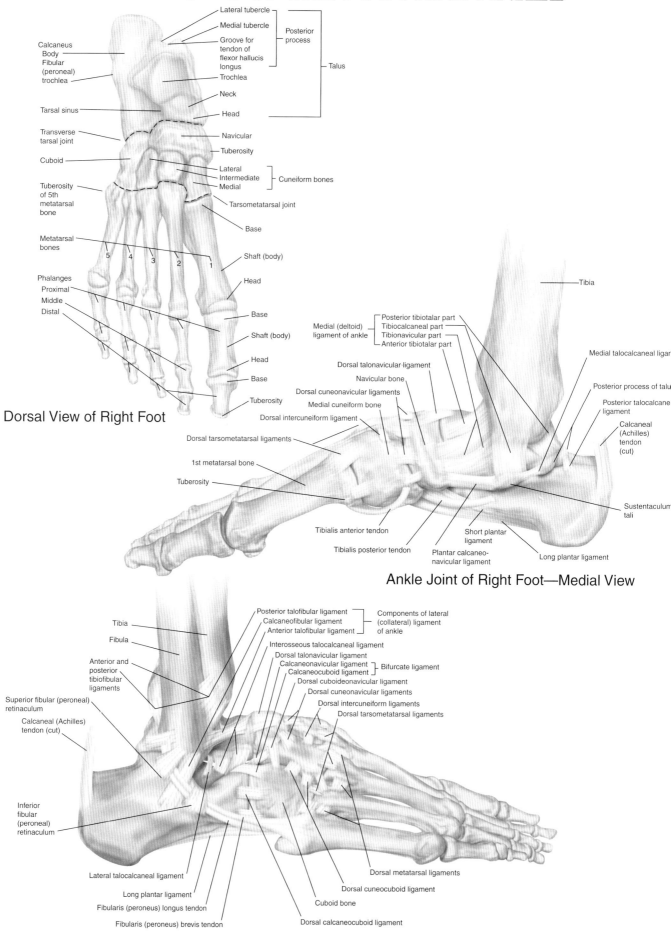

Dorsal View of Right Foot

Labels (Dorsal View):
- Lateral tubercle
- Medial tubercle
- Groove for tendon of flexor hallucis longus
- Posterior process
- Calcaneus
- Body
- Fibular (peroneal) trochlea
- Talus
- Trochlea
- Neck
- Head
- Tarsal sinus
- Transverse tarsal joint
- Navicular
- Tuberosity
- Cuboid
- Lateral
- Intermediate
- Medial
- Cuneiform bones
- Tuberosity of 5th metatarsal bone
- Tarsometatarsal joint
- Base
- Metatarsal bones
- 5 4 3 2 1
- Shaft (body)
- Head
- Phalanges
- Proximal
- Middle
- Distal
- Base
- Shaft (body)
- Head
- Base
- Tuberosity

Ankle Joint of Right Foot—Medial View

Labels (Medial View):
- Tibia
- Medial (deltoid) ligament of ankle
- Posterior tibiotalar part
- Tibiocalcaneal part
- Tibionavicular part
- Anterior tibiotalar part
- Medial talocalcaneal ligament
- Posterior process of talus
- Posterior talocalcaneal ligament
- Calcaneal (Achilles) tendon (cut)
- Dorsal talonavicular ligament
- Navicular bone
- Dorsal cuneonavicular ligaments
- Medial cuneiform bone
- Dorsal intercuneiform ligament
- Dorsal tarsometatarsal ligaments
- 1st metatarsal bone
- Tuberosity
- Tibialis anterior tendon
- Tibialis posterior tendon
- Plantar calcaneo-navicular ligament
- Short plantar ligament
- Long plantar ligament
- Sustentaculum tali

Ankle Joint of Right Foot—Lateral View

Labels (Lateral View):
- Tibia
- Fibula
- Posterior talofibular ligament
- Calcaneofibular ligament
- Anterior talofibular ligament
- Components of lateral (collateral) ligament of ankle
- Anterior and posterior tibiofibular ligaments
- Interosseous talocalcaneal ligament
- Dorsal talonavicular ligament
- Calcaneonavicular ligament
- Calcaneocuboid ligament
- Bifurcate ligament
- Dorsal cuboideonavicular ligament
- Dorsal cuneonavicular ligaments
- Dorsal intercuneiform ligaments
- Dorsal tarsometatarsal ligaments
- Superior fibular (peroneal) retinaculum
- Calcaneal (Achilles) tendon (cut)
- Inferior fibular (peroneal) retinaculum
- Lateral talocalcaneal ligament
- Long plantar ligament
- Fibularis (peroneus) longus tendon
- Fibularis (peroneus) brevis tendon
- Dorsal metatarsal ligaments
- Dorsal cuneocuboid ligament
- Cuboid bone
- Dorsal calcaneocuboid ligament

Bones of the Foot and Ankle

Overview of the Foot and Ankle

The foot differs from the rest of the body in that it is the only site that is confined to a closed and possibly constricting space—the shoe. During standing and gait, the foot provides support, shock absorption, adaptation to uneven surfaces, balance, power, and direction. During more complex motions such as running and jumping, the functions provided by the foot and ankle increase. Therefore, it is not surprising that more than 20% of musculoskeletal problems affect the foot and ankle. Most of these disorders can be treated in the office setting.

The key to the successful diagnosis of foot and ankle pathology is to find the exact location of the problem because most of the problematic structures lie in close proximity to each other, as in the case of the posterior tibial tendon and the posterior tibial nerve. Identifying the precise location of the problem requires an understanding of the anatomy of the foot and ankle. Furthermore, certain systemic illnesses such as diabetes mellitus, peripheral vascular disease, neuropathy, and inflammatory arthritis can affect the foot and therefore should be evaluated in the medical history. A history of bilateral foot pain should prompt a search for a possible systemic or spinal etiology.

Most patients with foot problems report pain. Chronic pain (> 2 weeks' duration) is more common than acute pain. A fracture, sprain, or infection should be suspected if the patient presents with acute pain. Always consider a stress fracture when a patient reports recent onset of pain over the metatarsals, especially in the distal aspects of the second or third metatarsals.

Foot problems can result from overuse, trauma, congenital abnormalities, systemic illness, or ill-fitting shoes. The standard radiographic views of the foot for all these problems are the AP, lateral, and 45° oblique views; these radiographs should always be obtained weight bearing if the patient's condition allows.

Forefoot Problems

Forefoot problems occur nine times more often in women than in men, a fact that is directly attributable to women wearing high-heeled and ill-fitting shoes. Shoe modification (lower heels, wider shoes) is always the first line of treatment. Bunions, hammer toes, claw toes, ingrown toenails, metatarsalgia, and interdigital neuromas account for most instances of forefoot pain. These problems are detailed in later chapters in this section.

Other common problems in the forefoot are hallux rigidus (arthritis of the metatarsophalangeal [MTP] joint of the great toe) and stress fractures. Limited extension (dorsiflexion) of the great toe is consistent with hallux rigidus. Pain and tenderness directly over the second or third metatarsals suggest a stress fracture. Synovitis of the lesser MTP joints is common in patients with hallux valgus (caused by pressure from the great toe against the second MTP joint) and inflammatory disorders. Synovitis of the MTP joint causes pain over the affected joint and is often confused with the pain of an interdigital neuroma (pain in the web space).

Midfoot Problems

Chronic dorsal pain at the midfoot most commonly occurs secondary to degenerative arthritis involving one or more of the midfoot joints. Patients are often able to pinpoint the exact location of the pain. A bony prominence, or osteophyte, referred to as dorsal bossing, can be palpated and corresponds to the underlying arthritic joint. Pain on the plantar aspect of the midfoot, which is unusual, occurs with plantar fasciitis, medial plantar nerve entrapment (jogger's foot), or plantar fibromas.

Hindfoot Problems

Plantar heel pain secondary to plantar fasciitis is the most common problem in the hindfoot. The pain associated with this condition is often severe with the first few steps taken in the morning; patients normally are pain free during rest. Patients have focal tenderness directly over the plantar medial heel (the origin of the plantar fascia); often, on examination, considerable pressure must be applied in this area to duplicate the patient's symptoms. It is very important to differentiate plantar fasciitis from Baxter nerve entrapment or distal tarsal tunnel syndrome, which also cause plantar heel pain, because the treatment modalities are different. Both of these problems present with consistent nerve-related pain, which usually continues in the resting period.

Posterior heel pain may be related to irritation from shoes or associated with a prominent superior process of the calcaneus (Haglund deformity) and/or pathology in the Achilles tendon at its insertion. Often an associated superficial bursitis of the posterior heel is present. When evaluating a patient with posterior heel pain, make sure that the problem is not more proximal within the Achilles tendon; otherwise, a partial or even complete rupture of the tendon might be missed. A palpable bump inside the tendon should alert the physician to the presence of tendinosis or delayed rupture.

A commonly overlooked problem in the hindfoot is posterior tibial tendon dysfunction. This condition is characterized by pain and tenderness posterior and distal to the medial malleolus in the region of the posterior tibial tendon. Progressive dysfunction results in an acquired unilateral flatfoot. In the later stages of the disease, patients usually start to experience more pain on the lateral side of the ankle as the medial-sided pain subsides with further collapse of the arch and impingement of the structures under the fibula and calcaneocuboid joint.

Ankle Problems

More than 25,000 ankle sprains occur each day in the United States. Acute anterolateral ankle pain, swelling, and, frequently, ecchymosis are the hallmarks of this condition.

A history of the ankle "giving way" suggests a diagnosis of ankle instability. Patients with this history often report pain only when the ankle gives way and not at other times. However, patients with chronic ankle pain, which commonly occurs at the anterolateral aspect of the ankle, may have constant low-grade pain. Chronic pain and swelling on the posterolateral aspect of the ankle are consistent with injury to the peroneal tendons. Sural neuritis can result from recurrent ankle inversion injuries caused by traction. An acute osteochondral fracture (osteochondritis dissecans) or occult osteochondral edema with chondral injury of the ankle joint can present with diffuse ankle pain and an intra-articular effusion. Subtalar synovitis or arthritis also can present in a similar fashion.

Arthritis of the ankle is most often secondary to previous trauma. Rheumatoid arthritis can also affect the ankle. Tarsal tunnel syndrome can cause chronic medial ankle pain but almost always is associated with neurologic symptoms and pain that radiates into the plantar aspect of the foot.

Musculoskeletal Conditioning of the Foot and Ankle

A conditioning program consists of three basic phases: strengthening exercises, to improve muscle power; stretching exercises, to improve range of motion; and proprioception, to enhance balance and agility. In addition, the exercise session should begin with an active warm-up, and plyometric exercises can be added for power after basic strength and flexibility have been achieved. Patient handouts are provided here and on the website for the strengthening and stretching exercises. Advanced proprioceptive exercises and plyometric exercises should be done under the supervision of a rehabilitation specialist or other exercise professional.

The goal of a conditioning program is to enable people to live a fit and healthier lifestyle by being more active. A well-structured conditioning program also will prepare the individual for participation in sports and recreational activities. The greater the intensity of the activity in which the individual wishes to engage, the greater the intensity of the conditioning that will be required. If the individual participates in a supervised rehabilitation program that provides instruction in a conditioning routine—instead of using only an exercise handout such as provided here—the focus should be on developing and committing to a home exercise fitness program. A conditioning program for the body as a whole that includes exercises for the shoulder, hip, knee, and spine as well as the foot and ankle is described in Musculoskeletal Conditioning: Helping Patients Prevent Injury and Stay Fit, the in General Orthopaedics section of this publication.

The foot is the first part of the lower kinetic chain to hit the ground during weight-bearing activities and is therefore the first input to the neuromuscular system of the lower kinetic chain. Dynamic joint stability is critical for injury prevention and improved performance during typical daily activities and sports activities. Whether an individual experiences a single-episode lateral ankle sprain or whether chronic ankle instability develops most likely depends on rehabilitation of the individual's proprioception.

Strengthening Exercises

Strengthening exercises for the foot and ankle include calf raises, ankle dorsiflexion/plantar flexion, and ankle inversion/eversion exercises.

Stretching Exercises

Perform stretching to maintain or increase flexibility. Heel cord stretches performed with the knee both straight and bent are good stretching exercises for the gastrocnemius-soleus muscle complex.

Toe Strengthening Exercises

The toe strengthening program can be helpful for patients with the particular conditions listed, including bunions, hammer toes, plantar fasciitis, and toe cramps.

Proprioceptive Exercises

Optimizing the proprioceptive system is important in preventing injuries such as ankle sprains in both athletes and nonathletes. Balance, or postural control, is the result of the integration of visual, vestibular, and proprioceptive afferent inputs. The goal of proprioceptive training is to enhance the activity of the proprioceptors, thereby improving their ability to protect the ligaments of the foot and ankle. Several commercial devices, such as tiltboards and proprioceptive disks, are available for proprioceptive training. Perturbation training is another way to optimize the proprioceptive system, especially in athletes. Perturbation exercises are performed on an unstable surface with perturbing forces applied in all directions. Perturbation training and advanced balance training should be performed under the supervision of a rehabilitation specialist or other exercise professional.

Plyometrics

Explosive power is necessary for a high level of athletic performance. Plyometrics facilitate the development of power. Examples of plyometric exercises are jumping rope and jumping from side to side over a 6-inch–high barrier. More advanced exercises should be performed under the supervision of a rehabilitation specialist or other trained exercise professional.

Home Exercise Program for Foot and Ankle Conditioning

- Performing active warm-up exercises before athletic activities is important for optimal neuromuscular control and for maintaining normal range of motion.
- Before beginning the conditioning program, warm up the muscles of the lower extremities by riding a stationary bicycle or jogging for 10 minutes and performing leg swings as follows: While standing, swing one leg forward/backward 10 times and then side-to-side 10 times. Repeat with the opposite leg. Place one hand against a wall for balance if needed.
- Perform the exercises indefinitely or as directed by your physician. Contact your physician if the exercises cause pain.
- The following exercise program is introductory only, and progression of this program will vary based on your specific injury, symptoms, and baseline level of fitness. For further progression of this routine, your physician may recommend evaluation and treatment by a physical therapist or other exercise professional.

Strengthening and Stretching Exercises for the Foot and Ankle

Exercise	Muscle Group	Number of Repetitions/Sets	Number of Days per Week
Strengthening			
Calf raise	Gastrocnemius-soleus complex	10 repetitions/3 sets	3 to 4
Ankle dorsiflexion/plantar flexion	Anterior tibialis Gastrocnemius-soleus complex	10 repetitions/3 sets	3 to 4
Ankle eversion/inversion	Posterior tibialis Peroneus longus and peroneus brevis	10 repetitions/3 sets	3 to 4
Stretching			
Heel cord stretch	Knee straight: Gastrocnemius Knee bent: Soleus	4 to 5 repetitions/2 to 3 sets	Daily

Toe Strengthening Exercises

Exercise	Condition Recommended For	Repetitions or Duration	Number of Days per Week
Toe squeeze	Hammer toe, toe cramp	10 repetitions	Daily
Big toe pull	Bunion, toe cramp	10 repetitions	Daily
Toe pull	Bunion, hammer toe, toe cramp	10 repetitions	Daily
Golf ball roll	Plantar fasciitis, arch strain, foot cramp	2 minutes	Daily
Marble pickup	Pain in ball of foot, hammer toe, toe cramp	Until all marbles have been picked up	Daily
Towel curl	Hammer toe, toe cramp, pain in ball of foot	15 to 20 repetitions	Daily

Strengthening Exercises

Calf Raise

- Stand with your weight evenly distributed over both feet. Hold on to the back of a chair or the wall for balance.
- Lift one foot so that all your weight is on the other foot.
- Then lift the heel off the floor as high as you can.
- Work up to 3 sets of 10 repetitions.
- Repeat on the other side, switching sides between sets.
- Perform the exercise 3 to 4 days per week.
- If you are unable to perform 10 repetitions on one leg, keep both feet on the ground and lift both heels simultaneously and increase the number of sets before attempting to perform with one leg as described above.

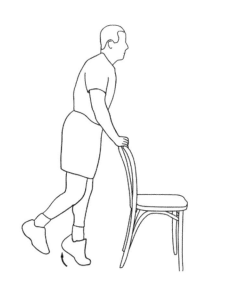

Essentials of Musculoskeletal Care 5   *© 2016 American Academy of Orthopaedic Surgeons*

Ankle Dorsiflexion/Plantar Flexion

- Find a position in which your weight is off your feet, such as lying on a bed or on the floor with your legs straight out in front of you.
- For dorsiflexion, wrap an elastic band or tubing around your foot and anchor the other end to a door or bedpost or have someone hold it. Pull your toes toward you, then return slowly to the starting position. Repeat 10 to 15 times.
- For plantar flexion, wrap an elastic band or tubing around your foot and hold the other end in your hand. Gently point your toes, then return slowly to the starting position. Repeat 10 to 15 times.
- Perform 3 sets of 10 repetitions, 3 to 4 days per week.

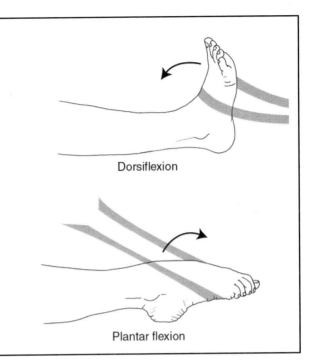

Dorsiflexion

Plantar flexion

Ankle Eversion/Inversion

- Find a position in which your weight is off your feet, such as lying on a bed or on the floor with your legs straight out in front of you.
- For inversion, wrap an elastic band or tube around the inside of your foot and anchor the other end to a door or bedpost or have someone hold it. Pull your foot inward against the resistance, then return slowly to the starting position. Repeat 10 to 15 times.
- For eversion, wrap an elastic band or tube around the outside of your foot and anchor the other end to a door or bedpost or have someone hold it. Pull your foot outward against the resistance, then return slowly to the starting position. Repeat 10 to 15 times.
- Perform 3 sets of 10 repetitions, 3 to 4 days per week.

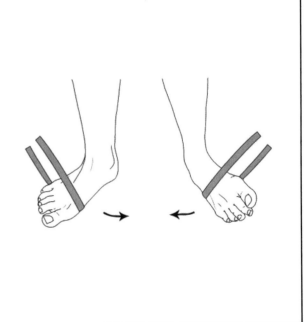

SECTION 7 FOOT AND ANKLE

Stretching Exercise

Heel Cord Stretch

- Stand facing a wall with one foot in front and the toes of both feet pointing forward.

  Stretch with knee straight: Keep your back leg straight and your heel flat on the ground. Move your hips toward the wall until you feel a stretch in the back of the calf of your left leg.

  Stretch with knee bent: Start in the same position, but allow the back knee to bend. Move your hips toward the wall until you feel a stretch in the back of the calf of your left leg.

- Hold the stretch for 30 seconds, then relax for 30 seconds.
- Repeat 4 to 5 times.
- Perform 2 to 3 times per day.

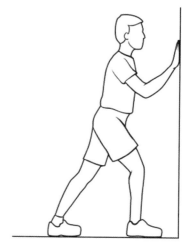

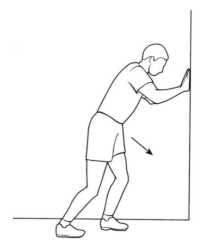

Toe Strengthening Exercises

Toe Squeeze

- Place small sponges or corks between the toes.
- Squeeze and hold for 5 seconds.
- Repeat 10 times.

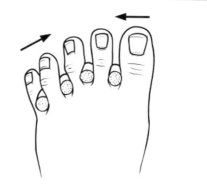

Big Toe Pull

- Place a thick rubber band around both big toes and pull the big toes away from each other and toward the small toes.
- Hold for 5 seconds.
- Repeat 10 times.

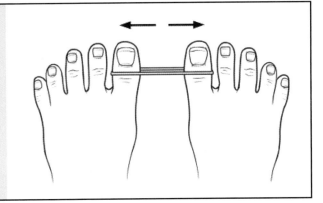

Toe Pull

- Put a thick rubber band around all your toes and spread them.
- Hold this position for 5 seconds.
- Repeat 10 times.

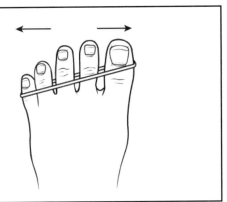

Golf Ball Roll

- Roll a golf ball under the ball of your foot for 2 minutes to massage the bottom of the foot.

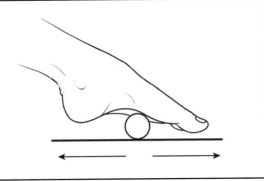

SECTION 7   FOOT AND ANKLE

Marble Pickup

- Place 20 marbles on the floor. Using your toes, pick up one marble at a time and put each in a small bowl.
- Repeat until you have picked up all 20 marbles.

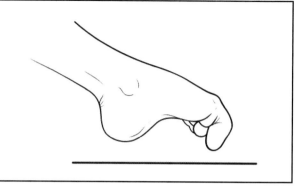

Towel Curl

- Place a small towel on the floor and curl it toward you, using only your toes. You can increase the resistance by putting weight on the end of the towel.
- Relax and repeat 15 to 20 times.

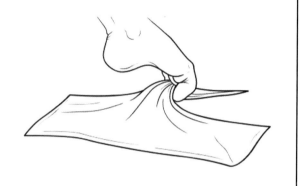

www.aaos.org/essentials5/footandankle

Physical Examination of the Foot and Ankle

Inspection/Palpation

No matter which part of the foot or ankle you are examining, the maximum point of tenderness is the most valuable finding. You can ask the patient to point to this spot using one finger, or the spot can be localized during the physical examination.

Anterior View, Standing

Observe the anterior aspect of both feet. Inspect the foot and ankle from the front. Observe the alignment of the great and lesser toes, the position of the foot in relation to the limb, and the medial curvature of the forefoot (metatarsus adductus). Any noticeable swelling should be identified, as well. The anterior tibial tendon should be identified as an indentation, especially at its attachment to the medial cuneiform. Failure to identify the tendon should alert you to possible anterior tibial tendon rupture. Forefoot abduction can be observed in Lisfranc injuries and midfoot arthritis.

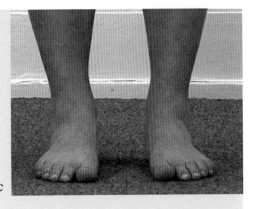

Medial View

Observe the medial aspect of both feet. Inspect for a high arch (cavus foot), flatfoot posture (pes planus), or undue prominence of the medial midfoot (accessory navicular). The arches of both feet should be symmetric.

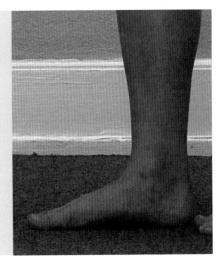

Lateral View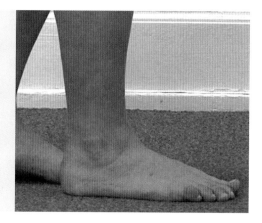

Observe the lateral aspect of both feet. Inspect for callosities, ankle swelling, or prominence of the posterior calcaneus.

Posterior View

Observe the posterior aspect of both feet. Assess heel alignment. Normal alignment is neutral or slight valgus (turned-out heel), with no more than one or two lateral toes visible from behind. A patient with an acquired flatfoot from posterior tibial tendon dysfunction will have increased valgus of the calcaneus and more than two visible toes ("too many toes" sign). A varus calcaneus (turned-in heel) occurs with a cavus foot.

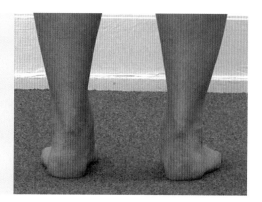

Standing on Toes

With the patient standing on the toes, look to see that the heels move into a normal varus (inward) position. A patient with an acquired flatfoot secondary to posterior tibial tendon dysfunction will not be able to rise up on the toes of the affected foot, and the heel will not be able to turn to neutral and remain in valgus.

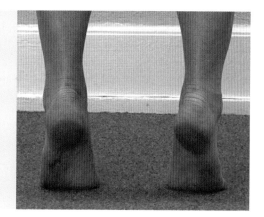

Gait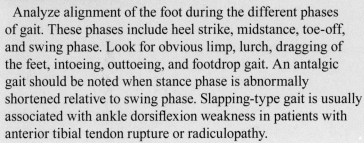

Gait is best observed with the patient barefoot. Have the patient walk across the room as you observe from the side. Look for deviations from normal while the patient walks. Normal gait demonstrates equal stride length, foot position, and weight distribution. At heel strike, the heel everts and the ankle plantar flexes. The weight transfers along the lateral side of the foot. Pronation occurs in the foot with dorsiflexion of the ankle and internal rotation at the leg, knee, and hip. As the body and leg move forward, supination begins with plantar flexion of the ankle.

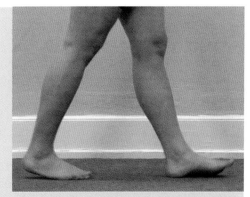

Analyze alignment of the foot during the different phases of gait. These phases include heel strike, midstance, toe-off, and swing phase. Look for obvious limp, lurch, dragging of the feet, intoeing, outtoeing, and footdrop gait. An antalgic gait should be noted when stance phase is abnormally shortened relative to swing phase. Slapping-type gait is usually associated with ankle dorsiflexion weakness in patients with anterior tibial tendon rupture or radiculopathy.

Angle of Gait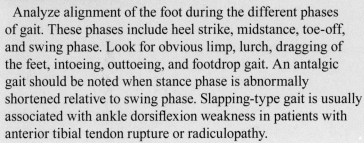

Assess the angle of gait, which is the angle of the foot in relation to the axis of the limb when the patient is walking, to identify problems of intoeing and outtoeing. When walking, the foot is normally positioned in 0° to 20° of external rotation. Because tibial torsion is typically asymmetric, one foot is normally positioned in more external rotation.

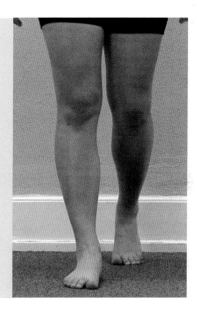

SECTION 7   FOOTANDANKLE

Anterior View, Supine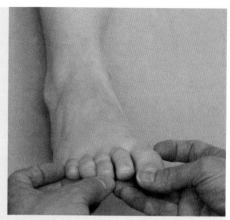

With the patient supine, inspect the top of the foot for a bunion and associated hallux valgus at the great toe metatarsophalangeal joint or a bunionette at the fifth metatarsophalangeal joint. Inspect the lesser toes for abnormalities in alignment such as hammer toe, mallet toe, or claw toe. Claw toe, in which the metatarsophalangeal joint is extended and the proximal interphalangeal and distal interphalangeal joints are flexed, commonly occurs in patients with diabetes mellitus, rheumatoid arthritis, Charcot-Marie-Tooth disease, or cavus foot deformities. Multiple toes tend to be involved, and often a hard callus (corn) is apparent over the proximal interphalangeal joint. A corn or callus develops where a deformity rubs against a shoe. Inspect the toenails for poor techniques in trimming and signs of infection from an ingrown toenail.

Spread Toes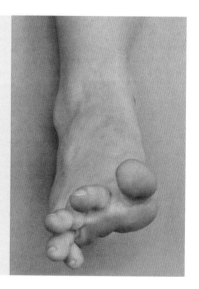

Ask the patient to spread or fan the toes as widely as possible. Look for soft corns or ulcerations between the toes. Inability to actively spread the toes can indicate loss of intrinsic muscle function. Beware of any suspicious lesions, because melanoma does occur in the foot.

Plantar Surface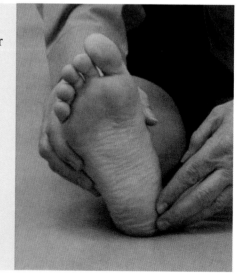

With the patient supine, inspect the bottom of the foot for plantar warts, which usually do not occur beneath the metatarsal head; a plantar callus, which occurs beneath the metatarsal head; prominence of the metatarsal heads; ulceration (especially in diabetic feet); or a thin fat pad.

Medial Malleolus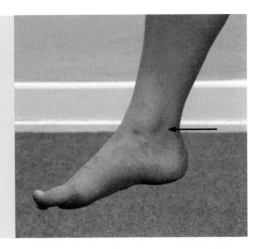

Palpate the area posterior and inferior to the medial malleolus in the region of the tibial nerve. In patients with tarsal tunnel syndrome, percussion over the nerve should reproduce symptoms, often described as "shooting" pains (paresthesias) in the heel and plantar aspect of the foot. Patients with posterior tibial tendon dysfunction will have swelling and tenderness along the course of the tendon in this region.

Posterior Heel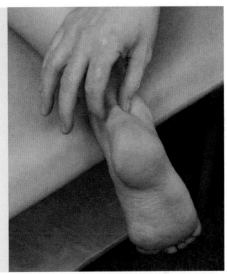

Palpate both sides of the Achilles tendon insertion to identify swelling or tenderness, which are signs of retrocalcaneal bursitis, a condition that is often associated with a prominence of the posterior superior calcaneus (pump bump, or Haglund deformity). Swelling and tenderness of the Achilles tendon at its insertion is associated with tendinitis or calcific tendinosis.

Peroneal Tendons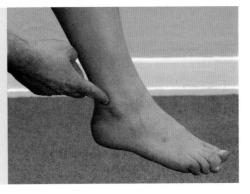

Palpate behind and below the fibular malleolus for tenderness or swelling associated with peroneal tenosynovitis or for subluxation of the tendons during active eversion, dorsiflexion, and plantar flexion of the ankle. Sural neuritis can be identified with a positive Tinel sign (pain on tapping the nerve trace).

Anterior Ankle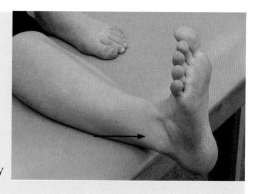

Palpate over the anterior talofibular ligament and then the calcaneofibular ligament for tenderness associated with a sprain, often the result of an acute inversion injury. In patients with chronic ankle pain, palpate at the anterolateral corner of the ankle joint (soft junction of the tibia, fibula, and talus) for synovitis. Take care to differentiate pain in the anterolateral corner of the ankle from pain in the sinus tarsi, which is more distal and anterior and may indicate inflammation or pathology of the subtalar joint.

Plantar Fascia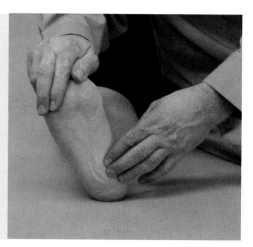

Palpate the plantar fascia for tenderness or swelling or nodules from the heel to the ball of the foot. With proximal plantar fasciitis, tenderness is noted with considerable pressure over the medial proximal aspect of the plantar fascia at its origin from the calcaneus. If the patient's point of tenderness is 1 cm to ½ inch distal and proximal to this point, you should suspect Baxter nerve entrapment. Rupture of the plantar fascia is associated with tenderness and swelling in the middle third of the plantar fascia. Plantar fibromatosis causes swelling and thickening of the plantar fascia, typically beginning in the middle portion.

Sesamoid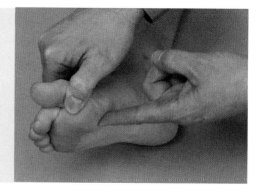

Palpate the area beneath the first metatarsal head for tenderness. If the sesamoids are the source of the pain, the tender spot will move as the toe is flexed and extended. The medial sesamoid is more commonly injured or inflamed than is the lateral sesamoid.

Metatarsophalangeal Joint

Palpate the top of the foot for tenderness and swelling of the metatarsophalangeal joints, which can be present with rheumatoid arthritis, idiopathic synovitis, Freiberg infraction, or metatarsalgia. With hallux rigidus, dorsal osteophytes are present at the great toe metatarsophalangeal joint.

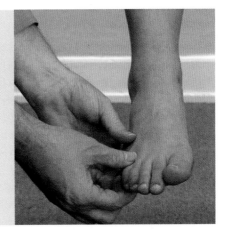

Range of Motion

Patients with hyperelasticity always show more range of motion compared with patients who have a standard level of flexibility. This should not be assessed as hypermobility or instability, and the patient should be tested for hyperelasticity prior to range of motion examination of the foot and ankle.

Ankle Motion: Zero Starting Position

To evaluate ankle motion, a goniometer is needed. With the patient supine, the patient's foot should be perpendicular to the tibia (zero starting position). Ankle dorsiflexion is movement of the foot toward the anterior surface of the tibia, and ankle plantar flexion is movement of the foot in the opposite direction. Passive and functional ankle motion typically is greater than active motion. Normal active ankle dorsiflexion is 10° to 20°, and normal plantar flexion is 35° to 50°.

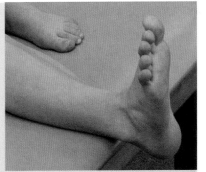

As the foot moves from dorsiflexion to plantar flexion, much of the motion occurs at the ankle joint, but other joints in the foot also contribute to this movement. Distinguishing the dorsiflexion/plantar flexion motion that occurs at the ankle joint from that at other joints is difficult; fortunately, it is not critical. From a functional standpoint, the total arc of motion is more important. Therefore, it is understood that clinical measurements of ankle motion also record motion of other joints of the foot. Align the goniometer with the axis of the leg and the lateral side of the plantar surface of the foot. To relax the gastrocnemius, measure ankle motion with the knee flexed approximately 90°. To assess heel cord tightness, measure ankle dorsiflexion with the knee fully extended.

SECTION 7   FOOTANDANKLE

Inversion and Eversion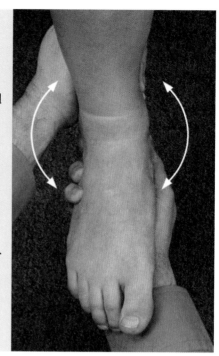

Inversion (turning the heel inward) and eversion (turning the heel outward) primarily reflect motion at the subtalar (talocalcaneal) joint. Precise measurements are difficult with standard techniques; therefore, in the clinical setting, these motions usually are estimated visually. With the patient seated, place the patient's ankle in 0° of plantar-/dorsiflexion. This position limits lateral motion at the ankle joint, and therefore provides better assessment of talocalcaneal mobility.

Use one hand to grasp the distal leg around the malleoli, and place your other hand under the heel to maintain the neutral ankle position, passively, manually turning the heel inward and outward several times. Restricted motion may be seen in patients following an acute ankle sprain and with subtalar arthritis, end-stage posterior tibial tendon dysfunction, or tarsal coalition (bony connection between talus and calcaneus).

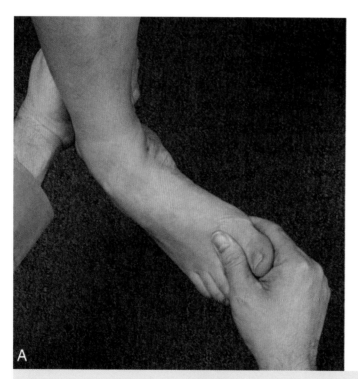

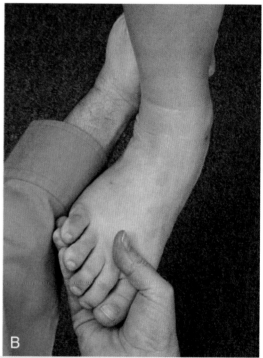

Supination and Pronation

Supination and pronation refer to rotation of the foot about an anterior/posterior axis. Supination (**A**) includes inversion of the heel, as well as adduction and plantar flexion of the midfoot. Pronation (**B**) is the opposite motion and includes eversion of the heel and abduction and dorsiflexion of the midfoot. Manually supinate and pronate the foot. Supination and pronation of the foot are difficult to quantify. Compare motion of the affected foot with that on the unaffected side for the most useful information.

Great Toe: Zero Starting Position

To evaluate the motion of the great toe, the patient is seated or supine, with the toe in the zero starting position. This position aligns the great toe with the plantar surface of the foot. Motion at the metatarsophalangeal and interphalangeal joints occurs in the dorsiflexion/plantar flexion plane. Dorsiflexion (extension) is the primary motion of the metatarsophalangeal joint, but this range of motion is virtually nonexistent at the interphalangeal joint.

Reduced motion at the first metatarsophalangeal joint can indicate hallux rigidus or gout. Pain with plantar flexion of the great toe is usually the first sign of hallux rigidus.

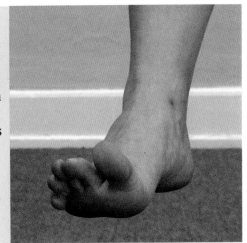

Muscle Testing

Posterior Tibialis

To test the strength of the posterior tibialis muscle or integrity of the posterior tibial tendon, stabilize the lateral aspect of the leg with the foot in plantar flexion so as to eliminate activity of the tibialis anterior. Use your other hand on the medial aspect of the distal first metatarsal to resist the patient's attempt to invert the foot. Weakness indicates injury or dysfunction of the posterior tibialis or a lesion involving the posterior tibial nerve or L5 nerve root.

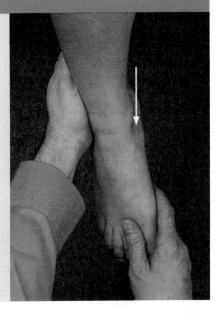

Essentials of Musculoskeletal Care 5

Anterior Tibialis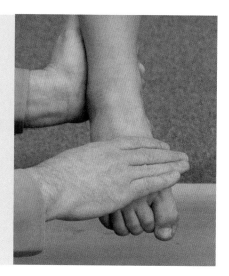

To test the strength of the anterior tibialis muscle, grasp the posterolateral aspect of the leg with one hand and apply resistance to the dorsal medial aspect of the foot. Ask the patient to flex the toes (to eliminate activity of the toe extensors) and then invert and dorsiflex the foot against your resistance. Weakness indicates a lesion involving the L4 nerve root or deep peroneal nerve.

Peroneus Longus and Brevis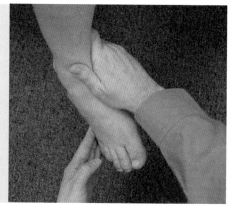

To test the strength of the peroneus longus and brevis muscles, grasp the anteromedial aspect of the leg with one hand and apply resistance to the lateral aspect of the fifth metatarsal. Position the foot in plantar flexion (to eliminate activity of the lateral toe extensors). Resist the patient's attempt to evert the foot. The peroneus longus function can be separated from that of the brevis by plantar flexing the first ray while attempting to evert the foot. Weakness indicates injury or dysfunction of the peroneal tendons or a lesion involving the superficial peroneal nerve.

Extensor Hallucis Longus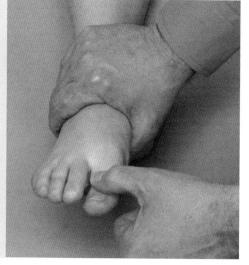

Test the strength of the extensor hallucis longus muscle by grasping the dorsal and plantar aspect of the midfoot medially with one hand and applying resistance to the dorsal aspect of the great toe. Maintain the ankle in a neutral position and have the patient extend the great toe against resistance. Weakness indicates deep peroneal nerve dysfunction, with weakness of the extensor hallucis longus muscle. Note that the extensor hallucis longus is the easiest and most specific muscle to assess for L5 nerve root dysfunction.

Flexor Hallucis Longus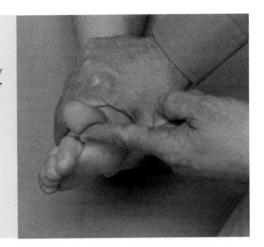

Test the strength of the flexor hallucis longus muscle by grasping the dorsal and plantar aspect of the midfoot medially with one hand and applying resistance to the plantar aspect of the great toe. Maintain the ankle in a neutral position and ask the patient to flex the great toe against resistance. Weakness indicates tibial nerve dysfunction. The flexor hallucis is the easiest and most specific muscle to assess for S1 nerve root dysfunction.

Special Tests

Anterior Drawer Test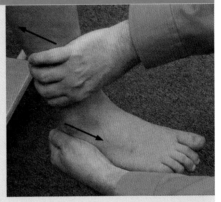

The anterior drawer test assesses the stability of the anterior talofibular ligament. With the patient seated and the knee flexed approximately 90°, place the ankle in approximately 20° of plantar flexion. Stabilize or provide a slight posterior force to the anterior aspect of the distal tibia with one hand, cup the palm of the other hand around the posterior aspect of the calcaneus, and attempt to bring the calcaneus and talus forward on the tibia. Normally, you should be able to translate the foot slightly forward on the ankle before reaching a relatively firm end point provided by the anterior talofibular ligament. Absence of this firm end point with asymmetric or excessive motion indicates moderate to severe injury to the anterior talofibular ligament and/or chronic ankle laxity. When performing this test, always compare the affected ankle with the opposite (normal) side. If this test elicits pain, the results may be unreliable due to an inability of the patient to relax the muscles that provide dynamic support to the ankle. If the test is inconclusive, patients can be tested under mini C-arm fluoroscopy, and comparative views can be obtained.

Varus Stress Test

With the tibia stabilized and the ankle in neutral, grasp the calcaneus and invert the hindfoot. Excessive or asymmetric motion will occur with chronic laxity of the calcaneofibular ligament. When performing this test, always compare the affected ankle with the opposite (normal) side. If the patient has pain during this test, the results may be unreliable.

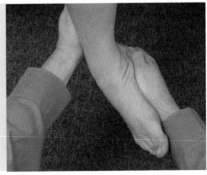

SECTION 7　FOOTANDANKLE

SECTION 7 FOOTANDANKLE

Metatarsophalangeal Joint Instability

With the patient sitting, stabilize the foot from the distal metatarsal shaft. Then grasp the proximal phalanx of each toe and move the joint in a dorsal (up) direction (also called the anterior drawer or the shock test). This is an apprehension test; in a patient with active synovitis, this test can be quite painful. Instability is often present after chronic synovitis or a long-standing claw toe deformity. The second toe is most often affected.

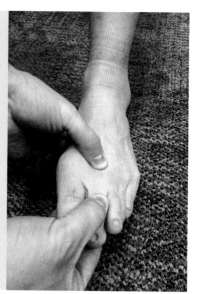

Interdigital (Morton) Neuroma Test

To evaluate the patient for interdigital neuroma, apply upward pressure between adjacent metatarsal heads and then compress the metatarsals from side to side with the free hand. The upward pressure places the neuroma between the metatarsal heads, allowing it to be compressed during side-to-side compression. Interdigital neuromas are most commonly located between the third and fourth metatarsal heads, occasionally between the second and third metatarsal heads, and rarely between the other metatarsal heads. Sometimes you will hear or, more likely, feel a click (Mulder sign) at the painful site, which is usually diagnostic.

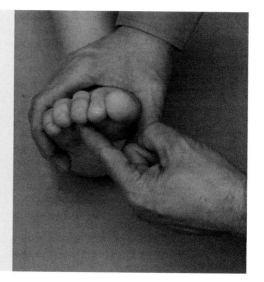

Kleiger Test (External Rotation Test)

With the patient seated and the knee flexed approximately 90° and the ankle relaxed, use one hand to grasp and stabilize the leg from behind, making sure not to compress the fibula and tibia together. Use your other hand to fully dorsiflex the ankle and then externally rotate the foot. If this causes pain, determine the specific location of the pain. Pain over the location of the anterior inferior tibiofibular ligament is indicative of a syndesmosis sprain. Depending on the severity, the interosseous membrane may be involved, and pain can be radiated further up between the distal fibula and tibia. This test is also sensitive for fractures of the fibula.

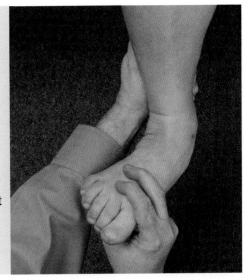

Distal Tibia and Fibular Squeeze Test

With the patient supine, squeeze the mid diaphyseal portion of the tibia and fibula together. Resulting pain is indicative of distal syndesmosis injury.

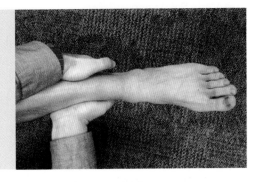

Thompson Test

With the patient prone and relaxed, use your fingers and thumb to squeeze the medial and lateral aspect of the mid calf together. If the foot does not plantar flex, the test is positive for an Achilles tendon rupture.

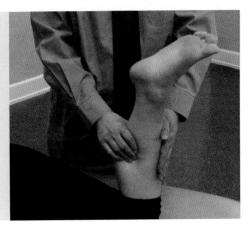

Essentials of Musculoskeletal Care 5

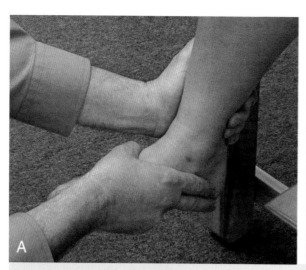
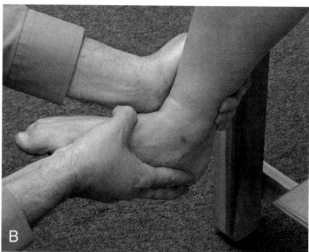

Eversion Stress Test

The eversion stress test evaluates the integrity of the deltoid ligament. With the patient seated and the knee flexed approximately 90°, place the ankle in neutral. Use one hand to stabilize the lateral aspect of the leg just above the lateral malleolus (**A**). Place your other hand somewhat inferomedial on the calcaneus and evert the hindfoot. Pain over the deltoid ligament and increased eversion as compared to the uninvolved side indicates possible injury to the mid portion of the deltoid or a possible avulsion fracture of the medial malleolus. This test should be repeated while holding the ankle in full dorsiflexion (**B**) to evaluate the posterior aspect of the deltoid and then repeated again in plantar flexion to evaluate the anterior aspect of the deltoid ligament. When performing this test, always compare the affected ankle with the opposite side.

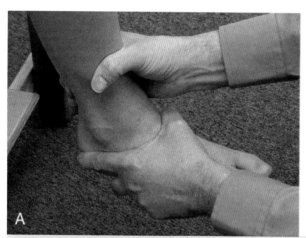
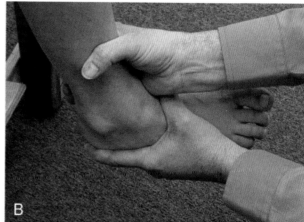

Inversion Stress Test

The inversion stress test evaluates laxity of the calcaneofibular ligament. With the patient seated and the knee flexed approximately 90°, use one hand to stabilize the medial aspect of the leg just above the medial malleolus. Place your other hand somewhat inferolateral on the calcaneus (**A**) and invert the hindfoot (**B**). An end point should normally be appreciated upon reaching full inversion, and absence of one indicates moderate to severe injury to the calcaneofibular ligament. Excessive or asymmetric motion will occur with chronic laxity of the calcaneofibular ligament. When performing this test, always compare the affected ankle with the opposite side. If the patient has pain during this test, the results may be unreliable.

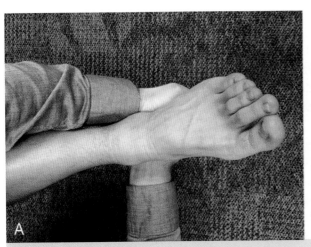
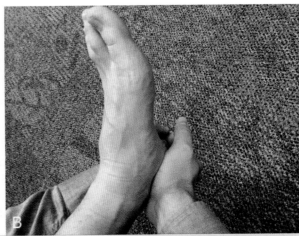

Calcaneal Squeeze Test

With the patient supine, squeeze the calcaneus from both sides using two hands. Pain associated with this maneuver is usually indicative of a calcaneal stress fracture.

Sensitivity Test 📷

To evaluate the sensitivity in the foot, use a 5.07-mm monofilament (equivalent to 0.10-g force) to identify lack of protective sensation in a patient with diabetes mellitus or other diseases associated with a peripheral neuropathy.

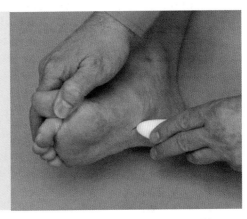

Achilles Tendon Tear

Synonyms

Achilles tendon rupture
Heel cord rupture

Definition

Disruption of the Achilles tendon (heel cord) usually occurs 5 to 7 cm proximal to the insertion of the tendon on the calcaneus. This condition commonly affects middle-aged men who play quick, stop-and-go sports such as tennis and basketball, as well as so-called weekend warriors. Partial tears of the tendon can also occur at the calcaneal insertion or the midsubstance.

Clinical Symptoms

The sudden, severe calf pain typically is described as a "gunshot wound" or as a "direct hit from a racquet." Partial tears can be described as strains or a "calf pull." The severe, acute pain can resolve quickly, and the injury may be misdiagnosed as an ankle sprain. When the rupture is missed, substantial weakness develops, impairing ambulation.

Tests

Physical Examination

Swelling in the lower calf is common. The patient often has difficulty bearing weight and often has a palpable defect in the tendon. With the patient lying prone and the foot hanging off the edge of the table, the foot with a ruptured Achilles tendon will rest at a 90° angle to the tibia, whereas a foot with an intact Achilles tendon will rest in slight plantar flexion because of the resting tension in the tendon. Perform the Thompson test by placing the patient prone with the knee and ankle at 90°. The test also can be done with the patient kneeling on a chair. Squeezing the calf normally results in passive plantar flexion of the ankle; a positive test result is the absence of plantar flexion. The Thompson test is most reliable within 48 hours of the rupture. Inability to plantarflex with the toes in extension also indicates tendon rupture.

Diagnostic Tests

None usually are needed.

Differential Diagnosis

- Achilles tendinitis or tendinosis (thick, tender Achilles tendon or crepitus may be noted on palpation)
- Deep vein thrombosis (no history of injury, negative Thompson test)
- Medial gastrocnemius tear (pain on palpation over the medial head of the gastrocnemius-soleus complex)

- Plantaris rupture (pain but little loss of function)
- Stress fracture of the tibia (constant pain over a localized area of the tibia)

Adverse Outcomes of the Disease

Weakness during the stance phase of gait and decreased athletic function are possible. Patients note that when they are walking, they feel as if they are on soft sand.

Treatment

Nonsurgical treatment consists of a program of gradual casting or bracing in plantar flexion with subsequent casting in a lesser degree of plantar flexion until the foot reaches a neutral position. Surgical repair typically requires a brief period of immobilization as well to allow the wound to heal. The surgeon may elect to use a tapered heel lift for several weeks following the immobilization. Rehabilitation may be necessary if full range of motion and balance are not attained by 6 months after surgery, but by this time almost all patients attain full range of motion, especially dorsiflexion. The decision whether to treat the patient surgically or nonsurgically is based on the degree of tendon retraction as well as the patient's activity level, age, medical condition, and surgical risk. A recently published study indicated no differences between surgical and nonsurgical treatment. When either treatment is delayed beyond a few days, Achilles tendon rupture becomes substantially more complicated to treat because retraction of the proximal muscle widens the gap. Whatever treatment modality is selected, a progressive strength and conditioning program is recommended during the rehabilitation phase, followed by a gradual return to sports.

Rehabilitation Prescription

An Achilles tendon rupture can be very painful and debilitating. The type of rehabilitation depends on the extent of the tendon tear. For both severe and minor tears, pain-free immobilization and rest, ice, compression, and elevation (RICE) are indicated for the first 5 or 6 days postinjury. Use of crutches is also helpful to prevent further injury. The home exercise program for minor tears can be started on day 7. Minor tears usually do well with gentle active mobilization. Stretching can be initiated on day 14. The stretch should be pain free. If the patient has difficulty achieving pain-free ankle range of motion, formal rehabilitation may be ordered. This evaluation should include assessment of the mobility of the tendon, the ankle, and the subtalar and midtarsal joints. The therapist should be careful to respect the stage of soft-tissue healing. Early management of swelling and gentle strengthening of the entire lower kinetic chain can facilitate early pain control. Progression of weight-bearing status should be directed by the physician and based on interval healing of the tendon.

Adverse Outcomes of Treatment

Surgical risks include infection and wound problems such as delayed healing. A second rupture can occur with either type of treatment but is more common after nonsurgical treatment.

Referral Decisions/Red Flags

A history of a sudden pop with pain and swelling in the calf indicates probable rupture of the Achilles tendon and the need for further evaluation within 24 hours.

Home Exercise Program for Minor Achilles Tendon Tear

- Begin gentle ankle range of motion on day 7 after the injury.
- Add the towel stretch, heel cord stretch, and calf raise on day 14 after the injury. Before stretching, warm up the tissues by applying moist heat or riding a stationary bicycle for 10 minutes.
- To prevent inflammation, apply a bag of crushed ice or frozen peas to the heel for 20 minutes after exercising.
- You should not experience pain with the exercises. If you are unable to perform the exercises because of pain or stiffness, or if your symptoms do not improve in 3 to 4 weeks, call your doctor.
- The following exercise program is introductory only, and progression of this program will vary based on your specific injury, symptoms, and baseline level of fitness. For further progression of this routine, your physician may recommend evaluation and treatment by a physical therapist or other exercise professional.

Home Exercises for Minor Achilles Tendon Tear

Exercise	Muscle Group	Number of Repetitions/Sets	Number of Days per Week	Number of Weeks
Ankle range of motion	Dorsiflexors Plantar flexors Invertors Evertors	2 sets	Daily	2 to 3
Towel stretch	Gastrocnemius-soleus complex	4 repetitions/2 to 3 sets	6 to 7	3 to 4
Heel cord stretch	Gastrocnemius-soleus complex	4 repetitions/2 to 3 sets	6 to 7	3 to 4
Calf raise	Gastrocnemius-soleus complex	10 repetitions/2 to 3 sets	Daily	3 to 4

Ankle Range of Motion

- Sit on a chair or the edge of a bed so your feet do not touch the floor.
- Leading with the big toe, write each letter of the alphabet in the air. Keep your knee flexed.
- Perform 2 sets per day, for 2 to 3 weeks.

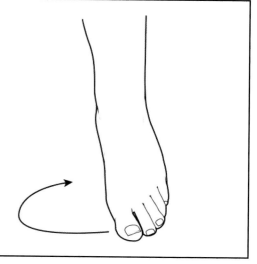

Towel Stretch

- Sit on the floor with the affected leg straight.
- Loop a towel around the ball of your foot.
- Grasp the ends of the towel and pull toward you, keeping the knee straight.
- Hold this stretch for 30 seconds and then relax for 30 seconds. Repeat 4 times.
- Perform this exercise 2 to 3 times per day, 6 to 7 days per week, for 3 to 4 weeks.

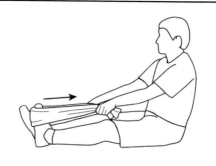

Heel Cord Stretch

- Stand facing a wall with the knee of the unaffected limb bent for support, the affected limb straight, and the toes pointed in slightly.
- Keeping the heels of both feet flat on the floor, lower your hips toward the wall.
- Hold this stretch for 30 seconds and then relax for 30 seconds. Repeat 4 times.
- Perform this exercise 2 to 3 times per day, 6 to 7 days per week, for 3 to 4 weeks.

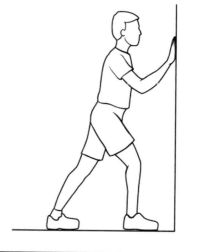

Calf Raise

- Stand on a flat surface with your weight evenly distributed over both feet.
- Hold on to the back of a chair or place your hands against a wall for balance.
- Raise the heel off the floor as high as you can, using your body weight as resistance. Repeat 10 times.
- Perform 2 to 3 sets per day for 3 to 4 weeks.
- If you are unable to perform 10 repetitions on one leg without pain, keep both feet on the ground and increase the number of sets before attempting to perform with one leg as described above.

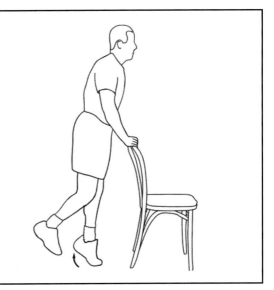

SECTION 7 **FOOT AND ANKLE**

Ankle Sprain

Synonyms

Inversion injury
Lateral collateral ligament tear of the ankle

Definition

More than 25,000 ankle sprains occur every day in the United States. Ankle sprains are not always simple injuries. Residual symptoms occur in up to 40% of patients. The lateral ligaments (anterior talofibular and calcaneofibular) are the only structures injured in most ankle sprains, but other ligament tears can occur with an inversion injury (**Figure 1**). Additional injury to the anterior tibiofibular syndesmosis, the thick ligaments connecting the distal tibia and fibula, also can occur. This combined injury, referred to as a "high" ankle sprain, increases recovery time. Injury to the subtalar joint is commonly associated with a severe ankle sprain. The most common injury to the subtalar joint after an inversion injury is a tear of one of the interosseous ligaments. Associated injuries to the medial deltoid ligament also occur but are less common.

Clinical Symptoms

Pain over the injured ligaments, swelling, and loss of function are common. A severe sprain is more common in patients who report feeling a pop, followed by immediate swelling and the inability to walk. Determine whether the patient has a history of ankle sprains and giving way to identify whether an acute injury is superimposed on chronic ankle instability.

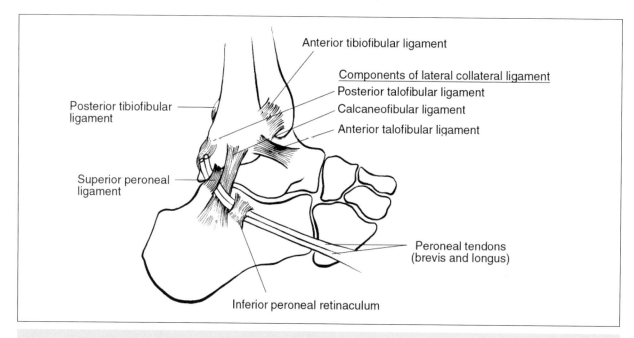

Figure 1 Illustration of ligaments of the ankle.

Tests

Physical Examination

Examination often reveals ecchymosis and swelling around the entire ankle joint, not just the lateral side. Tenderness on palpation over the anterior talofibular and calcaneofibular ligaments can help identify which ligaments are injured. Palpate the lateral and medial malleoli and the base of the fifth metatarsal; crepitus or tenderness suggests a fracture. Injury to the tibiofibular syndesmosis is suggested by two tests: the squeeze test (**Figure 2**) and the external rotation test. The squeeze test is performed by compressing the tibia and fibula at the mid calf. The external rotation test is performed by placing the ankle in dorsiflexion and then externally rotating the foot. A positive result is the presence of pain over the distal tibiofibular syndesmosis. After an injury to the subtalar joint, tenderness over the sinus tarsi is present; ecchymosis also may be observed on the medial aspect of the heel.

Diagnostic Tests

When tenderness is present over the distal fibula, ankle joint, tibiofibular syndesmosis, or other bony structure, radiographs of the ankle and/or foot are needed to rule out a fracture or syndesmosis disruption. Radiographs also are indicated when the patient has marked swelling and cannot bear weight on the affected extremity. The Ottawa ankle rules provide a guideline on when to obtain radiographs of the ankle.

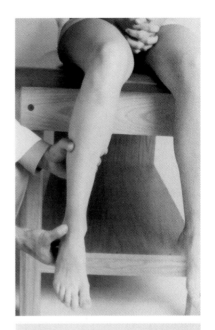

Figure 2 Clinical photograph shows the squeeze test for injury to the tibiofibular syndesmosis. Pain over the distal tibiofibular syndesmosis when the examiner squeezes the tibia and fibula at the mid calf is a positive result.

Differential Diagnosis

- Fracture of the calcaneus, talus, lateral malleolus, or base of the fifth metatarsal (focal tenderness over the fractured anatomic structure, evident on radiographs)
- Fracture of the lateral process of the talus (also known as the snowboarder fracture) (focal tenderness, swelling below the fibula)
- Fracture of the proximal fibula (Maisonneuve fracture associated with tear of deltoid and disruption of syndesmotic ligament) (focal tenderness, crepitus over the proximal fibula)
- Osteochondral fracture of the talar dome (evident on ankle radiographs, bone scan, or MRI)
- Peroneal tendon tear or subluxation (retrofibular tenderness and swelling)
- Sural neuritis or damage (neuroma) (positive Tinel sign along the nerve in the posterior subfibular margin, shooting pain and sensation loss in the sural distribution)

Adverse Outcomes of the Disease

An untreated severe sprain can result in chronic pain, instability, and the possibility of ankle arthritis. Chronic pain can result from subtalar stiffness. Chronic instability is most common after incomplete rehabilitation.

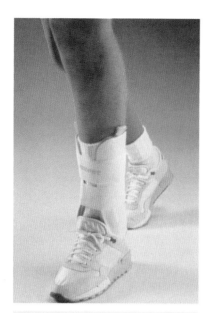

Figure 3 Photograph of an air stirrup–type ankle brace.

Treatment

The goal of treatment is to prevent chronic pain and instability. A three-phase treatment program is recommended.

Phase 1 consists of NSAIDs, rest, ice, compression, and elevation (RICE). The use of a functional ankle brace or air stirrup is indicated for protection and to promote soft-tissue healing (**Figure 3**). Encourage weight bearing as tolerated, with crutch use as needed. For severe sprains or sprains in children, the use of a cast or cast boot for 2 to 3 weeks may facilitate walking and healing.

Phase 2 begins when the patient can bear weight without increased pain or swelling, usually 2 to 4 weeks after the injury. Continue use of the air stirrup or functional ankle brace. Begin exercises to increase peroneal and dorsiflexor strength; also, the Achilles tendon should be stretched. Continue this phase until the patient has full range of motion and 80% of normal ankle strength. Plantar flexion exercises are not included in the exercise program because they place the ankle in a position of minimal stability.

Phase 3 usually begins 4 to 6 weeks after injury. This phase of functional conditioning includes proprioception, agility, and endurance training. Exercises that are helpful for proprioception include standing on the sprained ankle with the opposite foot elevated and the eyes closed. Balance boards are very useful during this phase of treatment. Running in progressively smaller figures-of-8 is excellent for agility and peroneal strength. During this time, the patient should be weaned from the air stirrup or functional ankle brace.

This three-phase treatment program may take only 2 weeks to complete for minor sprains, or up to 6 to 8 weeks for severe injuries. For athletes with moderate to severe sprains who are returning to sports, the use of a functional ankle brace or air stirrup, or taping on a long-term basis, will help prevent recurrent injury. The use of a brace is particularly indicated for athletes in sports associated with a high risk for ankle sprains such as basketball, volleyball, and soccer. Long-term exercises should include peroneal strengthening in both dorsiflexion and plantar flexion, as well as continued Achilles tendon stretching.

Rehabilitation Prescription

The most important part of early rehabilitation is to control the inflammation with RICE for the first 5 or 6 days postinjury. Use of crutches during this same period can be helpful to control further damage to the healing ligament. Early mobilization of the ankle can begin as part of a home program of active pain-free exercises beginning on day 7. If the patient continues to have pain and limited mobility of the ankle after 2 to 3 weeks on a home exercise program, formal rehabilitation may be ordered. This evaluation by the rehabilitation specialist should include assessment of the mobility of the ankle and subtalar joints. Strengthening exercises combined with balance training can be initiated at the discretion of the rehabilitation specialist.

Adverse Outcomes of Treatment

In 2015, the FDA strengthened its warning linking NSAIDs with the risk of heart attack or stroke, even in the first weeks of use of an NSAID. Casting and ankle immobilization for more than 3 weeks may cause stiffness and a slower return to normal activity. Incomplete rehabilitation is the most common cause of chronic instability after an ankle sprain. Subtalar stiffness can result in persistent anterolateral pain.

Referral Decisions/Red Flags

Fractures of the foot and ankle, tears or subluxation of the peroneal tendons, nerve injury, a history of repeated giving way (chronic instability), and failure to improve in 6 weeks with appropriate treatment all indicate serious injury and the need for further evaluation.

SECTION 7 FOOT AND ANKLE

Home Exercise Program for Ankle Sprain (Initial Program)

- To minimize inflammation, apply a bag of crushed ice or frozen peas to the ankle for 20 minutes after performing the exercises.
- You should not experience pain with the exercises.
- If you continue to experience pain or limited mobility of the ankle after performing the exercises for 2 to 3 weeks, call your doctor.
- Progression of the rehabilitation program beyond ankle range of motion, ankle dorsiflexion/plantar flexion, and ankle eversion/inversion should occur after 2 to 4 weeks and may include standing on one leg and heel raise exercises.
- The following exercise program is introductory only, and progression of this program will vary based on your specific injury, symptoms, and baseline level of fitness. For further progression of this routine, your physician may recommend evaluation and treatment by a physical therapist or other exercise professional.

Home Exercises for Ankle Sprain (Initial Program)

Exercise	Muscle Group	Number of Repetitions/Sets	Number of Days per Week	Number of Weeks
Ankle range of motion	Dorsiflexors Plantar flexors Invertors Evertors	2 sets	Daily	3 to 4
Ankle dorsiflexion/ plantar flexion	Anterior tibialis Gastrocnemius-soleus complex	10 to 15 repetitions/2 to 3 sets	Daily	3 to 4
Ankle eversion/inversion	Posterior tibialis Peroneus longus and peroneus brevis	25 repetitions/3 sets, progressing to 45 repetitions/3 sets	Daily	2 to 3
Standing on one leg	All muscles of the foot and calf	5 repetitions/3 sets	Daily	3 to 4
Heel raise	Gastrocnemius-soleus complex Posterior tibialis	10 to 15 repetitions/3 sets	Daily	3 to 4

Ankle Range of Motion

- Sit on a chair or the edge of a bed so your feet do not touch the floor.
- Leading with the big toe, write each letter of the alphabet in the air. Keep your knee flexed.
- Perform 2 sets per day, for 3 to 4 weeks.

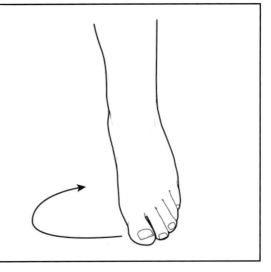

Ankle Dorsiflexion/Plantar Flexion

- Find a position in which your weight is off your feet, such as lying on a bed or on the floor with your legs straight out in front of you.
- For dorsiflexion, wrap an elastic band or tubing around your foot and anchor the other end to a door or bedpost or have someone hold it. Pull your toes toward you, then return slowly to the starting position. Repeat 10 to 15 times.
- For plantar flexion, wrap an elastic band or tubing around your foot and hold the other end in your hand. Gently point your toes, then return slowly to the starting position. Repeat 10 to 15 times.
- Perform 2 to 3 sets per day, for 3 to 4 weeks.

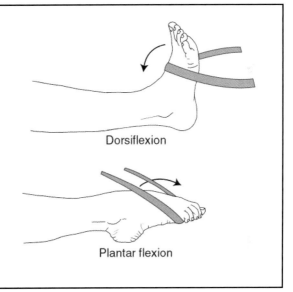

Dorsiflexion

Plantar flexion

SECTION 7   FOOT AND ANKLE

SECTION 7   FOOT AND ANKLE

Ankle Eversion/Inversion

- Find a position in which your weight is off your feet, such as lying on a bed or on the floor with your legs straight out in front of you.
- For inversion, wrap an elastic band or tube around the inside of your foot and anchor the other end to a door or bedpost or have someone hold it. Pull your foot inward against the resistance, then return slowly to the starting position. Repeat 25 times.
- For eversion, wrap an elastic band or tube around the outside of your foot and anchor the other end to a door or bedpost or have someone hold it. Pull your foot outward against the resistance, then return slowly to the starting position. Repeat 25 times.
- Perform 3 sets of each exercise per day, progressing to 3 sets of 45 repetitions per exercise per day, for 2 to 3 weeks.

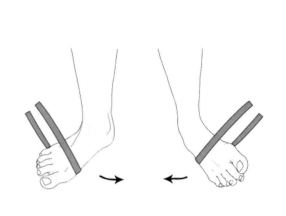

Standing on One Leg

- Stand facing the back of a chair or other stable surface.
- Lift one foot and try to balance on the other foot without using your hands. Keep your hands close to the back of the chair for safety.
- Hold the position for up to 20 seconds.
- Perform 5 repetitions, 3 times per day, for 3 to 4 weeks.
- If balance allows, perform the exercise while standing on foam or on a pillow.

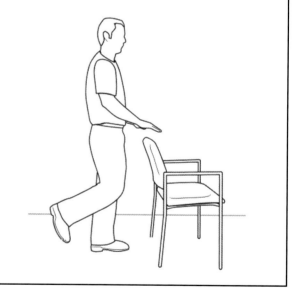

Heel Raise

- Stand with your feet shoulder width apart, and use the back of a chair for balance support if needed.
- Slowly raise up onto your toes, with your weight evenly distributed between both feet. Hold the position for 3 seconds.
- Slowly lower back down to the starting position.
- Perform 10 to 15 repetitions, 3 times per day, for 3 to 4 weeks.
- The exercise may be gradually progressed to standing on one foot as strength allows.

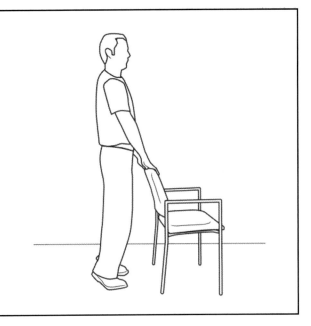

Arthritis of the Foot and Ankle

Synonyms
Osteoarthritis
Posttraumatic arthritis

Definition
The most common types of arthritis of the foot and ankle are osteoarthritis (degenerative arthritis) and posttraumatic arthritis. Frequent locations of arthritis in the foot and ankle are the first metatarsophalangeal (MTP) joint (MTP joint of the great toe) (hallux rigidus), the midfoot (tarsometatarsal joint), the talonavicular joint, the subtalar (talocalcaneal) joint, and the ankle (talonavicular) joint (**Figure 1**).

Clinical Symptoms
Patients with arthritis of the first MTP joint report pain, loss of dorsiflexion, and swelling of the great toe joint. Midfoot osteoarthritis commonly is idiopathic in older women and also occurs after a Lisfranc (tarsometatarsal) dislocation. The patient usually reports diffuse aching in the midfoot that worsens with prolonged walking or standing as well as difficulty pushing off with the foot.

Talonavicular arthritis causes focal pain over the joint (medial aspect of the hindfoot). This is a common site for rheumatoid arthritis.

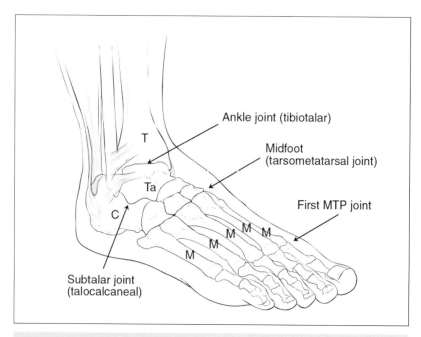

Figure 1 Illustration of common sites of foot and ankle arthritis. C = calcaneus, M = metatarsal, MTP = metatarsophalangeal, T = tibia, Ta = talus.

Subtalar arthritis produces pain over the subtalar joint and frequently follows calcaneal fractures. Pain and difficulty walking on uneven surfaces (such as sand or rocky terrain) results because the motion of this joint primarily involves inversion and eversion of the foot.

Most patients with ankle arthritis have a history of trauma. Pain, swelling, and stiffness in the anterior ankle are common symptoms. Patients with ankle arthritis have difficulty flexing and extending the ankle and therefore tend to walk with the leg externally rotated.

Tests

Physical Examination

With hallux rigidus, loss of motion in the first MTP joint noted at the start of dorsiflexion and difficulty pushing off with the great toe are common. Patients also describe hallux rigidus as a newly formed painful bunion and have difficulty wearing shoes. Pain in the middle of the flexion-extension arc is usually diagnostic. In patients with midfoot arthritis, palpation reveals tenderness and often a dorsal bump on the midfoot. Pain can be elicited by a midfoot pronation and supination maneuver. The piano key test is helpful to determine which tarsometatarsal joints are mainly involved. In the piano key test, individual distal metatarsal heads are pressed down as if pressing on piano keys; pain in each metatarsal is noted. Patients with talonavicular or subtalar arthritis may show a loss of inversion and eversion of the hindfoot compared with the opposite foot; however, ankle joint motion is relatively normal. The heel should be kept in neutral position during range-of-motion testing. Patients with ankle joint arthritis have swelling around the ankle joint and loss of ankle motion mainly in dorsiflexion, and they often walk with the leg externally rotated.

Diagnostic Tests

Weight-bearing radiographs reveal the typical signs of degenerative or posttraumatic arthritis, including osteophytes (spurs) and joint space narrowing. The first MTP joint usually shows dorsal osteophytes protruding from the metatarsal head. The osteophyte usually starts in the lateral portion of the joint and extends in a superior and medial direction. In midfoot arthritis, joint space narrowing is especially evident at the second tarsometatarsal joint (**Figure 2**). Talonavicular arthritis is best viewed on an AP radiograph of the foot. With subtalar arthritis, the lateral view of the foot reveals loss of the normal talocalcaneal joint space. Ankle joint arthritis usually causes loss of joint space, which can be seen on both AP (**Figure 3**) and lateral ankle views, as well as spur formation anteriorly and posteriorly. A weight-bearing Harris heel view is helpful to determine the heel varus or valgus. Recently, weight-bearing CT has gained popularity because it can be done quickly in the clinical setting and it has radiation exposure similar to that of conventional radiography.

When the extent of arthritis is uncertain, CT can be helpful, especially in the midfoot, where the bony anatomy is sometimes difficult to view on plain radiographs. More recently, single photon

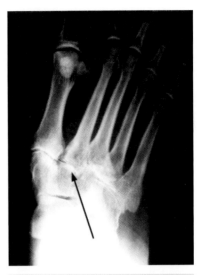

Figure 2 AP radiograph demonstrates primary degenerative arthritis of the midfoot. Note the joint space narrowing at the second tarsometatarsal joint (arrow). (Reproduced from Beaman DN, Saltzman CL: Arthritis of the midfoot, in Mizel MS, Miller RA, Scioli MW, eds: *Orthopaedic Knowledge Update: Foot and Ankle*, ed 2. Rosemont, IL, American Academy of Orthopaedic Surgeons, 1998, p 294.)

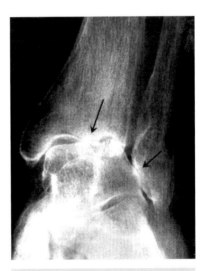

Figure 3 AP radiograph of an ankle demonstrates ankle arthritis with asymmetric loss of joint space (arrows).

emission computed tomography (SPECT)-CT (CT combined with nuclear imaging) gained popularity in cases in which it is difficult to diagnose the source of the patient's pain because of the multiple areas involved.

Differential Diagnosis

- Charcot arthropathy (history of diabetes mellitus, swelling that is disproportionate to symptoms)
- Gout (positive history) (redness and swelling)
- Tendinitis (normal radiographs)

Adverse Outcomes of the Disease

Pain and difficulty with ambulation are common with untreated foot and ankle arthritis.

Treatment

Initial therapy consists of shoe modifications, orthotic inserts, and NSAIDs. A stiff-soled shoe with a rocker bottom will help relieve symptoms in patients with hallux rigidus. If nonsurgical measures fail, débridement of the first MTP joint with cheilectomy (early-stage disease) or arthrodesis (late-stage disease) should be performed.

Midfoot arthritis can be treated nonsurgically with a rigid custom orthotic insert or a steel shank inserted into the sole of the shoe and with repetitive corticosteroid injections done under fluoroscopic guidance. Patients with refractory symptoms will need surgical midfoot fusion. Symptoms of talonavicular and subtalar arthritis can be improved with a medial longitudinal arch support or the more rigid UCBL (University of California Biomechanics Laboratory) orthoses. Corticosteroid injections and NSAIDs may be helpful. Predictable pain relief can be obtained with subtalar arthrodesis (fusion), which retains ankle motion.

Ankle arthritis is treated initially with a custom-molded ankle-foot orthosis and NSAIDs. Injection of a corticosteroid also may be beneficial. In mild to moderate cases, débridement of the joint may defer the need for fusion. Ankle arthrodesis will benefit patients with refractory symptoms. An ankle fused in a neutral position functions well, and the function of the surrounding joints is preserved. For patients older than 60 years with mild to moderate deformity, total ankle replacement surgery has recently gained popularity; results are better than or comparable to those for ankle fusion.

Adverse Outcomes of Treatment

In 2015, the FDA strengthened its warning linking NSAIDs with the risk of heart attack or stroke, even in the first weeks of use of an NSAID. Infection, nonunion, and persistent pain can occur after foot and ankle fusions.

Referral Decisions/Red Flags

Persistent and disabling pain requires further evaluation. Chronic symptoms can be relieved by surgical débridement or fusion.

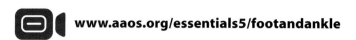

www.aaos.org/essentials5/footandankle

Procedure: Ankle Joint Injection

Materials
- Sterile gloves
- Bactericidal skin preparation solution
- Two 5-mL syringes
- One 21-gauge needle
- 4 mL of 1% lidocaine
- 2 mL of 40 mg/mL corticosteroid preparation without epinephrine
- Sterile adhesive dressing

Step 1
Wear protective gloves at all times during this procedure and use sterile technique.

Step 2
Cleanse the skin with a bactericidal skin preparation.

Step 3
Palpate the soft spot over the ankle joint just medial to the anterior tibial tendon (**Figure 1**). This spot usually is 1 cm proximal to the tip of the medial malleolus. Using a 5-mL syringe with a 21-gauge needle, inject 2 mL of the 1% lidocaine anesthetic into the subcutaneous tissue of the soft spot.

Step 4
Advance the needle into the joint by directing it slightly laterally and superiorly. Inject the last 2 mL of the 1% lidocaine anesthetic. If the needle is in the joint, injection of the fluid meets no resistance. Leave the needle in place and exchange the syringe.

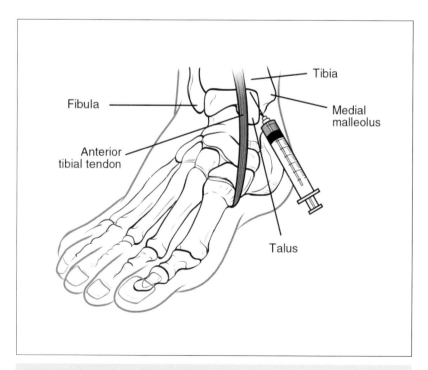

Figure 1 Illustration of the proper location for ankle joint injection.

Step 5
Inject 2 mL of 40 mg/mL depocorticosteroid preparation. Injection of the fluid should meet no resistance. Withdraw the needle.

Step 6
Dress the puncture site with a sterile adhesive dressing.

Adverse Outcomes
Injury to the distal branch of the saphenous nerve is possible. Slow atrophy at the site of the injection is possible secondary to subcutaneous steroid deposition.

Aftercare/Patient Instructions
Remind the patient that one third of patients experience a flare-up of symptoms, with increased joint pain for 1 to 2 days. NSAIDs or analgesics may be given during this period. Ice may be helpful for the first 24 hours.

SECTION 7   FOOT AND ANKLE

Bunionette

Synonym
Tailor's bunion

Definition
A bunionette, sometimes referred to as a tailor's bunion, is a deformity of the fifth metatarsophalangeal (MTP) joint that is analogous to a bunion (hallux valgus) deformity of the great toe. A bunionette is characterized by prominence of the lateral aspect of the fifth metatarsal head and medial deviation of the small toe. A bunionette is usually associated with frequent wearing of tight, narrow, pointed-toe shoes, but it can also result from an angular deformity of the fifth metatarsal bone.

Clinical Symptoms
Patients report pain and problems finding comfortable shoes.

Tests

Physical Examination
Deformity is evident on physical examination. An overlying hard corn is frequently present.

Diagnostic Tests
Weight-bearing AP radiographs will show medial deviation of the fifth proximal phalanx and lateral deviation of the fifth metatarsal shaft and/or a prominence on the lateral aspect of the fifth metatarsal head (**Figure 1**). The joint usually is normal.

Differential Diagnosis
- Cavovarus foot deformity (excessive weight bearing on the lateral side of the foot and pain over the fifth metatarsal noted on physical examination)
- Inflammatory arthropathy (painful, swollen fifth MTP joint with deviation of the small toe often noted)

Adverse Outcomes of the Disease
The most common problem is persistent pain aggravated by shoe wear. Patients also may have associated hard and soft corns, with possible ulceration and infection.

Treatment
Patients should be advised to select proper shoes with a soft upper and a roomy toe box. A shoe repair shop can stretch the shoe in the area over the bunionette. A modified metatarsal pad also can help shift pressure off the fifth metatarsal head. Pads can be applied to

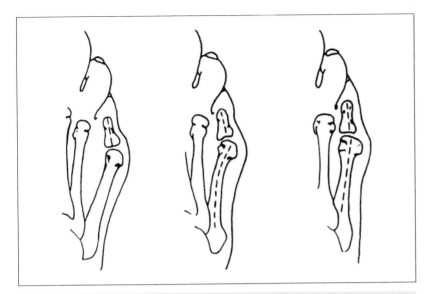

Figure 1 Illustrations of typical deformities associated with a bunionette. *Left,* Increased intermetatarsal angle between the fourth and fifth metatarsals. *Middle,* Lateral angulation of the fifth metatarsal shaft distally. *Right,* A larger metatarsal head and associated soft-tissue bulge on the outside. (Reproduced from Coughlin MJ: Etiology and treatment of the bunionette deformity. *Instr Course Lect* 1990;39:37-48.)

the lateral aspect of the toe box to float the painful fifth metatarsal head. A medial longitudinal arch support can help a patient who has a flexible flatfoot. This orthotic device rotates the forefoot slightly, which decreases direct pressure over the bunionette prominence.

With continued symptoms, surgical excision of the bunionette with or without realignment osteotomy of the fifth metatarsal bone may be required.

Adverse Outcomes of Treatment

Pain may persist despite the application of a metatarsal pad. Surgical risks include persistent pain, infection, incomplete correction, painful surgical scar, and neuroma formation from injury to the cutaneous nerves in the surgical field.

Referral Decisions/Red Flags

Failure of nonsurgical treatment indicates the need for further evaluation.

Procedure: Application of a Metatarsal Pad

Materials

- Felt, silicone, or gel metatarsal pad
- Temporary marker (lipstick, eyeliner)

Step 1

Ask the patient to mark the painful spot on the bottom of the foot with a material that transfers easily, such as lipstick or eyeliner (**Figure 1, A**). The mark should be approximately 0.5 cm².

Step 2

Instruct the patient to stand in a shoe without wearing a sock, to transfer the mark to the inside of the shoe.

Step 3

Place a metatarsal pad in the shoe approximately 10 mm proximal to (toward the heel), not directly under, the mark (**Figure 1, B**). This ensures that the painful area is suspended by the proximally placed pad. Prefabricated, off-the-shelf felt or gel pads are easy to use, inexpensive, and effective, and they come in different sizes to accommodate different-size lesions and feet.

Aftercare/Patient Instructions

If the pad is effective, continue the use of the pad and replace when worn. If the patient cannot comply with use of the pad or complains of slippage of the pad inside the shoe, a custom-made insole with an embedded metatarsal pad can be fabricated and can be transferred from shoe to shoe.

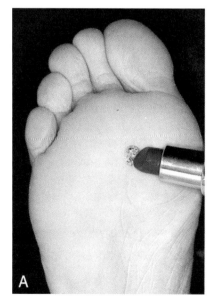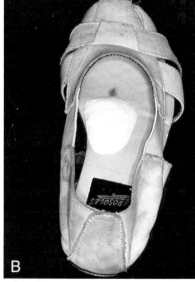

Figure 1 Clinical photographs show application of a metatarsal pad. **A,** Marking the painful area. **B,** Proper placement of the metatarsal pad in the shoe.

Chronic Lateral Ankle Pain

Definition

Chronic pain on the lateral aspect of the ankle is a common symptom that often follows an inversion injury. Several conditions may cause chronic lateral ankle pain after an inversion injury to the ankle, and they should be considered in the differential diagnosis.

Clinical Symptoms

Patients typically report pain on the lateral aspect of the ankle. Episodes of giving way and repeated sprains are typically associated with instability. Between sprains, however, the patient will have periods that are symptom free. In contrast, patients with a bone, cartilage, or tendon lesion often report constant, dull pain over the involved area.

Tests

Physical Examination

Asking the patient to identify focal tenderness using one finger is the key element of the examination and can often identify the source of the problem. Identify any area of swelling. Range of motion should be assessed for both the ankle and subtalar joints. Assess laxity of the ankle and subtalar joints. Test sensation of the sural and superficial peroneal nerves.

Lidocaine injections can be very helpful in differentiating the source of a patient's symptoms. An intra-articular injection of 5 mL of 1% lidocaine into the ankle joint, for example, should provide transient pain relief in a patient with anterolateral impingement syndrome. Other common areas for differential injection include the subtalar joint and peroneal sheath.

Diagnostic Tests

AP, lateral, and mortise radiographs of the ankle joint are obtained for suspected ankle pathology. AP, lateral, and oblique radiographs of the foot are obtained for suspected foot pathology. If ankle or subtalar joint laxity is suspected, varus and anterior stress radiographs are helpful and should often include comparison stress views of the opposite, uninjured side. If the radiographs are normal and occult bony pathology is suspected, technetium Tc-99m bone scanning, limited to AP and lateral views of both feet and ankles, will identify the lesion. Although the bone scan is not specific, it is very sensitive and will detect most bony lesions, including occult fractures, arthritic changes, and tumors. If the bone scan is abnormal and an occult fracture is suspected, CT with thin cuts through the area in question should be diagnostic. If a soft-tissue or tendon injury is suspected (such as tenosynovitis, a partial tear, or rupture of a tendon), MRI is appropriate. In these cases, the radiologist should be directed to the specific area of the tendon in question.

Differential Diagnosis

Anterolateral Impingement Syndrome of the Ankle

Anterolateral impingement of the talus with inversion (lateral gutter syndrome) occurs after an inversion ankle sprain. The borders of the lateral gutter of the ankle include the talus medially, the fibula laterally, and the tibia superiorly. Following a sprain, chronic scar tissue in the lateral gutter causes the anterolateral impingement. Patients with Bassett ligament (accessory slip of anterior inferior tibiofibular ligament) are more prone to developing this problem even without an evident injury. This condition is common in athletes, who often report pain and tenderness along the anterolateral aspect of the ankle. The pain is absent at rest and present with activities (especially dorsiflexion). These patients usually do not report buckling or giving way and do not show any signs of instability. Examination reveals tenderness and swelling along the anterior talofibular ligament and lateral gutter. Radiographs, MRIs, technetium Tc-99m bone scans, and CT scans appear normal, so this condition is often overlooked. An intra-articular injection of lidocaine will provide transient pain relief. Initial treatment should include an anti-inflammatory medication, rehabilitation, and possibly a steroid injection. Arthroscopic débridement of the lateral gutter provides definitive treatment.

Chronic Ankle/Subtalar Instability

Following an inversion sprain, chronic instability of the ankle and/or the subtalar joint can develop. These patients report frequent giving way and generalized weakness in the ankle and an inability to return to full sports or daily activities. The cause may be inadequate rehabilitation or inadequate healing, with subsequent attenuation of one or more ligaments. After a moderate to severe inversion injury, a patient will often lose proprioception, range of motion, and muscle strength. A mild contracture of the Achilles tendon also may develop. Six weeks of rehabilitation, directed specifically at increasing proprioception and range of motion, will often benefit these patients. The use of an ankle brace during sports activities also can be of significant benefit. If symptoms persist, further evaluation is required. The anterior drawer test and the varus stress test should be administered. Stress radiographs can be helpful but are not required; patients with functional instability can have negative stress views. The benchmark for surgical management is anatomic Broström repair. In the absence of adequate tissue, nonanatomic reconstructions using autograft or allograft methods have also been described.

Nerve Injury

Injury by direct blow, stretch, entrapment, or even transection of the superficial peroneal or sural nerves can be a cause of chronic lateral ankle pain. Repetitive stretching or nerve compression typically causes symptoms over the site of a fascial band or bony ridge. Patients report diffuse, dull, achy pain on the lateral aspect of the ankle, and burning, tingling, or radiating pain in the nerve distribution. Plantar flexion and inversion of the ankle and foot will often aggravate the symptoms. Focal tenderness and radiating paresthesia with percussion over the site of nerve injury (Tinel sign) is diagnostic. A more generalized neurologic examination should include an evaluation of the L4, L5, and S1 nerve roots to rule out a proximal nerve lesion. Electromyography and nerve conduction velocity studies often are not helpful in the diagnosis of superficial peroneal or sural nerve lesions. Many of these injuries resolve spontaneously, but some require surgical intervention.

Occult Bony Pathology

Routine radiographs identify most fractures in the foot and ankle, but osteochondral lesions of the talus, avulsion fractures of the calcaneus, lateral process fractures of the talus, and stress fractures of the fibula may not be obvious. A bone scan or single photon emission computed tomography-CT is an excellent initial study if these injuries are suspected. Once diagnosed, an occult bony lesion often can be treated with 4 to 6 weeks of immobilization. For persistent symptoms, excision of a loose bone fragment, arthroscopic débridement of an osteochondral lesion, or surgical fusion of an arthritic joint may be required.

Peroneal Tenosynovitis/Peroneal Tendon Subluxation

A common cause of chronic lateral ankle pain is tenosynovitis from a tear or subluxation of one of the peroneal tendons. The peroneus brevis is most commonly affected by a tear, usually just posterior to the tip of the fibula. Patients usually report chronic retromalleolar swelling, pain, and tenderness. Recurrent subluxation of the peroneal tendons over the lateral ridge of the fibula also can be associated with this condition. MRI is helpful in the evaluation of peroneal pathology, but it is difficult to obtain the optimal view of the peroneal tendons where they curve around the fibular tip. Recently, dynamic ultrasonography was shown to be more effective in diagnosing tears and subluxations. Simple tenosynovitis may be treated with cast immobilization for 4 to 6 weeks. A tear or chronic subluxation of the tendon, however, usually requires surgical treatment.

Subtalar Joint Arthritis

Early arthritis of the subtalar joint may be difficult to identify. These patients present with chronic lateral ankle pain that is aggravated by standing and walking, particularly on uneven terrain. Examination reveals limited inversion and eversion compared with the unaffected side. Special radiographic views and/or diagnostic injections may be required to confirm early arthritis in this joint.

Subtalar Joint Synovitis/Subtalar Impingement Lesion

Similar to anterolateral impingement syndrome, subtalar joint synovitis/subtalar impingement lesion (STIL) is characterized by a chronic synovitis of the subtalar joint, often following an inversion injury. The interosseous ligaments of the ankle that insert on the floor of the sinus tarsi tear, creating thick scar tissue and impinging in the subtalar joint. Examination reveals focal pain over the lateral entrance to the sinus tarsi, which is the lateral entrance to the subtalar joint.

Patients often have slight restriction and discomfort with passive subtalar motion. Diagnostic studies usually are normal, although MRI may detect chronic inflammation or fibrosis within the subtalar joint. A diagnostic anesthetic injection with relief of symptoms can be very helpful. The treatment is similar to that for anterolateral impingement syndrome. Surgical débridement of the subtalar joint usually produces good results.

Corns and Calluses

Synonyms

Callosity
Clavus
Heloma durum
Heloma molle

Definition

A callus is a hyperkeratotic lesion of the skin that forms in response to excessive pressure over a bony prominence. When the callus forms on a toe, it is called a corn. When it forms elsewhere (as under a metatarsal head), it is called a callus (**Figure 1**). A persistent callus on the sole of the forefoot also is referred to as intractable plantar keratosis.

A callus usually occurs beneath the metatarsal heads and is associated with metatarsalgia, a general term for pain overlying one or several of the metatarsal heads. Pain can be caused by the callus itself or by some other manifestation of chronic pressure overload of the metatarsal head, such as synovitis of the joint, attritional tearing of the metatarsophalangeal (MTP) ligaments, or claw toe deformity. Pressure overload also can be secondary to a cavus foot, long toe (typically, the second), or wearing high-heeled shoes.

Corns usually are the result of toe deformities—hammer toe, bunionette, claw toe—caused by inappropriately tight footwear. Hard corns (heloma durum) occur over exposed bony prominences, whereas soft corns (heloma molle) develop between the toes in the web space as well as over bony prominences (**Figure 2**). Periungual corns are small but painful lesions that occur at the edge of a nail, often in association with a mallet toe or improper shoe fit.

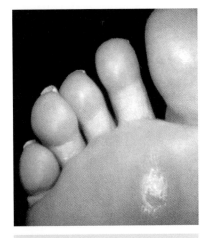

Figure 1 Photograph shows the clinical appearance of a diffuse callus beneath the second metatarsal head.

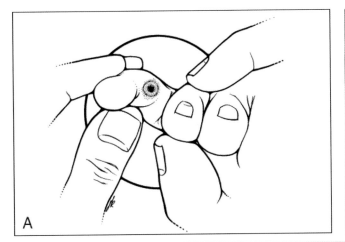
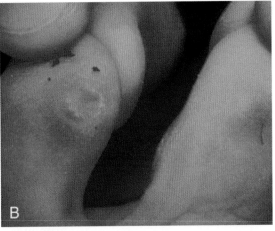

Figure 2 A, Illustration of a soft interdigital corn on the medial aspect of the small toe. **B,** Photograph of a corn on the plantar aspect of the small toe.

Clinical Symptoms

Patients with corns and calluses typically report pain with walking or when wearing shoes.

Tests

Physical Examination

The pared surface of a callus has a uniform, waxy appearance. Warts and calluses generally can be distinguished by palpation. Warts are tender when pinched from side to side, whereas corns and calluses are tender with direct pressure. Plantar warts usually do not develop over a bony prominence. Corns occur over or between the toes.

When tenderness exists over the dorsal surface of the MTP joint, the MTP instability test should be performed to assess joint instability.

Diagnostic Tests

None

Differential Diagnosis

- Foreign body (history of penetrating wound)
- Interdigital (Morton) neuroma (location between the third and fourth metatarsal heads or second and third metatarsal heads, no callus)
- Plantar warts (occur on non–weight-bearing areas, can have a nearby satellite lesion, pared surface has multiple tiny points of hemorrhage near the base)
- Synovitis of the MTP joint (tenderness over the dorsal MTP joint, no plantar callus, painful MTP instability test)

Adverse Outcomes of the Disease

Persistent pain or ulceration of the skin can develop. Metatarsalgia, when caused by plantar plate rupture or MTP synovitis, can result in gradual subluxation of the joint and deformity of the toe.

Treatment

Paring and pressure relief are the principal treatments. Paring involves shaving the lesion layer by layer with a scalpel after the skin has been prepared with alcohol or iodine. The goal is to remove enough of the avascular keratin to restore a more normal contour to the skin without drawing blood. When performed gradually and with care, this can be accomplished using a No. 15 blade, without anesthetic. Paring also provides excellent short-term pain relief. Patients then should be instructed in self-care, using a pumice stone or callus file to regularly débride the lesion after soaking the foot or after a shower.

Treatment of metatarsalgia includes use of a metatarsal pad, trimming the callus/corn, and correction of associated problems, such as improper shoe fit and claw toe deformities. Pressure is relieved by wearing roomier shoes, using commercially available silicone cushions, or inserting small foam donut pads or metatarsal pads to shift pressure from the lesion. For soft corns, a small amount of lamb's wool or a silicone spacer between the toes can wick away moisture and help cushion the area.

When nonsurgical measures fail, surgical treatment to remove the underlying bony prominences is indicated, such as removing the prominent condyles of both adjacent phalanges in the setting of a soft corn or, in cases of intractable plantar callus, performing plantar condylectomy of the involved metatarsal head.

Adverse Outcomes of Treatment

Infection and bleeding can occur from excessively deep paring. Paring a soft corn can be especially difficult because of its awkward location in the web space. Medicated keratolytic corn pads often cause maceration and can result in infection; therefore, these pads are probably best avoided.

Referral Decisions/Red Flags

Failure to respond to nonsurgical treatment and presence of ulceration and/or infection are indications for further evaluation of hyperkeratotic lesions. Deformity or persistent metatarsalgia also requires further evaluation.

Procedure: Trimming a Corn or Callus

Materials

- Sterile gloves
- Scalpel with No. 15 or No. 17 blade

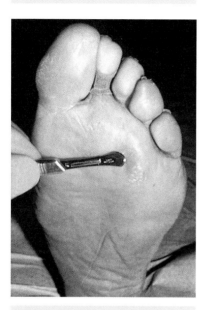

Figure 1 Clinical photograph shows trimming of a callus.

Step 1

Wear protective gloves at all times during the procedure, and use excellent lighting and sterile technique.

Step 2

Anesthesia is not required to trim a corn or callus; however, before the procedure, the patient should soak the foot in water for several minutes to soften the skin.

Step 3

Holding the blade almost parallel to the lesion, shave the excess skin (**Figure 1**). Bleeding should not occur.

  Note: Take special care with a corn on the toe because the skin is thin and may be fragile. Shell out several millimeters of the hard central core of a plantar callus with the sharp tip of the blade.

Adverse Outcomes

Paring down a corn or callus too deeply can expose subcutaneous tissue. If bleeding occurs, the corn or callus has been trimmed too deeply. A wart, however, tends to bleed because of its hypervascularity.

Aftercare/Patient Instructions

Instruct the patient to continue to pare down the lesion with a pumice stone or nail file daily after a shower or bath.

Dance Injuries to the Foot and Ankle

Definition

Dancing emphasizes flexibility, repetition, and technique, and great demands are placed on the foot and ankle. Poor technique and overuse can lead to injury.

Most dancers are girls and young women. Although many of the physical demands placed on dancers are similar to those of other athletes, several are unique. Unique to dance are the turned-out, demi-pointe, and en pointe foot positions (**Figure 1**). These positions place considerable stress on the anatomic structures of the foot and ankle and, particularly if improper technique is used or the individual has preexisting conditions, can lead to injuries and conditions commonly seen in dancers.

Management of injuries in dancers can be difficult because dancers are required to perform repetitive movements and move the joints through extreme ranges of motion as part of their training. Also, dancers often ignore injuries, especially during times of rehearsal or performance, until they become chronic.

Common injuries of the foot and ankle as seen in dancers are described in this chapter. For a more complete discussion of these conditions as seen in the general population, see the following

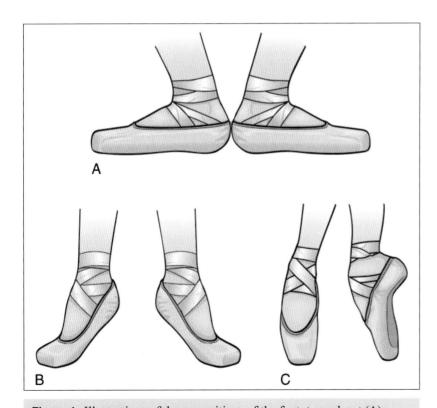

Figure 1 Illustrations of dance positions of the foot: turned-out (**A**), demi-pointe (**B**), en pointe (**C**).

chapters: Ankle Sprain, Hallux Rigidus, Hallux Valgus, Posterior Heel Pain, Sesamoiditis, and Stress Fractures of the Foot and Ankle.

Differential Diagnosis

Hallux Valgus and Hallux Rigidus

Dancing en pointe does not cause hallux valgus, but it can cause an existing hallux valgus to progress. Similarly, hallux rigidus can be made worse by a dancer's efforts to rise into the demi-pointe position. A dancer with hallux rigidus will "sickle," or abduct the forefoot, while attempting to assume the demi-pointe position. The proper demi-pointe position will be difficult if not impossible to achieve because it requires the great toe to be capable of at least 90° of flexion. Treatment of hallux valgus is usually limited to symptomatic care, if possible, until the end of the dancer's career, as surgery may limit the range of motion of the great toe. Treatment of hallux rigidus can be successful in many dancers. Ballet dancers are an exception because a full range of motion is necessary for the demi-pointe position, and this will most likely not be achieved with surgery.

Sesamoiditis

Sesamoiditis in dancers can result from excessive stress on the sesamoids caused by poor technique when landing from jumps, which puts excessive stress on the sesamoids. An ideal landing in ballet includes a small plié (bending of the knees) to absorb the forces of landing, whereas a poor landing is usually audible. On examination, the dancer will have pain on palpation over the involved (usually the medial) sesamoid. With dorsiflexion of the great toe, the point of maximal tenderness will move with the sesamoids and their soft-tissue attachments. Treatment includes using proper landing technique. If it fits in the shoe, a small felt pad can be added to the ballet shoe to relieve pressure on the sesamoid.

Stress Fractures

The most common site of stress fractures of the foot is at the neck of the second metatarsal, followed by the base of the second metatarsal. The second metatarsal is the longest metatarsal and is where the body weight of a dancer is centered when in the demi-pointe position. Although stress fractures can occur in any bone of the foot and ankle, the distal fibula, the sesamoids, the talus, the calcaneus, and the navicular bone are most commonly involved. On examination, the dancer with a stress fracture will have swelling and pain to palpation over the injured bone. Occasionally, crepitus will be present as well.

Treatment of stress fractures is conservative. Because dancers, like athletes, want to heal and return to participation as quickly as possible, non–weight-bearing ambulation on crutches, followed by a gradual return to dance, may be recommended.

Osteophytes at the Anterior Ankle

Extreme plantar flexion of the ankle places stress on the anterior joint capsule. This may result in thickening of the capsule or traction osteophytes off the distal tibia. The thickened capsule or the osteophytes impinge, limit range of motion, and cause pain with dorsiflexion. On examination, a dancer with anterior impingement of the ankle will have maximal tenderness over the anterior osteophytes or the hypertrophied anterior ankle joint capsule. Pain will be exaggerated with dorsiflexion of the ankle, and occasionally dorsiflexion will be limited on the involved side.

The condition is initially treated with rest and, if that fails, surgical débridement of the thick anterior capsule and/or anterior osteophytes.

Ankle Sprain

The most common acute injury in dancers is an inversion sprain of the ankle (lateral collateral ligament injury). If the sprain occurs while the dancer is in demi-pointe, the injury can be quite severe. Care should be taken to examine and perform a stress test on each ligament. It is extremely important in a dancer to perform comparison stress tests on the opposite, uninjured side, as a dancer's range of motion can be exceptional compared with that of the general population. Most ankle sprains are treated nonsurgically, with the dancer returning to dance 2 to 4 weeks postinjury.

Retrocalcaneal Bursitis

The retrocalcaneal bursa can be compressed between the posterior aspect of the calcaneus and the Achilles tendon when the dancer rises up on the ball of the foot. Such compression results in the bursa becoming inflamed and painful. On physical examination, the patient will experience pain with side-to-side compression of the bursa, just anterior to the Achilles tendon. Most cases of retrocalcaneal bursitis resolve with rest, ice, NSAIDs, a heel lift worn in street shoes, or injection of the bursa (sparing the Achilles tendon). If the dancer ignores the pain, the problem can become chronic and require surgical excision of the bursa.

Posterior Impingement Syndrome

The posterior lateral tubercle of the talus (also known as the Stieda process) varies greatly in size and configuration. In 10% of people, the tubercle does not fuse with the body of the talus and is called the os trigonum, which projects into the posterior aspect of the ankle. Impingement of this bone on the soft tissue of the ankle, especially as the dancer assumes the en pointe and demi-pointe positions, results in posterior impingement syndrome. This syndrome is characterized by pain at the back of the ankle when rising up on the toes. Examination reveals tenderness at the posterior aspect of the ankle, deep behind the flexor tendons. Pain increases as the foot is placed into plantar flexion, compressing the soft tissues at the posterior aspect of the ankle.

Conservative treatment includes rest, NSAIDs, and, if these measures do not relieve the pain, an injection of local anesthetic and cortisone into the posterior aspect of the ankle can be done under fluoroscopic or ultrasound guidance. If these measures do not provide relief, surgical excision of the posterior lateral tubercle or os trigonum is recommended.

Tendinitis of the Flexor Hallucis Longus Tendon

For dance positions requiring a turned-out foot position, turnout should take place at the hip because when the femur is externally rotated the greater trochanter of the femur clears the pelvis, allowing the leg to abduct. Some dancers, however, using poor technique, turn out only the feet. This causes the feet to roll into an everted position and puts stress on the medial side of the foot, which can lead to tendinitis of the flexor hallucis longus (FHL) tendon.

The FHL tendon passes through a fibro-osseous tunnel posterior to the talus as it travels to its insertion at the great toe. With chronic overuse, inflammation and fibrosis of the tendon can result in a nodular thickening. The inflamed, thickened tendon can catch and cause the great toe to trigger. FHL tendinitis will cause pain and occasionally clicking over the course of the tendon. The pain may increase when the FHL tendon travels through the fibro-osseous tunnel behind the talus. Pain may also increase when the dancer rises up on the toes or completes a grande plié, which puts tension on the FHL tendon.

Examination should include palpating the entire course of the FHL tendon while passively moving the great toe. Check for crepitus or a click in the fibro-osseous tunnel posterior to the talus.

Nonsurgical treatment includes ice, NSAIDs, rest, and an injection of a local anesthetic agent into the fibro-osseous tunnel. If conservative treatment fails, surgical release of the fibro-osseous tunnel and a tenosynovectomy may be recommended. Posterior arthroscopic débridement enables the dancer to return to his or her original activity level sooner with less incision and scar tissue formation compared with release.

Tests

Clinical and diagnostic tests depend on the specific condition. Pain elicited on the posterior side of the ankle with passive plantar flexion usually is a sign of posterior impingement, whereas pain that increases with resisted active flexion of the great toe is a sign of FHL tendinitis. A lateral view of the ankle in plantar flexion is recommended to examine for posterior impingement syndrome of the ankle. This view will reveal not only the position and size of the posterior lateral process of the talus (and os trigonum) but also any visible impingement. A lateral view with the ankle in full dorsiflexion is also recommended to evaluate for anterior impingement.

Adverse Outcomes of the Disease

Some conditions, such as hallux rigidus, can end a dancer's career because full range of motion of the great toe will most likely not be achieved, even with proper treatment.

Treatment

The goal of treatment is to return the dancer to a preinjury level of dance. This usually includes a sequence of rehabilitation, barre work, return to class, and then return to performance. This should be gradual and include consultation with the rehabilitation specialist, the dance instructor, and the dancer.

Adverse Outcomes of Treatment

In 2015, the FDA strengthened its warning linking NSAIDs with the risk of heart attack or stroke, even in the first weeks of use of an NSAID.

Referral Decisions/Red Flags

Further evaluation is indicated in any patient with an overuse injury that does not respond within 72 hours to ice, anti-inflammatory medication, and rest; an injury that is associated with a pop, click, or other audible sound; triggering of the great toe; any fracture; or any loss of range of motion.

SECTION 7   FOOT AND ANKLE

The Diabetic Foot

Synonyms

Charcot arthropathy
Neuropathic foot

Definition

Diabetes is a group of metabolic disorders characterized by high blood glucose levels. The four major categories are type 1 diabetes mellitus (insulin-dependent), type 2 diabetes mellitus (non–insulin-dependent), gestational diabetes mellitus, and diabetes secondary to other conditions. Types 1 and 2 are the most common forms, with approximately 5% to 10% of all cases of diabetes in the United States identified as type 1 and 85% to 90% as type 2.

Diabetic foot problems are a major health problem in the United States and are a common cause of hospitalization and amputation. Patients present with skin ulceration, infection, and/or Charcot arthropathy. The primary etiology is peripheral nerve impairment that results in loss of protective sensation, autonomic dysfunction, and/or motor impairment. With inadequate sensory feedback, repetitive trauma is not perceived and skin breakdown results. Vascular insufficiency also can contribute to foot problems in patients with diabetes.

Patients with autonomic dysfunction have dry, scaly, and cracking skin, a condition that predisposes the skin to ulceration.

Motor neuropathy leads to weakness of the intrinsic muscles of the foot, claw toe deformities, subluxation or dislocation of the metatarsophalangeal joints, abnormal plantar positioning of the metatarsal heads, increased pressure on the sole of the foot, skin breakdown, ulcers, deep infections, and osteomyelitis. Extrinsic forces, such as tight shoes, can contribute to skin breakdown.

Charcot arthropathy results from repetitive stress in a patient in whom pain and proprioceptive sensation is not perceived normally. Recent studies have shown that synovial tissue is the primary tissue involved. The result is progressive disruption of joint stability and severe bony deformities (**Figure 1**).

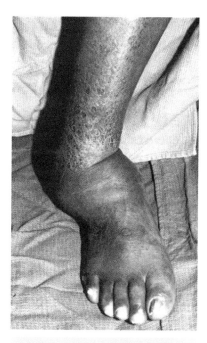

Figure 1 Clinical photograph shows severe deformity from Charcot breakdown of the ankle joint. (Reproduced from Harrelson JM: The diabetic foot: Charcot arthropathy. *Instr Course Lect* 1993;42:141-146.)

Clinical Symptoms

Patients may have no symptoms or they may report foot pain at night, characterized as burning and tingling, secondary to neuritis. With abnormal areas of pressure, skin breakdown follows, leading to a painless ulcer. Deep infections and osteomyelitis can subsequently develop, usually with a sudden increase in swelling, redness, and drainage, and sometimes pain.

Patients with Charcot arthropathy have noticeable swelling, warmth, and redness, even though pain is only mild or absent. Charcot arthropathy may be misdiagnosed as cellulitis, osteomyelitis, or gout.

Tests

Physical Examination

A thorough evaluation of the feet is essential when examining patients with diabetes. A substantial number of amputations can be avoided by simple preventive measures and early treatment of skin lesions. Light touch should be tested. Protective foot care, including wearing well-cushioned shoes, is particularly necessary in patients below the protective sensation threshold, that is, those who cannot feel a 10-g (5.07-mm) nylon filament applied to the plantar aspect of the foot (**Figure 2**).

Diabetic ulcers are insensate and can be easily inspected and probed to determine depth and size. If bone can be probed, osteomyelitis is likely to be present.

Examination of a Charcot joint reveals a hot, red, swollen joint with intact skin. Pulses usually are strong in patients with Charcot arthropathy. A Charcot foot elevated above the heart for 1 minute will lose its redness, whereas a foot affected by cellulitis, soft-tissue abscess, and/or osteomyelitis will not.

Diagnostic Tests

Radiographs are necessary to help rule out osteomyelitis and Charcot arthropathy (**Figure 3**). Vascular studies are appropriate when pulses are absent or when the patient has a nonhealing ulcer. MRI reports usually misidentify Charcot arthropathy as osteomyelitis; even though MRI can help confirm a deep abscess, this diagnostic study usually is not necessary. Combined technetium-iridium bone scans have been used in difficult cases to differentiate Charcot arthropathy from osteomyelitis.

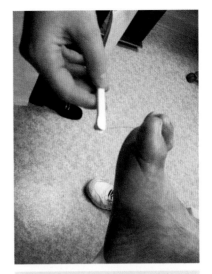

Figure 2 Clinical photograph shows testing for protective sensation using a nylon filament applied to the plantar aspect of the foot. (Reproduced from Pinzur MS: Ankle fractures in patients with diabetes mellitus, in Nunley JA, Pfeffer GB, Sanders RW, Trepman E, eds: *Advanced Reconstruction: Foot and Ankle*. Rosemont, IL, American Academy of Orthopaedic Surgeons, 2004, p 427.)

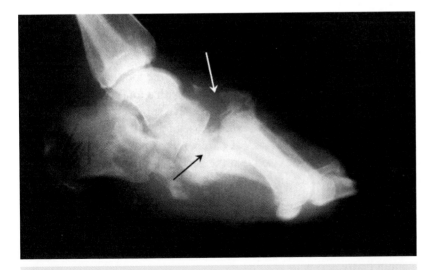

Figure 3 Lateral radiograph demonstrates Charcot degeneration of the midfoot (arrows). (Reproduced from Harrelson JM: The diabetic foot: Charcot arthropathy. *Instr Course Lect* 1993;42:141-146.)

Differential Diagnosis

- Cellulitis (most likely associated with skin breakdown)
- Gout (painful lesion, increased serum uric acid)
- Osteomyelitis (usually beneath an open skin ulcer)
- Other neuropathies (Charcot-Marie-Tooth disease, alcoholic neuropathy, spinal cord neuropathy)

Adverse Outcomes of the Disease

Skin ulceration, Charcot joint, chronic osteomyelitis, and gangrene all occur in the diabetic foot. Amputation may be necessary.

Treatment

The goal of treatment is patient education and prevention. Control of serum glucose is paramount. Once neuropathy occurs, it is irreversible. When a problem exists, aggressive treatment is needed to avoid a more serious and debilitating situation. A callus, which indicates a pressure point, is the first phase of a diabetic ulcer and signals the need for adaptive footwear (cushioned shoes and soft, molded insoles) and close follow-up.

Treatment of a diabetic ulcer requires removing the pressure causing the ulcer, allowing the ulcer to heal, and prescribing optimal footwear to prevent recurrence. Accommodative footwear, an orthotic device, and total contact casting can be used for superficial ulcerations. For deeper ulcerations, these measures are often inadequate, and surgery may be required. An associated equinus contracture should be corrected by serial casting or percutaneous heel cord lengthening.

Treatment of a deep infection must be aggressive and prompt. The infection is often polymicrobial. Skin swab cultures are inaccurate. Bone biopsy provides more definitive cultures to direct antibiotic therapy. Any abscess should be considered an emergency and drained surgically. Osteomyelitis can be treated surgically with débridement of the affected bone. Digit or ray (toe plus metatarsal) amputation is often needed to eradicate osteomyelitis of the toes or metatarsal heads.

In the initial stage of Charcot arthropathy, the foot and ankle need to be unweighted and stabilized, usually with a total contact cast. After the acute swelling and erythema have subsided, the patient can begin bearing weight with continued use of a cast or a customized clamshell-type short leg brace (Charcot restraint orthotic walker). The patient must be advised that the period of immobilization may be lengthy, often up to 12 months, and that a permanent brace might be required for ambulation. When Charcot arthropathy is properly recognized and treated, acceptable limb salvage can be achieved. Occasionally, surgical resection of a bony prominence or reconstruction by arthrodesis is needed for severe deformity that cannot be treated with bracing.

Adverse Outcomes of Treatment
The adverse outcomes of treatment are the same as those for diabetes and, in addition, include surgical complications of infection, ischemia, and death.

Referral Decisions/Red Flags
Unexplained pain in a diabetic foot, sudden onset of swelling and pain, and nonhealing ulcerations all signal the need for further evaluation.

Acknowledgment
Information regarding the sensory testing nylon filament was provided by the Filament Project, 5445 Point Clair Road, Caryville, LA 70721.

Procedure: Care of Diabetic Feet

Care of the Feet

1. Never walk barefoot; always wear shoes or slippers.
2. Wash feet daily with mild soap and water.
   - Always test the water temperature with your hand or elbow before putting your feet in the water.
   - After washing, pat your feet dry; do not rub vigorously.
   - Use only one thickness of towel to dry your feet, especially between the toes.
   - Use a skin moisturizing lotion to prevent skin from getting dry and cracked; however, do not use these lotions between the toes.
3. Inspect your feet daily for puncture wounds, bruises, pressure areas and redness, and blisters.
   - Puncture wounds—Have you stepped on any nails, glass, or tacks?
   - Bruises—Feel for swelling.
   - Pressure areas and redness—Check the six major locations for pressure on the bottom of the foot:
     a. Tip of the big toe
     b. Base of the little toe
     c. Base of the middle toes
     d. Heel
     e. Outside edge of the foot
     f. Across the ball of the foot (metatarsal heads)
   - Blisters—Check the six major locations on the bottom of the foot for blisters, plus the tops of the toes and the back of the heel. Never pop a blister!
4. Seek treatment by a physician for any foot injuries or open wounds.
5. Do not use Lysol disinfectant, iodine, cresol, carbolic acid, kerosene, or other irritating antiseptic solutions to treat cuts or abrasions on your feet. These products will damage soft tissue.
6. Do not use sharp instruments, drugstore medications, or corn plasters on your feet. Always seek the advice of your physician for any condition that needs such care.
7. Protect your feet.
   - Wear loose bed socks while sleeping.
   - Avoid frostbite by wearing warm socks and shoes during cold weather.
   - Do not use a heating pad on your feet.
   - Do not place your feet on radiators, furnaces, furnace grills, or hot water pipes.

- Do not hold your feet in front of a fireplace, circulators, or heaters.
- Do not use a hair dryer on your feet.

8. Place thin pieces of cotton or lamb's wool between your toes if there is maceration of the skin between your toes or if your toes overlap.

9. Do not sit cross-legged; this position can decrease circulation to your feet.

10. Take care of your toenails in the following manner:
    - Soak or bathe feet before trimming nails.
    - Make sure that you trim your toenails under good lighting.
    - Trim toenails straight across.
    - Never trim toenails into the corner.
    - If toenails are thick, see your physician for evaluation of the cause and advice on routine nail care.
    - Consult your physician when there are any signs of an ingrown toenail. Do not treat an ingrown toenail with drugstore medications; however, you can place a thin piece of cotton or waxed dental floss under the toenail.

Socks and Stockings

1. Wear clean, dry socks daily. Make certain that there are no holes or wrinkles in your socks or stockings.

2. Wear thin, white cotton socks in the summer; cotton is more absorbent and porous than synthetic materials. Change them if your feet sweat excessively.

3. Wear square-toe socks; they will not squeeze your toes.

4. Wear pantyhose or stockings with a garter belt. It is important that you do not wear or use the following:
    - Elastic-top socks or stockings, or knee-high stockings
    - Circular elastic garters
    - String tied around the tops of stockings
    - Stockings that are rolled or knotted at the top

Shoe Wear

1. Always wear proper shoes. Check the following components daily to ensure that your shoes fit properly and will not damage your feet:
    - Shoe width—Make sure that the shoes are wide and deep enough to give the joints of your toes breathing room. Shoes that are too narrow will cause pressure bruises and blisters on the inside and outside edges of your foot at the base of the toes.
    - Shoe length—Shoes that are too short will cause pressure and blisters on the tops of your toes. Make sure to measure your shoe size regularly. If your second toe is longer than your big toe, you should measure your shoe size in regard to your second toe; otherwise, your second toe can curl under and result in hammer toe deformity.
    - Back of shoe—Looseness at the heel will cause blisters at your heels.

SECTION 7 FOOT AND ANKLE

- Bottom of heel—Make sure there are no nails. The presence of holes indicates that there are nails in the heels.
- Sole—Make sure that the sole is not broken. A break in the sole will allow nails or other sharp objects to puncture the skin. Flexible shoes with thick soles are preferred.

2. Be careful about the type of new shoes you purchase. Use the following guidelines:
   - Buy new shoes in the evening to allow for swelling in your feet.
   - Inspect your feet once per hour for the first few days you wear a new pair of shoes. Look for red areas, bruises, and blisters.
   - Do not wear your new shoes for more than a half day for the first few days.
   - The following features are desirable:
     a. Laces or adjustable closure
     b. Soft leather tops (to allow feet to breathe; they mold to the feet)
     c. Crepe soles (to provide a good cushion for walking)
   - Avoid the following features:
     a. Elastic across the tops of the shoes
     b. Pointed-toe styles (they constrict the toes)
     c. High heels
     d. Shoes made of plastic (they retain moisture and do not allow the feet to breathe)

3. Put your shoes on properly.
   - Inspect the inside of each shoe before putting it on. Make sure to remove any small stones or debris. Be certain that the inside of the shoe is smooth.
   - Loosen the laces before putting on or taking off your shoes. Make sure that the tongue is flat, with no wrinkles.
   - Be certain that you do not tie your laces either too tightly or too loosely.

Fracture-Dislocations of the Midfoot

Synonym

Lisfranc fracture-dislocation

Definition

Fracture-dislocations of the midfoot, commonly called Lisfranc fracture-dislocations, are traumatic disruptions of the tarsometatarsal joints. Injury to these joints occurs as a result of significant trauma or from an indirect mechanism, as can occur in athletics or as a result of tripping. The critical injury involves the second tarsometatarsal joint. The second metatarsal wedges into a slot in the cuneiforms and is key to stabilizing the other tarsometatarsal joints.

Clinical Symptoms

Patients often report a "sprain." Pain is localized to the dorsum of the midfoot. The swelling may be relatively mild.

Tests

Physical Examination

This injury is easily missed and is sometimes misdiagnosed as a foot or ankle sprain. Examination reveals maximum tenderness and swelling over the tarsometatarsal joint rather than the ankle ligaments. An acute injury to this joint usually presents with ecchymosis in the plantar arch. During examination, stabilize the hindfoot (calcaneus) with one hand and rotate and/or abduct the forefoot with the other hand (**Figure 1**). This maneuver produces severe pain with a Lisfranc injury but only minimal pain with an ankle sprain.

Diagnostic Tests

AP, lateral, and oblique radiographs of the foot should be obtained. Spontaneous reduction after complete dislocation can occur. Subtle injuries may be more apparent on weight-bearing radiographs. The medial aspect of the middle cuneiform should line up with the medial aspect of the second metatarsal on an AP radiograph (**Figure 2**). The oblique view should show the medial aspect of the fourth metatarsal aligned with the medial aspect of the cuboid. Comparison views of the uninjured foot may be helpful.

When the AP radiograph shows that the second metatarsal base has shifted laterally, even by only a few millimeters, a Lisfranc fracture-dislocation has occurred (**Figure 3**). Lateral deviation of the second metatarsal base associated with a small avulsion fracture between the base of the first and second metatarsals indicates disruption of the ligament connecting the base of the second metatarsal and the medial

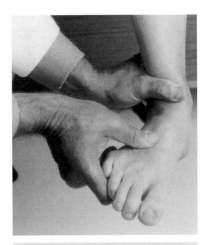

Figure 1 Clinical photograph shows how to test for a Lisfranc fracture-dislocation; stabilize the hindfoot with one hand and rotate and/or abduct the forefoot with the other.

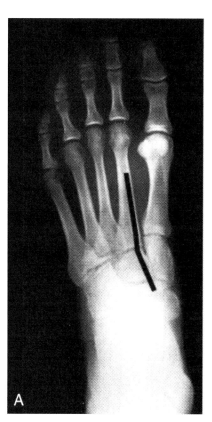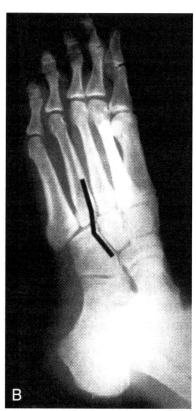

Figure 2 The normal radiographic relationship of the metatarsals and cuneiforms. **A,** AP view. Note the relationship of the second metatarsal and the middle cuneiform. **B,** Oblique view. Note the unbroken line at the medial fourth metatarsal base and the medial cuboid. (Reproduced from Lutter LD, Mizel MS, Pfeffer GP, eds: *Orthopaedic Knowledge Update: Foot and Ankle.* Rosemont, IL, American Academy of Orthopaedic Surgeons, 1994, p 261.)

cuneiform (Lisfranc ligament) and instability of the tarsometatarsal joints.

When radiographs are normal but physical examination suggests injury to the tarsometatarsal joints, stress radiographs of the midfoot under local anesthetic or sedation may be indicated. If confusion still exists, CT or MRI is helpful in confirming the diagnosis and localizing the joints involved.

Differential Diagnosis

- Ankle fracture (bony tenderness over the malleolus)
- Ankle sprain (focal tenderness over the lateral ankle ligament)
- Metatarsal fracture (focal tenderness over the metatarsal) (proximal metatarsal fractures can mimic Lisfranc injuries but lack displacement at the tarsometatarsal joints)
- Midfoot arthritis (chronic pain and tenderness, no recent history of trauma)
- Navicular fracture (focal tenderness over the navicular)

Adverse Outcomes of the Disease

Adverse outcomes include midfoot instability, deformity, and arthritis. Compartment syndrome with subsequent ischemic contracture, claw toes, and sensory impairment also can occur.

Treatment

Nondisplaced injuries are treated with 6 to 8 weeks of non–weight-bearing cast immobilization, followed by use of a rigid arch support for 3 months. A fracture or fracture-dislocation with any displacement requires surgical open reduction and internal fixation of the involved joints or arthrodesis in case of severe damage to the articular surfaces. Temporary immobilization for 2 to 3 weeks in a splint or controlled-ankle motion walker is usually needed to decrease the swelling before surgery. Use of a bandage impregnated with zinc oxide cream (Unna Boot [Hartmann USA]) is very effective in decreasing resistant edema.

Adverse Outcomes of Treatment

If the tarsometatarsal articulations are not well reduced, posttraumatic arthritis may develop.

Referral Decisions/Red Flags

Because these injuries are frequently missed, further evaluation and diagnostic testing is warranted if there is even a slight suspicion of their presence. Even a minimally displaced fracture-dislocation requires surgical reduction. Any possibility of compartment syndrome requires immediate surgical evaluation.

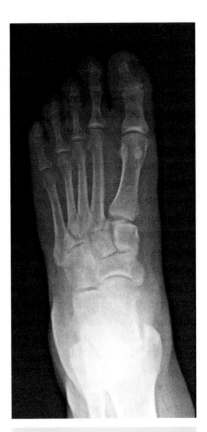

Figure 3 AP radiograph of a left foot demonstrates a Lisfranc fracture-dislocation. Note the small fracture fragment at the base of the second metatarsal and lateral deviation of the second and third metatarsal base, with slight medial deviation of the first metatarsal base.

Fractures of the Ankle

Definition

Ankle fractures include injuries to the lateral malleolus (distal fibula), the medial malleolus, the posterior lip of the tibia (posterior malleolus), the collateral ligamentous structures, and/or the talar dome. Stable fractures involve only one side of the joint (such as a fracture of the distal fibula without injury to the medial deltoid ligament) (**Figure 1**). Unstable ankle fractures involve both sides of the ankle joint and can be bimalleolar or trimalleolar. Bimalleolar injuries are either fractures of the lateral and medial malleolus or a fracture of the distal fibula with disruption of the deltoid ligament. Trimalleolar injuries include a fracture of the posterior malleolus (**Figure 2**). A more severe and unstable variant of a posterior malleolar fracture with extension to the tibial plafond has also been described. Posterior dislocation of the ankle also may be present with a trimalleolar fracture. This injury is described as a trimalleolar fracture-dislocation. Stable injuries may be treated nonsurgically. Unstable injuries, however, are vulnerable for displacement and subsequent posttraumatic arthritis and usually require surgical management.

Clinical Symptoms

Patients usually report acute pain following trauma. The etiologies of ankle fractures are as varied as the circumstances, but usually some element of rotation or twisting has occurred.

Tests

Physical Examination

Medial, lateral, and/or posterior swelling accompanies most ankle fractures. Marked tenderness is evident at the fracture site. A palpable gap may be apparent on the medial side. External rotation or lateral displacement of the foot from the tibia may be present as well.

A fracture of the distal fibula (lateral malleolus) with tenderness over the medial deltoid ligament is presumed to be an unstable bimalleolar injury.

Palpate the proximal fibula for tenderness because tenderness in this area, coupled with swelling of the medial ankle, may indicate a Maisonneuve fracture, an unstable external rotation injury that includes fracture of the proximal fibula, a tear of the medial deltoid ligament, and a disruption of the tibiofibular syndesmotic ligaments.

Assess circulatory status and posterior tibial, superficial peroneal, and deep peroneal nerve function distal to the fracture. Lacerations over the fracture site can indicate an open fracture and should be assessed carefully.

Diagnostic Tests

AP, lateral, and mortise (AP view with the ankle internally rotated, usually 15°) views will reveal most fractures. The relationships of the

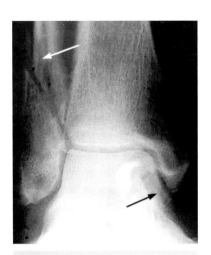

Figure 1 Mortise radiograph demonstrates minimally displaced fracture of the lateral malleolus (white arrow). Note the small chip off the medial malleolus (black arrow).

tibia, fibula, and talus are clearest in the mortise view (**Figure 3**). AP and lateral views should include the proximal fibula and tibia when there is tenderness in that area.

Minimally displaced fractures may not be apparent on initial radiographs; therefore, when such a fracture is suspected, radiographs should be repeated in 10 to 14 days, when callus will usually be evident.

With a rotational injury, an osteochondral fracture of the lateral articular surface of the talus can occur. This is best seen on the mortise view. CT may be required for evaluation of complex fractures.

Differential Diagnosis

- Ankle sprain (history of inversion injury, lateral tenderness, normal radiographs)
- Charcot arthropathy (diffuse swelling, erythema, minimal tenderness)
- Fracture of the base of the fifth metatarsal (focal tenderness)
- Maisonneuve fracture (widening of syndesmosis, tenderness over the proximal fibula)
- Osteochondral fracture of the talar dome, lateral process of the talus, or anterior process of the calcaneus (focal tenderness over the fracture site)

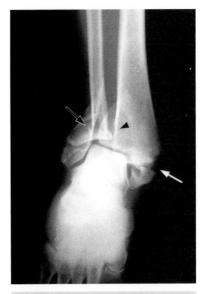

Figure 2 AP radiograph demonstrates displaced trimalleolar ankle fracture. Note the fracture of the lateral malleolus (black arrow), posterior malleolus (black arrowhead), and medial malleolus (white arrow). This fracture requires immediate reduction. (Reproduced from Grantham SA: Trimalleolar ankle fractures and open ankle fractures. *Instr Course Lect* 1990;39:105-111.)

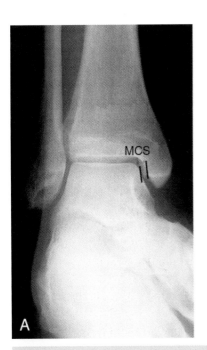
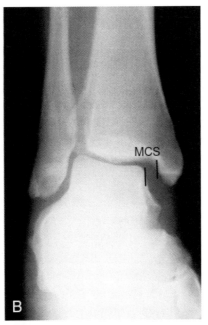

Figure 3 Mortise radiographs of the ankle. **A,** Uninjured ankle demonstrates normal medial clear space (MCS). **B,** Ankle with lateral fibular fracture and deltoid disruption, resulting in widening of the MCS (>5 mm). (Reproduced from Stiehl JB: Ankle fractures with diastasis. *Instr Course Lect* 1990;39:95-103.)

SECTION 7   FOOT AND ANKLE

Adverse Outcomes of the Disease

Posttraumatic arthritis, instability, deformity, complex regional pain syndrome, nerve injury, and compartment syndrome are possible.

Treatment

Stable fractures of the distal fibula can be treated with a weight-bearing cast or brace for 4 to 6 weeks. Unstable but nondisplaced fractures require a non–weight-bearing short or long leg cast and more prolonged immobilization. Unstable, displaced fractures require either closed or open reduction. In most cases, open reduction provides better restoration of joint function. Osteochondral fragments of the talus should be removed. If the fragment is large and there is viable bone on both the fragment and the base, the fracture can be reduced and pinned. The outcome of this procedure usually is good only in young patients. Concomitant dislocation should be reduced as soon as possible to relieve pressure on the skin and neurovascular structures. Open fractures require immediate surgical débridement. Rehabilitation is indicated in elderly patients or if full range of motion and balance are not achieved by 3 months after the fracture has healed.

Adverse Outcomes of Treatment

Joint stiffness and atrophy from casting may occur.

Referral Decisions/Red Flags

Patients with unstable fractures or osteochondral fractures of the talus need further evaluation. All open fractures or open joint injuries require immediate evaluation.

Fractures of the Calcaneus and Talus

Synonyms
Aviator's fracture (talus)
Heel fracture

Definition
Fractures of the two bones of the hindfoot, the talus and calcaneus, usually occur as a result of severe trauma, such as a motor vehicle accident or a fall from a height. The two fractures seldom occur together, however. Most fractures of the talus or calcaneus involve the articular surface and are serious injuries.

Clinical Symptoms
Patients often report acute pain and inability to bear weight.

Tests

Physical Examination
Examination reveals swelling and tenderness. Function of the superficial peroneal, deep peroneal, sural, and medial and lateral plantar nerves distal to the fracture should be assessed. With swelling, the pulses might not be palpable. Capillary refill of the toes should be checked.

Compartment syndrome is difficult to evaluate with calcaneal and talar injuries; however, notable swelling in the area of the arch is suggestive of a plantar compartment syndrome.

Falls that result in fracture of the calcaneus or talus may be associated with a compression fracture of the lumbar spine or other injuries to the ipsilateral lower extremity. Palpate the spine and the entire lower extremity for pain and tenderness.

Diagnostic Tests
AP and lateral radiographs of the hindfoot (**Figure 1**) and Harris heel views are indicated, along with AP, lateral, and mortise views of the ankle. AP and lateral views of the spine should be obtained if spinal tenderness is present. Coronal CT scans should be obtained for further evaluation of the subtalar or calcaneocuboid joints in the presence of an intra-articular fracture pattern or tendon entrapment between the fracture fragments (**Figure 2**).

Differential Diagnosis
- Ankle fracture (ankle swelling or deformity) (evident on radiographs)
- Associated lumbar spine fracture (pain and tenderness in the lower back)

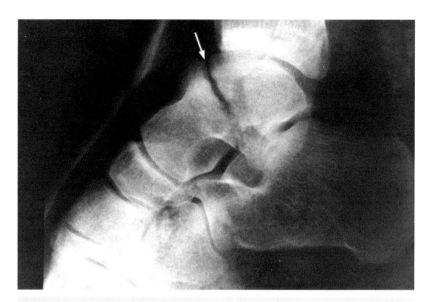

Figure 1 Lateral radiograph of the foot demonstrates a displaced fracture of the anterior talar body (arrow). (Reproduced from Johnson TS, Steinbach LS: *Essentials of Musculoskeletal Imaging.* Rosemont, IL, American Academy of Orthopaedic Surgeons, 2004, p 606.)

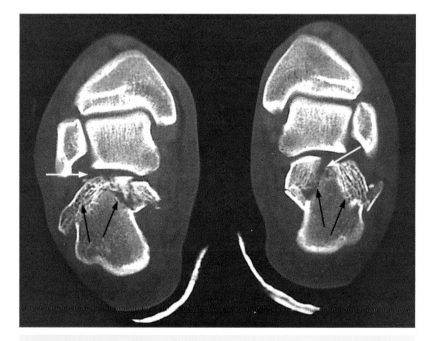

Figure 2 Coronal CT scan of the calcaneus shows bilateral displaced, comminuted, intra-articular fractures (black arrows) and depression of the posterior facet (white arrows). (Reproduced from Johnson TS, Steinbach LS: *Essentials of Musculoskeletal Imaging.* Rosemont, IL, American Academy of Orthopaedic Surgeons, 2004, p 587.)

- Medial or lateral ankle ligament injury (swelling and tenderness over involved ligaments)
- Talocalcaneal dislocation (deformity of the hindfoot)

Adverse Outcomes of the Disease

The adverse outcomes of either type of fracture are potentially severe and disabling, and treatment is difficult. Fractures of the talus often interrupt the blood supply to the body of the talus and can lead to osteonecrosis. Chronic pain, posttraumatic arthritis, osteonecrosis of the talus, deformity, tarsal tunnel syndrome, complex regional pain syndrome, or plantar compartment syndrome may result from either a calcaneal or a talar fracture.

Treatment

Immediate treatment consists of splinting with a well-padded posterior splint from the toe to the upper calf. The extremity should be elevated above the level of the heart, and ice should be applied for 20 minutes every 1 to 2 hours.

  Many of these fractures with associated displacement require surgical reduction and fixation to minimize later complications. Rehabilitation to obtain range of motion of the subtalar joint is indicated after clinical healing of the fracture has occurred.

Adverse Outcomes of Treatment

Stiffness and atrophy are adverse outcomes of treatment.

Referral Decisions/Red Flags

Patients with fractures of the calcaneus or talus or a dislocation of the talocalcaneal joint need further evaluation immediately upon diagnosis.

SECTION 7 FOOT AND ANKLE

Fracture of the Metatarsals

Synonym
Forefoot fracture

Definition
Most fractures of the metatarsal bones heal with nonsurgical treatment; however, a zone 2 fracture of the proximal diaphysis of the fifth metatarsal (classic Jones fracture) requires more extensive immobilization, and a zone 3 fracture (usually a stress fracture) of this bone may result in nonunion or delayed union (**Figure 1**).

Clinical Symptoms
Swelling and pain on weight bearing are common. Stress fractures usually occur after a sudden increase in activity, such as a new training regimen (increase in intensity or distance), change in running surface, or even prolonged walking.

Tests
Physical Examination
Examination reveals swelling, ecchymosis, and tenderness over the fractured metatarsal.

Diagnostic Tests
AP, lateral, and oblique radiographs of the foot may demonstrate the fracture. A stress fracture of a metatarsal may not show up on radiographs for 2 to 3 weeks. Follow-up radiographs are necessary if a stress fracture is suspected.

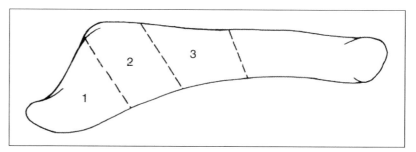

Figure 1 Illustration of the three anatomic zones at the base of the fifth metatarsal. Zone 1 includes the articular surface of the fifth metatarsocuboid joint; zone 2 encompasses the articulation of the proximal fourth and fifth metatarsals; zone 3 extends 1.5 cm distal to zone 2. (Reproduced from Dameron TB Jr: Fractures of the proximal fifth metatarsal: Selecting the best treatment option. *J Am Acad Orthop Surg* 1995;3[2]:110-114.)

Differential Diagnosis

• Interdigital (Morton) neuroma (plantar pain and tenderness between the metatarsal heads)
• Lisfranc dislocation or sprain (location at the tarsometatarsal joint)
• Lisfranc fracture (location at the tarsometatarsal joint)
• Metatarsalgia (plantar pain and tenderness over the metatarsal head)

Adverse Outcomes of the Disease

Both malunion and nonunion are possible; however, nonunion is uncommon except in association with a fracture in zone 2 or 3 of the proximal fifth metatarsal. Malunion of a metatarsal shaft or neck fracture can result in metatarsalgia with a plantar callus. Compartment syndrome may develop after severe trauma or multiple metatarsal fractures.

Treatment

Treatment of nondisplaced metatarsal neck and shaft fractures includes the use of a short leg cast, fracture brace, or wooden-soled shoe. The device that requires the minimum amount of immobilization while providing adequate comfort should be selected. Weight bearing is permitted as tolerated. In most cases, radiographs should be repeated after 1 week to identify any displacement, and again at 6 weeks to confirm healing. Tenderness at the fracture site will diminish as the fracture heals. A fracture of the first metatarsal is often the result of a high-impact injury and may require surgery (**Figure 2**).

Multiple metatarsal fractures and fractures with more than 4 mm of displacement or an apical angulation of more than 10° (seen on the lateral view) may require either closed or open reduction to reestablish a physiologic weight-bearing position of the metatarsal head.

Fractures of the proximal fifth metatarsal can be easy or difficult to manage. Avulsion fractures of the base of the fifth metatarsal (zone 1) or proximal metaphyseal fractures (zone 2) do well with nonsurgical treatment. Immobilization with an air stirrup, wooden-soled shoe, or fracture brace is continued until symptoms subside. Acute fractures in zone 2 are more difficult to treat. Most cases will heal with cast immobilization, but treatment of these injuries should start with non–weight-bearing ambulation in a short leg cast for 6 to 8 weeks. Early internal fixation may be considered for some patients, such as athletes. Fractures in zone 3 often resemble a stress fracture with prodromal symptoms suddenly exacerbated by an inversion injury. These require surgical intervention to avoid nonunion or delayed union.

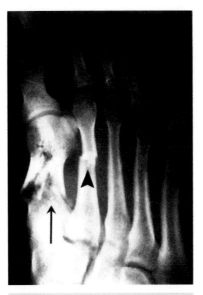

Figure 2 AP radiograph demonstrates fractures of the first metatarsal (arrow) and second metatarsal (arrowhead). (Reproduced from Shereff MJ: Fractures of the forefoot. *Instr Course Lect* 1990;39:133-140.)

Adverse Outcomes of Treatment

Malunion with painful plantar callosities under the metatarsal heads or transfer lesions under the neighboring metatarsal heads can occur if there is displacement or shortening of the metatarsal.

Referral Decisions/Red Flags

Multiple metatarsal fractures, a metatarsal fracture with more than 4 mm of displacement or more than 10° of angulation, possible compartment syndrome, and proximal fifth metatarsal fracture in zones 2 or 3 are all indications for further evaluation. Displaced or comminuted fractures of the first metatarsal also require further evaluation. Open fractures require immediate surgical intervention. Patients with a stress fracture nonunion should be evaluated for possible vitamin D deficiency or associated overloading resulting from a mechanical issue (such as heel varus causing a nonhealing fifth metatarsal fracture).

Fracture of the Phalanges

Synonym
Broken toe

Definition
A phalangeal fracture, commonly known as a broken toe, usually involves the proximal phalanx and is caused by direct trauma. These fractures rarely result in major disability. The fifth (little) toe is the most commonly affected.

Clinical Symptoms
Patients have pain, swelling, or ecchymosis.

Tests
Physical Examination
Examination can reveal deformity of the toe, but local bony tenderness, swelling, and ecchymosis are often the only principal findings.

Diagnostic Tests
Radiographs usually confirm the diagnosis (**Figure 1**).

Differential Diagnosis
- Freiberg infraction (osteonecrosis of the metatarsal head seen on radiographs)
- Ingrown toenail/paronychia (inflammation of the fold of tissue around the toenail noted on physical examination)
- Metatarsalgia (plantar tenderness over the metatarsal head)
- Metatarsophalangeal (MTP) synovitis (tenderness over the MTP joint)

Adverse Outcomes of the Disease
Chronic swelling and deformity of the toe are possible. Permanent deformity is an uncommon possibility.

Treatment
Phalangeal fractures are treated by buddy taping the fractured toe to an adjacent toe, usually the toe medial to the one fractured (**Figure 2**). A gauze pad can be placed between the toes to absorb moisture and prevent maceration of the skin from sweating. The tape and gauze should be changed as often as needed to maintain a clean, dry environment.

 Closed reduction under a digital block or open reduction and pinning is rarely necessary but should be considered in several circumstances: for markedly angulated fractures, or for fractures

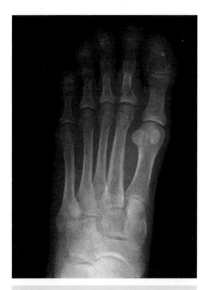

Figure 1 AP radiograph of the foot demonstrates a fracture of the proximal phalanx of the second toe.

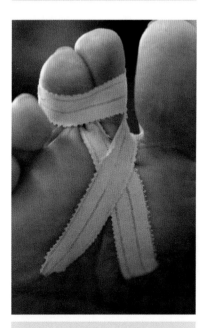

Figure 2 Photograph shows buddy taping of a fractured toe to an adjacent toe.

involving the articular surface of the MTP joints of all toes or the interphalangeal joint of the great toe.

Adverse Outcomes of Treatment

The skin can become macerated from moisture under the tape.

Referral Decisions/Red Flags

Patients with an open fracture or a displaced intra-articular fracture (especially at the MTP joint) need further evaluation.

Fracture of the Sesamoid

Definition

The first metatarsophalangeal (MTP) joint has two sesamoids, one medial and one lateral (**Figure 1**). The plantar aspect of each sesamoid is surrounded by the fibers of the flexor hallucis brevis and the plantar plate, and the dorsal aspect of the sesamoid has a facet that articulates with the metatarsal head. Because of its more protected position in the lateral soft tissues, the lateral, or fibular, sesamoid is less susceptible to fracture than is the medial sesamoid. Sesamoid fractures can occur secondary to avulsion forces, such as hyperdorsiflexion of the first MTP joint; repetitive stress; or, more commonly, from direct trauma. The repetitive stress from running or dancing can result in either a stress fracture or an avulsion fracture. Accessory sesamoids also can be found under any of the lesser metatarsal heads. The most common location is under the second metatarsal head on the tibial side. Although fractures of the sesamoids of the MTP joint (**Figure 2**) are the most common, sesamoids under any metatarsal head may fracture.

A bipartite sesamoid is a normal variant (**Figure 3**). It is important to distinguish this normal condition from a fracture.

Clinical Symptoms

Patients report pain under the first metatarsal head. Swelling and, rarely, ecchymosis may be present. The patient may have a history of direct trauma, a hyperdorsiflexion injury (resulting in an avulsion fracture), or a history of repetitive stress such as running, jumping, or dancing.

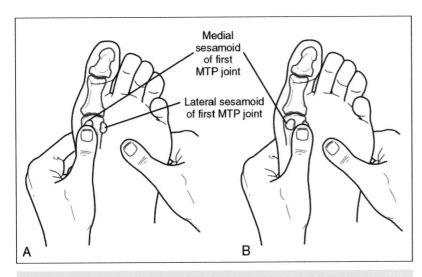

Figure 1 Illustration of the method of palpating the sesamoids of the first metatarsophalangeal (MTP) joint.

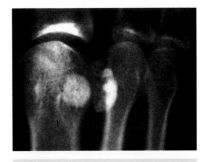

Figure 2 AP radiograph of the foot shows a fracture of the lateral sesamoid of the MTP joint.

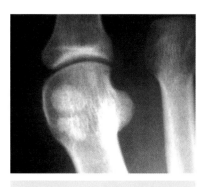

Figure 3 AP radiograph of a right foot shows a bipartite lateral sesamoid.

Tests

Physical Examination

Patients report pain localized over the fractured sesamoid. The painful spot will move with the sesamoid as the great toe is flexed and extended. The pain may increase with dorsiflexion of the first MTP joint, as tension is applied to the flexor tendon complex. Range of motion of the first MTP joint may be restricted, especially in dorsiflexion, due to pain or guarding.

Diagnostic Tests

AP, lateral, and axial views should be obtained to establish the diagnosis. The lateral sesamoid is best visualized on an internal oblique view. A technetium Tc-99m bone scan can help differentiate an acute fracture or stress fracture from a bipartite sesamoid and is considered to be 100% sensitive. A fractured sesamoid will demonstrate increased uptake on a bone scan, whereas a bipartite sesamoid will show no increased activity. MRI can help differentiate a fracture from a bipartite sesamoid or osteonecrosis. In the presence of a fracture, MRI will show marrow edema. MRI can also help evaluate the plantar plate, the intersesamoid ligament, and the flexor tendons.

Differential Diagnosis

- Bipartite sesamoid (smooth, sclerotic edges on radiographs) (negative bone scan) (may be bilateral)
- Osteonecrosis (sclerotic appearance of entire sesamoid or irregularity with fragmentation seen on radiographs)
- Plantar plate disruption (turf toe) (proximal migration of sesamoid noted on physical examination and radiographs)

Adverse Outcomes of the Disease

The patient with an untreated sesamoid fracture will usually demonstrate pain and a limp. A nonunion can occur following an acute fracture.

Treatment

The recommended treatment for an acute sesamoid fracture is a removable short leg fracture brace or a stiff-soled shoe with a rocker bottom. Usually at 4 weeks, as the symptoms improve, the patient is allowed to wear a stiff-soled shoe with a high toe box. After the fracture is clinically healed, a felt pad to suspend the metatarsal head is recommended for 6 months. If the fracture is associated with a plantar plate rupture, surgical open repair of the plantar plate with sesamoid reduction and internal fixation is indicated.

Adverse Outcomes of Treatment

Healing of this fracture can take 6 to 12 months, resulting in limited dorsiflexion of the first MTP joint.

Referral Decisions/Red Flags

Persistent pain is an indication for further evaluation. In more severe cases, the fractured sesamoid may have to be removed surgically.

Procedure: Digital Anesthetic Block (Foot)

Materials

- Sterile gloves
- Bactericidal skin preparation solution
- Ethyl chloride spray
- 10-mL syringe
- 18-gauge needle
- 25-gauge, 1½″ needle
- 10 mL of 1% lidocaine or 0.5% bupivacaine, both without epinephrine
- Adhesive dressing

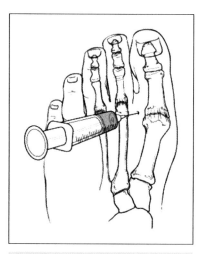

Figure 1 Illustration of the location of needle insertion for a digital anesthetic block.

Step 1
Wear protective gloves at all times during the procedure and use sterile technique.

Step 2
Use the 18-gauge needle to draw 10 mL of the local anesthetic into the syringe; then switch to the 25-gauge needle to preserve sterility.

Step 3
Cleanse the dorsal surface of the foot with bactericidal solution on either side of the metatarsal heads.

Step 4
Freeze the dorsal skin with ethyl chloride spray.

Step 5
Insert the 25-gauge needle into the soft-tissue space on either side of the metatarsal head until it just begins to tent the plantar skin (**Figure 1**). Remember that the sensory nerves travel along the plantar side of the metatarsal.

Step 6
Withdraw the needle approximately 1 cm or until the tip rests at the level of the plantar aspect of the metatarsal head.

Step 7
Inject 3 mL of anesthetic, then an additional 2 mL while the needle is withdrawn. Make certain that some of the anesthetic is deposited subcutaneously around the dorsal sensory nerves.

Step 8
Repeat the procedure on the other side of the metatarsal of the toe that is to be anesthetized. Within 1 to 2 minutes, the involved toe should become numb.

Step 9
Dress the puncture site with a sterile adhesive dressing.

Adverse Outcomes

Although rare, infection is possible. Necrosis of a digit is possible if epinephrine is used in the anesthetic solution.

Aftercare/Patient Instructions

Advise the patient that a collection of fluid on the plantar aspect of the foot may appear but that the fluid will dissipate within several hours after the block.

Hallux Rigidus

Synonyms
Great toe arthritis
Hallux limitus
Metatarsus primus elevatus

Definition
Hallux rigidus, or degenerative arthritis of the metatarsophalangeal (MTP) joint of the great toe, is the most common manifestation of arthritis in the foot. The principal symptoms are pain and stiffness, especially as the toe moves into dorsiflexion. Hallux rigidus is the second most common malady of the great toe behind hallux valgus and is the most common arthritis of the foot.

Clinical Symptoms
Patients have pain in the great toe joint with activity, especially in the toe-off phase of gait as the MTP joint goes into extension. The osteophytes start to develop on the lateral side of the joint but are more pronounced on the dorsum of the toe and may cause the overlying soft tissue to become red and irritated with shoe wear (**Figure 1**). The dorsal sensory nerves of the great toe may be irritated by the associated swelling.

Tests
Physical Examination
Stiffness of the great toe with loss of extension at the MTP joint is the hallmark of hallux rigidus. Osteophytes develop primarily on the dorsal portion of the first metatarsal head (**Figure 2**). The toe is usually in normal alignment, unless the patient has had hallux valgus

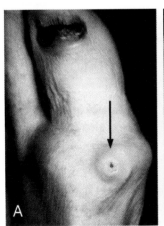 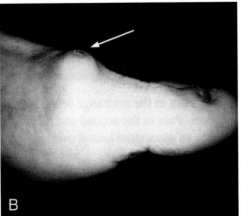

Figure 1 Photographs show a foot with dorsal prominence from an underlying bony osteophyte (arrow). **A,** Top view. **B,** Lateral view. (Reproduced from Mann RA: Hallux rigidus. *Instr Course Lect* 1990;39:15-21.)

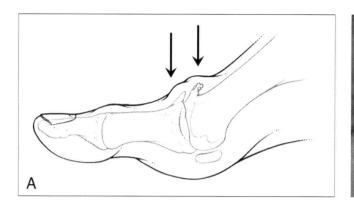 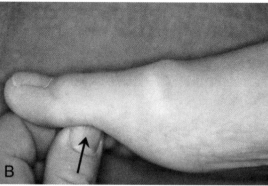

Figure 2 **A,** Illustration of hallux rigidus osteophytes (arrows). **B,** Clinical photograph of loss of extension, which is the hallmark of this condition. (Part B reproduced from Alexander IJ: *The Foot: Examination and Diagnosis.* New York, NY, Churchill Livingstone, 1990, p 65.)

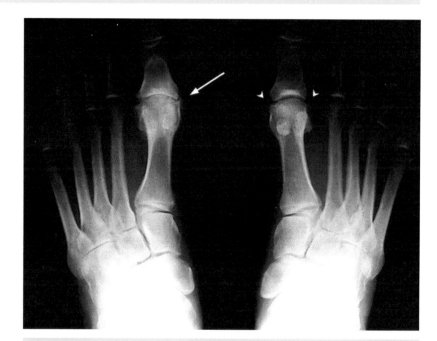

Figure 3 Weight-bearing AP radiograph of the feet of a patient with hallux rigidus. Note the advanced arthritic changes (white arrow) in the left foot and the small medial and lateral spurs (white arrowheads) in the right foot.

before. Pain in the midrange of the motion arc indicates a more severe problem. Pain in the second and third MTP joints is also common if there is an associated lateral overload.

Diagnostic Tests

AP and lateral radiographs show narrowing of the MTP joint of the great toe and osteophytes, predominantly on the dorsal and lateral aspects of the great toe (**Figure 3**).

Differential Diagnosis

- Gout (recurrent episode of erythema and swelling, positive clinical history)
- Hallux valgus (bunion and valgus angulation of the great toe)
- Turf toe (history of injury, pain on the plantar aspect of MTP joint exacerbated by extension of the toe)
- Sesamoiditis or sesamoid osteonecrosis (pain on the plantar side of the joint over the sesamoids without involving the MTP joint line)

Adverse Outcomes of the Disease

Pain aggravated by walking is common. Weight is transferred to the lateral side of the foot, especially during toe-off, causing increased stress and overuse on the lateral side of the foot.

Treatment

Nonsurgical treatment consists of wearing a shoe with a large, soft toe box to decrease pressure on the toe. A stiff-soled shoe modified with a steel shank or rocker bottom limits dorsiflexion of the great toe and decreases pain caused by motion in the arthritic joint. An off-the-shelf or custom-made Morton extension that limits motion of the first MTP joint can also be helpful. Patients should be advised to avoid wearing high-heeled shoes. NSAIDs, ice, and contrast baths also can help decrease inflammation and control symptoms for a short time.

Surgical treatment consists of either excision of the dorsal osteophytes with oblique osteotomy (cheilectomy) or fusion of the joint (arthrodesis). Resection of the joint (Keller procedure) should be reserved for older and lower-demand patients. An artificial joint implant is not recommended.

Adverse Outcomes of Treatment

NSAIDs can cause gastric, renal, or hepatic complications. In 2015, the FDA strengthened its warning linking NSAIDs with the risk of heart attack or stroke, even in the first weeks of use of an NSAID. No other adverse outcomes of treatment have been reported, other than the usual surgical complications.

Referral Decisions/Red Flags

Failure of nonsurgical treatment is an indication for further evaluation.

Hallux Valgus

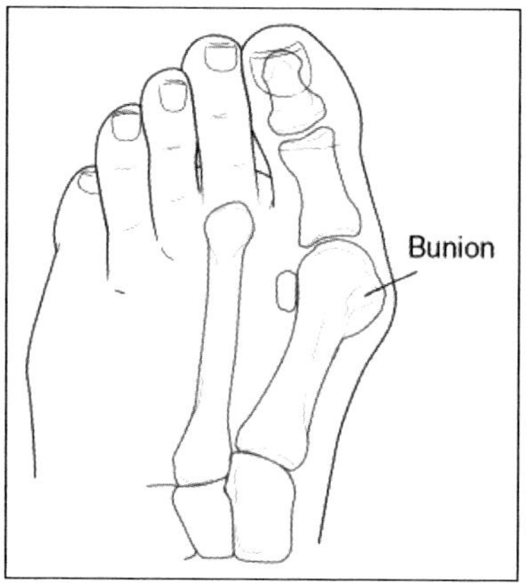

Synonyms

Bunion
Metatarsus primus varus

Definition

Hallux valgus is lateral deviation of the great toe at the metatarsophalangeal (MTP) joint that may lead to a painful prominence of the medial aspect of the first metatarsal head, known as a bunion (**Figure 1**). The female-to-male ratio of symptomatic hallux valgus occurrence is approximately 10:1.

Clinical Symptoms

Pain and swelling, aggravated by shoe wear, are the principal symptoms. A hypertrophic bursa can occur over the medial eminence of the first metatarsal. The great toe may pronate (rotate inward), with resultant callus on the medial aspect. Irritation of the medial plantar sensory nerve can cause numbness or tingling over the medial aspect of the great toe.

Tests

Physical Examination

Assess the valgus angulation at the MTP joint (normal valgus at the MTP joint is < 15°). Measure the range of motion at the MTP joint. Most patients with hallux valgus have relatively normal MTP motion (60° to 90° of extension and 30° of flexion). Evaluate the lesser toes for associated deformities. A second toe that overrides the laterally deviated great toe is a common problem (**Figure 2**). Other lesser toe problems include corns, calluses, hammer toes, and bunionettes (bunion-like prominences on the lateral side of the fifth MTP joint). Assess motion of the affected first tarsometatarsal and compare it with the unaffected, opposite foot. Excessive motion is usually an indication of hypermobility. Assess other joints of the body for generalized hyperelasticity of the joints.

Diagnostic Tests

The severity of a bunion deformity is graded by measuring certain forefoot angles on weight-bearing AP radiographs of the foot. The hallux valgus angle is measured between the first metatarsal and the proximal phalanx. Normal is less than 15°. A normal 1-2 intermetatarsal (IM) angle formed between the first and second metatarsals is less than 10° (**Figure 3**). Radiographs also are used to assess lateral subluxation of the sesamoids, the shape of the metatarsal head, degenerative changes in the MTP joint, valgus at the interphalangeal (IP) joint, and lesser toe abnormalities. A weight-bearing lateral radiograph of the foot is less helpful but is important

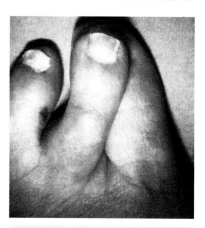

Figure 1   Illustration of anatomy of hallux valgus.

Bunion

Figure 2   Photograph shows severe hallux valgus with dislocation of the second toe.

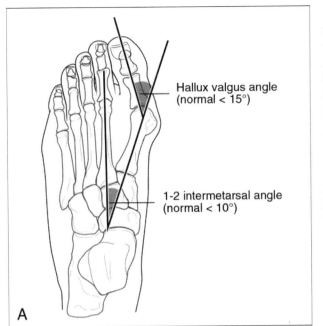
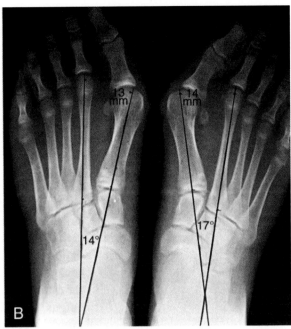

Figure 3 Hallux valgus severity is assessed by measuring the hallux valgus angle and the intermetatarsal (IM) angle on a weight-bearing AP radiograph of the foot. **A,** Diagram shows the hallux valgus angle and the IM angle. **B,** AP radiograph of the feet of a patient with hallux valgus demonstrates valgus angulation of 14° in the left foot and 17° in the right foot.

for evaluating any lesser toe subluxation or arthritic changes of the great toe MTP joint.

Differential Diagnosis

- Gout (articular and periarticular inflammation and tenderness on physical examination)
- Hallux extensus (cock-up toe, or extension of the great toe) (seen on physical examination)
- Hallux interphalangeus (lateral deviation of the great toe at the IP joint) (seen on physical examination or radiographs)
- Hallux rigidus (osteoarthritis of the first MTP joint) (limited dorsiflexion of the great toe)
- Hallux varus (medial deviation of the great toe at the MTP joint seen on physical examination)

Adverse Outcomes of the Disease
Chronic pain is the primary symptom.

Treatment
When bunions occur in children, they are generally managed with observation rather than surgery because surgical intervention frequently results in recurrence with continuing growth. In adults, the initial treatment is patient education and shoe wear modifications. Nonsurgical treatment is usually successful in mild to moderate

SECTION 7   FOOT AND ANKLE

cases. Recommended shoes have adequate width at the forefoot, soft uppers, and no stitching patterns over the bunion. An orthotist or skilled shoemaker can stretch the shoe directly over the bunion. High heels increase the pressure under the ball of the foot and over the bunion deformity and therefore should be avoided. Rehabilitation, splints, and bracing are not helpful, although a medial longitudinal arch support can decrease pressure on a bunion associated with a pronated flatfoot.

The first question to ask the patient when determining whether treatment of hallux valgus is needed is if he or she has pain. No treatment is needed for asymptomatic hallux valgus, even if the deformity continues to progress. Competitive athletes should avoid surgical correction of hallux valgus deformities until after their competitive careers are over, as surgery can affect performance. For patients who have continued disability despite nonsurgical treatment, several well-established surgical procedures are available. Indications for different procedures are based on the severity of the hallux valgus, the IM angle, and joint congruity. Joint arthroplasty should be avoided because of the high complication rate.

Adverse Outcomes of Treatment
Surgical treatment can result in recurrence, undercorrection, overcorrection (hallux varus), decreased function, stiffness, pain, malunion or nonunion of an osteotomy, and transfer lesions (metatarsalgia).

Referral Decisions/Red Flags
Persistent pain despite shoe modifications indicates the need for further evaluation. Patients with persistent pain may benefit from surgical correction.

Ingrown Toenail

Synonyms
Infected toenail
Onychocryptosis
Paronychia

Definition
With an ingrown toenail, the distal margin of the nail grows into the adjacent skin, causing irritation, inflammation, and possibly secondary bacterial or fungal infection. The condition is mostly limited to the great toe. Ingrown toenails are associated with improper trimming of the toenail, tight shoes, hereditary predisposition, subungual pathology, congenital incurved nail, thickened nail, direct trauma, or any combination of these factors (**Figure 1**).

Unlike fingernails, toenails should not be cut in a curved fashion because this allows the sharp edge of the nail to grow into the more prominent skin margins (nail fold) found at the end of toenails. Properly trimmed toenails are cut straight across to keep the lateral margin of the toenail beyond the nail fold. Some people have toenails that have a naturally incurved shape. Ingrown toenails can occur in these patients even with proper trimming techniques. Soft-tissue hypertrophy over a normal nail plate secondary to trauma or tight shoes also can cause an ingrown toenail. Skin breakthrough creates a portal of entry for a secondary bacterial or fungal infection.

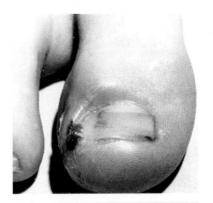

Figure 1 Photograph shows an ingrown toenail. (Reproduced from Lutter LD, Mizel MS, Pfeffer GB, eds: *Orthopaedic Knowledge Update: Foot and Ankle*. Rosemont, IL, American Academy of Orthopaedic Surgeons, 1994, p 54.)

Clinical Symptoms
Stage I (inflammation) is characterized by induration, swelling, and tenderness along the nail fold. In stage II (abscess), the patient has purulent or serous drainage, increased tenderness, and increased erythema. In stage III (granulation), granulation tissue grows onto the nail plate, inhibiting drainage. This stage is less painful than stage II.

Tests
Physical Examination
The diagnosis is clinical; visual inspection is the basis for staging the condition.

Diagnostic Tests
Radiographs of stage II and stage III ingrown toenails can be obtained to rule out a subungual exostosis (cartilage-capped projection from bone) and osteomyelitis.

Differential Diagnosis
• Felon (deep abscess on the plantar aspect of the toe)
• Onychomycosis (fungal infection of the nail)
• Osteomyelitis (bone infection with changes on radiograph)

- Paronychia (superficial abscess on the base of the toenail)
- Subungual exostosis (osteochondroma beneath the nail, noted radiographically)

Adverse Outcomes of the Disease

Progressive pain, paronychia, felon, nail plate deformity, and osteomyelitis are all possible. Hematogenous seeding of other organs can occur but is very uncommon.

Treatment

- Stage I: Warm soaks, proper nail trimming, accommodative shoe wear, and clean socks are recommended. With a blunt instrument, insert cotton or waxed dental floss beneath the nail to lift the edge of the nail from its embedded position. Exchange packing daily until the nail has grown out sufficiently. Nonconstrictive shoes or sandals prevent extrinsic irritation of the inflamed skin.
- Stage II: Initial treatment should include foot soaks along with broad-spectrum oral antibiotics (cephalosporin). Partial excision of the nail under digital block should be performed when the patient has severe pain, when there is a risk of secondary infection to a prosthetic joint, or when a course of oral antibiotics fails to treat associated infection. Partial nail excision is preferred. Complete nail excision increases the risk of deformity of the nail bed, resulting in clubbing. An avulsed nail requires 3 to 4 months to regrow. Spring coil application to the sides of the nail has been described; this method applies continuous elevation force to the sides of the nail. It is most commonly used in Europe and Japan. These springs can be attached to the nail under local anesthesia or can be glued to the nail. They usually remain in place for approximately 2 to 3 months and have been shown to decrease or reverse the curving or clubbing of the sides of the nail, which could result in a permanent cure.
- Stage III: Partial or complete nail plate excision with or without ablation of the germinal matrix of the nail is indicated.

Adverse Outcomes of Treatment

Adverse outcomes include recurrence (50% to 70% with excision alone), nail plate deformity, upturned nail or clubbed nail after complete nail plate excision, and poor cosmetic result.

Referral Decisions/Red Flags

Failure of nonsurgical treatment or the presence of stage III disease is an indication for further evaluation.

Procedure: Nail Plate Avulsion

Anatomy

A recurrent ingrown toenail or paronychial infection, which usually occurs in the great toe, makes it necessary to remove a portion of the nail plate. The lateral and/or medial margins of the nail may be involved.

Removal of the entire nail plate is described here. Because this risks nail bed deformity, however, partial removal should be performed whenever possible. Partial removal involves elevating one third of the nail on the affected (lateral or medial) side with a small scissors or hemostat, cutting the nail longitudinally with strong small scissors or an anvil nail cutter, and avulsing the freed portion of the nail adjacent to the nail fold.

Step 1
Wear protective gloves at all times during the procedure, and use sterile technique.

Step 2
Cleanse the toe with a bactericidal solution.

Step 3
Follow the steps in the procedure titled Digital Anesthetic Block (Foot) to administer a digital block.

Step 4
Wrap a ¼" Penrose drain or strip of rubber around the base of the toe to act as a tourniquet and control bleeding (optional).

Step 5
Using a small scissors or hemostat, elevate the nail plate from the underlying nail bed (**Figure 1**).

Step 6
Separate the proximal cuticle (nail fold) from the nail plate.

Step 7
Grasp the free portion of the nail plate with a hemostat and avulse it (**Figure 2**), then palpate the nail bed to ensure that no spikes of nail tissue remain.

Step 8
If a tourniquet was used, remove it and apply compression to stop local bleeding.

Step 9
Apply nonadherent sterile gauze over the exposed nail bed and wrap the entire toe with a sterile dressing.

Materials

- Sterile gloves
- Bactericidal skin preparation solution
- ¼" Penrose drain or a strip cut from a rubber glove (optional)
- Materials to administer a digital block (ethyl chloride spray; 10-mL syringe; 18-gauge needle; 25-gauge, 1½" needle; 10 mL of 1% lidocaine or 0.5% bupivacaine, both without epinephrine; adhesive dressing)
- Strong small scissors or anvil nail cutter
- Small hemostat
- Nonadherent sterile gauze
- Sterile dressing material

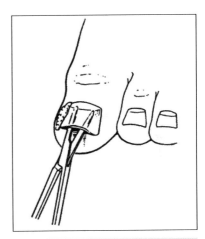

Figure 1 Illustration of nail plate avulsion: elevating the nail plate from the nail bed.

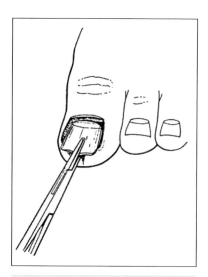

Figure 2 Illustration of nail plate avulsion: avulsing the nail plate.

Adverse Outcomes

Recurrence of the ingrown toenail is common after nail plate avulsions. Permanent ablation of the nail matrix may be required.

Permanent Ablation

This procedure may be necessary and can be performed by curettage and/or phenol ablation of the nail matrix.

Interdigital (Morton) Neuroma

Synonyms
Intermetatarsal neuroma
Morton neuroma
Plantar neuroma

Definition
A plantar interdigital neuroma, also referred to as a Morton neuroma, is not a true neuroma but rather a perineural fibrosis of the common digital nerve as it passes between the metatarsal heads. The fibrosis is secondary to repetitive irritation of the nerve. The condition most commonly occurs between the third and fourth toes (third web space) (**Figure 1**). Interdigital neuromas occur less frequently in the second web space (between the second and third toes) and rarely in either the first or fourth intermetatarsal space. The simultaneous occurrence of two neuromas is extremely uncommon. Interdigital neuroma has a female-to-male ratio of 5:1, probably related to compression of the nerve by tight shoes.

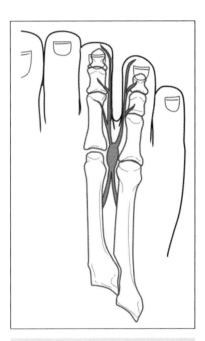

Figure 1 Illustration of interdigital neuroma between the metatarsal heads.

Clinical Symptoms
Plantar pain in the forefoot is the most common presenting symptom. Dysesthesias into the affected two toes or burning plantar pain that is aggravated by activity also is common. Occasionally, patients report numbness in the toes adjacent to the involved web space. Night pain is rare. Many patients state that they feel as though they are "walking on a marble" or that there is "a wrinkle in my sock." Relief often is obtained by removing the shoe and rubbing the ball of the foot. Symptoms are aggravated by wearing high-heeled or tight, restrictive shoes.

Tests
Physical Examination
Isolated pain on the plantar aspect of the web space is consistent with an interdigital neuroma. Apply direct plantar pressure to the interspace with one hand and then squeeze the metatarsals together with the other hand (compression test). If an interdigital neuroma is present, this maneuver will cause increased tenderness and pain radiating to the toes. The Mulder sign is considered positive if the examiner feels a click or grinding sensation of the metatarsal heads during lateral squeeze.

Inspect the plantar surface for calluses. Then palpate dorsally along the metatarsal shafts and plantarly over the metatarsal heads to evaluate for stress fractures or metatarsalgia, respectively. Evaluate sensory function of the digital nerves. Stress each tarsometatarsal joint by grasping the midfoot with one hand and moving each metatarsal dorsally and then plantarly (piano key test) to rule out midfoot arthritis. Similarly, grasp the metatarsal shaft and, while keeping the toe parallel to the metatarsal, try to displace the digit dorsally, then plantarly. Pain or excess motion with this maneuver indicates synovitis or inflammation of the metatarsophalangeal (MTP) joint.

Diagnostic Tests
Radiographs are normal in patients with interdigital neuroma. MRI and ultrasonography sometimes detect neuromas, but these modalities are unreliable for this purpose and their use is not commonly indicated.

Differential Diagnosis
- Hammer toe (flexion deformity of the proximal interphalangeal joint noted on physical examination)
- Metatarsalgia (plantar tenderness over the metatarsal head noted on physical examination)
- MTP synovitis (tenderness and swelling directly over the MTP joint noted on physical examination)
- Stress fracture (dorsal metatarsal tenderness noted on physical examination)

Adverse Outcomes of the Disease
Chronic, intermittent pain and the need for shoe and activity modifications are possible.

Treatment
Patients should be advised to wear a low-heeled, well-cushioned shoe with a wide toe box. A well-cushioned sandal is another option. In addition, pain relief may be obtained using metatarsal pads to spread the metatarsal heads and take pressure off the nerve.

Locate the neuroma on the plantar aspect of the foot in the soft tissue between the involved metatarsal heads. Ask the patient to mark the painful spot on the bottom of the foot with a material that transfers easily, such as lipstick or eyeliner. Instruct the patient to stand, without socks, in a shoe to transfer the mark to the inside of the shoe. Place the pad in the shoe just proximal to the mark, to suspend the painful area. This also ensures that the metatarsal heads are kept apart and away from the neuroma when the patient is bearing weight. Felt or gel pads are inexpensive and effective. They come in different sizes to accommodate shoes and feet of different sizes. Advise the patient that, if the pad is effective, a more permanent orthosis can be fabricated that can be transferred from shoe to shoe. Avoid using a rigid orthosis, as it can aggravate the neuroma.

A mixture of 1 to 2 mL of lidocaine without epinephrine and 1 mL (10 mg/mL) of corticosteroid injected just proximal to the metatarsal heads can be both diagnostic and therapeutic. Multiple injections should be avoided.

If symptoms persist or recur, surgical excision of the neuroma or release of the plantar nerve by division of the transverse metatarsal ligament is indicated.

Adverse Outcomes of Treatment
Symptoms may persist or recur after nonsurgical treatment. Symptoms may recur or become worse after surgical excision of the neuroma if a painful stump of nerve develops.

Referral Decisions/Red Flags
Persistent pain despite shoe or insert modifications or injection of corticosteroid indicates the need for further evaluation.

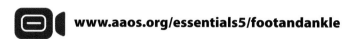
Procedure: Interdigital (Morton) Neuroma Injection

Materials

- Sterile gloves
- Bactericidal skin preparation solution
- Ethyl chloride spray
- 5-mL syringe
- 18- and 21-gauge needle
- 2 mL of 10 mg/mL corticosteroid preparation
- 2 mL of 1.0% lidocaine or 0.5% bupivacaine, both without epinephrine
- Adhesive dressing

Step 1

Wear protective gloves at all times during the procedure and use sterile technique.

Step 2

Use the 18-gauge needle to draw 2 mL of the 10 mg/mL corticosteroid preparation and 2 mL of the local anesthetic into the syringe; then switch to the 21-gauge needle to preserve sterility.

Step 3

Cleanse the dorsal skin between the metatarsal heads with bactericidal solution.

Step 4

Freeze the dorsal skin with ethyl chloride spray.

Step 5

Place the needle in line with the metatarsophalangeal joint, which is approximately 1 to 2 cm proximal to the web of the toe (**Figure 1**).

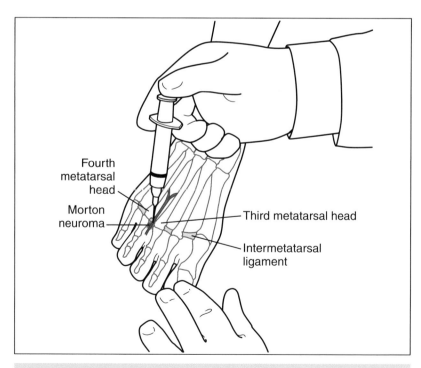

Figure 1 Illustration of the proper location for injection for interdigital (Morton) neuroma.

Step 6
Insert the needle through the dorsal tissues until the tip barely tents the skin of the plantar aspect of the foot. Withdraw the needle approximately 1 cm so that the tip is where the neuroma is found, at the level of the plantar metatarsophalangeal joint.

Step 7
Inject the corticosteroid-anesthetic mixture around the neuroma, taking care not to inject into the plantar fat pad.

Alternative Injection Location
Alternatively, the same injection can be done from the interdigital area, aiming toward the affected web space.

Metatarsalgia

Synonym
Forefoot pain

Definition
Metatarsalgia is a general term indicating forefoot pain localized under one or more of the lesser metatarsals. Abnormal metatarsal length with alteration of weight-bearing forces is one cause of metatarsalgia. Toe deformities such as claw or hammer toe also can lead to metatarsalgia by causing displacement of the plantar fat pad and loss of cushioning under the metatarsal heads. Atrophy of the metatarsal fat pad, which occurs with increasing age, contributes to the pain. Callus formation occurs, and this thickened skin may be a major component of the patient's symptoms. A persistent callus on the sole of the foot is called intractable plantar keratosis.

Clinical Symptoms
Activity-related pain is localized to the plantar aspect of the forefoot directly over the metatarsal heads. The patient may complain about the diffuse callus formation. Patients usually indicate that they feel as though they are walking on pebbles.

Tests
Physical Examination
Observe the alignment of the toes. Evaluate swelling, range of motion, and stability of the metatarsophalangeal (MTP) joints. Palpate for swelling or masses along the plantar and dorsal aspects of the metatarsals as well as adjacent interspaces. Note the extent of any callus and whether it is discrete or diffuse. A discrete callus is tender with direct pressure. Evaluate digital nerve function. A callus that presents in a line formation usually indicates overload of the metatarsal head.

Diagnostic Tests
Weight-bearing AP and lateral radiographs of the foot should be obtained to assess metatarsal and toe alignment. The anterior drawer test (shock test) is usually positive if there is associated MTP joint instability or plantar plate tear.

Differential Diagnosis
- Claw toe–related pain (plantar displacement of the metatarsal heads and fat pad noted on physical examination)
- Interdigital neuroma (numbness in the involved web space)
- Intractable plantar keratosis (persistent callus on sole of foot)
- Metatarsal stress fracture (localized tenderness over the fracture site, radiographic findings)

Essentials of Musculoskeletal Care 5

- MTP synovitis (swelling of the joint, dorsal tenderness)
- Plantar wart (tender with circumferential pressure)
- Diffuse callus formation with or without callus on the heel (usually indicates a dermatologic condition rather than an orthopaedic problem)

Adverse Outcomes of the Disease
Patients may experience progressive pain and difficulty walking.

Treatment
Accommodative shoes, a metatarsal pad, or an orthotic device is the key to treatment. A thickened callus can be shaved. Nonsurgical treatment usually is successful, but if these measures fail, surgery to realign the toes and/or metatarsal head can be considered. Removal of the metatarsal head should be avoided. A localized callus under a metatarsal head can be treated with plantar condylectomy. Plantar plate repair has been shown to be effective if metatarsalgia is associated with plantar plate rupture.

Adverse Outcomes of Treatment
Inadequate pain relief, delayed union, nonunion, transfer lesions (stress with resultant pain transferred to the adjacent metatarsal), stiffness of the MTP joint, and cock-up toe deformity (also called floating toe) are possible complications of surgical treatment.

Referral Decisions/Red Flags
Symptoms that persist despite nonsurgical care indicate the need for further evaluation.

Nail Fungus Infection

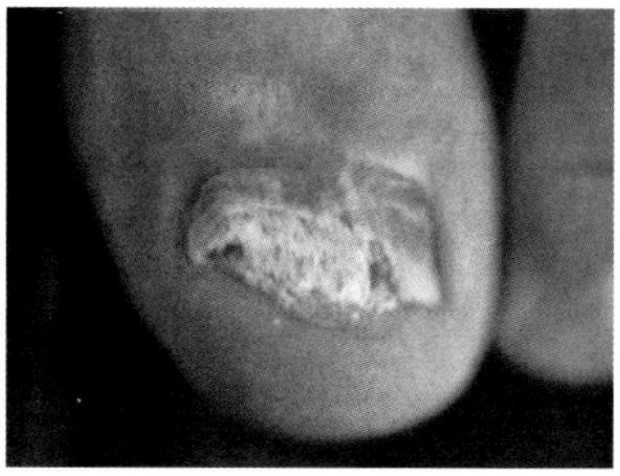

Figure 1 Photograph of a toenail with fungal infection.

Synonyms

Dermatophytic onychomycosis

Tinea ungulum

Definition

Fungal infection of the nail (onychomycosis) occurs four times more frequently in the toes than in the fingers. *Trichophyton rubrum* and *Trichophyton mentagrophytes* cause 90% of these infections. Approximately 50% of patients are older than 70 years. The problem can be primarily cosmetic, or the nail may become so hypertrophic that it interferes with shoe wear and is painful.

Clinical Symptoms

Patients report discoloration, thickening, and difficulty trimming the nails.

Tests

Physical Examination

Thickening and chalky yellow or white discoloration of the nail is observed (**Figure 1**).

Diagnostic Tests

Diagnosis is made by microscopic examination of nail scrapings and potassium hydroxide slide preparation.

Differential Diagnosis

- Onychogryphosis (severe nail deformity, curling at the edge of the nail)
- Repetitive trauma (ridges and cracking of the nail with thickening)

Adverse Outcomes of the Disease

A thickened nail can make shoe wear difficult.

Treatment

Treatment options include observation with periodic trimming of the thickened nail, removal of the nail, and/or medications. Topical medications are less effective than oral agents because topical medications cannot penetrate the thickened nail. Oral agents such as itraconazole, fluconazole, ketoconazole, and terbinafine have been shown to be effective in the treatment of onychomycosis. For example, itraconazole 200 mg per day given continuously or as a pulse dose (200 mg twice daily for 1 week per month for 3 consecutive months) has been reported to achieve a mycologic cure of 64% at 12 months, with 88% of patients showing marked improvement. Elderly patients with reduced mobility must be seen by a podiatrist for planned nail care to avoid further problems.

Adverse Outcomes of Treatment

Oral therapy is costly and can elevate hepatic enzyme levels. These levels should be tested periodically (especially in patients with a history of hepatic dysfunction). Rare cases of hepatobiliary dysfunction have been reported.

Essentials of Musculoskeletal Care 5

Orthotic Devices

Definition

Proper shoe fit, shoe modifications, inserts, pads, and orthoses can substantially relieve symptoms caused by common foot problems. An orthosis can support an area of collapse, cushion an area of pressure, accommodate fixed deformity, limit motion, equalize limb length, and reduce shear of the foot in the shoe. The appropriate use of shoe orthoses, commonly referred to as orthotics, depends on an adequate physical examination and a basic understanding of foot alignment and functions. For a fixed deformity or problem, an accommodative orthosis is used. If the deformity is flexible or correctable, a corrective orthosis is used.

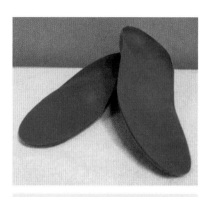

Figure 1 Photograph of custom orthoses.

Foot Types and Functions

During gait, the normal foot changes from a supple, shock-absorbing structure to a rigid lever for push-off. At heel strike, the foot is supple, allowing shock absorption and accommodations to uneven ground. During midstance, the foot is converted to a rigid lever that supports full body weight while allowing continued progression of the limb (rollover).

A cavus (highly arched) foot is rigid, cannot unlock during early stance, and lacks shock absorption. A pes planus (flatfoot) foot is extremely supple and often does not supinate effectively to form a rigid lever for push-off.

Many types of simple off-the-shelf orthotic devices can be dispensed directly from the physician's office or are available at drugstores, sporting goods stores, and shoe stores. Custom orthoses (**Figure 1**) should be prescribed by a physician and made by a certified orthotist; these orthoses are used for more complex problems or after off-the-shelf devices fail to correct the problem.

Types of Orthotic Devices

Pads/Inserts

1. Full-contact (full-length) insert: A prefabricated rubber or silicone insert that reduces shock by absorbing normal and shear forces.
2. Full-contact orthosis: An orthosis that is molded to the shape of the patient's foot. These are often posted with a wedge that redistributes weight to improve foot alignment and biomechanics, accommodate a deformity, and/or cushion the foot.
3. Soft orthosis: An orthosis that is used primarily for cushioning but offers little control of foot motion.
4. Semirigid orthosis: The most common type of orthosis; it provides reasonable strength and durability and is made to help control alignment of the foot during gait.
5. Rigid orthosis: An orthosis that offers maximum durability and support but requires a precise fit because it provides little flexibility.

6. Heel insert (such as felt, foam, gel, rubber, or silicone): Prefabricated, shock-absorbing device available over the counter (**Figure 2**).
7. Heel wedge: A device that is tapered to support varus or valgus hindfoot.
8. Scaphoid pad (arch cookie): A medial longitudinal arch pad that provides support for a flatfoot.
9. Metatarsal pad: A pad that is fixed to an insert or the bottom of the shoe (**Figure 3**).
10. Toe crest: An insert that elevates a toe to relieve pressure at the tip (for mallet toe).
11. Toe separator: A pad that is placed between toes to decrease friction. It is used for calluses and corns.
12. UCBL (University of California Biomechanics Laboratory) orthosis: A type of full-contact orthosis that stabilizes the hindfoot by using medial and lateral vertical supports (**Figure 4**). Custom molded by a certified pedorthotist, this is used for subtalar arthrosis, midfoot plantar fasciitis, or a moderate pes planovalgus foot.

Shoes/Modifications

1. Extra-depth shoe: A shoe with increased depth that accommodates forefoot problems, such as a hammer toe, and allows room for inserts.
2. Shoe lift: A device that partially or fully corrects limb-length discrepancy. Typically, ¼″ of lift can be accommodated inside the shoe. Any elevation of ½″ or more must be added to the outside of the shoe.
3. Metatarsal bar: An internal or external transverse bar that unloads the forefoot (for metatarsalgia).
4. Rocker-bottom sole: Sole of shoe that is contoured to simulate the rollover phase of gait and therefore reduce forces on the plantar surface of the foot during walking (**Figure 5**).
5. Solid ankle–cushion heel (SACH): Soft material that replaces the posterior portion of the shoe's heel to reduce shock at heel strike.
6. Running shoes: Shoes that are designed for shock absorbency. Typically, 50% of shock absorbency is lost at 300 to 500 miles, so running shoes should be replaced at least every 6 months.
7. Shoe fit: Measure the foot by tracing the width of the forefoot while standing barefoot. The forefoot width of the shoe should be wider than this measurement. The end of the longest toe should be approximately ½″ from the end of the shoe.
8. Thomas heel: Medial extension of the heel to support flatfoot.

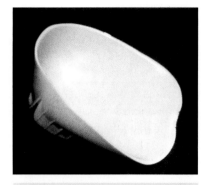

Figure 2 Photograph of a heel insert.

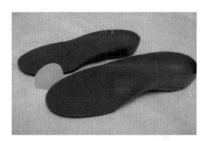

Figure 3 Photograph of custom orthoses and metatarsal pad.

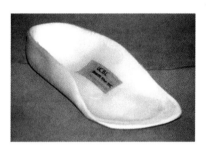

Figure 4 Photograph of the University of California Biomechanics Laboratory orthosis.

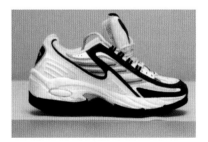

Figure 5 Photograph of an over-the-counter shoe with a rocker-bottom sole.

SECTION 7 FOOT AND ANKLE

Table 1

Recommended Orthotic Treatment for Specific Diagnoses

Diagnosis	Orthotic Therapy
Bunions and/or bunionettes	Wide toe box, stretch shoes, soft seamless uppers, "bunion shield" type pad
Cavus foot (rigid)	Soft orthotic accommodative cushions to distribute pressures evenly
Flatfoot (adult)	Asymptomatic: No special orthotic or shoe treatment indicated
	Symptomatic: Semiflexible insert or longitudinal arch pad, medial heel wedge, extended medial heel counter
Flatfoot (child)	No special orthotic or shoe treatment indicated; normal in infancy, with more than 97% correcting spontaneously
Hallux rigidus	Full-length prefabricated stiff insert, Morton extension inlay, rocker-bottom sole, stiff (stable) midsole
Hammer toe or claw toe	Accommodative shoe wear, toe crest
Interdigital (Morton) neuroma	Wide toe box, metatarsal pad with neuroma positioning
Metatarsalgia	Wide shoes, metatarsal pads, metatarsal bars, or rocker-bottom sole; wide toe box, metatarsal pad with neuroma positioning
Neuropathic ulceration	Full-contact cushioned orthosis, extra-depth or custom shoes, rocker-bottom sole to unload forefoot
Plantar fasciitis	Prefabricated heel insert and medial longitudinal arch support (silicone, rubber, or felt) if associated with pes planus

Application of Orthotic Devices and Shoe Modifications

The types of orthotic therapy recommended for specific foot conditions are listed in **Table 1**.

Plantar Fasciitis

Synonyms

Heel pain syndrome
Heel spur
Plantar heel pain

Definition

The plantar fascia arises from the medial tuberosity of the calcaneus and extends to the proximal phalanges of the toes (**Figure 1**). The plantar fascia provides support to the foot, and as the toes extend during the stance phase of gait, the plantar fascia is tightened by a windlass mechanism, resulting in elevation of the longitudinal arch, inversion of the hindfoot, and a resultant external rotation of the leg.

Plantar fasciitis is the most common cause of heel pain in adults. The etiology is probably a degenerative tear of part of the fascial origin from the calcaneus, followed by a tendinosis-type reaction. Chronic degenerative changes in the fibers of the plantar fascia are the predominant histologic finding. Plantar fasciitis affects women twice as often as men and is more common in overweight persons. It is not associated with a particular foot type.

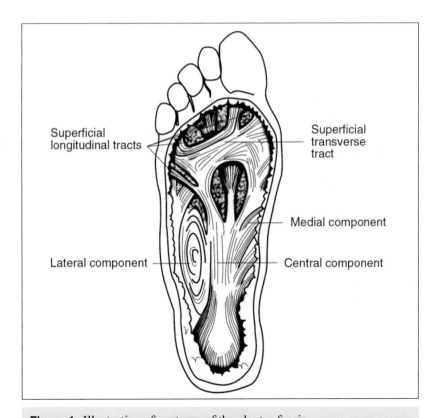

Figure 1 Illustration of anatomy of the plantar fascia.

Clinical Symptoms

Onset of symptoms is usually insidious and not related to a fall or twisting injury. Patients report focal pain and tenderness directly over the medial calcaneal tuberosity and 1 to 2 cm distally along the plantar fascia. Pain is usually most intense when the patient rises from a resting position, especially in the morning. This occurs because the foot is usually in plantar flexion during rest and the first few steps stretch the plantar fascia. Prolonged standing and walking also increase the pain. Sitting typically relieves symptoms.

Tests

Physical Examination

Examination reveals tenderness directly over the plantarmedial calcaneal tuberosity and 1 to 2 cm distally along the plantar fascia. Often, considerable pressure must be applied to this area during the examination to reproduce weight-bearing stress and the patient's symptoms. Patients may have tightness in the Achilles tendon. Passive dorsiflexion of the toes (windlass mechanism) can cause increased pain.

Diagnostic Tests

Radiographs are not necessary as part of the initial evaluation if the patient's history and examination are consistent with a diagnosis of plantar fasciitis. Weight-bearing lateral radiographs should be obtained before an injection of corticosteroid or for patients who continue to have symptoms after 6 to 8 weeks of nonsurgical treatment. Weight-bearing lateral radiographs also may be indicated for patients with systemic symptoms or pain at rest.

A heel spur (enthesophyte) develops in the origin of the flexor brevis muscle just superior to the plantar fascia in approximately 50% of patients with plantar fasciitis (**Figure 2**). The spur is not a source of

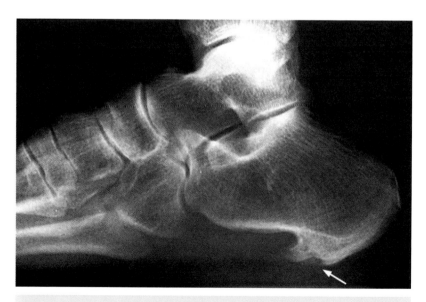

Figure 2   Radiographic appearance of a plantar heel spur (arrow).

pain, however, and is present in 20% of similar-age adults who do not have plantar fasciitis.

Although not necessary for diagnosis, a bone scan may show increased uptake at the medial calcaneal tuberosity. MRI, which also is not necessary for diagnosis or treatment, will often show thickening of the origin of the plantar fascia, as well as marrow edema in the calcaneal tuberosity.

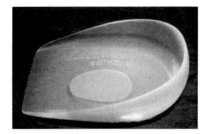

Figure 3 Photograph of an orthotic heel pad.

Differential Diagnosis

- Acute traumatic rupture of the plantar fascia (ecchymosis, tenderness, swelling over the proximal plantar fascia)
- Baxter nerve entrapment (the first branch of the lateral plantar nerve innervating the abductor digiti minimi [ADM]) muscle) (pain is 1 cm superior to the classic location of plantar fasciitis and usually not associated with activity) (in long-standing cases, loss of ADM strength can be observed) (can also be seen together with plantar fasciitis and usually needs to be treated surgically)
- Calcaneal stress fracture (rare, tenderness with medial and lateral pressure of the calcaneus)
- Calcaneal tumor (rare, pain at rest, night pain)
- Fat pad atrophy/contusion (tenderness over an abnormally prominent calcaneal tuberosity)
- Sciatica (radicular symptoms)
- Seronegative spondyloarthropathy (typically bilateral enthesitis of the plantar fascia, other sites of enthesitis, arthralgic joints involved)
- Tarsal tunnel syndrome (paresthesia and numbness on the plantar aspect of the foot)

Adverse Outcomes of the Disease

Patients may experience chronic heel pain and a substantial alteration in daily activities. Altered gait can aggravate forefoot, knee, hip, or back problems.

Treatment

More than 95% of cases of plantar fasciitis can be managed satisfactorily with nonsurgical treatment. Patients should be informed that it commonly takes 6 to 12 months for symptoms to resolve. Avid walkers and joggers should be counseled concerning alternative exercise regimens, such as use of a stationary bike.

Initial treatment should include an over-the-counter orthotic device, such as a silicone, rubber, or felt heel pad (**Figure 3**), along with a home program of stretching exercises. Shock-absorbing shoe wear is advised. Some studies suggest that a night splint should be used as part of initial treatment if the patient experiences increased pain on rising from a resting position in the morning. The night splint holds the ankle and foot in slight dorsiflexion, which maintains the Achilles tendon and plantar fascia in a stretched position during sleep. Patient compliance in proper use of the splint is very low, however.

Contrast baths, ice, NSAIDs, and/or shoes with shock-absorbing soles also can be used to decrease inflammation in the painful heel.

If symptoms persist despite nonsurgical management, injection of corticosteroid into the heel may be indicated. A formal rehabilitation consultation may be necessary to help direct the patient's continued stretching program. Repeat injections should be avoided because this can cause plantar fascia rupture.

Successful outcomes have been reported with the use of shock wave therapy and botulinum toxin type A injection.

If symptoms persist, the use of a custom orthotic device should be considered. Surgical treatment typically consists of partial release of the plantar fascia and should not be attempted until after 6 months of unsuccessful nonsurgical treatment.

Rehabilitation Prescription

Early rehabilitation is directed at controlling pain and increasing the range of motion of the ankle. Heel cord stretching is an important part of a home exercise program. Use of a night splint and limited weight bearing may also be beneficial. If the symptoms do not respond to these measures, formal rehabilitation may be ordered. The rehabilitation professional should include evaluation of the foot and ankle mechanics during gait. If overpronation is present, the use of foot orthoses can result in substantial improvement. Continued stretching and pain-relieving modalities may be used as deemed appropriate by the treating practitioner.

Adverse Outcomes of Treatment

NSAIDs can cause gastric, renal, or hepatic complications. In 2015, the FDA strengthened its warning linking NSAIDs with the risk of heart attack or stroke, even in the first weeks of use of an NSAID. Fat pad necrosis or rupture of the plantar fascia can develop from improper injection of corticosteroids. Surgical treatment may not improve symptoms and also can cause complete disruption of the plantar fascia or pain resulting from lateral overload if excessive release has been done.

Referral Decisions/Red Flags

Patients whose symptoms do not respond to nonsurgical treatment require further evaluation. Surgical release should be considered only after 6 to 12 months of intense nonsurgical management. Preliminary data indicate that radial or focal shock wave treatment may be a good option in some patients whose symptoms do not respond to initial nonsurgical treatment.

Home Exercise Program for Plantar Fasciitis

- Apply moist or dry heat to the painful area of the foot during the exercises.
- To prevent inflammation, apply a bag of crushed ice or frozen peas to the heel for 20 minutes after performing the exercises.
- You should not experience pain with the exercises. If you are unable to perform the exercises because of pain or stiffness or if your symptoms do not improve after performing the exercises for 3 to 4 weeks, call your doctor.
- The following exercise program is introductory only, and progression of this program will vary based on your specific injury, symptoms, and baseline level of fitness. For further progression of this routine, your physician may recommend evaluation and treatment by a physical therapist or other exercise professional.

Home Exercises for Plantar Fasciitis

Exercise	Muscle Group	Number of Repetitions/Sets	Number of Days per Week	Number of Weeks
Heel cord stretch	Gastrocnemius-soleus complex	4 to 5 repetitions/2 to 3 sets	Daily	3 to 4
Plantar fascia massage	Plantar fascia	60 to 90 seconds/2 to 3 sets	Daily	3 to 4

Heel Cord Stretch

- Stand facing a wall with the knee of the unaffected limb bent, the affected limb straight, and the toes pointed in slightly.
- Keeping the heels of both feet flat on the floor, lower your hips toward the wall.
- Feel the stretch in the back of your calf and hold for 30 seconds and then relax for 30 seconds.
- Repeat 4 to 5 times.
- Perform this exercise 2 to 3 times per day, for 3 to 4 weeks.

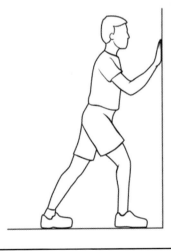

Plantar Fascia Massage

- Sit on a chair with your feet touching the floor.
- Place a tennis ball under the affected foot.
- Roll the foot back and forth and side to side over the tennis ball, applying pressure to the ball to achieve a greater massage, for 60 to 90 seconds. (This exercise might cause slight discomfort but should not be painful. If you experience pain, reduce the pressure on the tennis ball.)
- Perform the exercise 2 to 3 times per day, for 3 to 4 weeks.

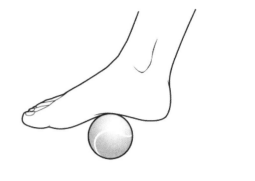

Procedure: Plantar Fasciitis Injection

Step 1

Wear protective gloves at all times during the procedure and use sterile technique.

Step 2

Use the 18-gauge needle to draw 2 mL of 40 mg/mL corticosteroid preparation and 2 mL of the local anesthetic into the syringe; then switch to the 21-gauge needle to preserve sterility.

Step 3

Prepare the medial aspect of the heel.

Step 4

Spray ethyl chloride onto the heel to freeze the skin.

Step 5

Measure the soft-tissue thickness beneath the calcaneus directly on the radiograph.

Step 6

Using the measurement from the radiograph as a guide, palpate the calcaneus medially where it begins to curve upward. Insert the 21-gauge needle into this area, which is approximately 2 cm from the plantar surface of the foot (**Figure 1**).

Step 7

Advance the needle down to the calcaneus until it hits the bone. Walk the tip of the needle distally along the bone to the plantar surface of the calcaneus. The needle should be immediately superior (deep) to the plantar fascia.

Step 8

Advance the needle to its hilt and inject 3 mL of the anesthetic-corticosteroid mixture. Inject the remaining 2 mL of the preparation while withdrawing the needle 2 cm; then withdraw the needle completely. Make certain that you do not inject the anesthetic-corticosteroid preparation into the medial subcutaneous tissue or the fat pad of the heel that is superficial to the plantar fascia.

Step 9

Dress the puncture wound with a sterile adhesive bandage.

Materials

- Sterile gloves
- Bactericidal skin preparation solution
- Ethyl chloride spray
- Lateral radiograph of the heel
- 5-mL syringe
- 18-gauge needle
- 21-gauge, 1″ to 1½″ needle
- Mixture of 2 mL of 10 to 40 mg/mL of corticosteroid preparation and 2 mL of 1% lidocaine, without epinephrine
- Adhesive dressing

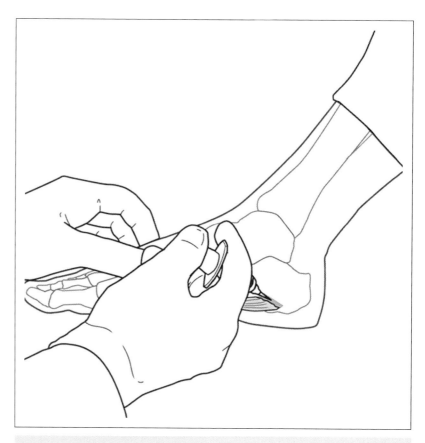

Figure 1   Illustration shows the proper location for injection for plantar fasciitis.

Adverse Outcomes

Injection of a corticosteroid into the superficial fat pad can cause fat necrosis, with loss of cushioning of the plantar heel. The injection may cause rupture of the plantar fascia.

Aftercare/Patient Instructions

Advise the patient that transient numbness of the heel can occur. Also explain that heel pain might return in a few hours when the anesthetic agent wears off and that 30% of patients experience increased pain for 2 to 3 days. Corticosteroids might take a few weeks to have an effect on the symptoms.

Plantar Warts

Synonym
Verruca vulgaris

Definition
Plantar warts are hyperkeratotic lesions on the sole of the foot caused by human papillomavirus. The peak incidence is in the second decade of life. Plantar warts are more commonly observed in athletic youngsters.

Clinical Symptoms
Patients have painful, slightly raised lesions on the sole of the foot. These lesions can occur in clusters known as "mosaic warts."

Tests
Physical Examination
Warts usually appear on non–weight-bearing areas on the sole of the foot. Normal papillary lines of the skin (fingerprint pattern) cease at the margin of the lesion (**Figure 1**). The lesions usually are very tender if pinched side to side, a finding not observed with a corn or callus. By contrast, a corn is tender with direct pressure. A plantar wart can occur anywhere on the sole, whereas a callus is associated with a bony prominence. Superficial paring of a wart with a scalpel reveals punctate hemorrhage and a fibrillated texture. A callus is avascular and on paring has a uniform texture that resembles yellow candle wax. The plantar wart typically starts with a single lesion, but satellite lesions can be seen in different locations of the foot, including the heel and toes, if the primary lesion is left untreated.

Diagnostic Tests
When doubt exists, histopathologic examination of a specimen confirms the diagnosis. This type of testing is seldom necessary, however, given the characteristic gross appearance after superficial paring.

Differential Diagnosis
- Callus (hyperkeratotic lesion that forms in response to a bony prominence)
- Foreign body (history and examination)
- Plantar fibromatosis (location beneath the skin)

Adverse Outcomes of the Disease
Plantar warts are often persistent; they can spread to other areas of the foot, grow larger, and leave scars on the sole of the foot.

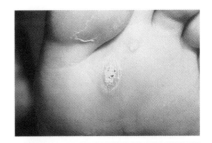

Figure 1 Photograph shows the clinical appearance of a plantar wart. (Reproduced with permission from California Pacific Medical Center, San Francisco, CA.)

Treatment

Most lesions resolve spontaneously within 5 to 6 months, so aggressive treatment should be reserved for unusually large, painful, or persistent lesions. Initial treatment commonly includes superficial paring, followed by the use of a keratolytic agent, such as salicylic acid in liquid or salve form. The lesion should then be covered with occlusive tape to ensure that the medication stays within the desired area and débrides the necrotic layers of tissue upon removal of the tape. Medication should be applied twice daily for 1 month.

Warts that are resistant to initial treatment will sometimes respond to intralesional injection of approximately 1 mL of local anesthetic with epinephrine. Electrocautery, cryotherapy with liquid nitrogen, laser ablation, or curettage can be performed under local anesthetic. Care should be taken to avoid causing necrosis of the deep dermis, which can produce intractable, painful scarring on the sole of the foot. In curettage, for example, the subcutaneous fat should not be visible when the procedure is finished. Intralesional injections of bleomycin and radiation therapy also have been described for severe, recalcitrant lesions, but these options are best performed by specialists with experience in their use.

Adverse Outcomes of Treatment

Secondary infection can occur after treatment. Intractable scarring from excessively deep ablation is also a significant risk.

Referral Decisions/Red Flags

Persistent or recurring warts warrant further evaluation.

Posterior Heel Pain

Synonyms
Achilles tendinosis
Haglund syndrome
Insertional Achilles tendinitis
Pump bump
Retrocalcaneal bursitis

Definition
Pain in the posterior heel around the insertion of the Achilles tendon can originate from one or more of the following structures: the insertion of the Achilles tendon onto the calcaneus (insertional Achilles tendinosis); the retrocalcaneal bursa (retrocalcaneal bursitis); a prominent process of the calcaneus impinging on the retrocalcaneal bursae and/or Achilles tendon (Haglund syndrome); or inflammation of the bursa between the skin and the Achilles tendon (pre-Achilles bursitis). The exact etiology may be confusing because frequently more than one of these areas is involved (**Figure 1**).

Clinical Symptoms
Patients with a prominent process of the calcaneus initially develop a bursa that is irritated by shoe wear and causes a pump bump (**Figure 2**). This bump is different from the Haglund deformity and is found in the posterolateral aspect of the heel. In older patients, insertional tendinosis with enthesopathy, calcification, and degenerative tears of the Achilles tendon are most often seen. A limp and pain with start-up or activity are common. Shoe wear may be difficult because of the direct pressure on the posterior heel prominence.

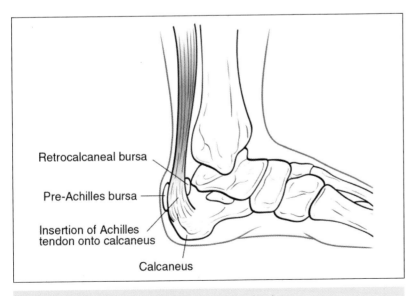

Figure 1 Illustration of sites of posterior heel pain.

Retrocalcaneal bursa
Pre-Achilles bursa
Insertion of Achilles tendon onto calcaneus
Calcaneus

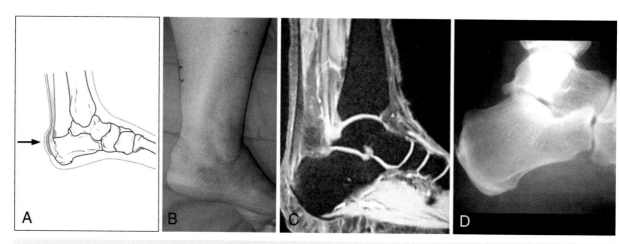

Figure 2 **A,** Illustration of the area of involvement. **B,** Photograph shows the clinical appearance. **C,** Sagittal T2-weighted MRI shows thickening of the Achilles insertion and fluid within the insertion of the tendon. **D,** Lateral radiograph demonstrates prominent Haglund deformity.

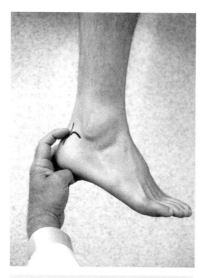

Figure 3 Clinical photograph of the foot of a patient with posterior heel pain. Pain on palpation on either side of the retrocalcaneal bursa, anterior to the Achilles tendon insertion, is indicative of retrocalcaneal bursitis.

Tests

Physical Examination

Examination reveals swelling and tenderness at the posterior heel. If a calcaneal prominence is present, it is usually larger on the lateral side of the heel. A superficial bursa (pump bump) may be present and may be inflamed by shoe wear.

If Achilles tendinosis is present, pain is present directly over the Achilles tendon and is increased by squeezing the tendon. The tendon may be thickened and have a nodule. Retrocalcaneal bursitis can cause swelling, redness, and pain anterior to the Achilles tendon; this pain is increased by squeezing the bursa from side to side and just anterior to the Achilles tendon (**Figure 3**).

Diagnostic Tests

Lateral radiographs of the heel may show calcification of the Achilles tendon and spur formation. A prominent posterosuperior process of the calcaneus also might be apparent.

Differential Diagnosis

- Achilles tendon avulsion (palpable defect in the tendon, positive Thompson test)
- Os trigonum syndrome (posterolateral pain increased with forced dorsiflexion)
- Plantar fasciitis (pain below the calcaneus)
- Stress fracture of the calcaneus (midcalcaneal bony tenderness and pain upon lateral squeeze of the calcaneus)

Adverse Outcomes of the Disease

Difficulty with shoe wear and sports activities can result, as well as chronic pain and limping. Rupture or avulsion of the Achilles tendon can be seen in long-standing insertional tendinitis.

Treatment

A heel lift or open-back shoes will minimize pressure on the inflamed area. Ice massage and contrast baths will decrease inflammation. Achilles tendon stretching exercises should be started after the inflammatory phase has passed. Casting for 4 to 6 weeks may alleviate symptoms. Surgical intervention will remove the inflamed bursa, prominent bone, and diseased tendon. Corticosteroid injection of the tendon should be strictly avoided because it can cause rupture or avulsion of the tendon. Ultrasound-guided decompression of the retrocalcaneal bursa can be helpful in patients with identifiable fluid collection.

Rehabilitation Prescription

A home exercise program of heel cord stretching with the toe pointing in and the knee bent will isolate and stretch the soleus muscle; heel cord stretching with the leg straight and calf eccentrics will stretch the gastrocnemius-soleus complex. A heel lift in the shoe can be helpful in resting the tendon. If these measures are not successful, formal rehabilitation can be ordered. The evaluation should include a biomechanical assessment of the foot and ankle during ambulation. If overpronation is present, foot orthoses can be very helpful in relieving the symptoms. In addition, guided activity modification/return-to-play recommendations, manual therapy techniques, and pain-relieving modalities may be used as deemed appropriate by the treating practitioner.

Adverse Outcomes of Treatment

Surgical removal of bone and débridement of the Achilles tendon can predispose the tendon to rupture.

Referral Decisions/Red Flags

Recalcitrant pain or failure to respond to nonsurgical management indicates the need for further evaluation.

Home Exercise Program for Posterior Heel Pain

- Apply moist or dry heat to the heel while exercising, and to prevent inflammation, apply a bag of crushed ice or frozen peas to the heel for 20 minutes after performing the exercises.
- You should not experience pain with the exercises.
- If your symptoms do not improve after performing the exercises for 3 to 4 weeks, call your doctor.
- The following exercise program is introductory only, and progression of this program will vary based on your specific injury, symptoms, and baseline level of fitness. For further progression of this routine, your physician may recommend evaluation and treatment by a physical therapist or other exercise professional.

Home Exercises for Posterior Heel Pain

Exercise	Muscle Group	Number of Repetitions/Sets	Number of Days per Week	Number of Weeks
Heel cord stretch with knee bent	Soleus	4 repetitions/2 to 3 sets	Daily	3 to 4
Heel cord stretch	Gastrocnemius-soleus complex	4 repetitions/2 to 3 sets	Daily	3 to 4
Calf eccentrics	Gastrocnemius-soleus complex	10 to 15 repetitions/2 to 3 sets	Daily	3 to 4

Heel Cord Stretch With Knee Bent

- Stand facing a wall with the unaffected limb in front and with the knee bent for support, the affected limb in back and with the knee also bent, and the toes pointed in slightly.
- Keeping the heels of both feet flat on the floor, lower your hips toward the wall.
- Stretching should be felt in the Achilles region or ankle.
- Hold for 30 seconds and then relax for 30 seconds.
- Perform 2 to 3 sets of 4 repetitions per day, for 3 to 4 weeks.

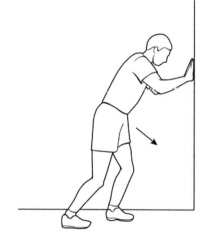

Heel Cord Stretch

- Stand facing a wall with the knee of the unaffected limb bent, the affected limb straight, and the toes pointed in slightly.
- Keeping the heels of both feet flat on the floor, lower your hips toward the wall.
- Feel the pull in the posterior calf region of the back leg.
- Hold the stretch for 30 seconds and then relax for 30 seconds.
- Perform 2 to 3 sets of 4 repetitions per day, for 3 to 4 weeks.

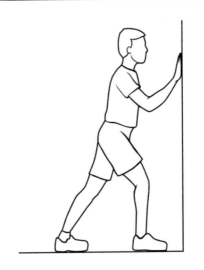

Calf Eccentrics

- Stand on the bottom step of a staircase with your heels extending off the step.
- Starting up on your toes, lower your heels slowly (5 count) as far as is comfortable. When you reach the lowest comfortable position, push back up to the starting position. Repeat 10 to 15 times.
- Perform the exercise 2 to 3 times per day, for 3 to 4 weeks.
- When you first perform this exercise, use both feet. As you get stronger and feel more comfortable, progress to using one foot at a time.

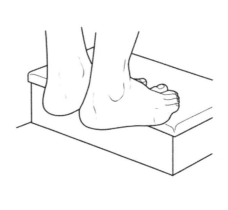

SECTION 7 FOOT AND ANKLE

Posterior Tibial Tendon Dysfunction

Synonyms

Acquired flatfoot
Posterior tibial tendon insufficiency
Posterior tibial tendon rupture

Definition

The posterior tibial tendon is one of the main supporting structures of the medial ankle and arch. Posterior tibial tendon dysfunction is the primary cause of medial ankle pain in the middle-aged patient. Demographically, the classic presentation is an overweight woman older than 55 years. Asymptomatic flexible flatfoot deformity, corticosteroid injections, diabetes mellitus, hypertension, and/or previous injury to the foot are other risk factors. The posterior tibial tendon is thickened and shows degenerative changes. As a result, the posterior tibialis muscle is ineffective, and its function of supporting the medial longitudinal arch is lost. Consequently, a painful flatfoot develops. Initially the foot is flexible, but over time the deformity becomes fixed, and arthritic changes can occur in the hindfoot and ankle.

Clinical Symptoms

Pain and swelling on the medial aspect of the ankle are the most common symptoms. Usually patients state that they have lost the arch and that the ankle rolls in. The onset of symptoms is insidious, and there usually is no history of trauma. Although pain and tenderness initially occur along the medial aspect of the foot, lateral pain ultimately develops as the collapsed flatfoot abuts the fibula or causes impingement in the sinus tarsi. Ankle pain can be the presenting symptom in late stages of the disease.

Tests

Physical Examination

Both feet should be examined from the knee down with the patient standing. Examination shows swelling and tenderness posterior and inferior to the medial malleolus, along the course of the posterior tibial tendon. The medial arch is decreased or completely flattened. The heel shows increased valgus, and with advanced changes, the forefoot is in abduction. When viewed from behind, more than two toes will be visible on the affected foot (the "too many toes" sign) because of forefoot abduction and hindfoot valgus (**Figure 1, A**). Also, the patient will not be able to rise on the toes of the affected foot (**Figure 1, B**).

Posterior tibial tendon strength is decreased on both manual muscle testing as well as functional maneuvers. Normally a patient with

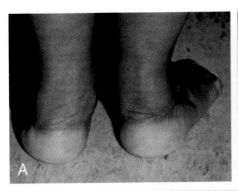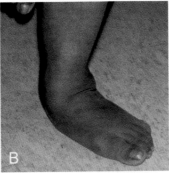

Figure 1 Clinical photographs show the feet of a patient with posterior tibial tendon dysfunction. **A,** Too many toes sign in the right foot, caused by forefoot abduction and hindfoot valgus typical of posterior tibial tendon dysfunction. **B,** Patient is unable to rise up on the toes of the affected left foot.

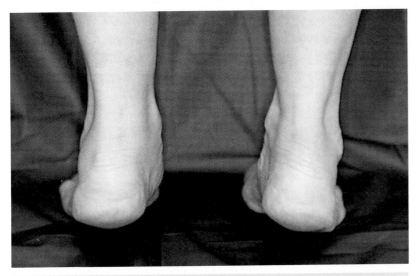

Figure 2 Photograph of the hindfeet of a patient with posterior tibial tendon dysfunction of the left foot shows that the left heel does not rotate inward (varus) when the patient stands on her toes.

both hands placed on a wall can perform a heel rise on one leg, and during this maneuver, the posterior tibial tendon will pull the heel into inversion. Patients with dysfunction or rupture of the posterior tibial tendon cannot perform a complete heel rise on the affected leg, and when this test is performed while standing on both legs, normal inversion of the heel does not occur (**Figure 2**).

In late stages of the disease, pain over the posterior tibial tendon either decreases or ceases with rupture of the tendon, and patients start to complain more of a lateral ankle pain over the peroneal tendons and calcaneocuboid joint. This is mainly due to decreased volume of the subfibular space and lateral overload upon hindfoot valgus and forefoot abduction.

Diagnostic Tests
Weight-bearing AP and lateral radiographs of the foot reveal flatfoot, with alignment changes at the talonavicular and other joints. MRI of the posterior tibial tendon may be useful in equivocal situations. It is very important to also obtain weight-bearing ankle radiographs to identify ankle valgus deformity, which can be seen in later stages of the disease as the result of deltoid ligament insufficiency.

Differential Diagnosis
- Congenital pes planus (bilateral, present since childhood if there has been no recent change)
- Lisfranc fracture-dislocation (history of trauma, pain in the midfoot)
- Medial ankle laxity (rare, abnormal ankle radiographs)
- Medial malleolus stress fracture (focal bony tenderness)
- Tarsal coalition (fixed deformity, onset as adolescent or young adult)
- Tarsal tunnel syndrome (burning pain even at rest)

Adverse Outcomes of the Disease
Progressive, painful flatfoot with gait disturbance is common. Severe flatfoot makes shoe wear or even bracing difficult. The deformity eventually affects the ankle joint and creates a valgus ankle with possible arthritis.

Treatment
Tenosynovitis of the tendon without flatfoot should be treated with a short leg cast or cast brace for 4 weeks, NSAIDs, and activity limitation. After the cast is removed, a molded ankle-foot orthosis can be used as the tendinitis resolves. A custom orthotic device with a medial longitudinal arch support and medial internal heel wedge is often recommended to help decrease the excursion of the tendon. Corticosteroid injection is not recommended because it can weaken the already pathologic tendon. When nonsurgical treatment fails, surgical débridement of the tendon may be indicated.

If flexible flatfoot develops, use of a custom orthotic device or ankle brace should be continued. A UCBL (University of California Biomechanics Laboratory) orthotic insert or Arizona brace also can be effective. Often, surgery is required. If the deformity is flexible, a tendon transfer combined with a realignment osteotomy is usually recommended. When rigid flatfoot develops, however, stabilization of the hindfoot by arthrodesis is the better alternative.

Adverse Outcomes of Treatment
In 2015, the FDA strengthened its warning linking NSAIDs with the risk of heart attack or stroke, even in the first weeks of use of an NSAID. Tendon transfer surgery may fail, requiring an arthrodesis of the hindfoot.

Referral Decisions/Red Flags

Patients with unexplained medial ankle pain require further evaluation because a medial ankle sprain is rare and therefore other, more serious, conditions must be considered. Patients with a recent onset of flatfoot deformity also require further evaluation.

Rheumatoid Arthritis of the Foot and Ankle

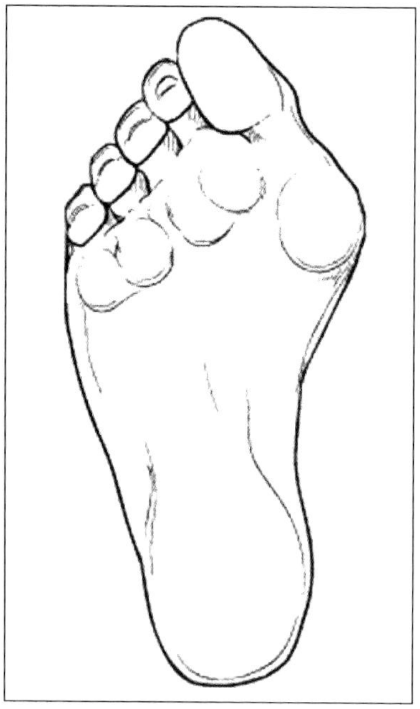

Definition

Ninety percent of patients with rheumatoid arthritis are estimated to have symptoms that are related to the foot or ankle; however, recent advances in drug therapy for rheumatoid arthritis have resulted in a decrease in foot and ankle involvement. The presence and severity of symptoms correlates with the longevity of the disease. Ninety percent of patients report symptoms in the forefoot and midfoot, and 67% report symptoms in the ankle and hindfoot. Chronic synovitis leads to stretching of the capsule and ligaments of the joints with subsequent malalignment of the joints, and ultimately to structural deformities such as hallux valgus, claw toes with subluxated or dislocated metatarsophalangeal (MTP) joints, and end-stage arthritis of the ankle or subtalar joint.

Clinical Symptoms

Patients present with loss of motion and pain on weight bearing. Metatarsalgia commonly occurs with subluxation/dislocation of the lesser toe MTP joints, claw toes, and distal migration of the fat pad (**Figure 1**). Severe hallux valgus often accompanies lesser toe deformities (**Figure 2**).

In the hindfoot, tenosynovitis of the posterior tibial tendon can produce medial ankle pain and swelling. Early arthritis of the talonavicular or subtalar joint also is common and typically occurs before ankle involvement.

The ankle is usually one of the last joints to be involved in rheumatoid arthritis.

Tests

Physical Examination

MTP synovitis, with focal pain and swelling over the MTP joints, may be the presenting symptom in patients with rheumatoid arthritis. Bilateral symptoms, multiple joint involvement, and the presence of nodules should lead to clinical suspicion of rheumatoid arthritis.

Diagnostic Tests

Laboratory tests reveal an elevated erythrocyte sedimentation rate and positive rheumatoid factor. Radiographs reveal soft-tissue swelling, osteopenia, subchondral erosions, and malalignment. Lateral drift occurs at the MTP joints and at the talonavicular joint (**Figure 3**).

Figure 1 Metatarsalgia develops as the fat pad is pulled distally and the metatarsal heads become more prominent, as shown in this illustration.

Differential Diagnosis

• Posterior tibial tendon dysfunction (swelling and tenderness over the posterior tibial tendon)
• Seronegative spondyloarthropathies (enthesitis present on physical examination with pain at the insertion sites of the plantar fascia and Achilles tendon)
• Traumatic arthritis (history of preceding trauma)

Adverse Outcomes of the Disease

Pain, progressive deformity, and metatarsalgia with plantar ulcerations are common if the condition remains untreated.

Treatment

Medical management can improve symptoms and slow the progression of disease. Disease-modifying agents (such as methotrexate and the newer pharmacotherapy agents such as disease-modifying antirheumatic drugs [DMARDs] that effect tumor necrosis factor alpha [TNF-α]) have been shown to decrease synovitis and slow progression of the disease. Corticosteroid injections can be helpful for inflamed joints and significant tenosynovitis.

An extra-depth accommodative shoe with a molded insole and rocker-bottom sole often relieves metatarsalgia. A UCBL (University of California Biomechanics Laboratory) orthosis can provide substantial pain relief for a patient who has a flexible hindfoot deformity. A molded ankle-foot orthosis can be used for more extensive disease involvement.

The most reliable surgery for forefoot deformity involves fusion of the first MTP joint with metatarsal head resections. Implant arthroplasty of the great toe should be avoided because this procedure has a very poor outcome.

Tenosynovectomy is only a temporizing procedure and is rarely indicated. Most patients with severe arthritis of the hindfoot joints require arthrodesis of the talocalcaneal, talonavicular, and/or calcaneocuboid joints. Patients still have dorsiflexion and plantar flexion through the ankle joint after a hindfoot arthrodesis.

Significant ankle arthritis can require arthrodesis in young and active patients. Patients with rheumatoid arthritis who have severe ankle destruction often have subtalar joint involvement. Injections into the joints can help determine which is more symptomatic. When both joints are involved, a hindfoot (tibiotalocalcaneal) fusion can be performed; this procedure acts as a biological prosthesis and has been shown to have worse functional outcome than a below-knee amputation. Recent results of total ankle replacement in patients with rheumatoid arthritis are encouraging, and this procedure can be used as an alternative treatment in less demanding patients who are older than 60 years. If the subtalar joint is also involved in these patients, subtalar joint fusion can be done, followed by ankle replacement.

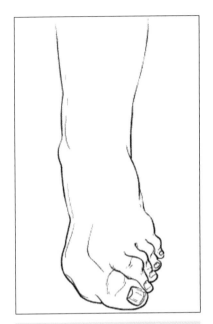

Figure 2 Hallux valgus and lesser toe deformities are associated with rheumatoid arthritis, as shown in this illustration.

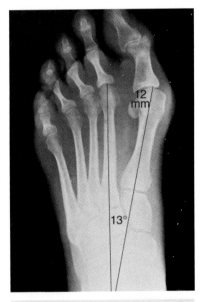

Figure 3 AP radiograph of the foot of a patient with rheumatoid arthritis demonstrates severe hallux valgus.

Adverse Outcomes of Treatment

Incomplete correction of the deformity, inadequate pain relief, delayed union, malunion, nonunion, or adjacent joint degeneration can complicate surgical treatment.

Referral Decision/Red Flags

Persistent pain despite medical management signals the need for further evaluation.

Sesamoiditis

Synonym
Dancer's toe

Definition
The sesamoid bones are embedded in the flexor hallucis brevis tendon beneath the first metatarsal head (plantar surface) (**Figure 1**). Sesamoid bones also may be present under any of the other metatarsal heads, but this is less common. Sesamoid disorders include inflammation, fracture, osteonecrosis, and arthritis. Sesamoiditis occurs from repeated stress of the sesamoid and the subsequent inflammation.

Clinical Symptoms
Pain under the first metatarsal head is noted, with or without swelling and ecchymosis. The usual stresses involve dancing or running, but sesamoiditis also can be caused by trauma from falls or more commonly by forced dorsiflexion of the great toe with acute onset of pain.

Tests
Physical Examination
With both sesamoiditis and sesamoid fractures, examination reveals focal tenderness at the sesamoid bone directly beneath the metatarsal head. The tender spot will move with the sesamoid as the great toe is flexed and extended. Dorsiflexion of the toe is painful, and range of motion may be restricted.

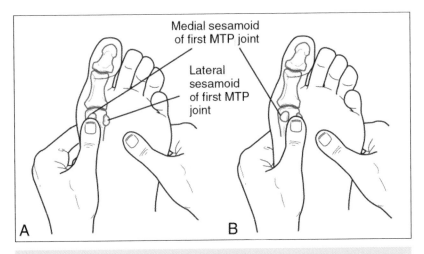

Figure 1 Illustration of the location of the medial sesamoid (**A**) and the location of the lateral sesamoid (**B**). MTP = metatarsophalangeal.

SECTION 7 FOOT AND ANKLE

Diagnostic Tests

AP, lateral, and axial radiographs of the sesamoid bones are indicated. An oblique view of the sesamoid also may be helpful in visualizing the entire bone and to rule out a fracture. Bipartite or multipartite sesamoid bones are common, occurring in 25% of the population. These normal variants have smooth margins and should not be confused with fractured sesamoids, which have irregular margins. Comparison views of the opposite foot or a bone scan may be helpful.

Differential Diagnosis

- Hallux rigidus (limited dorsiflexion, dorsal spur, dorsal tenderness)
- Hallux valgus (pain medially, lateral deviation of the great toe)
- Metatarsalgia (tenderness over the plantar aspect of a lesser metatarsal)
- Neuroma (pain and tenderness over the medial sensory nerve)

Adverse Outcomes of the Disease

Without treatment, the patient may have pain and a limp.

Treatment

Patients with sesamoiditis should be advised to avoid wearing high-heeled shoes. For more severe symptoms, relieving pressure on the sesamoids by taping the great toe in plantar flexion, using sesamoid pads (a felt pad used to relieve pressure on the sesamoid bone), wearing a stiff-soled or rocker-bottom shoe, or wearing a removable short leg fracture brace for 4 to 6 weeks can decrease inflammation. If these measures fail, excision of the sesamoid may be required.

Adverse Outcomes of Treatment

Hallux valgus or varus rarely develops following removal of a sesamoid.

Referral Decisions/Red Flags

Persistent pain is an indication for further evaluation.

Shoe Wear

Shoes protect and cushion the feet and in many cases serve a cosmetic purpose. Improperly fitted or improperly manufactured shoes are the cause of many foot deformities. Women who consistently wear high-heeled shoes with a narrow toe box have an increased incidence of bunions, hammer toes, corns, and—ultimately—foot surgery (**Figure 1**).

Foot size increases with age, but many men and women continue to buy the same size shoe throughout their adult lives without having their feet measured. Patients require instruction about the proper fitting of shoes.

Shoe Design and Lasting Techniques

The seven basic shoe styles are the pump, oxford, sandal, mule, boot, clog, and moccasin. Shoe designers create many variations of these styles, and unfortunately the design of some fashionable footwear indicates little regard for proper shoe function.

The three-dimensional form (either straight or curved) on which the base of the shoe is made is called the last. The shape of the toe box and instep and the curve of the shoe are determined by the last. The straighter the last, the straighter the shoe and the more medial support the shoe can provide. Common methods of lasting include slip lasting, board (or flat) lasting, and combination lasting. A slip-lasted shoe is constructed by sewing together the upper, like a moccasin, and then gluing it onto the sole. This method makes a lightweight, flexible shoe with no torsional rigidity. With board-lasting or

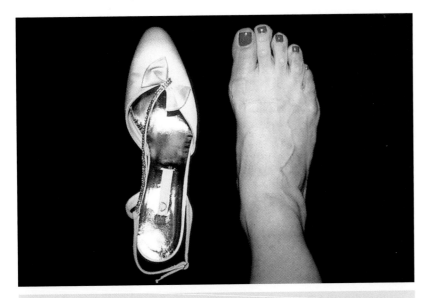

Figure 1 Clinical photograph of a high-heeled shoe with a narrow toe box next to the foot of the wearer. The foot takes the shape of the shoe. Common deformities include hallux valgus, hammer toes, corns, and calluses.

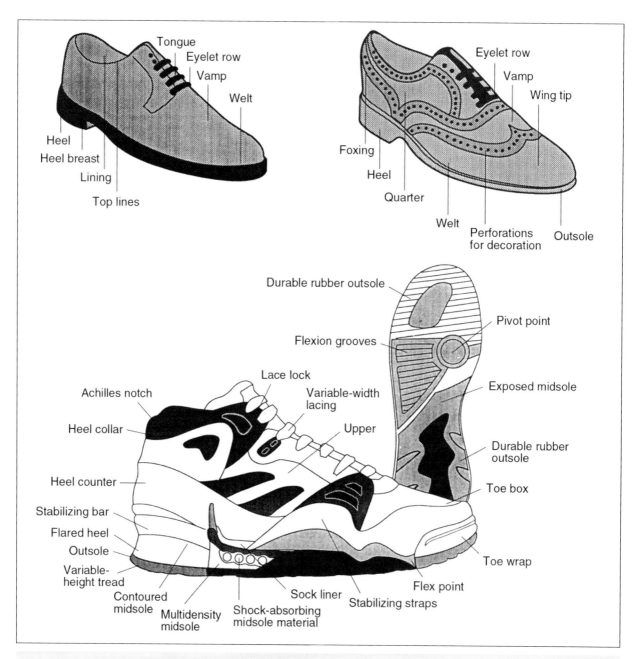

Figure 2 Illustration of the anatomy of several types of shoe.

flat-lasting techniques, the upper is fastened to the insole with tacks or staples. This construction makes a stable but less flexible shoe.

Combination lasting uses more than one technique for the same shoe. Shoes made in this way are typically board-lasted in the rear for stability and slip-lasted in the forefoot for flexibility.

Shoe Anatomy

The anatomy of several types of shoe is illustrated in **Figure 2**.

Outsole

The outsole makes contact with the ground and usually is attached to the midsole. Most athletic shoes have outsoles made of hard carbon rubber or blown rubber compounds. The outsole provides pivot points and can be designed with a herringbone pattern, suction cups, radial edges, or asymmetric studs. These design patterns enhance stability and traction.

Midsole and Heel Wedge
The midsole and the heel wedge are located between the inner sole and the outsole and are attached to both. These components provide cushioning, shock absorption, lift, and control.

Heel Counter
The heel counter is a firm cup built into the rear of the shoe that holds the heel in position and helps control excessive foot motion.

Toe Box
The toe box may include a stiff material inserted between the lining and outer surface in the toe area to prevent collapse and protect the toes.

Tongue
The tongue is designed primarily to protect the dorsum of the foot from dirt, moisture, and pressure.

Sock Liners, Arch Supports, and Inserts
The sock liner covers the insole and provides comfort and appearance. This liner acts primarily as a buffer zone between the shoe and the foot. Arch supports, heel cups, and other types of padding provide additional support, cushioning, and motion control.

Welt
The welt is a strip of leather or other material that joins the upper with the outer sole.

Shoe Analysis and Fit
With any foot or ankle problem, evaluation of the patient's shoes should be an integral part of the examination. Wear patterns are generally predictable, with the normal wear pattern on the outsole slightly medial at the toe and lateral at the heel (**Figure 3**). Abnormalities in the wear pattern indicate problems with alignment and gait. A tracing of the weight-bearing foot should be compared with a tracing of the shoe (**Figure 4**).

Shoe manufacturers have added extra eyelets to many shoes so that they can be laced for a custom fit. Most people can use a conventional technique, where the laces crisscross to the top of the shoe, aiming for a snug but comfortable fit. If foot or fit problems are present, other lacing techniques can be used (**Figure 5**).

Although proper fitting of shoes is not an exact science, relying on several easy-to-follow guidelines can help. Shoes always should be fit to the weight-bearing foot at the end of the day, when feet are at their largest. Shoes cannot be stretched to the shape of the foot. The upper should not wrinkle with flexion, and the foot should not bulge over the welt. The end of the longest toe of the larger foot should be

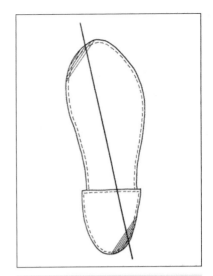

Figure 3 Illustration of the normal wear pattern of a shoe. (Reproduced from Yodlowski ML, Femino JE: Shoes and orthoses, in Mizel MS, Miller RA, Scioli MW, eds: *Orthopaedic Knowledge Update: Foot and Ankle*, ed 2. Rosemont, IL, American Academy of Orthopaedic Surgeons, 1998, p 57.)

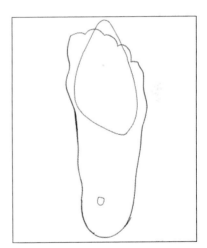

Figure 4 Illustration of the common finding of a large mismatch between the contour of a patient's foot and the shoe being worn. Note the compression of the forefoot and the very small contact area of the high heel. Such a tracing can often disclose the cause of a patient's foot pain.

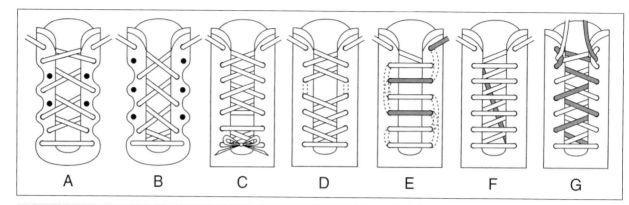

Figure 5 Illustration of lacing patterns. **A,** For narrow feet, use the eyelets set wider apart to bring up the sides of the shoe for a tighter fit. **B,** For wide feet, use the eyelets set closer to the tongue of the shoe. This has the same effect as letting out a corset. **C,** For a narrow heel and wide forefoot, use both sets of eyelets to achieve a custom fit. **D,** For dorsal pain from a bump on the top of the foot, a high arch, or pain from a dorsal nerve or tendon, leave a space in the lacing to alleviate pressure. **E,** For a high arch, avoid the normal crisscross pattern to avoid pressure points. **F,** For hammer toes, claw toes, corns, or toenail problems, lace as shown to allow the toe box to be lifted by pulling on the lace that runs from the toe to the throat of the shoe. **G,** For heel blisters, lock the laces at the throat of the shoe to prevent excess motion of the heel in the shoe.

within ⅜″ to ½″ of the end of the toe box. The forefoot should not be crowded, and the toes should easily extend. The shoe should provide a relatively snug grip at the counter above the heel. High heels should be avoided because this style exerts excessive pressure on the front of the foot. Both the left and the right shoe should be tried before buying because shoe size can differ from left to right. Athletic shoes should be bought according to the running and activity style as well as needed cushioning. Above all else, shoes should be comfortable from the moment they are tried on.

Adverse Outcomes From Poor Shoe Fit

Bunions, hammer toes, neuromas, corns and calluses, and ingrown toenails are all possible.

Soft-Tissue Masses of the Foot and Ankle

Synonyms
Fibromatosis
Ledderhose disease
Mucoid cyst
Nodular fasciitis
Plantar fibroma

Definition
Ganglia and plantar fibromas are the most common soft-tissue tumors in the foot and ankle. Other lesions are not discussed in this chapter. Malignant tumors of the soft tissues of the foot and ankle are very rare. A ganglion is a cystic tumor that contains gelatinous fluid and arises from a joint capsule or tendon sheath (**Figure 1**). Ganglia of the foot or ankle usually are small, 2- to 3-cm masses that arise on the top or side of the foot. A common site is the lateral aspect of the foot or ankle, with the ganglion cyst arising from the subtalar or ankle joint.

A plantar fibroma is a benign thickening of the plantar fascia that can vary in size from 1 to 6 cm in diameter. Plantar fibromas may evolve to plantar fibromatosis (nodular fasciitis of the plantar fascia), a condition that is similar histologically to Dupuytren disease of the palmar fascia. Compared with Dupuytren disease, plantar fibromatosis is less likely to cause severe deformities.

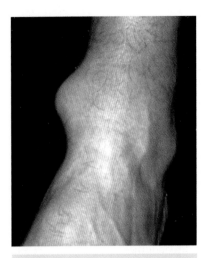

Figure 1 Clinical photograph of a ganglion cyst of the medial ankle.

Clinical Symptoms
A ganglion cyst can be seen in any location in the foot and ankle. It typically is a painless, soft nodule, but it may cause problems with aching, nerve compression, or shoe wear. A plantar fibroma is a firm mass that is usually seen on the medial aspect of the plantar fascia; it may be painful and is more likely to interfere with shoe wear.

Tests
Physical Examination
A ganglion cyst is a discrete mass that is usually movable with side-to-side pressure. A plantar fibroma can be focal or can have multiple, discrete masses that are hard (rubbery) and are part of the plantar fascial band.

Diagnostic Tests
Plain radiographs are typically normal. Aspiration of a ganglion with an 18-gauge needle will return a straw-colored, gelatinous material. Sophisticated diagnostic imaging generally is not necessary for either a ganglion cyst or a plantar fibroma.

Differential Diagnosis

- Giant cell tumor of the tendon sheath (solid mass, inability to aspirate soft core)
- Lipoma (subcutaneous fatty deposit) (pathology diagnosis)
- Malignant sarcoma (synovial sarcoma, fibrosarcoma) (pathology diagnosis)
- Neurofibroma (often tubular along the course of the nerve) (pathology diagnosis)

Adverse Outcomes of the Disease

Patients may report persistent discomfort and difficulty with shoe wear. Malignant degeneration of a plantar fibroma is possible, but the risk is small.

Treatment

The wall of the ganglion is pierced three or four times with an 18-gauge needle to release the gelatinous core and promote complete collapse of the cyst. Care should be taken to avoid any overlying sensory nerve. If the ganglion recurs and continues to be symptomatic, it should be excised. The efficacy of corticosteroid injection into a ganglion has not been proved. A plantar fibroma is best treated with shoe modifications and an orthotic device. The orthotic device should be cushioned and designed to float the fibroma. Surgical excision is indicated only in patients with significant persistent symptoms or if the fibroma has increased substantially in size.

Adverse Outcomes of Treatment

Surgical excision of a plantar fibroma should be avoided, if possible, because of the high rate of recurrence and potential for a painful plantar surgical scar.

Referral Decisions/Red Flags

If the diagnosis of the mass is not clear based on anatomy, examination, radiographs, and aspiration, further evaluation is required to rule out other etiologies. Recurrence of a ganglion following aspiration usually requires surgical excision.

Stress Fractures of the Foot and Ankle

Synonyms

Insufficiency fracture
March fracture

Definition

A stress fracture is caused by repetitive overloading. The bone fails
when the fatigue process exceeds the reparative process. Stress
fractures often result from an increased level of activity or after
beginning a different type of activity, such as military training
or exercise walking. Conditions that weaken the bone predispose
patients to stress fractures; therefore, these injuries are sometimes
referred to as insufficiency fractures. Young, athletic women
are at risk because of the female athlete triad of amenorrhea,
osteopenia, and disordered eating. Older women are at risk because
of osteoporosis. The metatarsals (especially the second metatarsal)
are the most common sites of a stress fracture, but these fractures
also can be seen in other bones of the foot and ankle including
the navicular, calcaneus, medial malleolus, and fibula (**Figure 1**).
Theoretically, any bone exposed to repetitive stress can sustain a
stress fracture.

Clinical Symptoms

Patients present with pain and swelling of insidious onset. The
pain increases with weight-bearing activity and is relieved by rest.
Metatarsal fractures present with a diffusely swollen dorsal forefoot,
whereas fibular fractures produce a swollen lateral ankle. Some
patients report hearing a crack or pop when the incomplete stress
fracture became a complete break.

Tests

Physical Examination

Localized point tenderness and concomitant swelling directly over
the fracture site are the most reliable physical signs. Ecchymosis
occasionally is observed.

Diagnostic Tests

Early radiographs (< 2 weeks from onset of symptoms) can be
normal, but after 3 to 4 weeks, radiographs show healing callus at
the fracture site. A bone scan is more sensitive than a radiograph and
can be positive by 5 days postinjury (**Figure 2**). MRI can confirm the
diagnosis but is not routinely used.

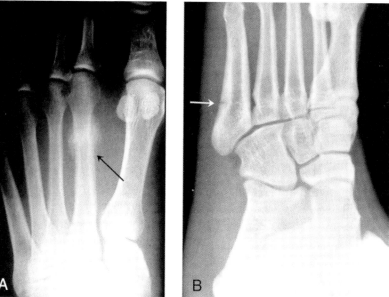

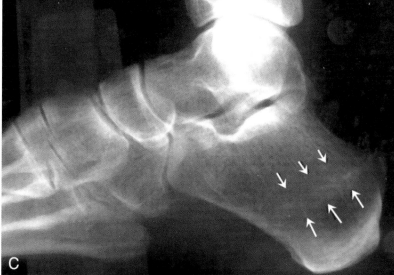

Figure 1   Radiographs demonstrate stress fractures. **A,** AP radiograph shows a healed stress fracture of the second metatarsal (arrow). **B,** Stress fracture of the fifth metatarsal (arrow). **C,** Calcaneal stress fracture seen as an area of increased density (between arrows).

Differential Diagnosis

- Gout (redness, erythema)
- Interdigital (Morton) neuroma (pain and tenderness in the intermetatarsal space)
- Metabolic bone disorders (multiple stress fractures)
- Neoplasm (pain at night or at rest)
- Synovitis of the second metatarsophalangeal joint (swelling and tenderness of the joint)
- Vitamin D deficiency

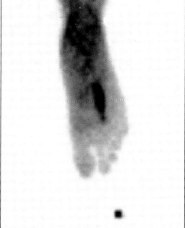

Figure 2   Bone scan shows area of increased uptake, indicative of a stress fracture of the third metatarsal.

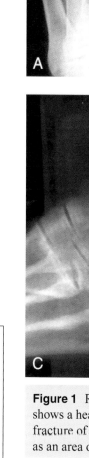

Adverse Outcomes of the Disease

Chronic stress fractures can require prolonged immobilization to heal. Displacement of fractures with continued unprotected activity can lead to malunion or nonunion that requires surgical procedures. This is more likely with fifth metatarsal (Jones fracture) and navicular stress fractures. Metatarsal stress fractures can displace in the sagittal plane and lead to a painful callus. An underlying cause such as vitamin D deficiency should be treated at the same time to avoid delay in healing or nonunion.

Treatment

Treatment for most patients is based on reduced activity and protective footwear. For metatarsal stress fractures, a stiff-soled shoe, wooden-soled postoperative sandal, or removable short leg fracture brace shoe is sufficient. Most patients with calcaneal and fibular fractures benefit from 2 to 4 weeks of immobilization in a short leg walking cast. Because of the high rate of nonunion, navicular and fifth metatarsal fractures both should be casted, and the patient should use crutches and avoid bearing weight on the involved limb. Internal fixation is often a better alternative for a stress fracture of the fifth metatarsal, especially in the athletic population. Underlying predisposing conditions such as heel varus (fifth metatarsal fractures) and heel valgus (fibular stress fractures) should also be treated in patients with nonunion. Patients may resume activity when they are asymptomatic and show healing radiographically. Time to healing is variable, depending on the bone involved.

Adverse Outcomes of Treatment

NSAIDs can slow osteogenesis and should be avoided during fracture healing. In 2015, the FDA strengthened its warning linking NSAIDs with the risk of heart attack or stroke, even in the first weeks of use of an NSAID.

Referral Decisions/Red Flags

Navicular, fifth metatarsal, and all fibular stress fractures require further evaluation early after diagnosis. Failure to heal by 4 to 6 weeks or recurrent fractures suggests the need for a metabolic workup.

Tarsal Tunnel Syndrome

Synonym
Tibial nerve entrapment

Definition
Tarsal tunnel syndrome describes the symptom complex associated with compression neuropathy of the tibial nerve or its branches posterior to the medial malleolus (**Figure 1**). Although an analogy to carpal tunnel syndrome of the upper extremity has been suggested, the only real similarity is the name. In contrast with carpal tunnel syndrome, tarsal tunnel syndrome is much less common, its symptoms are more vague and intermittent, and its diagnosis is more difficult. Numerous causes of tarsal tunnel syndrome have been reported, including compression from a ganglion or bony lesion, but most cases are of unknown etiology.

Clinical Symptoms
Most patients report diffuse, poorly localized pain along the medial ankle. Paresthesia (tingling) or dysesthesia (burning) along the medial ankle and into the arch is a common component of the symptom complex. The pain is often worse after walking or other exercise and also may occur at night.

Tests
Physical Examination
The physical examination reveals tenderness over the tarsal tunnel just posterior to the medial malleolus (**Figure 2**). Percussion over the tibial nerve should reproduce the symptoms (Tinel sign). Decreased

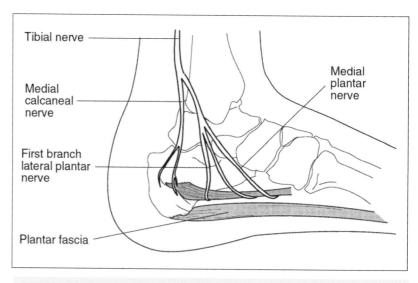

Figure 1 Illustration of the anatomy of the tarsal tunnel.

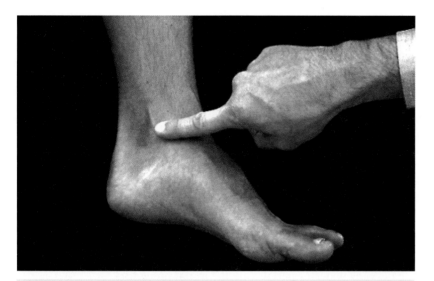

Figure 2 Clinical photograph shows testing for tenderness over the tarsal tunnel just posterior to the medial malleolus, which can be indicative of tarsal tunnel syndrome.

sensation in the distribution of the tibial nerve on the plantar aspect of the foot also may be present.

Diagnostic Tests

Radiographs of the foot and ankle usually are normal but are necessary to rule out bony pathology. MRI usually is normal but can be useful for determining the presence of a space-occupying lesion such as a ganglion. Electrodiagnostic testing can identify tibial nerve entrapment, but the test is not as accurate at the ankle level and below as in the upper extremity; however, it is beneficial for identifying underlying pathology such as neuropathy, for which surgical treatment would be useless. Furthermore, a positive or negative test does not always correlate with intraoperative findings or clinical outcomes.

Differential Diagnosis

- Baxter nerve entrapment (distal localization of the pain)
- Complex regional pain syndrome (discoloration of the foot, skin and temperature changes)
- Diabetic neuropathy (history of diabetes, bilateral loss of nerve function in a stocking distribution)
- Herniated lumbar disk (leg and thigh pain)
- Peripheral neuropathy (stocking distribution)
- Posterior tibial tendon dysfunction (pain associated with pes planus)

Adverse Outcomes of the Disease

Persistent pain and numbness are possible, and severe numbness can lead to plantar ulcers. Complex regional pain syndrome also may develop.

Treatment

For patients with flatfoot and substantial pronation, an orthotic device used to support the medial arch and decrease stretch along the tibial nerve can alleviate symptoms. Review of the surgical results shows a lower success rate for tarsal tunnel release than for carpal tunnel release. The distal tarsal tunnel should be released together with lateral and medial plantar nerve branches at the bifurcation deep to the deep abductor hallucis muscle fascia.

Adverse Outcomes of Treatment

Symptoms may not resolve completely if permanent nerve damage has occurred. Surgical nerve release can lead to increased scarring and increased symptoms. The results of revision tarsal tunnel surgery are extremely poor, especially when an adequate decompression of the nerve was performed during the initial procedure.

Referral Decisions/Red Flags

Further evaluation is required for patients who have one or more of the following conditions: severe or progressive symptoms; loss of motor strength; pain that radiates above the knee, which can indicate a herniated disk; or severe pain to light touch, which can indicate complex regional pain syndrome.

Toe Deformities

Synonyms
Claw toe
Hammer toe
Mallet toe

Definition
Deformities of the lesser toes are categorized as three types: claw toes, hammer toes, and mallet toes. These deformities are most commonly caused by tight, improperly fitting shoes. They also are caused by an imbalance of the intrinsic (arising from the foot) and extrinsic (arising from the leg) muscles. A claw toe has fixed extension of the metatarsophalangeal (MTP) joint and flexion of the proximal interphalangeal (PIP) joint (**Figure 1**). A flexion contracture of the distal interphalangeal (DIP) joint may be present as well. Claw toes usually affect all of the lesser toes of the foot and often are secondary to a neurologic disorder such as Charcot-Marie-Tooth disease, or an inflammatory arthritis such as rheumatoid arthritis. Patients with diabetes mellitus who have a peripheral neuropathy commonly develop claw toes. A hammer toe has a correctable extension deformity at the MTP joint, with flexion deformity of the PIP joint with no significant deformity of the DIP joint (**Figure 2**). The flexion deformity of the PIP joint causes passive extension of the MTP joint when the patient is standing, but the MTP joint is in neutral alignment when the foot is examined in a non–weight-bearing position. A mallet toe has a flexion deformity at the DIP joint with relatively normal alignment of the PIP and MTP joints (**Figure 3**). Hammer toes and mallet toes can be isolated to a single toe and are often caused by improper shoe wear. The second toe, especially if longer than the great toe, is most commonly affected.

The presence of an acute/traumatic sagittal extension deformity formation at the MTP joint level should raise suspicion for plantar plate rupture. Plantar plate rupture has been shown to be the primary cause of fixed extension deformity at the MTP joint level in the presence of a hammer toe deformity.

Clinical Symptoms
Pain, deformity, and difficulty with shoe wear are the common symptoms of patients with lesser toe deformities. A corn can develop on the dorsum of the PIP joint or the tip of the toe. These calluses are painful and can become infected. In patients with hyperextension of the MTP joint, the metatarsal head is displaced plantarly with resultant increased pressure, callus, and pain on the plantar side of the forefoot.

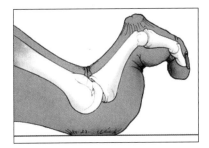

Figure 1 Illustration of the appearance of a claw toe.

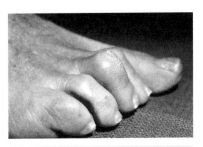

Figure 2 Photograph of the clinical appearance of a hammer toe.

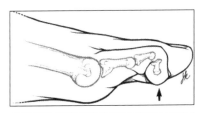

Figure 3 Illustration of the appearance of a mallet toe.

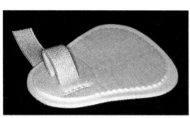

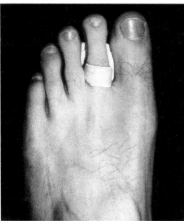

Figure 4 Photographs of the type of splint used for a claw toe.

Tests

Physical Examination

Examine the patient in both standing and sitting positions. Note alignment, the presence of corns, and flexibility and stability of the MTP, PIP, and DIP joints. Evaluate alignment and mobility of the ankle and hindfoot joints. Look for a cavus foot, which is associated with neurologic disorders. Evaluate sensory and motor function of the foot and lower extremities. The examiner should also evaluate for the presence of a plantar plate rupture using the anterior drawer (shock) test.

Diagnostic Tests

Radiographs are helpful only in planning surgery and to rule out osteomyelitis when ulceration of the toe has occurred. A neurologic workup may be indicated in patients with claw toes and a high arch.

Differential Diagnosis

- Neurologic or rheumatologic disorder (claw toes) (noted on physical examination)

Adverse Outcomes of the Disease

Without treatment, patients have difficulty with shoe wear and with persistent, painful corns and calluses. Ulceration may lead to infection and possible osteomyelitis.

Treatment

A shoe with a soft, roomy toe box to accommodate the deformity is the mainstay of treatment. A shoe repair shop can help by stretching shoes to accommodate single hammer and mallet toe deformities. Athletic shoes usually provide enough room to accommodate the deformity. Shoes with heels higher than 2¼″ should be avoided. Protective cushions sold over the counter are helpful when corns develop.

Commercially available splints to hold the toes in place can provide symptomatic relief (**Figure 4**). In addition, the patient can tape the toe into flexion at the MTP joint. With a narrow strip of tape, begin on the plantar aspect of the foot under the metatarsal head, looping over the dorsum of the proximal phalanx and crossing back to the starting point while holding the toe flexed at the MTP joint. Surgical correction may be necessary for fixed deformities or plantar plate ruptures. The goal of surgery is not cosmetic but the proper alignment of the toes to comfortably accommodate shoe wear. Surgical correction usually achieves toes that sit flat but do not have normal range of motion. Postoperative swelling tends to last for several months.

Rehabilitation Prescription

Stretching and strengthening of the toes helps to preserve flexibility. Toe strengthening exercises can help maintain normal range of motion in the toes and keep the intrinsic muscle of the foot strong to help prevent the condition from getting worse or recurring.

Adverse Outcomes of Treatment

Continued pain, corns, decreased range of motion, and recurrent deformity are possible.

Referral Decisions/Red Flags

Failure of nonsurgical treatment or persistent ulceration requires further evaluation. Patients with vascular insufficiency are poor candidates for surgical treatment.

www.aaos.org/essentials5/exercises

Home Exercise Program for Toe Strengthening

- The following exercise program is introductory only, and progression of this program will vary based on your specific injury, symptoms, and baseline level of fitness. For further progression of this routine, your physician may recommend evaluation and treatment by a physical therapist or other exercise professional.

Home Exercises for Toe Strengthening

Exercise	Condition Recommended for	Repetitions or Duration
Toe squeeze	Hammer toe Toe cramp	10 repetitions
Big toe pull	Bunion Toe cramp	10 repetitions
Toe pull	Bunion Hammer toe Toe cramp	10 repetitions
Golf ball roll	Plantar fasciitis Arch strain Foot cramp	2 minutes
Marble pickup	Pain in ball of foot Hammer toe Toe cramp	Pick up all marbles once
Towel curl	Hammer toe Toe cramp Pain in ball of foot	5 repetitions

Toe Squeeze
- Place small sponges or corks between the toes.
- Squeeze and hold for 5 seconds.
- Repeat 10 times.

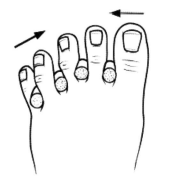

Big Toe Pull
- Place a thick rubber band around both big toes.
- Pull the big toes away from each other and toward the small toes.
- Hold for 5 seconds.
- Repeat 10 times.

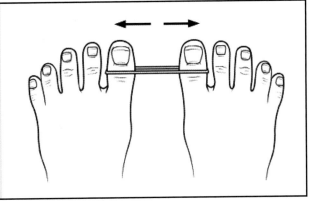

Toe Pull
- Put a thick rubber band around all your toes and spread them.
- Hold this position for 5 seconds.
- Repeat 10 times.

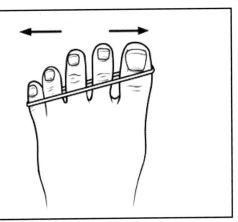

Golf Ball Roll
- Roll a golf ball under the ball of your foot for 2 minutes to massage the bottom of the foot.

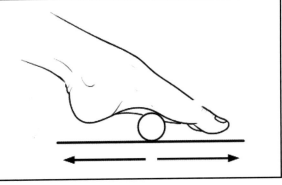

SECTION 7 FOOT AND ANKLE

SECTION 7 FOOT AND ANKLE

Marble Pickup

- Place 20 marbles on the floor.
- Pick up one marble at a time and put it in a small bowl.
- Repeat until you have picked up all 20 marbles.

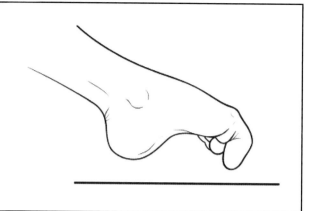

Towel Curl

- Place a small towel on the floor and curl it toward you, using only your toes. You can increase the resistance by putting weight on the end of the towel.
- Relax and repeat 5 times.

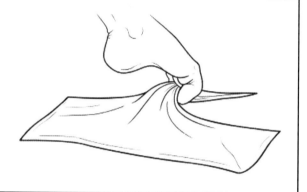

Turf Toe

Synonym

First metatarsophalangeal (MTP) joint sprain

Definition

Turf toe is a sprain of the first metatarsophalangeal (MTP) joint that most commonly occurs with hyperextension but can occur with any forced range of motion. The term turf toe was coined because the incidence of these injuries increased with the use of artificial turf on athletic playing fields. Turf toe injuries are associated with significant morbidity, and in some studies these injuries accounted for more missed playing time than did ankle sprains.

Clinical Symptoms

Patients usually report swelling, tenderness, and limited motion of the first MTP joint. A grade 1 sprain is a stretch injury of the capsule, with the athlete usually able to participate in sports with mild symptoms. A grade 2 sprain is a partial tear of the plantar ligamentous complex of the MTP joint. These patients have moderate swelling, ecchymosis, and decreased range of motion. A grade 3 sprain is a complete tear of the MTP ligamentous complex. Marked swelling, bruising, and limited motion occur with grade 3 injuries. The patient can neither compete athletically nor walk normally.

Tests

Physical Examination

Assess the degree of swelling, ecchymosis, range of motion, and gait.

Diagnostic Tests

Radiographs are useful to detect associated avulsion fractures, evaluate joint congruity, and rule out preexisting arthritic changes. When the diagnosis is in question, a bone scan or MRI can help exclude other possibilities such as sesamoid or metatarsal fractures.

Differential Diagnosis

• Hallux rigidus (limited range of motion of the first MTP joint)
• Sesamoid stress fracture (focal pain over the sesamoid)

Adverse Outcomes of the Disease

Instability and arthritis (hallux rigidus) of the first MTP joint can develop. Symptomatic loose bodies and osteochondritic lesions can occur.

Treatment

Nonsurgical treatment with rest, ice, compression, and elevation (RICE) usually is sufficient. Early range of motion is started as symptoms allow. After a grade 1 or 2 sprain, a stiff-soled or rocker-bottom shoe is recommended to restrict MTP joint motion and alleviate symptoms. Grade 3 injuries require protected weight bearing or immobilization for 1 to 2 weeks, with a 4- to 6-week period of rest from athletics. Taping, orthotic devices, or a stiff-soled or rocker-bottom shoe is then recommended. Surgical intervention is seldom necessary except in the case of displaced intra-articular or avulsion fractures or high-grade sprains.

Adverse Outcomes of Treatment

Delayed return to sports activities, hallux rigidus, and acquired hallux varus or valgus can occur.

Referral Decisions/Red Flags

Intra-articular fractures may require open reduction or excision. Urgent surgical intervention is necessary for an irreducible dislocation. Osteochondral lesions or loose bodies also require further evaluation.

PAIN DIAGRAM
Spine

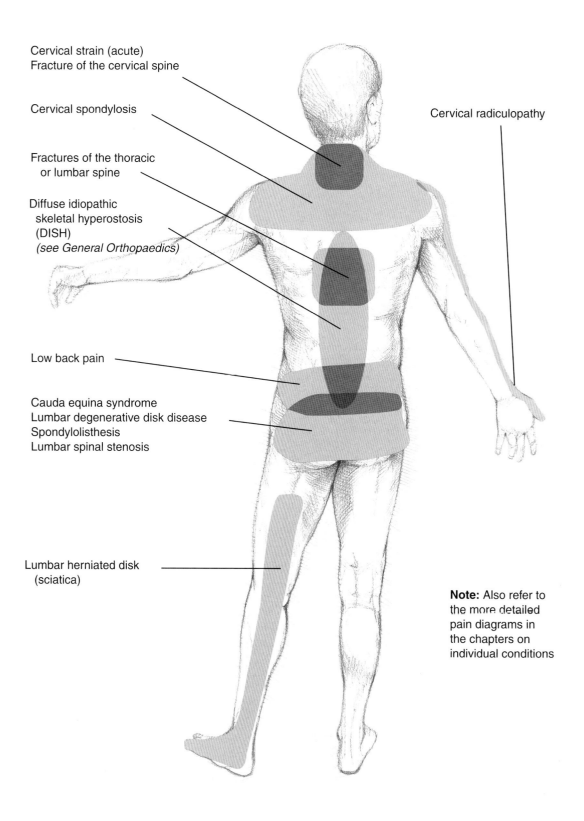

Cervical strain (acute)
Fracture of the cervical spine

Cervical spondylosis

Fractures of the thoracic
   or lumbar spine

Diffuse idiopathic
   skeletal hyperostosis
   (DISH)
   (see General Orthopaedics)

Cervical radiculopathy

Low back pain

Cauda equina syndrome
Lumbar degenerative disk disease
Spondylolisthesis
Lumbar spinal stenosis

Lumbar herniated disk
   (sciatica)

Note: Also refer to
the more detailed
pain diagrams in
the chapters on
individual conditions

Spine

Section Editor

Daniel T. Altman, MD, FACS

Associate Professor of Orthopaedic Surgery
Drexel University College of Medicine
Allegheny General Hospital
Pittsburgh, Pennsylvania

Contributor

Mark C. Hubbard, MPT

Physical Therapist
Bone and Joint Institute
Penn State Milton S. Hershey Medical Center
Hershey, Pennsylvania

ANATOMY OF THE SPINE

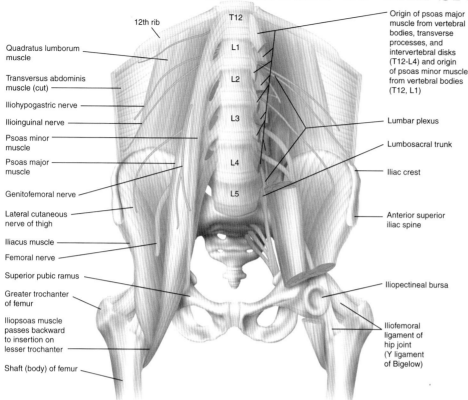

12th rib

T12

Quadratus lumborum muscle

Transversus abdominis muscle (cut)

Iliohypogastric nerve

Ilioinguinal nerve

Psoas minor muscle

Psoas major muscle

Genitofemoral nerve

Lateral cutaneous nerve of thigh

Iliacus muscle

Femoral nerve

Superior pubic ramus

Greater trochanter of femur

Iliopsoas muscle passes backward to insertion on lesser trochanter

Shaft (body) of femur

L1

L2

L3

L4

L5

Origin of psoas major muscle from vertebral bodies, transverse processes, and intervertebral disks (T12-L4) and origin of psoas minor muscle from vertebral bodies (T12, L1)

Lumbar plexus

Lumbosacral trunk

Iliac crest

Anterior superior iliac spine

Iliopectineal bursa

Iliofemoral ligament of hip joint (Y ligament of Bigelow)

Pelvis: Anterior Muscles

Bones of the Spine/Ribs and Pelvis

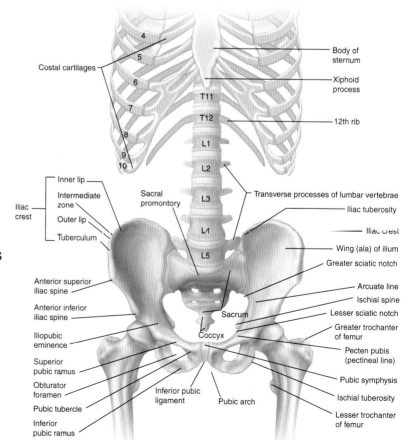

Costal cartilages

4

5

6

7

8

9

10

Body of sternum

Xiphoid process

T11

T12

L1

L2

L3

L4

L5

12th rib

Transverse processes of lumbar vertebrae

Iliac tuberosity

Iliac crest

Wing (ala) of ilium

Greater sciatic notch

Arcuate line

Ischial spine

Lesser sciatic notch

Greater trochanter of femur

Pecten pubis (pectineal line)

Pubic symphysis

Ischial tuberosity

Lesser trochanter of femur

Inner lip

Intermediate zone

Outer lip

Tuberculum

Iliac crest

Sacral promontory

Anterior superior iliac spine

Anterior inferior iliac spine

Iliopubic eminence

Superior pubic ramus

Obturator foramen

Pubic tubercle

Inferior pubic ramus

Sacrum

Coccyx

Inferior pubic ligament

Pubic arch

Overview of the Spine

Low back pain affects 60% to 70% of adults at some time in their lives; 15% to 30% of the population is affected at any one time. Low back pain may be related to overuse/strain or age-associated degenerative changes, or it may be caused by significant pathology, such as segmental instability, neural compromise, or spinal deformity. Many pathologic disorders associated with low back pain and pain of spinal origin can have a substantial and measurable effect on health-related quality of life. Low back pain and back injury are the leading causes of disability and missed work hours in persons 45 years and younger. More than 30 million visits were made to physicians' offices in 2002 because of back problems. Cost estimates vary, but in 2008, care related to back pain was estimated to be $86 billion. The actual number of patients seeking spine-related care has increased substantially in the past decade.

Most individuals with low back pain experience pain for only a brief time, with near-complete resolution of symptoms within 30 days. Some patients experience persistent symptoms that progress to chronic pain, usually lasting longer than 90 days. In other patients, symptoms resolve, but the patient then experiences bouts of recurrent pain.

A complete medical history and physical examination are essential in patients with low back pain symptoms. In the absence of red flags or significant physical findings, nonsurgical treatment can begin with NSAIDs and/or rehabilitation. Initial treatment efforts should be directed toward diminishing acute symptoms; rehabilitation should be initiated as acute symptoms resolve. Rehabilitation is not immediately effective in patients with marked paraspinous dysrhythmia, limited mobility, and marked pain. Following symptom resolution, however, active rehabilitation and patient education are important to reduce recurrence.

Most patients should be able to return to activities or work quickly, depending on presentation, but work modifications may be required. Patients unable to return to work quickly should undergo more extensive evaluation, including laboratory tests and advanced imaging studies to exclude infections, lumbar disk herniations, or other causes of pain. Other factors, such as litigation and workers' compensation claims, may considerably affect pain behavior and have an effect on the motivation to return to work rapidly. These issues become clear over time. Patient education is important and requires time and patience on the part of the physician and other healthcare providers.

The differential diagnosis for low back pain is wide-ranging, and the patient must be evaluated to ensure that no identifiable cause for the pain is overlooked (**Table 1**). Diagnoses include inflammation, infection, degenerative disorders, neoplasms (primary and metastatic), trauma, metabolic disorders, developmental defects, neurologic disorders, referred pain, psychologic problems, and rare conditions. Cauda equina syndrome is one of the more ominous

Table 1		
Common Presentations of Spinal Problems		
Problem	**Associated Signs and Symptoms**	**Possible Diagnosis**
Neck pain	Paravertebral discomfort relieved with rest and aggravated with activity	Acute neck strain; upper cervical disk herniation
	Limited motion or morning stiffness	Cervical spondylosis
Neck and arm pain	A younger patient with an abnormal upper extremity neurologic examination	Cervical radiculopathy due to herniated nucleus pulposus
	An older patient with limited motion and pain on extension	Cervical radiculopathy due to cervical spondylosis
	Urinary dysfunction with global sensory changes, weakness, and an abnormal gait	Cervical myelopathy secondary to cervical spondylosis or trauma; demyelinating disorder
	Shoulder pain and a positive impingement sign	Shoulder pathology; superior sulcus tumor of lung (uncommon)
	Positive Tinel sign and nondermatomal distribution of symptoms	Peripheral nerve entrapment
Back pain	Paravertebral discomfort relieved with rest and aggravated with activity	Acute low back strain
	Limited motion or stiffness	Degenerative disk disease; ankylosing spondylitis
	Unrelenting night pain and weight loss	Tumor; infection
	Fevers, chills, and sweats	Infection or intervertebral disk infection
Back and leg pain	A younger patient with an abnormal lower extremity neurologic examination	Lumbar radiculopathy due to herniated nucleus pulposus
	An older patient with poor walking tolerance and a stooped gait	Spinal stenosis
	Tenderness over the lateral hip and discomfort at night	Trochanteric bursitis

conditions that should be considered—early recognition and treatment are critical to provide the best chance for recovery. **Table 2** lists and compares several conditions commonly associated with back pain.

Types of Pain

Night pain that interrupts or prevents sleep, along with fever and weight loss, may be an ominous symptom that indicates a more serious problem such as malignancy or infection. Night pain also may be experienced by patients with significant lumbar spinal stenosis. Acute posttraumatic pain may indicate a fracture. Patients with advanced osteoporosis or chronic steroid use may experience acute pain and may sustain a vertebral compression fracture with minimal trauma or no history of trauma. Low back pain is uncommon in children and warrants a thorough evaluation. A pain diagram is a

Table 2

Conditions Commonly Associated With Back Pain

Condition	Age (Years)	Position Associated With Pain	Anatomic Area Affected	Flexion/ Extension	Night Pain/ Fevers
Intervertebral disk herniation	20-50	Sitting	Leg	Flexion	No
Discogenic pain	20-50	Sitting	Back	Flexion	No
Spinal stenosis	>50	Standing	Both	Extension	No
Neoplasia	>50	Constant	Back	Flexion	Yes
Infection	Any	Constant	Back	Flexion	Yes

useful tool for communication between the patient and physician in detailing the location and quality of pain that a patient may experience (**Figure 1**).

Location of Pain
Neck Pain
Pain from strain, overuse, or an acute cervical sprain (flexion-extension or whiplash injury) is common and usually self-limiting. Pain located in the neck, trapezial, and interscapular areas commonly occurs in association with degeneration or herniation of an intervertebral disk. If the herniation occurs above the C5-6 level, the patient may not experience radiculopathy but will report only neck, trapezial, and/or interscapular pain. When injury results from a motor vehicle accident, one method to approximate the degree of injury is to ask questions regarding the mechanism and severity of the crash. These patients require evaluation of the cervical spine with radiography and/or CT. If there is no pathology evident on radiographs or CT scan but pain persists, MRI may be indicated to evaluate the disk and soft tissues.

Neck and Radicular Arm Pain
When accompanied by pain that radiates into the arm, neck pain may be the result of an entrapment or compression of a cervical nerve root by a herniated disk or an osteophyte. For screening evaluation, see **Figure 1**. Many patients with a herniated cervical disk are more comfortable when they place the hand of the symptomatic arm on their head because this position reduces the tension on the nerve. In contrast, patients with intrinsic shoulder problems feel more comfortable with their arms at their sides. With peripheral nerve entrapment syndromes, such as carpal tunnel syndrome, patients may report arm pain and a lesser degree of neck pain. Other less common disorders also may cause neck and arm pain. For example, a superior sulcus tumor of the lung (Pancoast tumor) may cause neck, shoulder, and arm pain, typically in the distribution of the ulnar nerve. Clues to this less common condition include intrinsic hand weakness, Horner syndrome, and a long history of cigarette smoking. Transient

SECTION 8 SPINE

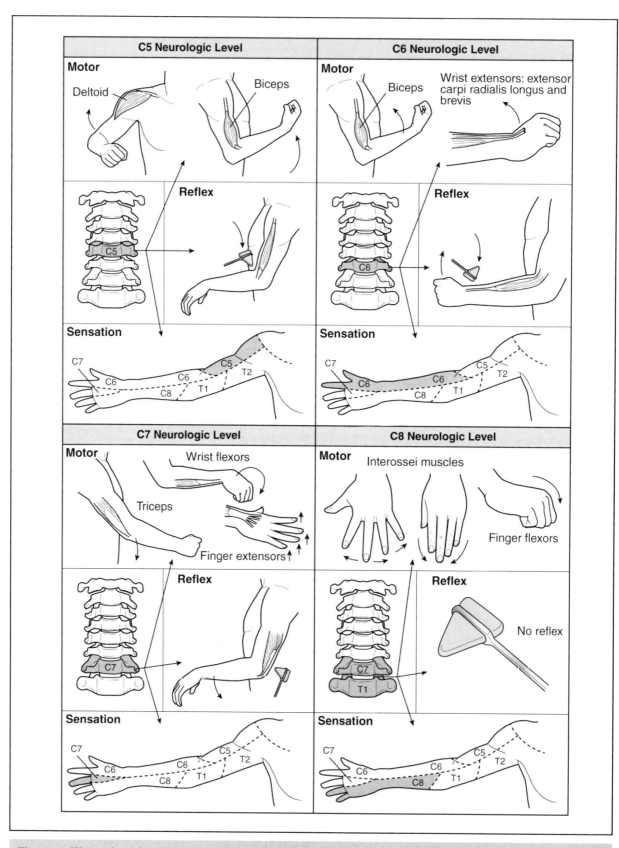

Figure 1   Illustration of neurologic evaluation of the upper extremity (C5, C6, C7, C8).

unilateral radicular symptoms (referred to as burners or stingers) can occur in persons who play contact sports.

Low Back Pain

In discussing low back pain in this section, a specific diagnosis is one that can be clearly diagnosed as a discrete entity through patient history, physical examination, imaging studies, or pathologic changes identified during surgical intervention. Conditions that meet these criteria include lumbar strain, herniated lumbar disk, lumbar spinal stenosis, degenerative spondylolisthesis, and others.

Low back pain typically occurs in the midline (axial) at approximately the L4 or L5 level and may radiate to the buttocks. Back disorders that affect patients between the ages of 20 and 40 years are often related to strains (affecting muscles) of the soft-tissue structures of the back, including the ligamentous support portion of the intervertebral disk. Young adults with spondylolysis and spondylolisthesis often report episodic axial back pain that may require further evaluation and treatment. Nonsurgical treatment should be tried initially; many of these patients ultimately require surgical treatment. Job modifications also may be advised, although many patients experience resolution of their symptoms and are able to continue rigorous physical work. With seronegative spondyloarthropathies (such as ankylosing spondylitis), patients often have back pain with morning stiffness that lasts longer than 30 minutes.

With aging and degeneration of the intervertebral disk, associated arthritis may develop in the facet joints and contribute to back pain in patients older than 40 years. In most patients with physiologic aging of the spine, significant symptoms that have an adverse effect on their quality of life do not develop. Back pain, with or without radiculopathy, may be associated with spinal stenosis. These symptoms are aggravated by spinal extension, as occurs during standing or walking upright or sleeping supine, and the symptoms can be relieved by flexion. Diffuse idiopathic skeletal hyperostosis (DISH), which primarily affects men, often becomes symptomatic after age 50 years.

Extraspinal causes of back pain include pancreatitis, inflammatory bowel disease, kidney stones, pelvic infections, retroperitoneal lesions, aortic aneurysms, and tumors or cysts of the reproductive tract.

Back and Radicular Leg Pain

Unilateral leg pain is common with herniation of an intervertebral disk, usually at the L4-5 or L5-S1 vertebral levels. Herniations at the L3-4 level generally cause pain that radiates into the thigh and/or groin area. The pain is typically worse with sitting and is associated with sciatic tension signs (straight leg raising test, supine and seated) as well as altered sensation, motor strength, and reflexes in the lower extremity (**Figure 2**). Patients with an L3-4 disk herniation may exhibit a positive reverse straight leg raising test (positive femoral

SECTION 8   SPINE

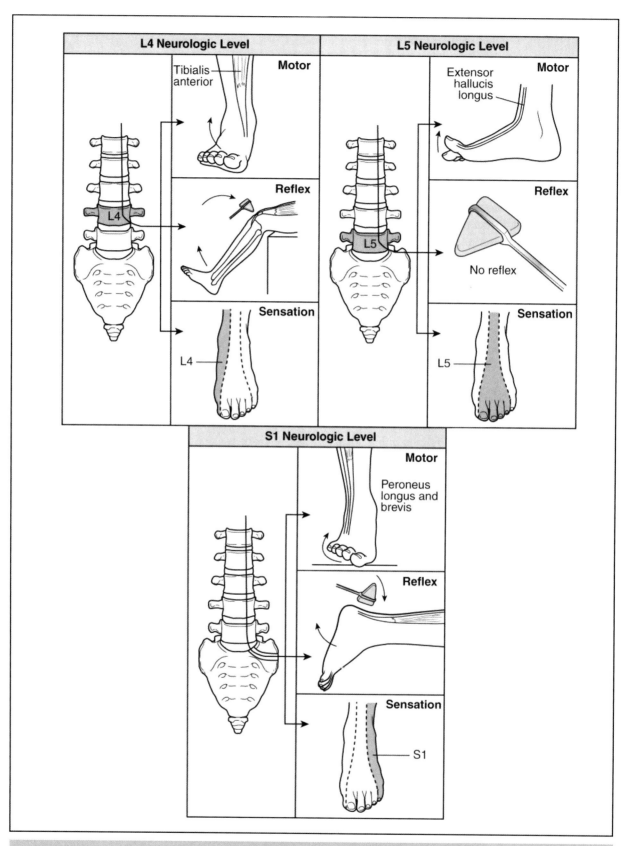

Figure 2 Illustration of neurologic evaluation of the lower extremity (L4, L5, S1).

nerve stretch sign) and a diminished quadriceps reflex. Trochanteric bursitis can mimic sciatica; these two diagnoses may coexist.

Bilateral leg pain may indicate spinal stenosis, a large central disk rupture, cauda equina syndrome, or spondylolisthesis, especially after age 40 years. In patients older than 40 years who present with back and leg pain, degenerative spondylolisthesis is much more common than isthmic spondylolisthesis. Patients with degenerative spondylolisthesis do not have spondylolysis. Exercise-induced leg pain (unilateral or bilateral) may indicate lumbar spinal stenosis; this pain is referred to as neurogenic claudication. Spinal stenosis occurs most commonly at the L3-4 and L4-5 interspaces.

Extraspinal causes of nerve root entrapment or irritation include hip disease, piriformis syndrome, ovarian cysts, and retroperitoneal lesions. Discerning a diagnosis between a hip disorder and a spinal etiology can be difficult because both disorders occur in an aging population and both disorders frequently occur in the same patient.

Deformity

Spinal deformity may affect the sagittal, coronal, and axial planes. Sagittal plane deformity or kyphotic deformities of the spine are best seen on physical examination from the side. Sagittal plane malalignment of the spine may involve any region of the spine but is most common in the thoracic and thoracolumbar spine and is common with aging. Scoliosis is defined by coronal plane deformity, but there is a concordant rotational deformity that is apparent on examination. Shoulder asymmetry, pelvic tilt, and asymmetric abdominal or flank creases are signs of deformity in the coronal plane. Trunk rotation or rib prominence on forward bending (Adam forward bend test) is a critical measure of axial plane deformity and may be apparent earlier than coronal deformity in patients with scoliosis. In younger patients, scoliosis is usually idiopathic, but in older patients it also may occur as a result of degenerative changes. Patients with a new onset of scoliosis or rapid progression of deformity should be evaluated for syndromes or diseases that may be a cause of spinal deformity such as neurofibromatosis, spinal cord lesions, or a tethered spinal cord. Spondylolisthesis (isthmic) usually occurs at the lumbosacral joint and is accompanied by tight hamstring muscles (inability to toe-touch). Onset of a spinal deformity in adulthood, or de novo degenerative scoliosis, is common and may be associated with aging, segmental instability, and osteoporosis. However, a rapid progression of deformity in the adult may be an indication of neoplasm or infection. These conditions may be accompanied by compromise of the spinal nerve roots and/or the spinal cord.

Trauma

All patients who sustain spinal trauma must be thoroughly evaluated, including appropriate radiographs. At many trauma centers, CT has replaced plain radiography as a screening modality. Some spinal injuries may be subtle, especially in the cervical spine.

Flexion-distraction injuries of the thoracolumbar spine also may be missed on radiographs because ligamentous injuries may occur without any bony injury. These injuries may be unstable, and early recognition is essential. The potential consequences of misdiagnosed spinal injuries can be devastating and include progressive deformities with or without neurologic deficits. Injuries to the spine are often associated with other life-threatening visceral, head, or skeletal injuries. For many reasons, some spinal injuries may be missed initially in the multiply injured patient, even after an appropriate evaluation.

Incidence by Sex

Women have an increased incidence of the following spinal conditions: scoliosis in adolescence, metastatic breast cancer, trochanteric bursitis in later adulthood, and osteoporosis with vertebral body fractures that may lead to an increased kyphosis following menopause.

Men have an increased incidence of the following spinal conditions: kyphosis in adolescence, ankylosing spondylitis in adulthood, and multiple myeloma and DISH in later adulthood. The most common metastatic spinal lesions in men include prostate and lung cancers.

Musculoskeletal Conditioning of the Lumbar Spine

The goal of a conditioning program is to enable people to live a more fit and healthy lifestyle by being more active. A well-structured conditioning program also will prepare the individual for participation in sports and recreational activities. If the individual participates in a supervised rehabilitation program that provides instruction in a conditioning routine—instead of using only an exercise handout such as provided here—the focus should be on developing and committing to a home exercise fitness program. A conditioning program for the body as a whole that includes exercises for the shoulder, hip, knee, and foot as well as the lumbar spine is described in the chapter Musculoskeletal Conditioning: Helping Patients Prevent Injury and Stay Fit.

Conditioning of the lumbar spine to prevent low back pain should include strengthening and stretching exercises to improve range of motion. The focus of conditioning should be on a daily home exercise program. In general, emphasis should be placed on aerobic exercise and active treatment rather than passive treatment.

Strengthening Exercises

The four muscle groups that protect the spine from daily overuse and trauma include the abdominals, the quadratus lumborum (two groups, one on each side of the spine), and the back extensors. The back extensors are important because poor endurance of these muscle groups has been found in patients with low back pain. Isometric exercises for these muscle groups, such as the bird dog exercise, have an important stabilizing effect on the spine.

The quadratus lumborum is an important lateral stabilizer of the trunk. A strengthening exercise for this muscle is the side bridge, which should be repeated on both sides for maximum and symmetric lateral stability. The abdominals are important to stabilization of the lumbar and thoracic spine. The four major muscle groups that make up the abdominals are the transverse abdominis, the internal and external obliques, and the rectus abdominis. The transverse abdominis muscle is a stabilizer of the lumbar spine through its attachment to the thoracolumbar fascia. Traditional sit-ups have been found to greatly increase the load on the lumbar disks and therefore should be avoided by patients with low back pain. A safe exercise is abdominal bracing, which activates all the abdominal muscles, including the transverse abdominis, and does not stress the lumbar spine. This exercise does not activate the transverse abdominis if a pelvic tilt is performed.

Stretching Exercises

Stretching exercises for the trunk and pelvis are helpful for improving range of motion. The cat back stretch and the kneeling back extension exercises are excellent stretching exercises for the spine in general. Flexibility of the hamstring muscles is essential for improving the mobility of the lumbar spine and reducing stress on the lumbar spine. The seat side straddle, modified seat side straddle, sitting rotation stretch, and leg crossover all are excellent stretching exercises for the lumbothoracic spine.

SECTION 8 SPINE

Home Exercise Program for Lumbar Spine Conditioning

- Perform the exercises in the order listed.
- If any of the exercises cause pain or increase your pain, discontinue the exercise and call your doctor.
- This exercise program may not be appropriate if back pain is severe or if substantial loss of range of motion of the spine is present.
- The following exercise program is introductory only, and progression of this program will vary based on your specific injury, symptoms, and baseline level of fitness. For further progression of this routine, your physician may recommend evaluation and treatment by a physical therapist or other exercise professional.

Strengthening and Stretching Exercises for the Lumbar Spine

Exercise Type	Muscle Group/Area Targeted	Number of Repetitions	Number of Days per Week	Number of Weeks[a]
Strengthening Exercises				
Abdominal bracing	Abdominals	5	Daily	3 to 4
Side bridges	Quadratus lumborum	5	Daily	3 to 4
Bird dog	Back extensors	5	Daily	3 to 4
Stretching Exercises				
Cat back stretch	Middle and low back	5	Daily	3 to 4
Low back extension and flexion stretch	Low back	5	Daily	3 to 4
Seat side straddle	Adductor muscles Medial hamstrings Semitendinosus Semimembranosus	5	Daily	3 to 4
Modified seat side straddle	Adductor muscles Hamstrings	5	Daily	3 to 4
Sitting rotation stretch	Piriformis External rotators Internal rotators	5	Daily	3 to 4
Leg crossover	Hamstrings	5	Daily	3 to 4

[a]These exercises can be performed indefinitely for the prevention of low back pain.

Essentials of Musculoskeletal Care 5 *© 2016 American Academy of Orthopaedic Surgeons*

SECTION 8 | SPINE

Strengthening Exercises

Abdominal Bracing

- Lie on your back on the floor with your arms at your sides, your knees bent, and your feet flat on the floor.
- Contract your abdominal muscles so that your stomach is pulled away from your waistband.
- Hold this position for 15 seconds while breathing normally. Do not hold your breath.
- Perform 5 repetitions once per day, continuing for 3 to 4 weeks.

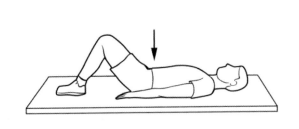

Side Bridges

- Lie on your side on the floor (for beginners, the knees may be bent 90°).
- With your elbow bent at 90°, lift your body off the floor as shown, keeping your body straight.
- Hold this position for 15 seconds and then repeat on the other side. The goal is to hold this position for 150 seconds total on each side.
- Perform 5 repetitions once per day, continuing for 3 to 4 weeks.

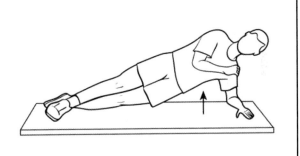

Bird Dog

- Kneel on the floor on your hands and knees.
- Lift your right arm straight out from the shoulder, level with your body, at the same time you lift your left leg straight out from the hip.
- Start by holding this position for 15 seconds. Gradually increase the hold time as tolerated, while maintaining proper body position. The goal is to hold this position for 150 seconds (30 years or older) or 170 seconds (younger than 30 years) total.
- Repeat with the opposite arm and leg.
- Perform 5 repetitions per day, continuing for 3 to 4 weeks.

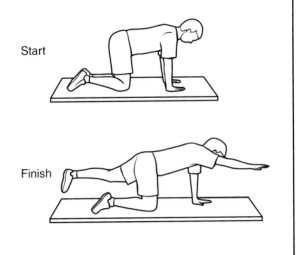

Start

Finish

SECTION 8 SPINE

Stretching Exercises

Cat Back Stretch

- Kneel on your hands and knees in a relaxed position.
- Raise your back up like a cat and hold for 30 seconds.
- Relax for 30 seconds.
- Repeat 5 times per day, continuing for 3 to 4 weeks.

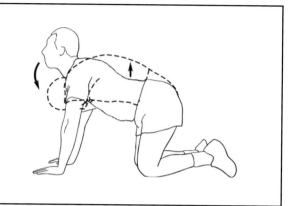

Low Back Extension and Flexion Stretch

- Lie on a firm surface, face down, and press up with your arms (position 1). Hold for 5 seconds.
- Extend your arms, rock back and sit on your bent knees, and tuck your head (position 2) until you feel a stretch in your back. Hold for 5 seconds.
- Repeat 5 times per day, continuing for 3 to 4 weeks.

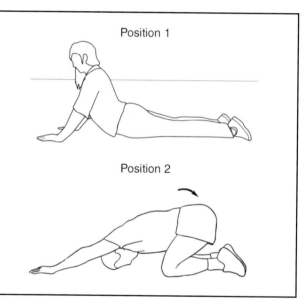

Position 1

Position 2

Seat Side Straddle

- Sit on the floor with your legs spread apart.
- Place both hands on the same ankle and bring your chin as close to your knee as possible.
- Hold the maximum stretch for 30 seconds and then relax for 30 seconds.
- Repeat on the other side.
- Repeat the sequence 5 times per day, continuing for 3 to 4 weeks.

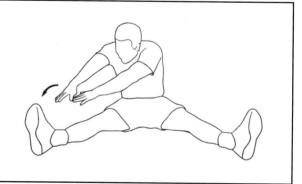

Modified Seat Side Straddle

- The modified seat straddle can be used if the aforementioned seat side straddle position is not tolerated. Sit on the floor with one leg extended to the side and the other leg bent as shown.
- Place both hands on the ankle of the extended leg and bring your chin as close to your knee as possible.
- Hold the maximum stretch for 30 seconds and then relax for 30 seconds.
- Reverse leg positions and repeat on the other side.
- Repeat the sequence 5 times per day, continuing for 3 to 4 weeks.

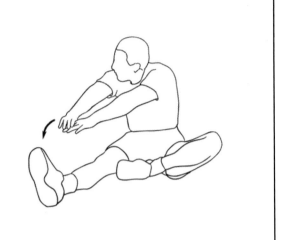

Sitting Rotation Stretch

- Sit on the floor with both legs straight out in front of you.
- Cross one leg over the other, place the elbow of the opposite arm on the outside of the thigh, and support yourself with your other arm behind you.
- Rotate your head and body in the direction of the supporting arm.
- Hold the maximum stretch for 30 seconds and then relax for 30 seconds.
- Reverse positions and repeat the stretch on the other side.
- Repeat the sequence 5 times per day, continuing for 3 to 4 weeks.

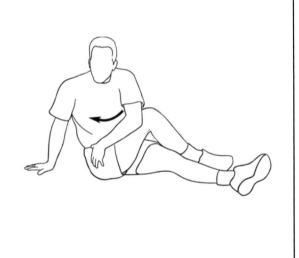

SECTION 8   SPINE

Leg Crossover

- Lie on the floor with your legs spread apart and your arms at your sides.
- Keeping the leg straight, bring your right toe to your left hand.
- Try to keep the other leg flat on the floor, but you may bend it slightly if needed for comfort.
- Hold the maximum stretch for 30 seconds and then relax for 30 seconds.
- Repeat with the left leg and the right hand.
- Repeat the sequence 5 times per day, continuing for 3 to 4 weeks.

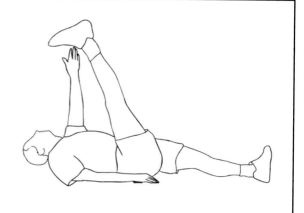

SECTION 8   SPINE

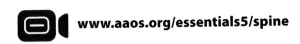

Physical Examination of the Spine

This examination is for patients who present with low back pain with or without radiculopathy.

Standing Examination

Posterior View

Inspect the spine for normal, straight alignment. Moderate to severe scoliosis will be obvious. Lesser degrees of scoliosis are best seen when the patient flexes forward. Also inspect for muscle atrophy. A lumbar list (lateral tilt) might be present in association with a herniated disk or other condition in which the patient will lean to one side to alleviate nerve root compression. In men younger than 40 years, measure chest expansion. Expansion of less than 1 inch suggests ankylosing spondylitis.

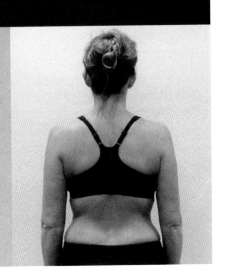

Lateral View

With the patient standing, inspect for deviations in normal cervical lordosis, thoracic kyphosis, and lumbar lordosis. Loss of cervical lordosis or lumbar lordosis may occur with painful conditions such as acute sprains, fractures, or infectious or neoplastic processes.

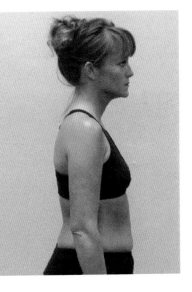

SECTION 8   SPINE

Pelvic Tilt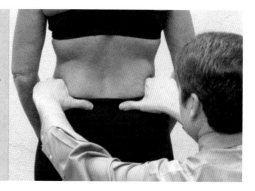

Observe the patient standing with the feet together and the knees straight. Inspect or palpate the top of the iliac crests. A pelvis that is not level may indicate a limb-length inequality, or it may be secondary to a spinal deformity.

Gait (Barefoot)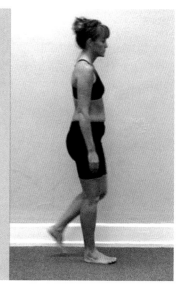

Evaluate the patient's gait with the patient barefoot. Have the patient walk across the room as you observe. Watch for a Trendelenburg lurch. If myelopathy is suspected, have the patient perform a heel-to-toe walk, and look for the inability or difficulty to maintain the weight on the heels or toes.

Trendelenburg Test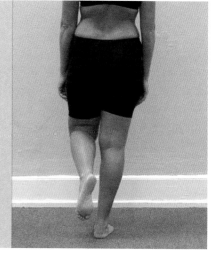

The Trendelenburg test is used to evaluate hip abductor strength, primarily the gluteus medius. Stand behind the patient to observe the level of the pelvis as you instruct the patient to stand on one leg. With normal hip abductor strength, the pelvis will remain level. If hip abductor strength is inadequate on the stance limb side, the pelvis will drop below level on the opposite side; this is a positive Trendelenburg test. Repeat the test on the other side.

SECTION 8   SPINE

Spinous Process Palpation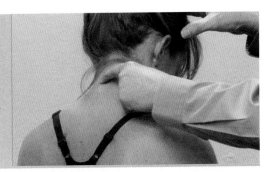

Palpate the spinous processes to define the alignment of the spine. With the patient standing, palpate each vertebra in turn, starting with C7, the most prominent cervical spinous process. In the anterior neck, the cricoid cartilage is parallel to the C6 vertebral body.

The top of the thyroid cartilage is at the level of the C4 vertebral body.

Flexion, Visual Estimation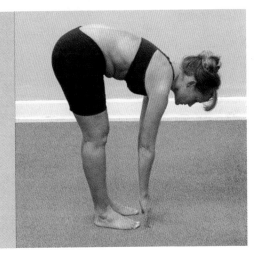

To evaluate lumbar flexion, ask the patient to stand with the hips and knees straight and the trunk in line with the lower extremities. The feet should be shoulder-width apart, and the arms should hang in a relaxed position. While viewing from the side, with the spine at maximum flexion, measure the distance between the fingertips and the floor. If at maximum flexion the fingertips are more than 10 cm from the floor, paraspinous spasm, hamstring tightness, nerve root compression, and/or symptom amplification should be considered. Pain reported on flexion is consistent with nerve root irritation from a disk herniation.

Extension, Visual Estimation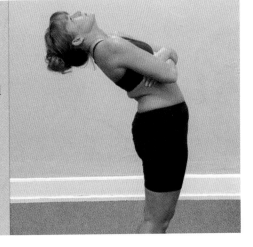

To evaluate lumbar extension, have the patient stand with the hips and knees straight and the trunk in line with the lower extremities. The feet should be shoulder-width apart to facilitate movement of the spine, and the arms should be folded comfortably across the chest. While observing from the side, have the patient bend backward. Pain on extension suggests spinal stenosis and/or spondylolisthesis.

SECTION 8 SPINE

Lateral Bending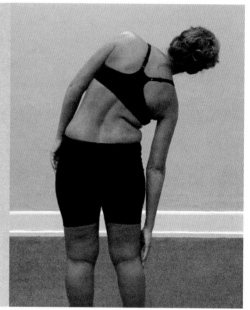

To evaluate lumbar lateral bending, have the patient stand with the hips and knees straight. The feet should be comfortably apart to facilitate movement of the spine, and the arms should hang in a relaxed position. Ask the patient to bend to the right and to the left. Estimate the maximum lateral bend on each side by observing how far down the thigh the fingertips reach. Note the location of pain or muscle spasm as the patient bends laterally, and then returns to the standing position. Pain reported on lateral bending may be due to muscle spasm, typically on the contralateral side, a facet joint irritation, or possibly nerve root irritation or disk herniation.

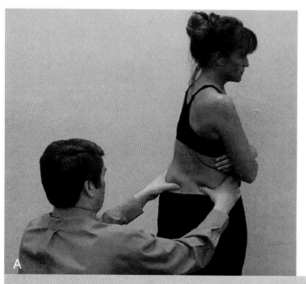
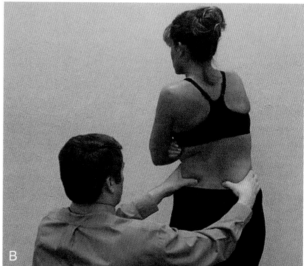

Lumbar Rotation

To evaluate lumbar rotation, have the patient stand with the hips and knees straight and the trunk in line with the lower extremities. The feet should be comfortably apart to facilitate movement of the spine, and the arms should be folded comfortably across the chest. Stabilize the pelvis with your hands on each iliac crest. Ask the patient to rotate to the right (**A**) and to the left (**B**). Observe the amount of rotation to each side. Note the location of pain or muscle spasm as the patient rotates and then returns to the neutral position. Pain reported on rotation may be due to muscle spasm or a facet joint irritation.

Heel Walking and Toe Walking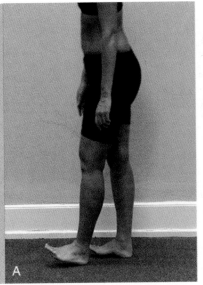

Heel walking and toe walking are used to evaluate spinal innervation. With the patient barefoot, have the patient walk first on the heels (**A**), and then on the toes (**B**), for a quick screen of the dorsiflexors (L4-L5 innervation) and plantar flexors (S1 innervation).

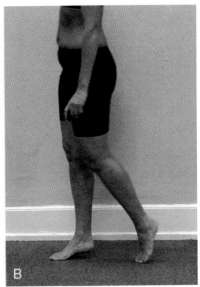

Seated Examination

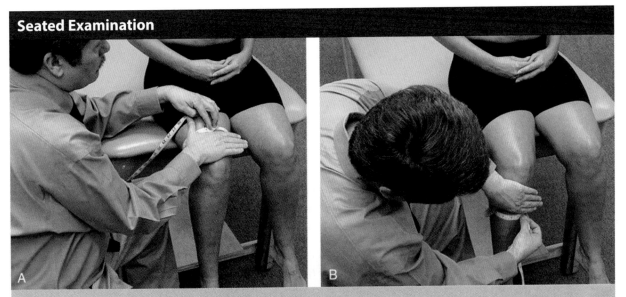

Calf and Thigh Circumference

To evaluate for calf and thigh atrophy, a cloth tape measure is needed. With the patient seated, measure the circumference of the thigh approximately 10 cm (or one hand breadth) above the patella (**A**) and the circumference of the calf approximately 10 cm below the patella (**B**). Atrophy may indicate chronic radiculopathy or disuse atrophy from a painful adjacent joint (knee or ankle).

SECTION 8   SPINE

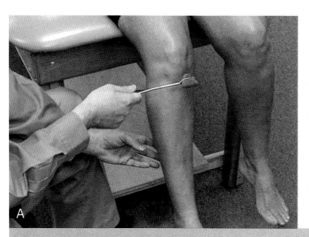
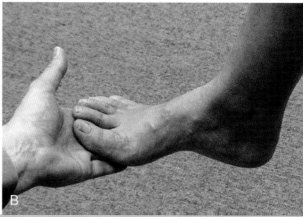

Deep Tendon Reflexes 📹

To assess deep tendon reflexes, a hammer is needed. With the patient seated, assess deep tendon reflexes at the knee. Tap the patellar tendon just below the patella (**A**). A decreased knee reflex is consistent with L3 or L4 nerve root compression. Assess deep tendon reflexes at the ankle (**B**). Tap the Achilles tendon just above the calcaneus. The ankle reflex may be diminished or absent with a decrease in function of the S1 root.

Dorsiflexion Strength Testing 📹

To assess the strength of the dorsiflexors, grasp the posterior aspect of the leg with one hand, and use your other hand on the dorsal aspect of the foot to resist the patient's attempt to dorsiflex the ankle. Weakness may indicate L4 nerve compression.

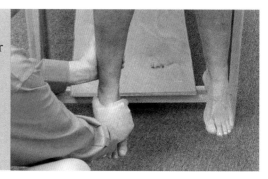

Extensor Hallucis Longus Strength Testing 📹

To assess the extensor hallucis longus, grasp the dorsal and plantar aspects of the midfoot medially with one hand to stabilize the foot in a neutral position, and apply resistance to the dorsal aspect of the great toe. Have the patient extend the great toe against your resistance. The extensor hallucis longus muscle is the easiest and most specific muscle to assess for L5 nerve root dysfunction.

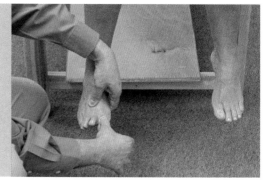

Quadriceps Testing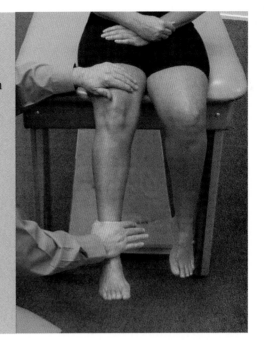

Evaluate the quadriceps muscle strength by asking the seated patient to extend the knee as you apply light resistance. Weakness in the quadriceps muscle may indicate compression on the L3 or L4 nerve root or perhaps pain inhibition from a knee disorder.

Hamstrings Testing

To evaluate the hamstrings, ask the patient to pull the leg toward the table as you apply light resistance. Weakness may indicate lumbar nerve root compression or pain inhibition from a knee injury.

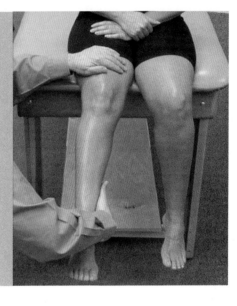

SECTION 8 SPINE

Iliopsoas Testing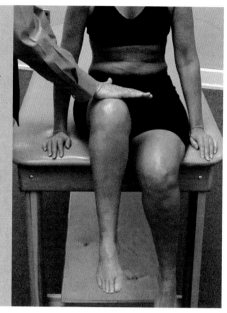

To evaluate the iliopsoas, ask the patient to flex the hip as you apply light resistance to the anterior aspect of the distal thigh. Weakness may indicate a primary hip disorder or an upper lumbar nerve root compression.

Seated Straight Leg Raising Test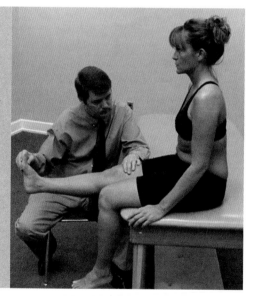

Use the seated straight leg test to evaluate sciatic tension. Distract the patient's attention away from the back by asking whether the patient has knee problems and then lift the foot and extend the knee. If straightening the knee to full extension on both sides does not cause the patient to lean back, no significant sciatic tension is present.

Meningeal Test (Slump Test of Maitland)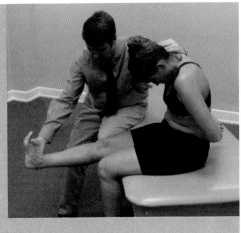

The slump test is a progressive test that is done bilaterally. The patient is questioned regarding symptoms at each step. Ask the seated patient to place his or her hands behind the back and then slump in a lumbar and thoracic flexed and relaxed position. Apply pressure over the shoulders, then apply light pressure to assist in cervical forward bending while the patient actively flexes the chin to chest. Apply slight pressure to the top of the head and then ask the patient to actively extend the knee fully. Then ask the patient to actively dorsiflex fully. As the examination has progressed to this step, impingement may be placed on the dura, spinal cord, or nerve roots, and this impingement may produce radicular symptoms in the area supplied by the sciatic nerve. Upon producing the symptoms at any of the preceding steps, the examination can be checked by seeing if cervical backbending, release of cervical flexion, and actively extending the head relieves the symptoms while extending the knee further.

Supine Examination

Palpation of Abdomen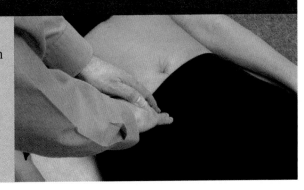

Examine the patient's abdomen. Palpate the abdomen for tenderness, masses, or enlarged organs. Consider referring female patients to a gynecologist for a pelvic examination, especially for chronic pain.

Supine Straight Leg Raising Test (Lasègue Sign)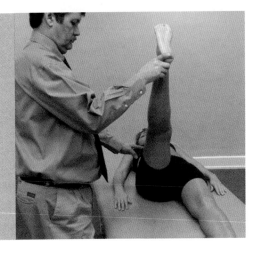

Passively raise the leg with the knee extended. Pain in the leg, not the back, is a positive sign and is suggestive of lumbar nerve root irritation or compression (typically from a herniated disk). A markedly positive test at 20° of elevation with a negative seated straight leg raising test is suggestive of symptom amplification rather than a true pathologic process.

SECTION 8   SPINE

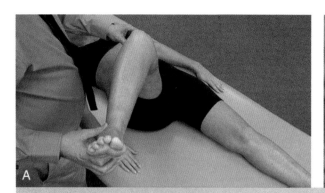

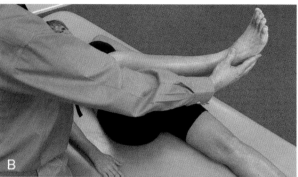

Internal-External Hip Rotation in Flexion

Flex the hip and knee to 90°, with the thigh held perpendicular to the transverse line across the anterior superior iliac spines. For internal rotation, rotate the tibia away from the midline of the trunk (**A**), thus producing inward rotation of the hip. For external rotation, rotate the tibia toward the midline of the trunk (**B**), thus producing external rotation of the hip. Pain in the groin or buttocks with this maneuver suggests hip irritability or pathology.

FABER Test

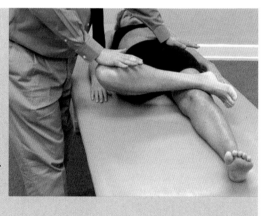

The FABER (flexion-abduction-external rotation) test, sometimes called the figure-of-4 test, the Patrick test, or the Jansen test, is a stress maneuver to detect hip and sacroiliac pathology. With the patient supine, place the affected hip in flexion, abduction, and external rotation, with the patient's foot on the opposite knee. Stabilize the pelvis with your hand on the contralateral anterior superior iliac spine and press down on the thigh of the affected side. If the maneuver is painful, the hip or sacroiliac region may be affected. Increased pain with this test also may be a nonorganic finding.

Sensory Examination

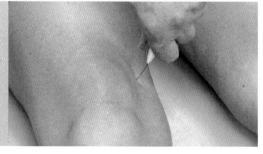

Using a zero-point, 10-g filament or a safety pin, test for pin-prick sensation over the lateral thigh and medial femoral condyle (L3 innervation), the medial leg and medial ankle (L4 innervation), the lateral leg and dorsum of the foot (L5 innervation), and the sole of the foot and lateral ankle (S1 innervation).

Babinski Sign (Flexor Plantar Response)

To evaluate the Babinski sign, stroke lightly upward on the plantar surface of the foot and look for great toe extension (withdrawal response) and fanning of the lesser toes as a sign of long-tract spinal cord involvement.

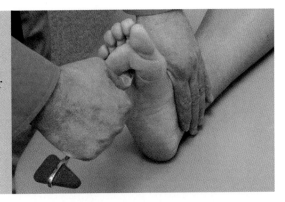

Ankle Clonus

To evaluate ankle clonus, dorsiflex the ankle suddenly and observe for rhythmic beating, noting the duration and the number of "beats." This is another sign of long-tract spinal cord involvement.

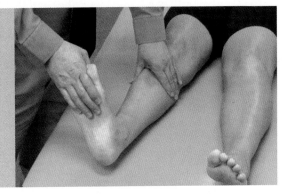

Brudzinski-Kernig Test

Ask the supine patient to cup his or her hands behind the head and then flex the head onto the chest. Then ask the patient to flex the hip and knee of one leg. Ask the patient to extend the flexed knee until pain is felt. If the patient then flexes the knee, and if pain disappears, it is a positive test. Pain may indicate meningeal irritation, nerve root involvement, or dural irritation.

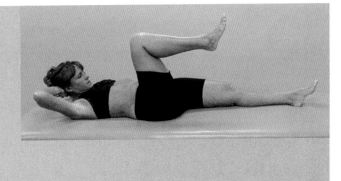

SECTION 8 SPINE

Prone Examination

Palpation of Lower Lumbar Area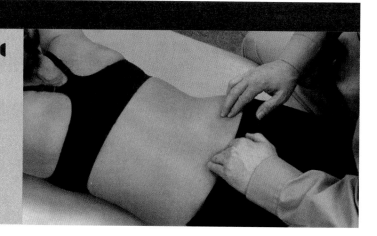

To evaluate the lower lumbar area, palpate the tissues over the lower lumbar area, looking for areas of tenderness, swelling, muscle spasm, or ecchymosis.

Reverse Straight Leg Raising Test (Femoral Nerve Stretch Test)

The reverse straight leg raising test is a traditional way to place the L1-L4 nerve roots under tension. With the patient prone, lift the hip into extension while keeping the knee straight. Pain over the anterior thigh suggests an upper lumbar disk problem, usually above L4-5. This test would also be markedly positive in a patient with a condition that involves inflammation of the iliopsoas, such as appendicitis.

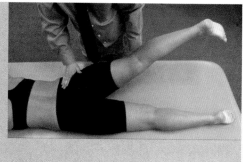

Findings Consistent With Nonorganic Pain (Waddell Signs)

The next four tests comprise the Waddell signs. In addition, the examiner should make a subjective evaluation of the entire history and physical examination to decide if the patient's pain behavior seems to be excessive. If the results of two or more of these tests, including the subjective evaluation, are positive, the examiner should be concerned that issues other than peripheral nociception are creating pain behavior.

Nonorganic Tenderness

To evaluate nonorganic tenderness, with the patient standing, lightly touch the tissues over the lower lumbar spine. This procedure should not cause pain. Marked pain behavior is a positive test.

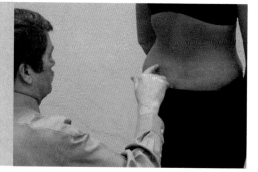

SECTION 8 SPINE

Axial Stimulation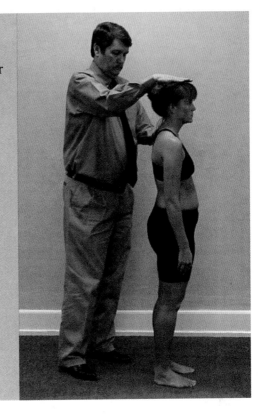

To evaluate axial stimulation, with the patient standing, apply light downward pressure on the patient's head. This maneuver should not cause pain in the lumbar spine. If the patient grimaces and moves, reporting pain, the test is positive.

Seated Straight Leg Raising Test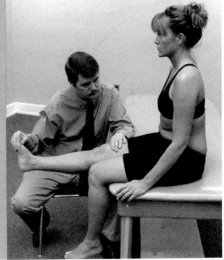

Use the seated straight leg test to evaluate sciatic tension. Distract the patient's attention away from the back by asking whether the patient has knee problems and then lift the foot and extend the knee. If straightening the knee to full extension on both sides does not cause the patient to lean back, no significant sciatic tension is present.

Sensory Examination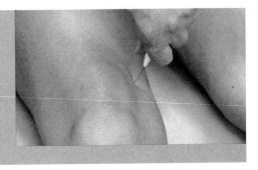

Using a zero-point, 10-g filament or a safety pin, test for pin-prick sensation over the lateral thigh and medial femoral condyle (L3 innervation), the medial leg and medial ankle (L4 innervation), the lateral leg and dorsum of the foot (L5 innervation), and the sole of the foot and lateral ankle (S1 innervation). Beware of a nonanatomic sensory (or motor) impairment.

Cervical Spine—Range of Motion

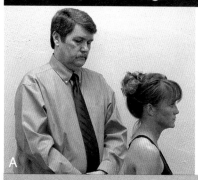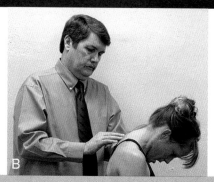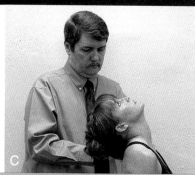

Flexion and Extension: Zero Starting Position 📷

To evaluate flexion and extension of the cervical spine, the patient is standing with the neck aligned with the trunk (**A**). Stabilize the trunk so that motion does not occur in the thoracic spine. Assess flexion with forward bending of the cervical spine (**B**), and extension with posterior inclination (**C**). Flexion and extension are typically estimated visually in degrees; however, limited flexion may also be measured as the distance between the chin and the sternum at maximum cervical flexion.

Lateral Bend 📷

To evaluate lateral bend, the nose is vertical and in line with the axis of the trunk. Stabilize the trunk so that motion occurs only at the neck. On lateral bend, the head is inclined toward the shoulder. Bend typically is measured as the degree of motion between the vertical axis and the mid axis of the face.

Inspect and palpate the supraclavicular fossae for tenderness and/or masses. Superior sulcus tumors of the lung (Pancoast tumors) sometimes present as neck pain and pain in the ulnar distribution.

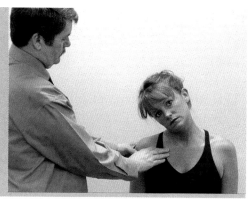

Rotation 📷

To evaluate neck rotation, the nose is vertical and in line with the axis of the trunk. Rotation is estimated in degrees. To estimate upper cervical vertebral rotation, measure rotation with the neck in maximum flexion.

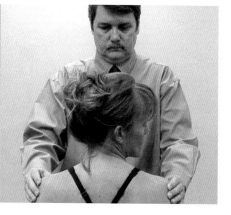

SECTION 8   SPINE

Spurling Test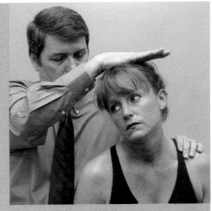

The Spurling test is used to help diagnose cervical disk herniations or cervical spondylosis. Performing this maneuver with incorrect technique can be harmful to the patient. You should perform the Spurling test only if you are confident in your ability to perform it correctly.

Ask the seated patient to rotate and laterally flex the head to the unaffected side first, then to the affected side. Use one hand to lightly compress downward on the head to axial load the cervical spine. If this is tolerated well, the test may be repeated with the neck extended. These maneuvers narrow the neural foramen and will increase or reproduce radicular arm pain associated with cervical disk herniations or cervical spondylosis.

Cervical Spine—Muscle Testing

C5—Deltoid Muscle (Seated)

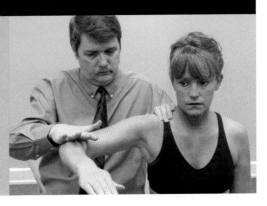

To evaluate the strength of the deltoid muscle, with the patient seated, abduct the shoulder to 90°. Push down on the arm to resist activity of the deltoid. A ratchety, giving-way motion more than likely is a nonorganic sign. Patients with true weakness exhibit a uniform ability to sustain resistance throughout the range of motion.

C5—Biceps Brachii

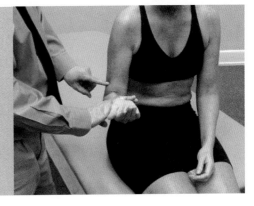

With the patient seated, ask the patient to flex the elbow in a supinated position as you apply resistance. The biceps brachii also is innervated by C6, but if C5 is intact, biceps strength should be at least grade 3. Test C5 sensation by assessing light touch on the lateral aspect of the arm.

SECTION 8 SPINE

C6—Radial Wrist Extensors

Flex the patient's fingers to eliminate wrist extension activity by the finger extensor muscles, and then ask the patient to extend the wrist in a radial direction as you apply resistance. Test C6 sensation by assessing light touch on the volar aspect of the thumb.

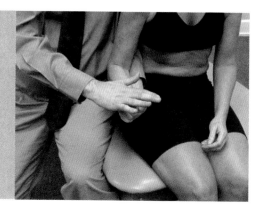

C7—Triceps Brachii

With the patient seated and the shoulder flexed approximately 90°, ask the patient to extend the elbow as you apply light resistance.

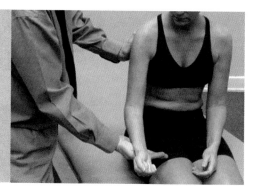

C7—Flexor Carpi Radialis

With the patient seated, place the fingers in extension to eliminate wrist flexor activity by the finger flexor muscles, and then ask the patient to flex the wrist in a radial direction as you apply resistance. Test C7 sensation by assessing light touch on the volar aspect of the long finger.

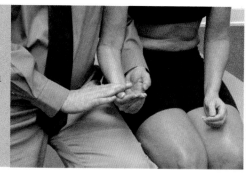

C8—Flexor Digitorum Superficialis to Ring Finger

Stabilize the long, index, and little fingers in extension and ask the patient to flex the fingers as you apply resistance. Test C8 sensation by assessing light touch on the volar aspect of the little finger.

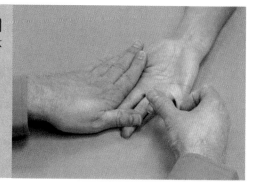

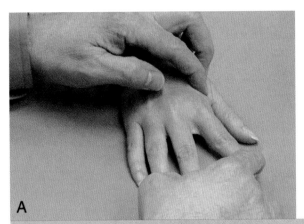

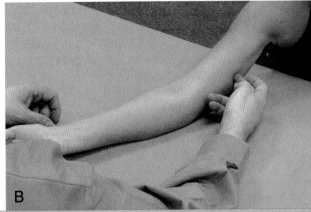

A

B

T1—First Dorsal Interosseous 🔲◀

Ask the patient to abduct the index finger as you apply resistance. Palpate the muscle belly of the first dorsal interosseous muscle to confirm activity (**A**). Test T1 sensation by assessing light touch on the medial aspect of the arm proximal to the elbow (**B**).

Hoffmann Reflex 🔲◀

To assess the Hoffmann reflex, with the patient seated and the patient's relaxed hand cradled in yours, flick the long fingernail and look for index finger and thumb flexion as a sign of long-tract spinal cord involvement in the neck.

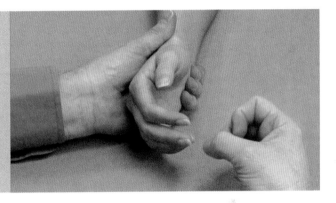

SECTION 8   SPINE

Cauda Equina Syndrome

Definition

The distal end of the spinal cord, the conus medullaris, terminates at the L1-2 level. Below this, the spinal canal is filled with the L2-S4 nerve roots, known as the cauda equina. Compression of roots distal to the conus causes paralysis without spasticity.

Cauda equina syndrome results from a sudden reduction in the volume of the lumbar spinal canal that causes compression of multiple nerve roots and leads to muscle paralysis. The sacral roots that control bladder and anal sphincter function (S2 to S4) are midline and are particularly vulnerable. Causes of cauda equina syndrome include a large central disk herniation, epidural abscess, epidural hematoma, and trauma to the spine with retropulsion of a portion of a vertebral burst fracture. Onset may be immediate (with a fracture) or may occur over a few hours or days (with other conditions). Cauda equina syndrome may require emergency surgery to relieve nerve root compression and to stop progression of neurologic deficit. Even with prompt recognition and immediate decompression, recovery of neurologic function may be incomplete and bowel and bladder function may be compromised.

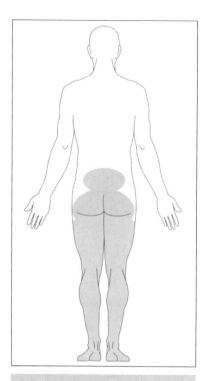

Figure 1 Illustration shows a typical pain diagram for cauda equina syndrome.

Clinical Symptoms

Radicular pain and numbness involve both legs; however, symptoms may be more severe in one extremity. The presence of perineal numbness in a saddle distribution is typical for most patients with cauda equina syndrome (**Figure 1**). Lower extremity pain may diminish as the paralysis progresses. Leg weakness may present as a stumbling gait, difficulty rising from a chair, or footdrop that is often symmetric. Patients may report difficulty voiding or loss of urinary and anal sphincter control.

Patients may have a history of preexisting spinal stenosis with a sudden increase in symptoms, or the history may reveal sudden onset of pain following lifting or recent spine surgery with subsequent onset of fever, chills, and increased back and leg pain.

Tests
Physical Examination
Watch the patient walk. Inability to rise from a chair without the assistance of armrests (quadriceps and/or hip extensor weakness) and inability to walk on the heels or toes (ankle dorsiflexor and plantar flexor weakness) suggest multiple nerve root dysfunction. Evaluate motor and sensory function of the lumbosacral nerve roots, including anal sphincter tone and/or perianal numbness. Patients seen in the emergency department for acute back pain may receive an injection of narcotics that may cause acute urinary retention and confuse the diagnosis of cauda equina syndrome.

Diagnostic Tests

Marked compression of the thecal sac on MRI of the lumbar spine or CT/myelogram (the latter if the patient cannot undergo MRI) will confirm the diagnosis of cauda equina syndrome. AP and lateral radiographs of the lumbar spine are important to identify structural problems such as a fracture and spondylolisthesis. A complete blood cell count, C-reactive protein level, and erythrocyte sedimentation rate can assist with the diagnosis of a suspected infection.

Differential Diagnosis

- Guillain-Barré syndrome (intact sensation possible, normal MRI)
- Herniated lumbar disk (unilateral radicular symptoms and motor weakness, normal rectal tone and perineal sensation)
- Metastatic tumor (lymphoma or leukemia) (abnormal blood studies, pathologic fracture)
- Multiple sclerosis (no history of trauma, patchy numbness, diplopia, facial and/or upper extremity numbness)
- Spinal cord tumor (positive Babinski sign, patchy numbness above L2, spasticity)

Adverse Outcomes of the Disease

Permanent paralysis and loss of bladder and anal sphincter function (urinary and anal) are possible. A possible error would be to relate the bladder symptoms to age-related conditions or female cystocele or male prostatism without considering the possibility of sphincter paralysis.

Treatment

Cauda equina syndrome is a surgical emergency. Immediate decompression is almost always necessary after the anatomic lesion has been defined.

Adverse Outcomes of Treatment

Wound infection and postoperative hematoma are possible.

Referral Decisions/Red Flags

Any unexplained neurologic deficit, loss of normal bowel or bladder function, increasing pain not controlled by simple analgesics, or decreasing pain in the face of increasing neurologic deficit is cause for concern.

SECTION 8 SPINE

Cervical Radiculopathy

Synonym
Herniated cervical disk

Definition
Cervical radiculopathy is referred neurogenic pain in the distribution of a cervical nerve root or roots, with or without associated numbness, weakness, or loss of reflexes. The usual cause in young adults is herniation of a cervical disk that entraps the root as it enters the foramen. In older patients, a combination of foraminal narrowing due to vertical settling of the disk space and arthritic involvement of the uncovertebral joint is the most common cause of lateral nerve root entrapment.

Clinical Symptoms
Neck pain and radicular pain with associated numbness and paresthesias in the upper extremity in the distribution of the involved root are common; these findings are often unilateral (**Figure 1**). Muscle spasms, or fasciculations, in the involved myotomes may occur. Other symptoms may include weakness, lack of coordination, changes in handwriting, diminished grip strength, dropping objects from the hand, and difficulty with fine manipulative tasks. Occipital headaches and pain radiating into the paraspinal and scapular regions also may occur.

Symptoms indicative of cervical myelopathy, such as trunk or leg dysfunction, gait disturbances, bowel or bladder changes, and signs of upper motor neuron involvement, occur more commonly with stenosis of the cervical spinal canal.

Patients may state that they can relieve the pain by placing their hands on top of their head, as this decreases tension on the involved nerve root.

Tests
Physical Examination
Cervical lordosis may be reduced, and the range of neck motion may be mildly restricted. Extension and axial rotation will often cause pain in the arm or shoulder. Assess motor and sensory function of the C5-T1 nerve roots as well as upper extremity reflexes and other upper motor neuron signs. Careful examination for signs of shoulder pathology, vascular disturbances, and peripheral nerve entrapment is necessary. A complete neurologic examination should be performed (**Table 1**).

Signs of upper motor neuron involvement suggest spinal cord compression.

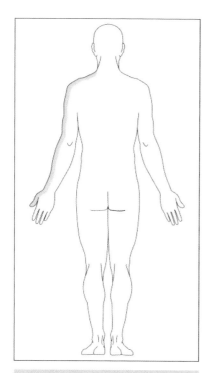

Figure 1 Illustration shows a typical pain diagram for a patient with cervical radiculopathy. Patients with root pressure above C5 may report scapular and interscapular pain with no extremity radiation.

Table 1

Clinical Features of Common Cervical Syndromes

Disk	Pain	Sensory Change	Motor Weakness Atrophy	Reflex Change
C4-5 (C5 root)	Base of neck, shoulder, anterolateral aspect of arm	Numbness in deltoid region	Deltoid, biceps	Biceps
C5-6 (C6 root)	Neck, shoulder, medial border of scapula, lateral aspect of arm, radial aspect of forearm	Dorsolateral aspect of thumb and index finger	Biceps, wrist extensors, pollicis longus	Biceps, brachioradialis
C6-7 (C7 root)	Neck, shoulder, medial border of scapula, lateral aspect of arm, dorsum of forearm	Index, long fingers, dorsum of hand	Triceps and/or finger extensors	Triceps

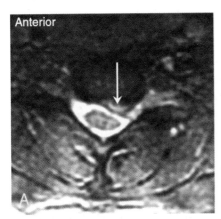
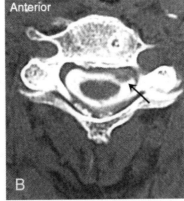

Figure 2 **A,** Axial MRI demonstrates a cervical disk herniation (arrow) in a younger patient. **B,** Axial CT scan with intrathecal contrast demonstrates a cervical disk herniation (arrow) in a younger patient.

Diagnostic Tests

Radiographs may identify regions of spondylosis or degenerative involvement of the disk and the facet joint. MRI or CT with intrathecal contrast (myelogram) confirms the diagnosis (**Figure 2**). Advanced imaging studies are necessary in patients who have not responded to nonsurgical management, in patients with profound neurologic deficits, or in patients who are considering surgical management. Symptoms must be correlated to imaging because there can be a high false-positive rate on MRI. Electromyography and nerve conduction velocity studies help in some instances to identify the location of neurologic dysfunction. These studies are valuable to differentiate radiculopathy from peripheral neuropathy and various nerve compression syndromes, such as carpal tunnel syndrome.

Differential Diagnosis

- Adhesive capsulitis of the shoulder (restricted passive and active motion)
- Demyelinating conditions (varying symptoms, intensity, and location)
- Myocardial ischemia (abnormal electrocardiogram or stress tests)
- Peripheral nerve entrapment (positive Phalen test, positive Tinel sign at elbow or wrist)
- Rotator cuff disease (painful wince with active shoulder abduction and circumduction movements)
- Thoracic outlet syndrome (distinctly uncommon; decrease in radial pulse with shoulder abduction and external rotation may be observed)

Adverse Outcomes of the Disease

Muscle paralysis, weakness, or chronic pain syndromes may develop. Rarely, the condition may progress to a myelopathy with spinal cord involvement.

Treatment

Spontaneous resolution of all or most symptoms occurs within 2 to 8 weeks in most patients. With radicular pain, a short course of anti-inflammatory medication coupled with cervical traction in a head halter is usually beneficial. Referral to a physical therapist/rehabilitation specialist is often more effective than use of a traction unit on its own. The physical therapist may treat the patient with appropriately selected exercises, manual therapy techniques, modalities, education regarding posture, avoidance of aggravating factors, and body mechanics. Narcotic medication is best avoided and seldom warranted. Manipulation of the cervical spine also is usually not indicated in patients with radiculopathy.

Adverse Outcomes of Treatment

Quadriparesis, herniation of an intervertebral disk, stroke, or vertebral fracture may follow manipulation of the cervical spine.

Referral Decisions/Red Flags

Patients in whom nonsurgical treatment fails or who develop atrophy, motor weakness, or signs of myelopathy may require surgical evaluation. Patients with any signs that suggest a demyelinating condition, infection, or tumor require further evaluation. If radicular symptoms are accompanied by intolerable pain, early specialty evaluation should be obtained.

Cervical Spondylosis

Synonyms
Cervical arthritis
Degenerative disk disease of the cervical spine

Definition
Cervical spondylosis is degenerative disk disease in the cervical spine. This condition is produced by the ingrowth of bony spurs (osteophytes), buckling or thickening of the ligamentum flavum, and/or herniation of disk material. These anatomic alterations may result in narrowing of the neural foramen and stenosis of the cervical spinal canal. Cervical spondylosis may cause neck pain, cervical radiculopathy, and/or cervical myelopathy.

Clinical Symptoms
The most common symptoms are limited mobility of the cervical spine and chronic neck pain that worsens with upright activity. Paraspinous muscle spasm can occur, as can headaches that appear to originate in the neck. Increased irritability, fatigue, sleep disturbances, and impaired work tolerance also may develop. Radicular symptoms and pain can occur in the upper extremities with lateral recess stenosis, causing nerve root entrapment. The resultant symptoms may be bilateral (**Figure 1**). Radiographs are of minimal value because many radiographic changes of spondylosis occur in patients who report no significant symptoms. Therefore, careful

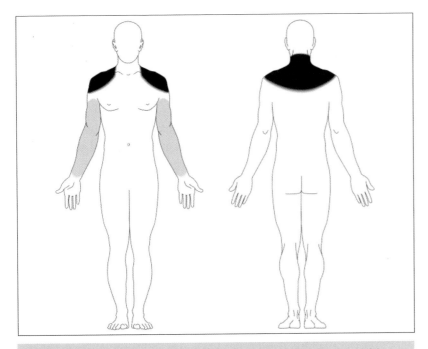

Figure 1 Illustration shows a typical pain diagram for a patient with cervical spondylosis.

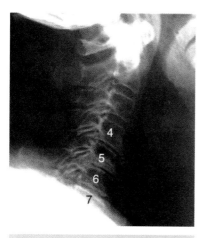

Figure 2 Lateral radiograph demonstrates advanced cervical spondylosis.

clinical evaluations are warranted to ensure that symptoms are linked to pathologic processes and not simply to physiologic changes of aging.

Narrowing of the spinal canal and resultant myelopathy are more common in older men. Typical symptoms of early cervical myelopathy may include palmar paresthesias in the upper extremities; difficulty with upper extremity dexterity, such as buttoning a shirt or blouse; and subtle gait disturbances that can usually be highlighted by asking the patient to perform a tandem walk (heel-to-toe walking). Urinary function may be abnormal as well. Loss of vibration and position sense (posterior column deficits) is more common in the feet than in the upper extremities. A concomitant radiculopathy in the upper extremity may be present; this finding is referred to as myeloradiculopathy. Additionally, because pain is frequently absent in patients with early cervical myelopathy, the subtle gait changes may be related to the lumbar spine, with the myelopathy being totally overlooked. The key physical findings in these patients include the presence of long-tract signs (signs that indicate an upper motor neuron lesion), subtle gait disturbances, and alterations in upper extremity dexterity. These changes are not related to the common stenosis that is seen in the lumbar spine because peripheral nerves, not the spinal cord, would be involved in lumbar stenosis unless the L1-L2 area is involved.

Tests

Physical Examination

Examination may reveal tenderness along the lateral neck or along the spinous processes posteriorly. Motion may be limited or painful. Assess sensory and motor function of the upper (C5-T1) and lower (L1-S1) nerve roots. Evaluate gait and tandem walking as well as bowel and bladder function. With myelopathy, flexion of the neck may produce electric shocks that travel down the spine, arms, or legs (Lhermitte sign). A Hoffmann reflex, clonus, hyperreflexia, and the Babinski sign (an extensor toe response) are possible, as are gait disturbances and global weakness.

Patients with radiculopathy may have signs that mimic a herniated cervical disk, including abnormal reflexes and motor and sensory function.

Diagnostic Tests

AP and lateral radiographs are useful. Findings on the lateral view include bony reactive changes in the vertebral end plates, with osteophytes projecting anteriorly (**Figure 2**). Osteophytes that emerge from the zygoapophyseal joints may also project into the neural foramina. In addition, osteophytes may develop on the posterior portion of the vertebral body and encroach into the spinal canal, producing stenosis of the cervical canal (**Figure 3**). Anterior subluxation of one vertebra onto the vertebra below (**Figure 4**) increases the likelihood of cervical stenosis and associated neurologic findings. Degenerative findings occur most commonly at the C5-6

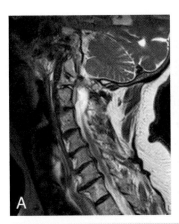 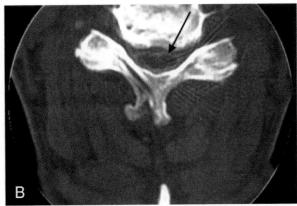 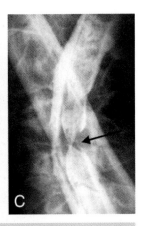

Figure 3 **A,** Sagittal T2-weighted MRI demonstrates multilevel cervical stenosis in a 70-year-old man. **B,** Axial CT myelogram of the midcervical spine demonstrates marked cervical spinal stenosis. Note the paucity of contrast material surrounding the deformed spinal cord (arrow). The anteroposterior dimension of the cervical spinal canal and the anteroposterior dimension of the cervical cord are both reduced. **C,** Lateral radiograph from a 72-year-old man with significant cervical spinal stenosis, with symptoms of cord compression and myelopathy found on examination. Note the marked narrowing of the column of contrast material (arrow).

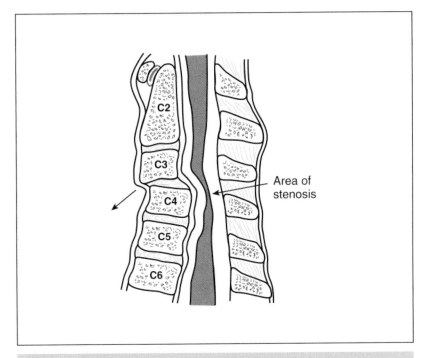

Figure 4 Illustration of degenerative disk changes and degenerative subluxations causing stenosis of the spinal canal. The arrow on the left indicates the forward slippage of C3 on C4.

and C6-7 disk spaces. For patients with progressive neurologic symptoms or myelopathic findings, MRI or CT myelography should be obtained to enable a more detailed evaluation of the canal pathology.

Differential Diagnosis

- Metastatic tumor (night pain that prevents sleep)
- Soft cervical disk herniation (generally seen in younger patients)
- Spinal cord tumor (extradural/metastatic, intradural/primary) (physical examination findings, confirmed by MRI and/or CT myelogram)
- Syringomyelia (loss of superficial abdominal reflexes, insensitivity to pain)
- Vertebral subluxation (in patients with advanced spondylosis or rheumatoid arthritis or following trauma)

Adverse Outcomes of the Disease

Chronic pain, myelopathy, or mixed myeloradiculopathy is possible. These sequelae of cervical spondylosis occur more commonly when the anatomic changes are more advanced.

Treatment

Supportive treatment and reassurance may be adequate, but symptoms may last several months or become chronic. NSAIDs are often adequate. Doxepin or amitriptyline, in minimal doses, may also be useful to help with sleep. Narcotic medication should be avoided. Management should also include a cervical pillow or cervical roll and rehabilitation. Referral to a physical therapist or rehabilitation specialist may be helpful.

Surgical decompression and fusion may be necessary for patients with intractable pain, progressive neurologic findings, or symptoms of cervical myelopathy and spinal cord compression.

Adverse Outcomes of Treatment

NSAIDs may cause gastric, renal, or hepatic complications. In 2015, the FDA strengthened its warning linking NSAIDs with the risk of heart attack or stroke, even in the first weeks of use of an NSAID. Sedation from tricyclic antidepressants may occur, and adverse reactions to monoamine oxidase inhibitors are possible. Narcotic dependence is also possible, especially with the early and prolonged use of stronger narcotic medication. Monoparesis or loss of specific nerve root function may occur, and, although uncommon, quadriparesis or quadriplegia may result from progressive cervical stenosis with spinal cord compression.

Referral Decisions/Red Flags

Intractable neck pain that is not responsive to treatment, neurologic symptoms that affect either the upper or lower extremities, lack of coordination, gait disturbances, and radicular symptoms related to neck motion all indicate the need for further evaluation and referral to a specialist.

Cervical Strain

Synonym
Neck sprain

Definition
Cervical strain is a common, usually self-limiting condition. By strict definition, an acute cervical strain is a muscle injury in the neck, whereas the term sprain generally refers to a ligamentous injury. These terms are often used interchangeably, however, by both the medical profession and the lay public. Moreover, because neither physical examination nor imaging can distinguish between muscle and ligament injuries in the deeply located soft-tissue structures of the neck, the term cervical strain includes ligamentous injuries of the facet joints and/or intervertebral disks. Regardless which soft-tissue structures have been injured, the diagnostic and treatment protocols are similar: Evaluate the patient to identify unstable injuries and/or neurologic deficits and then provide appropriate treatment.

A whiplash mechanism (acceleration-deceleration of the neck with rapid flexion-extension) occurs commonly as a result of motor vehicle accidents. The classic mechanism is a stopped car that is struck from behind by another vehicle. These injuries may cause prolonged disability despite no apparent pathologic process. The cause may be a combination of a ligament/muscle injury and symptom amplification. On occasion, severe injuries result in definite instability patterns and/or cervical disk displacements. The concept of symptom amplification should not be advanced until after a thorough history, physical examination, and appropriate imaging studies have been performed.

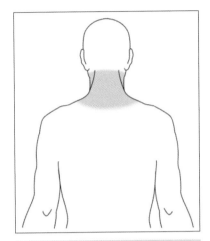

Figure 1 Illustration shows a typical pain diagram for a patient with an acute cervical strain.

Clinical Symptoms
Cervical pain may follow an incident of trauma or may be spontaneous in onset. Nonradicular, nonfocal neck pain, noted anywhere from the base of the skull to the cervicothoracic junction, is most common (**Figure 1**). Patients may also have pain in the region of the sternocleidomastoid muscles and/or the trapezius muscles. Pain is often worse with motion and may be accompanied by paraspinal spasm. Occipital headaches may occur in the early phase and may persist for months. Pain following trauma often persists longer than pain following strains or sprains of spontaneous onset. Patients may report increased irritability, fatigue, sleep disturbances, and difficulty concentrating. Work tolerance may be impaired.

Tests
Physical Examination
Examination may reveal areas of tenderness in the paraspinous muscles, trapezii, sternocleidomastoid muscles, spinous processes, interspinous ligaments, and/or the medial border of the scapula. Limited motion is common and may involve rotation, lateral bending,

and/or flexion and extension. Pain is often noted at the extremes of motions. The neurologic examination is usually normal.

Diagnostic Tests

AP, lateral, and open-mouth (odontoid) radiographs are necessary if the patient has a history of trauma or associated neurologic deficit or if the patient is elderly. All seven cervical vertebrae must be seen. Anterior displacement of the pharyngeal air shadow indicates soft-tissue swelling that may develop following spinal fracture, injury to the intervertebral disk or anterior longitudinal ligament, or injury at the occipitocervical level. The presence of precervical swelling mandates a specialty consultation to assess the numerous possible causes. In normal adults, the width of the prevertebral soft tissue at the level of C3 should not exceed one third the width of the C3 vertebral body. The normal lordotic curve of the cervical spine may be straightened or reversed as a result of muscle spasm, but this finding is also observed in approximately 10% of normal adults. Preexisting degenerative changes may be noted; they are most commonly age related and occur most frequently at C5-6 or C6-7.

If the patient has severe pain, the screening radiographs should be examined for signs of instability that include translation of a vertebral body of more than 3.5 mm and/or more than 11° of angulation of adjacent vertebrae. Routine flexion-extension radiographs of the cervical spine should not be ordered until the patient has been evaluated by a specialist because of the risk of increased neurologic damage from the maneuvers.

Differential Diagnosis

- Cervical disk herniation (neurologic abnormality and radicular pain)
- Cervical spine tumor or infection (night pain, weight loss, history, fever, chills, sweats)
- Dislocation or subluxation of the spine (usually evident on radiographs; however, on occasion a spontaneous reduction occurs, masking the severity of the injury)
- Inflammatory conditions of the cervical spine (rheumatoid arthritis with abnormal radiographs)
- Spinal fracture (abnormal radiographs)
- Symptom amplification/secondary gain (inconsistent or exaggerated findings)

Adverse Outcomes of the Disease

Symptoms resolve completely in most patients within the first 4 to 6 weeks. With whiplash, resolution typically is delayed, but most symptoms resolve within 6 to 12 months, with few residual symptoms.

Patients with subtle disk injuries superimposed on existing degenerative conditions of the cervical spine may have intractable pain. In some instances, radiculopathy due to lateral nerve root entrapment or myelopathy due to central spinal stenosis may develop.

Treatment

Providing the patient with reassurance about the natural history of these disorders represents an important first step. Acute care (1 to 2 weeks) involves appropriate pain medications and/or short-term NSAIDs and possible use of a soft cervical collar. Muscle relaxants may help if the patient has muscle spasm. Commercially available cervical pillows help with reestablishing a normal sleep pattern.

Appropriately applied rehabilitation may help, especially in the first 4 weeks. Mild narcotic medication may be useful initially but should be restricted to the first week or two following the injury. Doxepin or amitriptyline may also be helpful for sleep. Manipulation of the cervical spine is contraindicated in patients with acute cervical injuries.

Aerobic activities, such as walking, should be initiated as soon as possible. Add isometric exercises as the patient's comfort improves, preferably in the first 2 weeks. Encourage an early return to normal activities and work.

Rehabilitation Prescription

A home program of exercises may be provided. If the symptoms do not respond to the home program within 2 to 3 weeks, formal rehabilitation should be considered. The evaluation should include an assessment to determine specific segmental limitations and muscle involvement. Cervical spine traction and mobilization of the restricted segments may be added.

Adverse Outcomes of Treatment

NSAIDs may cause gastric, renal, or hepatic complications. In 2015, the FDA strengthened its warning linking NSAIDs with the risk of heart attack or stroke, even in the first weeks of use of an NSAID. If the patient's condition fails to improve, depression may develop. Chronic pain syndrome and drug dependence also may develop in these patients.

Referral Decisions/Red Flags

Patients with pain refractory to treatment, nerve root deficits, or myelopathy or who present a diagnostic dilemma must be evaluated thoroughly.

SECTION 8 SPINE

Home Exercise Program for Cervical Strain

- Perform the exercises in the order listed.
- Apply heat to the painful area for 20 minutes before performing the exercises.
- If the pain worsens or does not improve, call your doctor.
- The following exercise program is introductory only, and progression of this program will vary based on your specific injury, symptoms, and baseline level of fitness. For further progression of this routine, your physician may recommend evaluation and treatment by a physical therapist or other exercise professional.

Home Exercises for Cervical Strain

Exercise Type	Area Targeted	Number of Repetitions/Sets	Number of Days per Week	Number of Weeks
Head rolls	Cervical spine	3 repetitions (all directions)/3 sets	Daily	3 to 4
Cat back stretch	Upper back	10 repetitions	Daily	3 to 4

Head Rolls

- Sit in a chair or stand with your weight evenly distributed on both feet.
- Begin by gently bowing your head toward your chest.
- Stretch your right ear toward your right shoulder (1), then stretch your left ear toward your left shoulder (2).
- Next, gently roll your head in a clockwise circle three times (3).
- Switch directions and gently roll your head in a counterclockwise circle three times (4).
- Perform 3 sets per day for 3 to 4 weeks.

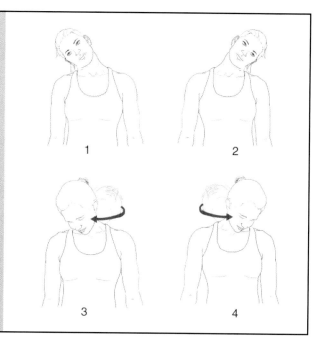

SECTION 8   SPINE

Cat Back Stretch

- Kneel on your hands and knees in a relaxed position.
- Raise your back up like a cat and hold for 5 seconds.
- Repeat 10 times.
- Perform the exercise every day for 3 to 4 weeks.

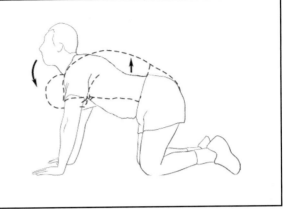

SECTION 8   SPINE

Fractures of the Cervical Spine

Definition
Cervical spine fractures and associated ligamentous injuries occur commonly as the result of high-energy trauma, such as a motor vehicle accident, a fall from a height, or a diving accident. These fractures must be suspected and either identified or excluded in all trauma patients who report neck pain. In addition, because in unconscious or intoxicated patients the history and physical examination are compromised, such patients must have appropriate imaging studies to evaluate the cervical spine. Most missed spinal injuries occur in patients who are obtunded from a closed head injury, unconscious, and/or intoxicated.

Clinical Symptoms
Severe neck pain, paraspinous muscle spasm, and/or point tenderness are the most common presenting symptoms. Pain that radiates into the shoulder or arm with associated numbness or tingling suggests nerve root impingement. Global sensory or motor deficits suggest spinal cord injury. In patients who have sustained multiple trauma, associated injuries may be so painful that the patient may not report every area of the body that is painful. Therefore, in these patients, the absence of neck pain on initial examination does not "clear" the patient or eliminate the possibility of a cervical spine injury.

Tests
Physical Examination
Inspect for swelling and contusions. Palpate for tenderness and paraspinal spasm. A gap or a step-off between spinous processes suggests an injury to the posterior ligamentous complex that is generally quite unstable. Evaluate motor and sensory function of the upper and lower extremities as well as the sensory status of the thoracic dermatomes. Perianal sensation, sphincter tone, and the bulbocavernosus reflex also should be assessed in any patient who is suspected of having a spinal injury.

Diagnostic Tests
Radiographs of the cervical spine should include AP and lateral views as well as an open-mouth view of the odontoid process (C2). In a multiply injured patient, however, the most important view is the cross-table lateral view of the cervical spine, to include C1 through T1. In most trauma centers, CT has replaced plain radiography as the initial imaging modality. The most commonly missed injuries are those at the upper and lower portions of the cervical spine. Lateral radiographs (if obtained instead of CT scan) must include the occiput superiorly and the top of T1 inferiorly. Occasionally, a swimmer's view is required to visualize the cervicothoracic junction.

The lateral radiograph should be evaluated for anterior soft-tissue swelling, height of the vertebral body, and alignment of the vertebral bodies, facet joints, and spinous processes. The odontoid view should be checked for odontoid fracture (often subtle), C1 lateral mass widening, and the position of the occipital condyles. The AP radiograph can show subtle malalignment of the spinous processes. This finding may indicate rotational malalignment secondary to facet fracture or dislocation.

Flexion-extension lateral views (if used to determine instability and possible ligamentous injury) should be obtained only after a three-view series has been cleared. Flexion-extension radiographs may not detect ligamentous instability if paraspinal spasm is present. Therefore, in the acute situation, other studies (such as CT or MRI) may be preferable to rule out a fracture or significant ligamentous injury.

Differential Diagnosis

- Acute disk herniation (normal radiographs with or without neurologic deficit)
- Cervical sprain (normal radiographs with muscle pain/tenderness)
- High thoracic fracture (evident on swimmer's view or thoracic radiographs)

Adverse Outcomes of the Disease

Severe injury may result in complete or incomplete quadriplegia. Nerve compression with radiculopathy may also occur. Chronic neck pain and fatigue may result from deformity or associated muscle injury.

Treatment

The cervical spine must be immobilized at the time of extrication of the patient from the accident scene. In addition, the cervical spine should be braced and a spine board used during transport of patients who sustain high-energy trauma or who have suspected neck injuries. Historically, intravenous steroids (a bolus of methylprednisolone 30 mg/kg of body weight followed by a continuous drip of 5.4 mg/kg/h for 23 hours) were used in patients with spinal cord injury. However, the use of high-dose methylprednisolone is now controversial and has been discontinued at many trauma centers.

Patients whose initial radiographs and neurologic examination are normal but who have persistent pain should wear a cervical collar for 7 to 10 days. The clinical examination and radiographs should be repeated if symptoms persist. If these radiographs are normal, flexion-extension lateral radiographs and an MRI should be obtained. If these studies are normal, the patient may start a neck stretching and strengthening rehabilitation program with scapular stabilization.

SECTION 8 SPINE

Adverse Outcomes of Treatment

Neurologic deficits may develop or worsen during treatment.

Referral Decisions/Red Flags

Patients with instability or with a fracture, dislocation, subluxation, or neurologic deficit require further evaluation. A high index of suspicion for occult injury should be maintained in patients who are intoxicated, uncooperative, or unconscious.

SECTION 8 **SPINE**

Fractures of the Thoracic or Lumbar Spine

Definition

Fractures of the thoracic or lumbar spine generally occur as a result of high-energy trauma such as motor vehicle accidents or falls from a height. They may also occur following minimal trauma in patients who have diminished bone strength from osteoporosis, tumors, infections, or long-term steroid use.

The fracture pattern usually determines fracture stability and likelihood of neural injury. Simple compression fractures involving only the anterior half of the vertebral body are generally stable, as are some burst fractures (compression fractures extending to the posterior third of the vertebral body). Flexion-distraction injuries that disrupt the posterior ligamentous complex are highly unstable. These injuries are often associated with abdominal injuries such as bowel lacerations.

Clinical Symptoms

Moderate to severe back pain related to a traumatic event is the most common presenting symptom. The pain is exacerbated by motion. Numbness, tingling, weakness, or bowel and bladder dysfunction suggest nerve root or spinal cord injury. In addition, decreased bowel motility may occur secondary to an ileus in patients with lumbar spine fractures.

Tests

Physical Examination

Inspect the trunk, chest, and abdomen for swelling and ecchymosis. Patients with lap belt (flexion/distraction) injuries often demonstrate ecchymosis or contusions over the anterior iliac spines. Tenderness to palpation or light percussion occurs at the level of injury. Hematoma formation and a step-off (forward shift) or gap between spinous processes with swelling are the hallmarks of an unstable flexion-distraction or burst fracture. Evaluate motor and sensory function of all nerve roots distal to the injury. Diffuse numbness, weakness, loss of reflexes, ankle clonus, or a positive Babinski sign indicates spinal cord injury. Examination of perianal sensation, sphincter function, and the bulbocavernosus reflex are particularly important with an associated spinal cord injury. Evaluate the abdomen and chest for possible associated injuries.

Diagnostic Tests

AP and lateral radiographs of the thoracic and lumbar spine are indicated; however, as with cervical spine trauma, CT is often the initial modality of choice. When a spine fracture is identified, the radiograph (or CT scan) should be scrutinized for adjacent or

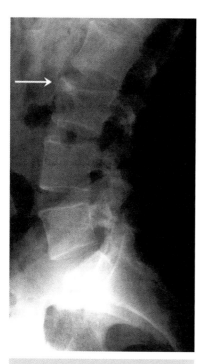

Figure 1 Lateral radiograph demonstrates a minimal compression fracture of the lumbar spine (arrow).

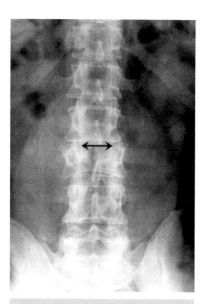

Figure 2 AP radiograph demonstrates a burst fracture of the lumbar spine with widening of the interpedicular distance (double-headed arrow).

nonadjacent fractures as well. CT scans with reconstructions offer the best information with respect to the need for surgical stabilization.

In the lateral view, compression and burst fractures show loss of height of the anterior wall of the vertebral body and resultant kyphotic deformity (**Figure 1**). Burst fractures involve an injury to the middle column, which can be best seen on a CT scan. Unstable flexion-distraction injuries show widening of the space between adjacent spinous processes on the AP and/or lateral view. The AP view may reveal transverse process fractures or widening of the interpedicular distance that also confirms an unstable burst fracture (**Figure 2**). Rotation of one vertebral body in relation to the one below also indicates instability. Any injury other than a simple compression fracture requires additional imaging studies.

Differential Diagnosis

- Herniated lumbar disk (no fracture, patient able to walk, single nerve root involvement)
- Thoracic or lumbar muscle strain (no neurologic findings or fractures)
- Visceral injuries (abnormal abdominal examination and radiographs, ultrasonogram, or CT scan)

Adverse Outcomes of the Disease

Loss of nerve or spinal cord function, persistent painful instability or deformity, and impaired function are serious sequelae of certain injuries to the spine.

Treatment

Preventing neurologic injury, restoring stability, and restoring normal function are the goals of treatment. Initial extrication, transportation, and evaluation in the emergency department require the use of spinal precautions, including a spine board and log rolling. If radiographs reveal no fracture or instability and no neurologic deficits are present, these precautions may be lifted after confirmation by a specialist.

Isolated transverse process fractures do not affect stability of the spine but do indicate substantial injury to adjacent muscles and possible injury to the kidneys. A thoracolumbar corset may be used to decrease symptoms.

Compression fractures with wedging of less than 20° and no posterior vertebral or posterior element involvement can be managed with a thoracolumbosacral orthosis for 8 to 10 weeks, to be worn during sitting and standing activities. Pain management may require short-term oral narcotics. Walking may be encouraged, but bending, stooping, twisting, and lifting more than 10 lb should be discouraged. Exercises to strengthen trunk flexor and extensor muscles can supplement walking after the brace is removed.

Other injuries usually require more aggressive treatment. Patients with unstable burst fractures, flexion-distraction injuries, or fracture-dislocations are usually treated with internal fixation and spinal fusion.

Adverse Outcomes of Treatment

Progressive collapse with kyphotic deformity may occur, resulting in chronic pain and/or neurologic compromise. Chronic muscle pain may also develop if the trunk muscles are not adequately strengthened after immobilization is discontinued.

Referral Decisions/Red Flags

Any neurologic deficit is a sign of substantial injury and requires further evaluation. Burst fractures, flexion-distraction injuries (or any injury to the posterior column of the spine), fractures with vertebral rotation, and fracture-dislocations all require further evaluation and treatment.

SECTION 8 SPINE

Low Back Pain: Acute

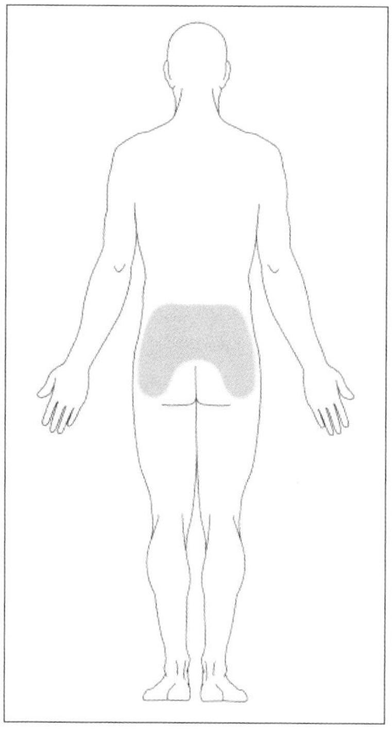

Synonyms

Low back strain
Lumbar sprain
Pulled low back

Definition

The term low back pain (LBP) more properly describes a symptom rather than a diagnosis. For more than 80% of patients with LBP, a more specific diagnosis is not possible.

LBP is the most frequent cause of lost work time and disability in adults younger than 45 years. Most symptoms, however, are of limited duration, with 80% of patients demonstrating substantial improvement and returning to work within 1 month. The 4% of patients whose symptoms persist longer than 6 months generate 80% to 90% of the costs to society for treating LBP.

A low back strain is an injury to the paravertebral spinal muscles. The term sprain is used to describe ligamentous injuries that may include the facet joints or anulus fibrosus. In persons with a ligamentous injury that involves the anulus fibrosus, the disk does not herniate into the spinal canal, but substances may leak from the nucleus pulposus that induce inflammation and cause irritation of the lumbosacral nerve roots. Because of the deep location of the lumbar soft tissues, however, localizing an injury to a specific structure is difficult, if not impossible. Furthermore, in this area, regardless which muscle or ligamentous structures have been injured, the treatment protocols are identical.

A history of repeated lifting and twisting or operating vibrating equipment may be associated with LBP. However, individuals who engage in little physical exertion may also report similar symptoms. Factors associated with reports of LBP include poor fitness, job dissatisfaction, smoking, and various psychosocial issues.

Clinical Symptoms

Patients report the acute onset of LBP, often following a lifting episode. The lifting may be a trivial event, such as leaning over to pick up a piece of paper. The pain often radiates into the buttocks and posterior thighs (**Figure 1**). Patients may have difficulty standing erect and may need to change position frequently for comfort. This condition may first be experienced in the early adult years.

Tests

Physical Examination

Examination reveals diffuse tenderness in the low back or the sacroiliac region. Range of motion of the lumbar spine, particularly flexion, is typically reduced and painful. The degree of lumbar flexion and the ease with which the patient can extend the spine are good

Figure 1 Illustration shows a typical pain diagram for a patient with low back pain.

parameters by which to evaluate progress. Lower extremity reflexes and the motor and sensory function of the lumbosacral nerve roots are normal.

Diagnostic Tests

Plain radiographs usually are not helpful in diagnosing acute LBP. In adolescents and young adults, there is little or no disk space narrowing, whereas in adults older than 30 years, there is variable disk space narrowing and/or spurs. These changes are widely prevalent and are not considered pathologic but rather physiologic signs of aging.

For patients with atypical symptoms, such as pain at rest or at night or a history of significant trauma, AP and lateral radiographs should be obtained. These views help to identify pathologic processes such as infection, neoplasms (visualize up to T10), fracture, and spondylolisthesis. In the absence of "red flag" symptoms, radiographs may be deferred for the first 4 to 6 weeks.

Differential Diagnosis

- Ankylosing spondylitis (family history, morning stiffness, limited mobility of the lumbar spine)
- Drug-seeking behavior (symptom amplification, inconsistent and nonphysiologic examination)
- Extraspinal causes (ovarian cyst, nephrolithiasis, pancreatitis, ulcer disease, aortic aneurysm, retroperitoneal tumors)
- Fracture of the vertebral body (major trauma or minimal trauma with osteoporosis)
- Herniated disk (unilateral radicular pain symptoms that extend below the knee and are equal to or greater than the back pain)
- Infection (fever, chills, sweats, elevated erythrocyte sedimentation rate)
- Multiple myeloma (night sweats, men older than 50 years)

Adverse Outcomes of the Disease

Functional impairment is the primary disability. This can be of great significance for any patient whose normal activities are strenuous and whose general health is otherwise excellent, but young adults in particular have difficulty accepting a condition that may impair function for several weeks.

Treatment

Before any treatment is begun, a complete history is obtained and the patient is evaluated to rule out any significant neurologic findings. If signs of neurologic deficits such as dorsiflexion weakness, plantar flexion weakness, or urinary frequency are found, a referral to a specialist is indicated.

For the patient with LBP with or without sciatic symptoms and with no significant neurologic deficits, treatment has two phases. The

SECTION 8 SPINE

initial phase focuses on symptomatic relief, and the second phase focuses on return to activity.

Phase one, or symptomatic treatment, should include avoidance of intense physical activity. Pain management can be initiated with aspirin, acetaminophen, or NSAIDs. Steroid dose packs, narcotic medication, or muscle relaxants are not recommended as primary pain management tools for most patients who present with acute LBP. It is important to inform the patient that in most cases the symptoms of acute LBP resolve quickly, with the patient able to return to work and other activities within a few days.

As the acute pain improves, phase two of treatment can begin, which focuses on helping the patient return to full activity. Initially, the patient may need lighter duty or shorter hours at work. Flexibility in allowing such arrangements benefits both the employee, in increased self-esteem, and the employer, in decreased costs. As pain diminishes and activity increases, the patient should be referred to a physical therapist for an exercise program focusing on an aerobic activity (walking, running, bicycling, swimming, using an elliptical machine) plus strengthening of trunk flexors and extensors. When the patient is established in this program, he or she may transition to a health club or a home exercise program such as the one described below. Patients who continue to exercise and remain fit have fewer recurrences of LBP.

A patient who is unable to return to work within 4 weeks should be referred to a specialist for further evaluation and treatment.

Rehabilitation Referral

The physical therapist or other rehabilitation specialist can have a role in both the early acute phase of back pain and in the development of a long-term strength and conditioning program. Usually, the physical therapist attempts to identify whether a specific movement deficit is present and attempts to identify any other postural or positional instigators of the patient's pain. Based on this information, repeated movements are often used to identify a directional preference. One common presentation in patients with recurrent, episodic back pain is that symptoms are made worse with sitting and bending forward and made better with walking. These patients often have limited back extension and can often reduce and resolve their symptoms with repeated lumbar extension when standing or in the prone position. An opposite presentation (limited lumbar flexion), or a limitation of side gliding or rotation, can also occur. A detailed examination and follow-up are required to ensure proper response to treatment and progression. Additionally, the therapist may employ gentle manual therapy techniques; modalities; and education regarding posture, avoidance of aggravating factors, and body mechanics. After symptoms are controlled, progression to a generalized flexibility, strengthening, and conditioning program is always indicated.

Adverse Outcomes of Treatment

NSAIDs may cause gastric, renal, or hepatic complications. In 2015, the FDA strengthened its warning linking NSAIDs with the risk of heart attack or stroke, even in the first weeks of use of an NSAID. Although uncommon, spinal manipulation may result in a lumbar disk herniation.

Referral Decisions/Red Flags

Neurologic abnormalities, constitutional symptoms, unresponsive pain syndromes, or an unusual clinical presentation indicates the need for further evaluation.

www.aaos.org/essentials5/exercises

Home Exercise Program for Acute Low Back Pain

- Perform the exercises in the order listed.
- Apply heat to the low back for 20 minutes before performing the exercises. If any of the exercises below cause your pain to increase or cause radiation of your pain down your leg(s), stop the exercise and try the next exercise on the list.
- If the pain worsens or if it does not improve after performing the exercises, call your doctor.
- The following exercise program is introductory only, and progression of this program will vary based on your specific injury, symptoms, and baseline level of fitness. For further progression of this routine, your physician may recommend evaluation and treatment by a physical therapist or other exercise professional.

Home Exercises for Acute Low Back Pain

Exercise Type	Muscle Group/ Area Targeted	Number of Repetitions/Sets	Number of Days per Week	Number of Weeks
Prone lying	Low back	Several times per day/5 to 10 minutes per repetition	Daily	3 to 4
Prone press up	Low back	10 repetitions/1 to 3 sets	Daily	3 to 4
Single knee to chest	Low back	10 repetitions/1 to 3 sets	Daily	3 to 4
Double knee to chest	Low back	10 repetitions/1 to 3 sets	Daily	3 to 4

Prone Lying
- Lie on a firm surface, face down, for 5 to 10 minutes. If lying flat on your stomach is not comfortable, place a folded pillow under your stomach. As you become more comfortable, remove the pillow and try lying flat.
- Use this position several times per day as required to keep pain minimized. Continue for 3 to 4 weeks.

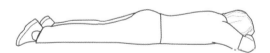

Prone Press Up

- Lie on a firm surface, face down, and press up with your arms until a gentle stretch/pressure is felt in the lower back.
- Hold this position for 3 seconds and repeat 10 times.
- Perform 1 to 3 sets per day for 3 to 4 weeks.

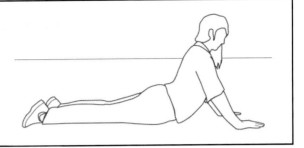

Single Knee to Chest

- Only perform this exercise if the first two exercises in this program are not effective at decreasing your pain.
- Lie on your back on a firm surface and bring one knee up to your chest.
- Pull on the knee with your hands until a gentle stretch is felt in the buttock/lower back region.
- Hold this position for 3 seconds and repeat 10 times.
- Perform 1 to 3 sets per day for 3 to 4 weeks.

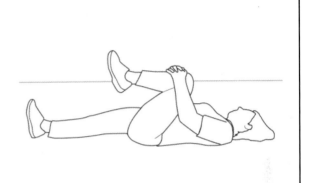

Double Knee to Chest

- Only perform this exercise if the first three exercises in this program are not effective at decreasing your pain.
- Lie on your back on a firm surface and bring both knees up to your chest.
- Pull on your knees with your hands until a gentle stretch is felt in the buttock/lower back region.
- Hold this position for 3 seconds and repeat 10 times.
- Perform 1 to 3 sets per day for 3 to 4 weeks.

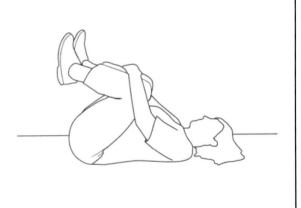

SECTION 8 SPINE

Low Back Pain: Chronic

Definition

Chronic low back pain (LBP) is used to describe LBP of more than 3 months' duration. Patients usually present between 30 and 60 years of age. Symptoms are typically recurrent and episodic, but in some patients the pain is unremitting. After chronic LBP has been identified, an evaluation is required to exclude causes such as cancer, stenosis, deformity, osteoporosis, infection, and abdominal conditions such as aneurysm, ulcer, or retroperitoneal tumor. All patients with chronic LBP should be evaluated by a spine specialist as well as by their internist, family practitioner, or, for women, their gynecologist.

Degeneration of the intervertebral disk is a physiologic event of aging and may be modified by factors such as injury, repetitive trauma, infection, heredity, and tobacco use. As the hydrophilic properties of the nucleus pulposus degrade, the disk loses height and the segmental ligaments develop laxity. Motions such as translation and twisting may create tears within the anulus fibrosus. Chronic LBP may develop.

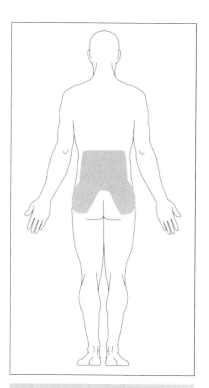

Figure 1 Illustration shows a typical pain diagram for a patient with chronic low back pain.

Clinical Symptoms

Low back pain that radiates to one or both buttocks is the hallmark symptom (**Figure 1**). The pain is often described as "mechanical" in that it is aggravated by activities such as bending, lifting, stooping, or twisting. Patients may report stiffness or have a history of intermittent sciatica (pain radiating down the back of the leg), but discomfort in the back is the predominant symptom. The pain is relieved with lying down or a night's rest. Some patients, however, have difficulty sleeping because of the symptoms.

Depression is not a primary cause of chronic LBP, but it can overlay the condition and complicate treatment. Early recognition will greatly assist with symptom resolution.

Tests
Physical Examination

Lumbar and sacroiliac tenderness is a common finding. Patients may also exhibit a side or forward list from muscle spasm. Motor and sensory function of the lower extremity nerve roots as well as the lower extremity reflexes are normal. Straight leg raising and spinal motion may be mildly restricted. Although not characteristic, nonorganic findings such as widespread sensitivity to light touch, nonanatomic localization of symptoms, inappropriate pain behaviors, and inconsistent actions may be seen with this condition.

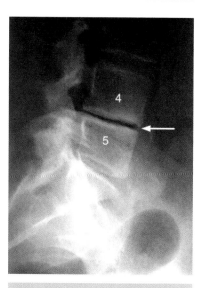

Figure 2 Lateral radiograph demonstrates marked degenerative changes affecting the disk between L4 and L5 (arrow). Note the extreme disk space narrowing.

Diagnostic Tests

AP and lateral radiographs often show age-appropriate changes, such as anterior osteophytes and reduced height of the intervertebral disks. Often there is a "vacuum sign," with apparent air (nitrogen) in the disk space (**Figure 2**).

Differential Diagnosis (Partial List)

- Degenerative disorders (imaging abnormalities)
- Developmental defects (abnormal radiographs)
- Infection (elevated erythrocyte sedimentation rate, C-reactive protein level, body temperature)
- Inflammation (other joint involvement, elevated erythrocyte sedimentation rate)
- Metabolic disease (abnormal laboratory studies)
- Neoplasms (weight loss, night pain, fatigue)
- Neurologic disorders (long tract signs)
- Psychosocial issues (depression, workers' compensation issues, positive Waddell signs)
- Referred pain (aortic aneurysm, pelvic tumor, renal disorders)
- Trauma (history of injury)

Adverse Outcomes of the Disease

In patients with more severe symptoms, vocational and recreational activities may be limited. Sleep disturbances, mood swings, and sexual dysfunction may occur, and concentration may be adversely affected. Deconditioning, which may be the result of reduced activity, is frequently associated with the condition and may aggravate the symptoms as well as increase any occupational dysfunction.

Treatment

Before treatment is initiated, the patient should have undergone a thorough clinical evaluation with appropriate laboratory tests and imaging studies to exclude processes other than physiologic aging. After these conditions have been ruled out, the term chronic benign LBP may be used.

Narcotic abuse is a cause for concern in this population. By definition, the patient with chronic LBP has experienced pain for a lengthy period and frequently has received a variety of medications, including addictive muscle relaxants and narcotics. In addition, many of these patients are deconditioned, depressed, unemployed, angry, and demanding, so management of the condition is often challenging. Referral to a comprehensive pain management program is warranted. These programs employ a wide range of strategies, including comprehensive evaluations with thorough psychologic testing, injections, biofeedback, cognitive/behavior conditioning programs, spinal cord stimulation, psychotherapy, and detoxification programs.

In addition, a return-to-activity program is also essential to overcome the deconditioning that is typical in the patient with chronic LBP. This can be initiated on an individual or group (class) basis and is typically overseen by a rehabilitation specialist. After a comprehensive management program has been developed, the primary care physician can follow the patient, emphasizing the need to maintain "well behavior." Pain relapses are common, and

SECTION 8 SPINE

referral to the pain management center may be necessary. Because of the complexity of evaluating and managing these patients, a comprehensive team approach is highly recommended for a successful outcome.

Rehabilitation Prescription

Chronic LBP is difficult to treat using any single approach. The first approach to chronic or episodic LBP is usually the same approach described earlier in the Low Back Pain: Acute chapter of this book. If the patient is able to reduce or resolve his or her pain with the described exercises, a progression to strengthening and stability program is usually advisable. Even in cases in which limited changes are made in the patient's chronic symptoms, an attempt to perform the stability program can be considered; however, the stability program should be progressed cautiously so as not to worsen the patient's symptoms. Aerobic or cardiovascular conditioning consistent with the patient's general health also is critical. If the patient's symptoms do not improve after adhering to the home program for 3 to 4 weeks, formal rehabilitation may be ordered. The rehabilitation specialist must conduct an extensive evaluation of the mobility and strength of the lumbar spine to determine a treatment approach. The use of pain modalities has limited efficacy with chronic LBP.

Adverse Outcomes of Treatment

NSAIDs may cause gastric, renal, or hepatic complications. In 2015, the FDA strengthened its warning linking NSAIDs with the risk of heart attack or stroke, even in the first weeks of use of an NSAID. Avoid labeling patients as "disabled" because this may negatively affect the patient's motivation. Narcotic dependency or abuse can become a problem for these patients.

Referral Decisions/Red Flags

Further evaluation is needed for patients who have fever, chills, unexplained weight loss, a history of cancer, significant night pain, or a history of pain for more than 6 to 12 months. Other indications for additional evaluation include the presence of pathologic fractures, obvious deformity, saddle anesthesia, loss of major motor function, bowel or bladder dysfunction, abdominal pain, or visceral dysfunction.

Home Exercise Program for Low Back Stability and Strength: Introductory

- Perform the exercises in the order listed.
- Apply heat to the low back for 20 minutes before performing the exercises.
- You should not experience pain with the exercises.
- This program should be performed in conjunction with a progressive cardiovascular training program that consists of exercise such as walking, cycling, or swimming for at least 30 minutes, 3 to 5 times per week.
- If the pain worsens or if it does not improve after performing the exercises for 3 to 4 weeks, call your doctor.
- The following exercise program is introductory only, and progression of this program will vary based on your specific injury, symptoms, and baseline level of fitness. For further progression of this routine, your physician may recommend evaluation and treatment by a physical therapist or other exercise professional.

Strength and Stability Exercises for Low Back Stability

Exercise Type	Muscle Group	Number of Repetitions	Number of Days per Week	Number of Weeks
Modified side bridges	Quadratus lumborum	10 to 20	Daily	4 to 6
Hip bridges	Back and hip extensors	10 to 20	Daily	4 to 6
Bird dog	Back extensors	10 to 20	Daily	4 to 6
Abdominal bracing	Abdominals	10 to 20	Daily	4 to 6

Modified Side Bridges
- Lie on your side on the floor with your knees bent.
- With your elbow bent at 90°, lift your body off the floor as shown, keeping your body straight.
- Hold this position for 5 seconds and then repeat on the other side.
- Perform 10 to 20 repetitions per day, for 4 to 6 weeks.

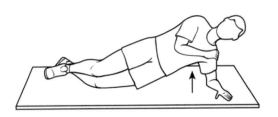

SECTION 8 SPINE

Hip Bridges

- Lie on your back on the floor with your arms at your sides, your knees bent, and your feet flat on the floor.
- Lift your pelvis so that your body is in a straight line from your shoulders to your knees.
- Hold this position for 5 seconds.
- Perform 10 to 20 repetitions per day, for 4 to 6 weeks.

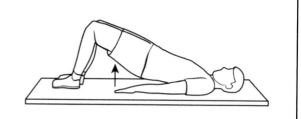

Bird Dog

- Kneel on the floor on your hands and knees.
- Lift your right arm straight out from the shoulder, level with your body, at the same time that you lift your left leg straight out from the hip.
- Hold this position for 5 seconds.
- Repeat with the opposite arm and leg.
- Perform 10 to 20 repetitions per day, for 4 to 6 weeks.

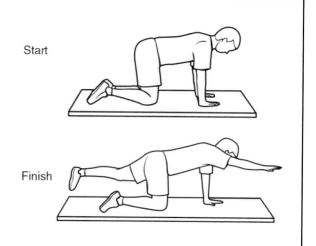

Start

Finish

Abdominal Bracing

- Lie on your back on the floor with your arms at your sides, your knees bent, and your feet flat on the floor.
- Contract your abdominal muscles so that your stomach is pulled away from your waistband. Do not hold your breath. Attempt to breathe normally.
- Hold this position for 5 seconds.
- Perform 10 to 20 repetitions per day, for 4 to 6 weeks.

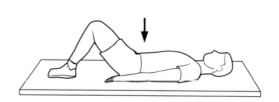

SECTION 8 SPINE

Essentials of Musculoskeletal Care 5

© 2016 American Academy of Orthopaedic Surgeons

Lumbar Herniated Disk

Synonyms
Herniated nucleus pulposus (HNP)
Lumbar radiculopathy
Neurogenic leg pain
Sciatica

Definition
The intervertebral disk is composed of the nucleus pulposus, a gel-like material containing type II collagen that cushions axial compression; the anulus fibrosus, a specialized ligamentous structure surrounding the nucleus pulposus that helps to stabilize the spine; and the superior and inferior cartilaginous end plates. Activities such as lifting and twisting increase pressure on the nucleus pulposus. Lumbar disk herniations develop over time as the weaker posterolateral portion of the anulus fibrosus develops fissures that permit the egress of other disk components that herniate into the lumbar canal adjacent to the exiting lumbar nerve root. The resultant herniated disk syndrome (commonly called sciatica) causes pain, numbness, and/or weakness in one or both lower extremities, depending on the anatomic location of the herniation. The pain results in part from direct mechanical compression of the nerve root and in part from chemical irritation of the nerve root by substances within the nucleus pulposus.

Lumbar disk herniation most commonly occurs at the L4-5 or L5-S1 levels, with subsequent irritation of the L5 or S1 nerve root. Herniations at more proximal intervertebral levels constitute only 5% of all lumbar disk herniations.

Lumbar disk herniations affect approximately 2% of the population. Even though only 10% of these patients have symptoms that persist longer than 3 months, the numbers are so great that this represents approximately 600,000 patients. Most of these patients improve with nonsurgical care, but those who remain symptomatic generally consider surgical management to improve their quality of life.

Clinical Symptoms
The onset of symptoms is often abrupt, but it also may be insidious. Unilateral radicular leg pain frequently follows the onset of acute low back pain. The theory is that the initial posterolateral disk bulge results in low back pain that then becomes sciatic pain as the herniation emerges past the anulus fibrosus to the spinal canal.

The pain is often severe and is exaggerated by sitting, walking, standing, coughing, and sneezing. Typically, the pain radiates from the buttock down the posterior or posterolateral leg to the ankle or foot (**Figure 1**). Patients have a difficult time finding a position of comfort.

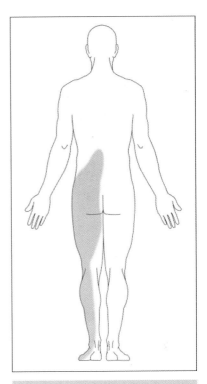

Figure 1 Illustration shows a typical pain diagram for lumbar radiculopathy.

SECTION 8 SPINE

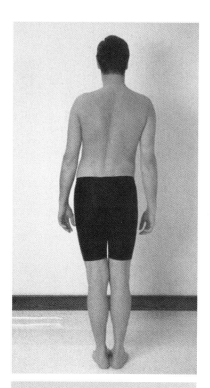

Figure 2 Photograph of the trunk shift, or "list," to the right, which is one finding in the patient with lumbar disk herniation.

Usually, lying on the back with a pillow under the knees or lying on the side in a fetal position provides some relief.

Upper or midlumbar radiculopathy (L1 to L4 nerve root compression) refers pain to the anterior aspect of the thigh and often does not radiate below the knee.

Tests

Physical Examination

As the patient stands, look for the presence of a trunk list to one side (**Figure 2**). The patient may also evidence limited forward flexion with dysrhythmia of the paraspinous muscles (that is, they contract asymmetrically). With the patient sitting, perform the seated straight leg raising test. As the knee is extended on the symptomatic side, a patient with true sciatic tension will lean back to relieve the pressure on the exiting nerve root. This sign has a high correlation with a herniated lumbar disk. Even more specific is the crossed straight leg raising sign: when the nonsymptomatic extremity is elevated, the patient reports buttock or sciatic pain on the symptomatic side. Evaluate motor and sensory function of the lumbosacral nerve roots as well as the deep tendon reflexes.

With the patient supine, perform supine straight leg raising on the involved and uninvolved limbs. This test places the L5 and S1 nerve roots on stretch. Ipsilateral restriction of straight leg raising is common with a variety of lumbar spine problems, but a positive crossed straight leg raising test (pain that occurs in the involved leg or buttock when the uninvolved leg is lifted) is highly specific for lumbar nerve root entrapment. To stretch the upper lumbar nerve roots, perform the reverse straight leg raising test. Classic findings (**Figure 3**) include the following:

- The L3-4 disk (L4 nerve root) may produce weakness in the anterior tibialis, numbness in the shin, pain in the thigh, and an asymmetric knee reflex. Approximately 5% of disk ruptures occur at this level.

- The L4-5 disk (L5 nerve root) may produce weakness in the great toe extensor, numbness on the top of the foot and first web space, and pain in the posterolateral thigh and calf. There is no predictable reflex test for a herniated lumbar disk at the L4-L5 level. Thus, checking the extensor hallucis longus is especially important because this may be the only sign to confirm an L5 radiculopathy.

- The L5-S1 disk (S1 nerve root) may produce weakness in the great toe flexor as well as in the gastrocnemius-soleus complex, with inability to sustain toe-walking, numbness in the lateral foot, pain and ache in the posterior calf, and an asymmetric ankle reflex.

Diagnostic Tests

Radiographs demonstrate age-appropriate changes with no specific findings. MRI should be ordered to confirm the diagnosis if symptoms persist longer than 4 weeks, if a substantial neurologic deficit is identified, or as a part of the preoperative evaluation (**Figure 4**). MRI is otherwise not necessary unless there are progressive neurologic changes or intolerable pain. In the setting

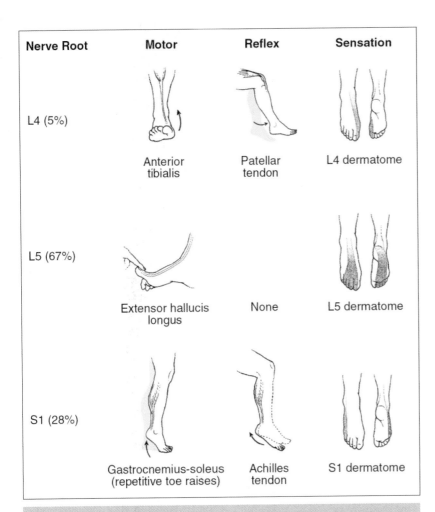

Nerve Root	Motor	Reflex	Sensation
L4 (5%)	Anterior tibialis	Patellar tendon	L4 dermatome
L5 (67%)	Extensor hallucis longus	None	L5 dermatome
S1 (28%)	Gastrocnemius-soleus (repetitive toe raises)	Achilles tendon	S1 dermatome

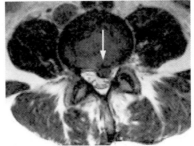

Figure 4 Preoperative axial MRI demonstrates herniated lumbar disk (arrow).

Figure 3 Illustration of typical motor, sensory, and reflex findings with common lumbar radiculopathies. (Adapted from Kasser JR, ed: *Orthopaedic Knowledge Update*, ed 5. Rosemont, IL, American Academy of Orthopaedic Surgeons, 1996, pp 609-624.)

of recurrent radicular symptoms after previous lumbar surgery, a contrast-enhanced MRI can be used to differentiate between a recurrent disk herniation and scar tissue.

Differential Diagnosis

- Cauda equina syndrome (perianal numbness, urinary overflow incontinence or retention, reduced anal sphincter tone, bilateral involvement)
- Demyelinating conditions (clonus)
- Extraspinal nerve entrapment (abdominal or pelvic mass)
- Hip or knee arthritis (decreased internal rotation of hip, knee deformity or effusion)
- Lateral femoral cutaneous nerve entrapment (sensory only, lateral thigh)
- Spinal stenosis (older population)

SECTION 8 SPINE

- Thoracic cord compression (clonus, spasticity, high sensory pattern, abdominal reflexes)
- Trochanteric bursitis (no tension signs, pain down lateral thigh and leg, exquisite tenderness over the trochanter)
- Vascular insufficiency (absent posterior tibial pulse, claudication, trophic changes)

Adverse Outcomes of the Disease

Cauda equina syndrome with permanent motor loss, urinary incontinence, and sensory numbness may develop. Specific root deficit, with permanent dysesthesia, pain, or weakness, may occur.

Treatment

NSAIDs may be used in the acute phase, along with 1 to 2 days of minimal activity. Narcotic medication may be helpful in the acute phase for selected patients but typically should not be prescribed for longer than 7 days. Patients should limit sitting, prolonged standing, or walking. Patients should be reassured that most disk herniations resolve without residual problems.

Most patients who have a lumbar disk herniation will improve within 3 to 4 weeks. If they do not, an evaluation by a specialist should be performed.

Rehabilitation as described for acute low back pain is also appropriate for patients with a lumbar herniated disk. Patients with true radiculopathy with a lumbar herniated disk take longer to recover, however, and usually require activity modification for at least 4 to 8 weeks. Both aerobic conditioning and trunk strengthening are essential for the best outcome. Patients whose symptoms do not improve and who experience a clear decrease in their quality of life are candidates for surgical diskectomy. Profound or progressive neurologic disorders, including cauda equina syndrome, require urgent surgery.

Epidural steroid injections (up to three in a 6-month period), which are usually administered under radiologic guidance, may be considered. These injections should be avoided in any patient who presents with a substantial neurologic deficit. Although the risk of substantial complications is low, epidural steroid injections should not be recommended without consideration of these risks. Also, if the patient experiences no relief of symptoms, repeating the injections later is not warranted.

The effectiveness of manipulative therapy, traction, or acupuncture for patients with a confirmed lumbar herniated disk remains unproved in level I studies.

Adverse Outcomes of Treatment

NSAIDs may cause gastric, renal, or hepatic complications. In 2015, the FDA strengthened its warning linking NSAIDs with the risk of heart attack or stroke, even in the first weeks of use of an

NSAID. Progression of neurologic deficit or persistent numbness and weakness may occur despite treatment.

Referral Decisions/Red Flags

Patients with any of the following conditions require further evaluation: cauda equina syndrome, urinary retention, perianal numbness, motor loss, severe single nerve root paralysis, progressive neurologic deficit, radicular symptoms that persist for more than 6 weeks, intractable leg pain, or recurrent episodes of sciatica that interfere with the patient's life activities.

SECTION 8   SPINE

Lumbar Spinal Stenosis

Synonym
Neurogenic claudication

Definition
Lumbar spinal stenosis is the narrowing of one or more levels of the lumbar spinal canal with subsequent compression of the nerve roots. Anatomically, lumbar stenosis affects as much as 30% of the population older than 60 years, yet only a portion of these individuals will have symptoms. In elderly patients, spinal stenosis is typically degenerative in origin. Younger patients with achondroplasia or other disorders that cause a small spinal canal may experience clinical symptoms in their 20s or 30s.

Degenerative lumbar spinal stenosis occurs most commonly at the L3-4, L4-5, and L2-3 levels. Although central lumbar stenosis is uncommon at L5-S1, lateral degenerative changes at this level may cause compression of the L5 (higher) nerve root.

Clinical Symptoms
The stenosis may be quite advanced before symptoms occur. Onset of symptoms may be insidious, or symptoms may develop quickly without any history of injury. A common pattern of presentation is neurogenic claudication that causes radicular symptoms (with or without associated back pain) in one or both legs (**Figure 1**). Neurogenic claudication differs from vascular claudication, but these conditions may coexist in elderly patients (**Table 1**). With neurogenic claudication, symptoms progress from a proximal to a distal direction. Walking or prolonged standing causes fatigue and weakness in the legs. Sitting or lying down generally relieves the pain. Vascular insufficiency may be difficult to differentiate from lumbar spinal stenosis.

Extension of the spine narrows the lumbar spinal canal, often worsening the symptoms, whereas flexion increases the canal diameter. Therefore, patients may obtain short-term relief by leaning forward (stooping). For example, these patients often lean on the cart while grocery shopping. The length of time that symptomatic relief lasts after sitting will vary. Patients may also awaken at night with back and/or leg pain after a few hours of sleep.

Lumbosacral pain occurs less commonly and is associated with walking or standing. A vague aching in the legs associated with leg weakness may also be reported. Spondylolisthesis (degenerative or spondylolytic), vascular insufficiency, and osteoarthritis of the hips are often coexisting pathologies seen in patients with spinal stenosis.

Tests
Physical Examination

True muscle weakness in the legs is uncommon. Proprioception may be impaired and result in a mildly positive Romberg test. Sensory changes are segmental if present but may involve more than one

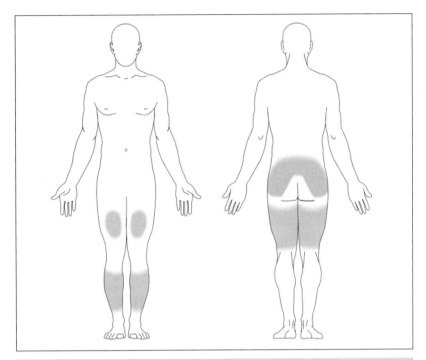

Figure 1 Illustration shows a typical pain diagram for a patient with spinal stenosis. Some patients may have severe stenosis but minimal thigh or leg pain.

Table 1

Comparison of Vascular and Neurogenic Claudication

Evaluation	Vascular	Neurogenic
Claudication distance	Fixed	Variable
Relief of pain	Standing	Sitting-flexed
Walk uphill	Pain	No pain
Bicycle ride	Pain	No pain
Type of pain	Cramp, tightness	Numbness, ache, sharp
Pulses	Absent	Present
Bruit	Present	Absent
Skin	Loss of hair, shiny	Normal
Atrophy	Rare	Occasional
Weakness	Rare	Occasional
Back pain	Uncommon	Common
Limitations of spinal movement	Uncommon	Common

(Reproduced from Herkowitz HN: Spinal stenosis: Clinical evaluation. *Instr Course Lect* 1992;41:184.)

SECTION 8 SPINE

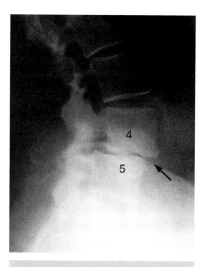

Figure 2 Lateral radiograph from a patient with degenerative spondylolisthesis at L4 on L5 (arrow).

spinal level. Reflexes may be diminished. The anterior and posterior tibial pulses will be normal unless the patient has concomitant vascular disease. Some patients will have a lumbar deformity. Bowel or bladder symptoms may be reported, but anal sphincter tone is rarely decreased. Because many patients have concomitant prostate disease or stress incontinence, genitourinary evaluation is necessary to differentiate these processes.

Diagnostic Tests
AP and lateral radiographs (including up to T10 in the lateral view) may show spondylolisthesis or significant narrowing of the intervertebral disk (**Figure 2**). Osteopenia may be present.

Differential Diagnosis
- Abdominal aortic aneurysm (palpable pulsatile mass)
- Arterial insufficiency (distance to claudication constant, recovery after rest, absent or diminished pulses)
- Diabetes mellitus (abnormal glucose metabolism, nonsegmental numbness, skin changes)
- Folic acid or vitamin B_{12} deficiency (confirmed by laboratory tests, anemia)
- Infection (mild temperature elevation, elevated erythrocyte sedimentation rate, elevated C-reactive protein level, intervertebral disk narrowing with reactive changes in the adjacent vertebral end plates)
- Tumor (patchy neurologic deficit, bone destruction, night pain)

Adverse Outcomes of the Disease
The rate of progression varies widely. Many patients tolerate this condition well and neurologic deficit never develops. However, pain and limited function may become significant and lead to an adverse quality of life with secondary depression. Standing erect may become impossible, forcing the patient to adopt a stooped posture. Claudication may develop after walking only a few feet. Although cauda equina syndrome must be considered, this syndrome is rare.

Treatment
Many patients with lumbar spinal stenosis are elderly and have comorbidities that require consideration when weighing treatment options. Initial treatment generally includes NSAIDs and physical activity. Water exercise therapy is a good initial activity for the elderly, deconditioned patient with mild symptoms. Narcotic medication is rarely required and should be avoided. Epidural steroid injections (up to three in a 6-month period), which are usually administered under radiologic guidance, may be considered. Epidural steroid injections improve symptoms in approximately 50% of patients, but the improvement usually lasts only 4 to 6 months.

Patients who are becoming nonambulatory and report a decreased quality of life are candidates for surgical management. The age of the patient is less important than comorbidities in predicting surgical outcomes. Patients with degenerative spondylolisthesis and/or scoliosis in addition to lumbar spinal stenosis may require spinal fusion in addition to decompression of the stenotic segments.

Adverse Outcomes of Treatment

Neural damage during decompression is possible but unlikely with improved techniques. Prolonged use of NSAIDs may cause renal failure, hepatotoxicity, and gastrointestinal ulcer disease. In 2015, the FDA strengthened its warning linking NSAIDs with the risk of heart attack or stroke, even in the first weeks of use of an NSAID. The chronic use of narcotics is associated with its own set of problems when these drugs are used inappropriately.

Referral Decisions/Red Flags

Any neurologic deficit, gait disturbance, or bowel and bladder dysfunction should be evaluated further. Because these changes may not improve following surgery, the goal of treatment is to prevent progression. If nonsurgical treatment is ineffective, specialty consultation is indicated. Night pain that disturbs sleep usually indicates advanced disease for which further evaluation is indicated.

SECTION 8 SPINE

Metastatic Disease

Definition

Malignant tumors involving the spine may be either primary (rare) or metastatic (common). Metastatic disease to the vertebrae occurs at some time in the clinical course of the disease in approximately 50% of all patients who have solid tumors. The highest incidence occurs with carcinoma of the breast, lung, prostate, colon, thyroid, and kidney.

Osseous involvement of the vertebrae is much more common than involvement of the spinal cord or dura. The most likely etiology is hematogenous spread, whereby neoplastic cells in the vertebral body are deposited through the Batson plexus, a unique venous plexus of the spine characterized by collateral connections to the inferior vena cava and a general lack of valves.

Metastatic disease may become clinically evident through one of several different presentations: (1) as an incidental finding in asymptomatic patients; (2) in patients with known primary tumors who are being evaluated for possible metastatic disease by bone scan, MRI, or CT; (3) as neurologic findings in patients with or without previous history of a primary tumor; or (4) as pain representing the primary presenting symptom of cancer in patients who were not aware they had a primary tumor.

Clinical Symptoms

Pain is the most common presenting symptom. The pain may be first noted following trivial trauma, is typically constant, and worsens progressively as the days or weeks pass. This pain is usually due to minor vertebral fractures secondary to the weakness created by the metastatic process. Weight-bearing activities (standing, sitting) aggravate the pain, whereas lying down typically results in relief. Pain that prevents sleep and persists through the night is highly suspicious for a neoplasm.

With compression of the nerve roots, the pain associated with cervical or lumbar tumors also radiates to the extremities. Similar nerve root entrapment by tumors in the thoracic spine causes a band-like distribution of pain around the chest. When the compression involves a nerve root, radicular symptoms and associated sensory loss and/or motor weakness are restricted to a single extremity. If more generalized sensory and motor dysfunction occurs, and especially if the patient reports bowel or bladder dysfunction or difficulty walking, cervical or thoracic cord compression or cauda equina syndrome may be present.

The rate of disease progression and neurologic dysfunction may be slow, evolving over weeks or months, or rapid in more aggressive tumors. Progression may be more difficult to identify in patients taking high dosages of pain medication for metastatic disease elsewhere. Acute onset of quadriplegia or paraplegia may occur (infrequently) with rapid enlargement of a soft-tissue tumor mass or following a pathologic fracture that compresses the spinal cord.

Tests

Physical Examination

An area of tenderness to palpation and/or percussion along the spinous processes is common. Tumors in the posterior elements (lamina, spinous process) may be palpable. A patient with a vertebral body collapse may develop increased kyphosis at the level of fracture. Assess motor and sensory function of all nerve roots distal to the lesion. Check deep tendon and other appropriate spinal cord reflexes. If the primary tumor has not been previously diagnosed, the patient will need a complete evaluation for staging purposes with particular emphasis on the thyroid, breasts, chest, kidney, and prostate. Consultation with an oncologist is warranted.

Diagnostic Tests

Initial radiographic evaluation requires high-quality AP and lateral radiographs. Cervical spine radiographs should also include odontoid views and show all vertebrae from the occiput to T1. Lumbar spine radiographs should include the bodies of T10 to the tip of the coccyx, with a spot lateral view of the lumbosacral junction if needed for clarity. A radiopaque marker placed next to an area of percussion tenderness helps identify the area of concern. The lateral view may show collapse with loss of height of the vertebral body or areas of bony destruction with lytic or blastic lesions in the vertebral body. Often the first radiologic sign of tumor involvement is loss of integrity of a pedicle, as seen on the AP view and commonly described as the "winking owl" sign because of the asymmetry of the involved and uninvolved pedicles (**Figure 1**).

A technetium Tc-99m bone scan is the best screening study to identify widespread metastatic disease because it evaluates the spine as well as other axial (pelvis) and appendicular (extremity) bones. This study will generally be negative in patients with multiple myeloma.

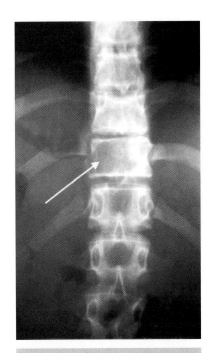

Figure 1 AP radiograph of the spine demonstrates a missing pedicle (arrow), which is indicative of a metastatic or a primary tumor (the "winking owl" sign).

SECTION 8 SPINE

Differential Diagnosis

- Degenerative arthritis (fracture rare, bone dense)
- Infection (loss of disk space, sclerosis)
- Multiple myeloma (men older than 50 years, fracture from trivial trauma)
- Osteoporotic fracture (generalized osteopenia, pedicles intact)
- Traumatic fracture (normal bone, widening of bone in AP and lateral views)

Adverse Outcomes of the Disease

Involvement of one area of the spine with metastatic disease usually does not change the overall survival rate, but spinal deformity and/or intractable pain poses considerable problems in patient care. Spinal involvement with neurologic deficit compromises quality of life and may shorten life span with complications of paraplegia. Quadriplegia and paraplegia are the most serious sequelae of pathologic fractures.

Treatment

Treatment of spinal tumors is based on the type of tumor, the degree of bony involvement, the type of symptoms, and physician/patient preference. Chemotherapy, hormone therapy, or radiation is appropriate for asymptomatic tumors detected during evaluation for metastatic disease. Radiation therapy is appropriate for painful metastases without serious deformity or neural compression. Alternative methods are considered in tumors that are insensitive to radiation (renal cell carcinoma). With pain and neurologic deficit, the most effective way to improve neural function and overall function is surgical decompression and stabilization, generally with adjunctive postoperative radiation therapy. Surgical intervention results in improved neurologic function in approximately 85% of patients.

Adverse Outcomes of Treatment

Neurologic deterioration persists in some patients, despite adequate decompression, because of recurrent tumor or tumor involvement in the vascular supply to the spinal cord. Surgical wound complications are more common when the surgery follows radiation therapy or the patient is taking oral steroids.

Referral Decisions/Red Flags

Patients with known prior malignancies and spinal symptoms or patients with intractable pain require evaluation by a specialist, as do patients in whom trivial trauma produces a spinal fracture, even in the presence of osteoporosis.

Scoliosis in Adults

Definition

Scoliosis is a lateral (coronal) curvature of the spine, but this condition also involves abnormalities of the axial and sagittal planes. In adults, scoliosis is classified as either a deformity that developed during childhood or a deformity that developed after skeletal maturity, usually secondary to degenerative spondylosis and/or degenerative spondylolisthesis. Changes that occur with aging, including osteoporosis, degenerative disk disease, spinal stenosis, and degenerative spondylolisthesis, may contribute to and/or confound the symptoms and progression of either condition.

Clinical Symptoms

The most common presenting symptom is pain localized to the region of the deformity. The most common overlapping syndrome is degenerative spondylosis, which may also cause lower lumbar pain. Because age-related changes in the spine are present in nearly everyone, a thorough evaluation is required to identify the most likely source of pain. Radicular pain is most commonly associated with compression of the L4 or L5 nerve root due to asymmetric hypertrophy of the facet joints, asymmetric disk degeneration, and mild rotatory subluxation. Neurologic changes are infrequent but most commonly involve the extensor hallucis longus muscle.

In some patients, the chief presenting symptom is a progressive spinal deformity. Some report that they are "getting shorter." These patients may also report that the "hump" on their back is getting bigger, or that they are leaning to the side more.

Cardiopulmonary decompensation rarely is evident in adult-onset scoliosis. Symptoms related to pulmonary compromise are associated with more severe thoracic curves, including both idiopathic and neuromuscular curves.

Tests

Physical Examination

The entire spine should be inspected and palpated with the patient standing. The relative height of the shoulders and iliac wings should be noted, as should any asymmetry at the waist. Decompensation is evaluated by measuring the distance a plumb line from C7 deviates to the right or left of the gluteal cleft. Forward bending also exaggerates the asymmetry of the posterior rib cage and thoracolumbar junction. Neurologic examination should include an evaluation of reflexes as well as motor and sensory function of the lumbosacral nerve roots. In addition, pathologic reflexes should be assessed and a gait analysis performed to examine for ataxia or evidence of spinal cord compression (myelopathy).

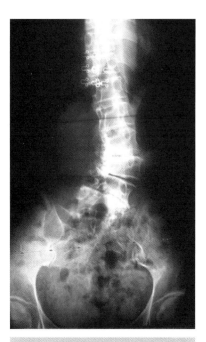

Figure 1 PA radiograph of the spine demonstrates advanced thoracolumbar kyphoscoliosis.

Diagnostic Tests
Weight-bearing full-length PA and lateral radiographs should be obtained on a 36-inch cassette (**Figure 1**). Electromyography is rarely indicated but occasionally may be helpful to distinguish radiculopathy from neuropathy.

Differential Diagnosis
- Congenital scoliosis (vertebral body abnormality, childhood or adolescent presentation)
- Degenerative disk disease with asymmetric disk space collapse (normal vertebral shape, sharp curve over few segments)
- Degenerative spondylolisthesis with accompanying lateral listhesis and disk degeneration (forward or backward slip of vertebral body)
- Neuromuscular scoliosis (neurologic abnormalities and weakness)
- Severe disk herniation with sciatic scoliosis and radiculopathy (unilateral neurologic signs, normal vertebral contour)
- Traumatic or pathologic vertebral fracture (wedge-shaped vertebral body, history of trauma)
- Vertebral osteomyelitis (fever, severe local pain, lysis of bone in vertebral body, narrowing of disk)

Adverse Outcomes of the Disease
Increased pain and deformity with diminished functional activity are possible. With increased cosmetic deformity, patients may become more introverted.

Treatment
Most cases of scoliosis in adults can be managed with NSAIDs and exercise. Exercise programs should begin with water therapy and progress to trunk strengthening as the symptoms decrease and the patient's tolerance increases. Aerobic activity is also recommended. Swimming is a particularly good exercise because it accomplishes trunk strengthening as well as aerobic conditioning.

Adverse Outcomes of Treatment
NSAIDs may cause gastric, renal, or hepatic complications. In 2015, the FDA strengthened its warning linking NSAIDs with the risk of heart attack or stroke, even in the first weeks of use of an NSAID. Complications of surgical management may include increased pain, increased deformity, infection, pseudarthrosis, instrumentation failure, and/or paralysis. The postoperative complication rate is much higher in adults than in adolescents. Patients must clearly understand the risks and benefits of this major surgery before undergoing the procedure. Elderly patients especially should be informed of the risks inherent in these surgeries in older patients. The physician should discuss the risks of both mortality and neurologic deficits.

Referral Decisions/Red Flags

Progressive neurologic deterioration requires emergency management. Patients who experience progressive pain and in whom the deformity progresses may be considered for major spinal fusion surgery. Patients who report that they cannot walk more than two blocks because of pain, respiratory dysfunction, or weakness require evaluation by a specialist. Any change in the deformity requires evaluation by a specialist as well.

SECTION 8 SPINE

Spinal Orthoses

Cervical

Soft Cervical Collar

This foam-covered orthosis is appropriate for short-term use in cervical sprains or intermittent use to alleviate pain in patients with cervical spondylosis. The most common error is selecting a soft cervical collar that is too wide, thus thrusting the neck into extension. A collar that positions the neck in approximately 10° of flexion maximizes the space for the nerve roots as they pass through the vertebral foramen. Patients should be on an isometric exercise program to avoid loss of intrinsic muscle support. Soft cervical collars worn at night can also be helpful.

Philadelphia Collar

This molded polystyrene brace provides better control of cervical rotation and is preferred for transport and initial immobilization of patients with suspected cervical fractures (**Figure 1**). Some physicians prefer this support to the cervical collar in the treatment of acute sprains. Unless rotational control is necessary (C1-2 injury), most patients prefer the greater comfort of a soft cervical collar.

Rigid Cervical Orthoses

A hard cervical collar limits flexion and extension better than a soft cervical collar. Greater restriction of neck motion is attained by a brace that extends from the neck to the midthoracic spine. For example, the Miami J orthosis (Össur, Paulsboro, NJ) is basically a Philadelphia collar that has a rigid plastic component extending to the middle of the chest. As such, it greatly restricts rotation that primarily occurs in the upper cervical spine as well as the flexion and extension and lateral bending that occur to a greater degree in the lower cervical spine.

Halo Brace

This brace provides superior immobilization of the cervical spine. The halo portion is rigidly secured to the head by four screws inserted into the outer table of the skull (**Figure 2**). Bars connect the halo to a plastic vest that surrounds the chest. Minimal cervical spinal motion occurs in a patient wearing this brace; however, this brace is cumbersome and may be poorly tolerated in elderly patients.

Thoracic

Thoracolumbosacral Corset

A standard lumbosacral corset with a proximal extension provides adequate support for patients with osteoporosis or acute thoracic sprains involving the lower thoracic spine (**Figure 3**). Some corsets are equipped with metal stays or plastic inserts that are bent to conform to the patient's spine. Women may not comply with this brace because breast irritation may occur. The orthotist may need to modify the brace to ensure patient compliance.

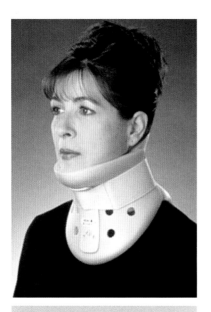

Figure 1 Photograph of the Philadelphia collar, which is used to support the cervical spine. (Reproduced with permission from Calabrese Group, Haddonfield, NJ.)

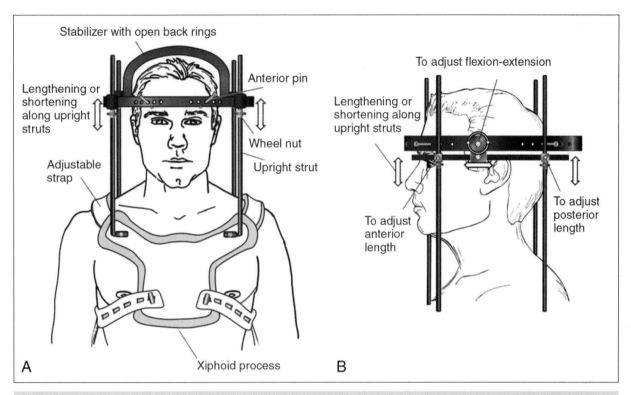

Figure 2 Illustration of the halo device. **A,** Frontal view of the components of the device in place. **B,** Side view of the upper components of the device in place. Angular (circular arrow), anteroposterior translational (left-to-right arrow), and axial lengthening and shortening (up-and-down arrow) adjustments can be made. (Reproduced from Bono CM: The halo fixator. *J Am Acad Orthop Surg* 2007;15[12]:728-737.)

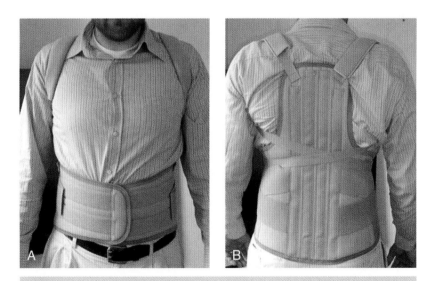

Figure 3 Photographs of the front (**A**) and back (**B**) views of a dorsal lumbar corset. (Reproduced from Agabegi SS, Asghar FA, Herkowitz HN: Spinal orthoses. *J Am Acad Orthop Surg* 2010;18[11]:657-667.)

Three-point Spine Orthosis

The basic principle of this type of orthosis is three-point fixation, with pressure over the sternum and pubis anteriorly and over the midspine posteriorly. Most are aluminum and bendable to fit the

SECTION 8   SPINE

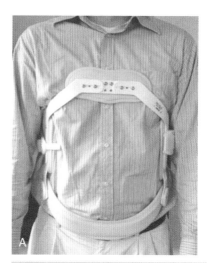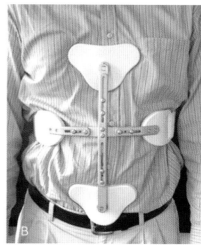

Figure 4 A, Photograph of the Jewett brace. **B,** Photograph of the cruciform anterior spinal hyperextension (CASH) brace. (Reproduced from Agabegi SS, Asghar FA, Herkowitz HN: Spinal orthoses. *J Am Acad Orthop Surg* 2010;18[11]:657-667.)

patient. These braces limit flexion and extension of the thoracic spine but provide limited rotational control. Because of their limited contact areas and light weight, these orthoses are well tolerated by patients. This type of orthosis is useful for patients with thoracic sprains or minimal compression fractures. The Jewett (**Figure 4, A**) and cruciform anterior spinal hyperextension (**Figure 4, B**) braces are examples of these three-point orthoses.

Thoracolumbosacral and Lumbosacral Orthosis

Thoracolumbosacral orthosis (TLSO) and lumbosacral orthosis (LSO) (**Figure 5**) braces are either prefabricated modules that are fitted based on patient measurements or are made from a plaster mold of the patient's torso. The orthosis made from a plaster mold provides better total contact and rotational control but is quite expensive. These braces usually are constructed of hard plastic anterior and posterior clamshells that are lined with a soft material and attach together on the sides. These braces are used primarily as definitive treatment in patients with stable fractures of the thoracolumbar spine or as a postoperative aid following spinal fusion.

Lumbar

Elastic Belts

These braces do not limit lumbar spine motion and probably do not prevent injury. With a mild lumbar strain, these braces do provide some abdominal support and can remind the patient to be careful during various activities.

Lumbosacral Corset

The standard lumbosacral corset can be worn with or without internal stays of metal or plastic. These devices provide very little restriction of motion and are most useful as an adjunct to pain control following

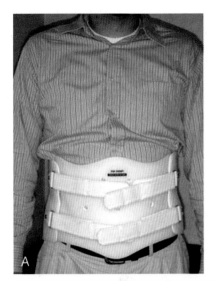
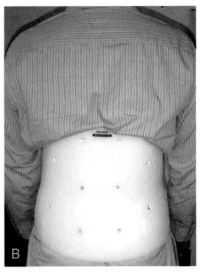

Figure 5 Photographs of the front (**A**) and back (**B**) views of a lumbosacral orthosis. (Reproduced from Agabegi SS, Asghar FA, Herkowitz HN: Spinal orthoses. *J Am Acad Orthop Surg* 2010;18[11]:657-667.)

a lumbar sprain or acute disk herniation. The time period of bracing should be short and accompanied by an exercise program after the acute pain has subsided.

Rigid Orthoses
See the descriptions for the three-point orthosis and the TLSO.

SECTION 8 SPINE

Spondylolisthesis: Degenerative

Synonym

Pseudospondylolisthesis

Definition

Degenerative spondylolisthesis is forward slippage of a lumbar vertebral body that is caused by degeneration and alterations in the facet joints in conjunction with degenerative changes in the intervertebral disk. By definition, the lamina and pars interarticularis are intact. This condition occurs most frequently between the fourth and fifth vertebral bodies. Degenerative spondylolisthesis is more common in women older than 40 years. These patients also tend to be mildly to moderately overweight.

Retrolisthesis is posterior slippage of a lumbar vertebral body on the vertebra below. This condition also develops secondary to degenerative changes.

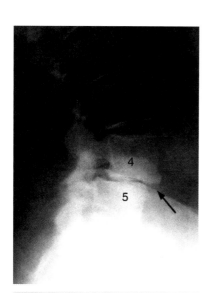

Figure 1 Lateral radiograph from a patient with degenerative spondylolisthesis at L4 on L5 (arrow).

Clinical Symptoms

Back pain that is aggravated by bending, lifting, or twisting activities is common. Narrowing of the lateral recesses may cause a radiculopathy. Narrowing of the central canal may cause neurogenic claudication or other symptoms of spinal stenosis.

Tests

Physical Examination

Inspect and palpate the spine for any curvature, loss of lordosis, or step-off of the spinous processes. Evaluate motor and sensory function of the L1-S4 nerve roots. Diminished knee and/or ankle reflexes are often present; however, these findings are common in elderly patients. Motor examination is usually normal, but strength testing after walking may reveal weakness in toe or heel walking or in great toe dorsiflexion strength.

Diagnostic Tests

AP and lateral radiographs are important. The lateral view will show slippage of one vertebra onto another, usually with the superior vertebra displaced several millimeters relative to the one below (**Figure 1**). The involved disk space frequently shows degeneration and narrowing.

Differential Diagnosis

- Iatrogenic instability (following diskectomy or decompression)
- Isthmic spondylolisthesis (pars defect) (findings on radiographs and single-photon emission CT [SPECT] scans)

- Pathologic fracture (from tumor)
- Posttraumatic instability (history of fracture)

Adverse Outcomes of the Disease

Disabling back pain or functional neurologic impairment associated with spinal canal stenosis or radiculopathy is possible.

Treatment

Initial management should include NSAIDs and exercise. Many patients with degenerative spondylolisthesis are overweight, and they should be counseled on the benefits of weight loss. Weight loss alone is unlikely to eliminate the patient's symptoms, however, because the forces generated by the trunk and spinal muscles will not be influenced by weight reduction. Patients may find an abdominal binder to be helpful occasionally, but more rigid braces are typically poorly tolerated and are seldom worn. Patients may engage in activities as tolerated because activity will not cause injury, although it may be uncomfortable. Nonsurgical management is often successful for several years in these patients, but they usually consider surgical management eventually.

Adverse Outcomes of Treatment

NSAIDs may cause gastric, renal, or hepatic complications and may interact with other medications. In 2015, the FDA strengthened its warning linking NSAIDs with the risk of heart attack or stroke, even in the first weeks of use of an NSAID.

Referral Decisions/Red Flags

Patients with symptoms of spinal stenosis (neurogenic claudication) after walking two blocks or less require further evaluation. Patients with cauda equina syndrome (perianal numbness and/or bowel or bladder impairment) require immediate evaluation.

Spondylolisthesis: Isthmic

Definition

Spondylolisthesis occurs when one vertebral body slips in relation to the one below. In children this usually occurs between L5 and S1. A defect develops at the junction of the lamina with the pedicle (pars interarticularis), leaving the posterior element without a bony connection to the anterior element. Most likely this condition represents a cyclic loading event (fatigue fracture) that evolves over time in the adolescent years and fails to heal. If only the defects are present, the patient has spondylolysis. When the vertebral body slides forward, producing the "slip" or "listhesis," the condition is called spondylolisthesis and classified as isthmic. Patients who participate in activities that place stress on this area, such as gymnastics and football, have a higher incidence of this condition. For example, the incidence of spondylolysis in female gymnasts is nearly sixfold the incidence in less active age-matched females.

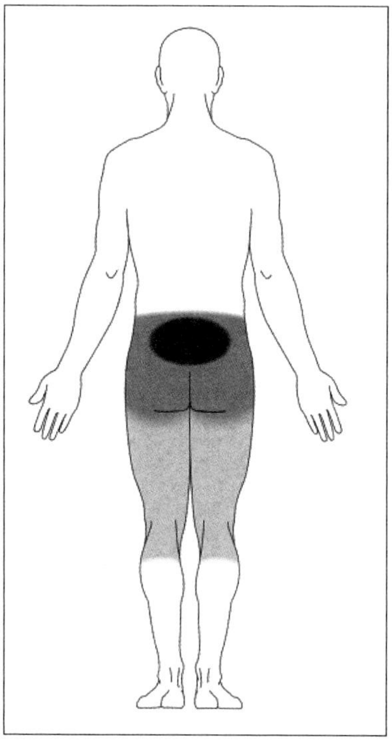

Clinical Symptoms

Spondylolisthesis may be asymptomatic or minimally symptomatic. However, in adolescent and adult patients, significant back pain that radiates posteriorly to or below the knees and worsens with standing may also develop (**Figure 1**). Frequently, patients report spasms in the hamstring muscles manifested by the inability to bend forward. In addition, markedly limited straight leg raising is demonstrated on examination. True nerve compression symptoms are rare, although the fibrocartilaginous tissue in the region of the pars interarticularis does compress the L5 nerve roots in patients with isthmic spondylolisthesis.

Tests

Physical Examination

Examination may reveal diminished lumbar lordosis and flattening of the buttocks. With significant spondylolisthesis, a step-off is noted, with the spinous process of the slipped vertebra that is "left behind" being more prominent than the one above. Hamstring spasm markedly limits the patient's ability to bend forward or the height to which the examiner can raise the patient's straight leg with the patient supine (straight leg raising test). Neurologic deficits are uncommon.

Diagnostic Tests

With forward slippage (spondylolisthesis), lateral radiographs demonstrate forward translation of L5 relative to S1 (expressed as a percentage of the AP width of the vertebral body) (**Figure 2**). A defect in the pars interarticularis (a "collar" on the "Scotty dog") is evident on the oblique views (**Figure 3**). This is the only radiographic abnormality if the condition is limited to spondylolysis. Increasing slippage can be evaluated with radiographs taken at 6-month intervals (or sooner if symptoms increase) until skeletal maturity is achieved.

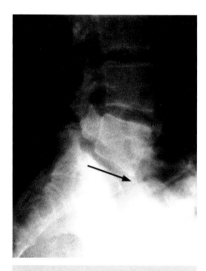

Figure 1 Illustration shows a typical pain diagram for a patient with isthmic spondylolisthesis. Distribution of leg symptoms will generally follow the L5 dermatome on one or both sides.

Figure 2 Lateral radiograph demonstrates a grade 2 to 3 spondylolisthesis at the lumbosacral junction (arrow).

Differential Diagnosis

- Intervertebral disk injury (no step-off or slip, no defect seen on plain radiograph)
- Intervertebral diskitis (elevated erythrocyte sedimentation rate, fever)
- Osteoid osteoma (night pain, abnormal bone scan, pain relieved with aspirin)
- Spinal cord tumor (sensory findings, upper motor neuron signs)
- Tethered spinal cord (pain, hamstring tightness, upper motor neuron signs)

Adverse Outcomes of the Disease

Progressive or complete slip of the vertebral body, chronic back pain and disability, paralysis of the lower lumbar nerve roots (usually L5), or bowel and bladder involvement (cauda equina syndrome) are possible.

Treatment

Isthmic spondylolisthesis differs from degenerative spondylolisthesis in that these patients are often skeletally immature at the outset of the condition; therefore, a single-photon emission CT (SPECT) scan should be performed in the young patient to assess metabolic activity in the area of the defect in the pars interarticularis. If the area of the defect is active and the patient is skeletally immature, rigid bracing is recommended. Surgical stabilization for refractory symptoms or high-grade slips may be indicated. When the patient has reached skeletal maturity, fixation of the defect is not warranted.

Skeletally mature patients need not be restricted from any activity. Marked progression of this condition (greater than 1 cm) in an adult is rare. Most cases of progression in adults occur in patients with spondylolisthesis following decompression surgery without spinal fusion.

In adults, nonsurgical treatment with NSAIDs and exercise is recommended. Surgery is recommended only in patients with a decreased quality of life whose symptoms have not responded to a well-planned and faithfully followed nonsurgical regimen.

Adverse Outcomes of Treatment

Despite treatment, progression of the forward slip may continue.

Referral Decisions/Red Flags

Patients with significant pain and/or obvious slippage require further evaluation.

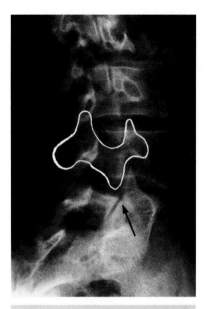

Figure 3 Oblique radiograph demonstrates a normal "Scotty dog" appearance to the lamina (outlined area). In the vertebra below, the Scotty dog has a "collar" (arrow), which is the site of the pars interarticularis defect of spondylolisthesis.

SECTION 8 SPINE

Pediatric Orthopaedics

Section Editors

Joseph A. Janicki, MD, MS
Assistant Professor of Orthopaedic Surgery
Northwestern University Feinberg School of Medicine
Attending Physician, Orthopaedic Surgery
Ann & Robert H. Lurie Children's Hospital
Chicago, Illinois

Kelly L. VanderHave, MD
Carolinas Medical Center
Levine Children's Specialty Center
Pediatric Orthopaedics
Charlotte, North Carolina

Contributor

Mark C. Hubbard, MPT
Physical Therapist
Bone and Joint Institute
Penn State Milton S. Hershey Medical Center
Hershey, Pennsylvania

Contributors from the American Academy of Pediatrics

Pooya Hosseinzadeh, MD
Assistant Professor
Department of Pediatric Orthopedics
Baptist Children's Hospital
Miami, Florida

Thomas G. McPartland, MD
Assistant Clinical Professor Orthopedic Surgery
Department of Orthopedic Surgery
Rutgers-Robert Wood Johnson Medical School
New Brunswick, New Jersey

Brien Rabenhorst, MD
Assistant Professor of Orthopaedic Surgery
University of Arkansas for Medical Sciences
Little Rock, Arkansas

Brian A. Shaw, MD
Associate Professor of Orthopaedic Surgery
Children's Hospital Colorado
University of Colorado School of Medicine
Colorado Springs, Colorado

Overview of Pediatric Orthopaedics

The often-quoted statement "Children are not just small adults" is particularly germane to pediatric disorders of the musculoskeletal system. Fractures, soft-tissue injuries, neurologic disorders, and infections all have unique features and different considerations in children versus adults. Furthermore, the effect of growth must always be considered, because it can have a positive or negative effect depending on the underlying diagnosis.

Common Presenting Symptoms in Children

Parental concern regarding the appearance of the child's stance, posture, or gait is a frequent cause for seeking medical advice. Pain from acute injuries is perhaps the most common symptom. Participation in athletics has increased both in frequency and intensity, resulting in symptoms from a host of overuse injuries. When a child presents with persistent pain and localized swelling and/or refuses to use a limb or bear weight on a lower extremity, a detailed evaluation is indicated.

Age and Sex

An understanding of normal growth and development is critical for the evaluation of children presenting with musculoskeletal complaints. Some so-called deformities in children are developmental in nature and normal for their age. Knowledge of the normal ranges of alignment and rotation of the limbs is essential to differentiate pathologic from physiologic factors. For example, genu varum (bowlegs) is normal in the first 2 years of life, but by the time a child reaches 3 years of age, a relatively large amount of genu valgum (knock-knee alignment) is typically seen.

Age and sex are important factors when evaluating children. For example, a boy between the ages of 4 and 8 years who has proximal thigh pain and a limp may have Legg-Calvé-Perthes disease. Similar symptoms in adolescent boys might suggest a slipped capital femoral epiphysis. Female infants are more likely than male infants to have hip dysplasia, whereas clubfoot is more common in males. Adolescent girls are more likely to have scoliosis, but kyphosis is more common in adolescent boys.

Growth

Skeletal growth may be beneficial in the management of certain musculoskeletal conditions. This is particularly true in the newborn period or during infancy, when a brace is used for a few months to treat a dysplastic hip and may result in a normal joint that functions well for a lifetime. Certain angular deformities in pediatric fractures also can remodel completely in young children, which allows for greater latitude in the closed management of fractures in children when compared with adults.

However, growth plate injuries have consequences that are unique to children. Fractures that damage the physis (growth plate) can cause progressive angulation and/or shortening of the limb. Progressive angulation of a weight-bearing bone (as seen in infantile tibia vara and rickets) can result from asymmetric growth on one side of the physis.

Neuromuscular Disorders

Many pediatric neuromuscular disorders such as cerebral palsy, myelomeningocele, and muscular dystrophy cause muscle weakness, spasticity, and/or imbalance (greater weakness on one side of the joint), which may result in limb deformities and impaired function. Normal longitudinal growth of the skeleton may be affected by muscle contractures, resulting in rotational and/or angular deformities. In a child with spastic cerebral palsy, the hip adductor and flexor muscles are often more involved and therefore stronger than the opposing hip abductors and extensors. With growth, this muscle imbalance can cause progressive contracture of the hip adductors and flexors as well as dysplasia of the acetabulum, valgus alignment of the proximal femur, and subluxation or dislocation of the hip.

Soft-Tissue Injuries

As children grow, their coordination and strength change. As a result, competitive sports require adaptation of the game to the age and size of the child. Although overuse injuries in the adult primarily manifest themselves as either microscopic tears or complete rupture at the musculotendinous junction (or within the substance of the tendon), the bone-tendon junction is the weak link in children and adolescents. Different types of overuse syndromes are seen in different age groups. For example, Osgood-Schlatter disease results from microscopic avulsion fractures at the insertion of the patellar tendon during development of the relatively weak secondary ossification center of the proximal tibia.

Infection and Arthritis

The higher incidence of acute hematogenous osteomyelitis (AHO) in children is related to the unique anatomy of the child's metaphyseal bone circulation. A child's spine is also more susceptible to discitis for similar reasons. Hematogenous septic arthritis also is more common in children. Chronic inflammatory diseases such as juvenile idiopathic arthritis present differently in children than adults.

Pediatric Physical Examination

Inspection/Palpation

Anterior View

With the patient standing, inspect frontal, side, and rotational alignment of the lower extremities. Conditions that can be easily recognized by inspection are genu valgum (knock-knee), genu varum (bowleg), internal femoral torsion (where the patellae point toward one another), external femoral torsion (where the patellae face away from each other and not straight ahead), and limb-length inequality (where the pelvis is not level). Also, look for increased angulation at the elbow or extreme shoulder height asymmetry. Look for asymmetry in the angle formed by the humerus and forearm (elbow carrying angle). It is normal for the elbow to be in slight valgus alignment. Unilateral deformity may indicate an acute injury or deformity from a congenital or traumatic growth disturbance.

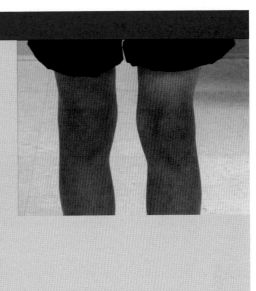

Palpation

A young child may not be able to verbalize the site of his or her pain. Initiate palpation by touching an area that is probably not involved, slowly moving to the suspected area of involvement. Even though the child may be apprehensive and crying, a change in discomfort can be identified as the tender area is palpated.

Range of Motion

Hip Internal Rotation

Measure hip internal rotation with the hip in extension for accurate measurement of femoral anteversion. With the patient prone and knees flexed to 90°, rotate the lower extremities outward. This maneuver positions the hip into internal rotation. With increased femoral anteversion, internal rotation will exceed external rotation by 30° or more.

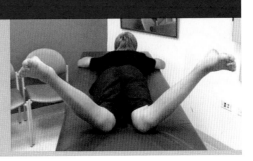

Hip External Rotation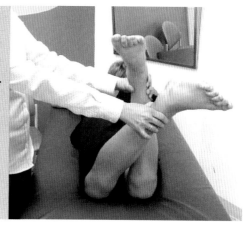

Assess hip external rotation with the child prone and the knees together. Rotate the lower extremities inward while stabilizing the pelvis. This maneuver positions the hip in external rotation. Compare the two sides. Rotation of the hips is typically symmetric.

Hip Abduction—Older Children

Assess hip abduction in older children with the hip in extension at the level of the pelvis. With the patient supine, place one hand on the contralateral anterior superior iliac spine. This hand will sense when the pelvis starts to tilt upward (limit of hip abduction). Abduct the hip until the pelvis starts to tilt and estimate the degree of movement. Asymmetric hip abduction should be considered pathologic and requires further evaluation.

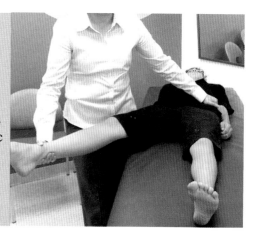

Special Tests

Limb-Length Discrepancy

Using a tape measure, measure each lower extremity from the anterior superior iliac spine to the inferior prominence of the medial malleolus. Compare the measurements of the two sides. Palpating the iliac crests with the patient standing can also help identify patients with limb-length discrepancy. In patients with iliac crests at different levels, different-sized wooden blocks can be placed under the shorter lower extremity. The thickness of the blocks under the lower extremity when the iliac crests are level indicates the amount of limb-length discrepancy.

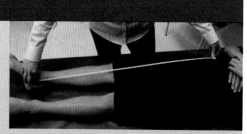

Scoliosis—Forward Bend Test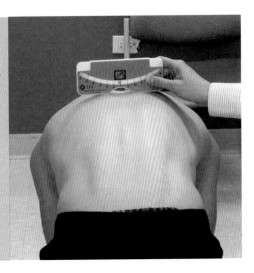

In a patient with scoliosis, the vertebral column rotates, causing a prominence on the convex side of the deformity. This posterior prominence is accentuated with the Adam forward bend test. Ask the patient to bend forward with the knees straight and with both arms hanging free. Examine the back from behind during the forward bend test. An asymmetric prominence indicates scoliosis. Measure the quantity of trunk asymmetry with a scoliometer.

Kyphosis

When assessing patients for kyphosis, inspect the thoracic spine from the side while the child is standing, looking for excessive rounding of the thoracic spine. Ask the patient to bend forward with the arms hanging free. If the patient is not able to touch the toes, consider the possibility of tight hamstrings associated with Scheuermann disease or spondylolisthesis in the lower lumbar spine.

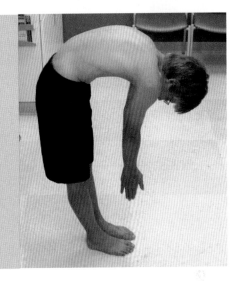

Wilson Test

The Wilson test is used to assess the presence of symptomatic osteochondritis dissecans. With the patient supine, flex the hip and knee 90° and internally rotate the tibia. Then, slowly extend the knee. The Wilson test is positive when the patient reports pain as the knee reaches full extension or near–full extension, and the pain is relieved with the external rotation of the tibia, while maintaining the same flexion angle. This maneuver causes the tibial spine to impact and then rotate away from an osteochondritis dissecans lesion located on the medial femoral condyle.

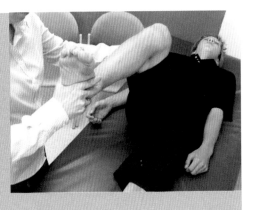

SECTION 9 PEDIATRIC ORTHOPAEDICS

Musculoskeletal Screening Examination

The musculoskeletal screening examination is used to clear young athletes (and others) for the musculoskeletal component of sports participation. It also can be used as part of a periodic musculoskeletal physical examination of a patient with no presenting symptoms.

The preparticipation physical examination (PPE) helps detect diseases, susceptibilities, or injuries that may preclude sports participation. It is important to remember, however, that the history and questionnaire have been shown to be the most sensitive in detecting medical issues or injuries. The examiner should question the patient about prior injuries and perform a more detailed examination of affected systems. The purpose of the musculoskeletal screening examination is to look for asymmetry, strength deficits, changes in muscle mass, or limitation of joint motion.

Make sure the patient is dressed appropriately to permit adequate examination of the spine and extremities. Ideally, males should be in shorts and should remove their shirt if they are comfortable doing so. Female patients can wear a tank top or a sports bra with shorts.

Gait

Observe the patient's gait. Assess for symmetry, antalgic gait, limb-length discrepancies, and abnormal mechanics. Assess for trunk shift by checking to see if the torso sways to one side. Ask the patient to walk on the toes, then the heels.

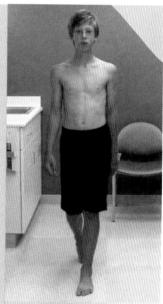

Spine

With the patient standing, inspect the spine. Observe the patient's posture to assess for normal thoracic kyphosis and lumbar lordosis. Check symmetry and height of the shoulders and hips. Perform the forward bend test and record the angle of trunk rotation (ATR).

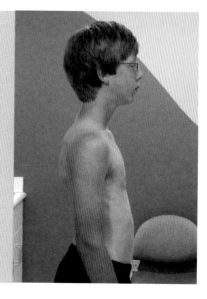

Cervical Spine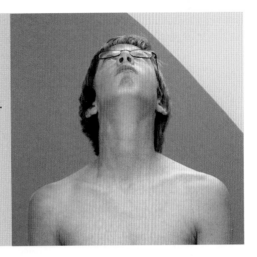

Inspect the cervical spine. Assess the patient's range of motion in each direction. Ask the patient to flex and extend the neck. Ask the patient to rotate the head laterally. Finally, have the patient bend the neck laterally, putting each ear to the shoulder.

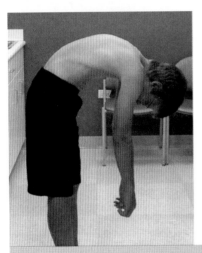 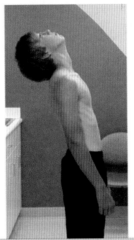 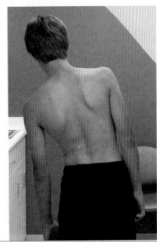 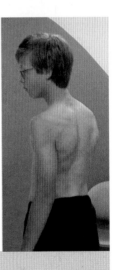

Thoracic and Lumbar Spine

Inspect the thoracic and lumbar spine. Observe for asymmetry. Ask the patient to avoid movement at the hips to ensure the assessment properly evaluates the spine. Assess range of motion by having the patient bend forward, bend backward, perform side bending, and rotation.

Upper Extremity

Begin with the patient standing and shoulders visible. Inspect for asymmetry and muscle atrophy.

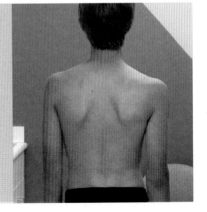

SECTION 9   PEDIATRIC ORTHOPAEDICS

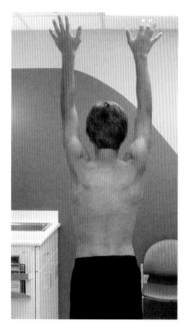
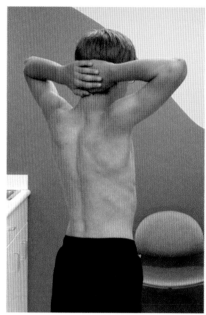
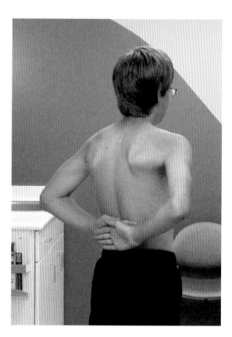

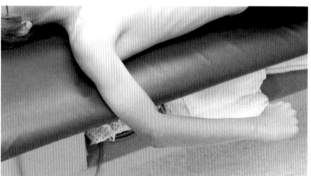
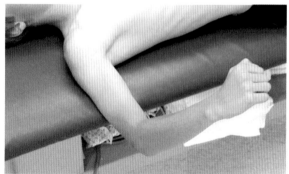

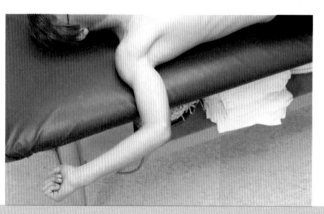

Shoulder Range of Motion

Evaluate shoulder forward flexion by asking the patient to lock the elbows and extend the arms fully overhead. Evaluate shoulder abduction by having the patient lock the elbows and then (like making a snow angel) bring the thumbs together overhead. Evaluate external and internal rotation by asking the patient to place the hands behind the head, palms facing in, and then to place the hands behind the back, with palms facing outward. Shoulder motion may be assessed with the patient supine, shoulder abducted to 90°, and elbow flexed 90° so the examiner can rotate the arm. Generally, external rotation is greater on the dominant side, particularly in a throwing athlete. Total arc of motion should be symmetric.

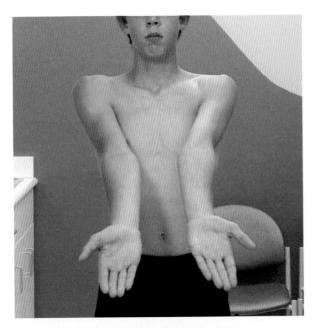
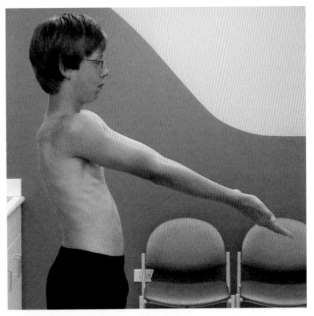
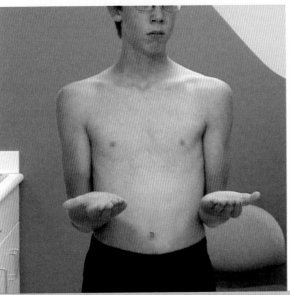
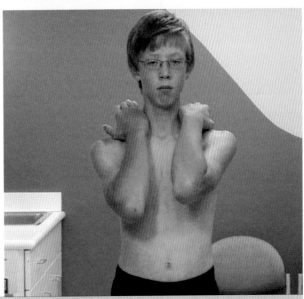

Elbows

Inspect the elbows. Ask the patient to raise the arms parallel to the floor. Inspect the elbows from the anterior and lateral aspects of the patient. Assess for cubitus varus and cubitus valgus. Have the patient extend and flex the elbows. Ask the patient to flex the elbows to 90° with the elbows at the side. Evaluate elbow pronation and supination.

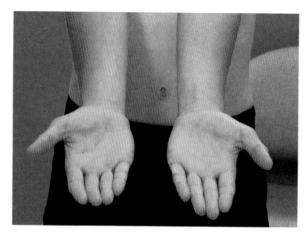

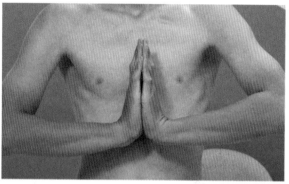
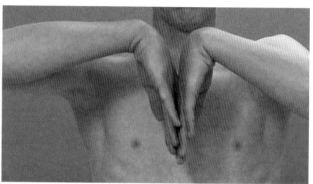

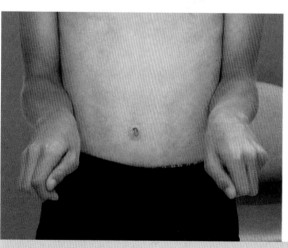
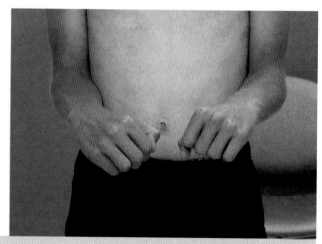

Wrists 🔲📹

Inspect the wrists. Look for asymmetry. Ask the patient to place the palms together, then the backs of the hands together, to check wrist extension and flexion. Ask the patient to bend the wrist inward and outward to assess for ulnar and radial deviation.

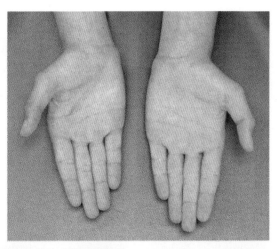

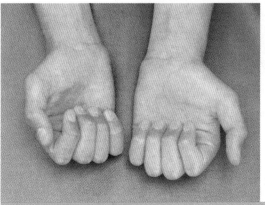
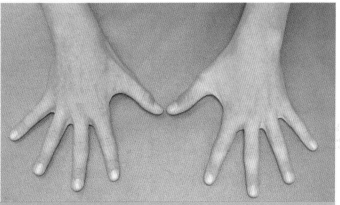

Hands

Inspect the hands. Look for asymmetry. Ask the patient to make a fist with the forearms supinated. Inspect the resting arc of the fingers. Have the patient open the hands and spread the fingers.

Hips

Inspect the hips. Ask the patient to put feet together, with hips abducted (the butterfly stretch position). Ask the patient to squat down, with knees out to the side, then stand.

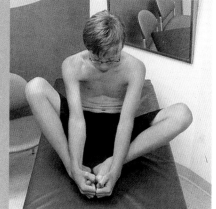
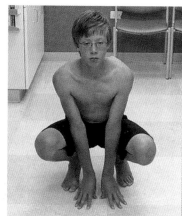

Knees

With the patient supine on the examination table, inspect for asymmetry. Assess knee flexion by having the patient fully flex the knees with the feet on the table.

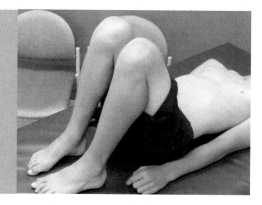

SECTION 9   PEDIATRIC ORTHOPAEDICS

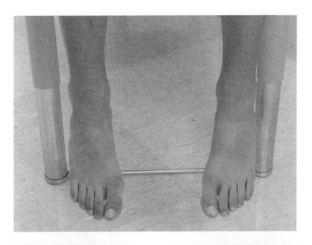

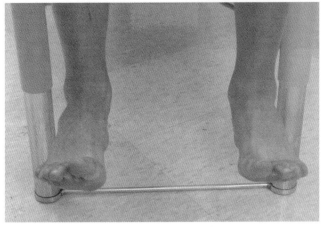

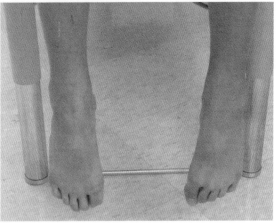

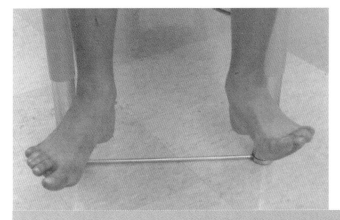

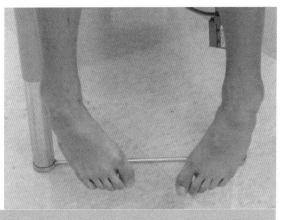

Ankles

Inspect the ankles. With the patient seated on the examination table with the legs flexed 90°, observe the position and alignment of the heels. Have the patient dorsiflex the ankles fully by pointing the feet upward, then plantar flex the ankles by pointing the feet downward. Then have the patient evert and invert the feet.

SECTION 9   PEDIATRIC ORTHOPAEDICS

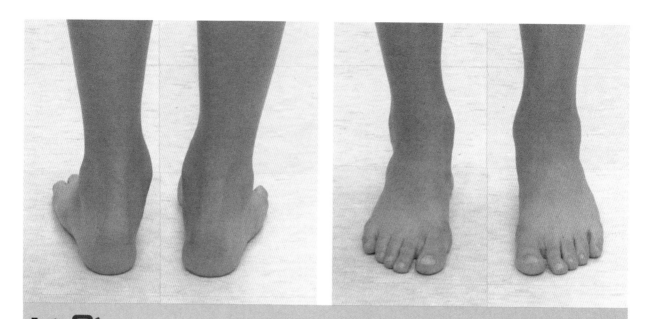

Feet 🔲📹

Inspect the feet for symmetry and normal alignment. Inspect the midfoot and forefoot. Inspect the number and appearance of the toes. Look for symmetry and normal alignment.

Anterior Knee Pain

Definition

Anterior knee pain is a common problem in active adolescents and preadolescents and is primarily the result of repetitive stress. The most common cause is patellar maltracking. Anterior knee pain caused by altered patellofemoral forces secondary to growth and changing patellar tracking in the trochlear groove of the femur with growth and development is common; this pain has different names, including patellofemoral syndrome (PFS), miserable malalignment syndrome (**Figure 1**), and anterior knee syndrome.

Less common causes of anterior knee pain are pathologic plica and a symptomatic bipartite patella. A plica is a normal fold of the synovium that may become thickened and/or fibrotic secondary to repetitive stress. A bipartite patella is a failure of an ossification center of the patella to fuse, most commonly the superolateral corner (**Figure 2**). A bipartite patella is typically seen as an incidental finding on radiographs; however, it may become symptomatic as a result of a direct blow or following repetitive stress from flexion-extension exercises.

Clinical Symptoms

Patients with anterior knee pain typically report a history of aching peripatellar knee pain, which is frequently activity related. With PFS, the pain frequently increases with flexion-extension activities such as running, kicking, and jumping, as well as with squatting, walking downhill, descending stairs, or prolonged sitting. Giving way (falling) with these activities is occasionally reported. Swelling is rarely seen.

A bipartite patella may be asymptomatic until the patient falls on the knee, presumably altering the fibrous union between the unfused ossicle and the remainder of the patella. In the acute setting, tenderness and swelling are localized to the superolateral corner of the patella. In chronic cases, patients report pain after running and jumping activities.

Tests

Physical Examination

If asked to place one finger on the spot that hurts the most, adolescents with PFS often report that they cannot identify an exact spot but will state that their knee "hurts around the kneecap" and make a sweeping gesture over the front of the knee. In contrast, a patient with symptomatic plica or bipartite patella typically localizes the symptoms. Painful plica typically is localized to the medial side of the patella, whereas pain associated with bipartite patella occurs at the superolateral pole. The hip should be examined to exclude the possibility of hip pathology (slipped capital femoral epiphysis, Legg-Calvé-Perthes disease), which can present as thigh or knee pain.

The overall alignment of the extremity should be assessed. Patients

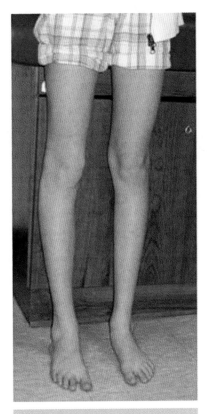

Figure 1 Photograph of a patient with miserable malalignment syndrome. Note the medial position of the patella caused by femoral anteversion, with outward position of the foot caused by external tibial torsion.

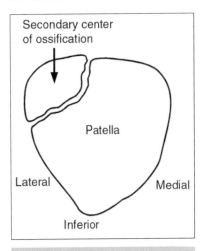

Figure 2 Illustration of the separate ossification center seen in bipartite patella.

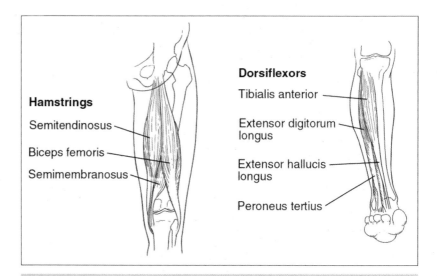

Figure 3 Illustration of the muscle groups that tend to lose flexibility during the adolescent growth spurt.

with PFS may have femoral anteversion, knee valgus, and foot pronation, resulting in excessive lateral tracking of the patella in the femoral groove. Strength of the abdominal and paravertebral muscles, as well as the muscles of the hip, should be evaluated, as should flexibility of the muscles of the lower leg (**Figure 3**). Weak muscles of the core and thigh can result in greater stress to the patellofemoral joint. A positive patellar apprehension sign implies true patellar instability rather than PFS. Patellar compression can cause pain but often is nonspecific. A thorough knee examination is required to rule out other causes of pain.

In patients with a symptomatic plica, examination may reveal a clicking sensation with knee flexion and extension. The tender plica occasionally can be palpated along the medial border of the patella.

Diagnostic Tests

Screening radiographs include AP, lateral, and skyline (Merchant) views of the knee. The skyline view shows both the location of the patella in the femoral groove and the thickness of the articular cartilage. Adolescents with PFS have a normal patellofemoral joint space. Special imaging studies such as CT or MRI may be required to further evaluate patients who have persistent pain.

Differential Diagnosis

- Articular cartilage defects (swelling, abnormal MRI)
- Infection (rare) (erythema, effusion, severe pain, elevated C-reactive protein level)
- Neoplasm (rare) (severe pain, night pain, abnormal bone scan)
- Osteochondritis dissecans (swelling, abnormal radiographs and MRI)
- Patellar subluxation or dislocation (marked positive apprehension sign, marked hypermobility of the patella)

Adverse Outcomes of the Disease

The long-term prognosis is good in patients treated nonsurgically for symptomatic bipartite patella, symptomatic plica, or PFS. The natural history of PFS, which is commonly seen in adolescents, is not well defined and continues to be studied. Most patients recover uneventfully. In the absence of true patellar subluxation or dislocation, progression to chondromalacia is rare.

Treatment

Symptoms associated with PFS improve with rest from aggravating activities, strengthening of the medial head of the quadriceps, and stretching of lower extremity muscles. Core strengthening exercises also are beneficial. Strengthening the hip, abdominal, and trunk muscles helps better position the body, increases agility, and diminishes the abnormal forces across the patellofemoral joint. A brace to help guide the patella more centrally in the groove (using a J sleeve or pad with window) may be beneficial. Orthoses (shoe inserts) can be used to decrease foot pronation, which can enhance apparent knee valgus. Surgical management of PFS is rarely recommended.

Treatment of symptomatic plica includes rest for 7 to 10 days with the knee in an extended position or, if symptoms are mild, activity modification. Occasionally, oral NSAIDs can help diminish symptoms. Applying ice to the area often provides relief. Arthroscopic excision of a symptomatic plica may be considered if a prolonged trial (3 to 6 months) of nonsurgical measures fails.

Treatment of a symptomatic bipartite patella is similar to that of symptomatic plica. Patients often recover after 5 to 7 days of rest or immobilization combined with a decrease in flexion-extension activities followed by quadriceps strengthening. In the unusual case of persistent pain over the fibrous junction of the ossicle with the patella, surgery to remove the unfused ossicle may be required.

Adverse Outcomes of Treatment

Persistent effusion of the knee may indicate inflammatory disease (for example, juvenile idiopathic arthritis) or infection (for example, Lyme disease). Pain, hypersensitivity to touch, and limited knee motion suggest the presence of complex regional pain syndrome.

Referral Decisions/Red Flags

Pain at rest or pain that increases at night requires further evaluation to rule out neoplastic processes. A joint effusion, increased generalized joint laxity, or joint line pain should raise concern for internal derangement. Locking and catching episodes reported by patients are also concerning for internal derangement. Marked apprehension with lateral deviation of the patella suggests patellar instability, and evaluation by a specialist may be warranted.

Back Pain

Synonyms

Axial back pain
Backache
Low back pain
Lumbar strain
Lumbar syndrome

Definition

The true prevalence of back pain in the pediatric population is unknown, but its prevalence varies and increases with age; by 18 years of age, the prevalence mirrors that of adults. Previously, it was believed that an extensive evaluation was required for most pediatric patients with back pain. Although it is true that back pain in infants and young children is likely to be the result of a specific etiology and requires a more extensive evaluation in most cases, in older children and adolescents, the likelihood of establishing a diagnosis is much lower, similar to that in the adult population. Two studies suggested that a definitive anatomic diagnosis was established in only 22% to 36% of older children and adolescents. All pediatric patients with back pain require a detailed history and physical examination, but the need for additional diagnostic tests (laboratory studies and advanced imaging) depends on the clinical findings and patient age.

Clinical Symptoms

The nature of onset, as well as the location, character, and radiation of the pain, should be determined. Back pain that occurs during or following physical activity and is relieved by rest suggests a mechanical cause. Back pain accompanied by neurologic signs and symptoms (such as radicular pain, muscle weakness, gait abnormalities, sensory changes, and bowel and bladder dysfunction) or systemic symptoms (such as fever, malaise, and weight loss) suggests an organic cause. Night pain often signals a more serious problem such as neoplasm.

Tests

Physical Examination

A comprehensive physical examination includes the spine, the nervous system, and other sources of referred pain such as the abdomen or pelvis. In adolescent females, a gynecologic examination may be helpful if a diagnosis has not been established, because an ovarian cyst, endometriosis, or other diagnoses can present with pain referred to the back. The spine should be examined with special emphasis on identifying any alterations in alignment or deformities, loss of motion, paraspinal muscle spasm, and areas of tenderness. Provocative tests also are important; spinal hyperextension loads the posterior elements in compression (spondylolysis), and spinal flexion loads the anterior column in compression (discitis, compression fracture). The straight leg raising test (and reverse straight leg raising test) are provocative tests for lumbar nerve root compression or stretch. The neurologic assessment includes motor and sensory function, deep tendon reflexes, and pathologic reflexes (Babinski sign or clonus). The superficial abdominal reflex is tested by lightly stroking the skin in a diagonal direction toward the umbilicus. A normal reflex is deviation of the umbilicus toward the side of the test in all four quadrants. Asymmetric abdominal reflexes may be the only finding in a child with syringomyelia or other spinal cord pathology; however, this reflex may be absent or asymmetric in healthy children. Neurologic deficits can develop as a late manifestation of a tumor or other pathology; thus, a normal neurologic examination does not rule out serious problems in the early stages of disease.

Diagnostic Tests

The extent of the evaluation depends on the duration and degree of symptoms as well as the results of the physical examination. No laboratory or radiographic studies are necessary if the examination is normal and symptoms are mild and of limited duration.

For symptoms in the thoracic and lumbar regions, weight-bearing PA and lateral radiographs of the entire spine are the initial study of choice. Radiographs of the lumbar spine are considered when spondylolysis is part of the differential diagnosis. Flexion-extension views of the cervical spine are indicated for patients with neck pain to rule out instability. The need for additional imaging studies (such as bone scanning, MRI, and CT) depends on the suspected etiology. The need for and sequencing of these tests depends on the differential diagnosis. Laboratory studies are considered in many cases, especially when systemic signs or symptoms are present, and may include a complete blood count with differential, erythrocyte sedimentation rate, and C-reactive protein level. Other tests to consider are rheumatoid factor, Lyme titer, antinuclear antibody, and HLA-B27.

Differential Diagnosis

The differential diagnosis of back pain in children is shown in **Table 1**. Muscle strain is the most common cause of thoracic and lumbar pain in children. Scheuermann kyphosis can present with pain in the thoracic and thoracolumbar regions, and spondylolysis and spondylolisthesis are common causes of pain in the lumbar and lumbosacral regions. Idiopathic scoliosis rarely causes pain in children, but scoliosis associated with syringomyelia, tethered spinal cord, or neoplasms can present as back pain.

Adverse Outcomes of the Disease

When back pain has an organic cause, failure to diagnose can result in progression of the condition. In certain conditions, such as

SECTION 9 PEDIATRIC ORTHOPAEDICS

Table 1

Differential Diagnosis of Back Pain in Children

Etiology	Condition
Congenital	Intraspinal anomalies (tethered cord, diastematomyelia)
	Upper cervical spine instability
Developmental	Scoliosis
	Kyphosis (Scheuermann disease)
	Syringomyelia
	Spondylolisthesis
Injury (acute or repetitive trauma)	Muscle strain
	Occult fractures
	Pathologic fractures (compression fractures)
	Spondylolysis
	Herniated disk or slipped vertebral apophysis
Infectious	Pyogenic (discitis or vertebral osteomyelitis)
	Granulomatous (tuberculosis, brucellosis)
	Epidural abscess
	Pyelonephritis
	Pancreatitis
Systemic	Chronic infection
	Storage diseases
	Juvenile osteoporosis
Inflammatory disease	Ankylosing spondylitis
	Juvenile idiopathic arthritis
	Psoriatic arthritis
	Reiter syndrome
Neoplastic	
Benign	Osteoid osteoma
	Osteoblastoma
	Aneurysmal bone cyst
	Langerhans cell histiocytosis
	Ganglioneuroma
Malignant	Spinal cord tumor
	Leukemia
	Lymphoma
	Neuroblastoma
	Osteogenic sarcoma
	Metastatic disease
Psychogenic	

instability of the upper cervical spine, tumors, or infections, failure to diagnose may result in spinal cord or peripheral nerve dysfunction.

Treatment

Treatment of back pain in children is specific to the diagnosis. Because of the extensive differential diagnosis for back pain, it is not possible to discuss all aspects of treatment here. For mild mechanical or activity-related discomfort, in the absence of worrisome signs or symptoms, observation with activity modifications and mild analgesics is appropriate initially. More extensive studies are necessary if the pain does not improve within 4 to 6 weeks, if the pain becomes worse, or if new symptoms and abnormal physical findings develop.

Adverse Outcomes of Treatment

Adverse outcomes of treatment also are specific to the diagnosis. The principal adverse outcome is lack of improvement or worsening of symptoms despite treatment.

Referral Decisions/Red Flags

The following factors suggest a treatable underlying etiology: (1) persistent or increasing pain; (2) night pain; (3) constant pain; (4) pain accompanied by systemic symptoms such as fever, malaise, or weight loss; (5) neurologic symptoms or findings; (6) bowel or bladder dysfunction; (7) onset of symptoms at a young age; and (8) a painful thoracic scoliosis. A more extensive evaluation is necessary in such cases.

SECTION 9 PEDIATRIC ORTHOPAEDICS

Elbow Pain

Synonyms
Little Leaguer's elbow
Overuse injury of the elbow

Definition
Elbow pain in children most often is caused by acute or chronic injury to the bone or soft tissues. Excessive throwing and the subsequent valgus stress can cause chronic elbow pain in children. The principal focus of this chapter is soft-tissue injuries. Fractures are discussed in other chapters.

Clinical Symptoms
Patients with acute conditions report pain, tenderness, swelling, and most often, a history of falling on an outstretched arm. For those with chronic pain, activity-related aching pain at the involved area is common.

Tests

Physical Examination
For patients with acute conditions, the status of the median, ulnar, and radial nerves should be evaluated distal to the injury. Radial and ulnar pulses must be assessed as well. With obvious deformity, the extremity is positioned or splinted for comfort and radiographs are obtained. When examining children with no obvious elbow deformity, the site of maximum tenderness should be sought and a gentle evaluation of elbow motion performed.

For children with chronic pain, the point of maximum tenderness is assessed. Mild swelling and limited motion may be present. The area should be palpated for a mass to exclude an atypical tumor.

Diagnostic Tests
AP and lateral radiographs of the elbow should be obtained for all acute injuries; medial and lateral epicondyle fractures or radial head and neck fractures may be better visualized with additional radiographic views. A fracture or dislocation can be obvious or subtle. The radial head should be directed toward the capitellum on all views. Comparison views of the uninjured elbow are helpful with subtle injuries.

With chronic pain, AP and lateral radiographs may be normal or may show fragmentation of the medial epicondyle (Little Leaguer's elbow), or irregularity of the capitellum.

Differential Diagnosis
The differential diagnosis and selected conditions are listed in **Table 1**.

Table 1

Differential Diagnosis for Elbow Pain in Children

Etiology	Condition
Acute Pain	
Traumatic	Dislocation
	Lateral condyle fracture
	Hemarthrosis
	Medial condyle fracture
	Medial epicondyle fracture
	Radial head fracture
	Occult fracture
	Olecranon fracture
	Sprain
	Subluxation of the radial head (nursemaid's elbow)
	Supracondylar humerus fracture
Infectious	
Chronic Pain	
Overuse	Osteochondritis of the capitellum
	Panner disease
	Little Leaguer's elbow
	Traction apophysitis
Neoplastic	

Occult Fractures About the Elbow

A posterior fat pad sign is associated with an occult fracture (80%) in a child. Overlying the distal humerus are anterior and posterior fat pads that are located within the elbow joint capsule. In a normal elbow, the anterior fat pad can be seen on a lateral radiograph, but the posterior fat pad usually is not seen. Any process that causes an elbow effusion will elevate the anterior and posterior fat pads and make both structures visible (**Figures 1** and **2**). In children who have a positive posterior fat pad sign and no evidence of fracture on initial radiographs, the likelihood of an occult bony injury is high. These findings have been confirmed in studies that include repeat AP, lateral, and oblique radiographs obtained 2 to 3 weeks after the injury.

A child with a posterior fat pad sign and no apparent fracture on initial radiographs or signs of septic arthritis should be assumed to have an occult, nondisplaced fracture. A posterior long arm splint or a long arm cast can be applied for 2 to 3 weeks. Bony injuries that demonstrate only a posterior fat pad sign at initial evaluation are usually nondisplaced fractures. If no tenderness is noted at the

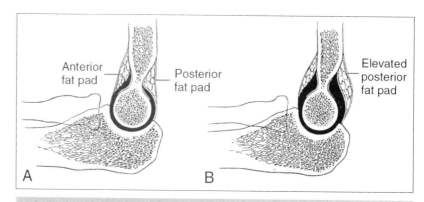

Figure 1 Illustration depicts normal anterior and posterior fat pads (**A**) and those elevated from an effusion (**B**). (Reproduced with permission from Skaggs DL, Mirzayan R: The posterior fat pad sign in association with occult fracture of the elbow in children. *J Bone Joint Surg Am* 1999;81:1429-1433.)

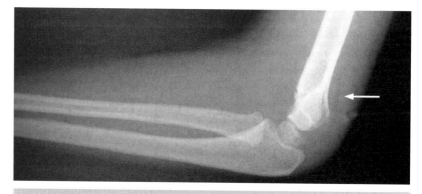

Figure 2 Lateral radiograph of the elbow demonstrates a posterior fat pad sign (arrow).

2- to 3-week evaluation, immobilization can be discontinued. In this situation, no evidence exists that repeat radiographs alter treatment.

Dislocation
Traumatic dislocation of the elbow is much less common in children than adults and is typically posterior. Associated injuries such as fracture of the medial epicondyle or other fractures can occur. A medial epicondyle fracture can be displaced and incarcerated in the joint or can entrap the ulnar nerve. Closed reduction usually is successful.

Sprains
Elbow sprains are uncommon in children because the bone is the weak link. Short-term immobilization is appropriate.

Subluxation of the Radial Head
Also called a "pulled elbow" or "nursemaid's elbow," subluxation of the radial head is the most common elbow injury in children younger than 5 years. This injury is associated with increased ligamentous laxity. The mechanism of injury is pulling on the forearm when the elbow is extended and the forearm is pronated. The annular ligament,

which wraps around the neck of the radius, slips proximally and becomes interposed between the radius and ulna.

Immediately after the injury, the child will react and cry, but the initial pain quickly subsides. Thereafter, the child is reluctant to use the arm but otherwise does not appear to be in great distress. The extremity is held by the side with the elbow slightly flexed and the forearm pronated. Tenderness over the radial head and resistance on attempted supination of the forearm are the only consistent findings. Radiographs are normal. To reduce the subluxation, the examiner's thumb is placed over the radial head and the forearm fully supinated. If this maneuver fails to produce the snap of reduction, then the elbow is flexed. Resistance may be perceived just before reaching full flexion. As the elbow is pushed through that resistance, the annular ligament will slip back into normal position and a snap may be perceived as the radial head reduces. Pronation of the forearm with elbow extension or flexion has been proposed as an alternative reduction strategy. If the reduction is successful, the child will begin to use the extremity normally in a few minutes. The exception is the child who presents 1 to 2 days after injury. At this time, swelling of the annular ligament may both obscure the snap that signals a successful reduction and also prevent immediate resumption of normal function. If the elbow has full flexion and supination, however, the radial head has been reduced. Immobilization may be used but is probably not necessary because parents report that slings are quickly discarded, except when discomfort persists. If reduction attempts are unsuccessful, splinting or casting is appropriate. Repeat evaluation, with radiographs, may reveal an occult fracture, or the child may have normal radiographs and return to full function after immobilization is discontinued. Failure of return of function warrants further investigation.

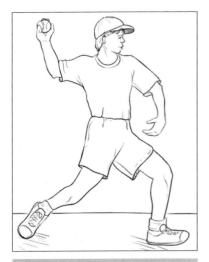

Figure 3 Illustration of the throwing motion. This motion imposes valgus stress on the elbow.

Infection

Infection (septic arthritis) as a cause of acute elbow pain is relatively uncommon; in one study of pediatric infections, the elbow accounted for only 12% of cases of septic arthritis. These conditions, however, should be considered when evaluating a child with elbow pain. The possibility of infection is more likely with an acute onset of pain, no history of injury, and an elevated temperature.

Chronic Pain

Chronic injuries may affect either the medial (tension) or lateral (compression) side of the humerus. Medial injuries can be acute (avulsion fracture of the medial epicondyle) or gradual in onset (traction apophysitis of the medial epicondyle, better known as Little Leaguer's elbow) (**Figure 3**). Lateral involvement is secondary to osteonecrosis of the capitellum. When children younger than 10 years are affected, the condition is called Panner disease and has a good prognosis. Chronic injuries generally are self-limited. Resting the arm, with no throwing for 3 to 6 weeks, is indicated followed by rehabilitation to restore elbow motion and upper extremity strength. Osteonecrosis of the capitellum in adolescents, called osteochondritis

SECTION 9   PEDIATRIC ORTHOPAEDICS

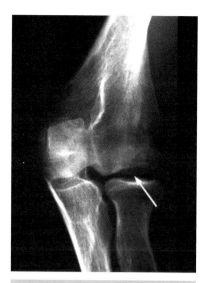

Figure 4 AP radiograph demonstrates radiolucency typical of osteochondritis dissecans of the capitellum (arrow). (Reproduced with permission from Peterson RK, Savoie FH III, Field LD: Osteochondritis dissecans of the elbow. *Instr Course Lect* 1999;48:393-398.)

dissecans, has a more guarded prognosis (**Figure 4**). This condition can result in an osteochondral loose body, which may cause a locking or catching sensation, and is more likely to cause residual symptoms. Surgical treatment should be considered. Surgical removal of loose bodies secondary to osteochondritis dissecans, along with débridement, is indicated if the loose bodies are causing pain and/or intermittent locking of the joint. Tumors, although very uncommon about the elbow in children, are more likely with chronic pain, no history of injury, pain at rest, night pain, and worsening pain.

Referral Decisions/Red Flags

Patients with pain that is constant or increasing, systemic signs or symptoms (fever, other pains), history of trauma, or chronic pain require further evaluation.

Foot and Ankle Pain

Definition
Foot and ankle pain in a child generally is caused by a specific clinical condition; however, trauma, infection, and tumors are other potential causes.

Clinical Symptoms
A history of a substantial injury combined with localized findings may suggest some type of trauma as the cause of pain. Children can sustain numerous minor injuries to the lower extremities and parents might attribute symptoms to a particular injury or episode when, in fact, the actual condition has nothing to do with trauma. Furthermore, injuries in younger children can occur without being observed by parents or others, and young children are typically unable to provide an exact account of how the injury occurred.

Determining whether the problem is acute or chronic provides information about its etiology. A recent onset of symptoms generally is associated with traumatic or infectious conditions.

Questions about systemic symptoms such as malaise, swelling, and fever are important with either acute-onset conditions or chronic symptoms. Fever and swelling are more likely to suggest infectious or possibly malignant conditions.

Tests
Physical Examination
Infections in the foot may be preceded by direct penetrating injuries such as a nail puncture wound. If the incident occurred within the preceding 24 to 72 hours, the diagnosis is most likely a soft-tissue cellulitis or abscess.

Physical examination can localize the area of tenderness to a specific anatomic site and is extremely helpful in determining the correct diagnosis. Ask an older child to point with one finger to the spot that hurts the most; this helps localize the anatomic site and greatly narrows the differential diagnosis.

The foot should be examined for areas of swelling, erythema, or ecchymosis. Whereas ecchymosis is generally a sign of traumatic injury, erythema suggests an inflammatory or infectious process. The ankle and subtalar joints should be evaluated for range of motion and pain with range of motion. Decreased inversion and eversion of the subtalar joint could suggest a tarsal coalition; painful range of motion of the joint can indicate an inflammatory or infectious process. Ligamentous stability should be evaluated as well.

Diagnostic Tests
Radiographs are needed when a fracture or chronic process is suspected. Physical examination will determine whether the problem is in the foot or ankle. If the problem is localized to the foot, AP, lateral, and oblique views of the foot are obtained; if localized to

SECTION 9   PEDIATRIC ORTHOPAEDICS

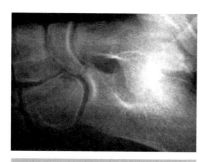

Figure 1 Oblique radiograph demonstrates calcaneonavicular coalition.

the ankle, AP, lateral, and mortise views of the ankle are ordered. If findings on radiographs could be a normal variant, comparison views of the opposite foot can be obtained.

Advanced imaging studies are sometimes necessary. A bone scan can be helpful if a stress fracture or infectious process is suspected. CT is generally best for benign bony lesions; MRI provides better information for soft-tissue lesions and malignant processes.

Differential Diagnosis
Hindfoot
Calcaneal Apophysitis (Sever Disease)
Calcaneal apophysitis is characterized by pain in the posterior aspect of the heel that occurs after activity and most commonly affects active, prepubertal children. Tenderness at the posterior aspect of the calcaneus is common. Radiographs typically are not needed. Short-term activity modification or restriction is indicated. Detailed information about calcaneal apophysitis is provided in the chapter Calcaneal Apophysitis.

Os Trigonum
The os trigonum is an accessory ossicle of the posterior talus that usually is a normal anatomic variant. This secondary center of ossification, however, may become symptomatic in older adolescents and adults, particularly those who participate in ballet or soccer. Patients commonly report posterior ankle pain that is activity related. Pain also develops secondary to posterior impingement of the os trigonum between the talus and tibia during plantar flexion. Relative rest and activity modification may relieve symptoms, although surgical excision may be required for refractory cases.

Osteochondral Lesion of the Talus
This lesion typically affects adolescents, particularly athletes. The pain is exacerbated by activity and is localized to the ankle region. Radiographs of the ankle usually confirm diagnosis, although MRI may be necessary in some cases. Osteochondritis dissecans of the talus may result in ankle pain with activity, swelling, and locking of the ankle joint. Treatment includes immobilization or sometimes surgery, depending on the size, location, and degree of displacement. Detailed information about osteochondral lesions of the talus is provided in the chapter Osteochondral Lesions of the Talus.

Tarsal Coalition
Tarsal coalition is a common cause of rigid flatfeet in children (**Figure 1**). Symptoms typically develop during the second decade of life. The onset of pain generally is insidious but can be associated with an injury or change in activity or perceived as recurrent ankle sprains. Hindfoot motion is markedly restricted, and spasm of the peroneal muscles is elicited by quickly inverting the foot. Talocalcaneal bars are difficult to see on routine radiographs; CT is necessary to confirm the diagnosis. Treatment depends on the presentation of symptoms.

Midfoot
Osteonecrosis of the Navicular

Osteonecrosis of the navicular, also called Köhler disease, primarily affects children (usually boys) 4 to 8 years of age. The patient limps, turns out the foot while walking, and may report pain and prominence in the medial arch. Radiographs show a dense, fragmented, thin navicular (**Figure 2**). A short leg walking cast for 4 to 8 weeks relieves pain, improves walking (less pain), and may speed resolution of the osteonecrosis. The eventual outcome, however, is good whether casting or activity modifications are chosen.

Accessory Navicular

Accessory navicular is an anatomic variant in which a secondary center of ossification forms at the medial aspect of the navicular and may become symptomatic during adolescence. Patients report pain and swelling on the medial side of the foot. Activity or shoe wear can exacerbate the pain. Radiographs may be necessary, depending on the presentation and history of symptoms. Treatment generally is limited to short-term activity restrictions or shoe modifications; however, a walking cast or surgical excision may be necessary.

Forefoot
Freiberg Infraction

Freiberg infraction is osteonecrosis that most commonly involves the head of the second metatarsal, most likely as a result of trauma, and typically affects adolescents. The pain is exacerbated by activity. Examination reveals tenderness under the involved metatarsal head, occasional swelling on the dorsal aspect of the metatarsal head, and pain at the extremes of dorsiflexion and plantar flexion. Radiographs usually show evidence of the condition within 2 to 3 weeks of the onset of symptoms (**Figure 3**). Treatment options include activity modifications, a metatarsal pad, or short-term casting. Occasionally, surgical treatment is required to remove loose bodies or to realign the metatarsal head.

Hallux Valgus

Hallux valgus can develop during adolescence. At this age, most patients are asymptomatic, but some may report pain. Asymptomatic cases are treated with a night brace; otherwise, treatment principles are similar to those for adults. The postoperative recurrence rate for hallux valgus is much higher in juvenile and adolescent patients than in adult patients; this higher recurrence rate should be considered when deciding whether to operate on symptomatic patients.

Other Foot Problems
Enthesitis

Enthesitis (pain and inflammation at a bone-tendon insertion) is uncommon in children. Disorders such as Achilles tendinitis or plantar fasciitis may be the presenting symptoms of a seronegative spondyloarthropathy.

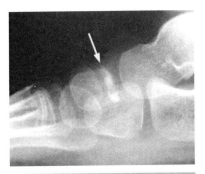

Figure 2 Lateral radiograph of the foot shows a condensed, fragmented navicular (arrow). (Reproduced from Ankle and foot: Pediatric aspects, in Kasser JR, ed: *Orthopaedic Knowledge Update*, ed 5. Rosemont, IL, American Academy of Orthopaedic Surgeons, 1996, pp 503-514.)

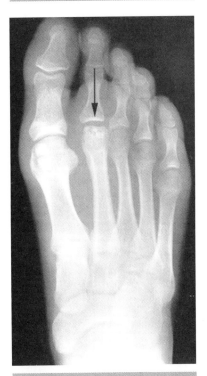

Figure 3 AP radiograph demonstrates Freiberg infraction. Note flattening and fragmentation at the head of the second metatarsal (arrow).

SECTION 9 PEDIATRIC ORTHOPAEDICS

Infection

Infection in the foot commonly is secondary to a direct penetrating injury, such as a nail puncture wound. If symptoms develop within 24 to 72 hours after the injury, cellulitis or abscess may be developing. If swelling and erythema develop several days after the injury, the infection may be the result of osteomyelitis secondary to *Pseudomonas aeruginosa*. Deep bone infection that is recalcitrant to antibiotics alone often must be managed with surgical débridement and intravenous antibiotic therapy.

Sprains, Strains, and Fractures

Sprains, strains, and fractures of the foot and ankle are relatively common. Most of these injuries in children can be managed nonsurgically. In a child who has a history of an inversion injury and tenderness over the distal fibular physis, the most likely diagnosis is a nondisplaced type I fracture of the distal fibular physis. This injury is treated with a walker boot or short leg cast.

Tumors

Tumors in the foot and ankle are uncommon at all ages. The most common benign bone tumor of the foot and ankle in children is a unicameral or aneurysmal bone cyst involving the calcaneus. Osteoid osteoma affecting the tarsal bones also occurs in children. Ewing sarcoma affecting the tarsal bones or diaphysis of metatarsals is the most common malignant bony lesion involving the foot. The pain, swelling, and radiographic findings in Ewing sarcoma can mimic osteomyelitis. Of the malignant soft-tissue lesions, synovial cell sarcoma is the most common in the foot. Typical symptoms include onset during the second decade of life and a slowly enlarging mass.

Growing Pain

Definition

Growing pain is a condition for which no specific diagnosis exists. Typically, the diagnosis is made after more specific pathologic conditions are excluded. Although its true etiology is unknown, growing pain or leg aches are often thought to be the result of overactivity (muscular strain or fatigue). The condition typically occurs in an otherwise healthy, active child. Growing pain is more common in boys, in children with ligamentous laxity, and in 2- to 5-year-old children. Older children, however, also may be affected. The pain or discomfort is commonly localized to the calf but may be perceived in the foot, ankle, knee, or thigh. The problem often is bilateral, but the patients may report that one leg seems to hurt more than the other or that one leg hurts some nights and the other leg hurts other nights.

Clinical Symptoms

Leg pain is described as mild to moderate, intermittent, and more noticeable in the evening or at night or following a day of increased activity or sport. Most children do not limp during the day. Parents report using warm or cold compresses, massage, or simple analgesics to relieve the symptoms. Constitutional symptoms such as fever, weight loss, appetite loss, or malaise are rarely reported.

Tests

Physical Examination

Examination of the affected extremity should focus on identifying any masses, inflammation, lymphadenopathy, abnormal joint movement, instability, muscle group atrophy, or neurologic deficits. With growing pain, the examination is normal in all aspects, although the affected extremity can be tender to deep pressure. Flexible flatfeet may be noted, but the gait and pattern of shoe wear is normal.

Diagnostic Tests

Radiographs should be considered in children who have a higher intensity of pain or more prolonged symptoms, a history of pain at rest that is not relieved by simple analgesics, or an associated abnormal clinical finding. Bone scanning, CT, or MRI is considered if a specific lesion, such as a bone or soft-tissue tumor, stress fracture, bone or joint infection, or tarsal coalition is suspected. Metabolic workup may be needed if the history and review of systems suggest conditions such as leukemia or endocrinopathy.

Differential Diagnosis

- Calcaneal apophysitis (heel pain with activity)
- Köhler disease (unilateral, pain with activity, foot turned out with walking)

SECTION 9 PEDIATRIC ORTHOPAEDICS

- Metabolic/systemic disease (history and review of systems that suggest leukemia, endocrine disorder, renal osteodystrophy, juvenile idiopathic arthritis, rheumatic disease)
- Subacute osteomyelitis (unilateral, activity-related symptoms)
- Trauma (unilateral, toddler's or stress fracture)
- Tumor (unilateral, pain more persistent and severe)

Adverse Outcomes of the Disease

Growing pain has a benign and self-limiting course, although the leg aches may occur intermittently for several months. Permanent long-term impairment has not been noted.

Treatment

An explanation of the natural history and expected outcome, reassurance, muscle stretches, and perhaps a recommendation about the use of simple analgesics usually are sufficient to allay parental fears and to avoid overtreatment. Short-term use of NSAIDs and/or a short period of rest or immobilization before resuming activities, as the level of pain allows, also can be recommended. Surgical treatment is not indicated.

Adverse Outcomes of Treatment

Overuse of pain medication with adverse psychologic and physical effects is possible. Unnecessary testing with its concomitant risk and costs also is possible.

Referral Decisions/Red Flags

Patients with a history of severe, persistent pain along with constitutional symptoms (such as fever, night sweats, malaise, poor appetite, weight loss) require further evaluation. Findings on physical examination that indicate masses, substantial inflammation, lymphadenopathy, circulatory compromise, neuropathy, or myopathy also are a concern. To make a diagnosis of growing pain or leg aches while overlooking the more specific underlying conditions listed in the differential diagnosis is a serious error.

Accessory Navicular

Definition

Accessory navicular is an anatomic variant in which a secondary center of ossification forms in the medial portion of the tarsal navicular bone at the attachment of the tibialis posterior tendon. During adolescence, this secondary center of ossification may become prominent and symptomatic by virtue of its size or as a result of repetitive sprains and microfractures at the attachment of the ossicle to the navicular. Symptoms are more common in girls. The disorder is common; one study observed a 14% incidence of symptoms during adolescence.

Clinical Symptoms

Patients report pain and swelling on the medial side (arch) of the foot. The pain is exacerbated with activity or with pressure from overlying shoes. Severe pain is uncommon.

Tests

Physical Examination

Tenderness and mild swelling over the medial aspect of the navicular (insertion of the tibialis posterior tendon) is typical. Inversion of the foot against resistance may be painful. A flexible pes planus may be present.

Diagnostic Tests

Radiographs are not necessary with a typical examination and mild symptoms. With persistent or severe symptoms, AP, lateral, and oblique radiographs of the foot will document the disorder and exclude other possibilities. The AP and lateral views should be weight-bearing views to best demonstrate pes planus or other alignment problems. The AP view often provides the best profile of the accessory ossicle (**Figure 1**). Some patients have a cornuate navicular (shaped like a horn), resulting from fusion of the accessory ossicle to the navicular.

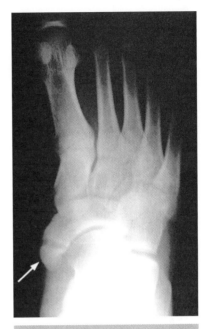

Figure 1 AP radiograph of the foot demonstrates accessory navicular (arrow).

Differential Diagnosis

- Flexible pes planovalgus (developmental or acquired)
- Posterior tibial tendinitis (swelling in the region of the tibialis posterior tendon)
- Tarsal coalition (restricted inversion, eversion of the heel)

Adverse Outcomes of the Disease

Patients may experience persistent pain or a limp.

Treatment

Most patients can be treated with short-term restriction of activities and/or shoe modifications to relieve pressure over the prominent navicular (soft material medial to the bump and/or stretching of the shoe). A short period of time in a walking cast may permit healing of the repetitive microfractures and resolution of symptoms. In most cases, the bump is not large and symptoms resolve with cessation of growth. Excision of the prominent portion of the navicular is the treatment of choice for patients with persistent, disabling symptoms.

Adverse Outcomes of Treatment

Postoperative infection and a tender medial scar that is irritated by shoe wear are both possible.

Referral Decisions/Red Flags

Persistent pain signals the need for further evaluation.

SECTION 9   PEDIATRIC ORTHOPAEDICS

Calcaneal Apophysitis

Synonym
Sever disease

Definition
Calcaneal apophysitis commonly affects active, prepubertal children and is characterized by pain in the posterior aspect of the heel that occurs after activity. This condition is caused by repetitive stress and microtrauma on the calcaneal apophysis. This weak link resolves when the apophysis fuses to the main body of the calcaneus, a process that occurs around 9 years of age in girls and 11 years of age in boys.

Clinical Symptoms
Patients have posterior heel pain and a limp that is activity related.

Tests
Physical Examination
Examination reveals little except tenderness at the posterior aspect of the calcaneus.

Diagnostic Tests
Radiographs are not diagnostic, and sclerosis at the secondary ossification center is common and normal (**Figure 1**). With bilateral involvement and a typical history, radiographs probably are not necessary. With unilateral involvement, a lateral view of the heel is necessary to rule out other problems, such as a bone cyst.

Differential Diagnosis
- Achilles tendinitis (can be associated with Reiter syndrome or other seronegative spondyloarthropathies)
- Infection (unilateral, elevated erythrocyte sedimentation rate, swelling)
- Tumor (unilateral, swelling, night pain)

Adverse Outcomes of the Disease
Pain, a limp, and activity modifications are possible, but there are no long-term sequelae.

Treatment
Treatment includes short-term modification or restriction of the precipitating activity. Shoe modifications that use a ¼″ heel lift or heel cushion and rehabilitation with Achilles tendon stretching can be helpful. Casting is needed only rarely but can be used for 4 to 6 weeks if the pain and limp are recalcitrant. Neither surgery nor steroid injection is indicated.

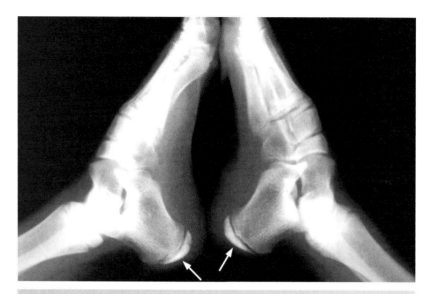

Figure 1 Lateral radiograph of the feet demonstrates irregular calcaneal apophyses (arrows), a normal finding. No radiographic findings exist that are diagnostic for or consistent with calcaneal apophysitis (Sever disease).

Adverse Outcomes of Treatment
There are no long-term sequelae.

Referral Decisions/Red Flags
Suspicion of tumor or osteomyelitis indicates the need for further evaluation. When treatment does not relieve discomfort, additional diagnostic studies are indicated to rule out infection or neoplastic disease.

Cavus Foot Deformity

Synonyms
High-arched foot
Pes cavus

Definition
Pes cavus is the term used to describe an abnormally high arch resulting from plantar flexion (equinus) of the forefoot or midfoot relative to the hindfoot. Cavovarus describes forefoot equinus in association with hindfoot varus (**Figure 1**), and equinocavovarus describes hindfoot equinus associated with hindfoot varus and forefoot equinus.

   Some cases of bilateral cavus or cavovarus feet are familial, but most children with these deformities have an underlying neurologic abnormality or neuromuscular disorder. A progressive unilateral cavus foot often is due to tethering of the spinal cord, and bilateral cavus feet are commonly seen in hereditary motor and sensory neuropathies such as Charcot-Marie-Tooth disease.

Clinical Symptoms
Progressive deformities may be associated with several symptoms, including problems with shoe wear, pain in the region of the metatarsal heads or forefoot (altered weight-bearing stresses) or in the region of the plantar fascia, and frequent ankle sprains. Calluses may develop underneath the prominent metatarsal heads or along the lateral border of the foot.

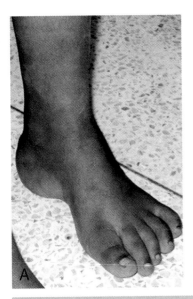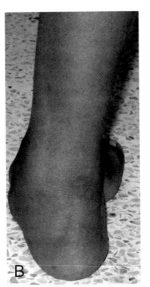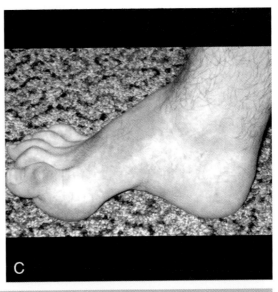

Figure 1 Photographs of cavovarus feet show high arch typical of a cavovarus foot (**A**), the hindfoot tilted into varus (**B**), and clawing of the toes (**C**), which is common.

SECTION 9 PEDIATRIC ORTHOPAEDICS

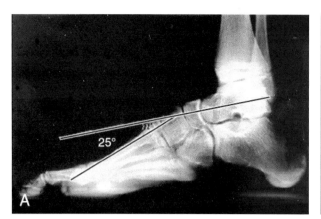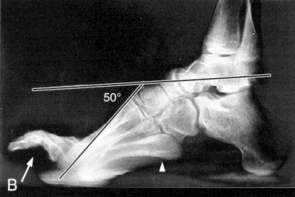

Figure 2 Lateral radiographs of cavus feet. **A,** Foot with a positive (25°) Meary angle caused by cavus foot and associated forefoot equinus. In a normal foot, a line drawn through the long axis of the talus would go through the first metatarsal. **B,** Foot with a more severe deformity (Meary angle = 50°). Note the claw toes (arrow) and the hypertrophy of the cortices of the fifth metatarsal (arrowhead) resulting from excessive lateral forefoot weight bearing.

Tests

History and Physical Examination

The history focuses on any symptoms, whether the changes in foot shape or alignment have been progressive, and whether any associated symptoms exist (back or leg pain, bowel or bladder dysfunction). Family members should be questioned regarding a family history of similar foot deformities or neuromuscular diseases. A thorough neurologic assessment is always required. For the musculoskeletal examination, the lower extremity should be inspected to evaluate the alignment of the ankle, heel, midfoot, and toes, and the plantar aspect of the foot checked for calluses. The spine is examined for curvature, paraspinal spasm, and midline defects such as dimpling or abnormal hairy patches and the upper extremity for weakness and atrophy of the intrinsic muscles of the hand.

Diagnostic Tests

Weight-bearing AP and lateral radiographs of the foot are obtained to evaluate alignment. On the lateral view of an unaffected foot, a line typically passes through the axis of the talus and first metatarsal. With a cavus foot, the first metatarsal is plantarflexed relative to the talus, resulting in an increase in the angle between the axis of the talus and the first metatarsal (the Meary angle) (**Figure 2**). Weight-bearing PA and lateral radiographs of the thoracolumbar spine should be considered; these may reveal abnormal curvatures, congenital anomalies, widening of the interpedicular distance (suggests diastematomyelia), or other abnormalities. Depending on the clinical findings, other diagnostic studies may be required, including electromyography, nerve conduction velocity studies, and MRI of the spine.

Differential Diagnosis
- Clubfoot (incomplete correction)
- Friedreich ataxia (gait abnormalities, autosomal recessive)
- Hereditary motor and sensory neuropathies (Charcot-Marie-Tooth disease) (peripheral neuropathy with abnormal nerve conduction velocity studies, autosomal-dominant is most common)
- Idiopathic (familial, a diagnosis of exclusion)
- Muscular dystrophy (previous diagnosis)
- Myelomeningocele (previous diagnosis)
- Neuromuscular conditions
- Poliomyelitis (previous diagnosis)
- Spinal cord tethering lesions (low-lying conus medullaris, spinal cord tumor, diastematomyelia, lipomyelomeningocele, other intraspinal anomalies)
- Trauma (residua of tendon laceration or fracture)

Adverse Outcomes of the Disease
Cavus deformities are often progressive and interfere with shoe wear and ambulation.

Treatment
Underlying neurologic or spinal cord pathology requires evaluation and possible surgical treatment (for example, release of a tethered spinal cord). The treatment of a cavus or cavovarus foot is based on the severity and flexibility of the deformity, as well as whether the deformity is expected to worsen (on the basis of the underlying diagnosis). Mild and flexible deformities can be accommodated by shoe modifications and arch supports, and rehabilitation can help with strengthening muscles and maintaining range of motion. An ankle-foot orthosis may be required to control the hindfoot and maintain ambulation. Surgical treatment is offered when these measures fail to accommodate the deformity and the symptoms are unacceptable to the patient. Various procedures, alone or in combination, may be required to restore range of motion and foot alignment, as well as muscle balance. These include soft-tissue releases (plantar fascia), tendon transfers (tibialis posterior and/or extensor hallucis longus), and osteotomies (medial cuneiform or first metatarsal, calcaneus) to realign the forefoot and often the hindfoot. A hindfoot fusion (triple arthrodesis) is reserved as a salvage procedure for rigid deformities in older patients.

Adverse Outcomes of Treatment
Most of these deformities occur in patients with progressive neuromuscular diseases, so recurrence or gradual progression of the foot deformity often is encountered even after surgical treatment. Additional treatment measures (surgery and/or bracing) may be required to maximize ambulatory potential. If a triple arthrodesis

SECTION 9 · PEDIATRIC ORTHOPAEDICS

was required to achieve correction, increased stresses at the ankle and midfoot joints may result in degenerative changes in ambulatory patients.

Referral Decisions/Red Flags

All patients with cavus feet should be referred for further evaluation.

Child Abuse

Synonyms
Nonaccidental trauma
Shaken baby syndrome

Definition
Approximately 3 million reports of child abuse are filed annually in the United States, and approximately 1,500 children die every year as a result of abuse or neglect. Most cases of abuse involve children younger than 3 years. Firstborn children, premature infants, stepchildren, and handicapped children are at a greater risk. Failure to recognize injuries of child abuse results in a child being returned to the environment, with a 25% risk of serious reinjury and a 5% risk of death.

A critical factor in identifying child abuse is to accurately determine whether the history given by the family adequately explains the child's injuries. Soft-tissue injuries such as bruises, burns, or scars are seen in most patients. It is normal for toddlers to have bruises over the chin, the brow, elbows, knees, and shins, but bruises on the back of the head, buttocks, abdomen, legs, arms, cheeks, or genitalia are suspicious for abuse. Fractures are common in child abuse cases, and these children are more likely to have additional injuries, including abdominal injury resulting from blunt trauma.

The Investigative Interview
The guiding principle for the conduct of the interview is to remain objective while calmly and methodically questioning family members. A single physical finding is seldom conclusive for a diagnosis of child abuse; additional injuries and risk factors in the home must be identified. Other guidelines for the investigative interview are listed in **Table 1**.

When obtaining the social history, unusual stresses on the family should be inquired about, such as recent loss of a job, separation or divorce, death in the family, housing problems, or inadequate funds for food. Alcohol abuse in the home is a risk factor for child abuse, and maternal cocaine use increases the risk of abuse fivefold.

If family members later change their account of how the injury occurred or any other aspect of the history, the original account should not be altered, but the revision dated and recorded as an addendum to the record.

Tests
Physical Examination
A head-to-toe physical examination of the child is conducted for any suspicious soft-tissue injuries. A thorough examination is important because in many cases of confirmed abuse, evidence of prior abuse will be identified. Any suspicious soft-tissue injuries should be

Table 1

Guidelines for Conducting an Investigative Interview

Interview individual family members in private.

Be attentive and nonjudgmental, and avoid leading questions during the history.

Carefully document the given history of injury verbatim, as well as its source.

Establish a scenario for the injury from each witness, noting carefully any inconsistencies.

Identify the person primarily responsible for feeding and disciplining the child.

Identify all family members and other individuals who have access to the child.

Identify individuals outside the family who have been with the child without family supervision.

Assess for risk factors: boyfriends, stepparents, babysitters, and even older siblings, as these individuals are often abusers.

Note any delay in seeking medical attention for injuries.

noted in detail. The face, spine, and upper and lower extremities are palpated for tenderness that suggests fracture and the abdomen examined for swelling and tenderness. Physical signs of sexual assault such as bruising or chafing of the genitalia are inspected for. Physical findings of sexual abuse may be subtle. A pediatric physician specializing in child abuse/sexual abuse may best be able to examine the child at this time.

Diagnostic Tests

If the child's mental status is abnormal, subdural hematoma and retinal hemorrhage secondary to violent shaking should be evaluated for. Bleeding studies are checked when bruising is evident and a toxicology screening ordered if there is a history of substance abuse or a mental status change in the family. CT of the abdomen is indicated if the head-to-toe examination shows abdominal tenderness or if liver function test levels are elevated.

AP and lateral radiographs of all long bones, the hands, the feet, the spine, and the chest, as well as a skull series, are standard for children age 2 years and younger. This examination is referred to as a skeletal survey. Clinically guided radiography is used in the examination of older children. A single radiograph, or so-called baby gram, does not provide adequate detail and may miss subtle fractures. No fracture pattern predominates in child abuse, but certain fractures are more suspicious for child abuse than others. Fractures considered highly specific for child abuse include posterior rib fractures, scapular fractures, fractures of the posterior process of the spine, and fractures of the sternum. Also, one type of fracture highly specific for child abuse is the "corner" or "chip" fracture of the metaphysis of long bones that avulses the edge of the metaphysis from the epiphysis as a

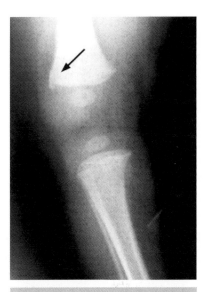

Figure 1 AP radiograph of the distal femur with a "corner" or "chip" fracture (arrow).

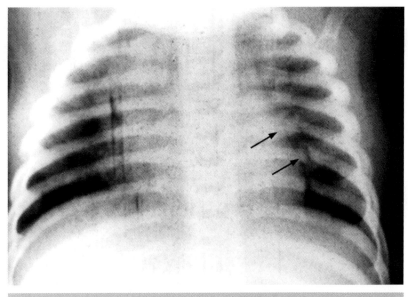

Figure 2 AP radiograph demonstrates rib fractures at various stages of healing (arrows).

result of downward traction or pull on the extremity (**Figure 1**). Other fracture patterns are more common but also occur frequently in accidental injuries. Inconsistency with the mechanism described by the caregiver should increase suspicion. Spiral fractures are caused by rotational injury, and transverse or oblique fractures are caused by a direct blow. Rib fractures also are common and, when healed, may appear only as fusiform thickening of the ribs. A bone scan can help detect rib fractures, but it may not show skull fractures or long-bone fractures near the epiphyseal growth plates.

Fractures considered moderately specific for abuse include multiple, especially bilateral, fractures; fractures of different ages; epiphyseal separations; vertebral body fractures; fractures of the fingers; and complex skull fractures. Multiple fractures at various stages of healing without explanation strongly suggest child abuse (**Figure 2**). In children of walking age, spiral fractures of the tibia and femur are much more likely to be the result of an accident than physical abuse.

The age of a fracture can be estimated by radiographic appearance. From 7 to 14 days after the injury, new periosteal bone and callus formation can be seen; from 14 to 21 days after the initial injury, loss of the definition of the fracture line and maturation of the callus with trabecular formation are evident. Callus that is more dense is seen 21 to 42 days after injury. As the bone remodels to a more normal status, fractures older than 6 weeks are distinguished by subtle fusiform sclerotic thickening that is best seen when compared with a normal contralateral bone.

It is important to avoid misdiagnosis of child abuse. Spiral fractures of the tibia, the so-called toddler's fracture, can occur in children 1 to 3 years of age as a result of a relatively trivial fall. Spontaneous

SECTION 9 PEDIATRIC ORTHOPAEDICS

fractures can occur with diseases such as osteogenesis imperfecta. The presence of osteopenia, a family history of osteogenesis imperfecta, as well as the presence of blue sclera would suggest this disease. Buckle fractures are rarely the result of abuse. Typically, they occur as the result of simple falls. Buckle fractures may present late because of the minimal associated pain, swelling, and dysfunction, which to many parents seems to be indicative of a minor injury. Pathologic fractures also are associated with osteomyelitis, benign and malignant tumors, rickets, neuromuscular disease, and other metabolic diseases.

Final Diagnosis

After pathologic fractures are excluded, the examiner must determine whether the child's fracture has been caused by accidental trauma or by inflicted trauma. Accidental trauma can be diagnosed when an acute injury is brought promptly to medical attention, has a plausible mechanism of injury, and lacks other risk factors for child abuse. Suspicious injuries must be reported as child abuse; the reporting physician does not need to prove abuse—just reasonable suspicion.

Reporting Child Abuse

In the United States, any physician who reports suspected child abuse in good faith is protected from both civil and criminal liability. Failure to report suspected child abuse exposes the physician to liability. Sexual abuse is a criminal offense and must be reported. Eliciting help from the hospital's child protection team is appropriate. In addition to making notes in the medical record, the physician may be asked to complete a notarized affidavit summarizing findings in the abuse case and stating that the child may be at risk for injury or loss of life if returned to the home environment. The child may then be removed from the home by the courts and placed elsewhere until an investigation is completed. The physician must be prepared to explain his or her findings in custodial hearings if the family challenges the actions of child protective services.

Clubfoot

Synonyms

Congenital clubfoot
Talipes equinovarus

Definition

Clubfoot, or talipes equinovarus, is a congenital deformity of the foot/ankle characterized by four clinical components: midfoot cavus (high arch), forefoot adduction, heel varus (adduction of calcaneus), and ankle equinus (plantar flexion) (or CAVE) (**Figure 1**).

Many theories exist about the etiology of clubfoot, but none has been proved correct. Most cases are idiopathic and occur in an otherwise healthy infant. A true idiopathic clubfoot is not fully correctable by passive manipulation. A positional clubfoot deformity may occur as a result of intrauterine molding. A positional clubfoot can be distinguished by inherent flexibility of the deformity, either spontaneous resolution or a rapid response to treatment, and the absence of calf atrophy or a difference in foot size. Clubfoot may be observed in association with various neuromuscular diseases such as myelomeningocele or arthrogryposis, as well as many syndromes (for example, congenital constriction band syndrome, diastrophic dysplasia). These secondary clubfeet tend to be more rigid and difficult to treat, as well as more susceptible to recurrence following initial treatment.

The incidence of clubfoot worldwide is approximately 1 in 1,000 live births; it is twice as common in boys as in girls. If a family has one child with clubfoot, the risk in subsequent siblings is 3% to 4%. If one parent and one child in a family have clubfoot, the risk in subsequent children is 25%.

Clinical Symptoms

In infancy, clubfoot is a visible deformity that is not associated with symptoms or physical limitations. Ambulatory patients with an

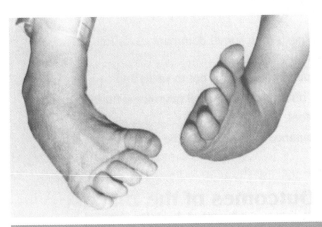
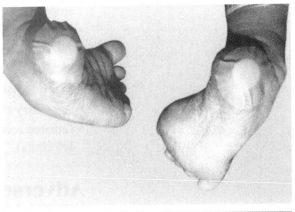

Figure 1 Photographs show bilateral congenital clubfoot in a newborn.

untreated clubfoot, or with recurrent or residual deformities, often have moderate to severe gait disturbance, have difficulties wearing standard shoes, and occasionally have pain.

Tests

Physical Examination

A comprehensive physical examination is required to rule out neuromuscular disorders or syndromes (nonidiopathic clubfoot). The extremities should be examined to rule out any contractures or deformities and to assess neuromuscular function. Assessment of motor function by observation or stimulation also is important because congenital absence of the anterior compartment muscles has been associated with clubfoot in rare instances. The spine should be examined for cutaneous manifestations of an underlying intraspinal anomaly. Abnormal neurologic findings also can indicate a spinal cord disorder such as tethering due to lipomyelomeningocele, diastematomyelia, or other cause. The foot examination should focus on characterizing the specific deformities (midfoot cavus, forefoot adduction, hindfoot varus, hindfoot equinus) and grading their rigidity or severity.

Diagnostic Tests

Radiographs are not usually required in infants with idiopathic clubfoot. Weight-bearing AP and lateral radiographs of the foot may be required in older children with recurrent or residual deformities following treatment, or with a neglected or untreated clubfoot. An MRI of the spine may be required to rule out intraspinal pathology. Rarely, electromyography and nerve conduction velocity studies may be needed in the diagnostic evaluation.

Differential Diagnosis

- Acquired equinovarus deformity
- Arthrogryposis (stiffness and weakness of multiple joints of the upper and/or lower extremities)
- Congenital constriction band syndrome (partial or circumferential bands of indented skin and underlying tissue, intrauterine amputations)
- Distal arthrogryposis (autosomal dominant condition, stiffness of the hands and feet)
- Metatarsus adductus (hindfoot is not in varus and equinus)
- Neuromuscular imbalance (abnormal neurologic findings)
- Secondary clubfoot
- Tethered cord (cutaneous lesions over the spine, recurrent deformity)

Adverse Outcomes of the Disease

Untreated clubfoot causes a substantial disability (**Figure 2**). Not only are walking and shoe wear severely impaired, possible

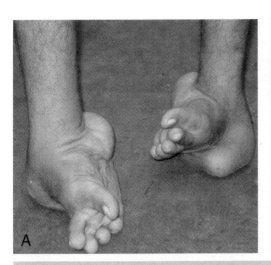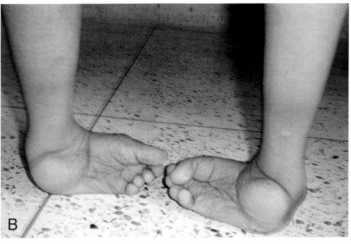

Figure 2 Anterior (**A**) and posterior (**B**) photographs of clubfoot in an older patient.

long-term consequences include pain and degenerative joint disease. The sociocultural implications are perhaps the greatest source of disability; in some societies, patients with a clubfoot are ostracized and thought to be "cursed." Even with adequate treatment, the affected foot will be smaller and less mobile than a normal foot. Calf atrophy is a normal finding in congenital clubfoot and will persist despite adequate treatment of the deformity. The difference is not as obvious with bilateral involvement but is readily apparent with unilateral involvement. The foot on the affected side is typically one half to a whole shoe size smaller than the unaffected foot.

Treatment

A recent paradigm shift has occurred in the treatment of clubfoot. Previously, most patients underwent extensive surgical release to achieve correction. Long-term studies have suggested that these extensive releases are complicated by stiffness and pain. The Ponseti method, which is minimally invasive, has become the treatment of choice in most centers in North America and in many others throughout the world. The initial phase involves serial casting with long leg casts using a specific technique and deformity correction that addresses the four clinical components of clubfoot represented by the CAVE mnemonic. All components except hindfoot equinus are typically corrected after four to seven casts; most patients require a percutaneous release of the Achilles tendon to treat the rigid hindfoot equinus. The tendon regenerates after 3 weeks in an infant, and there is no increased risk of Achilles tendon rupture later in life. After casting is completed, patients wear a foot abduction brace full time for 3 months, and then at night for 3 years. Recurrence of deformity can occur in approximately 30% of patients, is most common within the first 2 to 3 years of life, and is very rare after 5 to 7 years of age. Most recurrences can be treated using the same method, although some patients with a dynamic supination (foot inverts during swing phase of gait) from tibialis anterior overactivity will require a lateral transfer of the tibialis anterior tendon. Approximately 95%

PEDIATRIC ORTHOPAEDICS

SECTION 9

of infants with a clubfoot can be treated with this method, avoiding the need for an extensive surgical release. Older patients with a clubfoot are commonly seen in societies with underdeveloped health infrastructure, and it appears that the Ponseti method may be of benefit in children up to 8 years of age. Older patients and those with recurrent or persistent deformities may require other surgical interventions such as soft-tissue release, osteotomies, or triple arthrodesis.

Adverse Outcomes of Treatment

Continuing with serial casting in the setting of rigid hindfoot equinus can result in spurious correction of the equinus through the midfoot or transverse tarsal joints, creating a rocker-bottom foot (convex sole, flatfoot). Worsening of the deformity occurs when improper casting technique is used or with failure to modify technique in the case of a complex clubfoot. Recurrent or residual deformities may require additional evaluation and treatment. Complications of the more extensive soft-tissue release and/or osteotomies or fusions include undercorrection, overcorrection, muscle weakness (especially during push-off), joint stiffness and/or arthritis, and gait disturbance.

Referral Decisions/Red Flags

Patients with a clubfoot will require referral to an orthopaedic surgeon and also may require evaluations by other specialists (such as in neurology, genetics), depending on the history and physical examination findings.

Complex Regional Pain Syndrome

Synonyms

Causalgia
CRPS
Reflex sympathetic dystrophy
RSD

Definition

Complex regional pain syndrome (CRPS) describes a constellation of signs and symptoms of a dysfunctional, debilitating pain syndrome that is not anatomic in distribution and is disproportionate to the inciting injury. CRPS is classified as either type I (reflex sympathetic dystrophy [RSD]) or type II (causalgia). Type I CRPS is a pain syndrome that principally involves the extremities and is associated with varied degrees of autonomic dysfunction. Type I CRPS is more common in children and adolescents, particularly in children between 9 and 15 years of age. The diagnosis often is delayed because of the confusing clinical presentation of musculoskeletal, neurologic, and inflammatory symptoms.

Clinical Symptoms

An older child or adolescent with type I CRPS commonly presents after a minor injury or contusion. Signs and symptoms typically include excessive pain and hypersensitivity to light touch, cold intolerance, transient swelling, and skin discoloration in the extremity (most commonly the foot and ankle). Weight bearing, joint range of motion, and limb mobility may be severely restricted by pain, weakness, and joint stiffness.

Tests

Physical Examination

Type I CRPS is a diagnosis of exclusion. Early in the disease, the physical examination can be confusing and may delay the diagnosis. The patient may be unable to bear weight on an affected lower extremity or may refuse to move an affected upper extremity. Localized soft-tissue edema and skin hyperemia are visible. Active range of motion is limited, and attempts at passive range of motion elicit severe pain. Minor sensory stimuli, such as brushing against bedsheets, cause severe burning pain in a localized but nonanatomic distribution.

Diagnostic Tests

Radiographs, three-phase bone scans, and MRIs, along with laboratory studies such as erythrocyte sedimentation rate, C-reactive protein level, and other hematologic tests are most useful to eliminate the common differential diagnoses. In the early stages of type I CRPS, routine study results are within normal limits. Tests specific for type I CRPS such as thermography, cold testing, and sympathetic blockade (the preferred method) can help confirm the diagnosis in equivocal cases. In patients with long-standing symptoms, radiographs reveal limb osteopenia, and MRIs show edema of soft tissues and bones.

Differential Diagnosis
- Contusion (joint swelling, pain with motion)
- Inflammatory synovitis (joint swelling, pain with motion)
- Ligament sprain (history of trauma)
- Musculoskeletal infection (swelling, fever, constant pain that is increasing)
- Neoplasm (constant pain, night pain)
- Occult fracture (history of trauma)
- Spinal pathology (back pain)
- Tendinitis (history of repetitive activities, pain after activity)

Adverse Outcomes of the Disease
Long-term signs and symptoms are associated with dystrophic changes such as muscle wasting, joint contracture, thickening of the nails, and the appearance of coarse hair on the extremities. The most serious complications are chronic pain, limb dystrophy, and rare permanent limb dysfunction. Most patients, however, recover fully if diagnosed early and treated appropriately.

Treatment
Rehabilitation is the mainstay of treatment. Frequent sessions that focus on desensitization, joint mobility, and weight bearing can help to restore function within 4 to 6 weeks. Low doses of antidepressants (commonly amitriptyline) or anticonvulsants (commonly gabapentin) are effective in diminishing symptoms and facilitating rehabilitation in patients who initially are unresponsive to rehabilitation. Narcotics and other pain medications are best used under careful supervision in the earliest stages of type I CRPS and have a limited long-term role in children.

Paravertebral sympathetic chain blockade by selective injection or epidural infusion is necessary only if other treatment regimens fail. A specialized team approach to pain management enhances outcomes.

Adverse Outcomes of Treatment
Inability to resolve the pain ultimately can result in severe disability, including loss of limb function.

Referral Decisions/Red Flags
Early diagnosis and referral to a multidisciplinary pain team are most likely to result in complete resolution of the pain complex.

SECTION 9   PEDIATRIC ORTHOPAEDICS

Concussion

Definition

Participation in recreation and organized sports results in more than 2 million medically treated musculoskeletal injuries in children annually. The number of sports-related concussions in the United States has risen substantially over the past decade. This number may even be underestimated because many concussions go unreported. Concussions are included in the spectrum of closed head injuries but are not associated with substantial gross neuroanatomic disruptions. They are subdivided by severity, depending on whether any loss of consciousness, amnesia, or associated neurologic sequelae occur. Contact sports are associated with the highest risk for head injuries. Most concussions do not involve any loss of consciousness; however, confusion and/or posttraumatic amnesia are more common.

Clinical Symptoms and Patient Evaluation

Several classification systems define the degrees of cerebral concussions. The Cantu guidelines were published in 1986 and updated in 2001. Grade I is a closed head injury with no associated loss of consciousness and less than 30 minutes of posttraumatic amnesia. Grade II is a closed head injury in which a player loses consciousness for less than 5 minutes or experiences amnesia lasting from 30 minutes to 24 hours. Grade III is a closed head injury that includes loss of consciousness lasting longer than 5 minutes or amnesia lasting longer than 24 hours. Because of some inconsistencies identified in the use of the Cantu guidelines, the Acute Concussion Evaluation (ACE) system has been adopted for use by many on-field physicians (**Figure 1**).

Treatment

An athlete with a grade I (mild) concussion according to the Cantu classification may return to play after being asymptomatic for 1 week. Any subsequent grade I concussion necessitates the player be symptom free for 1 week and removed from play for at least 2 weeks. A CT scan should be obtained to rule out intracranial pathology. Termination of play should be strongly considered in the player who sustains three concussions in one playing season.

If an athlete sustains a Cantu grade II (moderate) concussion, he or she is removed from play for 2 weeks, with at least 1 week of that time symptom free. After the occurrence of a second moderate concussion, a head CT scan is warranted. If the CT scan is normal, the athlete may return to play after 1 month if he or she has been symptom free for at least 1 week of that time. An athlete who sustains a third moderate concussion should not return to play for the remainder of the season, and permanent restrictions from contact sports should be strongly considered.

ACUTE CONCUSSION EVALUATION (ACE)
PHYSICIAN/CLINICIAN OFFICE VERSION

Gerard Gioia, PhD[1] & Micky Collins, PhD[2]
[1]Children's National Medical Center
[2]University of Pittsburgh Medical Center

Patient Name:_____
DOB: _____ Age:_____
Date:_____ ID/MR#_____

A. Injury Characteristics   Date/Time of Injury_____   Reporter: __Patient __Parent __Spouse __Other_____

1. Injury Description _____
_____

1a. Is there evidence of a forcible blow to the head (direct or indirect)?   __Yes __No __Unknown
1b. Is there evidence of intracranial injury or skull fracture?   __Yes __No __Unknown
1c. Location of Impact: __Frontal __Lft Temporal __Rt Temporal __Lft Parietal __Rt Parietal __Occipital __Neck __Indirect Force
2. **Cause:** __MVC __Pedestrian-MVC __Fall __Assault __Sports (specify)_____Other_____
3. **Amnesia Before (Retrograde)** Are there any events just BEFORE the injury that you/ person has no memory of (even brief)?   __ Yes __No Duration
4. **Amnesia After (Anterograde)** Are there any events just AFTER the injury that you/ person has no memory of (even brief)?   __ Yes __No Duration
5. **Loss of Consciousness:** Did you/ person lose consciousness?   __ Yes __No Duration
6. **EARLY SIGNS:** __Appears dazed or stunned __Is confused about events __Answers questions slowly __Repeats Questions __Forgetful (recent info)
7. **Seizures:** Were seizures observed? No__ Yes__ Detail_____

B. Symptom Check List* Since the injury, has the person experienced any of these symptoms any more than usual today or in the past day?
Indicate presence of each symptom (0=No, 1=Yes).   *Lovell & Collins, 1998 JHTR

PHYSICAL (10)			COGNITIVE (4)			SLEEP (4)		
Headache	0	1	Feeling mentally foggy	0	1	Drowsiness	0 1	
Nausea	0	1	Feeling slowed down	0	1	Sleeping less than usual	0 1	N/A
Vomiting	0	1	Difficulty concentrating	0	1	Sleeping more than usual	0 1	N/A
Balance problems	0	1	Difficulty remembering	0	1	Trouble falling asleep	0 1	N/A
Dizziness	0	1	COGNITIVE Total (0-4) ___			SLEEP Total (0-4) ___		
Visual problems	0	1	EMOTIONAL (4)					
Fatigue	0	1	Irritability	0	1	**Exertion:** Do these symptoms worsen with:		
Sensitivity to light	0	1	Sadness	0	1	Physical Activity __Yes __No __N/A		
Sensitivity to noise	0	1	More emotional	0	1	Cognitive Activity __Yes __No __N/A		
Numbness/Tingling	0	1	Nervousness	0	1	**Overall Rating:** How different is the person acting compared to his/her usual self? (circle)		
PHYSICAL Total (0-10) ___			EMOTIONAL Total (0-4) ___			Normal 0 1 2 3 4 5 6 Very Different		
(Add Physical, Cognitive, Emotion, Sleep totals) Total Symptom Score (0-22) ___								

C. Risk Factors for Protracted Recovery (check all that apply)

Concussion History? Y ___ N___	√	Headache History? Y ___ N___	√	Developmental History	√	Psychiatric History	√
Previous # 1 2 3 4 5 6+		Prior treatment for headache		Learning disabilities		Anxiety	
Longest symptom duration Days__ Weeks__ Months__ Years__		History of migraine headache __ Personal __ Family		Attention-Deficit/ Hyperactivity Disorder		Depression	
						Sleep disorder	
If multiple concussions, less force caused reinjury? Yes__ No__		_____		Other developmental disorder_____		Other psychiatric disorder _____	

List other comorbid medical disorders or medication usage (e.g., hypothyroid, seizures)_____

D. RED FLAGS for acute emergency management: Refer to the emergency department with sudden onset of any of the following:
* Headaches that worsen   * Looks very drowsy/ can't be awakened   * Can't recognize people or places   * Neck pain
* Seizures   * Repeated vomiting   * Increasing confusion or irritability * Unusual behavioral change
* Focal neurologic signs   * Slurred speech   * Weakness or numbness in arms/legs   * Change in state of consciousness

E. Diagnosis (ICD): __Concussion w/o LOC 850.0 __Concussion w/ LOC 850.1 __Concussion (Unspecified) 850.9 __Other (854) _____
__No diagnosis

F. Follow-Up Action Plan   Complete ACE Care Plan and provide copy to patient/family.
___ No Follow-Up Needed
___ Physician/Clinician Office Monitoring: Date of next follow-up _____
___ Referral:
      ___ Neuropsychological Testing
      ___ Physician: Neurosurgery___ Neurology___ Sports Medicine___ Physiatrist___ Psychiatrist___ Other_____
      ___ Emergency Department

ACE Completed by:_____   © Copyright G. Gioia & M. Collins, 2006

This form is part of the "Heads Up: Brain Injury in Your Practice" tool kit developed by the Centers for Disease Control and Prevention (CDC).

Figure 1 Acute Concussion Evaluation form for use by on-field physicians in evaluating patients with suspected concussion. (Reproduced with permission from Centers for Disease Control and Prevention: Acute Concussion Evaluation [ACE]: *Heads Up: Brain Injury in Your Practice.* Available at: http://www.cdc.gov/concussion/headsup/pdf/ACE-a.pdf. Accessed July 14, 2015.)

SECTION 9 PEDIATRIC ORTHOPAEDICS

A concussion (or mild traumatic brain injury (MTBI)) is a complex pathophysiologic process affecting the brain, induced by traumatic biomechanical forces secondary to direct or indirect forces to the head. Disturbance of brain function is related to neurometabolic dysfunction, rather than structural injury, and is typically associated with normal structural neuroimaging findings (i.e., CT scan, MRI). Concussion may or may not involve a loss of consciousness (LOC). Concussion results in a constellation of physical, cognitive, emotional, and sleep-related symptoms. Symptoms may last from several minutes to days, weeks, months or even longer in some cases.

ACE Instructions

The ACE is intended to provide an evidence-based clinical protocol to conduct an initial evaluation and diagnosis of patients (both children and adults) with known or suspected MTBI. The research evidence documenting the importance of these components in the evaluation of an MTBI is provided in the reference list.

A. Injury Characteristics:

1. Obtain **description of the injury** – how injury occurred, type of force, location on the head or body (if force transmitted to head). Different biomechanics of injury may result in differential symptom patterns (e.g., occipital blow may result in visual changes, balance difficulties).
2. Indicate the **cause of injury**. Greater forces associated with the trauma are likely to result in more severe presentation of symptoms.
3/4. **Amnesia:** Amnesia is defined as the failure to form new memories. Determine whether amnesia has occurred and attempt to determine length of time of memory dysfunction – <u>before</u> (retrograde) and <u>after</u> (anterograde) injury. Even seconds to minutes of memory loss can be predictive of outcome. Recent research has indicated that amnesia may be up to 4-10 times more predictive of symptoms and cognitive deficits following concussion than is LOC (less than 1 minute).[1]
5. **Loss of consciousness (LOC)** – If occurs, determine length of LOC.
6. **Early signs.** If present, ask the individuals who know the patient (parent, spouse, friend, etc) about specific signs of the concussion that may have been observed. These signs are typically observed early after the injury.
7. Inquire whether **seizures** were observed or not.

B. Symptom Checklist: [2]

1. Ask patient (and/or parent, if child) to report presence of the four categories of symptoms since injury. It is important to assess all listed symptoms as different parts of the brain control different functions. One or all symptoms may be present depending upon mechanisms of injury.[3] Record "1" for Yes or "0" for No for their presence or absence, respectively.
2. For all symptoms, indicate presence of symptoms as experienced within the past 24 hours. Since symptoms can be present premorbidly/at baseline (e.g., inattention, headaches, sleep, sadness), it is important to assess <u>change</u> from their usual presentation.
3. **Scoring**: Sum total <u>number</u> of symptoms present per area, and sum all four areas into Total Symptom Score (score range 0-22). (Note: most sleep symptoms are only applicable after a night has passed since the injury. Drowsiness may be present on the day of injury.) If symptoms are new and present, there is no lower limit symptom score. Any <u>score > 0</u> indicates <u>positive symptom</u> history.
4. **Exertion:** Inquire whether any symptoms worsen with physical (e.g., running, climbing stairs, bike riding) and/or cognitive (e.g., academic studies, multi-tasking at work, reading or other tasks requiring focused concentration) exertion. Clinicians should be aware that symptoms will typically worsen or re-emerge with exertion, indicating incomplete recovery. Over-exertion may protract recovery.
5. **Overall Rating:** Determine how different the person is acting from their usual self. Circle "0" (Normal) to "6" (Very Different).

C. Risk Factors for Protracted Recovery: Assess the following risk factors as possible complicating factors in the recovery process.

1. **Concussion history:** Assess the number and date(s) of prior concussions, the duration of symptoms for each injury, and whether less biomechanical force resulted in re-injury. Research indicates that cognitive and symptom effects of concussion may be cumulative, especially if there is minimal duration of time between injuries and less biomechanical force results in subsequent concussion (which may indicate incomplete recovery from initial trauma).[4-8]
2. **Headache history:** Assess personal and/or family history of diagnosis/treatment for headaches. Research indicates headache (migraine in particular) can result in protracted recovery from concussion.[8-11]
3. **Developmental history:** Assess history of learning disabilities, Attention-Deficit/Hyperactivity Disorder or other developmental disorders. Research indicates that there is the possibility of a longer period of recovery with these conditions.[12]
4. **Psychiatric history:** Assess for history of depression/mood disorder, anxiety, and/or sleep disorder.[13-16]

D. Red Flags: The patient should be carefully observed over the first 24-48 hours for these serious signs. Red flags are to be assessed as <u>possible signs of deteriorating neurological functioning</u>. Any positive report should prompt strong consideration of referral for emergency medical evaluation (e.g. CT Scan to rule out intracranial bleed or other structural pathology).[17]

E. Diagnosis: The following ICD diagnostic codes may be applicable.

850.0 (Concussion, with no loss of consciousness) – Positive injury description with evidence of forcible direct/ indirect blow to the head (A1a); plus evidence of active symptoms (B) of any type and number related to the trauma (Total Symptom Score >0); no evidence of LOC (A5), skull fracture or intracranial injury (A1b).

850.1 (Concussion, with brief loss of consciousness < 1 hour) – Positive injury description with evidence of forcible direct/ indirect blow to the head (A1a); plus evidence of active symptoms (B) of any type and number related to the trauma (Total Symptom Score >0); positive evidence of LOC (A5), skull fracture or intracranial injury (A1b).

850.9 (Concussion, unspecified) – Positive injury description with evidence of forcible direct/ indirect blow to the head (A1a); plus evidence of active symptoms (B) of any type and number related to the trauma (Total Symptom Score >0); unclear/unknown injury details; unclear evidence of LOC (A5), no skull fracture or intracranial injury.

Other Diagnoses – If the patient presents with a positive injury description and associated symptoms, but additional evidence of intracranial injury (A 1b) such as from neuroimaging, a moderate TBI and the diagnostic category of 854 (Intracranial injury) should be considered.

F. Follow-Up Action Plan: Develop a follow-up plan of action for symptomatic patients. The physician/clinician may decide to (1) monitor the patient in the office or (2) refer them to a specialist. Serial evaluation of the concussion is critical as symptoms may resolve, worsen, or ebb and flow depending upon many factors (e.g., cognitive/physical exertion, comorbidities). Referral to a specialist can be particularly valuable to help manage certain aspects of the patient's condition. (Physician/Clinician should also complete the ACE Care Plan included in this tool kit.)

1. **Physician/Clinician serial monitoring** – Particularly appropriate if number and severity of symptoms are steadily decreasing over time and/or fully resolve within 3-5 days. If steady reduction is not evident, referral to a specialist is warranted.
2. **Referral to a specialist** – Appropriate if symptom reduction is not evident in 3-5 days, or sooner if symptom profile is concerning in type/severity.
   - <u>Neuropsychological Testing</u> can provide valuable information to help assess a patient's brain function and impairment and assist with treatment planning, such as return to play decisions.
   - <u>Physician Evaluation</u> is particularly relevant for medical evaluation and management of concussion. It is also critical for evaluating and managing focal neurologic, sensory, vestibular, and motor concerns. It may be useful for medication management (e.g., headaches, sleep disturbance, depression) if post-concussive problems persist.

Figure 1 (continued) Acute Concussion Evaluation form for use by on-field physicians in evaluating patients with suspected concussion. (Reproduced with permission from Centers for Disease Control and Prevention: Acute Concussion Evaluation [ACE]: *Heads Up: Brain Injury in Your Practice*. Available at: http://www.cdc.gov/concussion/headsup/pdf/ACE-a.pdf. Accessed July 14, 2015.)

When an athlete sustains a Cantu grade III (severe) concussion, he or she should undergo head CT and be restricted from play for a minimum of 1 month. The second severe concussion mandates termination for the season and results in strong consideration for no return to contact sports. Athletes with a severe closed head injury generally should not return to play. Although uncommon, death can result from second-impact syndrome without an initial loss of consciousness. For these reasons, the physician on the field must closely evaluate all athletes with head injuries and should be familiar with accepted return-to-play guidelines.

Referral Decisions/Red Flags

Even mild concussions can result in persistent postconcussion symptoms and cognitive deficits for up to 6 months after the initial injury. The athlete should be monitored and reevaluated for postconcussion signs and symptoms, which can include headache, confusion, nausea, vomiting, memory impairment, and disorientation. Other symptoms can be more related to mood, such as emotional lability, irritability, sensitivity to noise, depression, poor concentration, poor attention span, anxiety, and trouble with sleep. Return to play is contraindicated in athletes until neuropsychologic test results are normal.

Many closed head injuries can be prevented if safety guidelines and protective equipment are used. Parents consider their child's coaches and physician an important source of safety education.

Congenital Deficiencies of the Lower Extremity

Conditions

Longitudinal deficiency of the fibula (partial or complete) (fibular hemimelia)
Tibial deficiency (tibial hemimelia)
Longitudinal deficiency of the femur, partial (proximal focal femoral deficiency [PFFD])

Definition

Congenital deficiencies of the lower extremity are usually obvious at birth, and their appearance can be alarming to parents. Support and counseling provided by the physician can be critical while the parents are attempting to understand their child's condition. Treatment decisions are based on two issues: whether the foot is functional (or can be salvaged), and what the anticipated limb-length discrepancy will be at skeletal maturity. A search for anomalies in other organ systems also is required in some cases. With limb-length discrepancy, the degree of growth inhibition is constant, and although the discrepancy remains proportional, the absolute difference in limb lengths increases as the child grows. Considerable variability exists in the degree of growth inhibition. Whereas some children can be treated with a simple shoe lift or an epiphysiodesis, others will require one or more limb lengthening procedures. Patients in whom a large discrepancy is predicted will be best served by early amputation and prosthetic fitting. In these cases, it should be emphasized to the parents that their child can lead an active life with a prosthesis. Recent improvements in techniques for lower extremity reconstruction have made limb salvage a more viable option for more patients.

Early referral to a specialist is important because families need to understand the pros and cons of all treatment options. Although surgical treatment usually is not performed until the child is at least 9 to 12 months of age, formulating a comprehensive treatment plan takes time. Providing the parents with an opportunity to meet other affected children at a more advanced stage of growth and development is reassuring.

Longitudinal Deficiency of the Fibula

Fibular deficiency, sometimes called fibular hemimelia or congenital absence of the fibula, is a sporadic disorder of unknown etiology. Fibular deficiency is the most common long-bone deficiency (**Figure 1**). All patients require treatment of a limb-length discrepancy, but the magnitude of the projected discrepancy is quite varied.

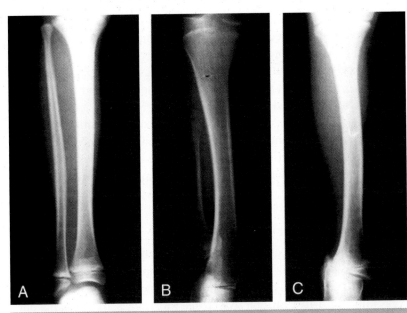

Figure 1 AP radiographs demonstrate three types of fibular deficiency using the Kalamchi classification. **A,** Type IA: minimal shortening of the fibula with a ball-and-socket ankle. **B,** Type IB: only partial fibula present. **C,** Type II: complete absence of the fibula.

Longitudinal deficiency of the fibula can be viewed as a "postaxial hypoplasia" because abnormalities may be noted along the lateral aspect of the limb. Coexisting problems include a common association with femoral deficiencies (congenital short femur with PFFD), patellar dysplasia, genu valgum due to hypoplasia of the lateral condyle of the femur, absent cruciate ligaments in the knee, partial or complete absence of the fibula, anteromedial bowing of the tibia, absence of the lateral rays of the foot, tarsal coalitions, and valgus alignment of the hindfoot. Attention often is focused on the degree of fibular involvement, but the morphology of the fibula does not necessarily correlate with the degree of growth inhibition or the amount of foot deformity and the associated clinical findings must be factored into the treatment plan.

The goal of treatment is a normal gait with an active lifestyle. In general, a foot with more than three rays is thought to be suitable for salvage, and in some cases, surgical soft-tissue release or other measures are required to achieve a plantigrade foot. The magnitude of limb-length discrepancy at skeletal maturity must be estimated. With a relatively small anticipated discrepancy and a functional foot (or one suitable for reconstruction), the treatment focuses on achieving a plantigrade foot and treating the limb-length discrepancy with a shoe lift and/or an epiphysiodesis (or a single limb lengthening). When the anticipated discrepancy is extremely large and/or the foot cannot be reconstructed, an early Syme disarticulation (occurring at the level of the ankle) or Boyd amputation (through the foot, but preserving part of the calcaneus) and prosthetic fitting are considered. The decision making is less straightforward for patients in whom the anticipated

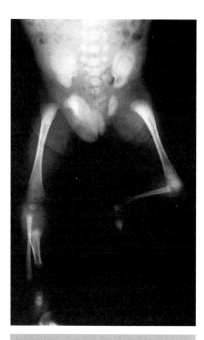

Figure 2 AP radiograph of an infant with bilateral tibial deficiency. The patient's right lower limb has incomplete absence of the tibia; the left tibia is completely absent.

discrepancy would require more than a single lengthening. Multiple factors must be weighed in the decision making: for example, the provision of a single straightforward procedure during infancy (amputation) versus multiple limb lengthenings and surgical procedures throughout the years of growth and development. With newer technologies and increased experience with limb lengthenings for severe discrepancies, limb salvage has become an option for more patients. A patient should not undergo multiple procedures to maintain a nonfunctional foot and equalize a large limb-length discrepancy, only to realize the leg must be amputated during adolescence.

Tibial Deficiency

Tibial deficiency, also called tibial hemimelia or congenital absence of the tibia, is characterized by partial or complete absence of the tibia (**Figure 2**). This is a rare, more severe anomaly, affecting approximately 1 in 1 million live births. Most cases are sporadic, but both autosomal dominant and autosomal recessive forms have been identified in a limited number of patients. Other disorders that may be associated with tibial deficiency include congenital heart disease, cleft palate, imperforate anus, hypospadias, hernias, and gonadal malformations. Hand anomalies can be seen in up to one third of patients.

In contrast to fibular deficiencies, which have coexisting abnormalities on the lateral side of the limb (postaxial), tibial deficiencies may be viewed as a preaxial hypoplasia, with involvement on the medial side of the limb. Femoral hypoplasia may be observed, as well as patellar dysplasia and absent cruciate ligaments. The fibula is bowed, and often a dislocation at the proximal tibiofibular joint exists with proximal migration of the fibula. The foot commonly has an equinovarus deformity, with absent medial rays, and tarsal coalition. The ankle joint is absent, and the distal fibula forms a rudimentary articulation with the lateral portion of the talus and/or calcaneus.

Involvement of the medial aspect of the foot commonly manifests as talipes equinovarus (clubfoot) and the absence of medial rays. Ironically, tibial deficiency also can be associated with polydactyly. Shortening of the involved limb is present and, with unilateral involvement, the anticipated discrepancy is typically large (8 to 16 cm). Knee flexion contracture exists when the tibia is totally absent or if the quadriceps is deficient, and the fibula may appear as a bony projection lateral to the lateral femoral condyle.

Treatment recommendations vary. In patients with complete absence of the tibia, the absence of both a knee and an ankle joint is associated with severe knee flexion contracture and absent quadriceps function, the anticipated limb-length discrepancy and the coexisting foot deformity are severe. These patients are treated at an early age with through-the-knee disarticulation and prosthetic fitting. In many cases, when a proximal tibia is present, the quadriceps muscle is functional and no knee flexion contracture exists. The proximal tibia anlage may not be ossified at birth, and an ultrasonogram or MRI may be required to evaluate the proximal tibial anatomy. The presence of quadriceps function and the absence of a fixed knee flexion contracture suggest that a proximal tibia is present. In such cases, the main concerns include absence of a stable knee and ankle, foot deformity, and a large projected limb-length discrepancy. Most of these patients undergo an early Syme disarticulation followed by a creation of a surgical synostosis between the proximal tibia and fibula to enhance prosthetic fit and wear.

Longitudinal Deficiency of the Femur

Longitudinal deficiency of the femur encompasses a spectrum of congenital abnormalities of the femur. PFFD is a sporadic condition of unknown etiology characterized by dysgenesis of the proximal femur with shortening of the femoral shaft. The incidence is between 1 in 50,000 and 1 in 200,000 live births; approximately 15% of cases are bilateral. The limb assumes a characteristic position with shortening of the femoral segment, and the thigh is flexed, abducted, and externally rotated. Shortening of the femur is marked, and the limb-length discrepancy at skeletal maturity ranges from 7 to 25 cm. Associated abnormalities occur in approximately 50% of patients and include hip dysplasia, hypoplasia of the lateral femoral condyle, absent cruciate ligaments, and longitudinal deficiency of the fibula. Associated deficiencies in other organ systems, including cleft palate and congenital heart defects, are less common.

Various classifications have been proposed, but none has been universally accepted. The Aitken classification describes the spectrum of plain radiographic findings, but it does not treat soft-tissue abnormalities, and it is less useful for treatment planning. The Aitken classification has four subtypes: type A (femoral head present but delay in ossification; subtrochanteric defect, which later ossifies), type B (femoral head and acetabulum present, subtrochanteric defect with discontinuity between the femoral head and shaft), type C (absent femoral head with short tapered femoral shaft, no acetabulum), and type D (absent proximal femoral shaft, small residual distal femur, no acetabulum).

The treatment is individualized, and a host of options are available depending on the anticipated limb-length discrepancy and the status of the hip and knee. Reconstruction procedures can include femoral osteotomy and bone grafting of the pseudarthrosis, soft-tissue rebalancing, and multiple femoral lengthenings. In cases that are not amenable to reconstruction, options include fitting with a custom prosthesis, knee fusion and Syme disarticulation (fit with a knee disarticulation prosthesis), and a Van Ness rotationplasty. In the Van Ness procedure, the knee is fused and the limb is rotated 180° so that the ankle is facing backward. The ankle joint then functions as the knee joint, and the patient can be fitted with a transtibial prosthesis. This procedure is rarely performed and is currently considered to be socially unacceptable.

Referral Decisions/Red Flags

All children with absence of toes or an obviously short limb should receive early consultation with an orthopaedic surgeon and appropriate additional testing for associated disorders.

SECTION 9   PEDIATRIC ORTHOPAEDICS

Congenital Deficiencies of the Upper Extremity

Conditions
Hypoplasia/absence of the thumb
Radial deficiency
Transverse deficiency of the forearm
Ulnar deficiency

Definition
Congenital deficiencies of the upper extremity may be either longitudinal (affecting one side of the extremity) or complete transverse deficiencies. A clinical evaluation is appropriate because some patients will have abnormalities in other organ systems. Deficiency of the thumb, radial deficiency, ulnar deficiency, and transverse deficiencies of the forearm are the most common. As a general principle, reconstructive surgery usually is not performed before the infant is 6 to 18 months of age; however, selected procedures may be required earlier. Early evaluation by a specialist helps allay anxiety of the parents and grandparents. Early consultation also allows time for parents to gain an understanding and develop realistic expectations of the anticipated function and appearance after surgical treatment. Some disorders will not benefit from surgical treatment, but early discussion concerning the principles of prosthetic management will be helpful.

Hypoplasia/Absence of the Thumb
The extent of the thumb deficiency varies. A hypoplastic thumb can be small, unstable, or thin because of deficient development of the thenar musculature. Other disorders are common, including congenital heart disease (Holt-Oram syndrome), craniofacial abnormalities, and vertebral anomalies (vertebral anomalies, anorectal atresia, tracheoesophageal fistula, and renal and vascular anomalies [VATER] association). Fanconi anemia also can develop in later childhood. Patients with untreated thumb deficiency adapt by using the pinch function between the index and long fingers to substitute for the deficient thumb. Patients with unilateral involvement generally have excellent overall function with minimal impairment.

Surgical management is based on the magnitude of the deficiency. Reconstruction is indicated when the hypoplastic thumb is of adequate size and the carpometacarpal joint is stable. Index pollicization (transfer of the index finger to the thumb position, leaving the hand with three fingers) is recommended for more severe deformities.

SECTION 9 PEDIATRIC ORTHOPAEDICS

Radial Deficiency

Radial deficiency, sometimes called radial hemimelia or radial clubhand, is characterized by radial deviation of the hand, variable presence and stiffness of the thumb and the index and long fingers, variable shortening and bowing of the forearm segment, and variable range of motion at the elbow. Associated disorders include congenital heart disease (Holt-Oram syndrome), craniofacial abnormalities, and vertebral anomalies (VATER association). Thrombocytopenia with absent radius (TAR) syndrome also is possible. The unique aspect of TAR syndrome is the presence of an essentially normal thumb. In other syndromes, the thumb is hypoplastic or absent.

Surgical management is designed to improve the alignment and appearance of the hand relative to the forearm. A centralization procedure ideally is performed between 6 and 18 months of age. Untreated patients can function surprisingly well. Surgical treatment, therefore, is contraindicated in patients with short forearms and/or limited elbow motion. These patients do better if the hand remains closer to the midline (for example, radially deviated).

Ulnar Deficiency

Ulnar deficiencies include various disorders involving either a partial or complete absence of skeletal and soft-tissue elements on the ulnar (postaxial) border of the forearm and hand. Conditions range from ulnar hypoplasia, in which the ulna is present but short, to total aplasia of the ulna, which may be associated with congenital fusion of the radius to the humerus (radiohumeral synostosis). Digital deficiencies are common and variable.

Unlike radial and thumb deficiencies, ulnar deficiencies are not associated with anomalies of other organ systems. Patients with ulnar deficiencies, however, are more likely to have disorders elsewhere in the skeletal system, including tibial deficiency and partial longitudinal deficiency of the femur (proximal focal femoral deficiency).

Surgical treatment is not commonly indicated for ulnar deficiency, except for associated digital deformities. Syndactyly release, web space reconstruction, and other procedures, when indicated, can improve hand function.

Transverse Deficiency of the Forearm

Transverse deficiency of the forearm, sometimes called congenital below-elbow deficiency, is characterized by complete absence of the hand and wrist and a hypoplastic or partially absent forearm. Elbow function is good, even if the radial head is dislocated. This disorder is sporadic, typically unilateral, and generally not associated with abnormalities in other organ systems, although patients may have congenital constriction band syndrome and other musculoskeletal anomalies.

Children with unilateral transverse deficiency of the forearm have minimal functional limitations. Bimanual activities are often performed using the medial aspect of the affected forearm to assist the opposite, uninvolved extremity (**Figure 1**). The principal deficit is cosmetic, which is particularly troublesome during the teenage years.

Surgical treatment is rarely necessary. Primitive digital remnants, if present, occasionally are removed to improve cosmetic acceptability. Prosthetic management is of great interest to families of infants with this condition. The best time to introduce the prosthesis is controversial, although many centers favor an aggressive "fit when they sit" protocol. This approach is based on the developmental principle that normal bimanual activities begin when an infant is able to sit independently, at approximately age 6 to 8 months. Other experts recognize that a prosthesis often impedes an infant's ability to crawl and favor the first fitting after an infant is able to stand and walk independently.

Prosthetic options include the standard body-powered design, consisting of a shoulder harness and a hook terminal device; a myoelectric design, consisting of a mechanical hand that is opened and closed by voluntary forearm muscle activity; and a passive design, consisting of a lightweight, durable, cosmetically appealing, nonmovable hand. The optimal design is based on several factors and is best determined on an individual basis.

The principal benefit of prosthetic management is cosmetic, which may be more important to the parents than the child before the teenage years. Function is not consistently improved by any of the prosthetic designs, resulting in a high rate of prosthetic rejection.

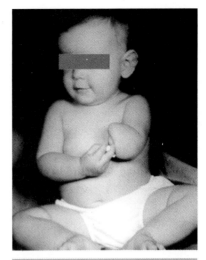

Figure 1 Photograph shows an infant with unilateral transverse deficiency of the forearm using the affected limb to assist the uninvolved extremity.

Congenital Deformities of the Lower Extremity

Conditions

Coxa vara
Congenital dislocation (hyperextension deformity) of the knee
Congenital dislocation of the patella
Posteromedial bowing of the tibia
Anterolateral bowing of the tibia
Calcaneovalgus foot
Congenital vertical talus
Congenital short first metatarsal
Congenital curly toe
Polydactyly

Definition

Congenital deformities of the lower extremity are present at birth and either may be truly congenital or may result from intrauterine molding. Some disorders, such as congenital dislocation of the patella, may not be apparent until the child is older.

Clinical Symptoms

Most of these conditions are noticed on examination of the infant, although symptoms such as pain, gait disturbance, or difficulties with shoe wear may develop during infancy and early childhood.

Tests

Physical Examination

Deviations from normal should evoke suspicion, although a range for normal exists. The lower extremities of a newborn have been compressed in the uterus, and a hip flexion contracture of 40° to 60° and a knee flexion contracture of 20° to 30° are normal in newborns. Similarly, in utero, the ankles and feet are pressed into a dorsiflexed position; therefore, calcaneovalgus posture of the foot is normal.

Disproportionate shortening of the upper and lower extremities or spine suggests a generalized skeletal dysplasia. Other organ systems should be evaluated to rule out other genetic and chromosomal disorders.

Diagnostic Tests

AP and lateral radiographs of the affected extremity are standard.

Coxa Vara

Coxa vara is a relatively uncommon hip disorder characterized by a decrease in the neck-shaft angle of the femur (**Figure 1**). Coxa vara can be congenital, acquired, and developmental. Congenital coxa vara is associated with a congenital short femur and proximal femoral

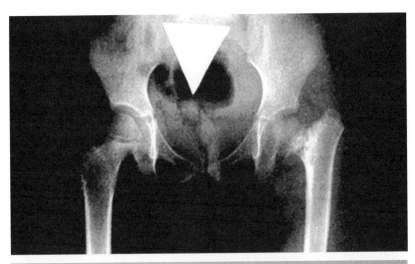

Figure 1 AP pelvic radiograph demonstrates congenital coxa vara in a 5-year-old child. (Reproduced from Hip, pelvis, and femur: Pediatric aspects, in Kasser JR, ed: *Orthopaedic Knowledge Update*, ed 5. Rosemont, IL, American Academy of Orthopaedic Surgeons, 1996, p 353.)

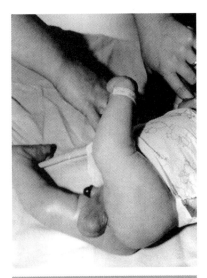

Figure 2 Photograph of a newborn with bilateral congenital dislocation of the knees. The patient also had associated bilateral dislocated hips and a left clubfoot.

focal deficiency. Acquired coxa vara is secondary to metabolic or traumatic conditions. Developmental coxa vara is an idiopathic condition that appears in early childhood. The diagnosis of congenital coxa vara often is made in infancy based on asymmetry in the lower extremities. Both acquired and developmental coxa vara present with gait disturbance in toddlers and young children. The bony deformity alters the mechanics of the hip and causes abductor muscle weakness, a Trendelenburg gait, and a limb-length discrepancy (unilateral disease). Untreated, the deformity and gait abnormality will progress. A realignment osteotomy can improve hip function and gait.

Congenital Dislocation of the Knee

Congenital dislocation, which results from intrauterine positioning, presents as a knee hyperextension deformity at birth. The spectrum of severity ranges from a mild positional deformity that responds readily to short-term splinting to a frank hyperextension/dislocation of the tibia on the femur that requires serial casting, and occasionally, open surgical reduction (**Figure 2**). Associated abnormalities such as hip dysplasia are common, and early ultrasonography should be considered even when the hip examination is considered normal.

Congenital Dislocation of the Patella

Congenital dislocation of the patella may not be apparent for several months after birth. Persistent flexion contracture of the knee and external rotation of the leg suggest this diagnosis. The patella may not be palpable in its dislocated lateral position. Ultrasonography helps confirm the diagnosis in a younger child whose patella has not started to ossify. Surgical treatment is necessary and involves releasing the tight lateral structures around the knee and essentially derotating the

PEDIATRIC ORTHOPAEDICS

SECTION 9

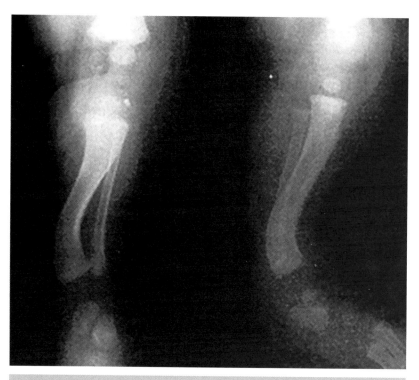

Figure 3 AP radiograph from an infant with congenital posteromedial bowing of the tibia. (Reproduced from Knee and leg: Pediatric aspects, in Kasser JR, ed: *Orthopaedic Knowledge Update*, ed 5. Rosemont, IL, American Academy of Orthopaedic Surgeons, 1996, p 441.)

quadriceps mechanisms; the insertion of the patellar tendon often is quite lateral and must be surgically relocated.

Posteromedial Bowing of the Tibia

Posteromedial bowing of the tibia is an idiopathic deformity that is most obvious and rather striking at birth (**Figure 3**) and is commonly associated with a calcaneovalgus foot, which often lies along the lateral aspect of the distal tibia. The calcaneovalgus foot often resolves spontaneously, but stretching and occasional splinting may be required. Posteromedial bowing of the tibia improves during growth and development, and a small subset of patients may require an osteotomy in late childhood or early adolescence if the deformity does not resolve. The major problem associated with posteromedial bowing is limb-length discrepancy, and almost all patients will require some form of treatment. Because the mean discrepancy is approximately 4 cm at skeletal maturity, most patients will require either a shoe lift or an epiphysiodesis.

Anterolateral Bowing of the Tibia

Anterolateral bowing of the tibia (**Figure 4**) is usually apparent during infancy and requires immediate referral to a specialist. A limited number of cases resolve spontaneously, but most represent a "prepseudarthrosis" of the tibia. A congenital pseudarthrosis of the tibia is extremely difficult to treat and often is associated

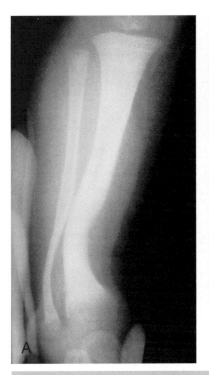
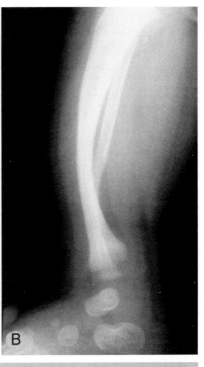

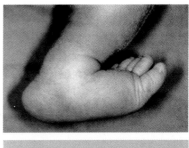

Figure 5 Photograph of a calcaneovalgus foot in a neonate.

Figure 4 AP (**A**) and lateral (**B**) radiographs demonstrate anterolateral bowing of the tibia.

with neurofibromatosis (genetically inherited disorders that cause tumors to grow in the nervous system), which must be ruled out. A clamshell orthosis is initially recommended in an attempt to prevent a fracture, and, although controversial, some authors recommend a prophylactic bypass graft for a prepseudarthrosis of the tibia. An established pseudarthrosis typically requires multiple surgical procedures to attempt to achieve union. Various surgical strategies have been successful in achieving union, including resection of the pseudarthrosis with bone grafting, intramedullary rodding, external fixation, and vascularized fibular bone grafting. Refracture is common, however, and multiple interventions are often required throughout childhood and adolescence. Even if union is achieved, patients usually require long-term bracing to prevent refracture. Some patients will elect to undergo amputation after multiple attempts to achieve union, often because of foot and ankle dysfunction.

Calcaneovalgus Foot

Calcaneovalgus foot is a common newborn positional abnormality or deformation characterized by marked dorsiflexion of the ankle and eversion of the foot, where the foot may be pressed against the tibia (**Figure 5**). Most cases resolve spontaneously, although stretching and/or several serial casts may be required in some patients. Rarely, this deformity results from deficient activity of the plantar flexors from an underlying neurologic disorder such as a lipomyelomeningocele.

SECTION 9 PEDIATRIC ORTHOPAEDICS

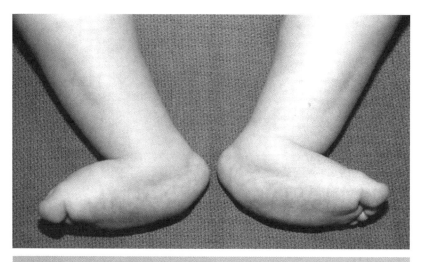

Figure 6 Photograph of the feet of a 9-month-old infant with bilateral congenital vertical talus. (Reproduced from Ankle and foot: Pediatric aspects, in Kasser JR, ed: *Orthopaedic Knowledge Update*, ed 5. Rosemont, IL, American Academy of Orthopaedic Surgeons, 1996, p 507.)

Congenital Vertical Talus

Congenital vertical talus is rare and appears as a flatfoot with a convex sole (rocker-bottom or "Persian slipper" foot), which is diagnosed shortly after birth or in infancy. The deformity is commonly rigid, and it does not resolve spontaneously (**Figure 6**). The condition may be idiopathic or familial, but most cases are associated with a neuromuscular disease or a genetic syndrome. In addition to prompt referral to an orthopaedic surgeon, referral to a neurologist and/or geneticist should be considered. The deformity is typically rigid and represents a dorsal dislocation of the medial column of the foot at the talonavicular joint, or of the entire midfoot on the hindfoot. A lateral radiograph of the foot obtained in maximum plantar flexion is diagnostic and determines whether the midfoot dislocation can be reduced. Because of the rigidity of the deformity, most patients require an extensive soft-tissue release for reduction. A new technique has been reported (the reverse Ponseti) that involves serial casting, followed by percutaneous release of the Achilles tendon. This method may reduce the need for more extensive surgical releases.

Congenital Short First Metatarsal

With congenital short first metatarsal, shortening of the great toe is obvious and often is associated with hallux varus or medial deviation of the great toe. Surgical treatment is warranted if problems with shoe wear develop. A short first metatarsal also can be seen in fibrodysplasia ossificans progressiva, a rare condition associated with progressive and diffuse ossification within various soft tissues.

Congenital Curly Toe

Congenital curly toe is an idiopathic condition characterized by flexion and medial rotation of the toe, often under the adjacent toe. Most children are asymptomatic. Strapping is ineffective. If problems develop with shoe wear, surgical treatment of the toe flexors often is successful.

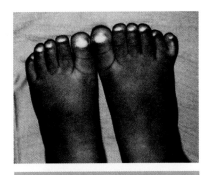

Figure 7 Photograph of the feet of a child with postaxial polydactyly of the right foot.

Polydactyly

Extra digits may be observed at the medial (preaxial polydactyly or duplication of the great toe) or the lateral (postaxial polydactyly) borders of the foot. In addition to cosmetic concerns, difficulties with shoe wear can occur (**Figure 7**). Extra digits should not be "tied off" in the newborn nursery. Surgical removal is best performed at around 10 months of age, before the child begins to walk. In some patients, soft-tissue reconstruction also may be required. An early consultation often helps the parents understand the rationale for the treatment, including the timing of surgery.

Referral Decisions/Red Flags

Calcaneovalgus foot and congenital vertical talus may look similar, but the rocker bottom and inability to plantarflex the foot, as well as lack of improvement over the first month of life, differentiates congenital vertical talus and should prompt referral to an orthopaedic surgeon for treatment.

SECTION 9 PEDIATRIC ORTHOPAEDICS

Congenital Deformities of the Upper Extremity

Conditions
Congenital dislocation of the radial head
Congenital radioulnar synostosis
Polydactyly
Syndactyly ("webbing")

Definition
Congenital deformities are, by definition, present at birth. Syndactyly and polydactyly are obvious; however, congenital dislocation of the radial head and congenital radioulnar synostosis usually are not identified until the child is 3 to 10 years of age.

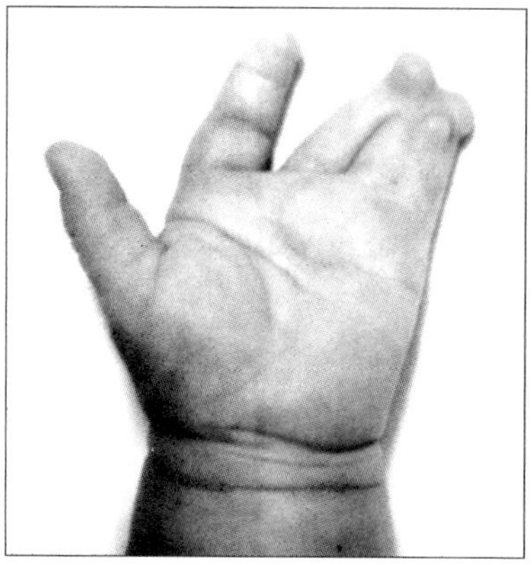

Syndactyly
Syndactyly is a condition characterized by the lack of normal separation between fingers or toes and occurs in approximately 1 in 200 live births (**Figure 1**). It can vary from simple syndactyly, in which only a skin bridge exists, to complex syndactyly, in which a bony fusion (synostosis) is located between the phalanges. The syndactyly is either complete (fingers joined to the tips) or incomplete. Other malformations occur in approximately 5% of patients, and a positive family history exists in 10% to 40% of cases. Syndactyly is associated with Apert syndrome and Poland syndrome in some cases.

Because the fingers differ in length, growth may cause progressive deviation of the conjoined fingers, especially the border digits (in which case earlier surgery is considered). Use of the digits is limited, and cosmesis is an issue for patients. Therefore, children with hand syndactyly should be assessed for surgical treatment. In most cases, a skin graft will be needed. Correction of syndactyly of the toes often is not required other than for cosmetic reasons.

Polydactyly
Polydactyly is the presence of extra digits in the hand or foot, usually adjacent to the thumb or great toe (preaxial) or lateral to the little finger (postaxial) (**Figure 2**). Extra digits can vary in appearance from a vestigial digit attached by a narrow bridge of skin to a normal-appearing digit with its own metacarpal/metatarsal. Radiographs usually are not needed for diagnostic purposes, only for prognosis and planning surgical treatment.

Polydactyly of the hand may not cause functional difficulties, but it is a substantial cosmetic deformity. Accessory digits of the foot frequently cause difficulty in shoe wear. Vestigial digits should not be ablated by application of a circumferential suture at the base of the skin bridge shortly after birth, but rather by formal excision. Removal

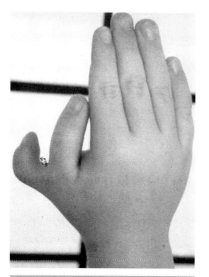

Figure 1 Photograph of the hand of a child with complex syndactyly of the ulnar three fingers. Note how the long finger is pulled toward the shorter ring and little fingers.

Figure 2 Photograph of the hand of a child with polydactyly expressed as a duplicated thumb.

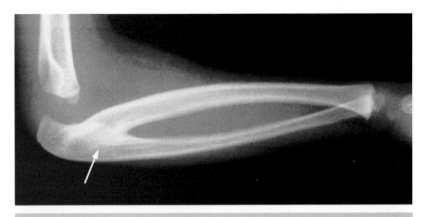

Figure 3 Lateral radiograph demonstrates radioulnar synostosis. Fusion of the proximal radius and ulna is apparent (arrow).

of extra digits is typically delayed until the child is at least 6 months old. Early consultation often helps the parents understand the treatment. Surgical deletion can be performed earlier if the extra digit interferes with function or if the parents have substantial concerns.

Congenital Radioulnar Synostosis

In congenital radioulnar synostosis, the proximal ends of the radius and ulna do not separate, resulting in an inability to pronate and supinate the forearm. Children substitute shoulder motion to place the hand in a pronated or supinated position. When the condition is unilateral, fewer symptoms occur because the normal opposite extremity can be used for many activities. This abnormality often is not detected until children are old enough to start using their hands in a purposeful manner.

Limited pronation and supination of the forearm can be readily detected, even during examination of the newborn. Because many young children have lax wrist ligaments, the distal end of the radius and ulna, not the hand, should be grasped and gently pronated and supinated to assess forearm rotation.

After ossification occurs, bony union of the proximal radius and ulna can be seen on radiographs (**Figure 3**).

No treatment is needed if the forearm is in a satisfactory position. Patients with bilateral involvement are more likely to have functional limitations. Surgery to divide the synostosis and restore motion has not been successful in most series. Surgical treatment usually is reserved for patients with disability secondary to a forearm positioned in either extreme pronation or supination. Osteotomy to realign the forearm can improve function. This procedure usually is not performed until the child is at least 4 years old and may be delayed until the adolescent or adult years if the degree of disability is questionable.

SECTION 9 PEDIATRIC ORTHOPAEDICS

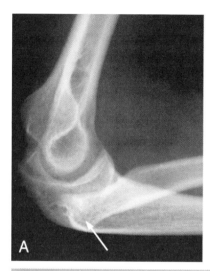
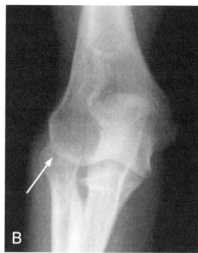

Figure 4 Radiographs demonstrate congenital dislocation of the radial head. **A,** The lateral view demonstrates that the radial head is dislocated posteriorly and does not articulate with the humerus (arrow). **B,** The AP view demonstrates that the normal concavity of the radial head is lost and is replaced by a convexity (arrow).

Congenital Dislocation of the Radial Head

Congenital dislocation of the radial head can occur in several directions but most commonly develops posteriorly; typically, it is bilateral. Elbow deformity and limited motion are the presenting symptoms, but these may not be noticed by the parents for several years. Occasionally, the child reports pain. The abnormality may also be discovered incidentally on radiographs following an injury; it is often mistaken for an acute radial head dislocation.

Examination reveals that elbow motion is limited. Rotation often is more limited than flexion and extension. The dislocated radial head often presents as a palpable prominence on the lateral side of the elbow.

Radiographs of the elbow demonstrate the dislocation (**Figure 4**) The radial head is dome-shaped (convex) instead of having a normal concave appearance, differentiating it from a traumatic radial head dislocation.

The deformity and limited elbow motion associated with this condition are often well tolerated. Attempts at open reduction in young children have had little success. Excision of the radial head, preferably after most growth is completed, can be considered for pain relief but usually does not improve motion.

Referral Decisions/Red Flags

Limitations in pronation or supination of the forearm should prompt radiographic evaluation and referral to an orthopaedic surgeon.

Concavity of a dislocated radial head suggests a traumatic dislocation amenable to surgical relocation and reconstruction, whereas a convex radial head indicates a congenital dislocation that is unlikely to be treated surgically.

SECTION 9 PEDIATRIC ORTHOPAEDICS

Developmental Dysplasia of the Hip

Synonyms

Congenital dislocation of the hip
Congenital dysplasia of the hip
Congenital subluxation of the hip
DDH

Definition

Developmental dysplasia of the hip (DDH) represents a spectrum of pathology related to the growth and development of the immature hip, varying from subluxation or dislocation of the hip (the femoral head is partially or completely displaced from the acetabulum) to deformity of the femoral head and/or acetabulum. The term congenital is too restrictive and is no longer used, except for cases in which a fixed dislocation is present at birth ("teratologic" or "syndromic" dislocation, associated with an underlying syndrome such as arthrogryposis). Most cases of nonsyndromic DDH are manifested by neonatal instability and are associated with abnormal physical findings after birth, but in some patients, physical findings after birth are normal (tests for instability are negative), and primary acetabular dysplasia is diagnosed later.

Risk factors for DDH are generally believed to be a positive family history, breech presentation, maternal oligohydramnios, first-born child, swaddling of the newborn's lower extremities, and female sex; of these factors, positive family history and female sex are most strongly associated. Approximately 10% to 20% of female babies with breech presentation will receive a diagnosis of DDH, although the term breech is poorly defined in the DDH literature (complete, partial, timing). DDH is more common in persons of northern European descent and in Native Americans, and the left hip is more commonly involved than the right (3:1 ratio). DDH may be more common in patients with so-called molding abnormalities as a result of intrauterine deformation, such as metatarsus adductus, congenital muscular torticollis, and hyperextension or dislocation of the knee. A careful screening physical examination is required in these patients, and consideration should be given to obtaining a hip ultrasonogram even when the examination is normal. Risk factors are thought to be cumulative.

Hip dysplasia is commonly observed in association with a host of diagnoses other than DDH. Neuromuscular hip dysplasia can be seen with diagnoses such as cerebral palsy, myelomeningocele, the muscular dystrophies, and conditions with flaccid weakness or paralysis such as spinal muscular atrophy or polio. The natural history and treatment of neuromuscular hip dysplasia varies with the underlying condition and usually differs from that of nonsyndromic DDH.

Clinical Symptoms

Neonates with DDH are asymptomatic, but infants and children will present with a limp or gait disturbance. Hip pain also can be observed in children or adolescents with subluxation, dislocation, acetabular dysplasia, or limb-length discrepancy.

Tests

Physical Examination

The examination in newborns and early infants focuses on detecting instability. The examination in older patients assesses for secondary adaptive changes associated with the hip dysplasia. Because most DDH occurs in the absence of known risk factors (except being female), the periodic hip physical examination for every child younger than 1 year is paramount for early detection of DDH.

Two maneuvers, the Barlow and the Ortolani, are helpful in detecting hip instability during the neonatal examination (**Figure 1**). The hip examination should be performed on a firm surface, and the infant must be relaxed. Each hip is examined separately with one hand while the pelvis is stabilized with the other hand. The Barlow maneuver is provocative; it attempts to displace the femoral head posteriorly from the acetabulum. To perform this test, the infant's hips and knees are flexed to 90° and the examiner's thumb is placed along the medial thigh and the long finger along the lateral axis of the femur. Gentle pressure is applied to the knee in a posterior direction while the femur is adducted. The Barlow maneuver is positive if a "clunk" occurs as the femoral head dislocates posteriorly over the acetabular margin. In contrast, the Ortolani maneuver attempts to relocate a dislocated hip. With the hips and knees flexed to 90°, the hip/thigh is manually abducted while the examiner applies gentle pressure from posterior to anterior with the long finger placed behind the greater trochanter. The Ortolani maneuver is positive when a "clunk" of reduction occurs as the femoral head

◨◀ Neonatal Hip Examination

◨◀ Barlow Maneuver- Animation

◨◀ Barlow Maneuver

◨◀ Ortolani Maneuver

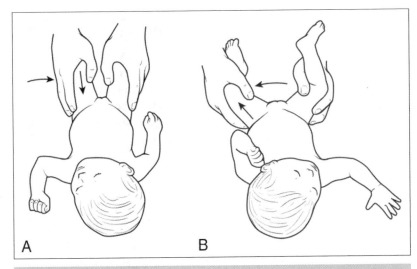

Figure 1 Illustration depicts the Barlow (**A**) and Ortolani (**B**) maneuvers used to assess for developmental dysplasia of the hip.

SECTION 9 PEDIATRIC ORTHOPAEDICS

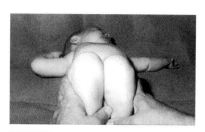

Figure 2 Clinical photograph of the Galeazzi sign, which indicates femoral shortening on the patient's left side. (Reproduced from Guille JT, Pizzutillo PD, MacEwen GD: Developmental dysplasia of the hip from birth to six months. *J Am Acad Orthop Surg* 2000;8[4]:232-242.)

◉◀ Galeazzi Sign

slides over the posterior lip and into the acetabulum. Of these two maneuvers, the Barlow is controversial because it almost always resolves spontaneously and therefore has little predictive value for future DDH. If performed too vigorously, it can actually create hip instability.

In older patients, the physical findings reflect the secondary changes that have developed as a result of a persistent subluxation or dislocation of the hip. The Ortolani maneuver becomes negative at approximately 3 months of age because of the development of fixed soft-tissue contractures that prevent manual relocation of a dislocated hip in an awake child. Instead, an adduction contracture develops in the child, preventing normal hip abduction as compared with the unaffected side. In infants, this condition is most easily detected by flexing the hips and knees to 90° and maximally abducting both hips. Asymmetric abduction suggests unilateral DDH; with bilateral disease, a symmetric loss of passive abduction (< 45°) may be seen, which makes diagnosis of bilateral DDH extremely difficult, often resulting in later diagnosis. Shortening of the involved extremity from the adduction contracture and/or superior migration of the femoral head from subluxation/dislocation results in a limb-length discrepancy. A unilateral subluxation or dislocation results in shortening of the thigh segment and is best demonstrated by the Galeazzi sign (**Figure 2**). Asymmetry in knee heights with the patient supine and the hips and knees flexed to 90° suggests shortening of one thigh (positive Galeazzi sign). In ambulatory patients, gait asymmetry commonly occurs as a result of a functional limb-length discrepancy.

Diagnostic Tests
Because the femoral head in a neonate is cartilaginous, hip radiographs can be difficult to interpret. The ossific nucleus of the proximal femur typically appears between 3 and 6 months of age, so plain radiographs are typically not obtained until patients are older than 4 to 5 months. Ultrasonography is especially useful during the first few months of life, before the femoral head has ossified, to establish the diagnosis and to monitor the effects of treatment (**Figure 3**), but should not be done prior to age 6 weeks because of the high false-positive rate associated with normal neonatal laxity. Ultrasonography has not been adopted as a routine screening tool for DDH in North America; most physicians recommend obtaining an ultrasonogram only if the infant is at increased risk for DDH or has an equivocal examination.

Differential Diagnosis
- Cerebral palsy (delay in motor development, increased muscle tone)
- Congenital femoral abnormalities (proximal focal femoral deficiency or congenital short femur)
- Developmental coxa vara (progressive decrease in femoral neck–shaft angle)

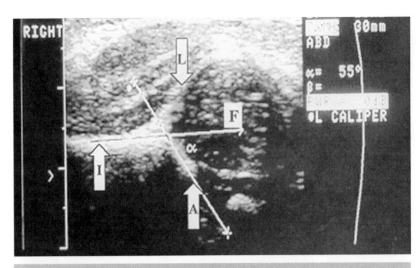

Figure 3 Ultrasonogram of a neonatal hip and measurements used to determine unstable hip. A = acetabulum, F = femoral head, I = ilium, L = labrum.

- Femur fracture (swelling, pain with limb motion)
- Neonatal septic arthritis of the hip (dislocation due to septic arthritis; Ortolani and Barlow maneuvers are painful)

Adverse Outcomes of the Disease

The longer the hip is dislocated, the less likely it is that closed reduction will be successful. If left untreated, DDH can result in premature degenerative joint disease (osteoarthritis), causing pain and limited function. Unilateral missed complete DDH can result in limb-length discrepancies, ipsilateral knee pain and valgus instability, and gait disturbances; bilateral missed complete DDH can result in back problems. Osteonecrosis is not an outcome of untreated DDH, as was previously believed.

Treatment

Swaddling of the lower extremities is the only modifiable risk factor for DDH and should be avoided in all newborns. Parents should be taught "safe swaddling" techniques. Treatment depends on the specific pathology and the age of the patient. The goal of treatment of instability in the neonate and infant is to achieve a concentric reduction of the femoral head and maintain the reduction while the acetabulum develops. If DDH is detected within the first few months, most hips will reduce with a dynamic positioning device, such as a Pavlik harness. The Pavlik harness is typically used in infants up to approximately 6 months of age. The anterior straps are tightened to hold the hips in flexion, and the posterior straps are adjusted to limit passive adduction. The posterior straps are never tightened to force the hips out in abduction, because excessive abduction may result in osteonecrosis. Another possible complication of the Pavlik harness is femoral nerve palsy from excessive hip flexion; this is

PEDIATRIC ORTHOPAEDICS

SECTION 9

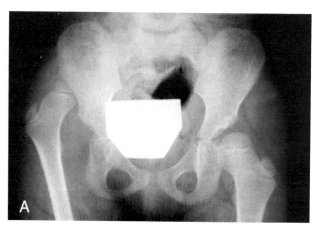

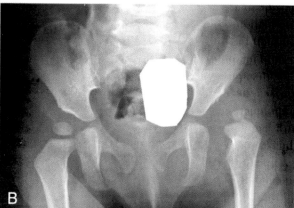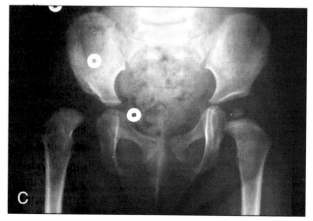

Figure 4 AP radiographs demonstrate developmental dysplasia of the hip, which is a spectrum of pathology. **A,** Dislocated hip. **B,** Severe subluxation with acetabular dysplasia. **C,** Dysplastic hip.

diagnosed by a lack of active knee extension. The nerve usually recovers with loosening of the anterior straps and decreasing the degree of hip flexion. If the hip is dislocated, a 2- to 3-week trial in the Pavlik harness can be followed up with ultrasonography to confirm reduction because leaving an unreduced hip in the harness for longer than this can result in deformation of the posterior rim of the acetabulum and a posterior capsular contracture. The Pavlik harness is typically worn full time for 6 to 12 weeks, followed by nighttime wear for a variable period. If the Pavlik harness fails to reduce the dislocation, the next options for treatment are closed reduction (open reduction if a closed reduction fails) and application of a spica cast, which are performed under general anesthesia. For hips that remain unstable despite an adequate trial with the Pavlik harness, there has been recent interest in splinting with a more rigid hip abduction orthosis before considering a closed reduction. In patients older than 18 to 24 months with a developmental dislocation, a more extensive procedure is typically required to reduce the hip, including open reduction and capsular repair, shortening proximal femoral osteotomy, or pelvic osteotomy. Even when the hip has been successfully reduced, patients may still require treatment of residual or progressive dysplasia of the proximal femur and/or acetabulum, most commonly realignment osteotomies on one or both sides of the joint (**Figure 4**).

Adverse Outcomes of Treatment

Failure of concentric reduction of the femoral head into the socket, persistent hip instability, and osteonecrosis of the femoral head are complications associated with treatment. Osteonecrosis can interfere with the growth of the proximal femur and the acetabulum, resulting in deformity of the proximal femur and progressive limb-length discrepancy. Osteonecrosis can also result in pain, arthritis, and joint replacement.

Referral Decisions/Red Flags

An infant with an abnormal periodic hip physical examination and/or substantial risk factors may require evaluation by a specialist. Parental concern regarding possibly abnormal hips should be investigated using careful physical examination and imaging, as indicated. A child with a positive Ortolani maneuver does not require hip ultrasonography prior to referral; the hip is, by definition, dislocated, and needs to be treated. A child with a positive Barlow maneuver may be followed by a primary care physician or referred to an orthopaedic surgeon, since most of these cases resolve without treatment. Asymmetric hip abduction and limited bilateral hip abduction are red flags requiring further investigation and/or referral. Indications for ultrasonographic or radiographic imaging of infants with positive risk factors but normal physical examination results are controversial, but the most recent clinical policy statements from the American Academy of Pediatrics and the American Academy of Orthopaedic Surgeons suggest that a lower threshold of substantial or additive risk factors are present, particularly hip dysplasia in a first-degree relative. These are not clearly defined because of the generally poor quality of the relevant literature. Finally, not all cases of DDH are detectable prior to walking age.

SECTION 9 PEDIATRIC ORTHOPAEDICS

Discitis

Definition

Discitis and vertebral osteomyelitis are bacterial infections involving the anterior elements of the spine. Discitis is most commonly seen in children younger than 5 years; vertebral osteomyelitis is diagnosed in older children and adolescents. This may be explained by age-dependent variations in the microcirculation within the vertebra and disk. In infants and young children, vascular channels communicate between the vertebral body and the disk space, allowing hematogenous seeding of the disk space. After those channels have closed, the bacteria typically settle within the vertebrae. Discitis can occur anywhere in the spine, but it most commonly affects the low thoracic and lumbar regions. The most common infecting organism is *Staphylococcus aureus*. Other organisms include *Kingella kingae*, group A streptococcus, and *Escherichia coli*.

Clinical Symptoms

A high index of suspicion is required to establish the diagnosis because the symptoms and findings are often nonspecific. Fever and malaise are common, and patients often experience back pain. Children who are able to communicate may be able to localize the pain to the back, but they also may perceive their pain to be in the abdominal region or thigh. Toddlers frequently are first seen with a limp or refusal to walk. The differential diagnosis is extensive and includes both infectious and noninfectious processes of the spine, the abdomen/pelvis, and the lower extremities.

Tests

Physical Examination

Children rarely appear systemically ill, although a fever, usually low grade, is common. Toddlers may refuse to walk or sit unsupported. Those who walk often lean forward and place their hands on their thighs for support (psoas sign). Percussion of the spinous processes may help localize the pain. The spine may be held in a rigid position to avoid spinal motion, and if both lower extremities are elevated simultaneously from the supine position, the back and hips are held in a rigid position. Passive spinal flexion, which compresses the anterior elements, is painful. A provocative test involves asking the patient to pick up an object from the floor; children with discitis will avoid bending forward and will not pick up the item. The single straight leg raise test also may have a positive result.

Diagnostic Tests

Laboratory studies should be obtained. The white blood cell count is within the normal range in many cases, but both the erythrocyte sedimentation rate and C-reactive protein level usually are elevated. Cultures of the blood and disk space are diagnostic in only 50% to 60% of cases. AP and lateral radiographs of the thoracolumbar spine

SECTION 9   PEDIATRIC ORTHOPAEDICS

are obtained as part of the initial assessment, recognizing that the plain radiographic findings such as irregularity of the vertebral end plates and narrowing of the disk are usually not apparent until 2 to 3 weeks after onset of symptoms. A three-phase bone scan can help establish the diagnosis and localize the pathology. MRI is the imaging study of choice (**Figure 1**). MRI not only confirms the diagnosis and clearly defines the extent of the process but also can help diagnose rare complications such as an epidural abscess. Because of the low diagnostic yield and the necessity for general anesthesia, CT-guided aspiration of the disk space is usually considered only in patients whose empiric treatment was not successful or when another diagnosis is likely, based on the clinical evaluation. A tuberculin skin test should be considered as well.

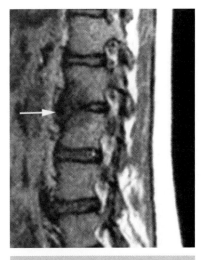

Figure 1 Sagittal T1-weighted MRI demonstrates signal intensity changes characteristic of discitis at L2-3 (arrow).

Differential Diagnosis

- Epidural abscess (rare, neurologic symptoms)
- Herniated disk or slipped vertebral apophysis (teenagers, radicular symptoms)
- Pyelonephritis (flank pain, pyuria)
- Retrocecal appendicitis (systemic symptoms, pain with hip extension)
- Retroperitoneal mass (may require MRI)
- Septic arthritis of the hip (marked pain on movement of the hip)
- Spinal tuberculosis (spares the disk, involves bone, usually thoracolumbar area)
- Spine tumor (neurologic abnormalities, may require MRI to differentiate)

Adverse Outcomes of the Disease

Although persistent disk space narrowing and spontaneous fusion of the adjacent vertebrae are common, these rarely result in any symptoms or problems.

Treatment

Most patients suspected of having discitis are treated empirically. Symptomatic treatment measures include bed rest or activity restriction, and analgesics. A spinal orthosis may provide considerable relief and is generally worn for 4 to 6 weeks. Antibiotics effective against *S aureus* are administered for a 6-week course in most patients. Intravenous administration is typically recommended for up to 2 weeks, and the transition to oral antibiotics is based on the clinical response.

A gradual return to activities is permitted. Surgical treatment, which rarely is required, usually involves either a biopsy with or without débridement or decompression of an epidural abscess. A biopsy is considered when the clinical response to empiric therapy is inadequate (especially if a CT-guided biopsy is nondiagnostic) or when another diagnosis is suspected.

SECTION 9   PEDIATRIC ORTHOPAEDICS

Adverse Outcomes of Treatment

Complications of intravenous antibiotics include line sepsis and an allergic reaction or intolerance to the agent selected.

Referral Decisions/Red Flags

A lack of response to empiric treatment suggests the need for additional workup and/or biopsy. Further evaluation also is indicated in the rare case in which neurologic symptoms are present, usually from an epidural abscess.

Evaluation of the Limping Child

Definition

Limping results from a host of causes. Differential diagnoses based on age are presented in **Tables 1**, **2**, and **3**. Several broad categories of gait disturbance exist in which the child may present with a limp. An antalgic gait is characterized by a shortened stance phase and is caused by pain in the extremity or spine. A Trendelenburg gait, or abductor lurch, is characterized by shifting the trunk or shoulders toward the affected side (stance phase) to compensate for weakness of the abductor muscles; it is associated with pathology localized to the hip. An equinus gait is characterized by foot contact with the floor by the front of the foot; it might be due to a heel cord contracture or to compensate for a limb-length discrepancy. A circumduction gait is characterized by swinging the entire leg out to the side in a circle during the swing phase, such as to allow clearance of a longer leg or because of spasticity. Although many conditions can result in limping, a history and physical examination, supplemented by appropriate imaging studies, will facilitate diagnosis in most cases.

Table 1	
Causes of Limping in Infants/Toddlers	
Diagnostic Category	**Differential Diagnosis**
Congenital	Limb-length discrepancies
Developmental	Hip dysplasia
	Developmental coxa vara
Traumatic	Toddler's fracture
	Nonaccidental injury
Infectious	Septic arthritis
	Osteomyelitis
	Pyomyositis
	Lyme disease
	Discitis
Inflammatory	Juvenile idiopathic arthritis
	Dermatomyositis
	Reactive arthritis
Neoplastic	Leukemia
	Neuroblastoma
Neurologic	Cerebral palsy
	Muscle diseases
	Neuropathies
	Tethered cord

Table 2	
Causes of Limping in Childhood	
Diagnostic Category	**Differential Diagnosis**
Congenital	Hypermobility syndromes
	Discoid meniscus
Developmental	Hip dysplasia
	Developmental coxa vara
	Spondylolysis or spondylolisthesis
Traumatic	Sprains or strains
	Fractures
	Overuse syndromes (Sever disease)
Infectious	Septic arthritis
	Osteomyelitis
	Pyomyositis
	Lyme disease
	Discitis
Inflammatory	Reactive arthritis
	Juvenile idiopathic arthritis (oligoarthritis, rheumatoid factor–negative polyarthritis, systemic arthritis, psoriatic arthritis, enthesitis-related arthritis)
	Rheumatic conditions (acute rheumatic fever, lupus, dermatomyositis)
Neoplastic	Leukemia
	Neuroblastoma
Neurologic	Cerebral palsy
	Muscle diseases
	Neuropathies
	Intraspinal anomalies (spinal cord tumor, tethered cord, diastematomyelia, lipomyelomeningocele, syrinx)
Other	Transient synovitis
	Legg-Calvé-Perthes disease
	Limb-length discrepancy
	Osteochondroses (Köhler disease, Freiberg infraction)

Unless an infection or other acute pathologic process is suspected, observation is appropriate for problems of short duration. Chronic problems, however, require further evaluation. Specific treatment strategies depend on the underlying diagnosis.

Diagnostic Evaluation
History
A history is essential, including the timing and location of any discomfort; the history of any injury (or chronic repetitive activities); the presence of systemic signs or symptoms; whether the limp is

Table 3

Causes of Limping in Adolescence

Diagnostic Category	Differential Diagnosis
Congenital	Tarsal coalition
	Discoid meniscus
Developmental	Slipped capital femoral epiphysis
	Spondylolysis or spondylolisthesis
Traumatic	Fractures, sprains/strains
	Stress fractures
	Overuse syndromes or repetitive microtrauma (Osgood-Schlatter disease, Sinding-Larsen–Johansson disease, Sever disease)
	Acetabular labral tears
	Apophyseal avulsion fractures
	Herniated disk or slipped vertebral apophysis
Infectious	Septic arthritis (*gonococcus*)
	Osteomyelitis
	Pyomyositis
	Lyme disease
	Vertebral osteomyelitis
Inflammatory	Reactive arthritis
	Juvenile idiopathic arthritis
	Rheumatic conditions (acute rheumatic fever, lupus, dermatomyositis)
Neoplastic	Malignant (osteogenic sarcoma)
	Benign (osteoid osteoma)
Neurologic	Cerebral palsy
	Muscle diseases
	Neuropathies
	Intraspinal anomalies (spinal cord tumor, tethered cord, diastematomyelia, lipomyelomeningocele, syrinx)
Other	Limb-length discrepancy
	Idiopathic pain syndromes (especially complex regional pain syndrome and fibromyalgia)
	Osteochondroses (Freiberg infraction, Köhler disease)

worsened by activities and relieved by rest; and the chronicity of symptoms (have they lasted for days, weeks, months, years?). A patient who has pain and is able to understand/cooperate should be asked to place one finger on the spot that hurts the most. Systemic signs or symptoms such as fever and malaise, weight loss, bruising, or other generalized symptoms increase the likelihood of an underlying infectious, inflammatory, or neoplastic process. Activity-related discomfort, which is relieved by rest, is characteristic for various overuse syndromes of childhood and adolescence. Pain that

SECTION 9 PEDIATRIC ORTHOPAEDICS

awakens a patient from sleep (night pain) is worrisome for infection or tumor. Stiffness when the patient wakes in the morning suggests an underlying inflammatory disease. A painless limp often relates to a congenital or developmental process, for example, Legg-Calvé-Perthes disease. A family history of musculoskeletal conditions (juvenile idiopathic arthritis or other inflammatory diseases, hip dysplasia) can suggest a similar disorder in the child.

Physical Examination

The assessment begins with obtaining measurements for height, weight, and vital signs. Has the child been losing weight? Is fever present? The gait is inspected by watching the patient walk (from the front, back, and side) down a long corridor, assessing the trunk/upper body, the hips, the knees, and the foot/ankle. Stance and alignment are inspected. The skin is examined for signs of bruising, erythema, or other abnormalities. The spine is examined for tenderness, spasm, deformity, and cutaneous signs of dysraphism. Palpation of muscles, bones, and joints should reveal any areas of tenderness, swelling, or synovitis. A neuromuscular examination should be performed. Muscle atrophy is an important finding, and limb girth is evaluated by measuring and comparing limb circumference at symmetric locations.

Diagnostic Tests

The extent to which additional studies are ordered depends on the chronicity of illness and the findings on history and physical examination. Rest, analgesics, and reevaluation may be indicated for the runner with a mild, activity-related limp of short duration, but an immediate inpatient evaluation is required for the child with night pain, fever, and multiple bruises. In most cases, the evaluation of a limping child can be conducted on an outpatient basis; a more extensive initial evaluation is justified in patients with chronic symptoms (lasting longer than 6 weeks) or when an infection or neoplastic process is in the differential diagnosis.

Radiographs are obtained when findings on the history and physical examination can be localized and should be the first imaging modality used. Orthogonal views (radiographs obtained at 90° to one another) of the area of interest must be obtained (for example, AP and lateral views); often, oblique views are also helpful. Specialized views such as a tunnel view may be required to rule out osteochondritis dissecans in an older child with knee pain and effusions. If the clinical examination is nonfocal, a three-phase bone scan may better localize the pathology. False-negative results can occur with this test. Leukemia may have a normal result or even a "cold" bone scan. When the location is known and radiographs are nondiagnostic, MRI, CT, or both can help establish the diagnosis. CT provides outstanding bony detail. MRI provides the most comprehensive evaluation, including excellent soft-tissue detail. MRI with intravenous contrast material should be ordered when an infection is in the differential diagnosis.

Laboratory studies are indicated if any suggestion of infection, neoplasia, or an inflammatory disease exists. Routine studies include a complete blood cell count with a manual differential, a C-reactive protein level, and an erythrocyte sedimentation rate. Other studies to consider are a Lyme titer and antinuclear antibody, rheumatoid factor, and antistreptolysin O tests.

Procedure: Hip Aspiration

Note: The approach for a hip aspiration in a child can be anterior, anterolateral, or medial. The medial approach is described here. This procedure should only be performed by an interventional radiologist under ultrasound guidance or by an orthopaedic surgeon in the operating room with fluoroscopy.

Step 1
Wear protective gloves during this procedure and use sterile technique.

Step 2
Place the patient supine with the hip flexed, maximally abducted, and externally rotated.

Step 3
Palpate the adductor longus.

Step 4
Cleanse the area with a bactericidal solution.

Step 5
Insert the syringe. Place the needle inferior to the proximal adductor longus tendon, aiming toward the femoral head–neck junction (**Figure 1**). Confirm placement on AP fluoroscopic imaging. Appropriate contrast material should be used to verify that the needle is intra-articular. Observe fluid for gross appearance and record it.

Step 6
Dress the puncture site with a sterile adhesive bandage.

Materials
- Sterile gloves
- Bactericidal skin preparation solution
- 10-mL syringe with a 22-gauge, ¼″ needle
- Adhesive bandage

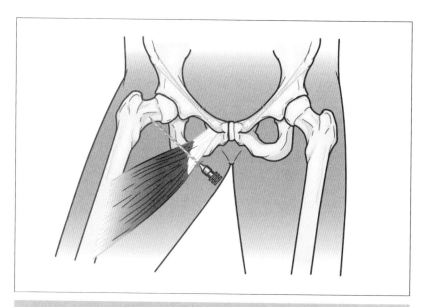

Figure 1 Illustration depicts the medial approach for hip aspiration.

Adverse Outcomes
Although rare, infection can occur.

Aftercare/Patient Instructions
Many pediatric patients undergoing this procedure are acutely, seriously ill. Many are inpatients. Aftercare includes activities as tolerated, depending on the clinical situation.

SECTION 9   PEDIATRIC ORTHOPAEDICS

Flatfoot

Synonyms

Flexible flatfoot
Peroneal spastic flatfoot
Pes planovalgus
Pes planus
Pronated foot

Definition

Flatfoot is defined as an abnormally low (or absent) longitudinal arch. In most cases, it is a normal variant. Flatfoot is common in infants and children. The longitudinal arch typically starts to develop around 4 years of age, maturing by 10 years of age. Flatfoot is present in up to 25% of the adult population, and patients often report a family history of flatfoot.

The most common diagnosis is a flexible flatfoot, which rarely is symptomatic and typically requires only reassurance. Flexible flatfoot in children is usually bilateral. Patients have a visible arch when they are not standing and have normal mobility of the subtalar joint (inversion and eversion of the hindfoot). Flexible flatfoot is sometimes associated with a contracture of the Achilles tendon, and this subset of patients is most likely to be symptomatic. A rigid flatfoot is uncommon, may be unilateral or bilateral, is more often symptomatic, and usually requires a diagnostic evaluation and treatment. Flattening of the longitudinal arch occurs in non–weight-bearing positions, associated with a restriction in subtalar motion. The etiology of a rigid flatfoot may be congenital (tarsal coalition, vertical talus), neuromuscular (cerebral palsy, hypotonia), or inflammatory (juvenile idiopathic arthritis). Idiopathic rigid flatfoot can be seen with obesity. In some of these cases, the flatfoot is initially flexible but becomes more rigid over time.

Clinical Symptoms

Flexible flatfoot usually is asymptomatic, although some patients may report activity-related discomfort in the medial hindfoot region (and under the longitudinal arch) and/or the ankles and legs. These children may think that they are unable to keep up with peers in running activities and that they become fatigued easily. Symptoms are much more common when the flatfoot is associated with an Achilles tendon contracture; these patients have mainly activity-related pain in the hindfoot region.

Tests

Physical Examination

The flexible flatfoot has a normal appearance when in a non–weight-bearing position. Findings in a weight-bearing position include loss of the longitudinal arch, valgus alignment of the hindfoot with

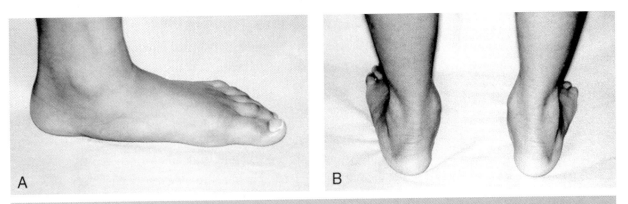

Figure 1 Photographs of medial (**A**) and posterior (**B**) views of flatfoot.

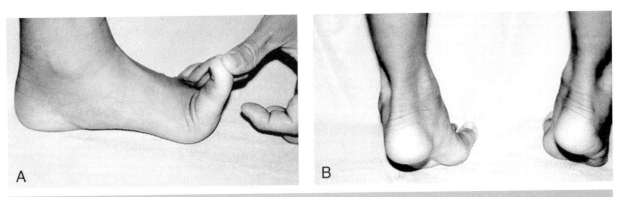

Figure 2 Photographs show elevation of the arches in flexible flatfeet using the Jack test (**A**) and by standing on the toes (**B**).

prominence of the medial malleolus, and abduction of the forefoot relative to the hindfoot (**Figure 1**). With severe pes planovalgus, the medial border of the foot is convex and the lateral border is concave. To identify an Achilles tendon contracture, ankle range of motion is assessed by dorsiflexing the foot; normal range of motion is more than 10°. During this test, the hindfoot is held in an inverted position to lock the subtalar joint and avoid "spurious" dorsiflexion through the hindfoot joints. Subtalar motion should always be assessed manually, and any restriction or asymmetry in motion between sides should be recorded. The Jack test, or great toe extension test, re-creates the arch during weight bearing in a flexible flatfoot. Hindfoot flexibility is assessed by asking the patient to stand on his or her tiptoes. In a flexible flatfoot, the medial longitudinal arch is restored, and the hindfoot rolls from valgus into varus in this position (**Figure 2**). The arch cannot be re-created by any means in a rigid flatfoot. A careful neurologic examination is required, as well as an assessment of connective tissue laxity.

Diagnostic Tests

Radiographs (weight-bearing AP and lateral views of the foot) are indicated only in children who are symptomatic. An oblique radiograph (and often a Harris heel view) of the foot also is obtained when the flatfoot is rigid.

Differential Diagnosis

- Calcaneovalgus foot (infancy, abnormal molding in utero)
- Flexible flatfoot associated with a connective tissue disease or syndrome (such as Down syndrome, Marfan syndrome, Ehlers-Danlos syndrome)
- Flexible flatfoot without Achilles tendon contracture (all ages, normal hindfoot motion)
- Rigid flatfoot associated with juvenile idiopathic arthritis
- Rigid flatfoot associated with neurologic diseases (such as cerebral palsy), connective tissue disorders, or syndromes
- Rigid flatfoot caused by congenital vertical talus (infancy and early childhood, rigid, underlying neuromuscular diagnosis or associated syndrome is common)
- Rigid flatfoot caused by tarsal coalition (adolescence, activity-related hindfoot pain)

Adverse Outcomes of the Disease

Flexible flatfoot is a normal variation of the shape of the foot that rarely causes disability or requires treatment. Pain, disability, and the need for treatment are more common in children with Achilles tendon contracture associated with flexible flatfoot. Rigid flatfeet are commonly symptomatic because of the altered kinematics of the hindfoot joints.

Treatment

Young children typically are asymptomatic, but the parents are often concerned about the appearance of the feet. Parents should be advised that flattening of the longitudinal arch usually improves and that corrective shoes and orthoses will not have a beneficial effect on the development of the longitudinal arch or the natural history. Furthermore, it helps to remind parents that adults with high arches (cavus feet) are more likely to have pain, and most adults with flatfeet are asymptomatic. Children should wear shoes with a flexible sole (rigid designs should be avoided), but time without footwear should also be encouraged. Arch supports may be tried, but patients with flexible flatfeet and heel cord contractures may experience pain from the supports and reject their use.

Orthoses are rarely indicated in the treatment of flexible flatfoot. Patients with symptomatic flexible flatfoot may obtain relief with a shoe insert. Generally, treatment is best begun with an over-the-counter orthosis; custom-molded devices can be used for refractory symptoms. Arch support is less important than controlling the hindfoot. For symptomatic deformities of greater severity, especially in patients with secondary flexible flatfoot, specific orthotic designs may be considered to achieve greater control of the hindfoot. A University of California Biomechanics Laboratory (UCBL) orthosis provides better control of the hindfoot. Rarely, a supramalleolar (trim lines extend above the malleoli) orthosis is required to control the hindfoot. Older children and adolescents with foot pain related to a contracted Achilles tendon may benefit from daily heel cord stretching exercises. Orthoses help control the hindfoot and prevent recurrence of the contracture, but the specific type or construction depends on the underlying etiology of the flatfoot and abnormal biomechanics.

Surgery is rarely indicated for flexible flatfoot. The exception is the older child with symptoms that persist despite a vigorous program of Achilles tendon stretching, orthosis use, and shoe modifications. Osteotomy to lengthen the lateral column of the foot, as opposed to arthrodesis, is generally accepted for management of this condition.

Surgical treatment is often required for rigid flatfoot. The procedure depends on the underlying diagnosis and findings. Achilles tendon lengthening can be considered if stretching fails to relieve symptoms associated with combined flexible flatfoot and Achilles tendon contracture. Symptomatic tarsal coalition may require excision of the connection (bone, cartilage, or fibrous tissue) between the tarsal bones in some patients, and a subset of these patients will be best managed with hindfoot fusion, often with realignment.

Adverse Outcomes of Treatment

Numerous surgical procedures have been developed to treat flexible flatfoot in young children. Almost all have been abandoned because of the benign natural history of the condition and because the various procedures have had inconsistent results and frequent complications.

Referral Decisions/Red Flags

Children with flexible flatfoot typically do not require referral unless they have persistent symptoms or an associated Achilles tendon contracture. Most patients with rigid flatfoot require further evaluation, particularly if symptoms are present.

SECTION 9 PEDIATRIC ORTHOPAEDICS

Fractures in Children

Fractures are more common in children than in adults, due in part to their play and in part to the different characteristics of their bone. The strength of bone gradually increases as a child grows, but a child's bone is not as strong as that of an adult until late adolescence. As a result, bone is the weak link in children, and ligamentous injuries are uncommon until late adolescence.

Fractures are uncommon in children younger than 3 years. Infants and young children usually are protected by their self-limiting activity, even though their bones are weaker. Nonaccidental trauma, however, is substantially higher in very young children, as described in the chapter on child abuse. In children older than 3 years, the incidence of fractures gradually increases until it peaks during adolescence. The incidence also is higher in boys and during the summer months.

Plasticity of bone (the modulus of elasticity) is greater in children—a child's bone can bend or deform without completely breaking. As a result, torus and greenstick fractures are common fracture patterns in children, but these injuries are rarely seen in adults.

Bone healing is more rapid in children. For example, a femur fracture in an adult requires 16 to 20 weeks of immobilization if treated by closed means. By comparison, the same fracture requires only 2 weeks of immobilization in an infant and 4 to 6 weeks of casting in young children. Because of more rapid healing, nonunion is extremely uncommon in children.

Fractures involving the growth plate or physis are unique to children, accounting for 15% to 20% of all pediatric fractures.

Bone remodeling is greater in children, and some postfracture malalignments will spontaneously self-correct. The potential for remodeling is greater in younger children, in fractures close to the physis, and in fractures angulated in the plane of motion (**Figure 1**). A fracture of the distal radius with 35° of volar or dorsal angulation in a 5-year-old child will completely remodel in 1 to 2 years ("a degree a month"), even if reduction is not performed. In this instance, the primary reason for reduction is to relieve pressure on adjacent soft tissues. Angular correction in other planes is less predictable, and rotational deformities typically do not correct.

Pediatric fractures present special considerations for diagnosis and management that deserve comment: A fracture might not be visible on routine radiographs when it involves only the physis and when the secondary ossification center has not ossified. Young children are also less tolerant of major blood loss, and a child with a displaced femoral fracture or multiple trauma must be monitored carefully.

Most displaced fractures in children are managed with closed reduction and casting, whereas displaced fractures in adults often require internal or external fixation devices (requiring surgery). The thick periosteum in children helps maintain the reduction. Pediatric fractures heal more rapidly than those in adults, which reduces

Essentials of Musculoskeletal Care 5

SECTION 9 PEDIATRIC ORTHOPAEDICS

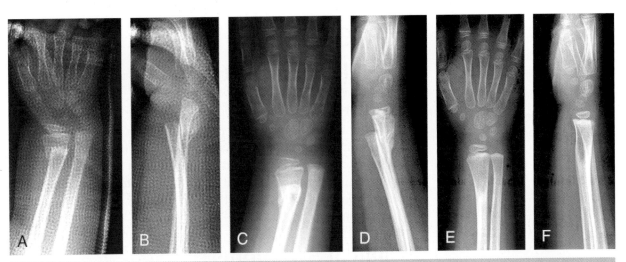

Figure 1 Radiographs demonstrate remodeling of a fracture of the distal forearm in a 5-year-old child. PA (**A**) and lateral (**B**) radiographs immediately postinjury. PA (**C**) and lateral (**D**) radiographs 3 weeks postinjury. PA (**E**) and lateral (**F**) radiographs 7 months postinjury.

the duration of and complications associated with immobilization. Furthermore, unlike adults, complications of prolonged bed rest such as pneumonia and thrombophlebitis are uncommon in children, so body casts can be used to treat complex pediatric fractures involving the spine, pelvis, and lower extremities.

Fractures of the Growth Plate

Definition

Any fracture that involves the epiphyseal growth plate (the physis) is called a physeal fracture. The Salter-Harris classification (**Figure 1**) is the system that has been most commonly used to describe these injuries, although some concern exists that a Salter-Harris type V fracture does not occur and that this system does not describe all fracture patterns.

Clinical Symptoms

Patients have acute pain and localized tenderness and swelling. They also may have localized deformity at the site of the injury and restricted motion of the involved site. There is typically a history of extremity trauma.

Tests

Physical Examination

Tenderness and swelling are localized and always present with maximum tenderness over the growth plate.

Diagnostic Tests

AP and lateral radiographs usually identify the fracture. Oblique views increase the ability to identify the fracture. Some nondisplaced fractures may show soft-tissue swelling only.

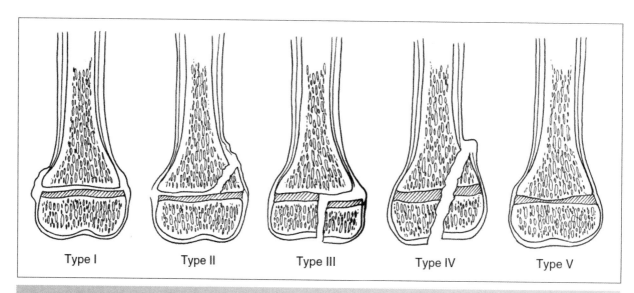

Figure 1 Illustration of the Salter-Harris classification of physeal fractures. (Reproduced from Kay RM, Matthys GA: Pediatric ankle fractures: Evaluation and treatment. *J Am Acad Orthop Surg* 2001;9[4]:268-278.)

Differential Diagnosis

- Contusion (swelling and ecchymosis near a joint, negative radiographs)
- Dislocation (evident on radiographs)
- Fracture of the metaphysis of a long bone (radiographs show no involvement of the physis)
- Infection
- Osteochondral fracture (involves articular surface but not the physis)
- Sprain (swelling, maximum tenderness over the ligament, negative radiographs)
- Tumor

Adverse Outcomes of the Disease

Premature growth arrest (partial or complete) results in diminished bone length (limb-length inequality) and angular deformity. Nonunion and overgrowth are rare.

Treatment

The goals are anatomic reduction, maintaining the reduction during the healing process, and avoiding growth arrest. These fractures heal rapidly, usually within 4 to 6 weeks.

Closed reduction and cast immobilization are indicated in Salter-Harris fracture types I and II. Minimally displaced fractures require only immobilization. In boys 15 years and older and girls 13 years and older, mild displacement can be acceptable because if premature arrest occurs, these patients have little growth remaining, minimizing the risk of limb-length discrepancy or angular deformity. Displaced fractures more than 7 days postinjury probably should not be reduced in children younger than 13 years because of the risk of growth plate reinjury causing arrest.

Salter-Harris fracture types III and IV involve the cartilage of both the growth plate and the articular surface. Therefore, anatomic reduction is required to ensure a congruous joint surface and to minimize the risk for bone bridge formation (physeal bar) between the epiphysis and metaphysis (**Figure 2**). In most instances, open reduction and internal fixation is necessary to obtain and maintain reduction. Open fracture requires immediate surgical attention. Physeal bars can develop after this injury and, if the patient has substantial growth remaining, reconstructive surgery may be required.

Adverse Outcomes of Treatment

Failure to recognize the fracture and its potential for growth arrest and failure to maintain anatomic reduction are the most common causes of a poor outcome. Physeal bars may not become evident for at least 3 months after fracture, and some not for many months.

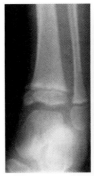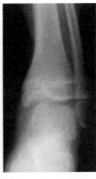

Figure 2 AP (left) and mortise (right) radiographs demonstrate a physeal bar. (Reproduced from Khoshal KI, Kiefer GN: Physeal bridge resection. *J Am Acad Orthop Surg* 2005;13[1]:47-58.)

SECTION 9 PEDIATRIC ORTHOPAEDICS

Follow-up for at least 1 year is mandatory, unless the patient reaches skeletal maturity earlier. Longer follow-up is needed for physeal fractures of the femur and tibia and for more complex injuries.

Referral Decisions/Red Flags

Displaced physeal fractures require reduction and maintenance of reduction. All patients require long-term follow-up.

Fractures About the Elbow

Definition

Fractures about the elbow are common in children. Injuries involving the distal humerus account for more than 80% of these fractures (**Table 1**).

Supracondylar fractures of the distal humerus are the most common elbow fractures in children, typically affecting children between 2 and 12 years of age. This fracture does not involve the physis. Most are extension type, with the distal fragment angulated and/or displaced posteriorly (**Figure 1**).

The next most common injury is a fracture of the lateral condyle of the distal humerus. Fracture of the medial condyle is uncommon; however, whether on the lateral or medial side, condylar fractures are serious because the fracture typically involves the growth plate of the distal humerus and the articular surface of the elbow (**Figure 2**).

Fracture of the medial epicondyle is the third most common elbow fracture (**Figure 3**), whereas fracture of the lateral epicondyle is uncommon. The epicondyles are secondary ossification centers at sites of muscle origin. Fractures of the medial or lateral epicondyle do not involve the articular surface and do not adversely affect growth. Medial epicondyle fractures are commonly seen in association with elbow dislocations. Epicondylar fractures of the distal humerus, even when displaced, can have limited consequences unless the elbow joint is concomitantly dislocated and the fragment is incarcerated in the joint. Instability under stress can result in pain, so surgical fixation may be preferred for athletes such as gymnasts and throwing athletes.

Table 1
Common Sites of Elbow Fractures in Children
Distal Humerus
Supracondylar
Lateral condyle
Medial condyle
Lateral epicondyle
Medial epicondyle
Distal humeral physis
Proximal Forearm
Radial neck
Olecranon

Figure 1 Lateral radiograph demonstrates a displaced supracondylar fracture. The humerus is outlined. (Reproduced from Sullivan JA, Anderson SJ, eds: *Care of the Young Athlete*. Rosemont, IL, American Academy of Orthopaedic Surgeons, 2000, p 317.)

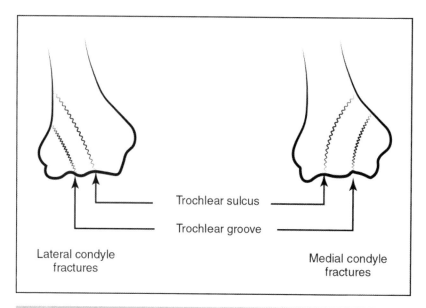

Figure 2 Illustration of typical fracture patterns of the lateral and medial condyles of the distal humerus in children.

Trochlear sulcus

Trochlear groove

Lateral condyle fractures

Medial condyle fractures

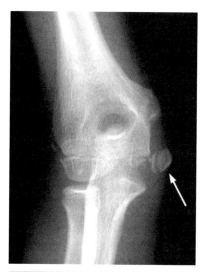

Figure 3 AP radiograph of the elbow demonstrates a displaced fracture of the medial epicondyle (arrow).

Exact criteria for repair of isolated displaced medial epicondyle fractures remains controversial.

Fractures across the entire physis (transphyseal) of the distal humerus are uncommon. These injuries occur most frequently in newborns, infants, and small children as a result of child abuse, and they may be either mistaken for elbow dislocations or completely missed because of the lack of ossification in the distal fragment.

In children, the metaphyseal portion of the radial neck is the weak link. Therefore, the valgus force that causes a fracture of the radial head in adults will result in a fracture of the radial neck in children. Olecranon fractures are uncommon in children. These injuries usually involve the articular surface and, when displaced, require an open reduction.

Clinical Symptoms

Patients have acute pain, tenderness, swelling, and most often a history of falling on an outstretched hand. The child often refuses to use the limb and holds it at the side with the elbow flexed. Swelling can be severe, but with nondisplaced or minimally displaced fractures, swelling may be mild.

Tests
Physical Examination

The status of the median, ulnar, and radial nerves distal to the injury are evaluated (**Figure 4**) and the distal pulses and capillary filling assessed. With obvious deformity, the limb is placed or splinted in a position of comfort and radiographs are obtained. In a child with

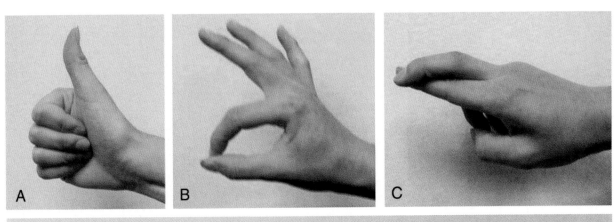

Figure 4 Photographs show how to test for radial (**A**), median (**B**), and ulnar (**C**) nerve function.

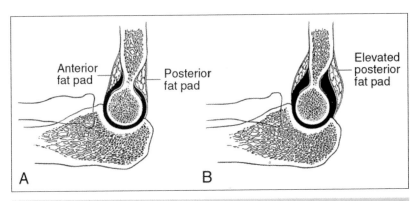

Figure 5 Illustration of normal anterior and posterior fat pads (**A**) and anterior and posterior fat pads elevated from an effusion (**B**). (Reproduced with permission from Skaggs DL, Mirzayan R: The posterior fat pad sign in association with occult fracture of the elbow in children. *J Bone Joint Surg Am* 1999;81:1429-1433.)

no obvious deformity at the elbow, the site of maximum tenderness should be found and elbow motion gently evaluated.

Diagnostic Tests

AP and lateral radiographs of the elbow are necessary. The fracture may be obvious or subtle. Oblique views and comparison radiographs of the opposite elbow are helpful with subtle injuries. The radial head should be directed toward the distal humerus (capitellum) on both AP and lateral views. An abnormal posterior fat pad sign is associated with fractures about the elbow, and the presence of this sign is particularly helpful with subtle or occult fractures. In an uninjured elbow, the anterior fat pad can be seen on a lateral radiograph, but the posterior fat pad is not visualized. Any process that causes an elbow effusion will elevate both anterior and posterior fat pads (**Figure 5**). The posterior fat pad is therefore often visible with elbow fractures in children (**Figure 6**), even when these injuries are not obvious on initial radiographs.

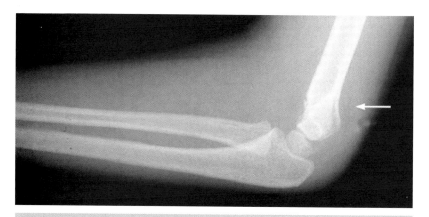

Figure 6 Lateral radiograph of the elbow demonstrates a posterior fat pad sign (arrow).

Differential Diagnosis

- Dislocation of the elbow (typically posterior, evident on radiographs)
- Hemarthrosis of the elbow (swelling, limited motion, no other positive findings)
- Infection
- Monteggia fracture-dislocation (fracture of proximal ulna and dislocation of the radial head)
- Sprain (swelling, tenderness over the involved ligament, no evidence of fracture)
- Subluxation of the radial head (typical history and age, tenderness over radial head, negative radiographs)
- Tumor

Adverse Outcomes of the Disease

Supracondylar fractures have the highest incidence of neurovascular problems. Median, ulnar, and radial nerve injuries are associated with this fracture, with anterior interosseous nerve palsy being the most common. The brachial artery may be injured, and compartment syndrome involving the volar forearm muscles can develop. Failure to recognize this problem in a timely fashion results in necrosis of forearm muscles and subsequent contractures (Volkmann ischemic contracture). Malunion with loss of the normal carrying angle (cubitus varus) can occur if displaced fractures remain untreated.

Condylar fractures can be missed, particularly in young children who have limited ossification of the distal humerus. In these children, only a thin wafer of metaphyseal fragment is apparent, with the rest of the fracture involving the cartilaginous physis and trochlea and, therefore, not visible on radiographs; oblique views in internal rotation (for the lateral condyle) or external rotation (for the medial condyle) may better visualize the fracture. Fractures displaced 2 mm or more are associated with delayed union, nonunion, or malunion (rotational and/or cubitus valgus). Condylar fractures of the humerus that are initially nondisplaced may become displaced, even when immobilized, by contraction of the forearm muscles attaching at the condyle. These injuries require close follow-up and repeat radiographs. Medial epicondyle fractures of the distal humerus may not cause residual problems, even when markedly displaced, unless associated with dislocation of the elbow and a fracture fragment that is not recognized as being trapped in the joint. Surgical fixation of isolated displaced medial epicondyle fractures is controversial, and surgery is most strongly considered to manage the dominant arm in an athlete who participates in a throwing sport or one that involves weight bearing in the upper extremity.

Fractures across the entire distal physis of the humerus have complications that are similar but typically less severe than supracondylar fractures. In addition, the potential for child abuse should be recognized and appropriately investigated.

Fractures of the radial neck that are angulated more than 30° to 45°, depending on patient age, may be associated with loss of forearm rotation, premature closure of the growth plate, and osteonecrosis of the radial head, so reduction is preferable to preserve motion.

Fractures of the olecranon with disruption of 2 mm or more of the articular surface require reduction to prevent progressive arthritic changes.

Treatment
Nondisplaced fractures are treated with splint or cast immobilization. Condylar fractures, in particular, require repeat radiographs in 3 to 5 days. Displaced fractures require reduction and, in most cases, pinning. Radial neck fractures with less than 30° to 45° of angulation in children younger than 10 years can also be considered for treatment with cast immobilization.

Adverse Outcomes of Treatment
Postoperative infection can develop.

Referral Decisions/Red Flags
Any displacement or angulation, an inability to extend all fingers of the affected hand, failure of over-the-counter medications to provide pain relief, and an absent or diminished radial pulse are signs that further evaluation is necessary.

SECTION 9   PEDIATRIC ORTHOPAEDICS

Fractures of the Clavicle and Proximal Humerus

Definition

The clavicle is a common site of fracture in children. Most clavicle fractures occur in the middle third, but they can occur at either end as well. Fractures close to the sternoclavicular joint can be serious because the great vessels are located just posterior to the joint. Fractures of the middle third of the clavicle (that is, the midshaft) generally heal rapidly in children and typically do not require surgery, even in cases of complete displacement. Distal clavicle fractures in older children and adolescents may involve disruption of the coracoclavicular ligaments, and more often require fixation.

Fractures of the proximal humerus account for approximately 5% of fractures in children. These fractures can occur in neonates during delivery (birth fracture) or in older children as a result of a fall. Metaphyseal fractures of the proximal humerus typically occur in children between 5 and 12 years of age; physeal fractures (those involving the growth plate) most commonly occur in children between 13 and 16 years of age. Metaphyseal fractures adjacent to the physis (Salter type II) are the most common pattern of physeal fracture.

Clinical Symptoms

Newborns with a fracture of the clavicle or proximal humerus may refuse to move the arm, a condition called pseudoparalysis. Clavicle fractures in children are characterized by acute pain, tenderness, swelling, and a palpable deformity. Fractures of the proximal humerus are less obvious because of the overlying deltoid muscle.

Tests

Physical Examination

The point of maximum tenderness is identified and the overlying skin checked for any tenting or blanching. Motor and sensory functions of the axillary, musculocutaneous, median, ulnar, and radial nerves should be assessed, as well as radial and ulnar pulses.

Diagnostic Tests

For suspected injury to the clavicle, an AP radiograph of the clavicle is obtained. AP and axillary views of the shoulder are necessary for suspected injury of the proximal humerus as well as to assess for shoulder dislocation (**Figure 1**).

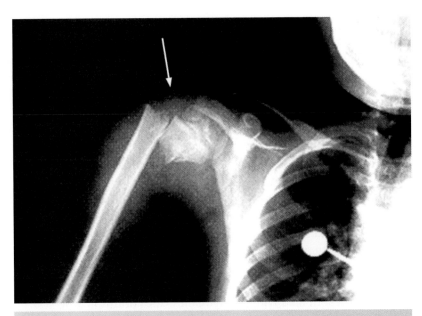

Figure 1 AP radiograph demonstrates a proximal humerus fracture (arrow) in a 5-year-old boy who fell from a tree.

Differential Diagnosis

- Cleidocranial dysostosis (absence of some or all of the clavicle, frontal bossing)
- Congenital muscular torticollis (asymmetric neck motion, plagiocephaly)
- Congenital pseudarthrosis of the clavicle (atrophic ends of bone at "fracture")
- Obstetric brachial plexus palsy (inability to spontaneously move fingers/wrist/elbow)
- Pathologic fracture (injury through a bone cyst or underlying bone disorder)
- Septic arthritis/osteomyelitis of the shoulder (no visible fracture, fever, pain with range of motion)
- Shoulder dislocation (evident on radiographs)
- Soft-tissue injury to shoulder (contusion)

Adverse Outcomes of the Disease

Malunion, physeal bar and growth arrest, neurologic or vascular compromise of the involved extremity, and/or osteomyelitis in an open fracture can occur.

Treatment

Newborns

Fractures in newborns and infants heal without incident and remodel well. For fractures of the clavicle, no treatment is needed. For fractures of the proximal humerus, the arm is immobilized for comfort by using a swathe or pinning the sleeve to the torso of the shirt.

Young Children

Fractures of the middle third of the clavicle in skeletally immature children, that is, in children with open physes (ages 0 to 12 years) do not require reduction; these fractures will remodel and straighten with time. Observation and immobilization in a sling or a figure-of-8 strap is satisfactory. Controversy exists regarding the amount of displacement that warrants surgery and the appropriate age for surgery among adolescent patients. Unless posterior displacement with involvement of the great vessels and/or respiratory difficulties is present, fractures of the proximal third also can be treated with a sling. Fractures of the distal third generally heal without reduction or surgery. Displacement and angulation of proximal humerus fractures are well tolerated. Nonsurgical treatment can be recommended to manage angulation measuring less than 70° in patients younger than 5 years, 40° to 70° in patients age 5 to 12 years, and less than 40° in patients older than 12 years. Fractures of the proximal humerus usually are best treated with a sling. Unless the child is nearing skeletal maturity, reduction usually is not needed regardless of angulation or displacement. A hanging arm cast is also commonly used.

Adolescents

Clavicle fractures in adolescents usually require only a sling or figure-of-8 strap unless the fracture is tenting or blanching the overlying skin. Shortening of more than 2 cm can indicate the need for surgical intervention, as in adults. Fractures of the proximal humerus in adolescents can be treated with a sling or a hanging arm cast, but such fractures may require reduction in the presence of more than 30° to 40° of angulation or fragments with less than 50% apposition. Rehabilitation is rarely required unless the patient has poor range of motion or atrophy several weeks after the fracture has healed.

Adverse Outcomes of Treatment

Recurrence, malunion, growth arrest of the physis, and resulting deformity are possible.

Referral Decisions/Red Flags

Neurovascular compromise, difficulty in breathing, skin tenting or blanching over the fracture site, open fractures, displacement of more than 50%, and/or angulation of more than 40° indicate the need for further evaluation.

Fractures of the Distal Forearm

Definition

The distal third of the forearm is the most common location for fractures in children, accounting for 20% to 40% of all pediatric fractures. Types of fractures, in order of relative severity, are listed in **Table 1**. Fractures of the distal forearm are uncommon in children younger than 4 years, but torus and greenstick fractures can occur in this younger age group. In children older than 10 years, fractures involving the growth plate of the distal radial physis are more common.

A torus fracture is characterized by buckling of the cortex on only one side of the bone; it is the least complicated forearm fracture (**Figure 1**). The most common torus fracture involves the dorsal surface of the distal radius. A metaphyseal fracture isolated to the distal radius typically is nondisplaced. In a greenstick fracture, the cortex is disrupted on the tension side but is intact or only buckled on the compression side. A Galeazzi fracture is a displaced fracture of the distal radius with a dislocation of the distal ulna or a fracture of the distal ulnar physis (**Figure 2**).

Clinical Symptoms

Patients typically report a fall on an outstretched hand. Acute pain, tenderness, and swelling are noted. With displaced fractures, the deformity is obvious. Symptoms following a torus fracture may not be immediately obvious.

Table 1
Types of Distal Radius Fractures in Children
Torus fracture (nondisplaced "buckle" fracture)
Metaphyseal fracture, complete
Greenstick fracture
Greenstick fractures of the distal radius and ulna
Complete fracture of the distal radius and greenstick fracture of the distal ulna
Complete fracture of the distal radius and ulna
Physeal fracture
Galeazzi fracture

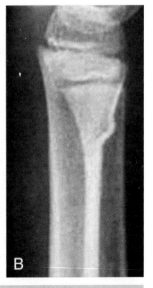

Figure 1 PA (**A**) and lateral (**B**) radiographs demonstrate a torus fracture of the distal radius.

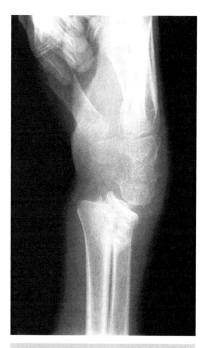

Figure 2 Lateral radiograph demonstrates a substantially displaced fracture of the distal radial physis in an 11-year-old boy who presented late. (Reproduced from Waters PM: Forearm and foot fractures, in Richards BS, ed: *Orthopaedic Knowledge Update: Pediatrics*. Rosemont, IL, American Academy of Orthopaedic Surgeons, 1996, pp 251-257.)

Tests

Physical Examination

The status of the median, ulnar, and radial nerves distal to the fracture is evaluated and the circulation at the fingertips assessed. The skin should be examined carefully; puncture wounds indicate a grade I open fracture.

Diagnostic Tests

AP and lateral radiographs of the forearm should show both the wrist and elbow joints. Comparison views are rarely needed with these injuries.

Differential Diagnosis

- Child abuse (multiple injuries)
- Osteomyelitis of the distal radius or ulna (no history of injury, fever, marked tenderness)
- Pathologic fracture through a bone cyst or other tumor (evident on radiographs)
- Septic arthritis of the wrist (subacute onset, no history of injury, fever, marked swelling)
- Wrist sprain (acute symptoms, uncommon in children)

Adverse Outcomes of the Disease

Malunion or crossunion (synostosis) with loss of forearm rotation, compartment syndrome (uncommon), and osteomyelitis (in open fractures) are possible.

Treatment

Most of these fractures heal without incident and can be treated by closed (nonsurgical) means. Residual angulation of 10° to 15° typically will remodel completely if 1 to 2 years of growth remain. The considerable remodeling potential of distal forearm fractures is related to the large amount of growth from the distal radial and ulnar physes, which contributes approximately 80% of forearm length. Fractures of the distal radial physis can result in growth arrest. If reduction is recommended, the number of attempts should be minimized. To minimize further injury to the physis, manipulation should be avoided more than 5 days after injury.

Torus fractures and nondisplaced fractures of the distal radius are stable but should be immobilized in a short arm cast or removable splint for comfort and to protect the bone from a second fall that could exacerbate the injury (**Figure 3**). Displaced fractures are treated initially by immobilization in a sugar-tong splint followed by casting; either short arm or long arm casts may be used, depending on physician preference and fracture type. The duration of immobilization depends on the age of the child and the extent of the injury.

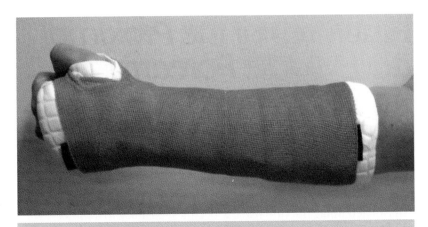

Figure 3 Photograph of a short arm cast.

For displaced fractures of the distal forearm, the acceptable degree of angulation depends on the plane of angulation and the amount of growth remaining. Loss of rotational alignment is the only absolute indication for both reduction and remanipulation. Distal forearm fractures that are angulated in the volar or dorsal plane remodel well in children, even if reduction was not performed. Completely displaced and overriding distal radius and/or ulnar fractures do not require reduction; such fractures will remodel in patients younger than 10 years. Mild radial or ulnar angulation can be gently corrected in a cast without vigorous manipulation. The principal reason for reduction is to relieve the pressure on adjacent soft tissues, including the median nerve if symptoms of compression exist. Unlike adults, most children with Galeazzi injuries can be treated by closed reduction.

Adverse Outcomes of Treatment

Reangulation is common in completely displaced fractures, particularly when reduction is incomplete. The decision to remanipulate the fracture depends on the age of the child (older), the degree of healing, and the plane of angulation. Substantial malunion with loss of functional wrist and forearm motion can occur but is relatively uncommon. Synostosis with loss of forearm pronation and supination is rare, but it is more common with open fractures. Physeal fractures may be complicated by an arrest of growth and resulting deformity at the wrist.

Referral Decisions/Red Flags

Inability to extend all fingers, pain not relieved by over-the-counter medications, neurologic dysfunction, dislocation of the distal ulna, and/or angulation of greater than 10° to 15° requires further evaluation.

Fractures of the Proximal and Middle Forearm

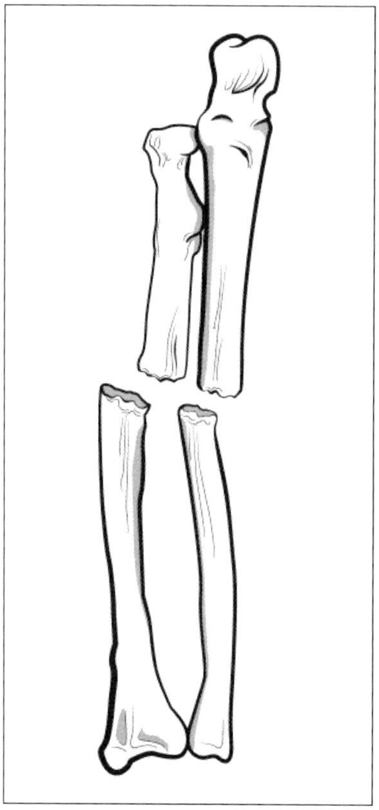

Definition

In children, fractures of the proximal or midportion of the forearm typically cause disruption of both the radius and the ulna (**Figure 1**). Other injury patterns include a Monteggia fracture-dislocation (radial head dislocation associated with a fracture of the ulna) (**Figure 2**), a both-bone forearm fracture, or an isolated fracture of the ulna. An isolated ulnar fracture usually occurs secondary to a direct blow as the child places the forearm in front of the face to deflect an oncoming blow.

Clinical Symptoms

Patients have acute pain, tenderness, and swelling, usually in association with a fall on an outstretched hand.

Tests

Physical Examination

Median, ulnar, and radial nerve function distal to the fracture site is assessed. Severe or inordinate pain on passive extension of the fingers should raise concern for possible compartment syndrome.

Diagnostic Tests

Full-length AP and lateral radiographs of the forearm that include the wrist and elbow are indicated. The radial head should align with the capitellum on both views. A Monteggia injury should be excluded if a fracture of the ulna is present. In a Monteggia injury, dislocation of the radial head is usually anterior but could be posterior or lateral.

Differential Diagnosis

- Child abuse (multiple injuries)
- Osteogenesis imperfecta (previous history, thin bony cortices)

Figure 1 Illustration of a fracture of the middle third of the forearm.

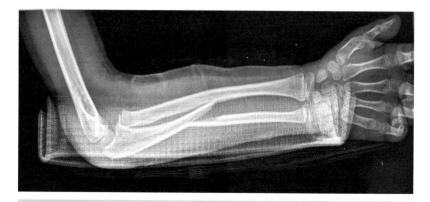

Figure 2 Lateral radiograph of a Monteggia fracture.

- Osteomyelitis of the proximal radius or ulna (fever, swelling)
- Pathologic fracture through a bone cyst or tumor (evident on radiographs)
- Septic arthritis of the elbow (fever, swelling, markedly restricted motion)

Adverse Outcomes of the Disease

If recognized early, a Monteggia fracture-dislocation in children can be treated by closed reduction. Failure to diagnose the injury in a timely fashion, however, will necessitate open reduction (surgery), reconstructive surgery, or acceptance of the deformity. Proximal forearm fractures are more likely to cause complications such as malunion, compartment syndrome, or loss of forearm rotation.

Treatment

Irrigation and débridement of open fractures is indicated. Both-bone forearm fractures that are angulated more than 10° and all Monteggia fracture-dislocations require closed reduction and immobilization in a long arm cast for 6 to 10 weeks. In adolescents, internal fixation may be required.

Adverse Outcomes of Treatment

Recurrence of the deformity, malunion, loss of forearm rotation, and compartment syndrome are possible. Both-bone fractures can develop a synostosis or bony bar connecting the radius and ulna.

Referral Decisions/Red Flags

Inability to extend all fingers, pain not relieved by over-the-counter pain medications, and angulation greater than 15° indicate the need for further evaluation.

SECTION 9   PEDIATRIC ORTHOPAEDICS

Fractures of the Femur

Definition

Fractures of the femur in children are the result of either high-energy or low-energy trauma, such as a car-pedestrian collision or a simple fall. Fractures can occur in any region of the femur (for example, femoral neck, intertrochanteric region, femoral shaft, supracondylar region, distal femoral physis) and can be transverse, oblique, spiral, or comminuted. Most involve the femoral shaft and heal without incident in 6 to 12 weeks. Closed treatment such as traction or spica casting was used more commonly but is giving way to surgical fixation in children older than 6 years and adolescents to enable early mobility and improved outcome.

Clinical Symptoms

Patients have acute pain, swelling, inability to bear weight, deformity, and a history of trauma.

Tests

Physical Examination

Pain and disability are immediate. Tenderness, deformity, or swelling may localize the fracture. Tibial and peroneal nerve function distal to the knee should be evaluated by testing the strength of the toe flexors and extensors and sensation over the plantar and dorsal aspects of the foot, as well as circulation at the ankle.

Diagnostic Tests

AP and lateral radiographs of the femur, including the hip and knee joints, should be obtained. Stress views may be necessary to identify physeal fractures of the distal femur.

Differential Diagnosis

- Child abuse (metaphyseal corner fractures or multiple fractures in various stages of healing; femoral shaft fractures in nonambulatory patients)
- Knee injury (especially collateral ligament tears)
- Osteogenesis imperfecta (multiple fractures after trivial trauma)
- Pathologic fracture through a cyst, bony tumor, or other lesion (evident on radiographs)
- Slipped capital femoral epiphysis (common in overweight adolescents)

Adverse Outcomes of the Disease

Malunion, either angular or rotational, along with growth derangement and limb-length discrepancy, is possible. Osteonecrosis of the femoral head may occur with a displaced or nondisplaced

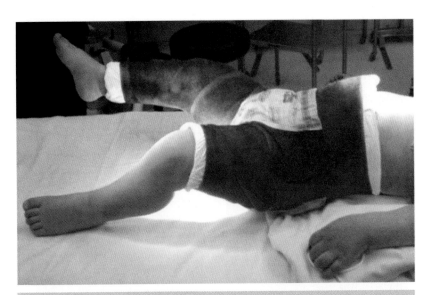

Figure 1 Photograph of a child in a spica cast following a fracture of the right femur.

fracture of the femoral neck. A fracture of the distal femoral physis can be misdiagnosed as a knee sprain and can result in growth arrest.

Treatment

The type of treatment depends on the location of the fracture in the femur, the fracture pattern, and the age of the patient. Immobilization with a spica cast or initial treatment by splint (posterior mold) traction followed by casting are effective modalities and are especially well suited to children 6 months to 5 years of age, who tolerate recumbency and heal rapidly (see AAOS Guidelines, *Treatment of Pediatric Diaphyseal Femur Fractures,* www.aaos.org/research/ guidelines/PDFFguideline.asp).

Nondisplaced femoral neck and intertrochanteric fractures can be treated with cast immobilization. These injuries should be monitored closely using radiographs for evidence of displacement. Displaced fractures should be treated with immediate reduction and fixation to minimize the risk of complications.

Femoral shaft fractures treated with immediate spica casting (**Figure 1**) or splint/bed rest/cast until early callus formation provide enough stability for the fracture to maintain alignment in a spica cast. This treatment is indicated for young children from 6 months to 5 years of age. Minor angulation will remodel without consequence.

Children 6 to 10 years of age and older children are candidates for surgery and fixation of the femoral shaft, which allows early mobility and earlier return to school. Supracondylar femur fractures and fractures of the distal femoral physis are difficult to reduce and hold in casts or splints and often require surgical fixation to maintain the reduction (**Figures 2** and **3**).

Adverse Outcomes of Treatment

These are similar to the adverse outcomes of the disease.

SECTION 9 PEDIATRIC ORTHOPAEDICS

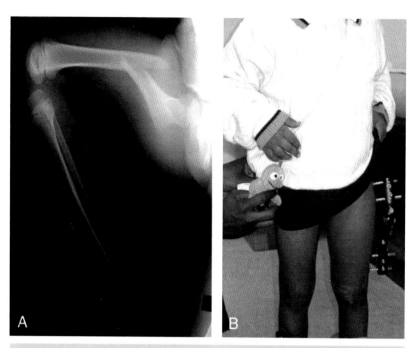

Figure 2 **A,** Preoperative AP radiograph demonstrates a femoral fracture of the right leg. **B,** Postoperative photograph of a child with a femoral fracture of the left leg treated with external fixation.

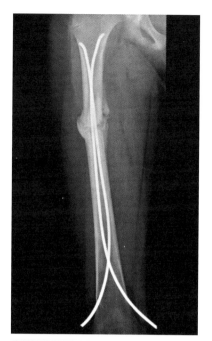

Figure 3 AP radiograph of flexible intramedullary nails used to treat a femoral fracture.

Referral Decisions/Red Flags

Virtually all femoral fractures require hospitalization. Open fractures and fractures with vascular compromise require urgent treatment. Children younger than 36 months with a diaphyseal femur fracture should be evaluated for child abuse. Typically, children younger than 1 year who are nonambulatory and have a femoral shaft fracture are also concerning for child abuse.

Fractures of the Tibia

Definition

Diaphyseal and proximal metaphyseal fractures of the tibia occur more commonly in younger children; growth plate and intra-articular fractures are more prevalent in older children. The tibia is a common site of fractures in children who are victims of child abuse. A list of various fracture types, age of peak incidence, and potential complications is provided in **Table 1**.

Clinical Symptoms

Most patients present with a history of injury causing an acute onset of pain and inability to walk. Toddler's fractures (minimally displaced spiral fractures of the diaphysis and/or metaphysis of the tibia), minimally displaced or incomplete metaphyseal fractures in older children, and stress fractures are characterized by a vague history of injury or insidious onset with minimal swelling or localizing signs and a limp.

Table 1

Types of Tibial Fractures

Fracture Type	Age of Peak Incidence	Pitfalls/Complications
Proximal		
Tibial spine fracture	Older child	Chronic laxity of knee
Tibial tubercle avulsion	Older child, adolescent	Growth arrest
		Compartment syndrome
Metaphyseal fracture	Younger child	Genu valgum
Diaphyseal		
Toddler's fracture	1 to 3 years	Failure to recognize
		Overdiagnosis
Stress fracture	Older child, adolescent	Failure to recognize
		Overdiagnosis
Complete fracture	Any	Varus malunion
		Compartment syndrome
Distal		
Physeal fracture	Older child, adolescent	Malunion
		Growth arrest
Triplane/Tillaux fractures[a]	Adolescent	Failure to recognize
		Degenerative arthritis

[a] Complex fracture of distal tibia occurring near end of growth.

SECTION 9   PEDIATRIC ORTHOPAEDICS

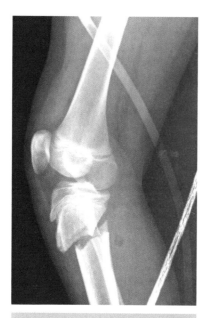

Figure 1 Lateral radiograph demonstrates a proximal tibia fracture.

Tests

Physical Examination

Superficial peroneal, deep peroneal, and posterior tibial nerve function is assessed and dorsalis pedis and tibialis posterior pulses, as well as capillary refill, evaluated. Possible compartment syndrome, particularly in proximal physeal (**Figure 1**) and midshaft fractures with muscle contusion, should be sought. The presence of any puncture wounds or abrasions could indicate an open fracture.

Diagnostic Tests

AP and lateral radiographs of the tibia that include the knee and ankle on both views are necessary. For injuries thought to involve the knee or ankle, the radiographs should be centered in these areas. Oblique radiographs and CT can help visualize complex fractures of the distal tibia, such as triplane or Tillaux fractures. A bone scan can help identify stress fractures or other occult injuries.

Differential Diagnosis

- Child abuse (multiple injuries, metaphyseal beak or corner fractures)
- Ligament injuries (unusual in prepubertal children)
- Osteogenesis imperfecta (previous history, thin bony cortices)
- Pathologic fracture through a bone cyst or tumor (evident on radiographs)
- Stress fracture (indolent onset)

Adverse Outcomes of the Disease

Early potential problems include compartment syndrome and vascular injuries, which require urgent evaluation. These complications are less common but may be more difficult to diagnose in children. Remodeling is unpredictable in deformities greater than 10°, and malunion with subsequent degenerative arthritis may occur. Growth arrest is common with distal tibial physeal injuries but less likely with proximal injuries.

Treatment

Treatment focuses on minimizing angular deformity, restoring joint congruity, and avoiding or identifying compartment syndrome or vascular injuries. Toddler's fractures, stress fractures, and certain nondisplaced fractures can be managed with immobilization in a short leg walking cast. Toddler's fractures also can be initially treated with a long leg cast. Displaced shaft fractures often require manipulative reduction and long leg casting. Patients with these fractures are best managed with hospital admission overnight for observation and elevation. Early splitting of the cast to accommodate swelling may be necessary. The duration of casting depends on the age of the child and the extent of the fracture.

Displaced intra-articular or physeal fractures require closed or open reduction and limited internal fixation supplemented by cast immobilization. All open fractures require surgical exploration and débridement.

Adverse Outcomes of Treatment
Infection may develop after open treatment.

Referral Decisions/Red Flags
Patients who report pain after immobilization that is not relieved by mild analgesics or over-the-counter medications require further evaluation. Patients who have lacerations or deep abrasions overlying the fracture site should be treated as if they have an open fracture. The acceptable angular deformity of tibial shaft fractures is 5° to 10°, depending on age. Inability to correct angular deformities to less than 10° is considered problematic. Proximal or distal tibial fractures that involve the physis or articular surface need further evaluation.

SECTION 9   PEDIATRIC ORTHOPAEDICS

Genu Valgum

Synonym
Knock-knees

Definition
Valgus alignment is inward angulation of the extremity in the frontal plane, with the tibia laterally deviated relative to the femur. The alignment of the lower limbs changes throughout infancy and childhood, and a wide physiologic range exists (values that lie within 2 SDs of the mean) (**Figure 1**). The extremities are aligned in 10° to 15° of varus (bowlegged) at birth and gradually straighten to neutral alignment by 12 to 18 months of age. The limb develops valgus alignment at or after 2 years of age, with maximal valgus (10° to 15°) observed between 3 and 4 years of age (**Figure 2**). This gradually improves to the adult mean of approximately 5° to 7° of valgus (normal range, 0° to 10°) by 11 years of age. Most patients presenting for the evaluation of knock-knees will have values within the physiologic range (**Figure 3**). The goal is to identify those few patients requiring further evaluation and treatment.

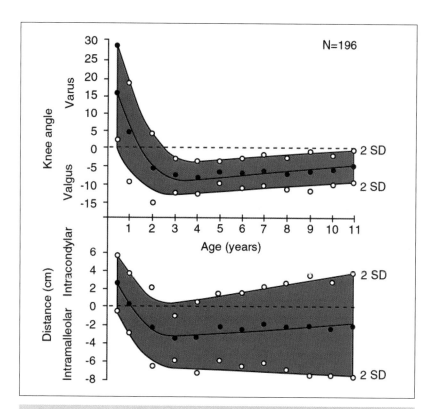

Figure 1 Illustration depicts normal values for the knee angle, shown in both degrees and intracondylar or intramalleolar distances. (Reproduced with permission from Heath CH, Staheli LT: Normal limits of knee angle in white children: Genu varum and genu valgum. *J Pediatr Orthop* 1993;13:259-262.)

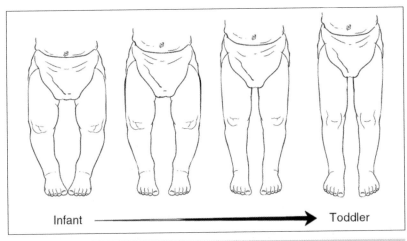

Figure 2 Illustration of normal progression from bowlegs of infancy through slow evolution to a physiologic valgus angle of approximately 12° at 3 years of age. (Reproduced from Gomez JE: Growth and maturation, in Sullivan JA, Anderson SJ, eds: *Care of the Young Athlete.* Rosemont, IL, American Academy of Orthopaedic Surgeons, 1999, pp 25-32.)

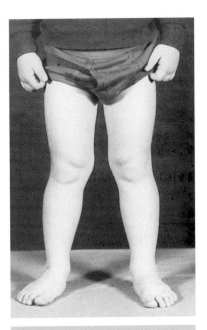

Figure 3 Photograph of a boy referred for evaluation of knock-knees. The patient was considered to be within normal limits. (Reproduced from Greene WB: Genu varum and genu valgum in children. *Instr Course Lect* 1994;43:151-159.)

Clinical Symptoms

Concern on the part of a parent or grandparent is the usual reason for the visit; children rarely have any pain or gait disturbance from variations in limb alignment. Most patients present for evaluation during the period of maximal valgus alignment, from 3 to 4 years of age. Children with obesity are at risk for worsening of genu valgum and should be evaluated regularly for progressive disease.

Tests

Physical Examination

The child's height and weight should be measured and plotted relative to normative data. The tibiofemoral angle can be measured using a goniometer, and the intermalleolar distance is measured as the distance between the medial malleoli with the patient standing with the medial femoral condyles touching. The lower extremity rotational alignment also should be evaluated.

Diagnostic Tests

Radiographs usually are not necessary, but should be considered when the valgus is more than 15° to 20°, or if the child is of short stature. A weight-bearing AP radiograph on a 36- × 43-cm cassette with the film centered at the knees and the patellae pointing straight ahead provides screening for rickets and skeletal dysplasia, as well as accurate measurement of the tibiofemoral angle. Laboratory studies should be ordered when a metabolic disease is suspected, for example with stature below the 5th percentile or when a more generalized disorder is suspected.

SECTION 9 PEDIATRIC ORTHOPAEDICS

Differential Diagnosis

- Epiphyseal dysplasia (multiple epiphyseal dysplasia or spondyloepiphyseal dysplasia)
- Posttraumatic (history of fracture, findings of asymmetric growth arrest on radiographs)
- Pseudoachondroplasia (short stature, limited range of motion, waddling gait)
- Renal osteodystrophy
- Rickets (such as nutritional, hypophosphatemic)

Adverse Outcomes of the Disease

Adults with excessive angulation in the frontal plane will experience asymmetric mechanical loading of the knee and can potentially be predisposed to early degenerative joint disease.

Treatment

Observation is the treatment of choice for an otherwise normal 3- to 4-year-old child with marked genu valgum. Shoe modifications are ineffective, and long leg braces are not indicated because spontaneous correction is achieved in most cases. In a small subset of older patients in whom the deformity is excessive and/or symptomatic, correction can be achieved either by growth modulation or with a realignment osteotomy, depending on the magnitude of the deformity and the age and skeletal maturity of the patient. Growth modulation by hemiepiphysiodesis is an option in patients with substantial growth remaining. A reversible hemiepiphysiodesis can be achieved by placing either a staple or a small metallic plate across the physis on the convex side of the deformity, which slows but does not eliminate the growth on that side. Normal growth on the concave side results in gradual correction of the deformity. The device can be removed when the deformity has been corrected and, ideally, symmetric growth is restored and alignment is maintained. In patients who are close to the end of their growth, a permanent hemiepiphysiodesis can be achieved by ablation of the convex portion of the growth plate. When the deformity is severe or when the patient has insufficient growth remaining for a hemiepiphysiodesis, an osteotomy is required to realign the limb.

Adverse Outcomes of Treatment

Reversible hemiepiphysiodesis requires removal of hardware. Undercorrection occurs if hemiepiphysiodesis is performed too close to skeletal maturity; substantial overcorrection is rare in closely monitored patients.

Referral Decisions/Red Flags

Patients of short stature and those with asymmetric or excessive genu valgum require further evaluation (more than 2 SDs from normal for their age). Patients with obvious genu valgum on clinical examination after age 11 years should be referred for evaluation to take advantage of the opportunity for guided growth and to avoid the need for corrective surgical osteotomy.

SECTION 9 PEDIATRIC ORTHOPAEDICS

Genu Varum

Synonym

Bowlegs

Definition

Genu varum (bowlegs) is an angular deformity at the knee with the tibia medially deviated (varus) in relation to the femur (**Figure 1**). Genu varum is normal at birth but should spontaneously correct to neutral by 12 to 18 months of age. The limb alignment evolves into valgus (maximal at 3 to 4 years of age) and ultimately is 0° to 10° of valgus at skeletal maturity. Most infants and young children have physiologic genu varum, and no treatment is required. A pathologic cause is more likely in older children and adolescents. Other causes include infantile or adolescent Blount disease, posttraumatic deformities, metabolic diseases, and skeletal dysplasias. The evaluation focuses on defining which patients have an alignment that lies outside the physiologic range, identifying the cause and location of the deformity, and instituting treatment when appropriate.

Clinical Symptoms

Parental concern is the usual reason for the visit, although children and adolescents with substantial varus deformity may present with activity-related pain in the medial aspect of the knee. Children with obesity are at risk for worsening of genu varum and should be regularly examined for progressive deformity.

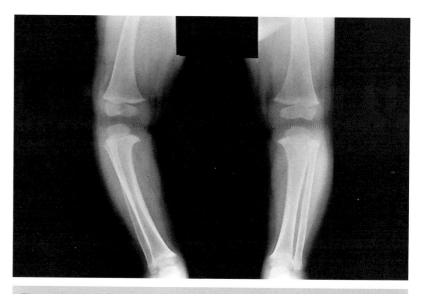

Figure 1 AP weight-bearing radiograph demonstrates genu varum in an 18-month-old girl. (Reproduced from Greene WB: Infantile tibia vara. *Instr Course Lect* 1993;42:525-538.)

Tests

Physical Examination

In infants and young children, the child's height and weight should be recorded and plotted on a nomogram. Limb alignment (angle between the femoral and tibial limb segments) is determined using a goniometer; this measurement is obtained with the limb placed with the patella facing upward (supine) or forward (standing). Whether the varus is localized (proximal tibia or other location) or generalized (involves both the femoral and the tibial segments) should be noted, as well as any asymmetry in alignment. The distance between the medial femoral condyles (intercondylar distance) should be measured with the patient standing and the medial malleoli apposed. It also is important to assess rotational alignment at both the femur and the tibia. Apparent varus can be seen in the standing position from the combination of external rotation at the hip and internal rotation below the knee (that is, internal tibial torsion). Observational gait analysis often demonstrates a lateral thrust at the knee during stance phase (varus thrust).

Diagnostic Tests

Radiographs are typically delayed until 2 years of age in patients suspected of having physiologic genu varum, but they may be obtained earlier if the child is below the 25th percentile for height, if the varus is relatively severe for the child's age, or if substantial asymmetry exists between the two extremities. For older patients, weight-bearing AP radiographs of the lower extremities are obtained on a 36- × 43-cm cassette with the film centered at the knees and the patellae facing forward. Measurements commonly obtained from the AP radiograph include the mechanical axis and the tibiofemoral angle. Leg lengths also can be evaluated, as well as the anatomy of the metaphyses and physes (which are widened in patients with rickets and certain skeletal dysplasias). Infantile tibia vara (Blount disease) and physiologic genu varum can be difficult to differentiate in children younger than 3 years. The metaphyseal-diaphyseal angle should be measured. Blount disease is likely with more severe bowing (**Figure 2**). Laboratory tests to rule out an underlying metabolic problem are considered, especially when the child is below the 5th percentile for height.

Differential Diagnosis

- Adolescent tibia vara (unilateral or bilateral, may or may not be overweight)
- Infantile tibia vara (children with obesity who begin walking at an early age; associated internal tibial torsion, depression of the medial aspect of the proximal tibial physis)
- Metaphyseal chondrodysplasia (short stature, widened physis, normal serum phosphorus level)
- Physiologic genu varum (spontaneous correction by 3 years of age)
- Postinfectious (sequelae of septic arthritis or osteomyelitis)

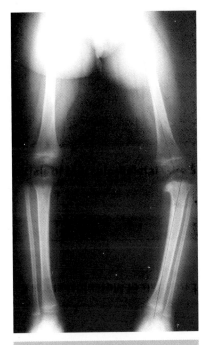

Figure 2 AP radiograph demonstrates medial depression of the tibial physis and increased bowing of the left leg, suggesting a high probability of Blount disease. A long leg brace was prescribed.

SECTION 9   PEDIATRIC ORTHOPAEDICS

- Posttraumatic (history of trauma, evidence of asymmetric growth arrest on radiographs)
- Rickets (short stature, widened physis, low serum phosphorus level)

Adverse Outcomes of the Disease

The principal adverse outcome is persistent varus deformity, which can result in abnormal loading at the knee and, in some cases, the development of premature degenerative joint disease.

Treatment

Physiologic bowing requires only reassurance. Patients diagnosed with infantile Blount disease, which causes a progressive varus deformity due to growth disturbance of the proximal posterior and medial tibial physes, usually require treatment. Bracing is controversial but can be considered in patients younger than 3 years with early stages of disease. Surgical realignment with an osteotomy is most successful if performed by 4 years of age. A high risk of recurrence accompanies any form of treatment in these younger patients. In the adolescent form of Blount disease, patients with milder deformities and sufficient growth remaining can be treated with hemiepiphysiodesis (staples or a plate are reversible; percutaneous physeal ablation is irreversible); those with deformities of great magnitude and/or who are skeletally mature require a tibial osteotomy.

Adverse Outcomes of Treatment

Bracing may not be tolerated by toddlers (or their families). Infantile Blount disease has a high risk of recurrence, even when treated appropriately. Reversible hemiepiphysiodesis requires the removal of hardware. Undercorrection can result if hemiepiphysiodesis is performed too close to skeletal maturity; overcorrection is rare in patients monitored closely during treatment.

Referral Decisions/Red Flags

The presence of disorders other than physiologic genu varum indicates the need for further evaluation. Obvious genu varum in a child older than 5 years should be monitored regularly for progression and referred before the prepubertal growth spurt to allow for hemiepiphysiodesis before skeletal maturity if necessary, or sooner if progressively worsening.

Intoeing and Outtoeing

Synonyms

Intoeing
Internal femoral torsion
Internal tibial torsion
Pigeon-toed
Outtoeing
External rotation contracture of infancy
External tibial torsion
Femoral retroversion

Definition

With intoeing gait, the child's foot turns in during walking and running activities. With outtoeing, the foot turns out. Parents perceive that turning in or out of any kind is not normal. Understanding the normal development of the lower extremities from infancy through adolescence allows the clinician to distinguish normal from abnormal. In most cases, intoeing and outtoeing are variations of normal development, and criteria are used to identify substantial deviations from the range of normal values.

Intoeing is more common than excessive outtoeing. Intoeing may be secondary to foot deformities, due to inward rotation of the femur or tibia, or the result of a combination of these. Internal tibial torsion is the most common diagnosis in toddlers. Internal femoral torsion (increased femoral anteversion) is most common in children older than 4 years. Both of these conditions improve with time, and nonsurgical treatment will not alter the natural history. Individuals with persistent intoeing rarely have functional problems, unless there is an underlying neuromuscular disorder, and very few patients ever require a derotational osteotomy for realignment. Education and reassurance are sufficient in most cases.

Because of intrauterine positioning, infants have an external rotation contracture of the hip and thigh that resolves over the first 1 to 2 years of life, and outtoeing may be noted when infants first stand and walk. Outtoeing in older children and adolescents may be due to external tibial torsion or external femoral torsion. External femoral or tibial torsion is unlikely to improve or resolve spontaneously, and in the few patients with chronic or disabling symptoms, the torsion can be corrected by derotational osteotomy.

Clinical Symptoms

Typically, medical attention is sought because parents or grandparents are concerned about how the child walks. Intoeing and outtoeing usually do not cause pain or interfere with development or stability in gait. With severe intoeing, children may stumble or trip when the foot in forward swing catches on the back of the trailing leg or the ground.

SECTION 9 PEDIATRIC ORTHOPAEDICS

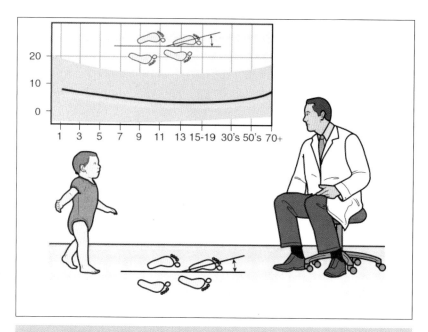

Figure 1 Illustration depicts the foot progression angle, which is estimated by observing the child walking. The normal range is shown in green.

With outtoeing, patients may have difficulty keeping up with their peers in running and certain sports.

Tests
Physical Examination
The examiner should recognize that a wide variation exists in what is considered normal. The physical assessment focuses on defining the magnitude and location of the intoeing or outtoeing. In addition, the family history should be reviewed. An assessment of the rotational alignment of the parents' limbs, conducted when they bring the child to the clinic, can provide helpful information to determine if any intoeing or outtoeing exists in the parents.

Measurements are compared with normative data; therefore, it is essential to know the normal range of values for these measurements for each age range. The normal rotation of an extremity about an axis is called version. A rotational value more than 2 SDs from the mean based on age-related normative data is called torsion. The examination documents a rotational profile, which includes measuring the foot progression angle, or the angle that the foot makes relative to the line of progression as the child walks (**Figure 1**); hip rotation, or femoral rotation (**Figure 2**); thigh-foot axis, or tibial rotation (**Figure 3**); and the foot alignment. Evaluation for possible neuromuscular disorders also is important.

The foot progression angle quantifies the magnitude of intoeing or outtoeing but does not identify the location of the problem. Hip rotation is used to estimate femoral version (rotational angle of the femoral head–neck relative to the distal epicondylar axis) and is tested with the patient prone (hips extended) and the knee flexed to

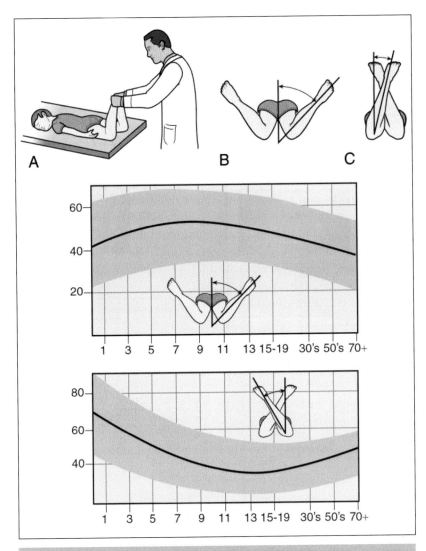

Figure 2 Illustration depicts hip rotation, which is assessed with the child prone (**A**). Internal (**B**) and external (**C**) rotation are measured. Normal ranges are shown in green.

90°. With one of the examiner's hands on the patients' buttocks to stabilize the pelvis, the lower leg is rotated outward to test internal (medial) rotation, and inward to test external (lateral) rotation. The degree of rotation is measured relative to the vertical axis (**Figure 4**). The mean range of hip rotation for a child older than 2 years is approximately 50° of internal rotation and 40° of external rotation. An excessive amount of internal rotation (more than 65°) coupled with a limited degree of external rotation indicates internal femoral torsion (excessive femoral anteversion). Internal femoral torsion is classified as mild (60° to 70°), moderate (70° to 90°), or severe (more than 90°). Femoral anteversion is approximately 40° at birth and decreases to approximately 15° in adults. Infants are born with an external rotation contracture at the hip, which allows 60° to 70° of external rotation and only 20° to 30° of internal rotation. This usually improves spontaneously. Persistent or excessive external rotation represents external femoral torsion (femoral retroversion).

Essentials of Musculoskeletal Care 5

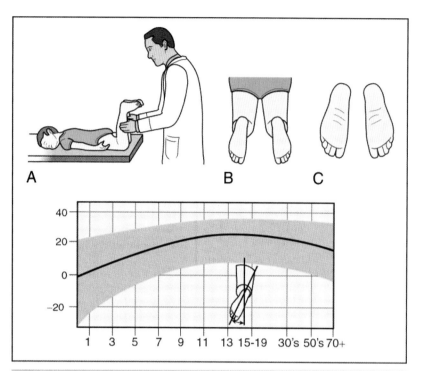

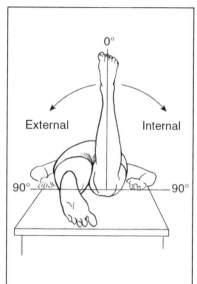

Figure 3 Illustration depicts assessment of rotational status of the tibia and the foot, which is best performed with the child in the prone position. **A,** Allow the foot to fall into a natural resting position. The thigh-foot axis (**B**) and shape of the feet (**C**) are readily determined. The range of normal is shown in green.

Figure 4 Illustration depicts hip rotation at the zero starting position. (Reproduced from Greene WB, Heckman JD, eds: *The Clinical Measurement of Joint Motion*. Rosemont, IL, American Academy of Orthopaedic Surgeons, 1994, pp 106-107.)

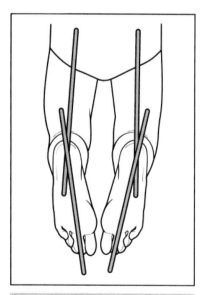

Figure 5 Illustration depicts bilateral internal tibial torsion.

The lower limb axis is assessed by measuring the thigh-foot angle and the alignment of the foot. With the patient in the prone position and the knee flexed to 90° (held in neutral at the ankle and subtalar joints), the axis of the foot is measured relative to the axis of the thigh. An internal thigh-foot angle greater than 10° to 15° indicates internal tibial torsion (**Figure 5**). Foot posture is assessed for metatarsus adductus, a possible cause of intoeing, as well as hindfoot alignment. Pes planovalgus can result in outtoeing. External tibial torsion can be associated with contracture of the iliotibial band; to assess for this, the Ober test should be performed. For the Ober test, the patient is placed in the lateral position and the downside leg is flexed so that the thigh is touching the abdomen. The other leg is then extended, internally rotated, and adducted. The test result may be positive for iliotibial band tightness if the upper leg cannot be adducted past neutral.

Patients with an underlying neuromuscular disorder can present for the evaluation of intoeing or outtoeing before the underlying disorder has been diagnosed. This is particularly common in patients with mild cerebral palsy. The patient should be assessed for appropriate motor milestones (**Table 1**) and examined for spasticity, muscle contractures, clonus, and a stiff walk or gait disturbance.

SECTION 9 PEDIATRIC ORTHOPAEDICS

Table 1	
Gross Motor Developmental Screens of Early Childhood	
Age (years)	**Activity**
2	Stairs, one step at a time
2½	Jumps
3	Stairs, alternating feet
4	Hops on one foot
5	Skips

(Adapted from Paine RS, Oppe TE: Neurologic examination of children, in *Clinics in Developmental Medicine*, Nos 20/21. London, England, William Heinemann Medical Books, 1966.)

Diagnostic Tests

Radiographs are rarely needed unless the child has evidence of short stature or if the possibility of hip dysplasia exists on history or physical examination. In a subset of patients, hip dysplasia is associated with increased femoral anteversion; occasionally, it is associated with true femoral torsion.

Differential Diagnosis

• External femoral torsion (femoral retroversion)
• Internal femoral torsion (excessive femoral anteversion)
• Metatarsus adductus (forefoot adducted)
• Neuromuscular disorders (cerebral palsy or others)
• Pes planovalgus (forefoot abducted, hindfoot valgus, results in external rotation during gait)
• Skeletal dysplasias (short stature)
• Tibial torsion (increased internal or external rotation of the tibia)

Adverse Outcomes of the Disease

Most children with intoeing or outtoeing do not have pain, and functional deficits are rare. Children with intoeing may trip more often than their peers, but this usually resolves with time. Compensatory external tibial torsion develops in some children with excessive femoral anteversion, resulting in so-called miserable malalignment syndrome. Children with miserable malalignment syndrome may require surgery in early adolescence for gait dysfunction and/or patellofemoral pain or subluxation refractory to nonsurgical treatment.

Treatment

Treatment focuses on education and reassurance for the family, as most cases will improve or resolve spontaneously. Shoe modifications, braces, and exercises do not alter the normal rotational development of the femoral and tibial axes. Foot deformities may

PEDIATRIC ORTHOPAEDICS

SECTION 9

require specific treatments, such as casting for persistent or rigid metatarsus adductus. Derotational osteotomy of the affected bone (femur or tibia) is reserved for the less than 1% of patients with severe torsional abnormalities. To allow for maximal spontaneous correction, a tibial osteotomy is usually not considered until 6 to 8 years of age, and a femoral osteotomy is delayed until at least 10 to 12 years of age. Chronic symptoms due to miserable malalignment syndrome are treated by correcting the rotational abnormalities at each level. In children with cerebral palsy and other neuromuscular disorders, abnormal femoral and tibial torsion persist in a much higher percentage of patients and are more likely to require surgical correction.

Adverse Outcomes of Treatment

Risks of surgery include failure to heal, infection, overcorrection or undercorrection of the deformity, and postoperative angular deformity. Risks of casting for metatarsus adductus are minimal.

Referral Decisions/Red Flags

Physicians who are familiar with the evaluation and examination of this problem can adequately reassure parents regarding the frequent resolution of these deformities. When metatarsus adductus persists in an infant older than 6 months, or when substantial rotational problems persist beyond 4 to 6 years of age, evaluation by a specialist is sometimes necessary to allay concerns of the parents or grandparents. Asymmetric intoeing can represent spasticity on the more severe side, although tibial torsion may be asymmetric; femoral anteversion should be symmetric, so asymmetry in hip rotation can represent spasticity or underlying bony abnormalities. Asymmetric outtoeing can be due to asymmetric tibial torsion, but outtoeing is a common position of comfort in the presence of injury, infection, or other bony abnormality; a full evaluation should be conducted for pain or limitations in joint range of motion and their potential etiologies.

Juvenile Idiopathic Arthritis

Synonyms

Juvenile chronic arthritis (JCA)
Juvenile rheumatoid arthritis (JRA)
Still disease

Definition

Formerly called juvenile rheumatoid arthritis (JRA) in North America and juvenile chronic arthritis (JCA) in Europe, juvenile idiopathic arthritis (JIA) is the term currently used for the various forms of chronic arthritis that affect children. At least seven types of arthritis occur in children (**Table 1**), but common to all JIA types is a chronic arthritis that persists for at least 6 weeks in a joint and begins in patients younger than 16 years.

Clinical Symptoms

All JIA is characterized by the classic symptoms of inflammatory arthritis: joint pain and swelling and inactivity stiffness (stiffness, usually on arising or after long periods of inactivity, such as after sleeping, that improves with activity). Small children may be unable to verbalize what or where the problem is, so they may just limp or

Table 1	
Types of Juvenile Idiopathic Arthritis	
Type	**Characteristics**
Systemic	Arthritis (any number of joints)
	High spiking fevers
	Rash
	Other systemic manifestations (lymphadenopathy, hepatosplenomegaly, pericarditis)
Oligoarticular	Arthritis in four or fewer joints
	High risk of asymptomatic uveitis
RF-negative polyarticular	Usually widespread polyarthritis in five or more joints
	RF not present
RF-positive polyarticular	Usually widespread symmetric polyarthritis in five or more joints
	Highly positive for RF
Psoriatic	Arthritis in any number of joints
	Associated with psoriasis, psoriatic nail changes, or first-degree relative with psoriasis
Enthesitis-related	Arthritis in any number of joints
	Associated with enthesitis, inflammatory spine arthritis, sacroiliitis
	Tendency to be HLA-B27 positive
Undifferentiated	Arthritis that does not fit into other classifications
RF = rheumatoid factor.	

be irritable when symptomatic. Each type of JIA has distinct ages of onset, associated symptoms, and sex predilection.

Systemic JIA is distinct from other types of JIA in that it is characterized by prominent systemic manifestations: daily spikes of high fever; evanescent (nonfixed) pink macular rash; and often liver, spleen, and/or lymph node enlargement, as well as serositis (usually pericarditis when it occurs). The arthritis may not be present initially in these patients, and when it is present, it can involve any number of joints. This disease affects boys and girls equally and can occur at any age; it is called Still disease in patients older than 16 years. Patients with systemic JIA are often quite ill and are anemic, with a very high white blood cell count, platelet count, erythrocyte sedimentation rate (ESR), and C-reactive protein (CRP) level. The ferritin level may be dramatically elevated.

Oligoarticular JIA (similar to what was formerly referred to as pauciarticular JRA) almost always occurs in girls and typically begins at a young age (younger than 6 years, and often at 2 years of age), with gradual onset of discomfort and swelling in one to four joints. The knee is the most commonly affected joint. The antinuclear antibody (ANA) test result may be positive; other blood tests results are almost always normal. Patients with oligoarticular JIA are at very high risk of the development of asymptomatic uveitis, so they must be screened every 3 months by an ophthalmologist. In some of these patients, more joint involvement may develop over the first 5 years; these patients are referred to as having extended oligoarticular JIA.

Rheumatoid factor (RF)–negative polyarticular JIA most commonly occurs in patients younger than 5 years, and usually by preadolescence. It is characterized by the gradual onset of polyarthritis involving five or more small and large joints. The pattern can be symmetric or asymmetric. Girls are three times more likely to be affected than boys. The ANA test may be positive and the ESR may be elevated, but in some patients, blood tests may be normal. RF-positive polyarticular JIA occurs in older children and adolescents, almost always older than 10 years. It is much more common in females. This aggressive, symmetric polyarthritis affects small and large joints and can be associated with rheumatoid nodules. RF-positive polyarticular JIA is virtually indistinguishable from adult rheumatoid arthritis. The ANA test and the anticyclic citrullinated peptide (CCP) antibody (anti-CCP) test result may be positive in these patients. The RF is positive by definition, usually in high titer. In active disease, the ESR is usually elevated.

Psoriatic JIA is arthritis associated with psoriasis and can affect any number of joints in a variable pattern (oligoarthritis, dactylitis, or polyarthritis). In children, the psoriasis can develop years after the arthritis, so a child with arthritis who has a strong family history of psoriasis or has nail changes (pitting or onycholysis) should be suspected of having this disorder. Chronic uveitis is common in this disease, so patients also need ophthalmologic screening three to four times per year.

Enthesitis-related JIA is arthritis associated with enthesitis (inflammation of tendons, fascia, or joint capsule insertions, especially around the heel). It can involve any number of joints but has a predilection for large weight-bearing joints. Boys are more often affected. Onset is usually at 6 years or older, and it occurs much more commonly in adolescents. A family history of spondyloarthropathies or inflammatory bowel disease often is present. Older children or adolescents may have inflammatory back pain and sacroiliitis, but these symptoms are often not present at onset. Most of these patients are HLA-B27–positive. Acute uveitis with sudden onset of a red, painful eye may occur. In some patients, spinal involvement can evolve into ankylosing spondylitis.

Undifferentiated JIA is chronic arthritis that occurs in patients younger than 16 years and that does not fit into one of the categories noted previously.

Tests

Physical Examination

A child with suspected arthritis or who has musculoskeletal pain or dysfunction should have all joints examined for possible arthritis because some children cannot verbalize their symptoms, and others may not report pain. Each joint should be (1) observed for obvious swelling, deformity, discoloration, surrounding muscular atrophy, and asymmetry with the opposite side; (2) palpated for warmth, tenderness, crepitus, and swelling and/or effusion; and (3) assessed for passive and active ranges of motion, including testing the ends of each arc of motion for even small amounts of loss of motion, and also assessed for pain at the ends of passive ranges of motion. The entheses around the heel and knee should be palpated for tenderness, and the spine and sacroiliac joints should be evaluated for tenderness and loss of motion. The temporomandibular joints may be affected even if they are asymptomatic, and they can become substantially deformed if untreated, so these should be examined carefully. The child's gait and strength should be evaluated. A general physical examination also should be performed because arthritis can be a sign/symptom of many other diseases that may have other physical findings or clues.

Diagnostic Tests

A general screening panel, including a complete blood cell count with differential, ESR and/or CRP level, comprehensive metabolic panel, and urinalysis should be ordered. In addition, depending on the type of arthritis the child may have (based on the history and examination), ferritin, RF, ANA, and HLA-B27 tests may be considered; however, it is important to remember that normal blood test results do not rule out JIA, and positive test results are not diagnostic. If the child appears to have a more acute form of arthritis, blood tests that detect other infectious and noninfectious causes should be ordered. Radiographs of involved joints should generally be obtained to exclude occult fractures, malignancy, or unsuspected bony dysplasias, but these will generally be normal in children with JIA of recent onset.

Differential Diagnosis

- Acute causes of arthritis (acute rheumatic fever, Lyme disease [Lyme arthritis], reactive arthritis, viral arthritis, especially parvovirus-associated arthritis)
- Enteropathic diseases (such as inflammatory bowel disease and celiac disease) (usually associated with abdominal pain, diarrhea, weight loss, poor growth)
- Hemophilic arthropathy (history of easy bruising or extreme bleeding)
- Leukemia and metastatic neuroblastoma (night pain, bone pain with refusal to bear weight, joint pain or effusion)
- Lupus and other rheumatic diseases (often associated with signs of other organ system involvement such as various rashes, fever, proteinuria/hematuria, weight loss, hypertension)
- Mechanical joint pain (occurs after increased activity and not after inactivity, symptoms of locking and "giving way," can be associated with hypermobility)
- Osteomyelitis (fever, severe pain with refusal to bear weight, toxic appearance and point tenderness of the involved bone)
- Septic arthritis (constant fever, usually single joint involvement, more severe pain, and refusal to move the joint)

Adverse Outcomes of the Disease

Contrary to popular belief, spontaneous remission is uncommon, although some types of JIA have a better prognosis than others. Most patients will have chronic arthritis into adulthood and may have substantial joint/bone deformities and limitations. Blindness can result from untreated uveitis. Persistent or untreated joint inflammation can result in progressive degenerative joint changes.

Treatment

Treatment depends on the type of JIA and the severity of the arthritis. NSAIDs are the first-line drugs. If only a few joints are involved, intra-articular steroids can be used. Unless arthritis is very mild, most patients are treated with disease-modifying antirheumatic drugs, primarily methotrexate, but also anti–tumor necrosis factor (TNF) agents such as etanercept, infliximab, and adalimumab. Infliximab and adalimumab also are useful in refractory uveitis. Other biologics used for JIA include abatacept (a T cell costimulation blocker), interleukin (IL)-1 blocking agents such as anakinra (especially for systemic JIA), anti–B cell antibodies such as rituximab (for RF-positive polyarticular JIA), and anti–IL-6. These treatments should be administered with the guidance of an experienced pediatric rheumatologist. Rehabilitation helps maintain joint motion and strength when the pain has diminished. Children should be encouraged to participate in as much physical activity as tolerated. Splinting is generally not helpful unless a substantial flexion contracture exists, and the splint should be used only at night. Orthoses can help maintain functional joint alignment. Regular ophthalmologic slit lamp examinations for uveitis are necessary, with the frequency of this examination dependent on the type of JIA, results of the ANA test, and the age of the child.

Adverse Outcomes of Treatment

NSAIDs can cause gastric, renal, or hepatic complications. Methotrexate requires regular safety monitoring and can cause centrally induced nausea. Increased susceptibility to infection is a concern with any biologic agent, but fungal and tuberculous infections are a particular concern with anti-TNF agents, so patients on these medications should be screened and monitored. Whether these agents can increase susceptibility to secondary malignancies is not known.

Referral Decisions/Red Flags

Atypical symptoms such as unexplained fever or severe pain and refusal to bear weight indicate the need for further evaluation. All patients suspected of having JIA should probably be referred to a pediatric rheumatologist if possible.

SECTION 9 PEDIATRIC ORTHOPAEDICS

Kyphosis

Synonyms
Juvenile kyphosis
Postural roundback
Scheuermann disease

Definition
Kyphosis is the normal spine profile of the thoracic region of the spinal column. It originates from the Greek word kyphos, meaning "humpbacked," and refers to a curve in the sagittal plane (the apex of the curve is posterior). The normal range of thoracic kyphosis is 20° to 50° (Cobb angle from T3 to T12), and values greater than 50° are considered hyperkyphotic. Conditions associated with hyperkyphosis in children are listed under Differential Diagnosis.

Postural kyphosis and Scheuermann disease are the most common causes of hyperkyphosis, and both present during adolescence. Postural kyphosis is a flexible deformity that is more common in girls, and patients are able to correct the kyphosis voluntarily. Scheuermann disease, in contrast, is more common in boys and is not passively correctable. Scheuermann disease is diagnosed radiographically as a hyperkyphosis associated with anterior wedging of more than 5° in at least three successive vertebrae, usually with disk space narrowing, irregularities of the vertebral end plates, and Schmorl nodes (herniations of disk material through the vertebral end plates). Congenital kyphosis implies a structural defect in vertebral formation and may become apparent in infants and toddlers. The other forms of kyphosis may be diagnosed throughout childhood and more commonly in adolescence.

Clinical Symptoms
Most patients are seen for cosmetic concerns, poor posture, and/or activity-related discomfort in the mid to low thoracic spine. Any discomfort is usually relieved by rest. Neurologic symptoms are very uncommon, except with congenital kyphosis.

Tests
Physical Examination
Hyperkyphosis is apparent when viewing the patient from the side, and the deformity worsens with the Adam forward bend test (**Figure 1**). Adolescents with Scheuermann disease and other pathologic causes of kyphosis usually have a sharp angulation at the apex of the kyphosis, whereas patients with postural kyphosis have a more gentle curvature. Patients with postural kyphosis have normal flexibility (that is, the spine flattens in the supine position). The neurologic examination is usually normal in postural hyperkyphosis and Scheuermann disease but may be abnormal with other forms of kyphosis, especially when the deformity is severe. Hamstring

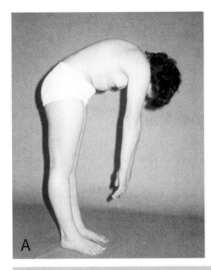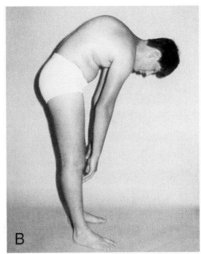

Figure 1 Photographs of the Adam forward bend test. **A,** Normal spine profile. **B,** Angulated spine profile seen in a patient with Scheuermann disease. (Reproduced from Staheli L, ed: *Pediatric Orthopaedic Secrets.* Hanley & Belfus, Philadelphia, PA, 1998, p 286.)

spasm and/or contracture are common with pathologic forms of hyperkyphosis.

Diagnostic Tests

AP and lateral radiographs of the entire spine should be obtained with the patient standing. The reviewer should look for congenital abnormalities as well as irregularities of the vertebrae, disk spaces, and the end plates. The curve magnitude is measured on the lateral radiograph using the Cobb method. When the upper thoracic vertebrae cannot be well visualized, kyphosis should be measured from T5 to T12. The angle is formed by the intersection of a line drawn along the superior end plate of T5 and a line drawn on the inferior end plate of T12. Kyphosis exceeding 50° is considered abnormal.

Differential Diagnosis

- Congenital
    - Failure of formation (hemivertebra)
    - Failure of segmentation (congenital fusion or wedge vertebra)
- Connective tissue diseases
    - Marfan syndrome (ligamentous hyperlaxity)
    - Osteogenesis imperfecta (frequent fractures, low bone mass)
- Dysplasias
    - Achondroplasia (short stature)
    - Mucopolysaccharidosis (short stature, neurologic symptoms)
    - Neurofibromatosis (café-au-lait spots, subcutaneous neurofibromas, inguinal and/or axillary freckling)
- Iatrogenic (history of steroid use, radiation, or surgery)

SECTION 9 PEDIATRIC ORTHOPAEDICS

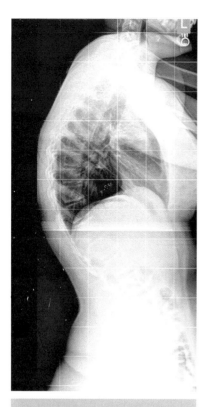

Figure 2 Lateral radiograph from a 15-year-old girl demonstrates development of a progressive and rigid posture problem associated with back pain. The radiograph demonstrates abnormalities that suggest thoracic Scheuermann disease. Although most patients with hyperkyphosis can be treated nonsurgically, this patient ultimately required an instrumented posterior spinal fusion.

- Infectious (fever, constant pain)
    Fungal (other fungal infections)
    Tuberculosis (Pott disease, other mycobacterial infections)
- Inflammatory
    Juvenile idiopathic arthritis requiring prolonged steroids (multiple joint involvement, osteopenia)
- Metabolic
    Gaucher disease (stress fractures due to other etiologies)
    Osteoporosis (chronic steroid use, idiopathic osteoporosis of childhood)
    Thalassemia (other anemias)
- Neoplastic (constant pain, signs of systemic illness)
    Eosinophilic granuloma (other infections)
    Leukemia (other infections)
- Neuromuscular (such as cerebral palsy, spinal muscular atrophy)
- Postural hyperkyphosis (patient can self-correct)
- Scheuermann disease (activity-related back pain)
- Traumatic (fractures or ligamentous injuries)

Adverse Outcomes of the Disease

The natural history of flexible or postural hyperkyphosis is benign, and these curves are unlikely to progress, but other forms of kyphosis present a substantial risk for progression. The consequences of a progressive kyphosis can include back pain; rarely, neurologic symptoms, usually seen with congenital kyphosis; and a decrease in pulmonary function, seen with curvatures greater than 90° to 100° (restrictive pattern).

Treatment

Postural kyphosis can be treated with an exercise program. Progressive curvatures due to Scheuermann disease in patients who are skeletally immature can be treated using a bracing program (full-time wear, Milwaukee brace or equivalent), and a subset of patients with progressive and symptomatic curvatures greater than 70° are candidates for a posterior or an anterior/posterior spinal fusion with instrumentation (**Figure 2**). Congenital kyphosis is much more likely to require surgical intervention, sometimes in the first few years of life. Bracing is not effective in patients with congenital deformities, and progressive deformities often require surgical stabilization.

Adverse Outcomes of Treatment

Bracing may not prevent progression. Surgical treatment can be complicated by progression of deformity above or below the fused levels (that is, proximal junction kyphosis [PJK]), nonunion of the fusion (pseudarthrosis), infection, implant-related complications such as loss of fixation or correction, medical problems such as pneumonia, and rarely, spinal cord injury.

Referral Decisions/Red Flags
Deformities of greater magnitude, especially those associated with a structural component and/or pain, require evaluation by a specialist.

PEDIATRIC ORTHOPAEDICS

SECTION 9

Legg-Calvé-Perthes Disease

Synonyms
Aseptic necrosis of the femoral head
Avascular necrosis of the femoral head
(Idiopathic) osteonecrosis of the femoral head
LCPD

Definition
Legg-Calvé-Perthes disease (LCPD) is an idiopathic osteonecrosis of the femoral head in children. It is most commonly diagnosed in boys between 4 and 8 years of age. Although numerous etiologic theories have been pursued, such as heritable coagulopathy and secondhand smoke, none has been proved. Most patients (90%) with LCPD are delayed in bone age, and one third may have a diagnosis of attention deficit hyperactivity disorder. A small percentage of patients have a history of transient synovitis of the hip, and 10% to 12% have bilateral disease. The physiology of the healing process in LCPD involves revascularization of the femoral head and replacement with viable bone that is initially relatively weak (woven bone), followed by remodeling of woven bone to normal lamellar bone. This biologic process occurs more rapidly and with greater consistency in children, but it still takes time. The clinical symptoms often last up to 18 months, and radiographic healing and remodeling may take 4 to 5 years. The prognosis is worse in older children (because they have less potential for joint remodeling) and in patients with greater degrees of epiphyseal involvement. In older patients with severe involvement, deformation of the femoral head and some incongruity between the femoral head and the acetabulum can result, which can result in premature arthritis.

Clinical Symptoms
Typically, the child has been limping for 3 to 6 weeks by the time of the initial visit. Activity worsens the limp, making symptoms more noticeable at the end of the day. If the child reports pain, it is typically an aching in the groin or proximal thigh. For knee pain, the hip should always be assessed.

Tests
Physical Examination
Range-of-motion testing will reveal restriction, especially in abduction and internal rotation, and there may be guarding at the extremes of motion. A flexion contracture also can develop. The gait examination will reveal an abductor lurch or Trendelenburg gait, and atrophy of the gluteal muscles also may be identified. Standing on the

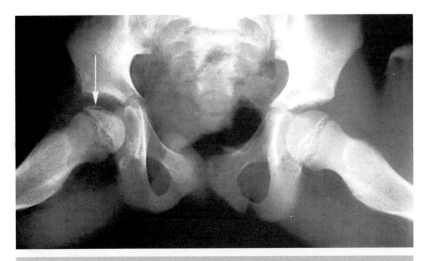

Figure 1 Frog-lateral radiograph from a 7-year-old boy with a 2-month history of right hip pain who was diagnosed with Legg-Calvé-Perthes disease. The subchondral fracture (arrow) extends through 75% of the femoral head. (Reproduced from Beaty JH: Legg-Calvé-Perthes disease: Diagnostic and prognostic techniques. *Instr Course Lect* 1989;38:291-296.)

affected limb will often show a Trendelenburg sign when compared with the opposite, unaffected limb.

Diagnostic Tests

AP and frog-lateral radiographs of the pelvis should be obtained; these may be normal very early in the disease course. MRI is not needed for all cases but can be useful when the diagnosis is elusive. Findings on plain radiographs evolve over 2 to 5 years, and various stages have been described. Initial findings include a decrease in the size of the ossific nucleus and an increase in density (sclerosis), usually during the first 6 to 9 months. The crescent sign, which represents a subchondral fracture, is seen on frog-lateral radiographs in many patients (**Figure 1**). Next is the fragmentation stage, with collapse of the epiphysis to a variable degree. This is followed by the reossification phase, when healing starts. The osteonecrosis often affects the physis, resulting in chronic changes in the alignment and morphology of the femoral head and neck, including shortening and widening of the femoral neck and valgus alignment of the proximal femur. Coxa magna, or enlargement of the femoral head, is a common finding as well. In patients with bilateral LCPD, the disease progression is typically metachronous (not synchronous) with both hips in different stages of the disease process (**Figure 2**). In a child with bilateral involvement and symmetric radiographic changes, screening AP radiographs of the hand, knee, and spine are needed to rule out an epiphyseal dysplasia, and laboratory studies should be obtained to rule out hypothyroidism.

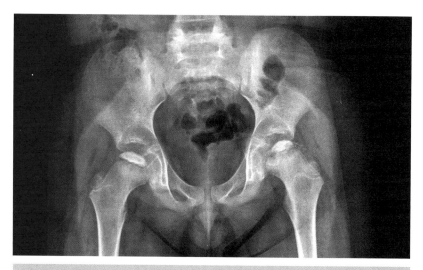

Figure 2 AP radiograph from a 6-year-old boy with bilateral Legg-Calvé-Perthes disease. The radiographic changes are typically asymmetric, and onset of symptoms may be months apart.

Differential Diagnosis

- Atypical septic arthritis (increasing pain and constitutional symptoms)
- Gaucher disease (osteonecrosis secondary to cerebroside and infarcts)
- Hypothyroidism (delayed development)
- Leukemia (constant pain, night pain)
- Multiple epiphyseal dysplasia (bilateral, mild short stature, autosomal dominant)
- Sickle cell anemia (osteonecrosis secondary to vascular infarcts)
- Spondyloepiphyseal dysplasia (bilateral, marked short stature)
- Stickler syndrome (bilateral, short stature)
- Transient synovitis (history of recent viral illness, mild limp)

Adverse Outcomes of the Disease

Residual deformity of the femoral head and incongruity between the femoral head and the acetabulum can result in premature degenerative changes in the hip (**Figure 3**). Limb-length discrepancy also is common.

Treatment

The treatment of LCPD has been a subject of much controversy, and it remains unclear what strategies will alter the natural history, especially in patients at high risk for a poor outcome (such as older patients with substantial involvement of the proximal femoral epiphysis). The overall goal of any treatment is to achieve an outcome in which normal sphericity of the femoral head and congruence is maintained between the femoral head and the acetabulum. During the early phases, the patient is treated with activity restriction

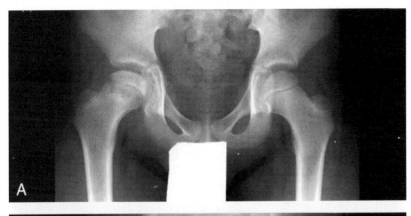

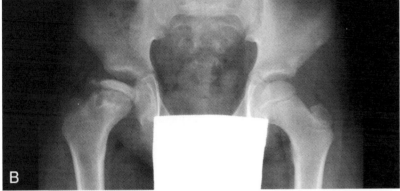

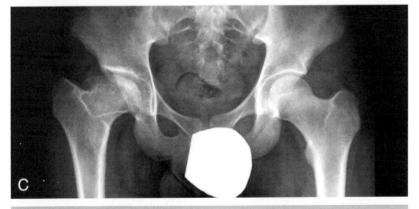

Figure 3 AP pelvis radiographs from a patient with right-sided Legg-Calvé-Perthes disease. **A,** Radiograph obtained on presentation demonstrates increased density in the entire epiphysis. **B,** Radiograph obtained during the fragmentation stage demonstrates progressive collapse of the epiphysis. **C,** Radiograph obtained at final healing several years later demonstrates enlargement of the femoral head (coxa magna) with asphericity and shortening/widening of the femoral neck. Note that the acetabulum also has remodeled, resulting in aspherical congruence.

(with or without short periods of bed rest) and anti-inflammatory drugs, and symptoms and range of motion are monitored closely. Rehabilitation may help to achieve and maintain motion. Patients younger than 5 years are more likely to have an excellent outcome without the need for more invasive treatment. Patients with persistent loss of motion may benefit from an examination under anesthesia with an arthrogram to evaluate the sphericity of the femoral head.

Concomitant release of the adductors is frequently performed to improve range of motion. Long leg casts with a spreader bar (Petrie casts) are then worn for 6 weeks. Patients who are considered to have a poor prognosis based on age and degree of involvement or in whom subluxation of the femoral head develops may be candidates for so-called containment treatment. Containment is achieved when the healing femoral head is completely within the acetabulum. Containment treatment can be nonsurgical (abduction bracing) or surgical (femoral osteotomy, pelvic osteotomy, combined osteotomy). The theory is that the contained femoral head has the best likelihood of spherical healing. Nonsurgical containment by full-time use of a long leg abduction brace is difficult to enforce and has not been shown to alter the outcomes, and thus it is rarely recommended. Currently, when containment is indicated, surgical intervention is recommended, although insufficient evidence exists to support one particular strategy over another.

Adverse Outcomes of Treatment

In addition to surgical complications (bleeding, infection, implant-related problems), the treatment may not alter the natural history of the disease. Treatment also can exacerbate limb-length discrepancy and/or gait disturbance.

Referral Decisions/Red Flags

Most children younger than 6 years who have substantial involvement of the femoral head or less than 40° of abduction require further evaluation. Children 6 years or older require further evaluation.

SECTION 9 PEDIATRIC ORTHOPAEDICS

Little Leaguer's Elbow

Synonyms

Medial epicondylar fracture or avulsion
Olecranon stress fracture
Osteochondritis dissecans (OCD) of the elbow
Panner disease
Traction apophysitis of the elbow
Valgus-extension overload syndrome

Definition

Little Leaguer's elbow is the name applied to several pathologic entities that share a common etiology (overuse in the overhead throwing athlete) and a common age group (range, 8 to 16 years). The term is too general, however; it is preferable and more accurate to use the name of specific pathologic entities when possible. These include injuries resulting from traction or tension (for example, traction apophysitis of the medial epicondyle or olecranon, medial epicondylar fragmentation or avulsion, olecranon avulsion, and ulnar collateral ligament sprains or tears) and injuries resulting from compression (such as osteochondritis dissecans [OCD] of the capitellum, Panner disease) (**Figure 1**).

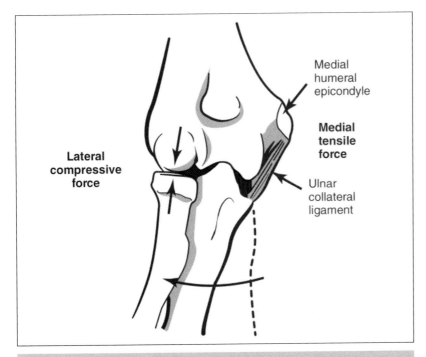

Figure 1 Illustration depicts forces at the elbow during overhead throwing. Compression forces occur on the lateral side, and tension forces occur on the medial side. Medial forces cause a medial humeral epicondyle stress fracture in the skeletally immature patient rather than an ulnar collateral ligament sprain, as seen in adults.

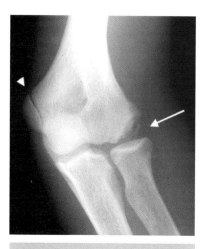

Figure 2 AP elbow radiograph from a left-handed baseball pitcher demonstrates osteochondritis dissecans lesion of the capitellum (arrow) with an open medial humerus epiphysis (arrowhead). (Reproduced from Hutchinson MR, Ireland ML: Overuse and throwing injuries in the skeletally immature patient. *Instr Course Lect* 2003;52:25-36.)

Traction apophysitis of the medial epicondyle is inflammation or injury to the unfused medial epicondyle that occurs as a result of overuse in the overhead throwing athlete who is skeletally immature. Fragmentation of the medial epicondyle can occur in the young athlete (range, 8 to 12 years), whereas avulsion of the medial epicondyle typically occurs in patients closer to physeal closure (range, 12 to 14 years). Similarly, traction apophysitis of the olecranon is an injury of the unfused olecranon physis in the young throwing athlete. Fragmentation of the olecranon epiphysis is rare, and avulsion is less common than with the medial epicondyle. Delayed or failed closure of the olecranon physis more commonly occurs as a result of overuse and can result in chronic pain.

Injuries of the ulnar collateral ligament are now recognized with increasing frequency in the adolescent overhead throwing athlete. This injury is more completely described in the chapter on ulnar collateral ligament injuries.

OCD occurs in adolescents (typically, older than 12 years) after the capitellum has ossified. This condition is characterized by focal osteonecrosis of the capitellum (but rarely the radial head) with varied degrees of subchondral separation and is frequently associated with overuse in the thrower (**Figure 2**). Osteochondral detachment and loose body formation is common, resulting in mechanical signs and symptoms.

Panner disease, which often is confused with OCD, is seen in children younger than 12 years and consists of a focal avascular lesion of the capitellum that typically is self-limited and has a good prognosis.

Clinical Symptoms

These conditions occur in the young overhead throwing athlete with a history of overuse, often a history of an excessive number of pitches per game, excessive number of innings pitched per week (or year), year-round participation in the throwing sport, and the premature use of the breaking ball (curveball or slider) before reaching adequate skeletal maturity. Pain, either chronic or acute, is the most common symptom.

Tests

Physical Examination

Tenderness to palpation is the most common physical finding and can be medial (medial epicondylar traction apophysitis, medial epicondylar fragmentation/avulsion, ulnar collateral ligament injuries), lateral (OCD, Panner disease), or posterior (olecranon traction apophysitis/avulsion). Flexion contractures are common. Instability may be seen in ulnar collateral ligament injuries or severe OCD with loss of capitellar lateral bony support.

Diagnostic Tests

Radiographs of the elbow help establish most of these diagnoses. Obtaining a comparison view of the contralateral side is essential to better visualize subtle changes. MRI often is necessary to confirm OCD, Panner disease, and ulnar collateral ligament injuries.

Differential Diagnosis

- Cubital tunnel syndrome/ulnar neuritis (rarely seen in this age group)
- Fractures of the radial head, olecranon, or supracondylar humerus (radiographs differentiate)
- Lateral epicondylitis/tendinosis (rarely seen in this age group)
- Medial epicondylitis/tendinosis (rarely seen in this age group)

Adverse Outcomes of the Disease

Persistent pain, inability to participate in sports, chronic instability, and loss of motion are possible. Medial epicondylar avulsion can result in late ulnar palsy. OCD can result in loose body formation and, in more severe cases, osteoarthritis.

Treatment

Because these conditions technically are overuse injuries, the most critical component of treatment is rest. At least 3 to 6 months of rest from throwing is appropriate for these problems. In OCD, abstaining from pitching for 1 year may be necessary. Rehabilitation is helpful during this time to help maintain strength and restore motion. Immobilization should be avoided, except for possible brief periods in the acute phase, given the likelihood of substantial and perhaps permanent loss of motion. Even with appropriate rest, the athlete may not be able to resume pitching, and a change in position or sport may be recommended. Nonsurgical care usually is appropriate, but surgical intervention is occasionally necessary to remove loose bodies.

Adverse Outcomes of Treatment

Surgery is associated with a small risk of infection, hardware failure, or neurovascular injury.

Referral Decisions/Red Flags

Further evaluation is needed if nonsurgical treatment fails.

Prevention

Given the increasing incidence of overuse injuries and the likelihood that results will be suboptimal even with appropriate care, prevention is emphasized. Education of athletes, parents, and coaches is critical, and governing bodies of youth baseball organizations must be willing to make rule changes for the long-term benefit of these athletes. Year-round pitching is not advised, and participation in baseball showcases should be restricted. Participation in other sports should

SECTION 9 PEDIATRIC ORTHOPAEDICS

Table 1	
Recommended Ages for Learning Various Pitches	
Pitch	**Recommended Age (years)**
Changeup	11 to 12 (or when sufficient velocity and control have been developed with the fastball)
Curveball	14.5
Slider	18

Table 2		
Recommended Pitching Limits		
Age (years)	**Maximum Number of Pitches Thrown per Game**	**Maximum Number of Innings Pitched per Week**
8-10	50	6
11-14	75	6
15-18	90 to 100	10

be encouraged. General physical conditioning and proper pitching mechanics should be emphasized. Current recommendations for pitchers are provided in **Tables 1** and **2**.

Metatarsus Adductus

Synonym
Metatarsus varus

Definition
Metatarsus adductus is a common foot deformity in infancy characterized by medial deviation (adduction) of the forefoot. It is most often due to deformation resulting from intrauterine positioning (**Figure 1**). The deformity is observed in approximately 13% of full-term infants. It resolves spontaneously in most patients. Some cases of rigid adductus of the forefoot or midfoot are caused by congenital bony abnormalities, and these deformities persist even with nonsurgical treatment. Metatarsus adductus is commonly associated with other intrauterine positional deformations such as congenital muscular torticollis, medial tibial torsion, and rarely, hip dysplasia.

Clinical Symptoms
Most patients are asymptomatic. Parental concern is the major reason for early referral. Pain is rarely reported.

Tests
Physical Examination
The patient presents with adduction of the forefoot relative to the hindfoot, with a convexity of the lateral border of the foot. The

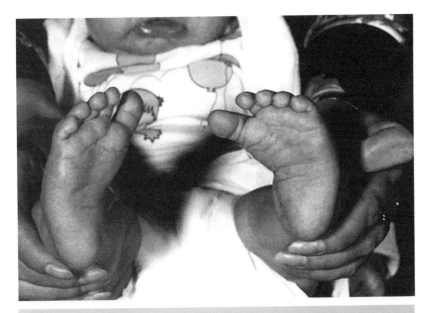

Figure 1 Photograph of a 3-month-old infant with obvious metatarsus adductus. The foot appears to be supinated; however, when the foot was placed in a weight-bearing position, the hindfoot alignment was normal. (Reproduced from Greene WB: Metatarsus adductus and skewfoot. *Instr Course Lect* 1994;43:161-177.)

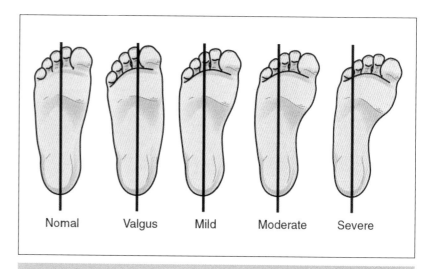

Nomal   Valgus   Mild   Moderate   Severe

Figure 2 Illustration depicts classification of metatarsus adductus using the heel bisector line described by Bleck. (Reproduced from Scaduto AA, Frost NL: Pediatric foot conditions, in Boyer MI, ed: *AAOS Comprehensive Orthopaedic Review,* ed 2. Rosemont, IL, American Academy of Orthopaedic Surgeons, 2014, p 690.)

hindfoot is in neutral or increased valgus and never demonstrates a varus posture. Normal ankle dorsiflexion also is present; these latter two findings are important because some children with severe metatarsus adductus may, at first inspection, appear to have a clubfoot deformity. Some patients also will have a mild plantar flexion deformity of the medial column of the foot, giving the appearance of an elevated longitudinal arch. An "atavistic" or "wandering" great toe (adduction of the great toe) also may be observed in association with the condition; it typically resolves over the first several years of life.

The severity of metatarsus adductus can be assessed using the heel bisector line (**Figure 2**). Normally, a line bisecting the heel passes through the second toe or the second and third toes. Metatarsus adductus is considered mild when the heel bisector crosses the third toe, moderate when the heel bisector crosses between the third and fourth toes, and severe when the heel bisector crosses between the fourth and fifth toes. The flexibility of the deformity determines the prognosis and helps identify the subset of patients who require treatment. Flexibility is assessed by first holding the hindfoot in varus to stabilize the subtalar joint, and abducting the forefoot relative to the hindfoot. If the foot can be abducted fully, the heel bisector will fall between the great toe and the second toe, demonstrating that the deformity is fully flexible and will likely resolve spontaneously. The foot also may be moderately flexible, where the alignment improves with stress but the heel bisector cannot be brought in line with the second toe. Truly rigid deformities are rare. The deformity can have a dynamic component from overactivity of the adductor hallucis, which makes the deformity more dramatic when the patient is walking.

Diagnostic Tests

Radiographs are rarely needed, but they are indicated when the deformity cannot be passively corrected or fails to respond to nonsurgical treatment. In such cases, obliquity of the medial cuneiform may be present, resulting in adduction of the great toe. Obtaining serial photocopies of the foot is a low-cost, no-risk method of charting the progression of metatarsus adductus (**Figure 3**). Hip ultrasonography may be indicated if the hip examination is abnormal or if the history and/or other physical findings (such as other intrauterine positional deformities) suggest a risk of hip dysplasia.

Differential Diagnosis

- Clubfoot (heel in varus, ankle in equinus)
- Hyperactive abductor hallucis (lateral border of the foot remains straight)
- Internal tibial torsion (foot rotated in, lateral border of the foot straight)
- Skeletal dysplasia (most common in diastrophic dwarfism)
- Skewfoot (Z or serpentine foot, valgus hindfoot and forefoot adduction)

Adverse Outcomes of the Disease

Cosmetic concerns and the inability to wear certain types of shoes are the most likely consequences of persistent metatarsus adductus. Abnormal shoe wear and discomfort are possible but much less likely.

Treatment

Most newborns do not require active treatment, because metatarsus adductus usually corrects spontaneously. Parents are advised to avoid positioning the infant prone with the feet turned in, a position that accentuates metatarsus adductus. If a structural component to the deformity exists (the foot does not passively overcorrect on physical examination), serial casting should be considered. Patients with structural deformities should be referred early, because correction is easiest to achieve during the first few months of life. Casts are applied for 2-week periods; usually, three or four casts will suffice. Casting can be successful in children from 1 to 3 years of age but is more difficult at these ages and is associated with a higher rate of failure. The cast should be applied in a manner that molds the forefoot into abduction without accentuating heel valgus. Neither stretching exercises nor nighttime splints (or outflare shoes) have proven value, but they are often considered as a supplement to casting for structural deformities. Very few cases of metatarsus adductus require surgical treatment. Soft-tissue releases have not been associated with favorable outcomes; thus, an osteotomy of the midfoot or the metatarsals is required to realign the foot. Dynamic hallux varus will resolve spontaneously and requires no specific treatment.

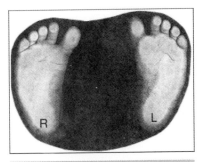

Figure 3 Photocopy of the feet of a 9-month-old infant with bilateral metatarsus adductus. (Reproduced from Greene WB: Metatarsus adductus and skewfoot. *Instr Course Lect* 1994;43:161-177.)

SECTION 9 PEDIATRIC ORTHOPAEDICS

Adverse Outcomes of Treatment

Recurrent deformity can occur even with serial casting. Complications of casting include increased heel valgus and the development of a flatfoot or skewfoot deformity. Degenerative changes at the tarsometatarsal joints have been noted after soft-tissue releases of the tarsometatarsal joints, and this procedure is no longer performed. Complications of osteotomies include undercorrection or overcorrection. Damage to the physis of the first metatarsal with subsequent shortening of that bone is a complication of a first metatarsal osteotomy.

Referral Decisions/Red Flags

Residual metatarsus adductus in an infant 3 to 6 months of age or a rigid metatarsus adductus in any infant signals the need for further evaluation.

SECTION 9   PEDIATRIC ORTHOPAEDICS

Neonatal Brachial Plexus Palsy

Synonyms

Obstetric brachial plexus palsy (OBPP)

Obstetric palsy

Definition

Neonatal brachial plexus palsy, sometimes called obstetric palsy, is a motor and sensory deficit of the upper extremity resulting from a stretch injury to the brachial plexus during labor and delivery. The incidence is between 0.4 and 4.0 per 1,000 live births. Three common patterns exist. The most common pattern is Erb palsy, affecting the nerves at C5-C6, which is seen in almost 50% of cases and results in weakness of elbow flexion and weakness of shoulder abduction, flexion, and external rotation. Patients with Erb palsy have the best prognosis for recovery. Klumpke palsy, a lesion of the lower plexus (C8-T1) that affects the hand and wrist, represents 30% of cases. Panplexus palsy involves the entire plexus and represents 20% of cases.

The spectrum of injury ranges from a minor stretch of the nerves (temporary conduction block) to a partial or complete rupture of the nerves or avulsion of the nerve root from the spinal cord. The prognosis is based on the severity of the injury. Most cases are transient, and spontaneous recovery of antigravity strength during the first 2 months predicts a high likelihood of full recovery. Patients who do not exhibit return to biceps function after 3 months of age rarely have a full recovery. Poor prognostic factors include involvement of the entire brachial plexus, Horner syndrome, and nerve root avulsions. Subtle long-term findings such as limb shortening and reduction in limb girth also may be of concern to patients.

Clinical Symptoms

Reduced spontaneous movement, or pseudoparalysis, is commonly observed. The patient may exhibit discomfort or irritability if an associated fracture of the clavicle or humerus is present.

Tests

Physical Examination

Examination findings vary depending on the pattern of nerve injury. They include diminished spontaneous movement of the upper extremity as well as impaired reflexes (Moro reflex, symmetric and asymmetric tonic neck reflexes). Initially, the upper extremity appears to be flail. Tenderness in the supraclavicular triangle may be present during the first few weeks after birth.

The classic appearance of a neonate with Erb palsy is the "waiter's tip" position (shoulder adducted and internally rotated, elbow

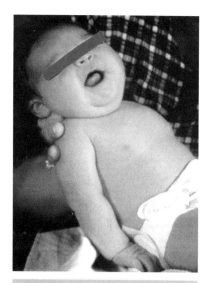

Figure 1 Photograph shows the typical posture ("waiter's tip" position) of a child with Erb palsy.

extended, forearm pronated, and wrist flexed) (**Figure 1**). It is important to determine whether the lesion is preganglionic (no potential for recovery) or postganglionic. Findings consistent with a preganglionic avulsion injury include involvement of the sympathetic chain (Horner syndrome), phrenic nerve paralysis, and involvement of other nerves coming off the plexus (long thoracic, dorsal scapular, suprascapular, and thoracodorsal).

Repeated examinations of muscle and sensory function are needed to correlate the physical findings with an anatomic location of injury and to assess the degree and rate of neurologic recovery. Failure to recover muscle balance results in contractures and limited motion, particularly at the shoulder and elbow.

Diagnostic Tests

Radiographs should be ordered if the physical examination results suggest a fracture of the clavicle or humerus. If the infant does not recover full function, electromyography and nerve conduction velocity studies can help guide decisions regarding surgical options. CT and MRI have been used to assess glenohumeral anatomy in patients with internal rotation contractures.

Differential Diagnosis

- Clavicle fracture (tenderness and deformity on palpation, pain on passive range of motion, possible pseudoparalysis that resolves in 1 to 2 weeks)
- Humerus fracture (swelling, deformity, and pain with range of motion of the arm, possible pseudoparalysis that resolves in 1 to 2 weeks)
- Proximal humeral osteomyelitis (cessation of normal motion, but infant may not appear toxic)
- Septic arthritis of the shoulder or elbow (cessation of normal motion, but infant may not appear toxic)

Adverse Outcomes of the Disease

The prognosis varies depending on the severity of the neurologic injury. Early evidence of recovery portends a good prognosis With Erb palsy, persistent weakness and muscle imbalance can result in progressive contractures (internal shoulder rotation), which is associated with early development of subluxation or dislocation in more than 60% of patients within the first 2 years. Radial head instability also may develop. Neurologic function may fail to improve sufficiently even with treatment. Permanent neurologic deficits can interfere with upper extremity function and may require reconstructive surgery. Bony deformities can develop and progress despite tendon transfers. Diminished overall growth potential of the extremity can occur.

Treatment

Initial treatment consists of rehabilitation to maintain joint range of motion; a supervised home exercise program may best accomplish this goal. Gentle passive range-of-motion exercise several times per day, with special attention to external rotation of the shoulder, is needed to prevent posterior subluxation of the shoulder. Motor function is evaluated at regular intervals. Early referral to a specialist is indicated if recovery is not observed within the first few weeks. The cornerstones of treatment are the detailed assessment and monitoring of neurologic function and recovery, the prevention of secondary deformities, and identifying the subset of patients who may benefit from surgical intervention to treat the neurologic impairment and/or the long-term musculoskeletal sequelae of muscle weakness/imbalance. Given the spectrum of pathology, surgical treatment needs to be individualized.

The procedures are varied and include microsurgical reconstruction (nerve grafts, nerve transfers), soft-tissue release/lengthening and/or derotational osteotomies, and tendon transfers. Although the field is advancing rapidly, many controversies remain, especially the timing and specific nature of interventions. Patients with Erb palsy who show evidence of recovery by 3 months are typically treated nonsurgically and have a good to excellent prognosis. The most recent information suggests that early microsurgical reconstruction (by 3 months) is increasingly favored in patients with global lesions and Horner syndrome, based on the poor prognosis without surgical intervention. The traditional approach to reinnervation included resection of scarred areas and nerve grafting (sural nerve), but recently, nerve transfer procedures have been performed with greater frequency. Nerve transfers, in which a viable nerve is anastomosed to one of the injured nerves, also can be performed in conjunction with nerve grafting procedures. Nerve transfers also have been used at a later time to improve motor strength in patients with partial recovery, whether or not early microsurgical reconstruction has been performed. Synthetic collagen nerve conduits also are under investigation as an alternative to nerve grafts.

Children with substantial muscle imbalance about the shoulder, elbow, and hand should undergo appropriate muscle releases and tendon transfers to provide a balanced upper extremity. The development of an internal rotation contracture at the shoulder can rapidly result in deformity of the glenohumeral joint, with progressive subluxation or dislocation, and early release can help stabilize the joint and prevent deformity. In older patients with substantial internal rotation contracture, a humeral derotational osteotomy will improve external rotation at the shoulder.

Referral Decisions/Red Flags

Referral is appropriate shortly after birth. Sepsis or skeletal trauma (child abuse) must be suspected if a sudden loss of function occurs in an extremity that moved well at birth.

SECTION 9 PEDIATRIC ORTHOPAEDICS

Osgood-Schlatter Disease

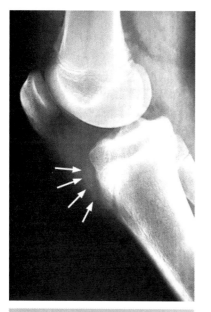

Figure 1 Lateral radiograph demonstrates symptomatic tibial tubercle ossicle (arrows) in a 13-year-old boy with Osgood-Schlatter disease. (Reproduced from Stanitski CL: Knee overuse disorders in the pediatric and adolescent athlete. *Instr Course Lect* 1993;42:483-495.)

Synonyms

Osteochondritis of the inferior patella
Osteochondritis of the tibial tuberosity
Tibial tubercle traction apophysitis

Definition

Osgood-Schlatter disease (or condition) is an overuse injury in the growing child that results from repetitive stress when a too-tight quadriceps "pulls" on the apophysis (secondary ossification center) of the tibial tubercle during a time of rapid growth (approximately age 11 to 13 years). Overuse explains the fivefold greater incidence in patients who are active in sports and the two to three times greater incidence in boys. Sinding-Larsen–Johansson disease is a similar disorder that occurs at the junction of the patellar tendon and the distal pole of the patella.

Clinical Symptoms

Patients report pain that is exacerbated by running, jumping, and kneeling activities. Pain also can occur after prolonged sitting with the knees flexed.

Tests

Physical Examination

Examination reveals tenderness and swelling at the insertion of the patellar tendon into the tibial tubercle in Osgood-Schlatter disease and at the inferior pole of the patella in Sinding-Larsen–Johansson disease. These conditions can occur in both knees simultaneously, but one side may be more symptomatic. Although knee motion usually is not restricted, kneeling is painful during the acute phase. The knee and patellofemoral joint are stable.

Diagnostic Tests

AP and lateral radiographs of the knee may be normal or show soft-tissue swelling. In Osgood-Schlatter disease, small spicules of heterotopic ossification can be seen anterior to the tibial tuberosity (**Figure 1**). In Sinding-Larsen–Johansson disease, elongation of the inferior pole of the patella can be apparent, along with fragmentation in the area, caused by repetitive stress on the growth center. Radiographs are rarely needed for patients with bilateral symptoms. In the patient with unilateral involvement, radiographs may be obtained to rule out tumor or bony abnormalities, or to manage a presentation that is refractory to typical nonsurgical management.

SECTION 9   PEDIATRIC ORTHOPAEDICS

Differential Diagnosis

- Infection (rare, elevated erythrocyte sedimentation rate)
- Neoplasm (rare, unilateral)
- Patellar sleeve fracture (acute onset, inability to perform straight leg raise)
- Tibial tubercle avulsion fracture (acute pain, inability to perform straight leg raise)

Adverse Outcomes of the Disease

The long-term prognosis for patients who undergo nonsurgical treatment is good, with minimal disability in adulthood. Some residual prominence of the tibial tubercle is common, particularly in patients who have fragmentation of the epiphysis and heterotopic ossification during the active phase of the disease. These patients occasionally report discomfort when walking. Rarely, an avulsion fracture through the tibial apophysis can occur with activity in symptomatic patients; therefore, these patients require rest from activity.

Treatment

Mild or moderate symptoms are often controlled adequately with intermittent use of ice after sports, coupled with occasional use of NSAIDs, use of a protective knee pad, and stretching exercises. Decreasing exercise for the muscles of the lower extremity to permit healing of the microscopic avulsion fractures is the key to treating severe symptoms.

Occasionally, immobilization is needed for severe or recalcitrant symptoms. This usually can be accomplished with a prefabricated knee immobilizer that is removed once per day for bathing and range-of-motion exercises. Another important aspect of treatment is helping the parents and patient understand how long sports activities may be restricted. In patients with Osgood-Schlatter disease, activity may need to be modified for an average of 2 to 3 months or more, until symptoms subside.

Surgical treatment is not commonly needed, except in the rare case of an avulsion of the ossification center or for excising a heterotopic ossification over the tibial tubercle.

Adverse Outcomes of Treatment

None.

Referral Decisions/Red Flags

Unilateral pain at rest or pain not directly over the tibial tubercle should raise concerns of a neoplasm or another disorder. Acute worsening of pain, inability to perform a straight leg raise while keeping the knee straight (patient should be able to lift his or her heel off the table without a lag, or bend, in the knee) suggests a disruption of the extensor mechanism at the patella or tibial tubercle that requires surgical fixation.

SECTION 9 PEDIATRIC ORTHOPAEDICS

Osteochondral Lesions of the Talus

Synonyms

Osteochondral fracture

Osteochondritis dissecans (OCD)

Definition

Osteochondral lesions of the hyaline cartilage and underlying subchondral bone of the weight-bearing surface of the talus can occur acutely after trauma (osteochondral fracture) or can develop secondary to idiopathic subchondral avascularity (osteochondritis dissecans [OCD] of the talus), appearing similarly to OCD of the knee. These abnormalities can cause fissuring and collapse of the joint surface of the talus, delamination of joint cartilage from the underlying bone, loose fragment formation, and hyaline cartilage defects within the ankle joint.

Clinical Symptoms

Patients present with ankle pain, swelling or recurrent effusion, a sensation of catching or popping, or occasional giving way. The symptoms can occur acutely after an injury or intermittently with vigorous activities over a period of weeks to months. A history of frequent ankle swelling, often misdiagnosed as a chronic ankle sprain, is not uncommon.

Tests

Physical Examination

Examination of the ankle reveals limited, painful active and passive range of motion, a palpable effusion, and tenderness along the anterior joint line. Ligamentous stress test results and subtalar joint mobility are normal.

Diagnostic Tests

Mortise views of the ankle (**Figure 1**) reveal an articular surface defect surrounded by a halo of lucent bone on the weight-bearing surface of the talus. Acute osteochondral lesions are often smaller and wafer-shaped and occur on the lateral talus; more chronic OCD lesions are deeper and cup-shaped and occur on the posteromedial talus. CT is useful for the staging of medial lesions. MRI best defines the extent of the cartilage surface disruption and its adjacent subchondral avascularity. Synovial fluid seen to be infiltrating between the OCD lesion and the adjacent bone of the talar body suggests an unstable lesion with little healing potential.

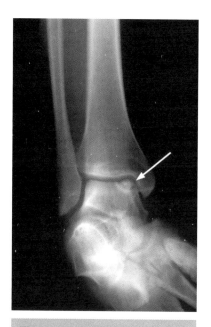

Figure 1 AP mortise radiograph of the ankle demonstrates nondisplaced osteochondritis of the talus (arrow).

Differential Diagnosis

- Acute osteochondral fracture (acute onset, hemarthrosis, pain)
- Erosive osteomyelitis (rare) (subacute, joint effusion, pain with motion)
- Neoplasm (rare) (insidious onset, night pain, joint swelling)
- Osteonecrosis of the talus (joint surface collapse from previous trauma, steroid use, sickle cell disease, delayed onset, decreased ankle motion)
- Septic arthritis of the ankle with resultant chondrolysis (rare) (pain, postinfection progressive decrease in ankle motion)

Adverse Outcomes of the Disease

Long-term complications include ankle pain, stiffness, synovitis of the ankle joint, and premature osteoarthritis. When large lesions do not heal, loose body formation and osteoarthritis of the ankle joint can develop.

Treatment

Osteochondral lesions in patients who have not reached skeletal maturity have the capacity to heal and should be evaluated for healing potential with immobilization. Osteochondral lesions in adolescents approaching skeletal maturity have a limited capacity for healing and, along with unstable lesions, usually require surgery.

Referral Decisions/Red Flags

Osteochondral lesions are best treated with early intervention and thus require early referral.

SECTION 9   PEDIATRIC ORTHOPAEDICS

Osteochondritis Dissecans

Definition

Osteochondritis dissecans (OCD) is osteonecrosis of subchondral bone. This disorder most commonly occurs in the knee but also can develop in other locations such as the elbow, talus, and distal humerus. The most common location in the knee is the posterolateral side of the medial femoral condyle (**Figure 1**), but OCD also occurs in other areas of the distal femur and, uncommonly, in the patella.

The lesion is thought to result from repetitive small stresses on the subchondral bone that disrupt the blood supply to an area of bone. The osteonecrotic bone becomes separated from surrounding viable bone by fibrous tissue. Over time, the resultant osteonecrosis weakens the involved area, and shear forces gradually fracture (dissect) the articular cartilage surface. Ultimately, the osteonecrotic section can completely fragment and become loose bodies in the joint.

Clinical Symptoms

Patients usually report a gradual onset of knee pain. They also may report knee effusions and catching or locking, particularly when the overlying articular cartilage has been disrupted. Walking with the foot rotated outward may relieve the pain.

Tests

Physical Examination

Examination reveals tenderness with palpation of the involved area. The most common site for OCD, on the medial femoral condyle, can be palpated with the knee flexed to 90°. Pressure is directed over the

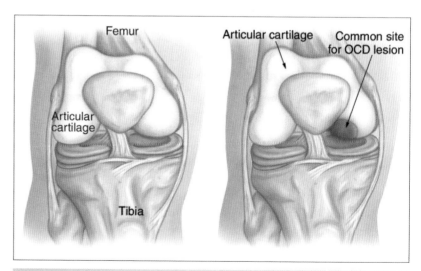

Figure 1 Illustration of the knee depicts the most common location for osteochondritis dissecans (OCD) of the knee, on the posterolateral aspect of the medial femoral condyle. (Reproduced from American Academy of Orthopaedic Surgeons OrthoInfo: *Osteochondritis dissecans.* Available at: http://orthoinfo.aaos.org/topic.cfm?topic=A00610.)

medial femoral condyle, just medial to the inferior pole of the patella. The Wilson test may be positive.

Diagnostic Tests

The lesion is best seen on tunnel (AP view obtained with the knee flexed) and lateral views of the knee, although it may be seen on an AP radiograph. MRI can help visualize the integrity of the overlying articular cartilage and in staging the lesion.

Differential Diagnosis

- Anterior knee pain (peripatellar pain, negative radiographs or finding of bipartite patella)
- Cruciate ligament injury (positive diagnostic tests, negative radiographs)
- Meniscal tear (joint line tenderness, negative radiographs)

Adverse Outcomes of the Disease

Untreated or unsuccessfully treated OCD lesions may fragment, forming loose bodies and leaving defects in the articular cartilage that can result in degenerative joint disease.

Treatment

The goal of treatment is to attain healing of the lesion. If shear forces are minimized, new bone formation can replace osteonecrotic bone. This process requires creeping substitution of new bone formation. Whether treated nonsurgically or surgically, OCD lesions take months to heal.

Nonsurgical treatment is appropriate when the overlying articular cartilage is intact; however, nonsurgical treatment is not likely to succeed after skeletal maturity. Nonsurgical treatment includes activity modifications to the point that symptoms are relieved, specifically, avoiding running and jumping activities and possibly a period of crutch ambulation. Immobilization is reserved for refractory symptoms or noncompliant patients.

Surgical treatment is necessary after skeletal maturity and in children in whom the lesion has progressed to the stage that the articular cartilage has partially or totally separated. If the lesion is intact (still in place), it is drilled to promote vascular ingrowth and creeping substitution. Unstable lesions require temporary internal fixation to promote healing. When the fragment is loose, treatment consists of removing the free fragment and débriding the articular surface defect.

Adverse Outcomes of Treatment

Possible complications of surgical treatment are infection or further damage to the joint caused by the hardware or by failure of the hardware.

SECTION 9 PEDIATRIC ORTHOPAEDICS

Referral Decisions/Red Flags

Children with lesions smaller than 1 cm wide usually do well with nonsurgical treatment; those with lesions larger than 2 cm usually have progressive problems. Children with lesions between 1 and 2 cm should be treated based on symptoms and radiographic findings. After the physis has closed, the prognosis for healing is substantially poorer, and these patients require further evaluation.

SECTION 9   PEDIATRIC ORTHOPAEDICS

Osteomyelitis

Synonym
Acute hematogenous osteomyelitis (AHO)

Definition
Osteomyelitis is a unique bone infection that usually develops in children as a result of hematogenous seeding (acute hematogenous osteomyelitis [AHO]); rarely, it is secondary to direct contamination, as from an open fracture or nail puncture wound. Substantial disability can result from osteomyelitis, especially if treatment is delayed and if the disease results in chronic infection.

The metaphysis of long bones is the most common location for AHO in children because small vessels are required to make a "U-turn" at the junction of the metaphysis and the physis, causing sluggish circulation in this area, where a nucleus of infection can take hold. The infection spreads through the medullary canal and penetrates the metaphyseal cortex, causing a subperiosteal abscess. Abscesses can result in local ischemia or osteonecrosis caused by an increase in intramedullary pressure and the loss of periosteal blood supply (elevation of the periosteum), which can result in one or more necrotic fragments of bone (sequestrae). If the periosteum remains viable, new bone (involucrum) will form to stabilize the area, and sequestrae may be partially or completely resolved. Sequestrae that persist can result in episodes of recurrence of acute infection (chronic osteomyelitis). Local or segmental bone loss can occur if substantial osteonecrosis exists and/or the host response is inadequate, or following inadequate treatment of the disease.

Subacute osteomyelitis presents in a more indolent fashion. It is typically caused by organisms of reduced virulence (bacteria, tuberculosis). The diagnosis often is delayed because symptoms are often vague, fever may not be present, and laboratory studies may have normal results. Some lesions have an aggressive (lytic) radiographic appearance that can mimic a tumor.

Chronic osteomyelitis develops when foci of necrotic and infected material remain within the bone, resulting in recurrent flare-ups of infection, and possibly, an intermittently draining sinus.

Clinical Symptoms
Pain, swelling, tenderness, erythema, increased localized warmth, and generalized malaise are associated with acute osteomyelitis. When the lower extremity, pelvis, or spine is involved, refusal to walk or limping is an early symptom, particularly in a young child. Pseudoparalysis (failure to use a limb despite normal neuromuscular structures) is observed when the upper extremity is affected. Subacute osteomyelitis can present with vague discomfort, but typically no fever or constitutional symptoms. Patients with chronic

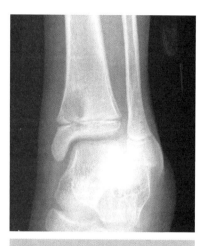

Figure 1 AP radiograph of the ankle of a patient with subacute osteomyelitis demonstrates a lytic area that extends across the physis and into the epiphysis.

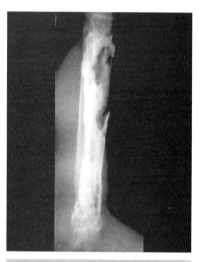

Figure 2 Lateral radiograph of the leg of a patient with chronic osteomyelitis demonstrates extensive involvement of the tibial diaphysis with areas of necrotic bone (especially anterior and superior sequestrae) and areas of new bone formation (posterior involucrum).

osteomyelitis present with periodic recurrence of sepsis and/or sinuses with chronic drainage.

Tests

Physical Examination

An elevated temperature of 100.4°F (38.0°C) or higher is typical for AHO, but patients with subacute or chronic osteomyelitis may have a normal temperature. Tenderness directly over the involved bone is common. Examination of the adjacent joint may be abnormal, and an effusion (reactive effusion or coexisting septic arthritis) is common. Pain with joint motion may be observed, as well as a mild restriction in range of motion, but not to the degree observed in septic arthritis.

Diagnostic Tests

Laboratory studies should include a complete blood cell count with differential, an erythrocyte sedimentation rate, and a C-reactive protein (CRP) level; the CRP level will be abnormal earliest, often within 8 hours of the onset of infection. These tests are not specific because they can be elevated in various other disease processes. The CRP level also is useful in monitoring the response to treatment. Neonates, children who are seen in the early stages of the disease, and those with an altered immune response may have normal laboratory study results and no fever or constitutional symptoms. A blood culture should be obtained because it will identify the infecting organism in 40% to 50% of patients. In patients clinically suspected of having AHO, aspiration along the metaphysis at the point of maximal tenderness should be considered. This can help identify a subperiosteal abscess, and the metaphysis itself can be aspirated as well. In most clinical settings, this practice has been abandoned in favor of imaging modalities such as MRI. When an effusion is present and septic arthritis is in the differential diagnosis based on clinical findings (instead of a reactive effusion), joint aspiration should be performed. A sterile or reactive effusion accompanies many cases of AHO, but a coexisting septic arthritis also is encountered in many cases. This is most common in joints in which the metaphysis is intra-articular (proximal femur, proximal humerus, proximal radius, and distal fibula).

AP and lateral radiographs of the suspected area are necessary, but they can be normal or show only soft-tissue swelling in the early stages of AHO, because bony changes such as periosteal elevation and/or destruction of bone may take 10 to 14 days to develop. In cases of subacute osteomyelitis, the lesions are most commonly lytic, have a thin sclerotic rim, and often cross the physis (**Figure 1**). In AHO, the physis is usually spared. A subset of cases of subacute osteomyelitis present with a more aggressive appearance, with periosteal reaction and/or bony destruction. The changes observed in chronic osteomyelitis are well delineated on plain radiographs (**Figure 2**). Additional imaging modalities also may be useful. MRI is currently the imaging modality of choice for diagnosing the early stages of AHO (**Figure 3**); technetium Tc-99m bone scanning also may be considered. MRI demonstrates not only signal intensity change within the bone but also coexisting findings such as abscesses, effusion, and soft-tissue changes (cellulitis, myositis). MRI should be obtained with intravenous contrast when an infection or tumor is suspected.

Differential Diagnosis

• Chronic recurrent multifocal osteomyelitis
• Infections

  Cellulitis (erythema and swelling of subcutaneous tissues)

  Pyomyositis (muscle pain and tenderness that gradually increases)

  Septic arthritis (joint swelling and severe restriction of motion)

• Inflammatory diseases (acute rheumatic fever, juvenile idiopathic arthritis, others)

  Lyme arthropathy (joint effusion, restriction of motion)

• Tumors

  Benign (eosinophilic granuloma)

  Malignant (leukemia, Ewing sarcoma, osteosarcoma)

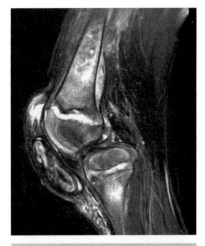

Figure 3 Sagittal MRI of early-stage osteomyelitis of the distal femur demonstrates increased signal intensity within the distal femoral metaphysis with a small subperiosteal abscess posteriorly.

Adverse Outcomes of the Disease

A host of potential sequelae are possible, depending on the timing of diagnosis and the response to treatment. These include persistent infection (chronic osteomyelitis), focal or segmental bone loss, pathologic fracture, angular deformity, involvement of the physis resulting in angular deformity and/or limb-length inequality, loss of motion at neighboring joints, and destruction of adjacent joints.

Treatment

When osteomyelitis is clinically suspected, empiric intravenous antibiotics should be started immediately after obtaining material for culture (or performing a biopsy). *Staphylococcus aureus* is the most common pathogen, and antibiotic selection should cover this organism in all age groups. Antibiotic selection also should cover group B streptococci and enteric rod organisms in neonates. In children ages 6 months to 4 years, *Haemophilus influenzae* also is covered if vaccination is incomplete. *Kingella kingae* may require polymerase chain reaction or specialized culture media. Consult with an infectious disease specialist to help identify epidemiologically and geographically relevant pathogens. The typical course of antibiotics is 6 weeks but can be longer depending on clinical response and laboratory values. The indication and time to switch from intravenous to oral antibiotics is currently controversial, but an early change to oral medication (after up to 7 days of intravenous therapy) is feasible in many patients, particularly those who present early.

Surgery for acute osteomyelitis consists primarily of draining a subperiosteal or intramedullary abscess and débriding any areas of bony destruction. A biopsy is required for diagnosis in most cases of

PEDIATRIC ORTHOPAEDICS

SECTION 9

subacute osteomyelitis, which often mimics a tumor, although some evidence exists to support empiric antibiotic therapy for lesions that have a characteristic appearance and the appropriate clinical history. Chronic osteomyelitis is very difficult to treat, often requiring staged surgical procedures. Removal of all infected material provides the best likelihood of disease eradication. Extensive débridement may be required, resulting in deficiencies in the soft-tissue envelope and/or local or segmental defects within the involved bone. Additional surgical procedures are often required, including skin grafting, local rotational flaps, or free-tissue transfers to achieve soft-tissue coverage, and bone grafting or bone transport to treat bony defects. Immobilization decreases pain and is considered for up to 3 to 6 weeks for comfort and to protect against a pathologic fracture. The bone is weaker not only because of the osseous destruction, but also because the woven bone that is initially formed in the healing process does not have the same strength as lamellar bone.

Adverse Outcomes of Treatment

The usual surgical risks, including infection, are possible.

Referral Decisions/Red Flags

Most patients with osteomyelitis benefit from a team approach.

Pediatric Sports Participation

Sports participation during childhood offers several potential benefits that result in lifelong habits of fitness. Children develop specific skills, learn the importance of teamwork, acquire leadership skills, and develop confidence. All of these attributes result in improved self-esteem. Physical activity also provides an appropriate outlet for releasing stress.

It is important to help children choose an activity routine that is fun, developmentally appropriate, and realistic given individual, family, and community resources. One method that is used in exercise prescriptions for adults is represented by the following mnemonic: frequency, intensity, time (duration), and type of activity (FITT). This can help create a physical activity prescription for children as well.

Suggestions for increasing physical activity can include walking or bicycling for transportation instead of riding in an automobile and planning physical activity rather than sedentary activities with friends. Many adolescents, especially girls, may not be active because they think organized sports are the only type of exercise that "counts." Therefore, it is important to provide education to adolescents to identify the physical activity they may already be getting (such as walking), as well as to reinforce the benefits of other lifetime activities such as bicycling, dancing, skating, and swimming.

Potential disadvantages of organized sports include burnout, injuries (acute and overuse), and an overemphasis on winning. Adults who lead children's sports activities should not forget that sports should be for the child and should be fun (**Table 1**).

Children are not merely small adults. They have unique needs that must be considered. For example, children are more heat-sensitive than adults and tend not to drink enough. They rarely will admit that they are tired. Therefore, practices should be scheduled during the cooler hours of the day and should include adequate breaks. Adults in charge should ensure that adequate amounts of fluids that children like to drink are readily available and are encouraged.

Readiness for Sports Participation

Overall readiness must be based on the individual child and his or her eagerness to participate, not parental preference. A variety of sport activities should be offered, and the child should be allowed to choose.

The attrition rate for youth sports participation is high: 35% annually. Many children drop out of sports because of burnout, not being able to participate, or because they are not matched to their level of skill. The developmental skills for sports and sports recommendations during childhood are listed in **Table 2**.

Sports programs to enhance motor development in infants and toddlers are limited, but aquatic programs for infants and toddlers

Table 1
Reasons Children Want to Play Sports
To have fun
To improve their skills
To learn new skills
To be with their friends
To make new friends
To succeed or win
To become physically fit
(Reproduced from Landry GL: Benefits of sports participation, in Sullivan JA, Anderson SJ, eds: *Care of the Young Athlete.* Rosemont, IL, American Academy of Orthopaedic Surgeons, pp 1-8.)

Table 2	
Developmental Skills and Sports Recommendations During Childhood	

Early Childhood (2 to 5 years)

Motor skills
  Limited fundamental skills
  Limited balance skills

Learning
  Extremely short attention span
  Poor selective attention
  Egocentric learning (trial and error)
  Visual and auditory cues are important

Vision
  Not fully mature before age 6 to 7 years (farsighted)
  Difficulty tracking and judging velocity of moving objects

Sports recommendations
  Emphasize fundamental skills with minimal variation and limited instruction
  Emphasize fun, playfulness, exploration, and experimentation rather than competition
  Activities: Running, swimming, tumbling, throwing, catching

Middle Childhood (6 to 9 years)

Motor skills
  Continued improvement in fundamental skills
  Posture and balance become more automatic
  Improved reaction times
  Beginning transitional skills

Learning
  Short attention span
  Limited development of memory and rapid decision making

Vision
  Improved tracking
  Limited directionality

Sports recommendations
  Emphasize fundamental skills and beginning transitional skills
  Flexible rules of sports
  Allow free time in practices
  Short instruction time
  Minimal competition
  Activities: Entry-level soccer and baseball

are popular. A recent policy statement developed by the American Academy of Pediatrics (available at http://www.aap.org) continues to encourage swim lessons for children 4 years and older; swim instruction for younger children is no longer discouraged because new evidence indicates that drowning risk is not increased, and may be decreased, as a result of such programs. The decision to pursue swim lessons at any age should be based on the child's development,

Table 2 (continued)

Developmental Skills and Sports Recommendations During Childhood

Late Childhood (10 to 12 years)

Motor skills

    Improved transitional skills

    Ability to master complex motor skills

    Temporary decline in balance control at puberty

Learning

    Selective attention

    Able to use memory strategies for sports such as football and basketball

Vision

    Adult patterns

Sports recommendations

    Emphasis on skill development

    Increasing emphasis on tactics and strategy

    Emphasis on factors promoting continued participation

    Activities: Entry-level for complex skill sports (such as football, basketball)

(Adapted with permission from Nelson MA: Developmental skills and children's sports. *Phys Sportsmed* 1991;19: 67-97.)

health, disabilities, and readiness to learn. Parents should be reminded that swim lessons do not eliminate all risk of drowning.

Children 3 to 5 years of age have developed the fundamental skills of crawling, walking, jumping, and running. Vision, however, is relatively imprecise. Children at this age have difficulty tracking moving objects. Therefore, the instruction to "keep your eye on the ball" is difficult to follow. Furthermore, children in this age group have shorter attention spans and are egocentric in their learning. Appropriate activities for this age include running, tumbling, and throwing, but team and competitive sports are inappropriate.

At 6 to 10 years of age, children begin the transition to adult skill development. Prior to this age they could throw, but now they are ready to work on accuracy. Some children at this age are proficient; others are not. At approximately 7 to 8 years of age, children begin to communicate and cooperate as a group effort; however, their attention span is still limited. Team sports in this group should be modified to ensure that practices are short and fun and that skills instruction is limited to 10 to 20 minutes. Egocentric activities should be included to practice the material taught and the rules modified to stress high scoring and full participation.

Adolescents develop complex sport skills that require rapid decision making. Certainly for some children, waiting until adolescence to become involved in competitive sports that require complex skills and interactions, such as football, wrestling, hockey, and basketball, prevents the burnout that occurs when these sports are pushed on the child at an earlier age. Adolescents also have fairly good attention spans, so chalk talks and the like can be used with this group.

SECTION 9 PEDIATRIC ORTHOPAEDICS

Preparticipation Physical Evaluation

Definition

The preparticipation physical evaluation (PPE) often is the only contact an older child or adolescent has annually with a physician. Therefore, although it is not intended to substitute for a routine annual physical examination, this examination should be as comprehensive as possible. The PPE has several objectives, as listed below:

Primary Objectives

- Screen for conditions that may be life-threatening or disabling
- Screen for conditions that may predispose to injury or illness

Secondary Objectives

- Determine general health
- Serve as an entry point to the healthcare system for adolescents
- Provide an opportunity to initiate discussion on health-related topics

Types of Evaluations

One of two types of PPE is appropriate. The first is an examination by the athlete's personal physician. This is the preferred method because it allows for continuity of care, regarding both past medical history and coordination of necessary referrals, as well as access to other aspects of preventive care. The second is the "station" method in which athletes move through several stations for different parts of the evaluation, all of which should be coordinated and supervised by the team physician. Specialists are often available to expedite consultations, but review of the history form and the physical examination should be performed by a single physician. A standard form can be used with either of these methods. The form developed by the American Academy of Family Physicians, American Academy of Pediatrics, American College of Sports Medicine, American Medical Society for Sports Medicine, American Orthopaedic Society for Sports Medicine, and the American Osteopathic Academy of Sports Medicine is reproduced on the following pages (**Figure 1**).

Components of the PPE

Timing and Interval

Optimal timing for the PPE is 6 weeks before the beginning of the athletic season. This allows adequate time for further consultation, diagnostic testing, or rehabilitation of identified problems. Comprehensive evaluations should be performed at every new school level (elementary school, middle school, high school, college) and every 2 years. On the intervening years, a comprehensive history should be obtained along with a focused evaluation of any identified issues.

■ PREPARTICIPATION PHYSICAL EVALUATION
HISTORY FORM

(Note: This form is to be filled out by the patient and parent prior to seeing the physician. The physician should keep this form in the chart.)

Date of Exam _____

Name _____ Date of birth _____

Sex _____ Age _____ Grade _____ School _____ Sport(s) _____

Medicines and Allergies: Please list all of the prescription and over-the-counter medicines and supplements (herbal and nutritional) that you are currently taking

Do you have any allergies? ☐ Yes ☐ No If yes, please identify specific allergy below.
☐ Medicines   ☐ Pollens   ☐ Food   ☐ Stinging Insects

Explain "Yes" answers below. Circle questions you don't know the answers to.

GENERAL QUESTIONS	Yes	No
1. Has a doctor ever denied or restricted your participation in sports for any reason?		
2. Do you have any ongoing medical conditions? If so, please identify below: ☐ Asthma ☐ Anemia ☐ Diabetes ☐ Infections Other: _____		
3. Have you ever spent the night in the hospital?		
4. Have you ever had surgery?		

HEART HEALTH QUESTIONS ABOUT YOU	Yes	No
5. Have you ever passed out or nearly passed out DURING or AFTER exercise?		
6. Have you ever had discomfort, pain, tightness, or pressure in your chest during exercise?		
7. Does your heart ever race or skip beats (irregular beats) during exercise?		
8. Has a doctor ever told you that you have any heart problems? If so, check all that apply: ☐ High blood pressure ☐ A heart murmur ☐ High cholesterol ☐ A heart infection ☐ Kawasaki disease Other: _____		
9. Has a doctor ever ordered a test for your heart? (For example, ECG/EKG, echocardiogram)		
10. Do you get lightheaded or feel more short of breath than expected during exercise?		
11. Have you ever had an unexplained seizure?		
12. Do you get more tired or short of breath more quickly than your friends during exercise?		

HEART HEALTH QUESTIONS ABOUT YOUR FAMILY	Yes	No
13. Has any family member or relative died of heart problems or had an unexpected or unexplained sudden death before age 50 (including drowning, unexplained car accident, or sudden infant death syndrome)?		
14. Does anyone in your family have hypertrophic cardiomyopathy, Marfan syndrome, arrhythmogenic right ventricular cardiomyopathy, long QT syndrome, short QT syndrome, Brugada syndrome, or catecholaminergic polymorphic ventricular tachycardia?		
15. Does anyone in your family have a heart problem, pacemaker, or implanted defibrillator?		
16. Has anyone in your family had unexplained fainting, unexplained seizures, or near drowning?		

BONE AND JOINT QUESTIONS	Yes	No
17. Have you ever had an injury to a bone, muscle, ligament, or tendon that caused you to miss a practice or a game?		
18. Have you ever had any broken or fractured bones or dislocated joints?		
19. Have you ever had an injury that required x-rays, MRI, CT scan, injections, therapy, a brace, a cast, or crutches?		
20. Have you ever had a stress fracture?		
21. Have you ever been told that you have or have you had an x-ray for neck instability or atlantoaxial instability? (Down syndrome or dwarfism)		
22. Do you regularly use a brace, orthotics, or other assistive device?		
23. Do you have a bone, muscle, or joint injury that bothers you?		
24. Do any of your joints become painful, swollen, feel warm, or look red?		
25. Do you have any history of juvenile arthritis or connective tissue disease?		

MEDICAL QUESTIONS	Yes	No
26. Do you cough, wheeze, or have difficulty breathing during or after exercise?		
27. Have you ever used an inhaler or taken asthma medicine?		
28. Is there anyone in your family who has asthma?		
29. Were you born without or are you missing a kidney, an eye, a testicle (males), your spleen, or any other organ?		
30. Do you have groin pain or a painful bulge or hernia in the groin area?		
31. Have you had infectious mononucleosis (mono) within the last month?		
32. Do you have any rashes, pressure sores, or other skin problems?		
33. Have you had a herpes or MRSA skin infection?		
34. Have you ever had a head injury or concussion?		
35. Have you ever had a hit or blow to the head that caused confusion, prolonged headache, or memory problems?		
36. Do you have a history of seizure disorder?		
37. Do you have headaches with exercise?		
38. Have you ever had numbness, tingling, or weakness in your arms or legs after being hit or falling?		
39. Have you ever been unable to move your arms or legs after being hit or falling?		
40. Have you ever become ill while exercising in the heat?		
41. Do you get frequent muscle cramps when exercising?		
42. Do you or someone in your family have sickle cell trait or disease?		
43. Have you had any problems with your eyes or vision?		
44. Have you had any eye injuries?		
45. Do you wear glasses or contact lenses?		
46. Do you wear protective eyewear, such as goggles or a face shield?		
47. Do you worry about your weight?		
48. Are you trying to or has anyone recommended that you gain or lose weight?		
49. Are you on a special diet or do you avoid certain types of foods?		
50. Have you ever had an eating disorder?		
51. Do you have any concerns that you would like to discuss with a doctor?		
FEMALES ONLY		
52. Have you ever had a menstrual period?		
53. How old were you when you had your first menstrual period?		
54. How many periods have you had in the last 12 months?		

Explain "yes" answers here

_____

_____

_____

_____

_____

_____

_____

_____

_____

I hereby state that, to the best of my knowledge, my answers to the above questions are complete and correct.

Signature of athlete _____ Signature of parent/guardian _____ Date _____

Figure 1 Preparticipation Physical Evaluation form.

SECTION 9 PEDIATRIC ORTHOPAEDICS

■ PREPARTICIPATION PHYSICAL EVALUATION
THE ATHLETE WITH SPECIAL NEEDS: SUPPLEMENTAL HISTORY FORM

Date of Exam _____

Name _____ Date of birth _____

Sex _____ Age _____ Grade _____ School _____ Sport(s) _____

	Yes	No
1. Type of disability		
2. Date of disability		
3. Classification (if available)		
4. Cause of disability (birth, disease, accident/trauma, other)		
5. List the sports you are interested in playing		
6. Do you regularly use a brace, assistive device, or prosthetic?		
7. Do you use any special brace or assistive device for sports?		
8. Do you have any rashes, pressure sores, or any other skin problems?		
9. Do you have a hearing loss? Do you use a hearing aid?		
10. Do you have a visual impairment?		
11. Do you use any special devices for bowel or bladder function?		
12. Do you have burning or discomfort when urinating?		
13. Have you had autonomic dysreflexia?		
14. Have you ever been diagnosed with a heat-related (hyperthermia) or cold-related (hypothermia) illness?		
15. Do you have muscle spasticity?		
16. Do you have frequent seizures that cannot be controlled by medication?		

Explain "yes" answers here

_____
_____
_____
_____
_____

Please indicate if you have ever had any of the following.

	Yes	No
Atlantoaxial instability		
X-ray evaluation for atlantoaxial instability		
Dislocated joints (more than one)		
Easy bleeding		
Enlarged spleen		
Hepatitis		
Osteopenia or osteoporosis		
Difficulty controlling bowel		
Difficulty controlling bladder		
Numbness or tingling in arms or hands		
Numbness or tingling in legs or feet		
Weakness in arms or hands		
Weakness in legs or feet		
Recent change in coordination		
Recent change in ability to walk		
Spina bifida		
Latex allergy		

Explain "yes" answers here

_____
_____
_____
_____
_____

I hereby state that, to the best of my knowledge, my answers to the above questions are complete and correct.

Signature of athlete _____ Signature of parent/guardian _____ Date _____

Figure 1 (continued) Preparticipation Physical Evaluation form.

■ PREPARTICIPATION PHYSICAL EVALUATION
PHYSICAL EXAMINATION FORM

Name _____   Date of birth _____

PHYSICIAN REMINDERS
1. Consider additional questions on more sensitive issues
   - Do you feel stressed out or under a lot of pressure?
   - Do you ever feel sad, hopeless, depressed, or anxious?
   - Do you feel safe at your home or residence?
   - Have you ever tried cigarettes, chewing tobacco, snuff, or dip?
   - During the past 30 days, did you use any chewing tobacco, snuff, or dip?
   - Do you drink alcohol or use any other drugs?
   - Have you ever taken anabolic steroids or used any other performance supplement?
   - Have you ever taken any supplements to help you gain or lose weight or improve your performance?
   - Do you wear a seat belt, use a helmet, and use condoms?
2. Consider reviewing questions on cardiovascular symptoms (questions 5–14).

EXAMINATION				
Height	Weight		☐ Male ☐ Female	
BP / (/) Pulse		Vision R 20/	L 20/	Corrected ☐ Y ☐ N

MEDICAL	NORMAL	ABNORMAL FINDINGS
Appearance • Marfan stigmata (kyphoscoliosis, high-arched palate, pectus excavatum, arachnodactyly, arm span > height, hyperlaxity, myopia, MVP, aortic insufficiency)		
Eyes/ears/nose/throat • Pupils equal • Hearing		
Lymph nodes		
Heart ª • Murmurs (auscultation standing, supine, +/- Valsalva) • Location of point of maximal impulse (PMI)		
Pulses • Simultaneous femoral and radial pulses		
Lungs		
Abdomen		
Genitourinary (males only)ᵇ		
Skin • HSV, lesions suggestive of MRSA, tinea corporis		
Neurologic ᶜ		
MUSCULOSKELETAL		
Neck		
Back		
Shoulder/arm		
Elbow/forearm		
Wrist/hand/fingers		
Hip/thigh		
Knee		
Leg/ankle		
Foot/toes		
Functional • Duck-walk, single leg hop		

ªConsider ECG, echocardiogram, and referral to cardiology for abnormal cardiac history or exam.
ᵇConsider GU exam if in private setting. Having third party present is recommended.
ᶜConsider cognitive evaluation or baseline neuropsychiatric testing if a history of significant concussion.

☐ Cleared for all sports without restriction

☐ Cleared for all sports without restriction with recommendations for further evaluation or treatment for _____
_____

☐ Not cleared
    ☐ Pending further evaluation
    ☐ For any sports
    ☐ For certain sports _____
      Reason _____
Recommendations _____

I have examined the above-named student and completed the preparticipation physical evaluation. The athlete does not present apparent clinical contraindications to practice and participate in the sport(s) as outlined above. A copy of the physical exam is on record in my office and can be made available to the school at the request of the parents. If conditions arise after the athlete has been cleared for participation, the physician may rescind the clearance until the problem is resolved and the potential consequences are completely explained to the athlete (and parents/guardians).

Name of physician (print/type) _____   Date _____
Address _____   Phone _____
Signature of physician _____   MD or DO

Figure 1 (continued) Preparticipation Physical Evaluation form.

SECTION 9 PEDIATRIC ORTHOPAEDICS

■ PREPARTICIPATION PHYSICAL EVALUATION
CLEARANCE FORM

Name _____ Sex ☐ M ☐ F Age _____ Date of birth _____

☐ Cleared for all sports without restriction

☐ Cleared for all sports without restriction with recommendations for further evaluation or treatment for _____
_____

☐ Not cleared

      ☐ Pending further evaluation

      ☐ For any sports

      ☐ For certain sports _____

      Reason _____

Recommendations _____
_____
_____
_____
_____
_____
_____

I have examined the above-named student and completed the preparticipation physical evaluation. The athlete does not present apparent clinical contraindications to practice and participate in the sport(s) as outlined above. A copy of the physical exam is on record in my office and can be made available to the school at the request of the parents. If conditions arise after the athlete has been cleared for participation, the physician may rescind the clearance until the problem is resolved and the potential consequences are completely explained to the athlete (and parents/guardians).

Name of physician (print/type) _____ Date _____

Address _____ Phone _____

Signature of physician _____, MD or DO

EMERGENCY INFORMATION

Allergies _____
_____
_____
_____
_____

Other information _____
_____
_____
_____
_____
_____
_____
_____
_____
_____

Figure 1 (continued) Preparticipation Physical Evaluation form.

Table 1

Cardiovascular Screening in Athletes

Condition	Cardiovascular Examination	Abnormality
Hypertension	Blood pressure	Varies with age–general guideline is >135/85 mm Hg in adolescents
Coarctation of aorta	Femoral pulses	Decreased intensity of pulse
Hypertrophic cardiomyopathy	Auscultation with provocative maneuvers (standing, supine, Valsalva)	Systolic ejection murmur that intensifies with standing or Valsalva maneuver
Marfan syndrome	Auscultation	Aortic (decrescendo diastolic murmur) or mitral (holosystolic murmur) insufficiency

(Adapted with permission from Maron BJ, Thompson PO, Puffer JC, et al: Cardiovascular screening of competitive athletes: A statement for health professionals from the Sudden Death Committee [clinical cardiology] and Congenital Cardiac Defects Committee [cardiovascular disease in the young], American Heart Association. *Circulation* 1996;94:850-856.)

History

The medical history is the most important piece in identifying relevant conditions. Often, the history given by adolescents is inaccurate or incomplete; therefore, parental input is preferable. Questions should emphasize symptoms related to the cardiovascular system such as dizziness or syncope with exercise, chest pain, shortness of breath, palpitations, and fatigability. Because many important cardiovascular conditions have a hereditary component, obtaining a family history also is critical. The family history should include details about any sudden death of a close relative younger than 50 years, Marfan syndrome, long QT syndrome, or other substantial cardiovascular conditions.

Additional aspects of the history should address musculoskeletal issues (prior injury, orthosis/brace use, cervical instability), asthma symptoms, infectious concerns (mononucleosis, methicillin-resistant *Staphylococcus aureus*, herpes), neurologic disorders (seizures; headaches; radiculopathy, especially in the upper extremity), solitary organs (for example, only one kidney), visual concerns, high-risk behaviors, and heat-related concerns (sickle cell disease or trait, muscle cramping, heat intolerance). In addition, in female patients, a menstrual history should be obtained.

Physical Examination

The examination component begins with a thorough general examination of all systems. The cardiovascular and musculoskeletal examinations are presented here in more detail.

Cardiovascular Examination

The cardiovascular examination includes evaluation of peripheral pulses, murmurs, and blood pressure. Important aspects of the screening cardiovascular examination are summarized in **Table 1**.

All diastolic murmurs and grade 3/6 systolic murmurs warrant further evaluation. Hypertrophic cardiomyopathy (HCM) can produce a systolic murmur that cannot be distinguished from an innocent murmur. The HCM murmur increases in intensity with standing (decreased ventricular filling, increased obstruction) and decreases with squatting or lying supine (increased ventricular filling, decreased obstruction); the aortic stenosis murmur can decrease with standing but worsens with squatting.

Blood pressures obtained during the PPE often are elevated; sometimes this is because the blood pressure cuff is too small, particularly for large adolescents. Sometimes a patient's blood pressure is recorded as elevated because reference was not made to a table of age-based norms. At times, however, the athlete's blood pressure is truly elevated. Hypertension is rarely severe enough to disqualify an athlete from participation, but it needs to be identified and followed by the athlete's regular physician.

Musculoskeletal Examination

The musculoskeletal examination is important because it typically accounts for 50% of the abnormal physical findings identified on the PPE. A general musculoskeletal examination may be acceptable for patients without symptoms, but in patients with prior injuries or symptoms, the examination should focus on those areas. Most musculoskeletal injuries are detected on the basis of the history alone. For a brief musculoskeletal screening examination that can detect problems in asymptomatic individuals, see the Musculoskeletal Screening Examination earlier in this section.

Some authorities recommend a sport-specific approach to the physical examination. This method emphasizes areas that are most commonly injured or diseased in each specific sport. For example, a swimmer's examination focuses on the shoulders and ears (otitis externa); a wrestler's examination emphasizes the skin, body fat composition, and the shoulders.

Diagnostic Tests

Recommendations regarding diagnostic screening tests for athletes are not provided because of the complexity of the issue. Additional tests such as electrocardiography, echocardiography, or musculoskeletal imaging should be ordered based on the history and physical examination.

Athletes With Special Needs

The PPE for athletes with physical or cognitive disabilities is the same except that additional aspects may be specific to the particular athlete's disability regarding history, physical examination, or possibly mandatory imaging.

Referral Decisions/Red Flags

Any history of the following physical findings indicates the need for further evaluation and possible consultation with a specialist.

- Best-corrected vision less than 20/40 in either eye
- Early fatigue, dizziness, syncope, chest pain, shortness of breath, palpitations with exercise, or unexplained seizures
- Family history of sudden death or substantial cardiovascular condition
- Murmur over left ventricular outflow tract
- Physical signs of Marfan syndrome
- Previous heat illness
- Substantial head or spinal injury or persistent postconcussion symptoms
- Substantial musculoskeletal problem or injury

After the PPE has been completed, a recommendation can be made for (1) unrestricted clearance, (2) clearance with recommendations for further evaluation or treatment, (3) "not cleared" but to be reconsidered after further evaluation or treatment, or (4) "not cleared" for some or all sports. Often these decisions will be made together with the athlete, parents, and consultants. Guidelines for cardiovascular system conditions can be found in "Eligibility Recommendations for Competitive Athletes With Cardiovascular Abnormalities," published in the *Journal of the American College of Cardiology.*

Blood pressure standards for children based on age, sex, and height are available from the National Institutes of Health (available at http://www.nhlbi.nih.gov/guidelines/hypertension/child_tbl.htm). Guidelines for most other conditions are presented in the *Preparticipation Physical Evaluation* monograph developed by the American Academy of Family Physicians, the American Academy of Pediatrics, the American College of Sports Medicine, the American Medical Society for Sports Medicine, the American Orthopaedic Society for Sports Medicine, and the American Osteopathic Academy of Sports Medicine, and published by the American Academy of Pediatrics (obtainable at AAP Publications: 1-888-227-1770 or www.aap.org/bookstore). The official Preparticipation Physical Evaluation forms can be accessed at http://www.aap.org/sections/sportsmedicine/PDFS/PPE-4-forms.pdf.)

Scoliosis

Definition

Scoliosis is a lateral curvature of the spine greater than 10° measured using the Cobb method; the curves can occur in the thoracic or the lumbar spine (occasionally in both). Scoliosis can be accompanied by abnormalities in sagittal alignment such as excessive kyphosis or lordosis. Idiopathic scoliosis is the most common diagnosis, with a prevalence of 2% to 3%. Other diagnoses associated with scoliosis are listed in **Table 1**. This chapter focuses on idiopathic scoliosis.

The etiology of idiopathic scoliosis is most likely multifactorial. Idiopathic scoliosis may be classified according to age at onset: infantile (birth to 3 years), juvenile (3 to 11 years), and adolescent (older than 11 years). For adolescent idiopathic scoliosis, the male-to-female ratio is almost equal for curves less than 20°, but girls are

Table 1	
Etiologic Classification of Structural Scoliosis	
Type	**Possible Cause**
Idiopathic	Genetic and environmental factors
Congenital	Failure of formation—hemivertebra or block vertebra
	Failure of segmentation—bony bar joining one side of two or more adjacent vertebrae
	Mixed anomalies
Neuromuscular	Cerebral palsy
	Muscular dystrophy
	Myelomeningocele
	Spinal muscular atrophy
	Friedreich ataxia (spinocerebellar degeneration)
	Poliomyelitis
	Myopathies
Vertebral disease	Tumor
	Infection
	Metabolic bone disease
Spinal cord disease or anomaly	Tumor
	Syringomyelia
	Spinal cord injury
Disease-associated	Neurofibromatosis
	Marfan syndrome
	Connective tissue disorders
Compensatory	Limb-length discrepancy

much more likely than boys to have a curve greater than 30°. The natural history depends on the magnitude of curvature and the degree of skeletal maturity. Thoracic curves greater than 80° to 90° can impair pulmonary function (restrictive pattern). Curves diagnosed during the infantile and juvenile years are much more likely to be progressive and require surgical treatment.

Neuromuscular scoliosis is associated with a host of diseases causing flaccid weakness or spasticity. The predominant effect of these deformities is a loss of sitting balance, but respiratory function also can be impaired. Patients with neuromuscular scoliosis typically have long thoracolumbar or lumbar curves.

Congenital scoliosis results from abnormalities in the shape and/or growth potential of vertebrae and can result from a failure of formation (part of the vertebra is absent) or a failure of segmentation (two or more vertebrae are partially or completely fused together); mixed anomalies are common. The risk of progression depends on the unique characteristics of each anomaly.

Clinical Symptoms

Idiopathic scoliosis is most commonly identified during a school screening program or routine examination, but it also may be noticed by family members. Pain is not common, and neurologic symptoms are very rare. Neuromuscular curves present as a loss of sitting balance. Congenital curves can present similar to idiopathic scoliosis.

Tests
Physical Examination

Idiopathic scoliosis is a diagnosis of exclusion, and a thorough history and physical examination is required to rule out other processes that may be associated with the deformity. In addition to the spinal examination, the trunk and lower extremities should be assessed for findings of potential etiologies: skin lesions such as café-au-lait spots, axillary freckling or lesions over the spine that can suggest neurofibromatosis or spinal disorders, respectively; cavus feet, which suggest neuromuscular disease or spinal cord anomaly; limb-length discrepancy; abnormal joint laxity associated with Marfan syndrome or connective tissue disorders; and neuromuscular abnormalities.

The patient's spine is inspected in an upright position. The Adam forward bend test is the most sensitive clinical method of screening for scoliosis. The patient is asked to bend forward with the feet together, knees straight, and the arms hanging free. The examiner looks at the back from behind and documents any rotational asymmetry. Spinal flexion accentuates rotation of the spine, causing elevation of the posterior hemithorax and/or prominence of the lumbar paravertebral muscle mass on the convexity of the curves. The deformity can be quantified in degrees using an inclinometer such as the scoliometer (**Figure 1**); values greater than 5° to 7° have been used in the past as a benchmark for referral. School screening programs, which are widespread in the United States, have been associated with a referral rate of 3% to 30%. The efficacy of school

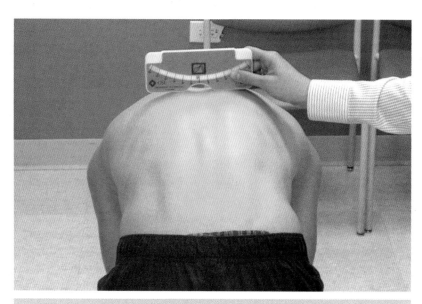

Figure 1 Photograph depicts using a scoliometer to quantify degree of scoliotic deformity. This patient demonstrates no deformity.

screening remains controversial. The flexibility of the deformity also is assessed clinically.

Diagnostic Tests

PA and lateral full-length radiographs should be obtained with the patient standing and the knees straight. The x-ray tube should be positioned 6′ from the cassette, using a 14″ × 36″ grid. Positioning the patients with their backs to the x-ray source and using modern image-enhancing equipment minimizes exposure of the thyroid, breasts, and reproductive organs. The Cobb angle is the standard method of quantifying the degree of curvature and is determined by measuring the angle between lines drawn perpendicular to the end plates of the highest and lowest vertebrae in the curve (**Figure 2**). By convention, radiographs of the spine are viewed, measured, and described as if the patient were being examined from behind. The indications for MRI of the spine in patients with presumed idiopathic scoliosis include (1) age (infantile or juvenile), (2) abnormal findings on the history or physical examination (chronic pain, neurologic symptoms or findings), and (3) selected plain radiographic findings (left-sided thoracic curve, excessive thoracic kyphosis, widening of the spinal canal, erosive vertebral changes or rib abnormalities). For patients with congenital spinal abnormalities that cause scoliosis or kyphosis, additional imaging studies include a renal ultrasonogram (40% have renal abnormalities), an MRI of the spine (20% have intraspinal anomalies), and an echocardiogram (15% have congenital heart abnormalities).

Differential Diagnosis

Differential diagnoses of potential etiologies for structural scoliosis are listed in **Table 1**. Limb-length discrepancy can cause an apparent scoliosis (resulting from spinal compensation for the tilt of the pelvis) or contribute to compensation or exacerbation of a structural curve; correcting the limb-length discrepancy by having the patient stand on a block resolves any compensatory curve and reveals the true degree of any underlying structural curve; radiographs can be obtained with the lift in place for confirmation.

Adverse Outcomes of the Disease

Progressive idiopathic curves are associated with cosmetic concerns. The small subset of patients with progressive thoracic curves greater than 80° to 90° can develop dyspnea from restrictive pulmonary disease. A reduced life expectancy from cardiopulmonary failure (cor pulmonale) is associated with severe curves, which most commonly occur in infantile/juvenile and congenital scoliosis. An increased risk of mild to moderate back pain in untreated idiopathic curves also exists, but overall, most patients do well throughout their lives. Disabling pain is more likely to develop in patients who have decompensated lumbar or thoracolumbar curves.

Treatment

Treatment recommendations are based on the natural history of the curve, which varies based on the underlying diagnosis, growth remaining, and other variables. Options include observation, bracing, and surgery. Observation is always appropriate for small and/or nonprogressive curves that are asymptomatic.

For progressive idiopathic scoliosis, physical therapy and electrical stimulation have not been shown to alter the natural history. Brace treatment is offered to selected patients with the goal of arresting progression of the deformity, typically in skeletally immature patients with progressive curves ranging from 25° to 45°. An underarm orthosis is appropriate for most curves; the recommended bracing time varies from 18 to 23 hours per day. Surgical treatment, which involves spinal fusion with instrumentation, usually is offered for skeletally immature patients with curves greater than 45° and for skeletally mature patients with curves greater than 50° to 60° (**Figure 3**). The spinal implants hold the spine in the maximally corrected position while the fusion mass develops, and usually no cast or brace is needed postoperatively. The goal is to achieve a well-balanced, stable spine while minimizing the number of vertebral segments fused (and therefore maximizing the number of mobile segments). Occasionally, an anterior spinal release (diskectomy) is required to achieve added mobility in large, rigid curves.

In neuromuscular scoliosis, deformities that do not interfere with sitting balance or function are observed. Progressive and symptomatic curves are often treated with a soft spinal orthosis. The softer materials used in this design are more comfortable, enhance the patient's sitting balance and upper extremity use, and are easy to care for. Bracing does not alter the natural history of neuromuscular scoliosis, but it can slow progression and delay the need for more definitive treatment. Surgical stabilization using an instrumented spinal fusion is required for progressive and symptomatic curves;

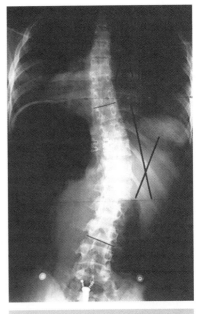

Figure 2 PA long-cassette radiograph of the entire spine demonstrates a scoliotic deformity and the Cobb method of measuring its magnitude.

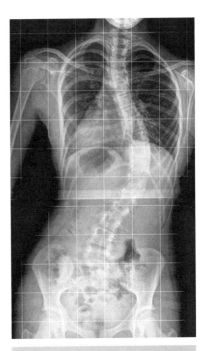

Figure 3 PA radiograph from a skeletally mature adolescent girl. She had a progressive right thoracolumbar curve despite bracing and ultimately underwent corrective surgery.

SECTION 9 PEDIATRIC ORTHOPAEDICS

the decision to operate is made on a case-by-case basis. The risk of complications is higher in patients with neuromuscular scoliosis.

For congenital scoliosis, bracing is ineffective. Given that surgical correction is associated with a higher risk of complications, preemptive spinal fusion is considered for curves with a poor natural history (high likelihood of substantial progression) before a substantial deformity has developed. Other surgical procedures such as anterior and posterior spinal fusion or excision of a hemivertebra may be considered in selected patients. Finally, progressive spinal deformities in young children are a particular challenge because definitive treatment (fusion) must be delayed until the pulmonary system has matured and, ideally, maximal trunk height has been achieved. Options to delay the need for fusion in this age group include bracing, serial casting followed by bracing, and surgical strategies such as growing rods. The growing rod program, which is essentially internal bracing, involves implantation of one or two rods to anchor points at the ends of the curve. The rods are lengthened periodically to maintain correction and delay the need for definitive fusion. Progressive curves in toddlers and young children, especially when associated with rib fusions or other anomalies of the chest wall, can result in a thoracic insufficiency syndrome, in which the chest wall is unable to support normal respiration. The vertical, expandable prosthetic titanium rib has been developed (and is FDA approved in the United States under the Humanitarian Device Exemption) to treat thoracic insufficiency syndrome. The device is attached between two ribs or between the upper thoracic ribs and the lumbar spine or pelvis and is sequentially distracted to maintain expansion of the hemithorax.

Adverse Outcomes of Treatment

Surgical procedures can be complicated by infection, neurologic injury, failure of the fusion to consolidate, and/or implant-related problems such as loss of fixation.

Referral Decisions/Red Flags

Patients with idiopathic scoliosis typically are referred for evaluation by a specialist. Patients with pain, neurologic symptoms or findings, unilateral foot deformity, or abnormal curve patterns require further evaluation to rule out intraspinal anomalies or other diagnoses.

Septic Arthritis

Synonyms
Infected joint
Pyarthrosis

Definition
Septic arthritis in children most often results from hematogenous seeding of the synovium from pneumonia, impetigo, or other skin infections. Septic arthritis also can be the result of direct extension from an adjacent metaphyseal osteomyelitis, or rarely, from penetrating wounds. Patients often have a history of viral illness in the days to weeks preceding the joint symptoms. Septic arthritis typically affects the large joints of the lower extremities (knee and hip), but it can occur in a variety of locations, including the sacroiliac joint. Early diagnosis and treatment are essential because damage to hyaline cartilage from the liberation of proteolytic enzymes by polymorphonuclear lymphocytes and synovial cells can be detected within 48 to 72 hours of inoculation.

Clinical Symptoms
Patients typically have an acute onset of guarding of the involved joint. The pain often is poorly localized initially. Children with lower extremity involvement often limp or refuse to walk; elbow or shoulder involvement may result in pseudoparalysis of the upper extremity. A history of mild trauma also is common. Systemic symptoms include malaise, fever, and loss of appetite.

Tests

Physical Examination
The patient typically appears ill at presentation. For comfort, the joint is held in a position that accommodates distention. When the hip is involved, patients prefer to hold the joint in a position of flexion, abduction, and external rotation. The elbow and knee are held in mild flexion. The child is apprehensive and resists attempts to examine the affected extremity. Joint movement is painful, typically throughout the range of motion. In contrast, patients with transient synovitis of the hip or Legg-Calvé-Perthes disease may only experience discomfort. Tenderness to palpation is common, as is joint swelling. An effusion may be identified on clinical examination in subcutaneous joints such as the knee, elbow, or ankle, but it may be impossible to appreciate clinically at the hip, shoulder, or sacroiliac joints.

Diagnostic Tests
Any suspected joint infection requires immediate aspiration and analysis of the joint fluid. The results are corroborated with the findings on physical examination and results of other laboratory tests (**Table 1**). Inflammatory markers are usually elevated. The

Table 1

Typical Laboratory Results Associated With Septic Arthritis

Condition	ESR	WBC Count	Synovial WBC Count	Blood Culture	Joint Culture
Septic joint	>30 mm/h in most patients; unpredictable in neonates	>15,000/mm³ (variable), often not elevated early	>50,000/mm³	Positive in 40% to 50% of patients	Positive in 50% to 60% of patients
Transient synovitis	<50 mm/h	Normal	Normal	Negative	Negative
Juvenile idiopathic arthritis	Variable	Normal	Variable, but usually <50,000/mm³	Negative	Negative

ESR = erythrocyte sedimentation rate, WBC = white blood cell.

white blood cell count is elevated in 40% to 60% of cases, especially in older children. The erythrocyte sedimentation rate (ESR) is commonly elevated, although there may be a delay of 24 to 48 hours following the onset of symptoms. The ESR lacks specificity and is elevated in many inflammatory or infectious disease processes. The C-reactive protein (CRP) level, which becomes elevated in 6 to 8 hours, is perhaps the most helpful marker. Blood cultures are positive in 40% to 50% of patients, and cultures of joint fluid are diagnostic in 50% to 60% of patients. Plain radiographs are rarely helpful in confirming the diagnosis early in the disease process, but they are useful in excluding other disorders. Initial radiographs are often normal but may reveal joint space widening. Ultrasonography will confirm the presence of a joint effusion, and aspiration may be performed at the same time. The absence of joint effusion on ultrasonography does not rule out a septic process.

Differential Diagnosis
- Hemophilia (history of bleeding)
- Infection
    Osteomyelitis (less pain with joint motion)
    Pyomyositis (muscle tenderness)
    Psoas abscess (pain similar to septic arthritis, negative hip ultrasound)
    Lyme disease (milder pain)
- Inflammatory diseases
    Juvenile idiopathic arthritis (pain is less severe, subacute presentation)
    Reactive arthritis (pain is less severe, subacute presentation)
    Rheumatic fever (pain is less severe, subacute presentation)
- Legg-Calvé-Perthes disease (intermittent limp, milder pain)

	Table 2	
Causative Organisms and Preferred Antibiotics for Pending Culture Results		
Age	**Organism**	**Empiric Antibiotic**
Neonates	*Staphylococcus aureus* Group B streptococci Gram-negative organisms *Streptococcus pneumoniae*	Antistaphylococcal antibiotic + cefotaxime[a]
1 mo to 3 y	*S aureus* *S pneumoniae* *Streptococcus pyogenes* *Kingella kingae*[b] *Haemophilus influenzae* type B (not immunized)	Antistaphylococcal antibiotic[a] ± cefotaxime/ceftriaxone[c]
>3 y	*S aureus* *S pneumoniae* *S pyogenes* *H influenza* type B (not immunized)	Antistaphylococcal antibiotic[a] ± cefotaxime/ceftriaxone[c]
Adolescence	*S aureus* *Neisseria gonorrhoeae* *S pneumoniae* *S pyogenes*	Antistaphylococcal antibiotic[a] ± cefotaxime/ceftriaxone[c]

[a]Antistaphylococcal penicillin types (oxacillin/nafcillin) are highly effective against *S aureus*, but vancomycin should be considered empirically if local rates of methicillin-resistant *S aureus* are high.

[b]*K kingae* has been increasingly reported in association with septic arthritis in this age group but still is relatively rare. Special culture media are required. Polymerase chain reaction is available.

[c]If the history suggests *H influenzae* (patient not immunized) or *N gonorrhoeae* (sexually active patient), cefotaxime or ceftriaxone should be added empirically.

- Neoplasia
    - Acute leukemia (constant pain, night pain)
    - Pigmented villonodular synovitis (painful joint swelling)
- Transient synovitis (milder pain, mild limp)
- Traumatic hemarthrosis (history of trauma)

Adverse Outcomes of the Disease

If untreated, septic arthritis causes damage to articular cartilage, which can result in progressive joint degeneration (arthritis). Capsular scarring and loss of motion also are observed. A delay in treating septic arthritis of the hip joint in a young child also can result in subluxation, dislocation, or osteonecrosis of the femoral head.

Treatment

An early diagnosis is essential. Prompt joint drainage, followed by intravenous antibiotic administration, is the treatment of choice. Empiric antibiotic therapy is directed against the most likely infecting organism (**Table 2**) and modified based on the culture results (**Table 3**).

SECTION 9 PEDIATRIC ORTHOPAEDICS

Table 3	
Preferred Antibiotics for Septic Arthritis Based on Causative Organism	
Organism	**Initial Intravenous Antibiotic**
Methicillin-sensitive *Staphylococcus aureus*	Oxacillin/nafcillin
Methicillin-resistant *S aureus*	Vancomycin
	Clindamycin
Streptococcus pyogenes or Group B streptococcus	Penicillin
Streptococcus pneumoniae	Ampicillin or cefotaxime/ceftriaxone
Kingella kingae	Penicillin
Neisseria gonorrhoeae	Cefotaxime/ceftriaxone
Haemophilus influenzae	Cefotaxime/ceftriaxone

When the diagnosis of septic arthritis (especially of the hip) is suspected on history and physical examination, immediate aspiration should be performed, often under ultrasonographic guidance. When the diagnosis is highly likely based on the clinical information, then it may be advisable to take the patient to the operating room for aspiration, followed by joint drainage and irrigation, even if the aspirate is equivocal. The duration and route of administration of antibiotics depends on various factors, including the severity of the infection, the virulence of the organism, and the initial response to either empiric or organism-specific antibiotics. Typically, patients are treated with intravenous antibiotics for several days to 2 weeks, followed by a course of oral antibiotics. MRI before or after emergency hip drainage is sometimes indicated to evaluate for concomitant osteomyelitis, but it should not delay surgical treatment. Repeat surgery is occasionally necessary if clinical progress is slow.

Referral Decisions/Red Flags

A high index of clinical suspicion is required to establish an early diagnosis. Patients suspected of having septic arthritis require emergent evaluation, and usually hospitalization. A multidisciplinary approach is helpful.

Seronegative Spondyloarthropathies

Synonyms

Ankylosing spondylitis
Psoriatic arthritis
Reiter syndrome

Definition

The seronegative spondyloarthropathies have the following characteristics in common: (1) inflammation of tendon, fascia, or joint capsule insertions (enthesitis); (2) pauciarticular arthritis, usually involving the lower extremity; (3) extra-articular inflammation involving the eye, skin, mucous membranes, heart, and bowel; and (4) association with HLA-B27.

Clinical Symptoms

Ankylosing Spondylitis

Ankylosing spondylitis is more likely to affect the joints of the lower extremities in children than in adults. Asymmetric pauciarticular arthritis involving the lower extremity in children 9 years or older, particularly boys, suggests the possibility of ankylosing spondylitis. The family history often is positive.

Reiter Syndrome

Reiter syndrome is characterized by the triad of conjunctivitis, enthesitis, and urethritis, although all three components of the disorder are not necessarily present in every patient, nor are they always present at the same time. In young children, it can be triggered by infectious diarrhea caused by *Yersinia, Campylobacter, Salmonella*, or *Shigella*. In adolescents, nongonococcal urethritis secondary to *Chlamydia* or trachoma may cause Reiter syndrome. The Achilles tendinitis or plantar fasciitis associated with Reiter syndrome can be extremely painful.

Psoriatic Arthritis

Psoriatic arthritis is considered uncommon in children, but in approximately one third of patients with this disease, especially girls, the onset is before the age of 15 years. Arthritis frequently antedates skin problems when this disorder occurs in childhood. A family history of psoriasis is a helpful clue when joint symptoms occur first.

Inflammatory Bowel Disease

Arthritis of inflammatory bowel disease, either ulcerative colitis or Crohn disease, typically causes symptoms in patients younger than 21 years, but the disease is diagnosed in only 15% of patients before age 15 years. Arthralgia without joint effusion is twice as common as arthritis with joint effusion.

SECTION 9   PEDIATRIC ORTHOPAEDICS

Tests

Physical Examination

A purplish discoloration around the joint is one of the distinguishing features of a juvenile spondyloarthropathy.

A child with ankylosing spondylitis may have an enthesitis, such as patellar tendinitis, Achilles tendinitis, or plantar fasciitis. Although children with ankylosing spondylitis may not have back pain, limited mobility of the spine can be present.

Mild conjunctivitis or an acute anterior uveitis causing painful red eyes and photophobia also are associated with Reiter syndrome. In psoriatic arthritis, monoarticular involvement of the knee is the most common presentation. Progression to other joints proceeds in an asymmetric fashion. Upper extremity involvement and tenosynovitis involving the digits and nail pitting is more common in psoriatic arthritis than in other spondyloarthropathies.

Pauciarticular arthritis of the lower extremity in inflammatory bowel disease is typically of short duration and either resolves spontaneously or with treatment of the bowel lesion. Progressive ankylosing spondylitis, however, can develop in some patients.

Diagnostic Tests

The presence of HLA-B27 and a positive family history for spondyloarthropathy support the diagnosis of ankylosing spondylitis. Sterile pyuria supports the diagnosis of Reiter syndrome.

Differential Diagnosis

- Juvenile rheumatoid arthritis (often younger age at onset, upper extremity joint commonly affected, synovitis more impressive)
- Overuse syndromes (localized and more often unilateral)

Adverse Outcomes of the Disease

Many lower extremity problems associated with childhood spondyloarthropathies resolve spontaneously, but persistent erosive arthritis may develop. Ultimately, changes in the sacroiliac joint develop in children with ankylosing spondylitis.

Treatment

NSAIDs, muscle strengthening, orthoses for the painful joint, and counseling about activity modifications are indicated.

Adverse Outcomes of Treatment

NSAIDs can cause gastric, renal, or hepatic complications.

Referral Decisions/Red Flags

Loss of function or inability to control pain indicates the need for further evaluation.

Shoes for Children

During the past several decades, clinical studies have clarified the role shoes play in a child's life. The accumulated body of data is now sufficiently large to establish recommendations for children's footwear.

Normal Foot Development

Clinical studies have consistently shown that in societies where going barefoot is common, the human foot has the following attributes: (1) excellent mobility; (2) thickening of the plantar skin to as much as 1 cm; (3) alignment of the phalanges with the metatarsals, causing the toes to spread; (4) variable arch height; and (5) an absence of most common foot deformities. These findings show that satisfactory foot development occurs in the barefoot environment.

Arch development has been documented in several studies. The arch develops spontaneously during a child's first 6 to 8 years, and the range considered as normal is broad. Approximately 15% to 25% of adults have flexible flatfoot, which is considered a variation of normal and typically are not associated with disability. The military no longer disqualifies individuals with flatfoot, as long as the flatfoot was not corrected and is asymptomatic.

Choosing Appropriate Shoes

The primary role of shoes is to provide protection for the foot. If shoes are not fitted properly, toe deformities are likely to develop.

Wearing shoes does not affect how soon a child will begin to walk. Infants do not require shoes, and socks or booties are just fine; soft shoes may be used for appearance or to protect the foot when outside. Soft, flexible shoes are best for the toddler. Nonslip soles help to provide traction on hardwood and tile floors. The shoes also should have breathable uppers to avoid excessive sweating. A wide toe box also is suggested to avoid constriction across the foot. If the toddler's foot is chubby, a high-top shoe can help keep the shoe on the foot, but this type of shoe does not affect the growth or development of the foot. High-top shoes also can be beneficial in children with ligamentous hyperlaxity or hypotonia.

Characteristics of a Good Shoe

For children, the features of a good shoe include the five Fs:

- Flexible. The shoe should allow as much free motion as possible. As a test, the examiner should make certain that the shoe can be easily flexed in his or her hand.
- Flat. High heels that force the foot forward, cramping the toes, should be avoided.
- Foot-shaped. Pointed toes or other shapes that are different from the normal foot should be avoided. A straight last shoe best approximates the child's foot.

- Fitted generously. Better too large than too short. Approximately a fingerbreadth of room for growth should be allowed.
- Friction like skin. The sole should have about the same friction as skin. Soles that are slippery or adherent can cause the child to fall.

The Corrective Shoe

Controlled prospective studies on the effect of shoe modifications on arch development showed no difference between treated and untreated feet. In essence, shoe inserts do not modify or alter intoeing, outtoeing, or flexible flatfoot. In fact, shoe inserts can be harmful. Adults who wore shoe modifications as children often remember the experience as negative and, in one study, were shown to have lower self-esteem than control subjects.

Shoe modifications that are not corrective but produce some immediate effect are useful. For example, shoe lifts for the short leg equalize limb length and improve walking. Shoe inserts for older children or adolescents with rigid foot deformities can redistribute weight-bearing forces and reduce discomfort or skin breakdown if sensation is impaired. Shock-absorbing footwear with cushioned soles can help in the management of overuse syndromes.

Current Problems

The design of shoes has improved over the past decade. The major problems continue to be the prevalence of constrictive and deforming shoes, including elevated heels, pointed toes, and tight fit, which can cause deformity (bunions) and instability, both of which can increase the risk of ankle injuries. Conversely, some adolescent children wear their shoes too loosely and with no fasteners, which counteracts some of the supportive elements of the shoe.

Recommendations

Shoes should be regarded as a form of clothing and should be designed to simulate the barefoot state.

- Walking and play in the barefoot condition in a safe environment is acceptable for infants and children.
- For most children, shoes should be flexible, flat, shaped like the foot, and have soles that provide friction similar to skin.
- Cushioning of the sole can reduce the risk of overuse conditions around the foot.
- Shoe modifications are not "corrective." Inserts are useful only for load redistribution and do not change the shape of the foot.
- Prescribing unnecessary shoe inserts and modifications is expensive for the family and society. More importantly, these can be uncomfortable and embarrassing for the child.

Slipped Capital Femoral Epiphysis

Synonym
Slipped epiphysis

Definition
Slipped capital femoral epiphysis (SCFE) is the result of progressive displacement of the upper portion of the femur relative to the capital femoral epiphysis. The slip occurs through the physis, typically during the adolescent growth spurt. The etiology is unknown and is likely multifactorial, involving an increase in shear stresses across a weakened physis. Anatomic variables that may predispose to SCFE include femoral retroversion, a greater inclination of the proximal femoral physis, and weakening of the perichondrial ring. Growth hormone treatment may increase this risk slightly. Mechanical factors also are important: Most patients are above the 95th percentile for weight. African Americans are more commonly affected than Caucasians or Hispanic Americans. SCFE is most common in boys from 13 to 15 years of age and in girls from 11 to 13 years of age. Patients who are outside the typical age ranges (younger than 11 years, older than 16 years) are likely to have an underlying endocrinologic or metabolic disorder (hypothyroidism or hyperthyroidism, panhypopituitarism, growth hormone deficiency, renal disease). Bilateral involvement is seen in 40% to 50% of patients who are followed to closure of the growth plate. SCFE can be classified according to time or duration of symptoms (acute is less than 3 weeks, chronic is more than 3 weeks; acute-on-chronic has exacerbation after several months of symptoms) or stability (stable patients can bear weight with or without crutches, unstable patients cannot).

Clinical Symptoms
Pain is the most common presenting symptom. It is usually localized to the groin or anterior thigh, but it also can occur in the distal thigh or knee. The pain is made worse by activity, and a limp is common. The slipped epiphysis develops gradually in most patients, although some may have acute onset of symptoms following an injury.

Tests
Physical Examination
Patients are typically in the upper ranges of weight and body mass index for age. An externally rotated limp is evident on the affected side. Patients with unstable SCFE are unable to ambulate even with crutches. Loss of hip internal rotation is the most sensitive and specific finding on physical examination. Hip flexion also should be tested because progressive flexion is usually accompanied by

SECTION 9   PEDIATRIC ORTHOPAEDICS

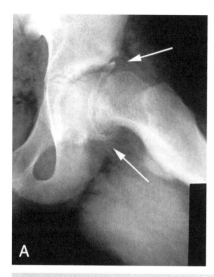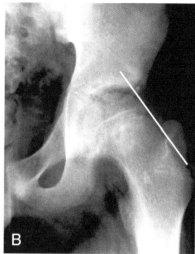

Figure 1 Radiographs of the pelvis demonstrate mild slipped capital femoral epiphysis (SCFE) of the left hip. **A,** Frog-lateral view demonstrates posterior displacement of the femoral head (arrows). **B,** AP view demonstrates mild degrees of medial displacement recognized by drawing a Klein line on the lateral aspect of the femoral neck. When SCFE is present, the line on the involved hip will either miss the femoral head or transect less of it than on the uninvolved hip.

obligatory external rotation of the hip. The affected extremity is shortened, often from 1 to 3 cm, depending on the severity of the slip.

Diagnostic Tests

AP and frog-lateral radiographs of the pelvis confirm the diagnosis (**Figure 1**). On rare occasions, in the so-called preslip phase, the radiographs are normal or demonstrate irregularity or subtle widening of the physis. MRIs can help confirm the diagnosis when radiographs are inconclusive. On the AP radiograph, SCFE is suspected if a line drawn along the superior femoral neck (the Klein line) does not intersect the lateral capital femoral epiphysis. The degree of displacement is best appreciated on the lateral view, and a prominence is usually seen along the anterior femoral neck. The severity of displacement is classified as mild, moderate, or severe as measured by the degree of angulation (mild, <30°; moderate, 30° to 50°; severe, >50°). If SCFE is clinically suspected but initial radiographs are normal, a true lateral view may reveal the slip.

Differential Diagnosis

- Acute fracture through the physis (Salter Harris type I) (history of acute trauma)
- Endocrinopathy (atypical age)
- Legg-Calvé-Perthes disease (in younger age range)
- Meralgia paresthetica (lateral femoral cutaneous nerve entrapment)
- Neoplasm (night pain, no restriction of hip internal rotation in flexion)
- Overuse injury

Adverse Outcomes of the Disease

Progressive slip may be accompanied by gait disturbance, and SCFE can predispose the hip to symptomatic degenerative changes. The prominence along the anterior femoral neck can impinge against the acetabulum, resulting in labral tears or other intra-articular pathology. The prognosis has been linked to stability of the physis: stable SCFE has a low likelihood (approximately 5%) of developing osteonecrosis, but unstable SCFE may be associated with osteonecrosis in up to 50% of patients.

Treatment

The goals of treatment of adolescents with SCFE are to stabilize the physis (promote closure of the physis), avoid complications such as osteonecrosis and chondrolysis, and maximize function. Most patients are treated with in situ stabilization with a single screw (**Figure 2**), although some surgeons prefer to treat unstable SCFE with two screws. This strategy has been shown to be effective and associated with few complications. Patients are typically allowed touch-down weight bearing (non–weight bearing for unstable SCFE) for the first 6 weeks, and activities are restricted until the physis has closed, typically for 6 to 9 months. Patients with greater degrees of deformity may require a realignment osteotomy, but this is only considered after the physis has stabilized and the patient has reached a plateau in function.

Several areas of controversy and continuing study remain, especially regarding the treatment of unstable SCFE and whether to prophylactically pin the other hip in patients with unilateral involvement. An unstable slip may be likened to a Salter-Harris type I fracture of the physis, and a subset of patients present with a history of an acute event. These unstable SCFEs are often stabilized as an emergency, and many surgeons decompress the hip joint to reduce intra-articular pressure. The role of manipulative reduction before pinning remains to be determined. Bilateral disease will develop in up to 60% of patients, and the need for routine prophylactic pinning of the contralateral hip remains a subject of debate. Families of patients with routine SCFE within the typical age range are counseled regarding the pros and cons of prophylactic pinning before making the final decision. Prophylactic pinning is indicated in patients with an underlying endocrinologic or metabolic diagnosis, and it is generally recommended in patients younger than 10 years.

Recently, interest has increased in open surgical dislocation of the hip to treat a variety of problems, including SCFE. This technique facilitates not only realignment of the proximal femur at the site of deformity, but also the treatment of any coexisting labral problems or intra-articular pathology. These strategies are currently under investigation in selected centers, and longer-term follow-up studies are required to define any role for these procedures.

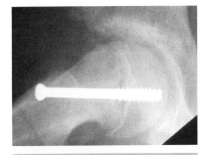

Figure 2 Radiograph demonstrates slipped capital femoral epiphysis treated in situ with surgical fixation using a single cannulated screw.

SECTION 9 PEDIATRIC ORTHOPAEDICS

Adverse Outcomes of Treatment

Patients are at risk for recurrent slippage until the physis closes. Chondrolysis and osteonecrosis also can occur.

Referral Decisions/Red Flags

Further evaluation for surgical treatment should occur immediately on diagnosis. Patients should be non–weight bearing after the diagnosis is made.

SECTION 9   PEDIATRIC ORTHOPAEDICS

Spondylolysis/ Spondylolisthesis

Definition

Spondylolysis refers to a unilateral or bilateral defect in the pars interarticularis, the region of bone lying between the superior and inferior articular facets. This condition is acquired. The process can start with a stress reaction, which results in a stress fracture and often an established pseudarthrosis (nonunion with fibrous tissue interposition). The most common level is L5, although spondylolysis can occur at higher levels in the lumbar spine and may be observed at more than one level. In up to 25% of patients with spondylolysis, a spondylolisthesis will develop.

Spondylolisthesis is anterior translation, or slippage, of one vertebra relative to the vertebral body below. The most common slip is L5 on S1, which represents more than 85% of cases (**Figure 1**). Most cases in children and adolescents are acquired (due to a stress fracture or spondylolysis); a small number of cases are congenital (or dysplastic) spondylolisthesis. Acquired spondylolisthesis, in which the amount of slip occurs through the defect in the pars interarticularis (which becomes filled with fibrocartilaginous material), is in contrast to congenital spondylolisthesis, in which elongation of the posterior elements often is associated with a dome-shaped sacrum. Higher grades of slip are often associated with kyphosis at the lumbosacral junction.

Clinical Symptoms

Activity-related low back pain that often radiates distally to the buttock and/or thigh is the most common symptom. Radiation to below the knee is uncommon and suggests lower lumbar

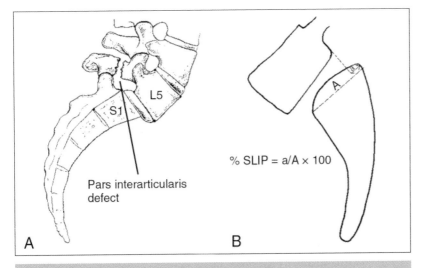

% SLIP = a/A × 100

Pars interarticularis defect

A   B

Figure 1 Illustrations depicts the lateral view of a grade I L5-S1 spondylolisthesis (**A**), and determination of slip percentage (**B**).

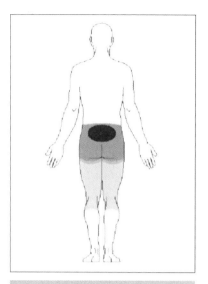

Figure 2 Illustration of a typical pain diagram for a patient with adolescent spondylolisthesis, highlighting buttock and posterior thigh pain.

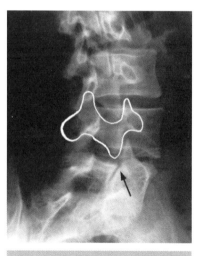

Figure 3 Oblique radiograph demonstrates a normal "Scotty dog" appearance in the outlined area. In the vertebra below, the Scotty dog has a "collar" (arrow), indicating the pars interarticularis defect of spondylolisthesis.

radiculopathy, which can occur with high-grade spondylolisthesis (**Figure 2**). Symptoms are more common with slips greater than 50%. Hamstring spasm/contracture is common and can result in limited forward bending. With higher grade lesions, neurologic abnormalities may be seen, such as nerve root symptoms (radiculopathy) from traction on the lower lumbar nerve roots, or bowel or bladder dysfunction (or symptoms of cauda equina syndrome) from compression (or traction) of the neural elements.

Tests

Physical Examination

Patients with substantial spondylolisthesis have a characteristic standing alignment, including mild flexion at the hips and knees, which compensates for backward tilting of the pelvis, and flattening of the normal lumbar lordosis (often a kyphosis at the lumbosacral junction). With marked levels of slip, a step-off can be palpated, and the spinous process of the vertebra below is more prominent than the one above. Patients often experience discomfort with hyperextension of the spine (loading the posterior elements in compression); the examiner should hold the spine in this position for 10 to 20 seconds to see if discomfort can be reproduced. This may be the first sign of a stress reaction or of spondylolysis. Manual pressure on the spinous processes may produce discomfort at the involved level. The popliteal angle should be tested to evaluate for hamstring contracture: With the patient supine and with one hip flexed to 90° and the other leg fully extended, the knee is extended and the angle between the tibia and the vertical plane is measured. The mean angle is 6° in toddlers and 25° in adolescents. A neurologic examination is essential, and other regions in which back pain may be referred (abdomen, pelvis, hips) must be evaluated as well.

Diagnostic Tests

AP and weight-bearing lateral radiographs of the lumbar spine are obtained, often supplemented by oblique radiographs. Established spondylolysis exhibits the so-called Scotty dog sign on oblique radiographs (**Figure 3**). When clinical suspicion of spondylolysis exists and plain radiographs are normal, a bone scan with single-photon emission CT (SPECT) images will help establish the diagnosis. CT with thin cuts through the pars region may be required to determine if a pars fracture has healed or progressed to nonunion. With spondylolisthesis, the lateral radiograph demonstrates forward translation of L5 relative to S1 for an L5-S1 slip (expressed as a percentage of the anteroposterior width of the vertebral body) (**Figure 4**). The degree of lumbosacral kyphosis, or flexion of the lumbar spine relative to the sacrum (the slip angle), also is measured. Lateral lumbar radiographs are occasionally obtained in flexion and extension to determine if excessive motion or instability between the involved segments occurs.

Differential Diagnosis

- Ankylosing spondylitis (HLA-B27–positive, sacroiliac joint changes)
- Intervertebral discitis (elevated erythrocyte sedimentation rate and fever, disk space narrowing on radiographs)
- Intervertebral disk injury or herniation (no step-off or slip and no defect seen on plain radiographs, radiculopathy occasionally present)
- Osteoid osteoma (night pain, abnormal bone scan, pain relieved by aspirin)
- Spinal cord tumor (sensory findings, upper motor neuron signs)

Adverse Outcomes of the Disease

The natural history of spondylolysis and spondylolisthesis is variable, and many patients will be asymptomatic and able to participate in activities as tolerated. Chronic back pain will develop in a subset, however, with or without radiculopathy, and bowel and bladder involvement or cauda equina syndrome (**Figure 5**) will develop in some patients with high-grade spondylolisthesis. Spondylolisthesis can progress in children and adolescents, so clinical and radiographic monitoring is required. The frequency of evaluation, typically every 6 to 12 months, depends on the amount of growth remaining, the degree of slip, and whether a patient is symptomatic. A weight-bearing spot lateral radiograph is usually adequate for periodic monitoring.

Treatment

Patients with a stress reaction or an early case of spondylolysis are treated with activity restriction, short-term analgesics or anti-inflammatory agents, and a thoracolumbosacral orthosis (TLSO) for 3 to 4 months, often supplemented by rehabilitation. Healing can be achieved using this approach in a subset of patients (especially those with unilateral pars defects), but in many patients, the spondylolysis ultimately progresses to a chronic pseudarthrosis or nonunion, which may or may not be symptomatic.

Asymptomatic spondylolysis requires no active treatment, and patients may participate in activities as tolerated. In patients with a symptomatic pseudarthrosis (limited or no healing potential), the goal of treatment is symptomatic relief rather than healing. Rehabilitation also is helpful and involves strengthening of the abdominal and paraspinal muscles, stretching the hamstring muscles, and postural adaptations. A TLSO also may be recommended for symptomatic relief in patients with chronic pain and an established pseudarthrosis, although the goal is symptomatic relief rather than healing of the stress fracture. For patients who have chronic symptoms despite an adequate trial of nonsurgical treatment, surgical options include repair of the pars defect (with instrumentation and bone grafting) or fusion of the involved segments. Fusion is typically recommended for

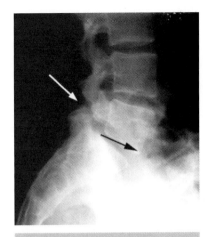

Figure 4 Lateral radiograph demonstrates a grade I L5-S1 spondylolisthesis. The black arrow indicates the direction of the slip; the white arrow indicates the defect.

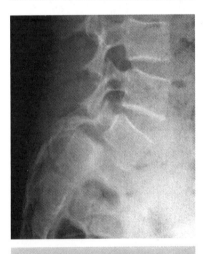

Figure 5 Lateral radiograph demonstrates a high-grade spondylolisthesis that required surgical stabilization.

SECTION 9 PEDIATRIC ORTHOPAEDICS

the less mobile L5-S1 articulation; repair is an option when higher levels of the spine are involved.

The treatment of spondylolisthesis depends on skeletal maturity, degree of deformity, and whether symptoms are present. Asymptomatic children with minimal amounts of slippage may continue with activities as tolerated, although follow-up at regular intervals will be required. Skeletally immature patients with a slip greater than 50% are candidates for spinal fusion (with or without instrumentation) with the goal of stabilizing the segment, as are those chronically symptomatic patients with a lower grade spondylolisthesis (less common). Patients with high-grade spondylolisthesis, especially with neurologic symptoms or findings, will require a neural decompression in addition to the spinal fusion, and either postural or instrumented reduction of the amount of slip is considered depending on the circumstances.

Adverse Outcomes of Treatment

In addition to the general complications of spine surgery such as bleeding and infection, surgical complications of spondylolysis repair include pseudarthrosis (nonunion); for spondylolisthesis, complications include nerve root or cauda equina injury, pseudarthrosis, implant failure, and chronic pain.

Referral Decisions/Red Flags

Patients with substantial or chronic back pain and/or a confirmed spondylolysis or spondylolisthesis require further evaluation.

Tarsal Coalition

Synonyms

Calcaneonavicular bar
Peroneal spastic flatfoot
Rigid flatfoot
Talocalcaneal bar

Definition

Tarsal coalition is an abnormal connection (fibrous, cartilaginous, or osseous) between two tarsal bones, most commonly the calcaneus and the navicular (calcaneonavicular coalition) or the talus and the calcaneus (talocalcaneal coalition). Rarely, more than one coalition is present. The condition is bilateral in approximately 50% of patients and may be found in other family members who are asymptomatic but have no hindfoot motion.

Clinical Symptoms

If symptoms develop, they usually occur during late childhood or adolescence. In some cases, the bar is initially cartilaginous and ossifies later, during early adolescence. Symptoms are the result of a restriction in hindfoot eversion and inversion. Calcaneonavicular coalitions generally become symptomatic in children between 9 and 13 years of age; symptoms from a talocalcaneal coalition generally develop later, between 13 and 16 years of age.

The onset of pain usually is insidious but can be associated with an injury or change in activity. Ankle sprains are frequent, and a limp is common. Pain from a talocalcaneal coalition usually is vague and located deep within the hindfoot. Pain from a calcaneonavicular coalition usually occurs laterally, over the area of the coalition.

Tests

Physical Examination

Patients with tarsal coalition typically have rigid flatfoot (hindfoot valgus, forefoot abduction); that is, the longitudinal arch is absent whether in a weight-bearing position or not. Hindfoot motion (inversion and eversion) is markedly restricted. Spasm of the peroneal muscles holds the foot in a stiff, everted position and may be demonstrated by attempting rapid passive inversion of the foot.

Diagnostic Tests

AP, lateral, and oblique radiographs of the foot can delineate a calcaneonavicular coalition (**Figure 1**). Talocalcaneal bars are difficult to see on these views, but they may be visualized on a Harris heel view. In most cases, CT is used to establish the diagnosis and better characterize the coalition. MRI evaluation of the foot can often visualize a coalition and rule out other cause of hindfoot pain.

SECTION 9   PEDIATRIC ORTHOPAEDICS

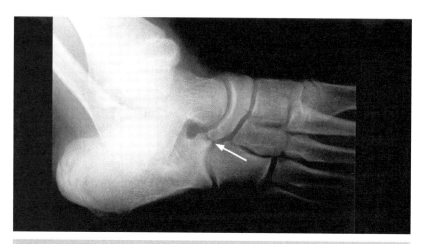

Figure 1 Oblique radiograph of a foot with a cartilaginous calcaneonavicular coalition (arrow).

Differential Diagnosis

- Accessory navicular (medial prominence and pain over the navicular)
- Congenital vertical talus (rigid flatfoot deformity noted in the infant or toddler)
- Flexible flatfoot (no restriction of subtalar motion, usually without pain)
- Juvenile idiopathic arthritis or other inflammatory disease (negative radiographs and CT, synovitis on MRI)

Adverse Outcomes of the Disease

Pain, restricted inversion and eversion of the foot, and limited walking and running are possible consequences.

Treatment

Treatment options include observation, short leg cast immobilization, resection of the coalition, and arthrodesis. Observation or activity modifications are appropriate for children who are asymptomatic or who have minimal symptoms. For more severe symptoms or for milder symptoms that persist, a 4- to 6-week trial in a short leg walking cast may be beneficial. For patients with persistent symptoms that do not respond to nonsurgical treatment, resection of the coalition with interposition of fat or muscle is the preferred treatment. Resection reduces pain in most patients, and this procedure is more reliable for calcaneonavicular coalitions. An osteotomy of the calcaneus also can be performed at the same time as coalition resection, when hindfoot realignment is needed. Hindfoot arthrodesis (joint fusion) is reserved for patients who have not responded to resection procedures or patients who are not candidates for coalition resection because the coalition is too large or arthritic changes are already present.

Adverse Outcomes of Treatment

Complications include cast sores, postoperative infection, failure of fusion, recurrence of the coalition, inadequate pain relief or persistent symptoms, and arthritic changes.

Referral Decisions/Red Flags

Substantial pain following nonsurgical treatment indicates the need for further evaluation.

PEDIATRIC ORTHOPAEDICS

SECTION 9

Toe Walking

Synonym

Habitual toe walking

Idiopathic toe walking

Definition

Idiopathic toe walking (or habitual toe walking) is toe walking in children who are otherwise healthy and have no underlying neurologic abnormalities. Toe walking can be a normal variation in children when they begin to walk. Toe walking that persists or develops after a child has been walking with the feet flat can indicate an underlying disease process. Symptoms are uncommon, and most patients respond to nonsurgical measures.

Clinical Symptoms

Parental concern is usually the reason for referral. Children with idiopathic toe walking generally are active and asymptomatic and have no functional difficulties or other medical problems. The patient may have occasional forefoot discomfort in the region of the metatarsal heads after prolonged activities. Discomfort in the hindfoot or posterior calcaneus also can occur if the child has an associated Achilles tendon contracture.

Tests

Physical Examination

Idiopathic toe walking is a diagnosis of exclusion, and pathologic causes must be ruled out. A thorough history is critical, particularly a detailed birth history, developmental history, and family history. Cerebral palsy is suggested by a delay in reaching motor milestones and a history of prematurity, low birth weight, hypoxia, or perinatal infection. Muscular dystrophy is suspected when a positive family history and proximal muscle weakness exists. The time of onset also is important. Patients with muscular dystrophy may be slightly delayed in achieving independent ambulation, and they typically walk with feet flat for a time before they begin to walk up on their toes. Children with idiopathic toe walking begin ambulation at the appropriate age and are up on their toes when they begin walking. Toe walking is common in children with speech and language delays, including autism spectrum disorders.

Ankle range of motion should be tested to quantify the degree of dorsiflexion. When assessing range of motion, the hindfoot should be inverted to lock the subtalar joint. Patients with less than 10° passive dorsiflexion have an Achilles tendon contracture. Toe walking varies in severity (**Figure 1**), but children with idiopathic toe walking generally can stand with their feet flat on the floor and can walk heel-to-toe if reminded. A subset of patients with idiopathic toe walking will also have Achilles tendon contracture. These patients may still be able to walk with the feet flat, but they will appear to have flatfoot when standing because dorsiflexion through the hindfoot joints compensates for a loss of dorsiflexion at the ankle. A thorough neurologic examination is essential, including evaluation for cutaneous lesions over the spine that can suggest occult spinal dysraphism.

Diagnostic Tests
Diagnostic tests should be ordered only if the history is unclear or if the examination reveals some abnormality that suggests another disorder.

Differential Diagnosis
- Autism spectrum disorder (other developmental/behavioral concerns)
- Cerebral palsy (delayed developmental milestones, spasticity of gastrocnemius-soleus complex)
- Intraspinal abnormality (cavus feet, unilateral or asymmetric involvement)
- Muscular dystrophy (proximal muscular weakness, positive family history)
- Occult hydrocephalus (upper motor neuron signs)

Adverse Outcomes of the Disease
The prevalence of long-term sequelae has not been documented; however, in some patients, persistent calluses and pain in the forefoot develop during late adolescence.

Treatment
Treatment depends on the age of the child and the severity of the problem. In the toddler who has just begun to walk, the condition often resolves spontaneously after 3 to 6 months. Observation is appropriate for older toddlers who walk on their toes only occasionally. Stretching exercises can be tried for young children with mild contractures. Children with autism spectrum disorders can benefit from physical therapy, occupational therapy, or other comprehensive interventional strategies.

Serial casting involving two to three short leg casts over a period of 6 weeks often is successful, especially with a coexisting Achilles tendon contracture. The degree of dorsiflexion is increased with each cast. Casting for several weeks results in atrophy of the Achilles tendon, which theoretically can help treat any habitual component, given that the child may find it difficult to stay up on the toes after the casts are removed, at least until the muscle regains its strength. Rehabilitation, possibly supplemented by nighttime splinting in dorsiflexion, can help prevent recurrent contracture. Some clinicians recommend using an ankle-foot orthosis to prevent recurrence. After

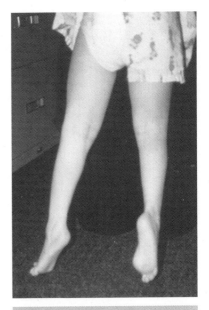

Figure 1 Photograph depicts idiopathic toe walking.

SECTION 9   PEDIATRIC ORTHOPAEDICS

casting, many of these children will walk heel-to-toe, but some will revert to their previous gait pattern.

Adverse Outcomes of Treatment

Observation and stretching exercises are complicated only by failure or recurrence. Recurrence and skin problems can occur with casting or with heel cord lengthening. Surgical overlengthening of the Achilles tendon can permanently affect push-off power.

Referral Decisions/Red Flags

Any child with persistent toe walking despite stretching and rehabilitation or with evidence of a neuromuscular impairment requires further evaluation. Surgical treatment typically is indicated for an older child with a fixed heel cord contracture when nonsurgical treatment is ineffective or poorly tolerated. Heel cord lengthening is considered after all nonsurgical measures have failed. Postoperatively, approximately 6 weeks of cast immobilization is required. Unilateral toe walking is never normal. In these instances, thorough examination is required to identify the underlying pathologic process. The most common causes of unilateral toe walking are limb-length discrepancy, cerebral palsy, and tethering of the spinal cord (intraspinal anomaly). Developmental evaluation of children with other developmental or behavioral concerns should be considered.

Torticollis

Synonyms
Acquired torticollis
Congenital muscular torticollis (CMT)
Wryneck

Definition
Torticollis describes a head position characterized by tilting (lateral bending) of the head to one side, often with rotation. It is a finding, not a specific diagnosis. Most cases that present at or shortly after birth represent congenital muscular torticollis (CMT). CMT is a unilateral contracture of the sternocleidomastoid (SCM) muscle and is diagnosed shortly after birth. The etiology remains unknown, but fibrosis and subsequent contracture can result from a localized compartment syndrome within the muscle caused by abnormal positioning in utero. Acquired torticollis presents later in infancy or in childhood. Acquired torticollis is associated with many conditions. It requires a detailed workup including advanced imaging studies, and often, consultations with a subspecialist. The differential diagnosis includes injuries, congenital anomalies, inflammatory or infectious disorders, neurologic abnormalities, ophthalmologic problems (nystagmus, superior oblique palsy), atlantoaxial rotatory displacement (AARD), posterior fossa brain tumors, and others. Torticollis in infants also can result from congenital anomalies within the cervical spine, either from a progressive congenital scoliosis at the cervicothoracic junction (**Figure 1**) or an anomaly at the occipitocervical junction. These deformities can present as a progressive tilt with or without substantial rotational deformity. Klippel-Feil syndrome involves a congenital fusion of two or more cervical segments, which commonly manifests as a restriction in cervical motion associated with a short neck, and is occasionally associated with head tilt.

Clinical Symptoms
Parental concern about head posture is the usual reason for the visit. Children with acquired torticollis can present with neck pain, fevers, or, rarely, neurologic abnormalities, depending on the underlying diagnosis. In CMT, contracture of the SCM muscle causes the head to tilt toward the affected side and rotate toward the unaffected side (**Figure 2**). CMT is commonly associated with plagiocephaly and facial asymmetry. A lump may be palpable within the midsubstance of the muscle during the first weeks of life, but this typically disappears within weeks to months. Associated findings may include positional foot deformities (metatarsus adductus, calcaneovalgus) and developmental dysplasia of the hip (5% to 8%).

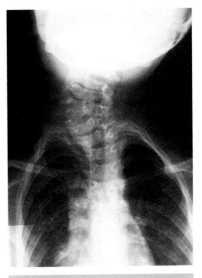

Figure 1 AP radiograph from an infant with torticollis caused by progressive congenital vertebral anomaly at the cervicothoracic junction.

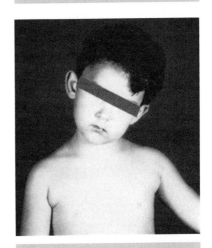

Figure 2 Photograph depicts a child with congenital muscular torticollis. The chin is rotated to the patient's right and the head is inclined to the left.

SECTION 9 PEDIATRIC ORTHOPAEDICS

Tests

Physical Examination

Infants with CMT hold the head in a so-called cock robin position. Contracture of the left SCM muscle results in tilting to the left side with rotation of the head to the right side, with associated facial/mandibular flattening on the left side and occipital flattening on the right side. In patients with CMT, a lump or swelling in the SCM muscle that disappears over the first few weeks to months may be noted. Patients with AARD hold the head in a similar position to those with CMT; however, spasm of the SCM usually occurs on the side opposite the tilt, in contrast to CMT. Range of motion should be evaluated; it can be limited as a result of contracture (CMT) or because of discomfort or muscle spasm. A complete neurologic examination is essential, as well as an ophthalmologic evaluation, to assess for ocular or neurologic disorders. A complete musculoskeletal examination also is required, because CMT can be associated with developmental dysplasia of the hip and intrauterine deformations.

Acquired torticollis requires a comprehensive evaluation. An ophthalmologic examination often is helpful because "ocular" torticollis can be a result of nystagmus or a superior oblique palsy. In such cases, the findings can resolve when the eyes are closed or vision is blocked. Neurologic causes of torticollis include tumors of the posterior fossa and cervical spine, as well as developmental conditions such as syringomyelia, and neurologic consultation (and MRI) is indicated in many patients. Infections such as discitis or vertebral osteomyelitis usually present with substantial pain and systemic signs or symptoms. Benign paroxysmal torticollis of infancy involves episodes of torticollis that can last from minutes to days; the side of involvement may alternate, and the condition usually resolves spontaneously. AARD represents a spectrum of abnormalities in the alignment and arc of motion between C1 and C2. Either subluxation or dislocation can be present, and the displacement is initially reducible but becomes fixed or irreducible over time. AARD can develop following minor trauma; in association with inflammatory disorders of the upper airway, neck, or pharynx (Grisel syndrome); or following surgical procedures of the ears, nose, or oropharynx.

Diagnostic Tests

The indications for screening radiographs of the cervical spine in patients with CMT are controversial; some authors advise obtaining radiographs when the typical clinical features of CMT are absent or the deformity does not respond appropriately to stretching. AP and lateral radiographs of the cervical spine should be obtained in all patients with acquired torticollis to rule out underlying congenital bony anomalies, and most patients in whom a cervical anomaly is diagnosed will require lateral radiographs in flexion and extension as well, to rule out instability. Patients with neurologic symptoms or findings also may require MRIs of the cervical spine in flexion and extension to rule out neurologic encroachment. Patients with a history of trauma should be imaged with more than two views of the cervical spine; an open-mouth odontoid view, and occasionally, oblique views.

Specialized imaging studies such as CT or MRI may be indicated as well. MRI of the brain and cervical spine often is required to rule out a brainstem tumor or other pathology. Open-mouth odontoid views should be obtained when AARD is suspected; however, this diagnosis is very difficult to establish using plain radiographs. CT scans of the cervical spine with the head in neutral and in maximal rotation (right and left) characterize the rotational alignment between C1 and C2 throughout the available range of motion and will clearly show any fixed subluxation or dislocation between C1 and C2. The study may be difficult to obtain if the patient has substantial pain or spasm.

Other imaging studies also may be considered, depending on the specific diagnosis. For example, screening hip ultrasonography is considered even when the physical examination is normal in patients with CMT. All patients with congenital vertebral anomalies should have coexisting visceral anomalies ruled out, typically by using a renal ultrasound, a cardiac evaluation with or without an electrocardiogram, and, often, MRI of the neural axis.

Differential Diagnosis for Acquired Torticollis

Present at or Shortly After Birth

- CMT (identified during first 2 months of life)
- Congenital vertebral anomalies or instabilities

    Klippel-Feil syndrome (short neck, low hairline, may have Sprengel deformity)

- Pterygium colli (skin webbing)
- Unilateral absence of SCM muscle

Acquired

- AARD (older patient, history of minor trauma, ear/nose/throat procedure, pharyngitis, late onset)
- Benign paroxysmal torticollis (infants, repeated episodes)
- Infectious or inflammatory

    Cervical lymphadenitis (lymphadenopathy)

    Discitis or vertebral osteomyelitis (pain with flexion)

    Juvenile idiopathic arthritis (multiple joint involvement, gradual onset)

    Soft-tissue infection in the neck/pharynx (localized tenderness in soft tissues)

- Neurogenic

    Cervical dystonia (increased muscle tone that fluctuates, history of developmental delay or cerebral palsy)

    Chiari malformation and/or syringomyelia (headaches, neurologic abnormalities)

SECTION 9 PEDIATRIC ORTHOPAEDICS

Ocular (nystagmus, superior oblique palsy) (ophthalmologic findings)

Posterior fossa tumor (headaches, constant and increasing pain, more gradual onset, neurologic findings)

- Posttraumatic

Muscle sprain, fractures (history of trauma)

- Other

Hysteria (rare, diagnosis of exclusion)

Sandifer syndrome (gastroesophageal reflux)

Adverse Outcomes of the Disease

The natural history of CMT includes persistent torticollis, facial asymmetry, and plagiocephaly. Untreated AARD results in fixed malalignment at the atlantoaxial joint, which can be associated with chronic pain and a risk of neurologic dysfunction. The natural history in other acquired cases of torticollis depends on the underlying diagnosis. Patients with Klippel-Feil syndrome are at risk of cervical spinal cord injury and should be restricted from participation in contact activities or those that involve sudden acceleration and/or deceleration.

Treatment

Congenital Muscular Torticollis

Nonsurgical treatment of CMT consists of frequent stretching exercises that tilt and rotate the head. Supervision by a rehabilitation specialist is helpful, but the parents themselves must actually perform the stretching exercises several times per day. In addition, the infant's bed and changing table can be positioned to encourage the infant to look away from the limited side. Nonsurgical treatment is successful in more than 90% of patients. If the problem persists after 12 to 18 months, surgical release/lengthening of the SCM can be considered, but the best results are obtained if surgery is performed after 4 years of age.

Acquired Torticollis

The treatment of acquired torticollis depends on the underlying etiology. Initial management of AARD is immobilization in a soft cervical collar and administration of analgesics for pain and low-dose benzodiazepines for muscle spasms. If restoration of motion and alignment does not occur in approximately 1 week, cervical traction with a head halter, coupled with analgesics and muscle relaxants, should be tried. Most cases resolve with this program, and patients are typically splinted in a collar or other device such as a pinless halo for several additional weeks. If this treatment fails, a period of halo traction should be considered to reduce the malalignment. AARD that persists for more than 1 month is less likely to respond to these treatment strategies, and some patients will ultimately require upper cervical fusion for relief of symptoms and restoration of alignment.

SECTION 9 PEDIATRIC ORTHOPAEDICS

Adverse Outcomes of Treatment

Unsightly scarring from halo pins or surgical incision, recurrence, incomplete correction, and cervical stiffness may occur.

Referral Decisions/Red Flags

Most infants with CMT are referred for rehabilitation and for evaluation by a specialist, recognizing that most cases will respond to nonsurgical measures. Referral should be considered for all patients with acquired torticollis, as well as those with head tilt and rotation to the same side.

SECTION 9 PEDIATRIC ORTHOPAEDICS

Transient Synovitis of the Hip

Synonyms

Coxalgia fugax

Toxic synovitis

Definition

Transient synovitis of the hip is a sterile effusion of the joint that resolves without therapy or sequelae, typically over 4 to 6 weeks, and is a common source of limping in children from 2 to 7 years of age. Boys are affected two to three times more often than girls. The etiology is unknown. Mild trauma can explain some cases, and many patients have a history of viral illness (upper respiratory or gastrointestinal) in the days to weeks preceding the onset of limping.

Clinical Symptoms

The child presents with a limp, which can be painless or associated with discomfort that is localized in the groin, proximal thigh, or knee. Some patients with more substantial symptoms will refuse to walk. The limp can be intermittent; typically, it worsens toward the end of the day and usually resolves over 1 to 2 weeks.

Tests

Physical Examination

Examination reveals a limp (typically an abductor lurch/Trendelenburg gait) and mild restriction of hip motion, particularly in abduction and internal rotation. There may be guarding at the extremes of hip rotation. Most children are afebrile.

Diagnostic Tests

Because transient synovitis is a diagnosis of exclusion, the extent of the evaluation process depends on the degree and duration of symptoms and the findings on physical examination. A short period of observation may be appropriate if the child has minimal symptoms, no systemic signs or symptoms, and no substantial pain with motion. In most patients with a limp and findings localized to the hip region, it is appropriate to order AP and frog-lateral radiographs of the pelvis and blood tests that include a complete blood count with a differential, an erythrocyte sedimentation rate, a C-reactive protein level, and an antistreptolysin O test. Other blood tests may be appropriate depending on the findings, such as a Lyme titer or rheumatologic tests. If any suspicion of septic arthritis exists or if the patient has substantial pain, any systemic signs or symptoms, or pain with short arc motion (midrange of motion rather than the extremes of motion), referral to the emergency department or hospital admission for further evaluation may be most appropriate.

Radiographs in patients with transient synovitis are usually normal, but they may show widening of the joint space due to effusion. If septic arthritis is suspected, hip ultrasonography is ordered urgently, and aspiration of the hip can be performed at the same time. MRI can be useful in selected cases to rule out other infections (osteomyelitis of the femur or pelvis, psoas abscess) or early Legg-Calvé-Perthes disease.

Differential Diagnosis

• Infections

  Lyme disease (similar presentation, may have swelling in other joints)

  Pelvic osteomyelitis (pain that is dull, constant, and increasing; fever)

  Proximal femoral osteomyelitis (pain that is dull, constant, and increasing; fever)

  Septic arthritis (pain that is dull, constant, and increasing; fever)

• Inflammatory diseases (juvenile idiopathic arthritis or other) (history of joint swelling)

• Injuries (sprain, strain, rarely occult fracture)

• Legg-Calvé-Perthes disease (boys age 4 to 8 years, similar presentation)

Adverse Outcomes of the Disease

No sequelae are associated with transient synovitis, and recurrence is uncommon. Legg-Calvé-Perthes disease subsequently develops in 1% to 3% of patients, but whether this disorder has any association with transient synovitis is unclear. A delay in diagnosing septic arthritis or another disease process is possible.

Treatment

Most children can be treated with activity restriction (bed rest acutely) and anti-inflammatory agents or mild analgesics. The limp typically improves within 3 to 14 days, but it may take 4 to 6 weeks for complete resolution. When the diagnosis is equivocal or the patient has substantial discomfort, hospitalization for observation and further investigation is indicated.

Referral Decisions/Red Flags

Patients with substantial pain and limping, with or without systemic signs or symptoms, require further evaluation. Consultation with a specialist is frequently obtained during the evaluation. Follow-up with a specialist is indicated if radiographs suggest Legg-Calvé-Perthes disease.

SECTION 9 PEDIATRIC ORTHOPAEDICS

Glossary

abduction The movement of a body part away from the midline.

acupuncture The insertion of needles into precisely defined points on the body; thought to realign imbalances of yin-yang and qi and thereby bring harmony to the "climate" of an individual.

adduction The movement of a body part toward the midline.

adhesive capsulitis Self-limiting condition resulting from any inflammatory process about the shoulder in which capsular scar tissue is produced, resulting in pain and limited range of motion; *also called* frozen shoulder.

aerobic exercise Exercise that uses oxidative metabolic pathways to provide energy.

allograft Biologic tissue from a cadaver that is used to surgically replace damaged tissue.

alternative medicine A wide spectrum of treatments—many finding support from collective anecdotal evidence—that is not considered standard therapy because of the lack of a scientific rationale, clinical evidence, or a favorable historic tradition.

anabolic steroid Testosterone, or a steroid hormone resembling testosterone, that stimulates anabolism in the body.

anaerobic exercise Exercise of short duration, not requiring the body's utilization of oxygen to make fuel available.

anaerobic metabolism Oxygen debt; when the cardiovascular system is unable to meet the needs of the working muscles, the anaerobic metabolism is activated.

analgesia The relief of pain.

ankylosing spondylitis An inflammatory disorder that affects the low back and pelvis and produces stiffness and pain.

ankylosis Marked stiffness of a joint typically observed with end-stage arthritis, following a complex intra-articular fracture, delayed treatment of septic arthritis, or severe rheumatoid arthritis.

anorexia nervosa A condition, common in young females, in which the patient takes in less food and may become seriously emaciated and malnourished; a manifestation of a severe underlying psychological disorder.

anterior compartment syndrome Increased soft-tissue pressure in the anterior compartment of the lower leg, resulting in pain, decreased sensation, and muscle paralysis.

anterior cruciate ligament (ACL) Ligament that passes from the lateral intercondylar notch of the femur to attach anteriorly on the articular surface of the tibia.

anterior superior iliac spine Blunt bony projection on the anterior border of the ilium, forming the anterior end of the iliac crest. Serves as the origin of the sartorius muscle.

anterior surface Surface at the front of the body, facing the examiner.

anterior talofibular ligament One of three lateral ligaments of the ankle; arises from the anterior border of the lateral malleolus to attach to the neck of the talus.

anterior tibial tendon Structure that arises in the anterior compartment of the leg and passes downward and medially to insert on the first cuneiform and the base of the first metatarsal.

anterior tibiofibular ligament Part of tibiofibular syndesmosis; it arises from the anterior calculi on the lateral side of the tibia and blends into the interosseous membrane above the ankle joint.

anterolateral rotatory instability Anterior internal rotational subluxation of the lateral tibial condyle on the femur, reflecting damage to the anterior cruciate ligament and lateral structures.

anteromedial rotatory instability When the medial plateau of the tibia rotates anteriorly and medial joint opening occurs, indicating disruption of the superficial tibia collateral ligament, medial and posteromedial capsular structures, and anterior cruciate ligament.

anteroposterior drawer test Test for anterior and posterior laxity in which the examiner holds the knee in 90° of flexion, stabilizes the thigh, and slowly draws the tibia forward on the fixed femur, noting the degree of displacement. The examiner then attempts to displace the tibia posteriorly on the femur. The test is positive if changes in anteroposterior displacement of the tibia are noted. The injured side should always be compared with the noninjured side. The Lachman test is done similarly but with the knee in 30° of flexion.

anulus fibrosus The outer ring of fibrous material surrounding the nucleus of the intervertebral disks.

apophysis A cartilaginous structure at the insertion of major muscle groups into bone that may be susceptible to overuse syndromes and acute fractures in pediatric athletes.

apophysitis Inflammation of an apophysis; injury from repetitive traction to the cartilaginous growth plate near the origin or insertion of muscle.

arcuate ligament Posterior third of the lateral capsule, which, together with the popliteus attachments, provides considerable stability to the posterolateral corner of the knee.

arthrocentesis Aspiration of a joint.

arthrodesis The surgical fusion of a joint. The procedure removes any remaining articular cartilage and positions the adjacent bones to promote bone growth across a joint. A successful fusion eliminates the joint and stops motion. The usual purpose is pain relief or stabilization of an undependable joint.

arthroplasty A procedure to replace or mobilize a joint, typically performed by removing the arthritic surfaces and replacing them with an implant. Total joint arthroplasty is replacement of both sides of the joint. Hemiarthroplasty replaces only one side of a joint.

arthroscopy A form of minimally invasive surgery in which a fiberoptic camera, the arthroscope, is introduced into an area of the body through a small incision.

aspiration Removal of fluids from a body cavity; often done to obtain specimens for analysis.

autograft Biologic tissue from the patient's own body that is used to surgically replace damaged tissue.

avascular necrosis The death of bone, often as a result of obstruction of its blood supply. *See also* osteonecrosis.

avulsion fracture A fracture that occurs when a ligament or tendon pulls off a sliver of the bone.

axis The second cervical vertebra (C2).

Bankart fracture A small chip fracture off the anterior and inferior rims of the glenoid that is seen after an anterior dislocation of the shoulder.

biceps brachii Muscle in the anterior arm, originating from two heads (hence biceps) from the anterior glenoid and the coracoid process of the scapula and inserting into the biceps tuberosity of the radius. It is a powerful flexor of the elbow and supinator of the forearm.

biceps muscle Large muscle that covers the front of the humerus; functions include forearm flexion and hand supination.

biceps tendinitis Inflammation of the biceps tendon in its subacromial location.

bone infarction Bone death that occurs as the result of ischemia.

bone remodeling A process that couples bone resorption by osteoclasts with deposition of osteoblasts (new bone cells).

bone scan A study used to identify lesions in bone such as fracture, infections, or tumor. A radioisotope is injected into a vein and allowed to circulate through the body. The distribution of radioactivity in the skeleton is measured by a special camera that can detect the emission of gamma rays. Lesions in bone with increased metabolic activity (eg, fracture, tumor, or infection) will show increased uptake of the radioisotope and appear as a dark area in the bone. *Also called* bone scintigraphy.

brachial muscle Originates on the humerus, extends anteriorly across the elbow joint, and attaches into the ulna; functions in forearm flexion.

brachial plexus Network of nerves that pass from the lower part of the cervical spine and upper part of the thoracic spine down the arm.

bucket-handle tear Complete longitudinal tear of the central segment of the meniscus with the torn fragment "flipped" into the joint like the handle of a bucket.

bunion Prominence of the first metatarsal head often associated with lateral shift of the great toe (hallux valgus deformity).

bursa A sac formed by two layers of synovial tissue that is located where there is friction between tendon and bone or skin and bone.

bursitis Inflammation of a bursa.

burst fracture A compression-type fracture of a vertebra that involves posterior displacement of the fragments, often into the spinal canal.

calcaneofibular ligament The longest of the three lateral ligaments of the ankle; inserts on the lateral surface of the calcaneus.

calcaneus Heel bone.

capsule A collagenous structure that surrounds a joint like a sleeve. The capsule allows motion of joints and protects the articular cartilage. The capsule, along with ligaments, tendons, and bony structure, provides stability of the joint.

carpal bones Bones of the wrist.

cartilage A cellular tissue that, in the adult, is specific to joints, but in children forms a template for bone formation and growth. Hyaline cartilage is a low-friction cellular tissue that coats joint surfaces. Fibrocartilage is tough with high collagen content, such as found in the meniscus of the knee, or the anulus fibrosus portion of the intervertebral disk.

cauda equina The terminal nerve roots of the spinal cord located within the vertebral canal; so named because they resemble the tail of a horse.

cavus Excessive height of the longitudinal arch of the foot.

cellulitis Inflammation of subcutaneous tissue. Can be caused by trauma or infection.

cerebellum The brain area located posteriorly and attached to the brainstem; functions with the cerebral cortex and brainstem to regulate movement and posture.

cerebrum A mass of nerve tissue that makes up the largest part of the brain.

cervical spine The upper seven vertebrae, which extend from the base of the occiput to the first thoracic vertebra.

chondroblasts The cells that form cartilage.

chondroitin sulfate An important class of glucosaminoglycans in articular proteoglycans; the oral form is thought to prevent degradation of joint cartilage and relieve symptoms.

chondromalacia Softening of the articular surface that results from exposure of normal cartilage to excessive pressure or shear.

chondrosarcoma A primary sarcoma formed from cartilage cells or their precursors but without direct osteoid formation.

chronic rotator cuff tear Tear of the rotator cuff of the shoulder resulting from degeneration within the rotator cuff tendon.

clavicle The collarbone.

clavicular epiphyseal fracture Fracture of the growth plate of the clavicle; may appear clinically as a dislocation, especially if some displacement is present.

claw toe Deformity involving hyperextension of the metatarsophalangeal joint and a hyperflexion of the interphalangeal joint.

closed fracture A fracture that does not disrupt the integrity of the surrounding skin.

closed reduction A procedure to restore normal alignment of a fractured bone or dislocated joint in which the fractured bones are simply manipulated and no incision is needed.

clubfoot A complex foot disorder that includes three separate deformities: metatarsus adductus, ankle equinus, and heel varus.

coccyx The three to five fused vertebrae distal to the sacrum.

collagen A triple helix protein that is the major structural macromolecule of the extracellular matrix of articular cartilage; found also in bone, tendon, and ligament.

Colles fracture Fracture of the distal radius, with dorsal displacement of the fragments; often caused by a fall on an outstretched arm with the hand extended.

comminuted fracture A fracture with more than two fragments.

common peroneal nerve Nerve lying below the head of the fibula that controls movement at the ankle and supplies sensation to the top of the foot.

compartment syndrome Ischemia of the nerves and muscles within a fascial compartment caused by elevated pressure within the compartment; frequently seen in association with tibial fractures.

compound fracture Any fracture in which the overlying skin has been penetrated.

computed tomography (CT) A radiographic modality that allows cross-sectional imaging from a series of x-ray beams. The x-ray tube is rotated 360° around the patient, and the computer converts these images into a two-dimensional axial image. CT is capable of imaging bone in three planes: coronal, sagittal, and oblique. This modality is particularly useful in evaluating fractures and bone tumors.

concentric contraction The shortening of a muscle during activation.

concentric exercises Exercises in which the muscle shortens while contracting against resistance.

concussion Traumatic brain injury caused by a sudden blow to the head or to the body that causes the brain to come in contact with the inside of the skull. Typically characterized by the rapid onset of short-lived impairment of neurologic function. Neuropathologic changes may occur, but the acute symptoms reflect a functional disturbance rather than a structural injury.

condyle A rounded process at the end of a long bone.

connective tissue Tissue that connects and supports the structures of the body.

contusion Bruise; injury to soft tissue without a break in the skin.

copper therapy An as-yet unproven therapy in which any of a number of copper devices are applied to the body to reduce pain and inflammation associated with joint and connective tissue problems.

coracoacromial ligament Ligament lying anteromedially and superior to the glenohumeral joint; defines the subacromial space.

coracoclavicular ligaments Strong stabilizers of the acromioclavicular joint, consisting of the conoid and trapezial ligaments.

coronal plane A coronal plane is any plane of section in the anatomic position that passes vertically through the body and is perpendicular to the median plane. It divides the body into anterior and posterior sections.

cortical bone Dense bone that is responsible for skeletal homeostasis.

corticosteroids Cortisone-like medicines that are used to provide relief for inflamed areas of the body. They reduce swelling, redness, itching, and allergic reactions. Often used for many diseases such as asthma or other autoimmune diseases.

costal arch Fused costal cartilage of the sixth to tenth ribs forming the upper border of the abdomen.

costovertebral angle Angle that is formed by the spine and the tenth rib; the kidneys lie beneath the back muscles in the costovertebral angle.

COX-1 Cyclooxygenase-1 enzyme; an enzyme that is present in most bodily tissues (including platelets and gastrointestinal mucosal tissues) and serves as a "housekeeping" enzyme to form prostaglandins.

COX-2 Cyclooxygenase-2 enzyme; an enzyme that is thought to be present in the body only when induced in response to injury and is responsible for the formation of prostaglandins that mediate pain and inflammation.

coxa valgus A valgus or abduction deformity of the hip. The neck/shaft angle is increased.

coxa magna A deformity of the hip in which the ball of the hip joint is enlarged. May be secondary to Legg-Calvé-Perthes disease or arthritis.

crepitus a grating or grinding sound.

cross-table lateral view Lateral view of the hip obtained by flexing the opposite hip and directing the x-ray beam "across" the table to image a true lateral view of the hip. Used in imaging hip fractures, when a frog lateral view (taken with the hip abducted and rotated) would cause patient discomfort.

crush injury An injury produced as a result of continuous pressure applied to a part of the body, usually an extremity.

cryotherapy The therapeutic use of cold.

cubital tunnel syndrome Compression of the ulnar nerve at the elbow.

cubitus (elbow) Cubitus varus is a bowing (or adduction) deformity of the elbow. Cubitus valgus is an elbow aligned in the opposite direction.

curettage The removal of growths from within cavity walls; in the treatment of musculoskeletal tumors, the scraping of tumor out of bone.

deep vein thrombosis (DVT) Venous clot formation caused by immobilization, hypercoagulation, obstructed venous flow, or endothelial injury, among others.

degenerative joint disease (DJD) Deterioration of the articular cartilage that lines a joint, which results in narrowing of the joint space and pain; osteoarthritis.

delayed union A delay in normal fracture healing; not necessarily a pathologic process.

deltoid The muscle that arises from the inferior surface of the lateral third of the clavicle, the acromion, and the spine of the scapula and inserts into the deltoid tuberosity of the humerus. The anterior fibers assist in flexing and medially rotating the arm, whereas the posterior fibers extend and laterally rotate the arm. Acting as a unit, the deltoid acts to abduct the arm at the glenohumeral joint.

deltoid ligament One of the major support ligaments of the ankle; originates on the medial malleolus and spreads to attach to the medial border of the talus.

dermatome A localized area of skin that has its sensation via a single nerve from a single nerve root of the spinal cord.

diaphysis The shaft of a long bone.

diphosphonates Potent inhibitors of osteoclasts and bone resorption. May be used to treat osteoporosis and Paget disease.

direct bone healing Method of healing of a fracture in which the approximated bone ends attach themselves to one another by laying down woven bone.

discoid meniscus A congenital deformity in which the meniscus is discoid in shape rather than semilunar.

diskectomy A surgical decompression procedure in which an intervertebral disk is removed.

dislocation Complete disruption in the normal relationship of two bones forming a joint (ie, no contact of the articular surfaces). The direction of the dislocation is described by the position of the distal bone (eg, with an anterior dislocation of the shoulder, the humerus is displaced anterior to the scapula).

displaced fracture A fracture that produces deformity of the limb.

distal Location in an extremity nearer the free end; location on the trunk farther from the midline or from the point of reference.

dorsal Toward the posterior surface of the body.

dorsalis pedis artery The continuation of the anterior tibial artery on the anterior surface of the foot.

dual-energy x-ray absorptiometry (DEXA or DXA) A diagnostic imaging technology that uses two different x-ray voltages to assess bone density.

dynamic strength The magnitude of isotonic or isokinetic contraction.

dysplasia A broad term that describes a condition affecting growth or development in which the primary defect is intrinsic to bone or cartilage.

dystrophy A condition resulting from defective or faulty nutrition, broadly construed to include nourishment of tissue by all essential substances, including those normally manufactured by the body itself.

eccentric contraction The lengthening of a muscle during activation.

eccentric exercises Exercises in which the muscle lengthens despite resisting a force, as in slowly lowering a weight.

ecchymosis Bruising or discoloration associated with bleeding within or under the skin.

edema Condition in which fluid escapes into the tissues from vascular or lymphatic spaces and causes local or generalized swelling.

effusion The presence of fluid within a joint.

electrical muscle stimulation (EMS) Treatment in which the biphasic current delivers stimulation to muscles in a variety of ways, including pulse, surged, or tetanizing contractions.

electromyography (EMG) A test that measures the electrical response of muscle contraction.

enchondral bone healing Process in which capillaries grow among mesenchymal cells, forming a fibrovascular tissue known as callus that bridges the gap between bone ends.

endochondral ossification The formation of bone within a cartilage model.

enthesopathy A disease process occurring at the insertion of muscle, tendon, or ligament into bone or a joint capsule.

epiphysis A part of a long bone developed from a center of ossification distinct from that of the shaft and separated at first from the latter by a layer of cartilage.

epiphyseal line The part of a long bone that produces growth.

equinus Plantar flexed position of the ankle.

Ewing sarcoma A primary sarcoma of the bone that usually arises in the diaphyses of long bones, ribs, and flat bones of children and adolescents.

exercise-induced compartment syndrome A condition in which exertion leads to relative muscle swelling within a restricted fascial compartment, resulting in compression of neurovascular structures, reduced circulation, muscle ischemia, bone death, and the painful buildup of lactic acid.

extensor A muscle, the contraction of which causes movement at a joint with the consequence that the limb or body assumes a more straight line, or so that the distance between the parts proximal and distal to the joint is increased or extended; the antagonist of a flexor.

extensor digitorum brevis Short toe extensor on the dorsum of the foot.

extensor digitorum longus Muscle in the anterior compartment of the muscles of the leg; divides and inserts on the dorsum of the small toes.

extensor hallucis longus Muscle in the anterior compartment of the leg that inserts on the dorsum of the great toe.

extensor mechanism Complex interaction of muscles, ligaments, and tendons that stabilizes the patellofemoral joint and acts to extend the knee.

extensor supinator muscle group Muscle group originating on the lateral epicondyle of the humerus and extending down the forearm dorsally into the wrist and hand that includes the extensor carpi radialis longus, the extensor carpi radialis brevis, and the supinator.

external fixation Stabilization of a fracture or unstable joint by inserting pins into bone proximal and distal to the injury that are then attached to an external frame.

fabella Sesamoid bone that is sometimes found in the lateral gastrocnemius muscle tendon.

fascia Sheet or band of tough fibrous connective tissue; lies deep under the skin and forms an outer layer for the muscles.

fascia lata Originates from the lateral crest region and continues over the lateral aspect of the knee, enveloping the lateral aspect of the thigh; iliotibial tract.

fasciculation Involuntary contractions, or twitchings, of groups (fasciculi) of muscle fibers, a coarser form of muscular contraction than fibrillation.

fast twitch muscle fibers Type II muscle fibers.

fat embolism syndrome Respiratory distress and cerebral dysfunction caused by droplets of marrow fat released at a fracture site and deposited in the lungs or brain.

fatigue fracture Microfracture that occurs when the bone is subjected to frequent, repeated stresses, such as in running or marching long distances, and the rate of bone breakdown exceeds the rate of bone repair.

fat pad Specialized soft tissue structure for weight bearing and absorbing impact.

fat pad sign A sign on a lateral view of the elbow with the elbow flexed 90° that indicates swelling within the joint, often from a fracture with hemorrhage.

felon Infection of the pulp of the distal phalanx of the finger.

female athlete triad The constellation of abnormal or absent menses, eating disorders, and osteoporosis/stress fractures seen in female athletes.

femoral condyles Two surfaces at the distal end of the femur that articulate with the superior surfaces of the tibia.

femoral head Proximal end of the femur: articulates with the acetabulum.

femoral neck The bone connecting the head and the shaft of the femur; fractures frequently occur in this area.

femur The thigh bone; extends from the pelvis to the knee and is the longest and largest bone in the body.

fibrochondrocytes Cells that are able to synthesize fibrous extracellular proteins and have the rounded appearance of chondrocytes.

fibula Outer and smaller of the two bones of the leg, extending from just below the knee to form the lateral portion of the ankle joint.

fibular collateral ligament Ligament that inserts from the femoral condyle to the fibular head.

flexibility The capacity of a muscle to lengthen or stretch.

flexor A muscle, the action of which is to flex or bend a joint.

flexor digitorum longus muscle One of the medial stabilizers of the ankle, located in the posterior compartment of the muscles of the leg, that flexes the lateral four toes.

flexor hallucis longus muscle One of the three muscles of the deep portion of the posterior compartment that flexes the great toe.

flexor pronator muscle group A muscle group with a primary role associated with the wrist and hand and a secondary role as elbow flexors.

floating ribs The eleventh and twelfth ribs, which do not connect to the sternum.

fluoroscopy A special type of radiograph that shows continuous motion of the structure, such as wrist motion.

fracture A disruption in the integrity of a bone.

fracture callus Bone developed after a fracture; initially formed from a hematoma at the bleeding edges of bone, it eventually forms a cartilage mass that is remodeled into mature bone.

fracture-dislocation A fracture of bone associated with a dislocation of its adjacent joint.

fracture reduction The realignment of fracture fragments to restore normal anatomy of the bone.

Freiberg disease An osteochondrosis or osteonecrosis of the metatarsal head.

frequency In strength training, the number of workouts completed per unit of time; also refers to number of workouts during 1 week.

frozen shoulder A condition characterized by restricted shoulder movement resulting from acute trauma or a periarticular biceps or rotator cuff tendon injury; *also called* adhesive capsulitis.

fusion (arthrodesis) The joining of two bones into a single unit, thereby obliterating motion between the two. May be congenital, traumatic, or surgical.

Galeazzi fracture Dislocated ulna with a fractured radius.

gamekeeper's thumb Rupture of the ligament on the ulnar side of the thumb metacarpophalangeal joint that helps to stabilize the joint during pinching.

ganglion A mass of nerve cell bodies usually found lying outside the central nervous system.

genu (knee) Genu valgum is knock-knee deformity; genu varum is bowleg deformity.

glenohumeral dislocation Injury in which the humeral head may displace from the joint; most of these dislocations are anterior and inferior to the glenoid rim.

glenohumeral joint True shoulder joint.

glenoid labrum A soft fibrous rim surrounding the glenoid fossa that deepens the socket and provides stability for the humeral head.

glenoid labrum tear Tear of the glenoid labrum; can result from acute trauma or overuse.

glucosamine sulfate A fundamental component in the synthesis of both hyaluronic acid and chondroitin that is thought to promote cartilage repair and synthesis; the oral form is taken as a dietary supplement to treat arthritis.

glycosaminoglycans Polysaccharides consisting of long-chain, unbranched, repeating disaccharide units, such as keratin and chondroitin sulfate.

gout An inflammatory arthritis associated with deposition of urate in the joint.

gracilis muscle One of the three hamstring muscles of the knee that make up the pes anserine and help protect the knee against rotatory and valgus stress (the others are the sartorius and semitendinosus).

greater trochanter Broad, flat process at the upper end of the lateral surface of the femur to which several muscles are attached.

greenstick fracture A fracture that disrupts only one side of the bone. This fracture pattern is seen in children because of the greater plasticity of their bones.

growth factors The molecules that stimulate cell growth or activation.

guarding Refusal to use an injured part because motion causes pain; involuntary abdominal muscular contraction reflecting inflammation and pain within the peritoneal cavity.

hallux The great toe.

hammer toe Flexion deformity of the distal interphalangeal joint of the foot.

hamstring One of the large muscle groups at the back of the thigh that flexes the knee.

hangman's fracture Fracture of the pedicles of the C2 vertebra.

head The upper or proximal portion of a structure; the head of a bone is the rounded end that allows joint rotation.

hemarthrosis The presence of blood in the joint.

hematoma A collection of blood resulting from injury.

herniated disk Rupture of the nucleus pulposus or anulus fibrosus of the intervertebral disk.

heterotopic ossification The formation of bone in any nonosseous tissue; often occurs following trauma.

Hill-Sachs lesion A wedge-shaped impaction fracture of the posterolateral portion of the humeral head seen following anterior dislocations of the shoulder.

hip pointer Painful injury caused by irritation or avulsion of the attachments of the abdominal and thigh muscles at the iliac crest.

homeopathy A system of therapy developed by Samuel Hahnemann based on the "law of similia," from the aphorism, *similia similibus curantur* (likes are cured by likes), which holds that a medicinal substance that can evoke certain symptoms in healthy individuals may be effective in the treatment of illnesses having similar symptoms, if given in very small doses.

ICES Acronym for ice, compression, elevation, and splinting.

iliofemoral ligament One of three extremely strong ligaments surrounding the hip joint anteriorly and posteriorly, which reinforce the capsule; the other two are the ischiofemoral and the pubofemoral ligaments.

iliopsoas bursa One of the two most important bursae (the other being the trochanteric bursa) about the hip joint; located between the capsule and the iliopsoas muscle anteriorly.

iliotibial band (ITB) Thickening of the iliotibial tract that inserts directly into the lateral tubercle of the tibia.

ilium One of the three bones (ilium, ischium, and pubis) that fuse to form the bony pelvis.

impacted fracture A fracture pattern in which the fragments are pushed together, thus imparting some stability.

impingement syndrome Shoulder pain caused by tendinosis of the rotator cuff tendon or irritation of the subacromial bursa. *See also* Rotator cuff impingement, external, and Rotator cuff impingement, internal.

infarct An area of tissue that is cut off from its blood supply, becomes ischemic, and dies.

inflammation Heat, redness, swelling, and pain that accompany musculoskeletal injuries; occurs when tissue is crushed, stretched, or torn.

infraspinatus Muscle of the rotator cuff that arises from the dorsal surface of the scapula and inserts on the greater tuberosity.

instability Looseness; unsteadiness.

intercondylar eminence Proximal tibial process; anterior and posterior to the intercondylar eminence are attachment sites for the cruciate ligaments' menisci.

intercondylar notch Bony notch that separates posteriorly the condyles of the femur.

intercondylar tubercles A lateral spur projecting upward from the intercondylar eminence.

internal fixation Surgical insertion of a device that stops motion across a fracture or joint to encourage bony healing or fusion.

internal impingement A condition in the shoulder of throwing athletes that results in tears of the underside of the rotator cuff and the posterior labrum.

interval throwing program A program for shoulder rehabilitation that allows the athlete to get a light workout several times per day at a submaximal level without fatiguing the arm.

intervertebral disk The structure located between two moving vertebrae that stabilizes the spine, helps maintain its alignment, allows motion between vertebral levels, absorbs energy, and distributes load applied to the spine.

intramedullary nailing or rodding A procedure for the fixation of fractures in which a nail or rod is inserted into the intramedullary canal of the bone from one of its two ends.

intramembranous ossification Bone formation characterized by the aggregation of undifferentiated mesenchymal cells, which differentiate into osteoblasts.

inversion injury Ankle injury resulting from landing on the lateral aspect of the foot.

involucrum In osteomyelitis, a sheath of live bone that forms around a piece of dead bone, the sequestrum.

iontophoresis Therapeutic modality that uses galvanic electrical current to drive ionized medications through the skin to injured tissues.

ischemic Lacking oxygen, usually as the result of partial or complete blockage of blood flow.

ischial tuberosity The bony prominence felt at the base of each buttock, near the crotch; the major attachment site for the hamstrings and the major weight-bearing structure for sitting.

ischiofemoral ligament One of three extremely strong ligaments surrounding the hip joint anteriorly and posteriorly, which reinforce the capsule; the other two are the iliofemoral and the pubofemoral ligaments.

ischium One of the three bones (ilium, ischium, and pubis) that fuse to form the bony pelvis.

isokinetic Literally, "same speed"; when applied to muscle action, it implies constant velocity of shortening.

isokinetic exercise In isokinetic contractions, the muscle contracts and shortens at constant speed.

isometric Literally, "same length"; when applied to muscle action, it implies that the muscle length is held constant even with varying loads. Accomplished by contracting the flexors and extensors of a joint at equal loads so that the joint does not move.

isotonic When applied to muscle action, the condition when a muscle shortens against a constant load, as in lifting a weight.

isotonic exercise Contraction of muscles concentrically or eccentrically against resistance with movement of the part so that the load remains constant.

jersey finger Traumatic rupture of the deep flexor tendon of the ring finger; so named because it often occurs as a result of grabbing an opponent's jersey.

joint Articulation, place of union, or junction between two or more bones of the skeleton.

joint mobilization A manually administered treatment modality in which joints are manipulated to improve flexibility and decrease pain.

Jones fracture Stress fracture of the proximal shaft of the fifth metatarsal; a fracture that frequently heals with difficulty.

jumper's knee Chronic tendinosis of the patellar tendon; frequently limited to the distal pole of the patella rather than being diffused throughout the tendon.

juvenile rheumatoid arthritis A chronic inflammatory disease in children that is characterized by pain, swelling, and tenderness in one or more joints and may result in impaired growth and development.

Kohler disease Osteochondrosis of the tarsal navicular.

kyphosis Curvature of the spine that is convex posteriorly.

lamellar bone Mature, well-organized form of cortical bone.

laminectomy A surgical decompression procedure in which part of the posterior arch of a vertebra is removed; allows access to the disk.

lateral Lying away from the midline.

lateral collateral ligament Ligament on the lateral side (outside) of three joints—the knee, the elbow, and the ankle.

lateral condyle Forms the lateral border of the upper surface of a joint.

lateral epicondylitis An irritation or partial tear of the extensor tendons of the wrist near their origin at the elbow; *also called* tennis elbow.

lateral ligament structure The three pairs of the lateral collateral ligament of the ankle: the posterior talofibular ligament, the calcaneofibular ligament, and the anterior talofibular ligament.

lateral malleolus Bony prominence at the end of the fibula that is part of the ankle joint.

lateral meniscus The lateral C-shaped fibrocartilaginous structure of the knee.

lateral view A view that passes from side to side at 90° to an AP or PA view.

latissimus dorsi A muscle of the trunk that originates on the spinous processes and supraspinous ligaments of all lower thoracic, lumbar, and sacral vertebrae; lumbar fascia; posterior third iliac crest; last four ribs (interdigitating with external oblique abdominis) and inferior angle of the scapula; inserting on the floor of the bicipital groove of the humerus after spiraling around the teres major. Extends, adducts, and medially rotates the arm. Costal attachment helps with deep inspiration and forced expiration.

lavage The irrigation or thorough washing of an infected joint with high-volume saline solution.

lesser trochanter Large medial prominence distal to the neck of the femur; the site of the insertion of the iliopsoas tendon.

ligament A collagenous tissue that connects two bones to stabilize a joint.

limb salvage Surgical removal of a tumor without amputation of the affected extremity.

Lisfranc fracture A fracture-dislocation of the tarsometatarsal joint.

longitudinal arch Arch along the long axis of the foot formed by the bones of the foot starting at the weight-bearing surface of the calcaneus and ending at the metatarsal heads.

lordosis Curvature of the spine that is convex anteriorly.

low-molecular-weight heparins (LMWHs) Anticoagulants that work by binding to antithrombin-III and catalyze its inactivation of factor Xa.

magnetic resonance imaging (MRI) An imaging modality that depends on the movement of protons in water molecules. When subjected to a magnetic field, protons that are normally randomly aligned become aligned. Radio waves directed at the tissue to be studied are used to change the alignment of these photons. When the radio waves are turned off, the protons emit a signal that is detected and processed by a computer into an image. In the musculoskeletal system, MRI is useful in diagnosing soft-tissue injuries, tumors, stress fractures, and infection.

mallet finger An injury often caused by direct contact with a ball in which the finger is forced into flexion against resistance and the extensor tendons attaching to the distal phalanx may rupture.

malunion Healing of a fracture in an unacceptable position.

maximal oxygen consumption (Vo_{2max}) Reflects the body's ability to maximally extract and use oxygen for aerobic metabolism; measures the lung's ability to extract oxygen.

mechanism of injury A representation of the patterns of energy that cause traumatic injuries.

medial Lying toward the midline.

medial capsular ligament Mid third of the true capsule of the knee joint; ligament extending from the femur to the midportion of the meniscus and then to the tibia.

medial collateral ligament Ligament on the medial aspect of the knee consisting of anterior, posterior, and oblique components and extending from the femur to the tibia.

medial condyle Forms the medial border of the upper surface of a joint.

medial malleolus The bony prominence at the end of the tibia that, together with the lateral malleolus, forms the sides of the ankle joint.

medial meniscus The medial C-shaped fibrocartilaginous structure of the knee.

medial patellar retinacula Extension of the vastus medialis that helps extend the knee joint.

medial retinaculum Structure composed of the aponeurosis of the vastus medial muscle itself; attaching along the medial border of the patella, its primary function is to hold the patella medially.

median nerve Nerve that controls sensation of the central palm, the thumb, and the first three fingers, as well as the ability to oppose the thumb to the little finger.

medullary canal The relatively hollow central core of a long bone that houses blood-forming cells.

meniscofemoral ligament With the meniscotibial ligament, it attaches the midportion of the medial meniscus peripherally to the tibia and the femur.

meniscotibial (coronary) ligament With the meniscofemoral ligament, it attaches the midportion of the medial meniscus peripherally to the tibia and femur.

menisci A fibrocartilage structure interposed between articular cartilage. In the knee, the medial and lateral menisci are semicircular structures on the periphery of the joint that act as protective buffers during walking and running activities.

Merchant view An axial view of the patella in which the patient lies supine on the x-ray table with the knee flexed 45°. The cassette is held perpendicular to the tibia approximately halfway between the knee and ankle. The x-ray beam is directed caudally through the patella at an angle of 60° from vertical. This view is useful to evaluate subluxation of the patella and patellofemoral arthritis.

metacarpal bones The five bones of the hand that extend from the wrist to the fingers.

metaphysis The broad portion of a long bone adjacent to a joint. In children, the broad portion of a long bone includes the epiphysis, the physis, and the metaphysis.

metastasis The transfer of disease from one part of the body to another; tumor metastasis usually occurs via the bloodstream or the lymphatic system.

metatarsus valgus Congenital deformity of the forefoot in which the forefoot is rotated laterally in relation to the hindfoot; also called metatarsus abductus.

metatarsus varus Congenital deformity of the forefoot in which the forefoot is rotated medially in relation to the hindfoot; also called metatarsus adductus.

microtrauma Destruction of a small number of cells caused by additive effects of repetitive forces.

midline Imaginary straight vertical line drawn from midforehead through the nose and the umbilicus to the floor.

modalities Physical agents that can create an optimum environment for injury healing, while reducing pain and discomfort.

monoarticular Affecting a single joint.

Monteggia fracture Dislocation of the radial head in association with an ulnar fracture.

mortise view A view of the ankle in which the ankle is rotated internally so that the medial and lateral malleoli are parallel with the plane of the film. This view is used to assess reduction of the ankle joint as well as joint space narrowing.

Morton foot Congenital abnormality characterized by a short first metatarsal, which shifts weight-bearing stresses to the second metatarsal head, often resulting in pain.

myelogram X-ray study of the spine carried out after injection of a contrast material into the spinal cord sheath; helpful in diagnosing ruptured or bulging disks.

myelopathy An abnormal condition of the spinal cord, whether through disease or compression. The usual consequences are spasticity, impairment of sensation, and impairment of bowel and bladder function.

myoblasts The embryonic cells that develop into skeletal muscle cells.

myofascial pain syndrome A painful musculoskeletal response that can follow muscle trauma.

myofibers The fibers that constitute a muscle.

myofibrils A slender thread within a muscle fiber that functions in muscle contraction.

myopathies A wide and varied group of primary muscle disorders characterized by weakness.

myositis ossificans Abnormal production of bone within muscle.

myotome A group of muscles innervated by a single spinal nerve root.

navicular bone Bone with which the head of the talus articulates on the medial side of the foot; also a bone in the wrist that articulates with the trapezium, trapezoid, and other carpal bones.

neck The constricted portion of a structure (eg, femoral neck).

nerve conduction studies Studies that test the speed by which motor, sensory, or mixed (combined motor and sensory) nerves transmit impulses.

neuralgia Pain along the course of a nerve.

neurapraxia A temporary loss of neural function.

neuritis Inflammation or irritation of a nerve.

neuroma A tumor composed of nerve cells.

neuropathic arthritis The chronic, progressive destruction of a joint that is caused by the loss of sensation from an underlying neurologic dysfunction; also known as Charcot arthropathy.

neuropathy An abnormal condition involving a peripheral nerve.

nociceptive Pain-sensing.

nondisplaced fracture Fracture in which there is no deformity of the limb.

nonlamellar (woven) bone Immature bone.

nonossifying fibromas Osteolytic and sometimes painful proliferative lesions composed of spindle (fibrous) cells.

nonsteroidal anti-inflammatory drugs (NSAIDs) Inhibitors of cyclooxygenase and therefore prostaglandin synthesis.

nonunion Failure of healing of a fracture or osteotomy. With continued motion through a nonunion, a pseudarthrosis will form.

nucleus pulposus The central core of gelatinous material within intervertebral disks.

oblique fracture A fracture in which the fracture line crosses the bone diagonally.

oblique view A view in which the x-ray beam passes at an angle somewhere between an AP or PA view and a lateral view.

odontoid view An open-mouth AP view of the C2 vertebra used to identify fractures of the odontoid (dens) process of C2.

olecranon bursa Bursa in the elbow that separates the skin from the underlying ulna; allows the soft tissue to glide smoothly over the olecranon process.

olecranon process Bony process of the proximal ulna that prevents hyperextension of the elbow.

open fracture A fracture in which the skin is broken, exposing the fracture site to the environment.

open reduction An open surgical procedure in which normal or near-normal relationships are restored to a fractured bone or dislocated joint.

open reduction and internal fixation (ORIF) A procedure that involves incising the skin and soft tissue to repair a fracture under direct visualization.

origin The more fixed end or attachment of a muscle.

osteitis pubis An inflammatory condition of the pubic bones caused by repetitive stress on the symphysis pubis.

osteoblasts The cells that synthesize the organic component of bone; also thought of as the bone-forming cells.

osteochondral fractures Injuries that disrupt articular cartilage and the underlying subchondral bone.

osteochondritis dissecans (OCD) A localized abnormality of a focal portion of the subchondral bone, which can result in loss of support for the overlying articular cartilage.

osteoclasts Large cells that resorb bone matrix when activated.

osteocytes The cells of established bone.

osteogenesis imperfecta A hereditary disorder of connective tissue caused by mutations in the gene for type I collagen.

osteoid osteoma A small, benign, but painful tumor usually found in the long bones or the posterior elements of the spine.

osteolysis Dissolution of bone, particularly as resulting from excessive resorption.

osteomalacia Softening of the bones due to impaired bone mineralization, usually caused by vitamin D deficiency.

osteomyelitis Infection of bone, either bacterial or mycotic.

osteonecrosis The death of bone, often as a result of obstruction of its blood supply. *See also* avascular necrosis.

osteophytes Overgrowth of bone, common in osteoarthritis and spinal stenosis.

osteosarcoma A primary sarcoma of the bone that is characterized by the direct formation of bone or osteoid tissue by the tumor cells.

osteosynthesis The process of bony union, as in fracture healing. It is a biologic welding process that is sometimes facilitated with grafts of bone from the iliac crest and insertion of fixation devices.

osteotomy Literally, cutting a bone. Used to describe surgical procedures in which bone is cut and realigned.

os trigonum A bony ossicle posterior to the talus.

overload principle States that strength, power, endurance, and hypertrophy of muscle can only increase when a muscle performs workloads greater than those previously encountered.

Paget disease A condition of abnormally increased and disorganized bone remodeling.

palmar The anterior surface of the forearm, wrist, and hand.

Panner disease Osteonecrosis of the capitellum seen in teenagers.

pannus A proliferation of synovium beginning at the periphery of the joint surface as seen in rheumatoid arthritis.

parasympathetic (craniosacral) nervous system A part of the autonomic nervous system that causes blood vessels to dilate, slows the heart rate, and relaxes muscle sphincters.

parathyroid hormone The major regulator of calcium homeostasis; promotes increased levels of serum calcium.

paresthesias Abnormal sensations such as tingling, burning, or prickling.

pars interarticularis Part of the vertebra posteriorly between the spinal arch and the pedicle.

patella Kneecap.

patellar ligament *See* patellar tendon.

patellar plica A synovial fold that may persist into adult life and cause medial knee pain in the absence of trauma.

patellar tendon The extension of the quadriceps mechanism from the patella to the tibia; also called patellar ligament.

patellectomy Surgical excision of the patella.

patellofemoral groove Groove that runs anteriorly between the condyles of the femur; the patella lies in the trochlear groove.

pathologic fracture A fracture caused by a normal load on abnormal bone, which is often weakened by tumor, infection, or metabolic bone disease.

patient-controlled analgesia (PCA) The intravenous or epidural delivery of narcotics via a pump that is controlled by the patient.

pectoralis major A muscle of the upper chest, originating from the anterior surface of the medial half of the clavicle and the anterior surface of the sternum, the superior six costal cartilages, and the aponeurosis of the external oblique muscle and inserting on the lateral lip of the intertubercular groove of the humerus, which adducts and medially rotates the humerus; draws the scapula anteriorly and inferiorly. Acting alone, the clavicular head flexes the humerus and the sternocostal head extends it.

pelvic cavity Space between the pelvis walls.

pelvis A bony ring, consisting of the sacrum, coccyx, and innominate bones, that connects the trunk to the lower extremities, supports the abdominal contents, and allows passage of the excretory canals.

percutaneous pinning Insertion of pins into bone through small puncture wounds in the skin for stabilization of a fracture or a dislocated joint that was realigned by closed reduction.

periosteum A sleeve of connective tissue that surrounds the shaft of the bone and contributes to fracture healing.

peritendinitis Inflammation of the tendon sheath, marked by pain, swelling, and, occasionally, local crepitus.

permeative margin An indistinct margin visible on radiographic images that signifies the hazy transition between growing tumors and normal bone.

peroneus brevis muscle Muscle in the lateral compartment of the leg that functions to evert the ankle; it passes distal and inferior to the lateral malleolus and inserts on the base of the fifth metatarsal; acts to plantar flex and abduct the foot.

peroneus longus muscle Muscle in the lateral compartment of the leg that functions to evert the ankle; it passes under the cuboid bone and inserts on the inferior surface of the medial cuneiform and base of the first metatarsal; it acts to plantarflex, abduct, and evert the foot.

pes planus Flattening of the arch of the foot.

phagocytosis The process by which white blood cells ingest debris or microorganisms.

phalanges Bones making up the skeleton of the fingers or toes.

phonophoresis The transdermal introduction of a topically applied medication (usually either an anti-inflammatory or analgesic) into soft tissue using ultrasound.

physis The growth plate. Specialized cartilaginous tissue interposed between the metaphysis and epiphysis in long bones in children. Provides growth in length of the bone.

pigmented villonodular synovitis A proliferative process of the synovial membrane of unknown etiology.

placebo effect The placebo effect is the measurable, observable, or felt improvement in health not attributable to treatment. This effect is believed by many people to be due to the placebo itself in some mysterious way. A placebo (Latin for "I shall please") is a medication or treatment believed by the administrator of the treatment to be inert or innocuous.

plantar The sole, or flexor surface, of the foot.

plantar calcaneonavicular ligament Sling ligament supporting the longitudinal arch.

plantar fascia Fibrous tissue band that runs from the calcaneal tuberosity to the phalanges and supports the talus.

plantar fasciitis Irritation of the plantar fascia, usually from overuse; the pain is most severe at the calcaneal tuberosity.

plyometric exercises Exercises that use explosive movements to increase athletic power.

polyarticular Affecting multiple joints.

polyneuropathies Neuropathies of several peripheral nerves simultaneously.

popliteal artery Continuation of the superficial femoral artery in the popliteal space (posterior surface of the knee); supplies the knee and the calf.

popliteal fossa The hollow area on the posterior surface of the knee; popliteal space.

popliteus muscle Muscle deep to the popliteal artery with three proximal insertions on the tibia; its primary function is internal rotation of the tibia on the femur.

portable transcutaneous electrical nerve stimulation (TENS) unit A portable therapeutic modality that uses electrical stimulation to attempt to modulate pain, strengthen muscles, and enhance soft-tissue healing.

posterior cruciate ligament (PCL) Ligament extending from the tibia to the medial surface of the intercondylar notch of the femur that functions with the anterior cruciate ligament in anteroposterior and rotatory stability of the knee.

posterior glenohumeral dislocation Disruption of the glenohumeral joint in a posterior direction.

posterior interosseous nerve The major terminal branch of the radial nerve that winds around the radius to the dorsal side of the forearm to provide motor and sensory function to the dorsal forearm and wrist.

posterior process That part of each vertebra that can be palpated, as it lies just under the skin in the midline of the back.

posterior sternoclavicular dislocation Disruption of the sternoclavicular joint posteriorly.

posterior talofibular ligament One of the three lateral ligaments of the ankle; the strongest of the three, it helps to resist forward dislocation of the leg on the foot.

posterior tibial artery Artery that is just posterior to the medial malleolus; supplies blood to the foot.

posterior tibial syndrome Pain along the posterior medial border of the tibia; thought to be secondary to a tight posterior tibial muscle "pulling" on the periosteum in this area; associated with running.

posterior tibial tendon One of the structures that creates a dynamic sling supporting the longitudinal arch; attaches directly on the tuberosity of the navicular bone and indirectly on the plantar surface of the navicular and middle cuneiform bones of the foot.

posterior tibiofibular ligament Part of the talofibular syndesmosis, arises from the posterior calculi on the lateral side of the tibia; helps to hold the fibula snug in its tibial groove.

posterolateral rotatory instability The lateral tibial plateau rotates posteriorly in relationship to the femur.

posteromedial rotatory instability The medial tibial plateau rotates posteriorly on the femur, with associated medial opening.

postmenopausal osteoporosis The most prevalent form of primary osteoporosis.

posttraumatic arthritis A form of secondary osteoarthritis caused by a loss of joint congruence and normal joint biomechanics.

preload Reflection of cardiac muscle quality; an elastic distensible ventricle propels more blood more rapidly than a stiffer, less distensible ventricle.

primary bone healing The end-to-end repair process that occurs when the bone ends are anatomically opposed and held together rigidly; no callus forms.

primary osteoarthritis Osteoarthritis without an identified cause; characterized by progressive loss of articular cartilage and reactive changes in the bone, leading to the destruction and painful malfunction of the joint.

proprioception A sense or perception, usually at a subconscious level, of the movements and position of the body and especially its limbs, independent of vision; this sense is gained primarily from input from sensory nerve terminals in muscles and tendons (muscle spindles) and the fibrous capsule of joints combined with input from the vestibular apparatus.

proteoglycans Complex macromolecules that consist of a protein core with covalently bound polysaccharide (glycosaminoglycan) chains.

proximal Describing structures that are closer to the trunk.

proximal patellar realignment Proximal soft-tissue reconstruction designed to align the muscle pull on the patella to enhance the action of the vastus medialis obliquus and to tighten the medial capsule.

pseudarthrosis A false joint produced when a fracture or arthrodesis fails to heal.

pseudofractures Lines of radiolucency that represent stress fractures with unmineralized osteoid.

pubic symphysis Firm fibrocartilaginous joint located anteriorly between the two innominate bones.

pubis One of the three bones (ilium, ischium, and pubis) that fuse to form the bony pelvis.

pulmonary embolism Migration of a thrombus from a large vein (often in the leg) to the lung, causing obstruction of blood flow, respiratory distress, or even death.

quadriceps angle (Q angle) An angle formed by the intersection of two lines: one line is drawn from the anterosuperior iliac spine to the midpatella; the second is drawn from the midpatella to the anterior tibial tuberosity. These lines parallel the quadriceps and patellar tendons.

quadriceps femoris Tendon located at the superior border of the patella, or kneecap.

quadriceps muscle Extensor muscle situated at the front of the thigh; composed of four components: the vastus medialis, vastus lateralis, vastus intermedius, and rectus femoris.

quadriceps tendon Convergence of the four muscles of the quadriceps—the rectus femoris, vastus intermedius, vastus medialis, and vastus lateralis; inserts in the superior pole of the patella.

radial artery One of the major arteries of the arm; it can be palpated at the base of the thumb.

radial nerve Nerve carrying sensation to the greater portion of the back of the hand and controlling extension of the hand at the wrist.

radial styloid Bony prominence felt on the lateral (thumb) side of the wrist.

radiculopathies A group of nerve root disorders often caused by nerve root compression or central or neuroforaminal stenosis.

radius Bone on the thumb side of the forearm.

range of motion (ROM) The amount of movement available at a joint.

reflex Fairly fixed pattern of response or behavior similar for any given stimulus; does not involve a conscious action.

rehabilitation Restoration, following disease, illness, or injury, of the ability to function in a normal or near-normal manner.

resection arthroplasty A procedure in which the surfaces of diseased bone are excised, allowing fibrocartilage to grow in its place.

revascularization A procedure to provide an additional blood supply to fractured bone.

rheumatoid arthritis A chronic inflammatory disease that is probably triggered by an antigen-mediated inflammatory reaction against the synovium in the joint.

rhomboid Muscle of the trunk that helps to stabilize and maneuver the shoulder girdle.

RICE method A method of treatment of acute injury that is used to counteract the body's initial response to injury; RICE is an acronym for rest, ice, compression, and elevation.

rickets The childhood form of osteomalacia.

rigid splint Splint made from firm material and applied to sides, front, and/or back of an injured extremity to prevent motion at the injury site.

Romberg test Used to test for deficits in the sensory systems that provide stability to the trunk. Standing with the feet together, the patient closes his or her eyes. Signs of swaying are a positive sign.

rotator cuff The rotator cuff is made up of four muscles and their tendons. These combine to form a "cuff" over the head of the humerus. The four muscles—the supraspinatus, infraspinatus, subscapularis, and teres minor—originate from the scapula and together form a single tendon unit that inserts on the greater tuberosity of the humerus. The rotator cuff helps to lift and rotate the arm and to stabilize the ball of the shoulder within the joint.

rotator cuff impingement, external Impingement of the rotator cuff on the acromion and the coracoacromial ligament; causes microtrauma to the cuff, resulting in local inflammation, edema, cuff softening, pain, and poor function of the cuff.

rotator cuff impingement, internal A condition in the shoulder of throwing athletes that results in tears of the underside of the rotator cuff and the posterior labrum.

sacroiliac joint The joint formed by the articulation of the sacrum and ilium.

sacrum One of the three bones (sacrum, coccyx, and innominate) that make up the pelvic ring.

saddle anesthesia Decreased sensation around the perineum.

saddle embolus A condition in which one or both of the major pulmonary arteries are totally occluded.

sarcolemma Muscle-cell membrane and its associated basement membrane.

sarcomeres The fundamental components of the contracting unit of the myofibril.

sarcopenia The loss of muscle mass and strength as a result of aging.

sarcoplasmic reticulum A continuous branching network of membrane, which is a specialized form of endoplasmic reticulum unique to muscle.

sartorius muscle One of the medial hamstring muscles that form the pes anserinus and help protect the knee against rotatory and valgus stress (the other pes anserinus muscles are the gracilis and semitendinosus).

scapula The shoulder blade.

scapular Y view A lateral view of the shoulder taken so that the blade of the scapula, the coracoid process, and the spine of the scapula form a "Y." Also called a transscapular view.

scapulothoracic joint Articulation in which the scapula is suspended from the posterior thoracic wall through muscular attachments to the ribs and spine.

Scheuermann disease Osteochondrosis of the vertebral epiphysis resulting in increased thoracic kyphosis in the preteen and early adolescent years.

Schwann cell A specialized support cell that encases nerve fibers.

sclerotic border A sharp, geographic margin visible on radiographic images that signifies the transition between inactive or slow-growing tumors and normal bone.

scoliosis Lateral curvature of the spine.

secondary bone healing The repair process that is characterized by the formation of fracture callus, which then remodels to form new bone.

secondary osteoarthritis Osteoarthritis resulting from known precipitants such as bone ischemia, trauma, and neuropathy.

secondary osteoporosis Osteoporosis characterized by conditions in which bone is lost because of the presence of another disease, such as hormonal imbalances, malignancies, or gastrointestinal disorders, or because of corticosteroid use.

second-degree burns Partial-thickness burns that extend down to the dermis; characterized by painful blistering of the skin.

selective estrogen receptor modulator (SERM) A class of drugs that is thought to provide the beneficial effects of hormone replacement therapy without some of its adverse effects.

semimembranosus muscle Muscle extending from the ischial tuberosity to the tibia that acts to flex the leg and extend the thigh; important stabilizing structure to the posterior aspect of the knee.

semitendinosus muscle One of the hamstring muscles that comprise the pes anserinus and help protect the knee against rotatory and valgus stress (the other pes anserinus muscles are the gracilis and sartorius).

senile osteoporosis Osteoporosis in which an age-related decline in renal production of active vitamin D is the probable cause of bone loss.

sensory nerve action potential (SNAP) The latency, amplitude, and conduction velocity recorded in sensory nerve conduction studies.

sensory nerves Nerves that carry sensations of touch, taste, heat, cold, pain, or other modalities to the spinal cord or brain.

septic arthritis Infection of a joint, either bacterial or mycotic.

sequestrum In osteomyelitis, the dead portion of bone inside and walled off by the involucrum. *See also* involucrum.

serratus anterior Muscle of the trunk that helps to stabilize and maneuver the shoulder girdle.

sesamoid bones Two small bones located beneath the first metatarsal head that function as extra weight-bearing structures and leverage points for the mechanics of the great toe.

sesamoiditis Inflammation of the sesamoid bones of the great toe.

Sever disease Osteochondrosis of the calcaneal apophysis seen in children aged 6 to 10 years.

shaft The long, straight, cylindrical midportion of a bone.

Sharpey fibers The small collagen fibers that attach tendon to bone; in the spine they connect the outer edges of intervertebral disks to the vertebral bodies.

shin splints Anterior or posterior tibial tendinitis.

short collateral ligament Ligament running parallel to the fibular collateral ligament and attaching to the fibular head posterior to the biceps tendon; also called fabellofibular ligament when it is attached to the fabella; reinforces the posterior capsule and contributes to the lateral stability of the knee.

shoulder dislocation *See* glenohumeral dislocation.

skeletal homeostasis The function of bone that supplies structural support and movement for the body.

skeletal survey Screening radiographs of the entire skeleton.

skeletal (voluntary) muscle Striated muscles that are attached to bones and usually cross at least one joint.

skeleton The skeletal system; the supporting framework of the human body, composed of 206 bones.

Slocum anterolateral rotatory instability test
Modification of the lateral pivot shift test in which the patient lies on his or her side with the uninvolved leg flexed at the hip and the examiner applies an internal rotation force to the proximal tibia and a valgus stress to the joint; at 20° of flexion the knee visibly, palpably, and audibly reduces.

Slocum external rotation test One of the tests for anteromedial-rotatory instability conducted with the hip flexed to approximately 45° and the knee to approximately 80°; a forward motion is applied to the thigh and the degree of anterior drawer is assessed.

slow twitch muscle fibers Type I muscle fibers.

smooth muscle Nonstriated, involuntary muscle that constitutes the bulk of the gastrointestinal tract and is present in nearly every organ to regulate automatic activity.

soleus muscle Muscle, extending from the proximal fibula to the calcaneus, that acts to extend and rotate the foot.

spinal column Central supporting bony structure of the body; vertebral column.

spinal cord Extension of the brain, composed of virtually all the nerves carrying messages between the brain and the rest of the body. It lies inside of and is protected by the vertebrae and the spinal column.

spinal stenosis Narrowing of the canal housing the spinal cord; commonly caused by encroachment of bone.

spine Column of 33 vertebrae extending from the base of the skull to the tip of the coccyx.

spinous processes Palpable prominences in the vertebrae.

spiral fracture A fracture caused by a twisting force that results in a helical fracture line.

splint Device used to immobilize part of the body.

sprain Partial or complete tear of a ligament.

static stretching The passive stretching of a given antagonist muscle by placing it in a position of maximal stretch and holding it there for an extended period.

stem cells Cells with the unlimited ability of self-renewal and regeneration; serve to regenerate tissue.

stenosis A stricture of any canal or orifice. In the spine, a narrowing of the spinal canal secondary to a combination of disk narrowing, thickening of the ligamentum flavum, and osteophytes from arthritis of the facet joints.

sternoclavicular dislocation Disruption of the articulation that lies between the clavicle and the sternum.

sternoclavicular joint Articulation between the sternum and the clavicle.

sternocleidomastoid Cervical muscle that produces rotation of the head.

sternum Breastbone.

straight lateral laxity Abnormal motion with lateral opening of the joint, or varus laxity; demonstrating injury to the fibular collateral ligament and lateral capsular structures.

straight medial laxity Abnormal motion with medial opening of the joint, or valgus laxity; reflecting damage to the tibial collateral ligament.

strain Partial tear of a muscle.

stress fracture An overuse injury in which the body cannot repair microscopic damage to the bone as quickly as it is induced, leading to painful, weakened bone.

Stryker notch view A special view of the shoulder used to demonstrate a Hill-Sachs lesion (a compression fracture of the humeral head on the posterolateral aspect of the articular surface) seen after recurrent anterior dislocations of the shoulder. This view is taken with the patient supine, the hand of the affected shoulder on the top of the head, and the x-ray beam directed 10° cephalad.

subacromial bursa Bursa that lies in the subacromial space and acts as the protective tissue between the cuff and the bony acromion.

subacute stage Time period between acute and chronic injury.

subluxation An incomplete disruption in the relationship of two bones forming a joint, that is, a partial dislocation. The joint surfaces retain partial contact.

supraspinatus The most superior muscle that arises from the dorsal surface of the scapula and inserts on the greater tuberosity; part of the rotator cuff.

sympathetic (thoracolumbar) nervous system Part of the autonomic nervous system that causes blood vessels to constrict, stimulates sweating, increases the heart rate, causes the sphincter muscles to constrict, and prepares the body to respond to stress.

symptom Evidence of change in body functions apparent to the patient and expressed to the examiner on questioning.

synapse A specialized site at which an electrical signal is transmitted chemically across a junction to produce a similar electrical impulse on the opposite side.

syndesmosis A form of fibrous joint in which opposing surfaces that are relatively far apart are united by ligaments; eg, the fibrous union between the radius and ulna (radioulnar syndesmosis).

synovial fluid The straw-colored fluid in the joint that is formed by filtration of capillary plasma.

synovial joint A joint formed by the articulation of two bones, the ends of which are lined with hyaline cartilage and are surrounded by a capsule that is lined with synovium.

synoviocytes Cells that form the synovial membrane, remove debris, and secrete hyaluronic acid.

synovitis A condition characterized by inflammation of the synovial lining.

synovium The thin membrane that lines a joint capsule. There are two types of synovial cells. Type A act as macrophages and type B produce synovial fluid for joint lubrication. Marked hypertrophy of the synovium occurs with an inflammatory arthritis.

tai chi A low-impact exercise program that is derived from the martial arts in China and was founded in accordance with the belief that chi (also called qi) is a vital life force flowing through the body.

talus One of the bones forming the ankle joint. It lies below and articulates with the distal tibia.

tarsal bones Seven bones that make up the rear portion of the foot.

tarsal coalition Fusion of two or more of the major tarsal bones (talus, navicular, calcaneus, and cuboid).

tarsal tunnel syndrome A neuritis of the posterior tibial nerve resulting in pain and/or numbness along the course of the nerve.

tendinitis Injury to a tendon or musculotendinous unit caused by the application of mechanical loads of high intensity or high frequency.

tendinosis lesion Asymptomatic tendon degeneration caused either by aging or by cumulative microtrauma without inflammation.

tendon A specialized type of collagenous tissue that attaches muscle to bone. Tendons transmit forces of muscular contraction to cause motion across a joint.

tennis elbow An irritation or partial tear of the extensor tendons of the wrist near their origin at the elbow; *also called* lateral epicondylitis.

tenocytes The cells in tendons.

tenosynovitis Inflammation of the thin inner lining of a tendon sheath.

tenosynovium The sheath surrounding a tendon that enhances movement or gliding of the tendon as it transmits muscle forces across joints.

teres minor The most inferior muscle that arises from the dorsal surface of the scapula and inserts on the greater tuberosity; part of the rotator cuff.

therapeutic ultrasound The use of high energy sound waves for healing purposes. Frequently used by physical therapists to reduce inflammation but increasingly used to heal enthesopathies, such as plantar fasciitis, lateral epicondylitis (tennis elbow), and impingement syndrome of the shoulder, as well as nonunions of fractures.

thoracic outlet syndrome A constellation of symptoms arising from compression of the vascular or neural components of the brachial plexus in the thoracic outlet.

thrombus A blood clot within a vessel.

tibia Shinbone; the larger of the two leg bones.

tibial collateral ligament One of the major ligamentous support structures of the knee; extends from the medial condyle of the femur to the medial condyle of the tibia and just slightly beyond.

tibialis anterior muscle Muscle located in the anterior compartment of the lower leg; inserts on the medial cuneiform and acts to flex and elevate the foot.

tibialis posterior muscle One of the three muscles of the deep portion of the posterior compartment of the muscles of the leg; one of the medial stabilizers of the ankle, it acts to invert the foot and extend the ankle.

tibial nerve Provides motor and sensory function to the lower leg; courses deep to the gastrocnemius muscle.

tibial plateaus The expanded upper ends of the tibia that articulate with the femoral condyles to form the knee joints.

tibial tubercle The bony prominence of the proximal tibia.

tibiofemoral joint Polycentric hinge joint that bears the body's weight during locomotion; joint between each tibial and femoral condyle.

tibiofibular syndesmosis One of the three groups of ankle ligaments; arrangement of dense fibrous tissues between the osseous structures just above the ankle joint that maintains the relationship of the distal tibia and fibula.

tidemark A wavy bluish line visible on histologic staining with hematoxylin and eosin that signifies the border between the deep zone and the zone of calcified cartilage.

Tinel sign Percussion of the median nerve at the wrist to demonstrate the degree of nerve irritability by reproducing symptoms of carpal tunnel syndrome.

tomography A radiographic modality that allows visualization of lesions or tissues that are obscured by overlying structures. Structures in front of and behind the level of tissue to be studied are blurred, which allows the object to be studied to be brought into sharp focus. Tomography has been used to evaluate the degree of fracture healing and to evaluate tumors such as osteoid osteoma. Increasingly, CT has replaced tomography as the imaging modality of choice in these circumstances.

tonic-clonic A generalized seizure involving rigid (tonic) muscular contractions and repetitive (clonic) muscular spasms.

tophi Chalky deposits of urate surrounded by inflammatory cells.

torus (buckle) fracture A fracture that only buckles one side of the cortex. Typically seen in children because of the greater plasticity of their bones.

traction Action of drawing or pulling on an object.

traction splint Splint that holds a lower extremity fracture or dislocation immobile; allows steady longitudinal pull on the extremity.

transcutaneous electrical nerve stimulation (TENS) Therapeutic modality in which electrical stimulation is applied to the body with an intact peripheral nervous system; can elicit either sensory or muscular responses by stimulating nerves when electrical current passes across the skin.

transverse fracture A fracture in which the fracture line is perpendicular to the shaft of the bone.

transverse plane Horizontal section of the body.

transverse processes Together with the posterior processes, the transverse processes allow the attachment of strong intervertebral ligaments that support the spine and also provide anchors for muscles attached to the spinal column.

trapezius Large diamond-shaped muscle lying posteriorly just beneath the skin of the shoulder girdle.

traumatic spondylolysis The condition in which one vertebra slips anterior to the one below it secondary to a trauma-induced defect in the right and left pars interarticularis.

triceps The muscle in the back of the upper arm that acts to extend the arm and forearm.

trochanter Prominence on a bone where tendons insert; specifically, two protuberances, greater and lesser, on the femur.

trochanteric bursa One of the two most important bursae about the hip joint located just behind the greater trochanter and deep to the gluteus maximus and tensor fascia latae muscle.

trochlea A groove in a bone that articulates with another bone, or serves as a channel for a tendon to track in.

T-score A score used to express the results of bone density tests derived from the difference between the bone density of the patient being tested and the peak bone density of a healthy, young adult population; a T-score is equivalent to one standard deviation above or below ideal bone mass.

tuberculosis A chronic granulomatous infection caused by the bacteria *Mycobacterium tuberculosis.*

tuberosity Prominence on a bone where tendons insert.

turf toe A hyperextension injury of the first metatarsophalangeal joint associated with athletic activity on hard surfaces.

type I muscle fibers (slow twitch) Muscle fibers identified by a slow contraction time and a high resistance to fatigue; helpful with slow movements such as running during a marathon.

type II muscle fibers (fast twitch) Muscle fibers identified by a fast contraction time and rapid fatigue; helpful in rapid movements such as sprints. Type II fibers are further divided into type II A and type II B. Type II B fibers have a moderate resistance to fatigue and represent a transition between the two extremes of the slow twitch and type II A fibers.

type B synoviocytes A type of synovial cell that secretes hyaluronic acid.

ulnar artery Artery originating from the brachial artery and supplying the forearm, wrist, and hand.

ulnar nerve Nerve originating from the brachial plexus and coursing down the ulnar side of the arm, adjacent to the medial condyle of the elbow and into the ulnar side of the forearm; controls sensation over the fifth and ulnar half of the ring fingers and controls much of the muscular function of the hand.

ulnar shaft The long cylindrical portion of the ulna between the olecranon proximally and the styloid distally.

ulnar styloid Bony prominence of the ulna felt on the medial (little finger) side of the wrist.

ultrasound (ultrasonography) An imaging modality in which images are created from high-frequency sound waves (7.5 to 10 MHz [1 MHz = one million cycles per second]) that reflect off of different tissues. The reflected sound waves are recorded and processed by a computer and then converted into an image. Ultrasound is used to evaluate infant hip disorders and tears of the rotator cuff.

valgus Angulation of a distal bone away from the midline in relation to its proximal partner. Genu valgum is a knock-knee deformity, with abduction of the tibia in relation to the femur. Can also be used to describe angulation of fractures or bony deformities.

varus Angulation of a distal bone toward the midline in relation to its proximal partner. Genu varum is a bowleg deformity, with adduction of the tibia in relation to the femur. Can also be used to describe angulation of fractures or bony deformities.

vastus intermedius A component of the quadriceps muscle that lies in the midline of the thigh and anterior to the femur.

vastus lateralis A component of the quadriceps muscle that lies lateral to the midline of the thigh and anterior and lateral to the femur.

vastus medialis A component of the quadriceps muscle that lies medial to the midline of the thigh and anterior to the femur.

vastus medialis obliquus (VMO) A smaller component of the vastus medialis muscle.

vertebral arch Part of the vertebra composed of the right and left pedicles and the right and left laminae; also called neural arch.

vertebral body compression Compression fracture of the vertebral body without damage to the ligamentous structures; the most common thoracic fracture; also called wedge fracture.

vertebral column Segmented spinal column composed of 24 movable vertebrae, 5 fixed sacral vertebrae, and 4 fixed coccygeal vertebrae.

vertebrochondral ribs Ribs that articulate directly with the sternum via their costal cartilages.

vertebrosternal ribs Ribs that connect the first 10 thoracic vertebrae to the sternum.

viscoelastic Having mechanical properties that depend on the loading rate of an applied force.

viscosupplements Intra-articular hyaluronic acid preparations commonly used to treat osteoarthritis; thought to increase joint lubrication.

volar Toward the anterior surface of the body.

Volkmann contracture A deformity of the hand, fingers, and wrist caused by injury to the muscles of the forearm. It is most commonly secondary to compartment syndrome after fracture or other trauma to the forearm. Also sometimes caused by inadvertent injection of caustic material (drugs) into the arterial system of the forearm.

voluntary (skeletal) muscle Muscle, under direct voluntary control of the brain, which can be contracted or relaxed at will.

warfarin An anticoagulant drug that reduces the synthesis of vitamin K–dependent clotting factors II, VII, IX, and X in the liver.

West Point axillary view An axillary view of the shoulder in which the patient is prone on the x-ray table with a pillow placed under the affected shoulder, the arm abducted 90°, and the forearm hanging off the edge of the table. The cassette is placed against the top of the shoulder, and the x-ray beam is then directed at the axilla, angled 25° toward the table surface and 25° toward the patient's midline. Useful to visualize potential damage to the anterior glenoid rim and Hill-Sachs lesions after an anterior dislocation. This view is often used to distinguish between anterior and posterior shoulder dislocation.

Wolff's law A law that states that the growth and remodeling of bone is influenced and modulated by mechanical stresses.

woven bone Primitive, less-organized form of cortical bone.

x-rays Radiant energy produced by exposing tungsten to a beam of electrons; useful in imaging many body parts.

yoga A variety of exercises designed to promote balance between mind and body and to bring practitioners into union with humankind and a higher power or life force.

Z-score Compares the patient's bone mineral density (BMD) with what is expected in someone of the same age and body size. Among older adults, however, low BMD is common, so comparison with age-matched norms can be misleading and therefore the T-score is more important.

Index

Felon, 478*f*, 479*f*. *See also* Fingertip, infections
  drainage of, 480*f*
Femoral anteversion, 1025*f*
Femoral condyle
  hypoplasia of, 1069
  osteonecrosis of, 724–726
    adverse outcomes of, 725
    adverse treatment outcomes in, 725–726
    clinical symptoms of, 724
    differential diagnosis of, 725
    imaging of, 724–725, 725*f*
    physical examination of, 724
    red flags in, 726
    treatment of, 725
  subchondral sclerosis, 724*f*
Femoral head
  core decompression in, 604
  loss of concavity in, 590*f*
  osteonecrosis in, 603*f*
Femoral neck
  displaced, treatment of, 1123
  fracture of, 579*f*, 585*f*
    adverse outcomes of, 586
    adverse treatment outcomes in, 587–588
    differential diagnosis of, 586
    imaging of, 139*f*, 586, 586*f*
    osteonecrosis after, 602
    physical examination of, 586
    in pregnancy, 631
    red flags in, 588
    risk factors, 585
    treatment of, 586–587
  stress fracture of, 627–629
    adverse treatment outcomes in, 629
    clinical symptoms of, 627
    definition of, 627
    differential diagnosis of, 628
    imaging of, 627–628, 628*f*
    physical examination of, 627
    red flags in, 629
    treatment of, 628–629
Femoral nerve stretch test, 950*f*
Femoral osteotomy, 1154
Femoral shaft
  displaced, treatment of, 1123
  fracture of, 578–580, 579*f*
    adverse outcomes of, 579
    adverse treatment outcomes in, 579
    clinical symptoms of, 578
    definition of, 578

differential diagnosis of, 579
imaging of, 578–579
physical examination of, 578
red flags in, 579
treatment of, 579
Femur
  anatomy of, 578*f*
  fracture of
    adverse outcomes of, 1122–1123
    in children, 1122–1124
    clinical symptoms of, 1122
    definition of, 1122
    differential diagnosis of, 1122
    imaging of, 1122
    physical examination of, 1122
    red flags in, 1124
    treatment of, 1123
  longitudinal deficiency of, 1069, 1070
Femur, distal aspect
  fractures of, 644, 1053*f*
    classification of, 707, 707*f*
  osteomyelitis, 145*f*, 1175*f*
Femur, proximal aspect. *See also* Hip, fracture of
  fracture of, 585–588
    adverse outcomes of, 586
    adverse treatment outcomes in, 587
    clinical symptoms of, 585–586
    definition of, 585
    diagnostic tests, 586
    differential diagnosis of, 586
    physical examination of, 586
    red flags in, 588
    treatment of, 586–587
  realignment osteotomy, 600
Fentanyl
  during reduction of dislocations, 350, 351
  transdermal patches, 173
Fibrodysplasia ossificans progressiva, 1078
Fibromyalgia syndrome (FMS), 109–114
  adverse outcomes of, 112
  adverse treatment outcomes in, 114
  causes of, 109*t*
  clinical symptoms of, 109–110, 111*t*, 112*t*
  conditions associated with, 111*t*
  definition of, 109–114

diagnostic tests, 112
differential diagnosis of, 112
medication for
  pramipexole, 114
  pregabalin (Lyrica), 113
myofascial pain syndrome and, 110, 111*t*
physical examination in, 110–112
posture in, 110
red flags in, 114
tender point sites, 110, 110*t*
treatment of, 113–114, 113*t*
trigger points for, 112*f*
Fibrous cortical defects, 256*t*
Fibrous dysplasia, 256*t*
Fibula, longitudinal deficiency of, 1066–1068
Fibular collateral ligament palpation, 666*f*
Fibular malleolus, examination of, 783*f*
Fight bites. *See* Human bite wounds
Fighter's fracture, 502
Figure-of-4-position, 695*f*
  fibular collateral ligament, 666*f*
Finger. *See also* Fingertip; Mallet finger; Trigger finger
  chronic instability of, 427
  flexor tendons injuries, 487*f*
  flexor tendons of, 486
  ganglion cyst of
    adverse outcomes of, 513
    adverse treatment outcomes in, 513
    differential diagnosis of, 512
    physical examination of, 512
    red flags in, 514
    treatment of, 513
  imaging of, 446
  index finger, T1 testing of, 955*f*
  little finger, loss of sensation, 428
  malrotation of, 505*f*
  oblique palmar view of, 490*f*
  physeal fracture of, 502
  physical examination of
    abduction, 433*f*
    adduction, 433*f*
    extension, 432*f*
    flexion, 432*f*
  range of motion in
    extension, 434*f*
    flexion, 434*f*
  ring finger
    fracture of the metacarpal neck, 504

Scoliometer, 1190*f*
Scoliosis
  adult, 999–1001
    adverse outcomes of, 1000
    adverse treatment outcomes
      in, 1000–1001
    clinical symptoms of, 999
    definition of, 999
    differential diagnosis of, 1000
    electromyography of, 1000
    imaging of, 1000, 1000*f*
    physical examination of, 999
    red flags in, 1001
    treatment of, 1000
  adverse outcomes of, 1191
  adverse treatment outcomes in,
    1192
  biologic sex and, 1011
  in children, 1188–1192
  classification of, 1188*t*
  clinical symptoms, 1189
  definition of, 931
  diagnosis of, 1188–1189
  differential diagnosis of,
    1190–1191
  growing rod program for, 1192
  imaging of, 1190
  physical examination of,
    1189–1190
    in children, 1015*f*
  red flags in, 1192
  treatment of, 1191–1192
"Scotty dog" sign, 1008, 1206,
  1206*f*
Scouring test, hip, 573*f*
Screw fixation
  failed, 588*f*
  femoral fracture, 587, 588*f*
Seat side straddle exercises
  for hip conditioning, 212*f*, 561*f*
  for lumbar spine conditioning,
    235*f*
Seat side straddle stretches
  for lumbar spine, 933, 936*f*, 937*f*
Segond fracture, 669
Selective estrogen receptor
  modulators (SERMs),
  163
Semitendinosus tendon insertion,
  646
Sensory examination
  in diabetic foot, 831*f*
  in spine, 948*f*
  Waddell signs in, 950, 950*f*–951*f*
Septic arthritis, 147–151

acute synovitis and, 367
adverse outcomes of, 149–150,
  1195
adverse treatment outcomes in,
  151
in children, 1012, 1035,
  1193–1196
clinical symptoms of, 147–148,
  1193
definition of, 147, 147*t*, 1193
diagnosis of, 3
diagnostic tests for, 148–149
differential diagnosis of, 149,
  1194–1195
elbow, 377*f*
  diagnostic tests in, 379
  red flags in, 380
  symptoms of, 378
knee, 645
laboratory tests in, 1193–1194,
  1194*t*
patient history, 148*t*
physical examination of, 148,
  1193
red flags in, 151, 1196
treatment of, 150*t*, 1195–1196
Septic tenosynovitis, 490, 491*f*
Seronegative spondyloarthropathies.
    See also Ankylosing
    spondylitis
  adult, 3, 53–57
    characteristics of, 3
    conditions, 53*t*
    definition of, 53
  in children, 1039, 1197–1198
    adverse outcomes of, 1198
    adverse treatment outcomes
      in, 1198
    clinical symptoms of,
      1197–1198
    definition of, 1197
    differential diagnosis of, 1198
    laboratory tests in, 1198
    physical examination of,
      1198
    red flags in, 1198
    treatment of, 1198
Serratus anterior muscle,
    examination of, 275*f*
Sesamoid
  fracture of, 851–853
    adverse outcomes of, 852
    adverse treatment outcomes
      in, 852
    differential diagnosis of, 852

imaging of, 851*f*, 852
physical examination of, 851*f*,
  852
red flags in, 853
treatment of, 852
  physical examination of, 784*f*
Sesamoid bones
  bipartite, 851, 852*f*, 900
  first metatarsal, 851*f*
  multipartite, 900
  palpation of, 851*f*
Sesamoiditis
  adverse outcomes of, 900
  adverse treatment outcomes in,
    900
  clinical symptoms of, 899, 899*f*
  definition of, 899
  differential diagnosis of, 826, 900
  imaging of, 900*f*
  physical examination of, 899
  red flags in, 900
  treatment of, 900
Shigella, reactive arthritis after, 54
Shin splints, 760–761
  adolescents and, 58
  adverse outcomes of, 760
  adverse treatment outcomes in,
    761
  clinical symptoms of, 760
  definition of, 760
  differential diagnosis of, 760
  imaging of, 760
  physical examination of, 760
  red flags in, 761
  treatment of, 760–761
Shock tests
  for metatarsalgia, 870
  for MTP instability, 790*f*
  plantar plate rupture, 914
Shock wave therapy, 880
Shoe inserts, efficacy of, 1102
Shoe lifts, 875
Shoe wear, 901–904
Shoes
  analysis, 903–904
  for children, 1199–1200
    characteristics of, 1199–1200
    corrective, 1200
    problems with, 1200
    recommendations of, 1200
    selection of, 1199
  custom, for rheumatoid arthritis,
    52
  design of, 901–902, 901*f*
  diabetic foot care and, 835–836

Essentials of Musculos.

Essent